Neonatology Questions and Controversies

ELSEVIER

Neonatology Questions and Controversies

Series Editor

Richard A. Polin, MD
William T. Speck Professor of Pediatrics
College of Physicians and Surgeons
Columbia University;
Director Division of Neonatology
New York Presbyterian
Morgan Stanley Children's Hospital
New York, New York

Other Volumes in the Neonatology Questions and Controversies Series

Neonatology Questions and Controversies

Third Edition

Istvan Seri, MD, PhD, HonD

Honorary Member
Hungarian Academy of Sciences,
First Department of Pediatrics
Semmelweis University
Faculty of Medicine
Budapest, Hungary;
Professor of Pediatrics (Adjunct)
Children's Hospital Los Angeles
USC Keck School of Medicine
Los Angeles, California

Martin Kluckow, MBBS, FRACP, PhD, CCPU (Neonatal)

Professor of Neonatology
University of Sydney;
Senior Staff Specialist
Department of Neonatology
Royal North Shore Hospital
Sydney, Australia

Consulting Editor

Richard A. Polin, MD

William T. Speck Professor of Pediatrics
College of Physicians and Surgeons
Columbia University;
Director Division of Neonatology
New York Presbyterian
Morgan Stanley Children's Hospital
New York, New York

ELSEVIER

ELSEVIER

1600 John F. Kennedy Blvd.
Ste 1800
Philadelphia, PA 19103-2899

HEMODYNAMICS AND CARDIOLOGY: NEONATOLOGY QUESTIONS
AND CONTROVERSIES, THIRD EDITION   ISBN: 978-0-323-53366-9

Notices

Previous editions copyrighted 2012 and 2008.

Library of Congress Cataloging-in-Publication Data

Names: Seri, Istvan (Pediatrician), editor. | Polin, Richard A. (Richard
   Alan), 1945- editor.
Title: Hemodynamics and cardiology : neonatology questions and controversies
   / [edited by] Istvan Seri, Martin Kluckow; consulting editor, Richard A. Polin.
Other titles: Neonatology questions and controversies.
Description: Third edition. | Philadelphia, PA : Elsevier, Inc., [2019] |
   Series: Neonatology questions and controversies | Preceded by Hemodynamics
   and cardiology : neonatology questions and controversies / [edited by]
   Charles S. Kleinman, Istvan Seri ; consulting editor, Richard A. Polin.
   2nd ed. c 2012. | Includes bibliographical references and index.
Identifiers: LCCN 2018013447 | ISBN 9780323533669 (hardcover)
Subjects: | MESH: Cardiovascular Diseases | Infant, Newborn | Infant,
   Newborn, Diseases | Neonatology--methods
Classification: LCC RJ421 | NLM WS 290 | DDC 618.92/12--dc23 LC record available at
https://lccn.loc.gov/2018013447

Content Strategist: Sarah Barth
Content Development Specialist: Lisa M. Barnes
Publishing Services Manager: Julie Eddy
Senior Project Manager: Rachel E. McMullen
Design Direction: Paula Catalano

Printed in United States of America

Last digit is the print number: 9   8   7   6   5   4   3

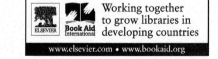

Working together
to grow libraries in
developing countries

www.elsevier.com • www.bookaid.org

Contributors

Timur Azhibekov, MD
Assistant Professor of Clinical Pediatrics
Fetal and Neonatal Institute;
Division of Neonatology
Children's Hospital Los Angeles;
Department of Pediatrics
Keck School of Medicine
University of Southern California
Los Angeles, California
Transitional Hemodynamics and Pathophysiology of Peri/Intraventricular Hemorrhage; Comprehensive, Real-Time Hemodynamic Monitoring and Data Acquisition: An Essential Component of the Development of Individualized Neonatal Intensive Care

Douglas Blank, MD
Newborn Research Centre
The Royal Women's Hospital;
The Ritchie Centre
Hudson Institute of Medical Research
Monash University
Melbourne, Victoria, Australia
Hemodynamic Significance and Clinical Relevance of Delayed Cord Clamping and Umbilical Cord Milking

Colm Riobard Breatnach, MB BAO BCh, MRCPI
Department of Neonatology
The Rotunda Hospital
Dublin, Ireland
Tissue Doppler Imaging

David J. Cox, MBChB, PhD
The Centre for the Developing Brain
Division of Imaging Sciences & Biomedical Engineering
King's College London
King's Health Partners
St. Thomas' Hospital
London, United Kingdom
Cardiac Magnetic Resonance Imaging in the Assessment of Systemic and Organ Blood Flow and the Function of the Developing Heart

Willem-Pieter de Boode, MD, PhD
Radboud University Medical Center,
Radboud Institute for Health Sciences,
Department of Neonatology
Amalia Children's Hospital
Nijmegen, The Netherlands
Assessment of Cardiac Output in Neonates: Techniques Using the Fick Principle, Indicator Dilution Technology, Doppler Ultrasound, Thoracic Electrical Impedance, and Arterial Pulse Contour Analysis; Comprehensive, Real-Time Hemodynamic Monitoring and Data Acquisition: An Essential Component of the Development of Individualized Neonatal Intensive Care

Koert de Waal, Dr, PhD
Department of Neonatology
John Hunter Children's Hospital
University of Newcastle
Newcastle, Australia
Speckle Tracking Echocardiography in Newborns; Assessment and Management of Septic Shock and Hypovolemia

Eugene Dempsey, FRCPI
Department of Paediatrics and Child Health
Irish Centre for Fetal and Neonatal Translational Research (INFANT)
University College
Cork, Ireland
Definition of Normal Blood Pressure Range: The Elusive Target

Karim Assaad Diab, MD, FACC, FASE
Medical Director,
Associate Professor
Department of Pediatrics
Rush University Medical Center
Chicago, Illinois
Catheter-Based Therapy in the Neonate With Congenital Heart Disease

Laura Dix, MD, PhD
Department of Neonatology
Wilhelmina Children's Hospital/
  University Medical Center Utrecht
Utrecht, The Netherlands
  *Clinical Applications of Near-Infrared
  Spectroscopy in Neonates*

Adré J. du Plessis
Chief
Division of Fetal and Transitional
  Medicine
Children's National Medical Center;
Professor of Pediatrics and Neurology
George Washington University School
  of Medicine and Health Sciences
Washington, District of Columbia
  *The Immature Autonomic Nervous
  System, Hemodynamic Regulation, and
  Brain Injury in the Preterm Neonate*

R.M. Dyson, PhD
Department of Paediatrics & Child
  Health
University of Otago
Wellington, New Zealand
  *Assessment of the Microcirculation in
  the Neonate*

**Afif Faisal El-Khuffash, MB, BCh,
BAO, BA(Sci), FRCPI, MD, DCE**
Department of Neonatology
The Rotunda Hospital;
Department of Paediatrics
Royal College of Physicians in Ireland
Dublin, Ireland
  *Tissue Doppler Imaging; Diagnosis,
  Evaluation, and Monitoring of Patent
  Ductus Arteriosus in the Very Preterm
  Infant*

Beate Horsberg Eriksen, MD, PhD
Children's and Youth Department of
  Ålesund,
Department of Paediatrics
Møre and Romsdal Hospital Trust
Ålesund, Norway
  *Assessment of Systemic Blood Flow and
  Myocardial Function in the Neonatal
  Period Using Ultrasound*

**Nicholas Evans, DM, MRCPCH,
CCPU (Neonatal)**
Clinical Associate Professor
Department of Newborn Care
RPA Hospital and University of Sydney
Sydney, Australia
  *Point of Care Ultrasound in
  the Assessment of the Neonatal
  Cardiovascular System; Hemodynami-
  cally Based Pharmacological Manage-
  ment of Circulatory Compromise in the
  Newborn*

Karen D. Fairchild, MD
Professor of Pediatrics
Division of Neonatology
University of Virginia School of
  Medicine
Charlottesville, Virginia
  *Heart Rate and Cardiorespiratory
  Analysis for Sepsis and Necrotizing
  Enterocolitis Prediction*

Erika F. Fernandez, MD
Associate Professor of Pediatrics/
  Neonatology
Department of Pediatrics
University of California, San Diego
San Diego, California
  *The Neonate With Relative Adrenal
  Insufficiency and Vasopressor Resistance*

Drude Fugelseth, MD, PhD
Professor
Institute of Clinical Medicine
University of Oslo;
Consultant
Department of Neonatal Intensive Care,
  Ullevål
Oslo University Hospital
Oslo, Norway
  *Assessment of Systemic Blood Flow and
  Myocardial Function in the Neonatal
  Period Using Ultrasound*

Gorm Greisen, MD, DrMedSci
Professor
Chairman of Paediatrics
Institute of Clinical Medicine
University of Copenhagen;
Consultant Neonatologist
Department of Neonatology
Rigshospitalet
Copenhagen, Denmark
  *Vascular Regulation of Blood Flow
  to Organs in the Preterm and Term
  Neonate; Methods to Assess Organ
  Blood Flow in the Neonate*

Alan M. Groves, MBChB, BSc, MD
Associate Professor of Pediatrics
Icahn School of Medicine at Mount Sinai
New York, New York
*Cardiac Magnetic Resonance Imaging in
the Assessment of Systemic and Organ
Blood Flow and the Function of the
Developing Heart*

**Samir Gupta, DM, MD, FRCPCH,
FRCPI**
Professor
Durham University;
Professor
Department of Paediatrics & Neonatology
University Hospital of North Tees
Stockton-on-Tees
Cleveland, United Kingdom
*Hemodynamics in the Asphyxiated
Neonate and Effects of Therapeutic
Hypothermia*

**Ziyad M. Hijazi, MD, MPH, FACC,
MSCAI**
Professor of Pediatrics and Medicine
Weill Cornell Medicine;
Chair
Department of Pediatrics,
Director, Sidra Cardiac Program,
Medical Director, International Affairs
    Office
Sidra Medicine
Doha, Qatar;
Editor-in-Chief
Journal of Structural Heart Disease
Honorary Professor
University of Jordan
Amman, Jordan
*Catheter-Based Therapy in the Neonate
with Congenital Heart Disease*

Stuart B. Hooper, BSc(Hons), PhD
Director
The Ritchie Centre
Hudson Institute for Medical Research;
Professor
Department of Obstetrics and
    Gynaecology
Monash University
Melbourne, Victoria, Australia
*Cardiorespiratory Effects of Delayed
Cord Clamping*

Amish Jain, MBBS, MRCPCH
Department of Paediatrics
University of Toronto;
Department of Paediatrics
Mount Sinai Hospital
Toronto, Canada
Tissue Doppler Imaging

Anup C. Katheria, MD, FAAP
Adjunct Assistant Professor of Pediatrics
Pediatrics
Loma Linda University
Loma Linda, California;
Director
Neonatal Research Institute
Sharp Mary Birch Hospital for Women
    and Newborns
San Diego, California
*Hemodynamic Significance and Clinical
Relevance of Delayed Cord Clamping
and Umbilical Cord Milking*

**Martin Kluckow, MBBS, FRACP, PhD,
CCPU (Neonatal)**
Professor of Neonatology
University of Sydney;
Senior Staff Specialist
Department of Neonatology
Royal North Shore Hospital
Sydney, Australia
*Cardiorespiratory Effects of Delayed Cord
Clamping; Pathophysiologically Based
Management of Persistent Pulmonary
Hypertension of the Newborn; Point of
Care Ultrasound in the Assessment of
the Neonatal Cardiovascular System;
Pathophysiology Based Management
of the Hemodynamically Significant
Ductus Arteriosus in the Very Preterm
Neonate; Cardiovascular Compromise
in the Preterm Infant During the First
Postnatal Day*

Satyan Lakshminrusimha, MBBS, MD
Dennis and Nancy Marks Chair of
    Pediatrics,
Professor of Pediatrics, UC Davis;
Pediatrician-in-Chief, UC Davis
    Children's Hospital
Sacramento, California
*Pathophysiology of Persistent Pulmonary
Hypertension of the Newborn–Cellular
Basis and Lessons from Animal Studies*

Petra Lemmers, MD, PhD
Department of Neonatology
Wilhelmina Children's Hospital/
    University Medical Center Utrecht
Utrecht, The Netherlands
    *Near-Infrared Spectroscopy and Its Use
    for the Assessment of Tissue Perfusion
    in the Neonate; Clinical Applications of
    Near-Infrared Spectroscopy in Neonates*

Bobby Mathew, MBBS MRCP (UK)
Assistant Professor of Pediatrics
University at Buffalo;
Associate Director
Neonatal Perinatal Medicine Fellowship
    Program
Oishei Children's Hospital
Buffalo, New York
    *Pathophysiology of Persistent Pulmonary
    Hypertension of the Newborn—Cellular
    Basis and Lessons from Animal Studies*

**Patrick Joseph McNamara, MB MCh,
BAO, MRCPCH MSc**
Professor of Pediatrics and Physiology
University of Toronto;
Staff Neonatologist
Department of Pediatrics
Hospital for Sick Children
Toronto, Ontario, Canada
    *Diagnosis, Evaluation, and Monitoring
    of Patent Ductus Arteriosus in the Very
    Preterm Infant; Surgical Management
    of Patent Ductus Arteriosus in the Very
    Preterm Infant and Postligation Cardiac
    Compromise*

Sarah B. Mulkey, MD, PhD
Assistant Professor
Department of Pediatrics and Neurology
George Washington University School
    of Medicine and Health Sciences;
Fetal-Neonatal Neurologist
Division of Fetal and Transitional
    Medicine
Children's National Health System
Washington, District of Columbia
    *The Immature Autonomic Nervous
    System, Hemodynamic Regulation, and
    Brain Injury in the Preterm Neonate*

Gunnar Naulaers, MD, PhD
Professor
Department of Development and
    Regeneration
KU Leuven
Leuven, Belgium
    *Clinical Applications of Near-Infrared
    Spectroscopy in Neonates*

Eirik Nestaas, MD, PhD
Institute of Clinical Medicine, Faculty of
    Medicine
University of Oslo,
Department of Cardiology and Center
    for Cardiological Innovation
Oslo University Hospital
Oslo, Norway;
Department of Paediatrics
Vestfold Hospital Trust
Tønsberg, Norway
    *Assessment of Systemic Blood Flow and
    Myocardial Function in the Neonatal
    Period Using Ultrasound*

Bassel Mohammad Nijres, MD
Division of Pediatric Cardiology
Department of Pediatrics
Chicago, Illinois
    *Catheter-Based Therapy in the Neonate
    With Congenital Heart Disease*

Shahab Noori, MD, MS CBTI
Associate Professor of Pediatrics
Fetal and Neonatal Institute
Division of Neonatology
Children's Hospital Los Angeles;
Department of Pediatrics
Keck School of Medicine
University of Southern California
Los Angeles, California
    *Principles of Developmental
    Cardiovascular Physiology and
    Pathophysiology; Transitional
    Hemodynamics and Pathophysiology
    of Peri/Intraventricular Hemorrhage;
    Assessment of Cardiac Output in
    Neonates: Techniques Using the Fick
    Principle, Indicator Dilution Technology,
    Doppler Ultrasound, Thoracic Electrical
    Impedance, and Arterial Pulse Contour
    Analysis; Comprehensive, Real-Time
    Hemodynamic Monitoring and Data
    Acquisition: An Essential Component
    of the Development of Individualized
    Neonatal Intensive Care; Diagnosis,
    Evaluation, and Monitoring of Patent
    Ductus Arteriosus in the Very Preterm
    Infant*

Markus Osypka, PhD, MSEE
President & CEO
Department of Research and Development
Osypka Medical
Berlin, Germany
*Assessment of Cardiac Output in
Neonates: Techniques Using the Fick
Principle, Indicator Dilution Technology,
Doppler Ultrasound, Thoracic Electrical
Impedance, and Arterial Pulse Contour
Analysis*

Nilkant Phad, MD
Neonatal Intensive Care Unit
Department of Neonatology
John Hunter Children's Hospital
University of Newcastle
Newcastle NSW, Australia
*Speckle Tracking Echocardiography in
Newborns*

Anthony N. Price, PhD
Centre for the Developing Brain and
    Department of Biomedical Engineering
Division of Imaging Sciences and
    Biomedical Engineering
King's College London
King's Health Partners
St. Thomas' Hospital
London, United Kingdom
*Cardiac Magnetic Resonance Imaging in
the Assessment of Systemic and Organ
Blood Flow and the Function of the
Developing Heart*

Jay D. Pruetz, MD
Associate Professor of Clinical Pediatrics
Department of Pediatrics
USC Keck School of Medicine;
Associate Professor of Clinical
    Obstetrics and Gynecology
Department of Clinical Obstetrics and
    Gynecology
USC Keck School of Medicine
Los Angeles, California
*Neonates With Critical Congenital Heart
Disease: Delivery Room Management
and Stabilization Before Transfer to the
Cardiac Intensive Care Unit*

**Chandra Rath, MBBS, MD, CCPU,
CFIN**
Senior Registrar
Department of Neonatology
King Edward Memorial Hospital
Perth, Australia
*Pathophysiologically Based Management
of Persistent Pulmonary Hypertension
of the Newborn; Pathophysiology Based
Management of the Hemodynamically
Significant Ductus Arteriosus in the Very
Preterm Neonate*

Istvan Seri, MD, PhD, HonD
Honorary Member
Hungarian Academy of Sciences,
First Department of Pediatrics
Semmelweis University
Faculty of Medicine
Budapest, Hungary;
Professor of Pediatrics (Adjunct)
Children's Hospital Los Angeles
USC Keck School of Medicine
Los Angeles, California
*Principles of Developmental
Cardiovascular Physiology and
Pathophysiology; Definition of Normal
Blood Pressure Range: The Elusive
Target; Transitional Hemodynamics and
Pathophysiology of Peri/Intraventricular
Hemorrhage; Comprehensive, Real-Time
Hemodynamic Monitoring and Data
Acquisition: An Essential Component
of the Development of Individualized
Neonatal Intensive Care; Cardiovascular
Compromise in the Preterm Infant
During the First Postnatal Day;
Assessment and Management of Septic
Shock & Hypovolemia*

Prakesh S. Shah, MD, FRCPC, MSc
Consultant Neonatologist
Department of Pediatrics
Mount Sinai Hospital;
Professor
Department of Pediatrics
University of Toronto
Toronto, Ontario, Canada
*Pharmacologic Management of Patent
Ductus Arteriosus in the Very Preterm
Neonate*

Yogen Singh, MBBS, MD, DCH, FRCPCH
Consultant Neonatologist and Expertise in Cardiology
Department of Pediatrics—Neonatology & Pediatric Cardiology
Cambridge University Hospitals;
Associate Lecturer
School of Clinical Medical
University of Cambridge
Cambridge, United Kingdom
Hemodynamics in the Asphyxiated Neonate and Effects of Therapeutic Hypothermia

Sadaf Soleymani, PhD
Senior Algorithm Development Engineer
Medtronic Diabetes
Los Angeles, California
Assessment of Cardiac Output in Neonates: Techniques Using the Fick Principle, Indicator Dilution Technology, Doppler Ultrasound, Thoracic Electrical Impedance, and Arterial Pulse Contour Analysis; Comprehensive, Real-Time Hemodynamic Monitoring and Data Acquisition: An Essential Component of the Development of Individualized Neonatal Intensive Care

M.J. Stark, PhD, FRACP
Women's and Children's Hospital,
Department of Neonatal Medicine
North Adelaide, South Australia, Australia;
Robinson Research Institute, School of Medicine
University of Adelaide
Adelaide, Australia
Assessment of the Microcirculation in the Neonate

Brynne A. Sullivan, MD
Assistant Professor of Pediatrics
Division of Neonatology
University of Virginia School of Medicine
Charlottesville, Virginia
Heart Rate and Cardiorespiratory Analysis for Sepsis and Necrotizing Enterocolitis Prediction

Linda Tesoriero, MD
Associate Professor of Pediatrics
Keck School of Medicine
University of Southern California;
Attending Neonatologist & Director MFC Liaison
Fetal and Neonatal Institute
Division of Neonatology
Children's Hospital Los Angeles
Los Angeles, California
Neonates With Critical Congenital Heart Disease: Delivery Room Management and Stabilization Before Transfer to the Cardiac Intensive Care Unit

Joseph Ting, MBBS, MPH
Clinical Assistant Professor
Department of Paediatrics
University of British Columbia;
Clinical Investigator
British Columbia Children's Hospital Research Institute;
Neonatologist
British Columbia Women's Hospital
Vancouver, British Columbia, Canada
Surgical Management of Patent Ductus Arteriosus in the Very Preterm Infant and Postligation Cardiac Compromise

Frank van Bel, MD, PhD
Professor Emeritus Neonatology
Director, Department of Neonatology
University Medical Center Utrecht/ Wilhelmina Children's Hospital
Utrecht, The Netherlands
Clinical Applications of Near-Infrared Spectroscopy in Neonates

Suresh Victor, MBBS, DCh, FRCPCH, PhD
Senior Lecturer and Honorary Consultant
Perinatal Imaging and Health
King's College London
London, United Kingdom
Near-Infrared Spectroscopy and Its Use for the Assessment of Tissue Perfusion in the Neonate

Jodie K. Votava-Smith, MD
Assistant Professor of Clinical Pediatrics
Keck School of Medicine
University of Southern California;
Pediatric and Fetal Cardiologist,
Associate Director
Fetal Cardiology Program
Division of Cardiology
Children's Hospital Los Angeles
Los Angeles, California
*Neonates With Critical Congenital
Heart Disease: Delivery Room
Management and Stabilization Before
Transfer to the Cardiac Intensive Care
Unit*

**Michael Weindling, MD, FRCP,
FRCPCH, Hon FRCA**
Professor of Perinatal Medicine
Department of Women's and Children's
Health
University of Liverpool;
Consultant Neonatologist
Neonatal Unit
Liverpool Women's Hospital
Liverpool, United Kingdom
*Near-Infrared Spectroscopy and Its Use
for the Assessment of Tissue Perfusion in
the Neonate*

Dany Weisz, BSC MD
Neonatal Intensivist
Newborn and Developmental
Paediatrics
Sunnybrook Health Sciences Centre
Toronto, Ontario, Canada
*Surgical Management of Patent Ductus
Arteriosus in the Very Preterm Infant
and Postligation Cardiac Compromise*

**Ian M.R. Wright, MBBS, DCH,
MRCP(Paeds) UK, FRACP**
Professor of Paediatrics and Child
Health Research
Illawarra Health and Medical Research
Institute
University of Wollongong
New South Wales, Australia
*Assessment of the Microcirculation in
the Neonate*

Tai-Wei Wu, MD
Assistant Professor of Clinical Pediatrics
Fetal and Neonatal Institute;
Division of Neonatology
Children's Hospital Los Angeles;
Department of Pediatrics
Keck School of Medicine
University of Southern California
Los Angeles, California
*Transitional Hemodynamics and
Pathophysiology of Peri/Intraventricular
Hemorrhage*

Preface

Neonatal cardiovascular compromise, defined as abnormal tissue oxygen delivery, clinically presents as inadequate systemic, organ, and peripheral blood flow often associated with decreased perfusion pressure. Cardiovascular compromise occurs in very preterm neonates primarily during the early transitional period and in critically ill preterm and term neonates with certain conditions, including but not limited to sepsis, necrotizing enterocolitis, ductal patency, pulmonary hypertension, perinatal asphyxia, and certain types of congenital heart disease. Neonatal cardiovascular compromise is associated with high mortality and increased rates of short- and long-term morbidities. Although definitive evidence is still lacking, it's generally accepted that timely diagnosis and pathophysiology-driven treatment of neonatal shock lead to improved outcomes. However, timely recognition of the early signs of cardiovascular compromise requires sophisticated and often complex bedside monitoring, and treatment demands a thorough understanding of developmental cardiovascular physiology, pathophysiology, and developmental pharmacology.

Since the publication of the second edition of *Hemodynamics and Cardiology* in the *Neonatology Questions and Controversies* series, advances have continued in the field of neonatal hemodynamics. To acknowledge these advances, the third edition has been completely redesigned with the practicing neonatologist in mind. Accordingly, there is only a two-chapter part on cardiology, addressing relevant aspects of the management of neonates with complex congenital heart disease that every neonatologist needs to be familiar with. Having redirected the focus to neonatology, the third edition now includes new parts and subsections reflecting this shift in target audience. In addition, the topics discussed in the previous edition and included in this book have been updated to accurately reflect the advances in neonatal hemodynamics over the past decade or so.

The five parts with their subsections and chapters have been carefully structured to allow the flow of the different interrelated topics to follow a distinct yet logical pattern.

The three updated chapters in the first part discuss the physiologic principles of developmental cardiovascular physiology and their relevance to clinical medicine.

The second part consists of six chapters and addresses the recent advances on postnatal transitional hemodynamics, the hemodynamic mechanisms and the clinical impact of delayed cord clamping/cord milking, the relationship between neonatal transition and brain injury, and the pathophysiology and treatment of persistent pulmonary hypertension of the neonate.

The third part focuses on the methods of hemodynamic monitoring and consists of four subsections. Chapters in the first three subsections provide detailed information on the different methods used for the assessment of cardiac function and systemic, organ, and peripheral blood flow. The methods discussed include but are not restricted to cardiac ultrasonography in general and tissue Doppler imaging and speckle tracking in particular, electrical impedance velocimetry, pulse waveform analysis, NIRS, magnetic resonance imaging, computed tomography, ^{133}Xe clearance, Laser Doppler imaging and flowmetry, and video-microscopy, as well as a description of the feasibility and clinical relevance of their use. The first chapter of the fourth subsection discusses the concept and use of comprehensive, real-time hemodynamic monitoring and data collection for predictive mathematical modeling as the first step in the development of precision medicine in neonatology. The second chapter in this subsection describes the development and clinical application of a heart-rate variability-based algorithm for the early prediction of neonatal sepsis, along with the decreased sepsis-specific mortality associated with the use of the model.

The fourth part consists of two subsections and addresses the most common clinical presentations and the treatment of neonatal cardiovascular compromise. The five chapters in the first subsection discuss the hemodynamic significance and the diagnosis, monitoring, and management of the patent ductus arteriosus (PDA), a condition that continues to remain a conundrum for the practicing neonatologist. These chapters also address the question of when to treat a patient with a PDA and describe the changing role of surgical ligation in the management of this condition. The chapters of the second subsection discuss novel aspects of pathophysiology-based management of neonatal cardiovascular compromise caused by abnormal postnatal transition in the very preterm neonate and sepsis, hypovolemia, and relative adrenal insufficiency in the preterm and term infant. Further chapters in this subsection review the use of cardiovascular medications in the management of neonatal shock, provide novel insights into the hemodynamics of the asphyxiated neonate, and discuss the impact of therapeutic hypothermia on the neonatal cardiovascular system.

The chapters of the final, cardiology-oriented, part focus on delivery room management of neonates with complex congenital heart disease and novel, catheter-based therapies the neonatologist should be aware of when managing patients with congenital heart disease.

In closing, we are grateful to the contributing authors whom we consider experts in their respective topics. We hope the reader finds the updated and restructured version of this popular series a comprehensive, thoughtful, and clinically relevant collection of novel information on developmental cardiovascular physiology and pathophysiology.

Istvan Seri, MD, PhD, HonD
Martin Kluckow, MBBS, FRACP, PhD, CCPU (Neonatal)

Series Foreword

Richard A. Polin, MD

"To study the phenomena of disease without books is to sail an uncharted sea, while to study books without patients is not to go to sea at all."

—William Osler

Physicians in training generally rely on the spoken word and clinical experiences to bolster their medical knowledge. There is probably no better way to learn how to care for an infant than to receive teaching at the bedside. Of course, that assumes that the "clinician" doing the teaching is knowledgeable about the disease, wants to teach, and can teach effectively. For a student or intern, this style of learning is efficient because the clinical service demands preclude much time for other reading. Over the course of one's career, it becomes clear that this form of education has limitations because of the fairly limited number of disease conditions one encounters even in a lifetime of clinical rotations and the diminishing opportunities for teaching moments.

The next educational phase generally includes reading textbooks and qualitative review articles. Unfortunately, both of those sources are often outdated by the time they are published and represent one author's opinions about management. Systematic analyses (meta-analyses) can be more informative, but more often than not the conclusion of the systematic analysis is that 'more studies are needed" to answer the clinical question. Furthermore, it has been estimated that if a subsequent large randomized clinical trial had not been performed, the meta-analysis would have reached an erroneous conclusion more than one-third of the time.

For practicing clinicians, clearly the best way to keep abreast of recent advances in a field is to read the medical literature on a regular basis. However, that approach is problematic given the multitude of journals, unless one reads only the two or three major pediatric journals published in the United States. That approach however, will miss many of the outstanding articles that appear in more general medical journals (e.g., *Journal of the American Medical Association, New England Journal of Medicine, Lancet,* and the *British Medical Journal*), subspecialty journals, and the many pediatric journals published in other countries.

Whereas there is no substitute to reading journal articles on a regular basis, the "Questions and Controversies" series of books provides an excellent alternative. This third edition of the series was developed to highlight the clinical problems of most concern to practitioners. The series has been increased from six to seven volumes and includes new sections on genetics and pharmacology. In total, there are 70 new chapters not included previously. The editors of each volume (Drs. Bancalari, Davis, Keszler, Oh, Baum, Seri, Kluckow, Ohls, Christensen, Maheshwari, Neu, Benitz, Smith, Poindexter, Cilio, and Perlman) have done an extraordinary job in selecting topics of clinical importance to everyday practice. Unlike traditional review articles, the chapters not only highlight the most significant controversies, but when possible, have incorporated basic science and physiological concepts with a rigorous analysis of the current literature.

As with the first edition, I am indebted to the exceptional group of editors who chose the content and edited each of the volumes. I also wish to thank Lisa Barnes (Content Development Specialist at Elsevier) and Judy Fletcher (VP, Content Development at Elsevier) who provided incredible assistance in bringing this project to fruition.

Contents

PART C • DIAGNOSIS OF NEONATAL CARDIOVASCULAR COMPROMISE: METHODS AND THEIR CLINICAL APPLICATIONS

SECTION C1

Assessment of Systemic Blood Flow and Cardiac Function: Ultrasound

SECTION C2

Assessment of Systemic Blood Flow and Cardiac Function: Other Methods

SECTION C3

Assessment of Organ and Peripheral Blood Flow

PART E • CARDIOLOGY

Corresponding color figures for select images are available on Expert Consult.

PART A • Developmental Cardiovascular Physiology and Pathophysiology

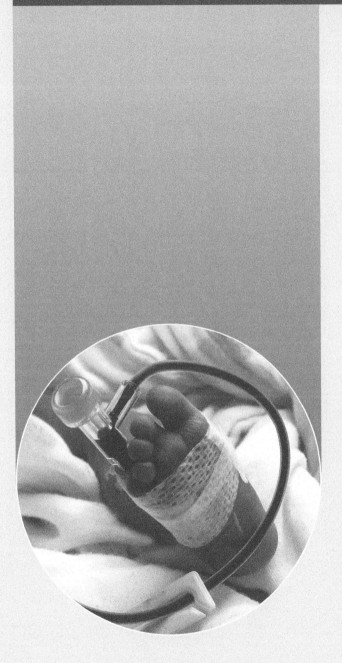

CHAPTER 1

Principles of Developmental Cardiovascular Physiology and Pathophysiology

Shahab Noori and Istvan Seri

- A successful hemodynamic transition from fetal to extrauterine life is a complex process that requires the interdependent sequential physiologic changes to take place in a timely manner.
- Immaturity- or pathophysiology-driven disturbances of the transitional process may have significant short- and long-term consequences.
- Timely diagnosis and pathophysiology-targeted management of neonatal shock pose difficult challenges for the clinician.
- Many questions remain unanswered, including, but not restricted to, the timely recognition of the subpopulation of neonates at high risk for the development of hemodynamic compromise in the transitional period, the definition of the individual patient-dependent blood pressure thresholds associated with inadequate tissue oxygen delivery, the role of physiologic cord clamping, and the recognition of the hemodynamic antecedents of peri-intraventricular hemorrhage.

Principles of Developmental Physiology

Fetal Circulation

The fetal circulation is characterized by low systemic vascular resistance (SVR) with high systemic blood flow and high pulmonary vascular resistance with low pulmonary blood flow. Given the low oxygen tension of the fetus, the fetal circulation allows for preferential flow of the most oxygenated blood to the heart and brain, two of the three "vital organs."[1] With the placenta rather than the lungs being the organ of gas exchange, most of the right ventricular output is diverted through the patent ductus arteriosus (PDA) to the systemic circulation. In fact, the pulmonary blood flow constitutes only approximately 7% to 8% of the combined cardiac output in fetal lambs.[2] However, Doppler and magnetic resonance imaging studies have shown that the proportion of combined cardiac output that supplies the lungs is significantly higher in the human fetus (11% to 25%), with some studies reporting an increase in this proportion with advancing gestational age to a peak approximately 30 weeks' gestation.[3–6] In fetal life, both ventricles contribute to the systemic blood flow, and the circulation therefore depends on the persistence of shunts via the foramen ovale and PDA between the systemic and pulmonary circuits, with the two circulations functioning in "parallel." The right ventricle is the dominant pumping chamber, and its contribution to the combined cardiac output is approximately 60%. The combined cardiac output is in the range of 400 to 450 mL/kg/min in the fetus, which is much higher than the systemic flow after birth (approximately 200 mL/kg/min). Approximately, one-third of the combined cardiac output (150 mL/kg/min) perfuses the placenta via the umbilical vessels. However, placental blood flow decreases to 21% of the combined cardiac output near term.[7] The umbilical vein carries the oxygenated blood from the placenta through the portal veins and the ductus venosus to the inferior vena cava (IVC) and eventually to the heart. Approximately 50% of oxygenated blood in the umbilical vein is shunted through the ductus venosus and IVC to the right atrium, where the oxygenated blood is preferentially directed to the left atrium through the patent foramen ovale. This percentage decreases as gestation advances. One of the unique characteristics of the fetal circulation is that arterial oxygen saturation (SaO$_2$) is different between the upper and lower body. Having the most oxygenated blood in the left atrium ensures supply of adequate oxygen to the heart and brain. Furthermore, in response to hypoxemia, most of the blood flow in the umbilical vein bypasses the portal circulation via the ductus venosus and again delivers the most oxygenated blood to the heart and brain.

Transitional Physiology

Transition from the fetal to the postnatal type of circulation is a complex process. In the past few years, research interest has again focused on cardiovascular and pulmonary adaptation at birth. Among others, animal and human studies have investigated the impact of the timing of cord clamping on cardiovascular and pulmonary transitional physiology. The findings of these studies have highlighted the importance of allowing for placental transfusion to take place and suggested that lung aeration should be established prior to umbilical cord clamping to ensure that the source of the left ventricular preload gradually changes over from the placenta to the lungs.[8] The maintenance of appropriate left ventricular preload during the immediate hemodynamic transition from the fetal to the postnatal circulation has been shown to attenuate the abrupt decrease in preload and systemic blood flow seen with the practice of immediate cord clamping[9] and is associated with improved postnatal hemodynamic stability and clinical outcomes (see Chapters 4 and 5). Among the clinical outcomes, improved postnatal transition, decreased need for blood transfusion, and lower incidence of intraventricular hemorrhage have been documented without significant untoward effects associated with delayed cord clamping in preterm infants.[10–12] In addition, a decreased need for blood transfusion has been observed in term neonates, albeit with higher rates of jaundice and polycythemia reported. As discussed in Chapter 5 in detail, these findings have led to a departure from the traditional approach of immediate cord clamping and a move to delayed clamping of the cord for all newborns who are vigorous at birth in the absence of conditions preventing placental transfusion.[13–15] Interestingly, cord milking seems to confer similar hemodynamic benefits to delayed cord clamping.[16,17] However, further studies are needed to provide convincing evidence that the two procedures indeed confer the same clinical benefits and are safe for the preterm infant.

After birth, the circulation changes from parallel to series, and thus the left and right ventricular outputs must become equal. However, this process, especially in very preterm infants, is not complete for days or even weeks after birth, due to the inability of the fetal channels to close in a timely manner. The persistence of the PDA significantly alters the hemodynamics during transition and beyond and has been associated with severe and even refractory hypotension.[18,19] The impact of the PDA on pulmonary and systemic blood flow in the preterm infant is discussed in Chapter 22. At birth, the removal of the low-resistance placental circulation and the surge in catecholamines and other hormones increases the SVR. On the other hand, the pulmonary vascular resistance drops precipitously due to the act of breathing air and exposure of the pulmonary arteries to higher partial pressure of oxygen as compared with the very low level in utero. Organ blood flow also changes significantly. In the newborn lamb, cerebral blood flow (CBF) drops in response to oxygen exposure.[20] A drop in CBF in the first few minutes after birth in normal term neonates was also reported.[21] This drop in CBF appears to be related, at least in part, to cerebral vasoconstriction in response to the increase in arterial blood oxygen content immediately after birth. In addition, the correlation between left-to-right PDA shunting and middle cerebral artery (MCA) flow velocity (a surrogate for CBF) suggests a possible role of the ductus arteriosus in the observed reduction in CBF.[21] Finally, especially in some very preterm neonates, the inability of the immature myocardium to pump against the suddenly increased SVR might lead to a transient decrease in systemic blood flow, which in turn could also contribute to the decrease in CBF (see Chapters 2 and 11).

Postnatal Circulation

Pressure, Flow, and Resistance

Poiseuille's equation ($Q = (\Delta P \times \pi r^4)/8 \mu L$) describes the factors that determine the movement of fluid through a tube. This equation helps us to understand how changes in cardiovascular parameters affect blood flow. Basically, flow *(Q)* is directly related to the pressure difference (ΔP) across the vessel and the fourth power of the radius *(r)* and inversely related to the length *(L)* of the vessel and the viscosity of the fluid *(μ)*. Therefore blood pressure (BP) is the driving force behind moving blood through the vasculature. Because there are several differences between laminar flow of water through a tube and blood flow through the body, the relationship between the previously mentioned factors in the body does not exactly follow the equation. In addition, because we do not measure all components of this equation, in clinical practice the interaction among BP, flow, and SVR is described by using an analogy of Ohm's law (cardiac output = pressure gradient/SVR). Therefore blood flow is directly related to BP and inversely related to SVR. Regulation of and changes in cardiac output and SVR determine the BP. In other words, systemic BP is the dependent variable of the interaction between the two independent variables: cardiac output (flow) and SVR. Of note is that, because cardiac output is also partly affected by SVR, in theory, cardiac output cannot be considered a completely independent variable.

Cardiac output is determined by heart rate, preload, myocardial contractility, and afterload. Preload can be described in terms of pressure or volume (i.e., central venous pressure or end-diastolic ventricular volume). Therefore preload is affected not only by the effective circulating blood volume but also by many other factors, such as myocardial relaxation and compliance, contractility, and afterload. The limited data available on diastolic function in the newborn in general and in preterm infants in particular suggest lower myocardial compliance and relaxation function. On the other hand, baseline myocardial contractility is high or comparable to older children, whereas the myocardial capacity to maintain contractility in the face of an increase in the afterload might be limited (see later). Afterload and SVR are related and usually change in the same direction. Yet, these two parameters are different and should not be used interchangeably. SVR is determined by the resistance of the vascular system and is regulated by changes in the diameter of the small resistance vessels, primarily the arterioles. In contrast, afterload is the force that the myocardium has to overcome to pump blood out of the ventricles during the ejection period. Wall tension can be used as a measure of afterload. Therefore, based on Laplace's law, left ventricular afterload is directly related to the intraventricular pressure and the left ventricular diameter at the end of systole and indirectly related to the myocardial wall thickness. Indeed, changes in SVR exert their effect on afterload indirectly by affecting BP.

Organ Blood Flow Distribution

Under resting physiologic conditions, blood flow to each organ is regulated by a baseline vascular tone under the influence of the autonomic nervous system. Changes in the baseline vascular tone regulate organ blood flow. Vascular tone is regulated by local tissue (e.g., H^+, CO_2, and O_2), paracrine (e.g., nitric oxide [NO], prostacyclin, and endothelin-1), and neurohormonal factors, as well as by the myogenic properties of the blood vessel. Under pathologic conditions such as hypoxia-ischemia, the relative organ distribution of cardiac output favors the "vital" organs (the brain, heart, and adrenal glands). In principle, vital organ designation is operational even in fetal life. However, the vascular bed of the forebrain (cortex) might only achieve the characteristic "vital organ" vasodilatory response to a decrease in perfusion pressure late in the second trimester (see further discussion later).

Microcirculatory Physiology (see Chapter 19)

Other than being the site of exchange of oxygen and nutrients and removal of metabolic byproducts, the microcirculation also plays a significant role in regulating systemic and local hemodynamics. The small arteries and arterioles are the main regulators of peripheral vascular resistance, and the venules and small veins play an important role as capacitance vessels. Coupling of oxygen supply and demand is one of the primary functions of the microcirculation. Oxygen delivery (DO_2) depends on blood flow and oxygen content. The total oxygen content of the blood (hemoglobin bound and dissolved) can be calculated based on the hemoglobin (Hb) concentration (g/dL), SaO_2, and partial pressure of oxygen (PaO_2; mm Hg) in the arterial blood ($[1.36 \times Hb \times SaO_2] + [0.003 \times PaO_2]$). Tissue blood flow is adjusted based on the oxygen consumption (VO_2) determined by the metabolic requirements. When the blood flow cannot be increased beyond a certain point, oxygen extraction is increased to meet the demand for VO_2. Therefore VO_2 is not affected by decreases in blood flow until the tissue's capacity to extract more oxygen is exhausted. At this point, VO_2 becomes directly flow dependent.[22]

In healthy term infants, localized peripheral (buccal) perfusion assessed by capillary-weighted saturation using visible light spectroscopy has only a weak correlation with central blood flow during the transitional period.[23] Therefore it is possible that under physiologic conditions, peripheral blood flow is not affected by the variability in the systemic blood flow. In other words, blood flow (cardiac output) is regulated to meet VO_2. In ventilated preterm infants, limb blood flow assessed by near-infrared spectroscopy showed no correlation with BP.[24] Along with the poor correlation of buccal SaO_2 with cardiac output in healthy term neonates, these findings suggest that regulation of the microcirculation and peripheral blood flow in relatively hemodynamically stable preterm and term neonates might be, at least to a certain point, independent from systemic blood flow.

Skin microcirculation has been more extensively studied in neonates. Orthogonal polarization spectral imaging studies of skin demonstrated that functional small vessel density, a measure of tissue perfusion and microcirculation, changes over the first postnatal month and directly correlates with hemoglobin concentration and environmental temperature in preterm infants.[25] In this study, functional small vessel density was also inversely related to BP. This finding indicates that evaluation of skin microcirculation may be useful in the indirect assessment of SVR. Findings of laser Doppler flowmetry studies of the skin indicate that the relationship between peripheral microvascular blood flow and cardiovascular function evolves during the first few postnatal days and that it depends on the gestational age and sex of the patient.[26–28] Indeed, the inverse relationship between microvascular blood flow and calculated SVR and mean BP immediately after delivery is no longer present by the fifth day of postnatal life.[26] Interestingly, male preterm infants are more likely to have peripheral vasodilation at 24 hours after birth, and this may be related to the different maturational pattern of the autonomic nervous system in male compared with female neonates.[27,28] A study found a higher sympathetic output at 6 hours after birth in male preterm infants compared with females; however, sympathetic tone tends to decrease in males and increase in females over time during the first 3 postnatal days.[27] Gestational age has an inverse relationship with microvascular blood flow during the first few postnatal days.[27] Among the most immature neonates (≤28 weeks), those who died during the transitional period had higher baseline microvascular blood flow (i.e., lower peripheral vascular resistance).[26] These findings suggest that developmental changes in the microcirculation also play a significant role in the regulation of transitional hemodynamics, and that microcirculatory maladaptation is associated with and/or may increase the risk of mortality.

Given the limited data available and inconsistency of the findings, further studies of the regulation of microcirculation are needed to improve our understanding of the physiology and pathophysiology of the microcirculation during development and postnatal transition and to better characterize its role in the regulation of systemic hemodynamics in the preterm and term neonate.

Myocardial Function—Developmental Aspects

There are significant differences in myocardial structure and function between the immature myocardium of the neonate compared with that of the older child and adult.[29,30] The immature myocardium of the preterm and term neonate has less contractile elements, higher water content, greater surface to volume ratio, and an underdeveloped sarcoplasmic reticulum. The immature myocardium primary relies on the function of L-type calcium channels and thus on extracellular calcium concentration for calcium supply necessary for muscle contraction. In children and adults, these channels serve only to trigger the release of calcium from its abundant intracellular sources in the sarcoplasmic reticulum. These characteristics of the immature myocardium explain the observed differences in myocardial compliance and contractility between preterm and term neonates and children and adults.

Echocardiographic studies have shown that the immature myocardium has a higher baseline contractile state and that contractility rapidly decreases in the face of an increase in afterload.[31] The sensitivity of the immature myocardium to afterload means that for the same degree of rise in the afterload, the myocardium of the neonate has a more significant reduction in contractility compared with children or adults. With the rise in SVR after birth, left ventricular afterload increases. This, in turn, may lead to a significant decrease in myocardial contractility with possible clinical implications (see discussion under Myocardial Dysfunction).

Impact of the Immature Autonomic Nervous System on Regulating Cardiac Function and Vascular Tone

Circulatory function is mediated at the central and local levels through neural, hormonal, and metabolic mechanisms and reflex pathways (Fig. 1.1). Integral to the regulation of cardiac function and vascular tone is the central nervous system. The medulla

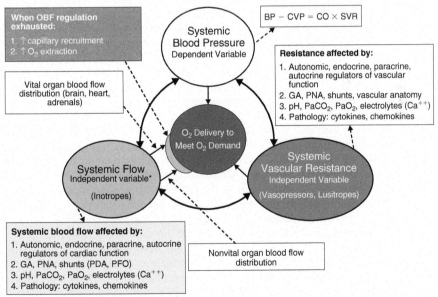

Fig. 1.1 To meet cellular metabolic demand, a complex interaction among blood flow, vascular resistance, and blood pressure takes place. Vascular resistance and blood flow are the independent variables, and blood pressure is the dependent variable in this interaction characterized by the simplified equation using an analogy of Ohm's law: BP − CVP = CO × SVR. *However, because cardiac output is also affected by SVR, it cannot be considered a completely independent variable. In addition to the interaction among the major determinants of cardiovascular function, complex regulation of blood flow distribution to vital and nonvital organs, recruitment of capillaries, and extraction of oxygen all play a fundamental role in the maintenance of hemodynamic homeostasis. *BP*, Blood pressure; *CBF*, cerebral blood flow; *CO*, cardiac output; *CVP*, central venous pressure; *GA*, gestational age; *OBF*, organ blood flow; *PaCO₂*, partial pressure of carbon dioxide in the arteries; *PaO₂*, partial pressure of oxygen in the arteries; *PDA*, patent ductus arteriosus; *PFO*, patent foramen ovale; *PNA*, postnatal age; *SVR*, systemic vascular resistance. See text for details. (Modified with permission from Soleymani S, Borzage M, Seri I: Hemodynamic monitoring in neonates: advances and challenges. *J Perinatol* 30:S38–S45, 2010.)

generates complex patterns of sympathetic, parasympathetic, and cardiovascular responses that are essential for homeostasis, as well as behavioral patterning of autonomic activity.[32,33] The balance between sympathetic and parasympathetic outflow to the heart and blood vessels is regulated by peripheral baroreceptors and chemoreceptors in the aortic arch and carotid sinus, as well as by the mechanoreceptors in the heart and lungs.[34] Although many of these pathways have been identified, much work remains to delineate the adaptation of cardiovascular control in the immature infant where the maturation of the many components of this complex system is at varying pace and has been shown to lead to instability in autonomic function and maintenance of adequate organ blood flow and BP. The effect of the dynamic nature of the developing system on cardiovascular function is unclear, but it may have short- and long-term implications for neonates born premature or with growth restriction.[35,36]

Heart rate variability analysis is a noninvasive tool used to assess the sympathetic and parasympathetic modulation of the cardiovascular system over a relatively short period of time.[37–39] This method has been found to be useful in conditions in which cardiac output has been impacted, such as in patients with sepsis (see Chapter 20).[40,41] Heart rate variability analysis holds promise to further characterize the autonomic control of cardiovascular function because the relationship among heart rate variability, sympathovagal balance, and the modulation of the renin-angiotensin-aldosterone system in various pathophysiologic states can be explored.

Developmental Cardiovascular Pathophysiology: Etiology and Pathophysiology of Neonatal Shock

To ensure normal cellular function and maintenance of structural integrity, delivery of oxygen must meet cellular oxygen demand. DO_2 is determined by the oxygen content of the blood and cardiac output (see earlier). However, cardiac output can deliver oxygen effectively only to the organs if perfusion pressure (BP) is maintained in a range appropriate to the given conditions of the cardiovascular system. Because BP is determined by the interaction between SVR and cardiac output (BP = SVR × systemic blood flow; see Fig. 1.1), the complex interdependence between perfusion pressure and systemic blood flow mandates that, if possible, both should be monitored in critically ill neonates (see Chapter 21).

Indeed, if SVR is too low, BP (perfusion pressure) may drop below a critical level at which cellular DO_2 becomes compromised despite normal or even high cardiac output. However, if SVR is too high, cardiac output and thus organ perfusion may decrease to a critical level so that cellular DO_2 becomes compromised despite maintenance of BP in the perceived normal range. Therefore the use of either the BP or cardiac output alone for the assessment of the cardiovascular status is misleading, especially under certain critical circumstances in preterm and term neonates. Unfortunately, although BP can be continuously monitored, there are only few, recently developed, and not yet fully validated invasive and noninvasive bedside techniques we can use to continuously monitor systemic perfusion, in absolute numbers in the critically ill neonate (see Chapter 21). Therefore in most intensive care units the clinician has been left with monitoring the indirect and rather insensitive and nonspecific measures of organ perfusion, such as urine output and capillary refill time (CRT) (see Chapter 26). Monitoring the time course of the development and cessation of lactic acidosis is the most specific indirect measure of the status of tissue perfusion, and it has become available from small blood samples, along with routine blood-gas analysis. However, this measure also has its limitations because elevated serum lactic acid levels may represent an ongoing impairment in tissue oxygenation or a previous event with improvement in tissue perfusion ("washout phenomenon"). Thus serum lactic acid concentration needs to be sequentially monitored and a single value may not provide appropriate information regarding tissue perfusion. Furthermore, when epinephrine is being administered, epinephrine-induced specific increases in lactic acid levels occur independent of the state of tissue perfusion.[42]

Because it is a common practice to routinely measure BP in neonates, population-based normative data are available for the statistically defined normal ranges of BP in preterm and term neonates.[43–45] It is very likely that the 5th or 10th percentiles of these gestational- and postnatal-age dependent normative data used to define hypotension do not represent BP values in every patient where autoregulation of organ blood flow or organ blood flow itself is necessarily compromised. Although findings have described the possible lower limits of BP below which autoregulation of CBF, cerebral function, and, finally, cerebral perfusion are impaired in very low birth weight (VLBW) preterm infants (Fig. 1.2),[46–48] the true impact of gestational and postnatal age, the individual patient's ability to compensate

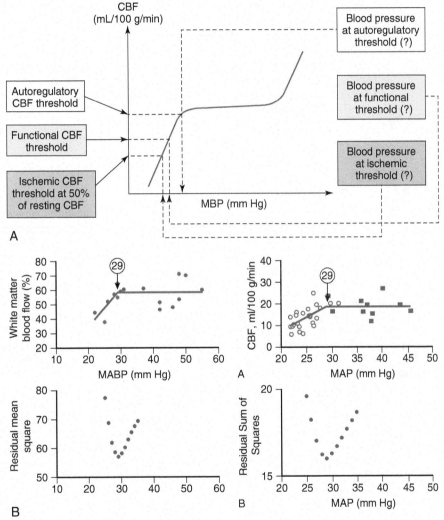

Fig. 1.2 (A) Definition of hypotension by three pathophysiologic phenomena of increasing severity: the "autoregulatory, functional, and ischemic thresholds" of hypotension. Cerebral blood flow (CBF) is compromised when blood pressure decreases to less than the autoregulatory threshold. With further decrease in blood pressure, first brain function is impaired followed by tissue injury as the ischemic threshold is crossed. (B) *Left panels.* Upper panel shows the relationship between cerebral white matter blood flow (expressed as the percentage of total CBF) and mean arterial pressure (MAP) in 13 preterm infants (16 measurements). A breakpoint in the relationship was identified at MBP of 29 mm Hg. *Lower panel* depicts the lowest residual mean square (best fit) with the breakpoint. *Right panels.* Serial measurements of CBF and MAP in a normotensive and untreated hypotensive ELBW neonates at 13 to 40 hours after birth. Note the breakpoint at 29 mm Hg in the CBF-MAP autoregulation curve (the same value obtained in the study shown on the left-hand side by Børch et al.). ([A] From McLean CW, Cayabyab R, Noori S, et al: Cerebral circulation and hypotension in the premature infant—diagnosis and treatment. In Perlman JM, editor: *Neonatology Questions and Controversies: Neurology,* Philadelphia, 2008, Saunders/Elsevier Co, pp 3–26. [B] Modified with permission from references Munro MJ, Walker AM, Barfield CP: Hypotensive extremely low birth weight infants have reduced cerebral blood flow. *Pediatrics* 114:1591–1596, 2004; and Børch K, Lou HC, Greisen G: Cerebral white matter blood flow and arterial blood pressure in preterm infants. *Acta Paediatr* 99:1489–1492, 2010.)

with increased cardiac output and appropriate regulation of organ blood flow, and the underlying pathophysiology on the dependency of CBF on BP in this population remain to be determined.[49–51] It is particularly interesting that two studies using different methods and patients with different gestational and postnatal age have found that the lower elbow of the CBF autoregulatory curve might be at 29 mm Hg of mean BP.[46,48] Yet, there is not sufficient evidence to recommend that mean BP in preterm neonates during the first postnatal days be kept greater than the breakpoint. Several epidemiologic studies have demonstrated that hypotension and/ or low systemic perfusion are associated with increased mortality and morbidity in the neonatal patient population. Other studies found an increase in mortality and morbidity in preterm infants who received treatment for hypotension. Due to the retrospective and uncontrolled nature of these studies, it is hard to tease out the cause of adverse outcome associated with hypotension. It is possible that the poor outcome associated with hypotension is multifactorial, and it may be due to the direct effect of hypotension on organ perfusion; the inappropriate use and titration of vasopressor-inotropes, inotropes, or lusitropes; coexistence of other pathologies with hypotension as a marker of disease severity; or a combination of all of these factors.[52]

Definition and Phases of Shock

Shock is defined as a condition in which supply of oxygen to the tissues does not meet oxygen demand. In the initial *"compensated" phase* of shock, neuroendocrine compensatory mechanisms and increased tissue oxygen extraction maintain perfusion pressure, blood flow, and oxygen supply to the vital organs (heart, brain, and adrenal glands) at the expense of blood flow to the rest of the body. This is achieved by selective vasoconstriction of the resistance vessels in the nonvital organs leading to maintenance of BP in the normal range and redistribution of blood flow to the vital organs. Low normal to normal BP, increased heart rate, cold extremities, delayed CRT, and oliguria are the hallmarks of this phase. Unfortunately, although these clinical signs are useful in detecting early shock in pediatric and adult patients, they are of limited value in neonates, especially in preterm infants in the immediate postnatal period. Indeed, in preterm infants immediately after birth, shock is rarely diagnosed in this phase, and it is usually only recognized in the second, "uncompensated," phase. In the *uncompensated phase* of shock, the neuroendocrine compensatory mechanisms fail and hypotension, decreased vital and nonvital organ perfusion, and DO_2 develop. These events first result in the loss of vital organ blood flow autoregulation and the development of lactic acidosis, and, if the process progresses, cellular function and then structural integrity become compromised. However, even in the compensated phase, recognition of shock may be delayed because of the uncertainty about the definition of hypotension in preterm infants.[53,54] Finally, if treatment is delayed or ineffective, shock progresses to its final *"irreversible" phase*. In this phase, irreparable cellular damage occurs in all organs and therapeutic interventions will fail to sustain life.

Etiology of Neonatal Shock

Neonatal shock may develop because of volume loss (absolute hypovolemia), myocardial dysfunction, abnormal peripheral vasoregulation, or a combination of two or all of these factors.

Hypovolemia

Adequate preload is essential for maintaining normal cardiac output and organ blood flow. Therefore pathologic conditions associated with absolute or relative hypovolemia can lead to a decrease in cardiac output, poor tissue perfusion, and shock. Although absolute hypovolemia is a common cause of shock in the pediatric population, in neonates in the immediate postnatal period it is rarely the primary cause. Neonates are born with approximately 80 to 100 mL/kg of blood volume, and only a significant drop in blood volume leads to hypotension. Perinatal events that can cause hypovolemia include a tight nuchal cord, cord avulsion, cord prolapse, placental abruption, fetomaternal transfusion, and birth trauma such as subgaleal hemorrhage. Fortunately, these perinatal events either do not result in significant hypovolemia and shock in most instances (e.g., placental abruption) or their occurrence is very rare (e.g., cord avulsion). Another cause of absolute hypovolemia is transepidermal water loss in extremely low birth weight (ELBW) infants in the immediate postnatal period. The potential role of early umbilical cord clamping in relative hypovolemia has recently been raised.

To explore the role of intravascular volume status in the occurrence of hypotension, several investigators have evaluated the relationship between blood volume and systemic arterial BP in normotensive and hypotensive preterm infants. Bauer et al. measured blood volume in 43 preterm neonates during the first 2 postnatal days and found a weak but statistically significant positive correlation between BP and blood volume.[55] However, there was no correlation between blood volume and BP until blood volume exceeded 100 mL/kg. Barr et al. found no relationship between arterial mean BP and blood volume in preterm infants and no difference in blood volume between hypotensive and normotensive infants.[56] Similarly, Wright and Goodall reported no relationship between blood volume and BP in preterm neonates in the immediate postnatal period.[57] Therefore absolute hypovolemia was for a long period thought to be an unlikely primary cause of hypotension in preterm infants in the immediate postnatal period. This notion was further supported by the fact that dopamine was shown to be more effective than volume administration in improving BP in preterm infants during the first days after delivery.[58,59]

On the other hand, delayed cord clamping and cord milking have been shown to confer short-term hemodynamic benefits, and, in addition to the improved maintenance of left ventricular preload during early hemodynamic transition, these beneficial hemodynamic effects are also thought to be the result of the associated increases in blood volume.[10,12,16,17,60] In summary, it is unclear at present to what extent and in which patients the hypovolemic component is a factor during hemodynamic transition.

Myocardial Dysfunction (see Chapter 26)

As discussed earlier, there are considerable differences in the structure and function of the myocardium among preterm and term infants and children. The significant immaturity of the myocardium of the preterm infant explains, at least in part, why these patients are prone to develop myocardial failure following delivery.[29,30]

The limited capacity to increase contractility greater than the baseline makes the immature myocardium prone to fail when SVR abruptly increases. This disadvantage associated with myocardial immaturity is especially important during the initial transitional period. As the low-resistance placental circulation is removed, SVR suddenly increases. This acute rise in the SVR and afterload may compromise left cardiac output and systemic blood flow. Indeed, superior vena cava (SVC) flow, used as a surrogate for systemic blood flow (left cardiac output), is low in a large proportion of VLBW infants during the first 6 to 12 postnatal hours.[61] The exaggerated decrease in myocardial contractility in response to increases in left ventricular afterload may play a role in development of low SVC flow.[62] However, this low flow state appears to be transient, because the majority of the patients recover by 24 to 36 hours after delivery. Similarly, findings of Doppler studies of CBF suggest an increase in CBF shortly after delivery.[63] Therefore, although the myocardium of the preterm neonate undergoes structural and functional maturation over many months, it appears that, after a transient dysfunction of varying severity immediately after delivery, it can relatively rapidly adapt to the postnatal changes in systemic hemodynamics.

In addition to the developmentally regulated susceptibility to dysfunction, a decrease in the oxygen supply associated with perinatal depression is a major cause of poor myocardial function and low cardiac output in preterm and term neonates immediately following delivery. During fetal life, despite being in a "hypoxic" environment by postnatal norms, neuroendocrine and other compensatory mechanisms and the unique fetal circulation enable the fetus to tolerate the "relative" hypoxemia and even brief episodes of true fetal hypoxemia. Indeed and as mentioned earlier, during fetal hypoxemia the distribution of blood flow is altered to maintain perfusion and oxygen supply to the vital organs, including the heart.[64–66] However, a significant degree of hypoxemia, especially when associated with metabolic acidosis, can rapidly exhaust the compensatory mechanisms and result in myocardial dysfunction. The critical threshold of fetal arterial SaO_2 below which metabolic acidosis develops varies depending on the cause of fetal hypoxia. In the animal model of maternal hypoxia-induced fetal hypoxia, fetal arterial oxygen saturations less than 30% are associated with metabolic acidosis. In addition, it appears that the fetus is more or less susceptible to hypoxia if the cause of hypoxia is umbilical cord occlusion or decreased uterine blood flow, respectively. Human data obtained by fetal pulse oximetry are consistent with the results of animal studies and indicate that the SaO_2 of 30% is indeed the threshold for the development of fetal metabolic acidosis.[67]

An increase in cardiac enzymes and cardiac troponin T and I are useful in the assessment of the degree of myocardial injury associated with perinatal asphyxia.[68–71] In addition, increases in cardiac troponin T and I have been shown to be helpful in diagnosing myocardial injury even in the mildly depressed neonate. Although cardiac troponin T and I may be more sensitive than echocardiographic findings in detecting myocardial injury,[72] the cardiovascular significance of the elevation of troponins in the absence of myocardial dysfunction remains unclear.

Modifications of the cardiac contractile protein myosin regulatory light chain 2 (MLC2) has also been implicated in the development of cardiac systolic dysfunction following newborn asphyxia. In a piglet model of perinatal asphyxia, a decrease in MLC2 phosphorylation and an increase in MLC2 degradation via nitration were observed, suggesting that these are potential targets for therapeutic interventions to reduce myocardial damage in perinatal depression.[73] Nevertheless, documentation of clinical relevance of these findings is necessary to determine the future utility of such therapies.

Tricuspid regurgitation is the most common echocardiographic finding in neonates with perinatal depression and myocardial dysfunction. In cases with severe perinatal depression and myocardial injury, myocardial dysfunction frequently leads to decreases in cardiac output and the development of full-blown cardiogenic shock.[74,75] Finally, if the myocardium is not appropriately supported by inotropes, the ensuing low cardiac output will exacerbate the existing metabolic acidosis (see Chapter 28).[76]

Cardiogenic shock due to congenital heart defect, arrhythmia, cardiomyopathy, and PDA is discussed in other chapters in this book.

Vasodilation

The regulation of vascular smooth muscle tone is complex and involves neuronal, endocrine, paracrine, and autocrine factors (Fig. 1.3). Regardless of the regulatory stimuli, intracellular calcium availability plays the central role in regulating vascular smooth muscle tone. In the process of smooth muscle cell contraction, the regulatory protein calmodulin combines with calcium to activate myosin kinase. This enzyme phosphorylates the myosin light chain, facilitating its binding with actin and thus resulting in contraction. As for vasodilation, in addition to the reduction in intracellular calcium availability, myosin phosphatase generates muscle relaxation by dephosphorylation of the myosin light chain.

Maintenance of the vascular tone depends on the balance between the opposing forces of vasodilation and vasoconstriction. The vasodilatory and vasoconstricting mediators exert their effects by inducing alteration in cytosolic calcium concentration and/or by direct activation of the enzymes involved in the process. Influx of calcium through cell membrane voltage-gated calcium channels and release of calcium

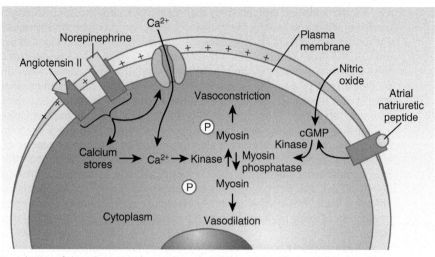

Fig. 1.3 **Regulation of vascular smooth muscle tone.** The steps involved in vasoconstriction and vasodilation are shown. Phosphorylation *(P)* of myosin is the critical step in the contraction of vascular smooth muscle. The action of vasoconstrictors such as angiotensin II and norepinephrine result in an increase in cytosolic calcium concentration, which activates myosin kinase. Vasodilators such as atrial natriuretic peptide and nitric oxide activate myosin phosphatase and, by dephosphorylating myosin, cause vasorelaxation. The plasma membrane is shown at resting potential (plus signs). cGMP, Cyclic guanosine monophosphate. (Modified with permission from Landry DW, Oliver JA: The pathogenesis of vasodilatory shock. *N Engl J Med* 345:588–595, 2001.)

from sarcoplasmic reticulum are the two sources responsible for the rise in cytosolic calcium required for muscle contraction.

The role of various potassium channels has been identified in the regulation of vascular tone. Among these, the adenosine triphosphate (ATP)-dependent potassium channel (K_{ATP}) emerged as the key channel through which many modulators exert their action on vascular smooth muscle tone. In addition, the K_{ATP} channel has been implicated in pathogenesis of vasodilatory shock.[77] K_{ATP} channels are located on the smooth muscle cell membrane, and opening of these channels leads to K^+ efflux with resultant hyperpolarization of the cell membrane. Cell membrane hyperpolarization in turn causes the closure of the voltage-gated calcium channels in the cell membrane and thus a reduction in cytosolic calcium and a decreased vascular tone. Under normal conditions the K_{ATP} channels are closed for the most part. However, under pathologic conditions a number of stimuli may activate these channels and thus affect tissue perfusion. For instance, via the associated reduction in ATP and the increase in H^+ concentration and lactate levels, tissue hypoxia activates K_{ATP} channels resulting in vasodilation and a compensatory increase in tissue perfusion.[78]

As mentioned earlier, a number of vasodilators and vasoconstrictors exert their effects through the K_{ATP} channels. For example, in septic shock, several endocrine and paracrine factors such as atrial natriuretic peptide, adenosine, and NO are released resulting in activation of K_{ATP} channels.[79,80] Thus K_{ATP} channels are thought to play an important role in pathogenesis of vasodilatory shock. Indeed, animal studies have shown an improvement in BP following administration of K_{ATP} channel blockers.[80,81] Inhibition of K_{ATP} channels can improve vascular tone in vasodilatory shock; however, because K_{ATP} channels are ubiquitously expressed and involved in a number of cellular and tissue functions, their inhibition can also lead to adverse effects.[82–84] A small human trial failed to show any benefit of administration of the K_{ATP} channel inhibitor glibenclamide in adults with septic shock.[85] Although the sample size was small and several problems have been identified with the methodology,[86] the findings of this study support the notion that the mechanism of vasodilation in septic shock is more complex than initially believed (see later).

Eicosanoids are derived from cell membrane phospholipids through metabolism of arachidonic acid by the cyclooxygenase or lipoxygenase enzymes and have a wide range of effects on vascular tone. For example, prostacyclin and prostaglandin E_2 (PGE_2) are vasodilators, whereas thromboxane A_2 is a vasoconstrictor. Apart from their involvement in the physiologic regulation of vascular tone, these eicosanoids also play a role in pathogenesis of shock. Both human and animal studies have shown a beneficial effect of cyclooxygenase inhibition in septic shock.[87,88] In addition, rats deficient in essential fatty acid and thus unable to produce significant amounts of eicosanoids are less susceptible to endotoxic shock than their wild-type counterparts. However, the role of eicosanoids in the pathogenesis of shock is also more complex and some studies suggest that, under different conditions, they may actually have a beneficial role. For example, administration of prostaglandin I_2 (PGI_2), PGE_1, and PGE_2 improves the cardiovascular status in animals with hypovolemic shock.[89,90] Another layer of complexity is revealed by the observation that production of both the vasodilator and vasoconstrictor prostanoids is increased in shock.[91,92]

NO is another paracrine substance, which plays an important role in the regulation of vascular tone. Normally, NO is produced in vascular endothelial cells by the constitutive enzyme endothelial NO synthase (eNOS). NO then diffuses to the adjacent smooth muscle cells, where it activates guanyl cyclase, resulting in increased cyclic guanosine monophosphate (cGMP) formation. cGMP then induces vasodilation by the activation of cGMP-dependent protein kinase and the different K^+ channels, as well as by the inhibition of inositol triphosphate formation and calcium entry into the vascular smooth muscle cells.

In septic shock (see Chapter 27), endotoxin and cytokines such as tumor necrosis factor alpha result in increased expression of inducible NO synthase (iNOS).[93–96] Studies in animals and humans have shown that the NO level significantly increases in various forms of shock, especially in septic shock.[97,98] This excessive and dysregulated production of NO then leads to severe vasodilation, hypotension, and vasopressor resistance (see Chapter 30). Because of the role of NO in the pathogenesis of vasodilatory shock, a number of studies have looked at the NO production pathway as a potential target of therapeutic interventions. However, studies using a nonselective NOS inhibitor in patients with septic shock have found significant side effects and increased mortality associated with this treatment modality.[99–101] The deleterious effects were likely due to inhibition of eNOS, the constitutive NOS that plays an important role in the physiologic regulation of vascular tone. Indeed, subsequent studies in animal models using a selective iNOS inhibitor found an improvement of BP and a reduction in lactic acidosis.[102,103] Finally, results of studies on the use of nonselective NOS inhibitors in adult humans with septic shock have also not been favorable.[104–107]

There has been a renewed interest in the cardiovascular effects of vasopressin.[108,109] Although in postnatal life and under physiologic conditions, this hormone is primarily involved in the regulation of osmolality, and there is accumulating evidence suggesting a role of vasopressin in the pathogenesis of vasodilatory shock. Vasopressin exerts its vascular effects through the two isoforms of V_1 receptors. V_{1a} receptor is expressed in all vessels, whereas V_{1b} is present only in the pituitary gland. The renal epithelial effects of vasopressin are mediated through V_2 receptors.

Postnatally and under physiologic conditions, vasopressin contributes little if any to the maintenance of vascular smooth muscle tone. However, under pathologic conditions such as in shock, the decrease in BP vasopressin production increases, attenuating the further decline in BP. However, with progression of the circulatory compromise, vasopressin levels decline as pituitary vasopressin stores become depleted. The decline in vasopressin production leads to further losses of vascular tone and contributes to the development of refractory hypotension.[77] Findings on the effectiveness of vasopressin replacement therapy in reversing refractory hypotension further support the role of vasopressin in the pathogenesis of vasodilatory shock.[110,111]

The vasoconstrictor effects of vasopressin appear to be dose dependent.[112] As mentioned earlier, excessive production of NO and activation of K_{ATP} channels are some of the major mechanisms involved in the pathogenesis of vasodilatory shock. Under these circumstances, vasopressin inhibits NO-induced cGMP production and inactivates the K_{ATP} channels, resulting in improvement in vascular tone. In addition, vasopressin releases calcium from sarcoplasmic reticulum and augments the vasoconstrictive effects of norepinephrine. As for its clinical use, vasopressin has been shown to improve cardiovascular function in neonates and children presenting with vasopressor-resistant vasodilatory shock after cardiac surgery.[113] However, the few published case series on preterm infants with refractory hypotension show variable effects of vasopressin treatment with improvement in BP and urine output only in some patients.[114,115] A pilot study showed similar efficacy of vasopressin to dopamine in improving BP and signs of shock in preterm infants.[116] Although vasopressin was associated with somewhat less tachycardia, the clinical significance of this finding is unclear. It is clear that more data are needed before vasopressin can be used routinely in the neonatal population.[117] In addition, a meta-analysis and trial sequential analysis concluded that vasopressin does not reduce mortality or intensive care unit stay in refractory shock and may increase the risk of ischemic injury in the pediatric population.[118]

In general, vasodilation with or without decreased myocardial contractility is the dominant underlying cause of hemodynamic disturbances in septic shock. However, there are very limited data on changes in cardiovascular function in neonates with septic shock. A study in preterm infants with late-onset sepsis found that the high cardiac output characteristic for the earlier stages of septic shock diminished and SVR sharply increased before death in nonsurviving patients, whereas there was only a mild increase in the SVR during the course of the cardiovascular disturbance in patients who survived. The authors also described a significant variability in hemodynamic response among the survivors.[119] In children, two distinct presentations of shock are seen: one with vasodilation (warm shock) characterized by high CO and low SVR and the other with vasoconstriction (cold shock) characterized by high SVR and low CO. A study in children with fluid resistant shock found different patterns of hemodynamic derangement in central venous catheter-related (CVCR) versus community-acquired (CA) infections. Low SVR and low cardiac output were the dominant pathophysiologic findings in patients with CVCR and CA septic shock, respectively. These findings suggest that the hemodynamic response may be different depending on the type of bacterial pathogen and/or represent the fact that patients with CA septic shock are usually diagnosed at a later stage and thus myocardial dysfunction might have already set in at the time of the diagnosis.[120] Although vasodilatory shock is thought to be the main presentation of neonates with septic shock, a recent study in preterm infants provided some evidence suggestive of the prevalence of vasoconstrictive type shock.[121] In older children, approximately 50% of patients with septic shock present with either systolic or diastolic dysfunction.[122] However, it is not known how common myocardial dysfunction is in the neonatal population with septic shock. The results of the previous studies underscore the importance of direct assessment of cardiac function by echocardiography and tailoring the treatment strategy according to the hemodynamic finding in each individual patient.

The case study presented next underscores this point and illustrates that the population-based BP values defining hypotension must be viewed as guidelines only and do not necessarily apply to an individual patient. This is explained by the fact that a number of factors including gestational and postnatal age, preexisting insults, partial pressure of carbon dioxide in the arteries and PaO_2 levels, acidosis, and the underlying pathophysiology all impact the critical BP value in the given patient at which perfusion pressure becomes progressively inadequate to first sustain vital organ (brain, heart, adrenal glands) perfusion and blood flow autoregulation, then brain function, and, finally, structural integrity of the organs.

CASE STUDY

A preterm infant (twin A) was born at 31 and 1/7 weeks' gestation (birth weight, 1180 g; eighth percentile) via cesarean section due to abnormal umbilical cord Doppler findings. There was no evidence of chorioamnionitis, and Apgar scores were 4 and 7 at 1 and 5 minutes, respectively. The patient was not requiring any respiratory support, and blood gases and CRT had been normal during the first 3 postnatal hours in the neonatal intensive care unit (NICU). However, the neonate's mean arterial BP had been low and, at 3 hours of age, it was 21 mm Hg with systolic and diastolic BPs at 34 and 14 mm Hg, respectively.

What would be the best course of action? Should one increase BP by increasing SVR and cardiac output using a vasopressor with inotropic property, such as dopamine or epinephrine? Or, is increasing cardiac output using a primarily inotropic agent such as dobutamine more appropriate in hypotensive preterm neonates during the early postnatal transitional period? Or, should one attempt to further increase preload by giving additional boluses of physiologic saline? Or, should we ignore the mean arterial blood pressure value because the clinical examination and laboratory findings were not suggestive of poor perfusion and there was no metabolic acidosis? Most neonatologists would choose one of the previously listed options, and, in the absence of additional information on the hemodynamic status, it is indeed impossible to know what to do and whether the treatment choice chosen was the right one.

Therefore, before choosing a treatment option, we obtained additional information on the cardiovascular status by assessing cardiac function, systemic perfusion, and CBF, using point of care ultrasonography (Fig. 1.4). Myocardial contractility, assessed by the shortening fraction, was 35% (normal, 28% to 42%) and left ventricular output was 377 mL/kg/min (normal, 150 to 300 mL/kg/min) in the presence of an equally bidirectional PDA flow. MCA blood flow, assessed by MCA mean velocity and flow pattern, was normal. Using the additional hemodynamic information obtained by echocardiography and ultrasonography, it was clear that the cause of the low BP was the low SVR with a compensatory increase in the cardiac output (BP = cardiac output × SVR). Given the normal myocardial contractility, the high cardiac output and the normal CBF, along with the lack of clinical or laboratory signs of systemic hypoperfusion, we opted to closely monitor the patient without any intervention to attempt to increase the BP. By 9 hours of age, mean BP spontaneously increased to 29 mm Hg and the repeat echocardiogram revealed a mild decrease in left ventricular output (LVO). Accordingly, a significant increase in the calculated SVR occurred (Fig. 1.5). After another 24 hours had passed, mean BP increased to 31 mm Hg and, because cardiac output did not change, calculated SVR continued to rise. The patient remained clinically stable during the entire hospital course and was discharged home without evidence of early brain morbidity.

This case study illustrates several important points. First, without appropriate assessment of systemic and organ blood flow while relying on BP and the indirect clinical and laboratory signs if tissue perfusion, it would have been impossible to ascertain the adequacy of systemic and brain perfusion *at the time of presentation*. Second, assessment of cardiac output and the calculation of the SVR did aid in choosing the most appropriate course of action. Third, in addition to the evaluation of cardiac output and calculation of SVR, information on systemic blood flow distribution to the organs, especially the brain, may help in formulating a pathophysiology-based treatment strategy in neonates with suspected hemodynamic derangement.

In this case, we chose to closely monitor the infants rather than to treat the hypotension because we documented a compensatory increase in cardiac output and one of the surrogate measures of CBF (MCA Doppler and flow pattern) was normal. In this case, it took 6 hours for the vascular tone to spontaneously improve to the degree where mean BP reached the lower limit of the population-based normal value. One may argue for the careful titration of low-dose vasopressor support even in this situation so that normalization of SVR can be facilitated and

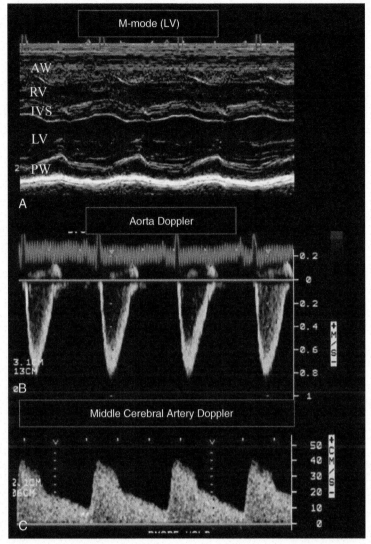

Fig. 1.4 **Direct assessment of the hemodynamics by ultrasound and Doppler.** (A) The changes in cardiac wall motions are shown in this M-mode image, note the normal motion of the IVS and PW resulting in normal shortening fraction. (B) The spectral Doppler at the aortic valve is shown here, which, along with the diameter of the aorta, is used to estimate the left ventricular output. (C) The middle cerebral artery flow Doppler depicts a normal pattern. *AW,* Anterior wall; *IVS,* intraventricular septum; *LV,* left ventricle; *PW,* posterior wall; *RV,* right ventricle.

hence mean BP would have "normalized" faster. However, in a patient with evidence of adequate systemic and CBF, the potential side effects of vasopressor use likely outweigh its benefits. This is especially true if vasopressors, when used, are not carefully titrated to achieve an appropriate hemodynamic target beyond the "normalization" of the BP. Because CBF autoregulation is impaired during hypotension, a significant and rapid rise in BP results in an abrupt increase in CBF with a potential for cerebral injury and possibly intracranial hemorrhage.[49] However, in patients for whom cardiac output does not compensate for the decreased SVR, hypotension will lead to decreased CBF with a potential for cerebral injury and possibly ischemic lesions especially in the white matter with or without a secondary hemorrhage.[49] In addition and as discussed earlier, because our ability to clinically assess the adequacy of the circulation is inaccurate,[123] it is very important that low BP values not be disregarded without additional direct assessment of systemic hemodynamics and CBF and close and careful monitoring of the patient.

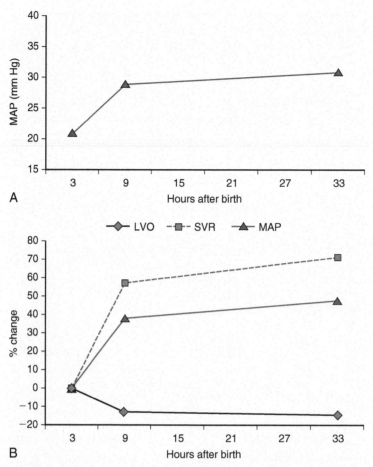

Fig. 1.5 The changes in hemodynamics are shown in these graphs. (A) Mean BP gradually increased from 21 to 31 mm Hg over 30 hours. (B) The 38% increase in mean BP at 9 hours after birth was the result of an increase in SVR (57%) and a mild decrease in LVO (13%). SVR continued to rise without a significant change in LVO at 33 hours. *BP,* Blood pressure; *LVO,* left ventricular output; *SVR,* systemic vascular resistance.

Adrenal Insufficiency (see Chapter 30)

The adrenal glands play a crucial role in cardiovascular homeostasis. *Mineralocorticoids* regulate intravascular volume through their effects on maintaining adequate extracellular sodium concentration. In cases of mineralocorticoid deficiency, such as the salt-wasting type of congenital adrenal hyperplasia, the renal loss of sodium is associated with volume depletion and leads to a decrease in circulating blood volume resulting in low cardiac output and shock. In addition to their role in the maintenance of circulating blood volume, physiologic levels of mineralocorticoids play an important role in the regulation of cytosolic calcium availability in the myocardium and vascular smooth muscle cells.[124] *Glucocorticoids* exert their cardiovascular effects mainly by enhancing the sensitivity of the cardiovascular system to catecholamines. The rapid rise of BP in the early postnatal period has been attributed to maturation of glucocorticoid-regulated vascular smooth muscle cell response to central and local stimulatory mechanisms, changes in the expression of the vascular angiotensin II receptor subtypes, and accumulation of elastin and collagen in large arteries.[125–127] Glucocorticoids play a role in the latter mechanism via their stimulatory effect on collagen synthesis in the vascular wall.[128] Given the importance of corticosteroids in cardiovascular stability, it is not surprising that deficiency of these hormones plays a role in the pathogenesis of certain forms of neonatal shock.

Preterm infants are born with an immature hypothalamic-pituitary-adrenal axis. Several indirect pieces of evidence suggest that immature preterm infants are only capable of producing enough corticosteroids to meet their metabolic demand and support their growth during a well state. When critically ill, a number of these patients cannot mount an adequate stress response. This condition has been referred to as relative adrenal insufficiency. However, the cause of this condition remains unclear. Hanna et al. reported normal adrenal responses to both corticotrophin-releasing hormone (CRH) and adrenocorticotropic hormone (ACTH) stimulation tests in ELBW infants, and these authors concluded that failure of mounting an adequate stress response in sick preterm neonates may be related to the inability if the immature hypothalamus to recognize stress and/or because of inadequate hypothalamic secretion of CRH in response to stress.[129] In contrast, Ng et al. reported a severely reduced cortisol (adrenal) response to human CRH in premature infants with vasopressor-resistant hypotension during the first postnatal week.[130] The same group of investigators using a CRH stimulation test also studied the characteristics of pituitary-adrenal response in a large group of VLBW infants.[131] Compared with normotensive infants, hypotensive patients receiving vasopressor inotropes had higher ACTH but lower cortisol responses. Similarly, Masumoto et al. found that, although cortisol precursors were elevated in preterm infants with late-onset circulatory collapse, their serum cortisol concentrations were similar to those of the control group suggesting immaturity of the adrenal gland.[132] In contrast to the findings of Hanna et al.,[129] the more recent data suggest that the pituitary gland of the VLBW infant is mature enough to mount an adequate ACTH response and that the primary problem of relative adrenal insufficiency is the immaturity of the adrenal glands.[131,132]

Although absolute adrenal insufficiency is a rare diagnosis in the neonatal period, as mentioned earlier, there is accumulating evidence that relative adrenal insufficiency is a common entity in preterm infants (see Chapter 30). Relative adrenal insufficiency is defined as a low baseline total serum cortisol level considered inappropriate for the degree of severity of the patient's illness. However, there is no agreement on what this level might be.[133,134] For the purpose of replacement therapy in adults, a cortisol level less than 15 mcg/dL is usually considered diagnostic for relative adrenal insufficiency.[135] The 2012 Surviving Sepsis Guidelines suggest a random cortisol level of less than 18 mcg/dL in adults with shock considered as evidence for adrenal insufficiency and for steroid therapy.[136] However, a recent study in children with acute respiratory distress syndrome and vasopressor-dependent shock did not find the less than 18 mcg/dL cutoff to be useful for diagnosis of adrenal insufficiency.[137] To establish the presumptive diagnosis of relative adrenal insufficiency for the neonatal patient population, some authors have suggested the use of a total serum cortisol cutoff value of 5 mcg/dL, whereas others have used the cutoff value established for adults earlier (15 mcg/dL).[138,139] However, use of an arbitrary single serum cortisol level to define relative adrenal insufficiency may not be appropriate especially in the neonatal period primarily because there is a large variation in total serum cortisol levels in neonates.[129,131,140–146] In addition, during the first 3 months of postnatal life, total serum cortisol levels progressively decrease with advancing postnatal age.[147,148] Furthermore, most studies have shown an inverse relationship between total serum cortisol levels and gestational age.[147–150] The study by Ng et al. discussed earlier has also demonstrated a gestational age–independent correlation between serum cortisol level and the lowest BP registered in the immediate postnatal period in VLBW infants.[131] These authors also found that serum cortisol levels inversely correlate with the maximum and cumulative dose of vasopressor inotropes. However, despite these correlations, they found an overlap of serum cortisol levels between normotensive and hypotensive VLBW infants, thus making it difficult to define a single serum cortisol level below which adrenal insufficiency can be diagnosed with certainty. A large prospective study of low-dose hydrocortisone therapy for prophylaxis of early adrenal insufficiency showed that low cortisol values at 12 to 48 hours or postnatal days 5 to 7 were not predictive of increased rates of morbidity or mortality.[151] This casts further doubt on the utility of a low cortisol level on a single random blood draw for the diagnosis of relative adrenal insufficiency.

Another important factor to consider is that free rather than bound cortisol is the active form of the hormone. Most of the circulating cortisol is bound to corticosteroid-binding globulin and albumin. Therefore, with changes in the concentrations of these binding proteins, total serum cortisol level may change without a significant change in the availability of the biologically active form (i.e., free cortisol).[152] In addition, the fraction of free cortisol is different in neonates from that of adults. In adults, free cortisol constitutes approximately 10% of total serum cortisol, but in neonates free cortisol is 20% to 30% of the total serum cortisol.[147] Finally, disease severity also appears to influence the ratio of free-to-total serum cortisol concentration as in critically ill adults, the percentage of free cortisol can be almost three times as high as in healthy subjects.[152] There is no information on the potential impact of a critical condition on the ratio of free-to-total serum cortisol concentration in neonates.

Irrespective of the pathogenesis of relative adrenal insufficiency, immaturity of the hypothalamus-pituitary-adrenal axis generally has been linked to susceptibility to common complications of prematurity such as PDA and bronchopulmonary dysplasia.[141,153,154] In addition, due to the role of corticosteroids in the regulation of BP and cardiovascular homeostasis, it is not surprising that adrenal insufficiency is commonly identified as a cause of hypotension especially when hypotension is resistant to vasopressor inotropes. Indeed, it has been demonstrated that more than half of the mechanically ventilated near-term and term infants receiving vasopressor inotropes have total serum cortisol levels below 15 mcg/dL.[139] In more immature preterm infants, an even larger proportion of patients have low serum cortisol levels. Korte et al. found that 76% of sick VLBW infants have serum cortisol levels less than 15 mcg/dL.[138] Several studies investigated the role of adrenal insufficiency in the pathogenesis of hypotension in preterm neonates following PDA ligation. These studies found that random and poststimulation cortisol levels prior to ligation do not predict hypotension.[155,156] However, after ligation, low cortisol levels in patients receiving vasopressor-inotrope therapy are associated with the development of vasopressor-resistant refractory hypotension and in need of hydrocortisone treatment.[157] Finally, studies demonstrating an improvement in the cardiovascular status in response to low-dose steroid administration in preterm and term neonates indirectly support the role of relative adrenal insufficiency in the pathogenesis of hypotension, especially in cases where the hypotension is resistant to vasopressor-inotrope treatment (see Chapter 30).[130,158–166]

Downregulation of Adrenergic Receptors

With exposure to agonists, stimulation of receptors generally results in desensitization, sequestration, and, finally, downregulation of the receptor. This process has been extensively studied in beta- and alpha-adrenergic receptors. For beta-adrenergic receptors, desensitization of receptor signaling occurs within seconds to minutes of the ligand-induced activation of the receptor. Desensitization involves uncoupling of the receptor-stimulatory G-protein compound caused by a conformational change of the receptor following phosphorylation of its cytoplasmic loops. If stimulation of the beta-adrenergic receptor is sustained, the process leads to endocytosis of the intact phosphorylated receptor (sequestration). Both receptor desensitization and sequestration are rapidly reversible. However, with continued prolonged exposure to its ligand, downregulation of the adrenergic receptor occurs. This process involves lysosomal degradation of the receptor protein. Recovery from downregulation requires biosynthesis of new receptor protein, takes several hours, and is enhanced in the presence of corticosteroids.[161,167]

Downregulation of adrenergic receptors has been implicated in the pathogenesis of vasopressor-resistant hypotension. Improvement in the cardiovascular status in patients with refractory hypotension following administration of

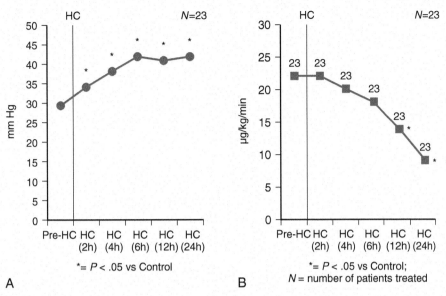

Fig. 1.6 (A and B) The increase in mean blood pressure and the decrease in dopamine requirement in response to low-dose hydrocortisone (HC) treatment in preterm infants with vasopressor-resistant hypotension. (Modified with permission from Seri I, Tan R, Evans J: Cardiovascular effects of hydrocortisone in preterm infants with pressor-resistant hypotension. *Pediatrics* 107:1070–1074, 2001.)

corticosteroids supports this notion because glucocorticoids upregulate adrenergic receptor gene function and result in enhanced expression of adrenergic receptors.[168,169] These *"genomic"* effects of corticosteroids may explain why vasopressor requirement decreases within 6 to 12 hours following corticosteroid administration (Fig. 1.6).[161,162] However, it is important to point out that the beneficial steroidal effects on the cardiovascular system are not limited to adrenergic receptor upregulation. Other genomic mechanisms include inhibition of iNOS and upregulation of myocardial angiotensin II receptors.[161,170–172] *"Nongenomic"* steroidal actions include the immediate increase in cytosolic calcium availability in vascular smooth muscle and myocardial cells, inhibition of degradation and reuptake of catecholamines, and inhibition of prostacyclin production.[161,171] The wide range of genomic and nongenomic effects of steroids explains the rapid and often sustained improvement in all components of the cardiovascular status (Fig. 1.7) of the critically ill neonate treated with low-dose hydrocortisone.[161,163]

Although downregulation of the cardiovascular adrenergic receptors is well described in critically ill adults and many clinical observations support its occurrence in neonates, findings of one study in the newborn rat question the importance of this phenomenon during the early neonatal period.[173] Obviously, more studies are needed to gain a better understanding of the potential developmentally regulated differences in the response of the cardiovascular adrenergic receptors to prolonged agonist exposure. Chapter 30 also addresses these questions in the context of relative adrenal insufficiency of the preterm and term neonate.

Summary

This chapter has reviewed the principles of developmental hemodynamics during fetal life, postnatal transition, and the neonatal period, as well as the etiology and pathophysiology of neonatal cardiovascular compromise. Although significant advances have recently been made in these areas, much more needs to be understood before we can accurately diagnose and appropriately treat preterm and term neonates with cardiovascular compromise during transition and beyond (see Chapters 26 to 30).

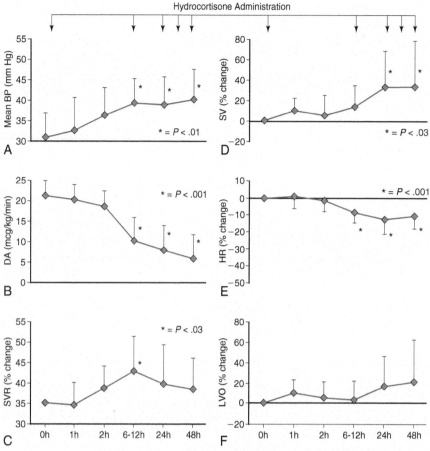

Fig. 1.7 **Changes in cardiovascular function in response to hydrocortisone in pressor-treated preterm neonates.** (A) and (B) depict changes in mean BP and dopamine dosage (DA), respectively. (C) through (F) demonstrate the percentage changes relative to baseline (0 hour) in SVR (C), stroke volume (SV) (D), heart rate (HR) (E), and LVO (F). *BP*, Blood pressure; *SVR*, systemic vascular resistance. (Modified with permission from Noori S, Friedlich P, Wong P, Ebrahimi M, Siassi B, Seri I: Hemodynamic changes following low-dose hydrocortisone administration in vasopressor-treated neonates. *Pediatrics* 118:1456–1466, 2006.)

REFERENCES

1. Kiserud T: Physiology of the fetal circulation, *Semin Fetal Neonatal Med* 10:493–503, 2005.
2. Rudolph AM: Distribution and regulation of blood flow in the fetal and neonatal lamb, *Circ Res* 57:811–821, 1985.
3. Sutton MS, Groves A, MacNeill A, et al.: Assessment of changes in blood flow through the lungs and foramen ovale in the normal human fetus with gestational age: a prospective Doppler echocardiographic study, *Br Heart J* 71:232–237, 1994.
4. Rasanen J, Wood DC, Weiner S, et al.: Role of the pulmonary circulation in the distribution of human fetal cardiac output during the second half of pregnancy, *Circulation* 94:1068–1073, 1996.
5. Mielke G, Benda N: Cardiac output and central distribution of blood flow in the human fetus, *Circulation* 103:1662–1668, 2001.
6. Prsa M, et al.: Reference ranges of blood flow in the major vessels of the normal human fetal circulation at term by phase-contrast magnetic resonance imaging, *Circ Cardiovasc Imaging* 7:663–670, 2014.
7. Kiserud T, Ebbing C, Kessler J, et al.: Fetal cardiac output, distribution to the placenta and impact of placental compromise, *Ultrasound Obstet Gynecol Off J Int Soc Ultrasound Obstet Gynecol* 28:126–136, 2006.
8. Bhatt S, et al.: Delaying cord clamping until ventilation onset improves cardiovascular function at birth in preterm lambs, *J Physiol* 591:2113–2126, 2013.
9. Kluckow M, Hooper SB: Using physiology to guide time to cord clamping, *Semin Fetal Neonatal Med* 20:225–231, 2015.
10. Baenziger O, et al.: The influence of the timing of cord clamping on postnatal cerebral oxygenation in preterm neonates: a randomized, controlled trial, *Pediatrics* 119:455–459, 2007.
11. Sommers R, et al.: Hemodynamic effects of delayed cord clamping in premature infants, *Pediatrics* 129:e667–e672, 2012.

12. Rabe H, Reynolds G, Diaz-Rossello J: A systematic review and meta-analysis of a brief delay in clamping the umbilical cord of preterm infants, *Neonatology* 93:138–144, 2008.
13. Wyckoff MH, et al.: Part 13: neonatal resuscitation: 2015 American Heart Association Guidelines Update for Cardiopulmonary Resuscitation and Emergency Cardiovascular Care, *Circulation* 132:S543–S560, 2015.
14. Katheria AC, Lakshminrusimha S, Rabe H, et al.: Placental transfusion: a review, *J Perinatol Off J Calif Perinat Assoc*, 2016, http://dx.doi.org/10.1038/jp.2016.151.
15. Committee Opinion No. 684: Delayed umbilical cord clamping after birth, *Obstet Gynecol* 129: e5–e10, 2017.
16. Hosono S, et al.: Blood pressure and urine output during the first 120 h of life in infants born at less than 29 weeks' gestation related to umbilical cord milking, *Arch Dis Child Fetal Neonatal Ed* 94:F328–F331, 2009.
17. Katheria AC, Truong G, Cousins L, et al.: Umbilical cord milking versus delayed cord clamping in preterm infants, *Pediatrics* 136:61–69, 2015.
18. Liebowitz M, Koo J, Wickremasinghe A, et al.: Effects of prophylactic indomethacin on vasopressor-dependent hypotension in extremely preterm infants, *J Pediatr*, 2016, http://dx.doi.org/10.1016/j.jpeds.2016.11.008.
19. Sarkar S, Dechert R, Schumacher RE, et al.: Is refractory hypotension in preterm infants a manifestation of early ductal shunting? *J Perinatol Off J Calif Perinat Assoc* 27:353–358, 2007.
20. Iwamoto HS, Teitel D, Rudolph AM: Effects of birth-related events on blood flow distribution, *Pediatr Res* 22:634–640, 1987.
21. Noori S, et al.: Transitional changes in cardiac and cerebral hemodynamics in term neonates at birth, *J Pediatr* 160:943–948, 2012.
22. Weindling AM: Peripheral oxygenation and management in the perinatal period, *Semin Fetal Neonatal Med* 15:208–215, 2010.
23. Noori S, Drabu B, McCoy M, et al.: Non-invasive measurement of local tissue perfusion and its correlation with hemodynamic indices during the early postnatal period in term neonates. *J Perinatol Off J Calif Perinat Assoc* 31:785–788, 2011.
24. Kissack CM, Weindling AM: Peripheral blood flow and oxygen extraction in the sick, newborn very low birth weight infant shortly after birth, *Pediatr Res* 65:462–467, 2009.
25. Kroth J, et al.: Functional vessel density in the first month of life in preterm neonates, *Pediatr Res* 64:567–571, 2008.
26. Stark MJ, Clifton VL, Wright IMR: Microvascular flow, clinical illness severity and cardiovascular function in the preterm infant, *Arch Dis Child Fetal Neonatal Ed* 93:F271–F274, 2008.
27. Corbisier de Meautsart C, et al.: Influence of sympathetic activity in the control of peripheral micro-vascular tone in preterm infants, *Pediatr Res* 80:793–799, 2016.
28. Stark MJ, Clifton VL, Wright IMR: Sex-specific differences in peripheral microvascular blood flow in preterm infants, *Pediatr Res* 63:415–419, 2008.
29. Anderson PA: The heart and development, *Semin Perinatol* 20:482–509, 1996.
30. Noori S, Seri I: Pathophysiology of newborn hypotension outside the transitional period, *Early Hum Dev* 81:399–404, 2005.
31. Rowland DG, Gutgesell HP: Noninvasive assessment of myocardial contractility, preload, and afterload in healthy newborn infants, *Am J Cardiol* 75:818–821, 1995.
32. Gilbey MP, Spyer KM: Physiological aspects of autonomic nervous system function, *Curr Opin Neurol Neurosurg* 6:518–523, 1993.
33. Spyer KM: Annual review prize lecture. Central nervous mechanisms contributing to cardiovascular control, *J Physiol* 474:1–19, 1994.
34. Segar J: *Fetal and neonatal physiology*, Philadelphia, 2004, Elsevier, pp 717–726.
35. Galland BC, Taylor BJ, Bolton DPG, et al.: Heart rate variability and cardiac reflexes in small for gestational age infants, *J Appl Physiol Bethesda Md 1985* 100:933–939, 2006.
36. Patural H, et al.: Autonomic cardiac control of very preterm newborns: a prolonged dysfunction, *Early Hum Dev* 84:681–687, 2008.
37. Pomeranz B, et al.: Assessment of autonomic function in humans by heart rate spectral analysis, *Am J Physiol* 248:H151–H153, 1985.
38. Heart rate variability: standards of measurement, physiological interpretation and clinical use: Task Force of the European Society of Cardiology and the North American Society of Pacing and Electrophysiology, *Circulation* 93:1043–1065, 1996.
39. Kleiger RE, Stein PK, Bigger JT: Heart rate variability: measurement and clinical utility, *Ann Noninvasive Electrocardiol Off J Int Soc Holter Noninvasive Electrocardiol Inc* 10:88–101, 2005.
40. Griffin MP, et al.: Heart rate characteristics: novel physiomarkers to predict neonatal infection and death, *Pediatrics* 116:1070–1074, 2005.
41. Fairchild KD, O'Shea TM: Heart rate characteristics: physiomarkers for detection of late-onset neonatal sepsis, *Clin Perinatol* 37:581–598, 2010.
42. Valverde E, et al.: Dopamine versus epinephrine for cardiovascular support in low birth weight infants: analysis of systemic effects and neonatal clinical outcomes, *Pediatrics* 117:e1213–e1222, 2006.
43. Seri I: Circulatory support of the sick preterm infant, *Semin Neonatol SN* 6:85–95, 2001.
44. Nuntnarumit P, Yang W, Bada-Ellzey HS: Blood pressure measurements in the newborn, *Clin Perinatol* 26:981–996, 1999.
45. Zubrow AB, Hulman S, Kushner H, et al.: Determinants of blood pressure in infants admitted to neonatal intensive care units: a prospective multicenter study. Philadelphia Neonatal Blood Pressure Study Group, *J Perinatol Off J Calif Perinat Assoc* 15:470–479, 1995.

46. Munro MJ, Walker AM, Barfield CP: Hypotensive extremely low birth weight infants have reduced cerebral blood flow, *Pediatrics* 114:1591–1596, 2004.
47. Victor S, Marson AG, Appleton RE, et al.: Relationship between blood pressure, cerebral electrical activity, cerebral fractional oxygen extraction, and peripheral blood flow in very low birth weight newborn infants, *Pediatr Res* 59:314–319, 2006.
48. Børch K, Lou HC, Greisen G: Cerebral white matter blood flow and arterial blood pressure in preterm infants, *Acta Paediatr Oslo Nor* 2010(99):1489–1492, 1992.
49. Tsuji M, et al.: Cerebral intravascular oxygenation correlates with mean arterial pressure in critically ill premature infants, *Pediatrics* 106:625–632, 2000.
50. Tyszczuk L, Meek J, Elwell C, et al.: Cerebral blood flow is independent of mean arterial blood pressure in preterm infants undergoing intensive care, *Pediatrics* 102:337–341, 1998.
51. Kissack CM, Garr R, Wardle SP, et al.: Cerebral fractional oxygen extraction in very low birth weight infants is high when there is low left ventricular output and hypocarbia but is unaffected by hypotension, *Pediatr Res* 55:400–405, 2004.
52. Noori S, Stavroudis TA, Seri I: Systemic and cerebral hemodynamics during the transitional period after premature birth, *Clin Perinatol* 36:723–736, 2009.
53. Seri I, Evans J: Controversies in the diagnosis and management of hypotension in the newborn infant, *Curr Opin Pediatr* 13:116–123, 2001.
54. Al-Aweel I, et al.: Variations in prevalence of hypotension, hypertension, and vasopressor use in NICUs, *J Perinatol Off J Calif Perinat Assoc* 21:272–278, 2001.
55. Bauer K, Linderkamp O, Versmold HT: Systolic blood pressure and blood volume in preterm infants, *Arch Dis Child* 69:521–522, 1993.
56. Barr PA, Bailey PE, Sumners J, et al.: Relation between arterial blood pressure and blood volume and effect of infused albumin in sick preterm infants, *Pediatrics* 60:282–289, 1977.
57. Wright IM, Goodall SR: Blood pressure and blood volume in preterm infants, *Arch Dis Child Fetal Neonatal Ed* 70:F230–F231, 1994.
58. Gill AB, Weindling AM: Echocardiographic assessment of cardiac function in shocked very low birthweight infants, *Arch Dis Child* 68:17–21, 1993.
59. Lundstrøm K, Pryds O, Greisen G: The haemodynamic effects of dopamine and volume expansion in sick preterm infants, *Early Hum Dev* 57:157–163, 2000.
60. Zaramella P, et al.: Early versus late cord clamping: effects on peripheral blood flow and cardiac function in term infants, *Early Hum Dev* 84:195–200, 2008.
61. Kluckow M, Evans N: Low superior vena cava flow and intraventricular haemorrhage in preterm infants, *Arch Dis Child Fetal Neonatal Ed* 82:F188–F194, 2000.
62. Osborn DA, Evans N, Kluckow M: Left ventricular contractility in extremely premature infants in the first day and response to inotropes, *Pediatr Res* 61:335–340, 2007.
63. Kehrer M, et al.: Development of cerebral blood flow volume in preterm neonates during the first two weeks of life, *Pediatr Res* 58:927–930, 2005.
64. Noori S, Friedlich P, Seri I: *Fetal and neonatal physiology*, Philadelphia, 2004, Elsevier, pp 772–778.
65. Reuss ML, Rudolph AM: Distribution and recirculation of umbilical and systemic venous blood flow in fetal lambs during hypoxia, *J Dev Physiol* 2:71–84, 1980.
66. Davies JM, Tweed WA: The regional distribution and determinants of myocardial blood flow during asphyxia in the fetal lamb, *Pediatr Res* 18:764–767, 1984.
67. Kühnert M, Seelbach-Göebel B, Butterwegge M: Predictive agreement between the fetal arterial oxygen saturation and fetal scalp pH: results of the German multicenter study, *Am J Obstet Gynecol* 178:330–335, 1998.
68. Güneś T, Oztürk MA, Köklü SM, et al.: Troponin-T levels in perinatally asphyxiated infants during the first 15 days of life, *Acta Paediatr Oslo Nor 1992* 94:1638–1643, 2005.
69. Trevisanuto D, et al.: Cardiac troponin I in asphyxiated neonates, *Biol Neonate* 89:190–193, 2006.
70. Gaze DC, Collinson PO: Interpretation of cardiac troponin measurements in neonates–the devil is in the details. Commentary to Trevisanuto et al: cardiac troponin I in asphyxiated neonates (Biol Neonate 2006;89:190-193), *Biol Neonate* 89:194–196, 2006.
71. El-Khuffash A, Davis PG, Walsh K, et al.: Cardiac troponin T and N-terminal-pro-B type natriuretic peptide reflect myocardial function in preterm infants, *J Perinatol Off J Calif Perinat Assoc* 28:482–486, 2008.
72. Szymankiewicz M, Matuszczak-Wleklak M, Hodgman JE, et al.: Usefulness of cardiac troponin T and echocardiography in the diagnosis of hypoxic myocardial injury of full-term neonates, *Biol Neonate* 88:19–23, 2005.
73. Doroszko A, et al.: Neonatal asphyxia induces the nitration of cardiac myosin light chain 2 that is associated with cardiac systolic dysfunction, *Shock Augusta Ga* 34:592–600, 2010.
74. Walther FJ, Siassi B, Ramadan NA, et al.: Cardiac output in newborn infants with transient myocardial dysfunction, *J Pediatr* 107:781–785, 1985.
75. Barberi I, et al.: Myocardial ischaemia in neonates with perinatal asphyxia. Electrocardiographic, echocardiographic and enzymatic correlations, *Eur J Pediatr* 158:742–747, 1999.
76. Seri I, Noori S: Diagnosis and treatment of neonatal hypotension outside the transitional period, *Early Hum Dev* 81:405–411, 2005.
77. Landry DW, Oliver JA: The pathogenesis of vasodilatory shock, *N Engl J Med* 345:588–595, 2001.
78. Quayle JM, Nelson MT, Standen NB: ATP-sensitive and inwardly rectifying potassium channels in smooth muscle, *Physiol Rev* 77:1165–1232, 1997.

79. Murphy ME, Brayden JE: Nitric oxide hyperpolarizes rabbit mesenteric arteries via ATP-sensitive potassium channels, *J Physiol* 486(Pt 1):47–58, 1995.
80. Vanelli G, Hussain SN, Dimori M, et al.: Cardiovascular responses to glibenclamide during endotoxaemia in the pig, *Vet Res Commun* 21:187–200, 1997.
81. Gardiner SM, Kemp PA, March JE, et al.: Regional haemodynamic responses to infusion of lipopolysaccharide in conscious rats: effects of pre- or post-treatment with glibenclamide, *Br J Pharmacol* 128:1772–1778, 1999.
82. Foster MN, Coetzee WA: KATP Channels in the cardiovascular system, *Physiol Rev* 96:177–252, 2016.
83. Sordi R, Fernandes D, Heckert BT, et al.: Early potassium channel blockade improves sepsis-induced organ damage and cardiovascular dysfunction, *Br J Pharmacol* 163:1289–1301, 2011.
84. Tinker A, Aziz Q, Thomas A: The role of ATP-sensitive potassium channels in cellular function and protection in the cardiovascular system, *Br J Pharmacol* 171:12–23, 2014.
85. Warrillow S, Egi M, Bellomo R: Randomized, double-blind, placebo-controlled crossover pilot study of a potassium channel blocker in patients with septic shock, *Crit Care Med* 34:980–985, 2006.
86. Oliver JA, Landry DW: Potassium channels and septic shock, *Crit Care Med* 34:1255–1257, 2006.
87. Fink MP: Therapeutic options directed against platelet activating factor, eicosanoids and bradykinin in sepsis, *J Antimicrob Chemother* 41(Suppl A):81–94, 1998.
88. Arons MM, et al.: Effects of ibuprofen on the physiology and survival of hypothermic sepsis. Ibuprofen in Sepsis Study Group, *Crit Care Med* 27:699–707, 1999.
89. Feuerstein G, Zerbe RL, Meyer DK, et al.: Alteration of cardiovascular, neurogenic, and humoral responses to acute hypovolemic hypotension by administered prostacyclin, *J Cardiovasc Pharmacol* 4:246–253, 1982.
90. Machiedo GW, Warden MJ, LoVerme PJ, et al.: Hemodynamic effects of prolonged infusion of prostaglandin E1 (PGE1) after hemorrhagic shock, *Adv Shock Res* 8:171–176, 1982.
91. Reines HD, Halushka PV, Cook JA, et al.: Plasma thromboxane concentrations are raised in patients dying with septic shock, *Lancet Lond Engl* 2:174–175, 1982.
92. Ball HA, Cook JA, Wise WC, et al.: Role of thromboxane, prostaglandins and leukotrienes in endotoxic and septic shock, *Intensive Care Med* 12:116–126, 1986.
93. Rubanyi GM: Nitric oxide and circulatory shock, *Adv Exp Med Biol* 454:165–172, 1998.
94. Liu S, Adcock IM, Old RW, et al.: Lipopolysaccharide treatment in vivo induces widespread tissue expression of inducible nitric oxide synthase mRNA, *Biochem Biophys Res Commun* 196:1208–1213, 1993.
95. Taylor BS, Geller DA: Molecular regulation of the human inducible nitric oxide synthase (iNOS) gene, *Shock Augusta Ga* 13:413–424, 2000.
96. Titheradge MA: Nitric oxide in septic shock, *Biochim Biophys Acta* 1411:437–455, 1999.
97. Doughty L, Carcillo JA, Kaplan S, et al.: Plasma nitrite and nitrate concentrations and multiple organ failure in pediatric sepsis, *Crit Care Med* 26:157–162, 1998.
98. Carcillo JA: Nitric oxide production in neonatal and pediatric sepsis, *Crit Care Med* 27:1063–1065, 1999.
99. Barrington KJ, et al.: The hemodynamic effects of inhaled nitric oxide and endogenous nitric oxide synthesis blockade in newborn piglets during infusion of heat-killed group B streptococci, *Crit Care Med* 28:800–808, 2000.
100. Mitaka C, et al.: Effects of nitric oxide synthase inhibitor on hemodynamic change and O2 delivery in septic dogs, *Am J Physiol* 268:H2017–H2023, 1995.
101. Grover R, et al.: An open-label dose escalation study of the nitric oxide synthase inhibitor, N(G)-methyl-L-arginine hydrochloride (546C88), in patients with septic shock. Glaxo Wellcome International Septic Shock Study Group, *Crit Care Med* 27:913–922, 1999.
102. Mitaka C, Hirata Y, Yokoyama K, et al.: A selective inhibitor for inducible nitric oxide synthase improves hypotension and lactic acidosis in canine endotoxic shock, *Crit Care Med* 29:2156–2161, 2001.
103. Pullamsetti SS, et al.: Effect of nitric oxide synthase (NOS) inhibition on macro- and microcirculation in a model of rat endotoxic shock, *Thromb Haemost* 95:720–727, 2006.
104. Bakker J, et al.: Administration of the nitric oxide synthase inhibitor NG-methyl-L-arginine hydrochloride (546C88) by intravenous infusion for up to 72 hours can promote the resolution of shock in patients with severe sepsis: results of a randomized, double-blind, placebo-controlled multicenter study (study no. 144-002), *Crit Care Med* 32:1–12, 2004.
105. López A, et al.: Multiple-center, randomized, placebo-controlled, double-blind study of the nitric oxide synthase inhibitor 546C88: effect on survival in patients with septic shock, *Crit Care Med* 32:21–30, 2004.
106. Howes LG, Brillante DG: Expert opinion on tilarginine in the treatment of shock, *Expert Opin Investig Drugs* 17:1573–1580, 2008.
107. Wong VWC, Lerner E: Nitric oxide inhibition strategies, *Future Sci OA* 1, 2015.
108. Rozenfeld V, Cheng JW: The role of vasopressin in the treatment of vasodilation in shock states, *Ann Pharmacother* 34:250–254, 2000.
109. Robin JK, Oliver JA, Landry DW: Vasopressin deficiency in the syndrome of irreversible shock, *J Trauma* 54:S149–S154, 2003.
110. Landry DW, et al.: Vasopressin deficiency contributes to the vasodilation of septic shock, *Circulation* 95:1122–1125, 1997.

111. Liedel JL, Meadow W, Nachman J, et al.: Use of vasopressin in refractory hypotension in children with vasodilatory shock: five cases and a review of the literature, *Pediatr Crit Care Med J Soc Crit Care Med World Fed Pediatr Intensive Crit Care Soc* 3:15–18, 2002.

112. Malay MB, et al.: Heterogeneity of the vasoconstrictor effect of vasopressin in septic shock, *Crit Care Med* 32:1327–1331, 2004.

113. Rosenzweig EB, et al.: Intravenous arginine-vasopressin in children with vasodilatory shock after cardiac surgery, *Circulation* 100:II182–II186, 1999.

114. Meyer S, Gottschling S, Baghai A, et al.: Arginine-vasopressin in catecholamine-refractory septic versus non-septic shock in extremely low birth weight infants with acute renal injury, *Crit Care Lond Engl* 10:r71, 2006.

115. Bidegain M, et al.: Vasopressin for refractory hypotension in extremely low birth weight infants, *J Pediatr* 157:502–504, 2010.

116. Rios DR, Kaiser JR: Vasopressin versus dopamine for treatment of hypotension in extremely low birth weight infants: a randomized, blinded pilot study, *J Pediatr* 166:850–855, 2015.

117. Shivanna B, Rios D, Rossano J, et al.: Vasopressin and its analogues for the treatment of refractory hypotension in neonates, *Cochrane Database Syst Rev* 3:CD009171, 2013.

118. Masarwa R, et al.: Role of vasopressin and terlipressin in refractory shock compared to conventional therapy in the neonatal and pediatric population: a systematic review, meta-analysis, and trial sequential analysis, *Crit Care Lond Engl* 21:1, 2017.

119. de Waal K, Evans N: Hemodynamics in preterm infants with late-onset sepsis, *J Pediatr* 156: 918.e1–922:922.e1, 2010.

120. Brierley J, Peters MJ: Distinct hemodynamic patterns of septic shock at presentation to pediatric intensive care, *Pediatrics* 122:752–759, 2008.

121. Saini SS, Kumar P, Kumar RM: Hemodynamic changes in preterm neonates with septic shock: a prospective observational study, *Pediatr Crit Care Med J Soc Crit Care Med World Fed Pediatr Intensive Crit Care Soc* 15:443–450, 2014.

122. Raj S, Killinger JS, Gonzalez JA, et al.: Myocardial dysfunction in pediatric septic shock, *J Pediatr* 164:72.e2–77.e2, 2014.

123. de Boode WP: Clinical monitoring of systemic hemodynamics in critically ill newborns, *Early Hum Dev* 86:137–141, 2010.

124. Wehling M: Looking beyond the dogma of genomic steroid action: insights and facts of the 1990s, *J Mol Med Berl Ger* 73:439–447, 1995.

125. Cox BE, Rosenfeld CR: Ontogeny of vascular angiotensin II receptor subtype expression in ovine development, *Pediatr Res* 45:414–424, 1999.

126. Kaiser JR, Cox BE, Roy TA, et al.: Differential development of umbilical and systemic arteries. I. ANG II receptor subtype expression, *Am J Physiol* 274:R797–R807, 1998.

127. Bendeck MP, Langille BL: Rapid accumulation of elastin and collagen in the aortas of sheep in the immediate perinatal period, *Circ Res* 69:1165–1169, 1991.

128. Leitman DC, Benson SC, Johnson LK: Glucocorticoids stimulate collagen and noncollagen protein synthesis in cultured vascular smooth muscle cells, *J Cell Biol* 98:541–549, 1984.

129. Hanna CE, et al.: Hypothalamic pituitary adrenal function in the extremely low birth weight infant, *J Clin Endocrinol Metab* 76:384–387, 1993.

130. Ng PC, et al.: Refractory hypotension in preterm infants with adrenocortical insufficiency, *Arch Dis Child Fetal Neonatal Ed* 84:F122–F124, 2001.

131. Ng PC, et al.: Transient adrenocortical insufficiency of prematurity and systemic hypotension in very low birthweight infants, *Arch Child Fetal Neonatal Ed* 89:F119–F126, 2004.

132. Masumoto K, et al.: Comparison of serum cortisol concentrations in preterm infants with or without late-onset circulatory collapse due to adrenal insufficiency of prematurity, *Pediatr Res* 63:686–690, 2008.

133. Ng PC: Is there a 'normal' range of serum cortisol concentration for preterm infants? *Pediatrics* 122:873–875, 2008.

134. Aucott SW: The challenge of defining relative adrenal insufficiency, *J Perinatol Off J Calif Perinat Assoc* 32:397–398, 2012.

135. Cooper MS, Stewart PM: Corticosteroid insufficiency in acutely ill patients, *N Engl J Med* 348: 727–734, 2003.

136. Dellinger RP, et al.: Surviving sepsis campaign: international guidelines for management of severe sepsis and septic shock, 2012, *Intensive Care Med* 39:165–228, 2013.

137. Yehya N, Vogiatzi MG, Thomas NJ, et al.: Cortisol correlates with severity of illness and poorly reflects adrenal function in pediatric acute respiratory distress syndrome, *J Pediatr* 177:212.e1–218.e1, 2016.

138. Korte C, et al.: Adrenocortical function in the very low birth weight infant: improved testing sensitivity and association with neonatal outcome, *J Pediatr* 128:257–263, 1996.

139. Fernandez E, Schrader R, Watterberg K: Prevalence of low cortisol values in term and near-term infants with vasopressor-resistant hypotension, *J Perinatol* 25:114–118, 2005.

140. Hingre RV, Gross SJ, Hingre KS, et al.: Adrenal steroidogenesis in very low birth weight preterm infants, *J Clin Endocrinol Metab* 78:266–270, 1994.

141. Watterberg KL, Scott SM: Evidence of early adrenal insufficiency in babies who develop bronchopulmonary dysplasia, *Pediatrics* 95:120–125, 1995.

142. Jett PL, et al.: Variability of plasma cortisol levels in extremely low birth weight infants, *J Clin Endocrinol Metab* 82:2921–2925, 1997.

143. Hanna CE, et al.: Corticosteroid binding globulin, total serum cortisol, and stress in extremely low-birth-weight infants, *Am J Perinatol* 14:201–204, 1997.

144. Ng PC, et al.: The pituitary-adrenal responses to exogenous human corticotropin-releasing hormone in preterm, very low birth weight infants, *J Clin Endocrinol Metab* 82:797–799, 1997.

145. Procianoy RS, Cecin SK, Pinheiro CE: Umbilical cord cortisol and prolactin levels in preterm infants. Relation to labor and delivery, *Acta Paediatr Scand* 72:713–716, 1983.

146. Terrone DA, et al.: Neonatal effects and serum cortisol levels after multiple courses of maternal corticosteroids, *Obstet Gynecol* 90:819–823, 1997.

147. Rokicki W, Forest MG, Loras B, et al.: Free cortisol of human plasma in the first three months of life, *Biol Neonate* 57:21–29, 1990.

148. Wittekind CA, Arnold JD, Leslie GI, et al.: Longitudinal study of plasma ACTH and cortisol in very low birth weight infants in the first 8 weeks of life, *Early Hum Dev* 33:191–200, 1993.

149. Goldkrand JW, Schulte RL, Messer RH: Maternal and fetal plasma cortisol levels at parturition, *Obstet Gynecol* 47:41–45, 1976.

150. Scott SM, Watterberg KL: Effect of gestational age, postnatal age, and illness on plasma cortisol concentrations in premature infants, *Pediatr Res* 37:112–116, 1995.

151. Aucott SW, Watterberg KL, Shaffer ML, et al.: PROPHET Study Group. Do cortisol concentrations predict short-term outcomes in extremely low birth weight infants? *Pediatrics* 122:775–781, 2008.

152. Hamrahian AH, Oseni TS, Arafah BM: Measurements of serum free cortisol in critically ill patients, *N Engl J Med* 350:1629–1638, 2004.

153. Watterberg KL, Scott SM, Backstrom C, et al.: Links between early adrenal function and respiratory outcome in preterm infants: airway inflammation and patent ductus arteriosus, *Pediatrics* 105:320–324, 2000.

154. Watterberg KL, et al.: Prophylaxis of early adrenal insufficiency to prevent bronchopulmonary dysplasia: a multicenter trial, *Pediatrics* 114:1649–1657, 2004.

155. El-Khuffash A, McNamara PJ, Lapointe A, et al.: Adrenal function in preterm infants undergoing patent ductus arteriosus ligation, *Neonatology* 104:28–33, 2013.

156. Clyman RI, et al.: Hypotension following patent ductus arteriosus ligation: the role of adrenal hormones, *J Pediatr* 164:1449–1455.e1, 2014.

157. Noori S, et al.: Catecholamine-resistant hypotension and myocardial performance following patent ductus arteriosus ligation, *J Perinatol Off J Calif Perinat Assoc* 35:123–127, 2015.

158. Helbock HJ, Insoft RM, Conte FA: Glucocorticoid-responsive hypotension in extremely low birth weight newborns, *Pediatrics* 92:715–717, 1993.

159. Fauser A, Pohlandt F, Bartmann P, et al.: Rapid increase of blood pressure in extremely low birth weight infants after a single dose of dexamethasone, *Eur J Pediatr* 152:354–356, 1993.

160. Gaissmaier RE, Pohlandt F: Single-dose dexamethasone treatment of hypotension in preterm infants, *J Pediatr* 134:701–705, 1999.

161. Seri I, Tan R, Evans J: Cardiovascular effects of hydrocortisone in preterm infants with pressor-resistant hypotension, *Pediatrics* 107:1070–1074, 2001.

162. Noori S, et al.: Cardiovascular effects of low-dose dexamethasone in very low birth weight neonates with refractory hypotension, *Biol Neonate* 89:82–87, 2006.

163. Noori S, et al.: Hemodynamic changes after low-dosage hydrocortisone administration in vasopressor-treated preterm and term neonates, *Pediatrics* 118:1456–1466, 2006.

164. Ng PC, et al.: A double-blind, randomized, controlled study of a 'stress dose' of hydrocortisone for rescue treatment of refractory hypotension in preterm infants, *Pediatrics* 117:367–375, 2006.

165. Baker CFW, et al.: Hydrocortisone administration for the treatment of refractory hypotension in critically ill newborns, *J Perinatol Off J Calif Perinat Assoc* 28:412–419, 2008.

166. Higgins S, Friedlich P, Seri I: Hydrocortisone for hypotension and vasopressor dependence in preterm neonates: a meta-analysis, *J Perinatol Off J Calif Perinat Assoc* 30:373–378, 2010.

167. Tsao P, von Zastrow M: Downregulation of G protein-coupled receptors, *Curr Opin Neurobiol* 10:365–369, 2000.

168. Davies AO, Lefkowitz RJ: Regulation of beta-adrenergic receptors by steroid hormones, *Annu Rev Physiol* 46:119–130, 1984.

169. Hadcock JR, Malbon CC: Regulation of beta-adrenergic receptors by 'permissive' hormones: glucocorticoids increase steady-state levels of receptor mRNA, *Proc Natl Acad Sci USA* 85:8415–8419, 1988.

170. Radomski MW, Palmer RM, Moncada S: Glucocorticoids inhibit the expression of an inducible, but not the constitutive, nitric oxide synthase in vascular endothelial cells, *Proc Natl Acad Sci USA* 87:10043–10047, 1990.

171. Wehling M: Specific, nongenomic actions of steroid hormones, *Annu Rev Physiol* 59:365–393, 1997.

172. Segar JL, et al.: Effect of cortisol on gene expression of the renin-angiotensin system in fetal sheep, *Pediatr Res* 37:741–746, 1995.

173. Auman JT, Seidler FJ, Tate CA, et al.: Are developing beta-adrenoceptors able to desensitize? Acute and chronic effects of beta-agonists in neonatal heart and liver, *Am J Physiol Regul Integr Comp Physiol* 283:R205–R217, 2002.

CHAPTER 2

Vascular Regulation of Blood Flow to Organs in the Preterm and Term Neonate

Gorm Greisen

- Multiple mechanisms operate to regulate blood flow to organs— these are also important in the newborn.
- Distribution of cardiac output is actively regulated.
- Cerebral autoregulation, that is, the ability to buffer the effects of blood pressure on cerebral blood flow, is developed even at the limits of viability.
- Cerebral autoregulation may best be described as a degree of capacity rather than an on-off phenomenon.
- A "diving" reflex-like response serves to prioritize vital organs during stress.
- The cerebral hemispheres may not be privileged, especially in the very preterm neonate.

In most organs, the principal role of perfusion is to provide substrates for cellular energy metabolism, with the final purpose of maintaining normal intracellular concentrations of the high-energy phosphate metabolites adenosine triphosphate (ATP) and phosphocreatine. The critical substrate is usually oxygen. Accordingly, organ blood flow is regulated by the energy demand of the given tissue. For instance, during maximal activation by seizures in the brain, cerebral blood flow (CBF) increases threefold, while in the muscle during maximal exercise, blood flow increases by up to eightfold. In addition, some organs, such as the brain, heart, and liver, have higher baseline oxygen and thus higher blood flow demand than others. Finally, in the kidney and skin, perfusion may be considerably above the metabolic needs to serve for glomerular filtration and thermoregulation, respectively. Indeed, during heating, skin blood flow may increase by as much as fourfold without any increase in energy demand.

In the developing organism, metabolic requirements are increased by as much as 40% due to the expenditures of growth. Since growth involves deposition of protein and fat, energy metabolism and, in particular, oxygen requirement are not increased as much as the requirements for protein and energy.

When blood flow is failing, there are several lines of defense mechanisms at the tissue level before the tissue is damaged. First, more oxygen is extracted from the blood. Normal oxygen extraction is about 30%, resulting in a venous oxygen saturation (Svo_2) of 65% to 70%. Oxygen extraction can increase up to 50% to 60%, resulting in a Svo_2 of 40% to 50%, which corresponds to a venous (i.e., end-capillary) oxygen tension of 3 to 4 kPa. This is the critical value for oxygen tension for driving the diffusion of molecular oxygen from the capillary into the cell and to the mitochondria (Fig. 2.1). Second, microvascular anatomy and the pathophysiology of the underlying disease process are both important for the final steps of oxygen delivery to tissue. When the cell senses oxygen insufficiency, its function is affected

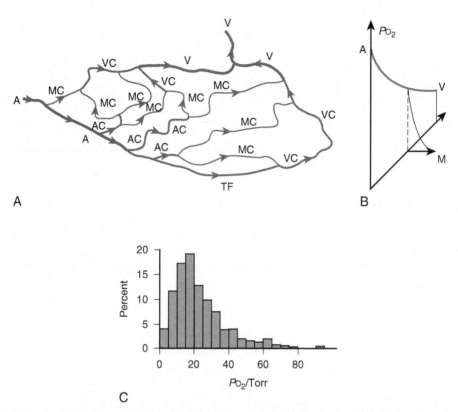

Fig. 2.1   (A) Draft of a capillary network. *A*, Arteriole; *AC*, arterial endcapillary; *MC*, middle endcapillary; *TF*, terminal flow; *V*, venule; *VC*, venous endcapillary. (B) A three-dimensional graph illustrating the Po_2 gradients from the arterial *(A)* to the venous *(V)* end of the capillaries and the radial gradient of Po_2 in surrounding tissue to the mitochondrion *(M)*. Y-axis: Po_2; X-axis: distance along the capillary (typically 1000 μm); Z-axis: distance into tissue (typically 50 μm). (C) The wide distribution of tissue Po_2 as recorded by microelectrode. Y-axis: frequency of measurements; X-axis: Po_2. Po_2 values in tissue are typically 10 to 30 Torr (1.5 to 4.5 kPa), but range from near-arterial levels to near zero. The cells with the lowest Po_2 determine the ischemic threshold, that is, the most remote cells at the venous end of capillaries. Microvascular factors, such as capillary density, and distribution of blood flow among capillaries are very important for oxygen transport to the tissue.

as growth stops, organ function fails, and, finally, cellular and thus organ survival are threatened (Fig. 2.2). *Ischemia* is the term used for inadequate blood flow to maintain appropriate oxygen delivery and thus cellular function and integrity. Since there are several steps in the cellular reaction to oxygen insufficiency, more than one ischemic threshold may be defined. It is even possible that newborn infants can be, at least, partly protected against hypoxic-ischemic injury by mechanisms akin to hibernation by "hypoxic hypometabolism."[1]

The immature mammal is also able to "centralize" blood flow during periods of stress. This pattern of flow distribution is often called the "diving reflex," since it is qualitatively similar to the adaptation of circulation in seals during diving, a process that allows sea mammals to stay under water for 20 minutes or more. Blood flow to the skin, muscle, kidneys, liver, and other nonvital organs is reduced to spare the oxygen reserve for the vital organs: the brain, heart, and adrenals. This reaction is relevant during birth with the limitations on placental oxygen transport imposed by uterine contractions and has been studied intensively in the fetal lamb. It has the potential of prolonging passive survival at a critical moment in the individual's life. For comparison, the "fight-or-flight" response of the mature terrestrial mammal supports sustained maximal muscle work.

Physically, blood simply flows toward the point of lowest resistance. While flow velocities in the heart are high to allow the kinetic energy of the blood to thrust forward, flow velocity is minimal in the peripheral circulation. Organs are perfused simultaneously and the blood flow through a given tissue is the result of the pressure gradient between the arteries and the veins, the so-called perfusion pressure.

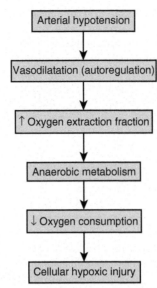

Fig. 2.2 **The lines of defense against oxygen insufficiency.** First, when blood pressure falls, autoregulation of organ blood flow will reduce vascular resistance and keep blood flow nearly unaffected. If the blood pressure falls below the lower limit of the autoregulatory elbow, or if autoregulation is impaired by vascular pathology, metabolic or respiratory acidosis, or immaturity, blood flow to the tissue falls. At this point, oxygen extraction increases from each milliliter of blood. The limit of this compensation is attained when the minimal Svo_2, or rather the minimal end-capillary oxygen tension, has been reached. This process is determined by microvascular factors as illustrated in Fig. 2.1. When the limits of oxygen extraction have been reached, the marginal cells resort to anaerobic metabolism (increase glucose consumption to produce lactate) to meet their metabolic needs. If this is insufficient, oxygen consumption decreases as metabolic functions related to growth and to organ function are shut down. However, in vital organs, such as the brain, heart, and adrenal glands, loss of function is life threatening. In nonvital organs, normal development may be affected if this critical state is long lasting. Acute cellular death by necrosis occurs only when vital cellular functions break down and membrane potential and integrity cannot be maintained. In newborn mammals, hypoxic hypometabolism is a mechanism that further reduces the sensitivity to hypoxic-ischemic injury.

Vascular resistance is composed of the limited diameter of blood vessels, particularly the smaller arteries and arterioles, and blood viscosity. The regulation of organ blood flow takes place by modifying arterial diameter, that is, by varying the tone of the smooth muscle cells of the arterial wall. Factors that influence vascular resistance are usually divided into four categories: blood pressure, chemical (Pco_2 and Po_2), metabolic (functional activation), and neurogenic. Most studies of vascular resistance have been done on cerebral vessels. Therefore, the following account refers to cerebral vessels from mature animals, unless stated otherwise.

Regulation of Arterial Tone

The Role of Conduit Arteries in Regulating Vascular Resistance

It is usually assumed that the arteriole, the precapillary muscular artery with a diameter of 20 to 50 μm, is the primary determinant of vascular resistance, while the larger arteries are more or less considered passive conduits. However, this is not the case. For instance, in the adult cat the pressure in the small cerebral arteries (150 to 200 μm) is only 50% to 60% of the aortic pressure.[2] Thus the reactivity of the entire muscular arterial tree is of relevance in regulating organ blood flow. The role of the prearteriolar vessels is likely even more important in the newborn than in the adult. First, the smaller body size translates to smaller conduit arteries. The resistance is proportional to length but is inversely proportional to the diameter to the power of 4. Therefore the conduit arteries of the newborn will make an even more important contribution to the vascular resistance. Second, conduit arteries, the largest arteries with an enhanced ability to stretch in response to pulsating flow, are very reactive in the newborn. The diameter of the carotid artery increases by

75% during acute asphyxia in term lambs, whereas the diameter of the descending aorta decreases by 15% when blood pressure drops.[3] Thus, the former response must indicate active vasodilation. For comparison, flow-induced vasodilatation in the forearm in adults is only in the order of 5%. As resistance is proportional to the diameter to the power of 4, the findings in asphyxiated lambs indicate a roughly 90% reduction of the arterial component of the cerebrovascular resistance coupled with a near doubling of the arterial component of vascular resistance to the lower body. Incidentally, these observations also suggest that blood flow velocity, as recorded from conduit arteries by Doppler ultrasound, may be potentially misleading in the neonatal patient population.

Arterial Reaction to Pressure (Autoregulation)

Smooth muscle cells of the arterial wall constrict in response to increased intravascular pressure in the local arterial segment to a degree that more than compensates for the passive stretching of the vessel wall by the increased pressure. The net result is that arteries constrict when pressure increases and dilate when pressure drops. This phenomenon is called the autoregulation of blood flow (Fig. 2.3). The response time in isolated, cannulated arterial segments is in the order of 10 seconds.[4] The cellular mechanisms of this process are now better understood. Vessel wall constriction constitutes an intrinsic myogenic reflex and is independent of endothelial function. Rather, pressure induces an increase in the smooth muscle cell membrane potential, which regulates vascular smooth muscle cell activity through the action of voltage-gated calcium channels. Although the precise mechanism of the mechanochemical coupling is unknown, several plasma-membrane-bound receptors are involved, including G-protein-coupled receptors and a class of transient potential receptors.[5] Furthermore, the calcium signal is modulated in many ways[6] but a detailed discussion of this topic is beyond the scope of this chapter. Suffice to mention that phospholipases and activation of protein kinase C are involved, and, at least in the rat middle cerebral artery, the arachidonic acid metabolite 20-HETE has also been implicated.[7] Furthermore, additional modulation of intracellular calcium concentration by alternative sources, such as the calcium-dependent K^+ channels, also exists.

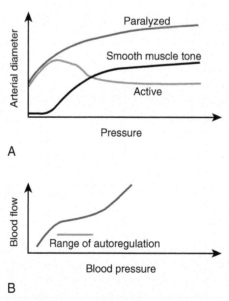

Fig. 2.3 **Increases in pressure lead to progressive dilatation of a paralyzed artery.** As pressure increases further, the elastic capacity is exhausted, and vasodilation decreases as collagen restricts further dilation limiting the risk of rupture (A). A certain range of pressures is associated with a proportional variation in smooth muscle tone. The precise mechanism of this mechanochemical coupling is not known, but it is endogenous to all vascular smooth muscle cells. As a result, in an active artery, the diameter varies inversely with pressure over a certain range. This phenomenon constitutes the basis of arterial "autoregulation" (B).

Local variations in the expression of these receptors and channels may, at least in part, explain the difference in responses to blood pressure in different vascular beds and the unique blood flow distribution between vital and nonvital organs.[8]

Interaction of Autoregulation and Hypoxic Vasodilatation

As described earlier, arterial smooth muscle tone is affected by a number of factors, all contributing to determine the incident level of vascular resistance. Among the vasodilators, hypoxia is one of the more potent and physiologically relevant factors. Vascular reactivity to O_2 depends, in part, on intact endothelial function ensuring appropriate local nitric oxide (NO) production. Hypoxia also induces tissue lactic acidosis. The decreased pH constitutes a point of interaction between O_2 and CO_2 reactivity (see later). In addition, hypoxia decreases smooth muscle membrane potential by the direct and selective opening of both the calcium-activated and ATP-sensitive K^+ channels in the cell membrane.[9] In the immature brain, adenosine is also an important regulator of the vascular response to hypoxia.[10] The membrane potential response to hypoxia is independent of the existing intravascular pressure.[11] However, at lower pressures, the decrease in membrane potential only leads to minimal further arterial dilation because, at low vascular tone, the membrane potential-muscular tone relationship is outside the steep part of the slope (Fig. 2.4). In other words, at low perfusion pressures, the dilator pathway has already been near maximally activated. Therefore, in a hypotensive neonate, a superimposed hypoxic event cannot be appropriately compensated due to the low perfusion pressure. The end result is tissue hypoxia-ischemia with the potential of causing irreversible damage to organs, especially to the brain. This is a clinically highly relevant point when providing care for the hypotensive and hypoxic neonate.

Interaction of Autoregulation and P_{CO_2}

Arteries and arterioles constrict with hypocapnia and dilate with hypercapnia. The principal part of this reaction is mediated through changes in pH, that is, H^+ concentration. Perivascular pH has a direct effect on the membrane potential of arterial smooth muscle cells since, mostly via activation of both the ATP-sensitive and calcium-activated K^+ channels, extracellular H^+ concentration is one of the main determinants of the potassium conductance of the plasma membrane in arterial

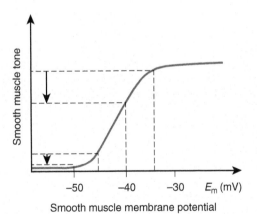

Fig. 2.4 **The relationship between smooth muscle cell membrane potential (E_m) and tone.** Pressure affects smooth muscle tone through membrane potential. Increased pressure increases membrane potential (i.e., makes it less negative), whereas decreased pressure induces hyperpolarization (i.e., membrane potential is more negative). Hyperpolarization induces relaxation and hence vasodilatation. The modifying effect of hypoxia is illustrated by the dashed lines and arrows. At high membrane potential (−35 mV), a decrease in membrane potential by 5 mV induces a marked reduction in muscular tone. Thus, at normal or high blood pressures, hypoxemia can be compensated by vasodilatation. However, at low membrane potential (hyperpolarization) a similar hypoxia-induced decrease in membrane potential has much less effect on muscular tone. This predicts that, at low blood pressure where there is a baseline low membrane potential to enable vasodilation keeping blood flow in the acceptable range, hypoxemia cannot be well compensated by further increases in blood flow. Many other factors may influence muscle tone by modifying membrane potential, and the magnitude of effects can be predicted to be interdependent.

smooth muscle cells regulating the outward K^+ current.[9] Therefore, when the pH decreases, the K^+ outflow from the vascular smooth muscle cell increases, resulting in hyperpolarization of the cell membrane and, via the closure of voltage-gated Ca^{++} channels, it causes vasodilatation. Furthermore, increased extracellular and, to a lesser degree, intracellular H^+ concentrations reduce the conductance of the voltage-dependent calcium channels, further enhancing vascular smooth muscle cell relaxation.[12]

Hypercapnic vasodilatation is reduced by up to 50% when NO synthase (NOS) activity is blocked in the brain of the adult rat.[13] The hypercapnic response is restituted by the addition of an NO donor.[14] This finding suggests that unhindered local NO production is necessary for the pH to exert its vasoregulatory effects. Indeed, it has been suggested that, although the calcium-activated and ATP-sensitive K^+ channels play the primary role in the vascular response to changes in P_{CO_2}, the function of these channels is regulated by local NO production.[15]

The role of prostanoids in mediating the vascular response to P_{CO_2} is less clear.[16,17] The fact that indomethacin abolishes the normal cerebral (or other organ) blood flow–CO_2 response in preterm infants is likely a direct effect of the drug independent of its inhibitory action on prostanoid synthesis.[18] This notion is supported by the finding that ibuprofen is devoid of such effects on the organ blood flow–CO_2 response.[19]

Interaction of Autoregulation and Functional Activation (Metabolic Blood Flow Control)

Several mechanisms operate to match local blood flow to metabolic requirements, including changes in pH, local production of adenosine, ATP and NO, and local neural mechanisms. It appears that, in the muscle, there is not a single factor dominating, since the robust and very fast coupling of activity and blood flow is almost unaffected by blocking any of these mechanisms one by one.[20] In the brain, astrocytes may be the central sites of regulation of this response in the neurovascular unit via their perivascular end-feet and by using many of the aforementioned cellular mechanisms, such as changes in K^+ ion flux and the local production of prostanoids, ATP, and adenosine.[21] Among these cellular regulators, adenosine has been proposed to play a principal role.[22] Adenosine also works by regulating the activity of the calcium-activated and ATP-sensitive K^+ channels.

Flow-Mediated Vasodilatation

Endothelial cells sense flow by shear stress and produce NO in reaction to high shear stress at high flow velocities. NO diffuses freely and reaches the smooth muscle cell underneath the endothelium. NO acts on smooth muscle K^+ channels using cyclic guanosine monophosphate (GMP) as the secondary messenger and then a series of intermediate steps. Since NO is a vasodilator, the basic arterial reflex to high flow is vasodilation. Thus when a tissue is activated (e.g., a muscle contracts), the local vessels first dilate, as directed by the mechanisms of the metabolic flow control described earlier, and blood flow increases. This initial increase in blood flow is then sensed in the conduit arteries through the shear stress-induced increase in local NO production, and vascular resistance is further reduced allowing flow to increase yet again. The action remains local as the generated NO diffusing into the bloodstream is largely inactivated by hemoglobin.

Sympathetic Nervous System

Epinephrine in the blood originates from the adrenal glands, whereas norepinephrine is produced by sympathetic nerve endings and extraadrenal chromaffin tissue. Sympathetic nerves are present in nearly all vessels, located in the adventitia and mixed in with the smooth muscle cells. Adrenoreceptors are widely distributed in the cardiovascular system located in the smooth muscle and endothelial cell membranes. Several different adrenoreceptors exist; alpha-1 receptors with at least three subtypes are present primarily in the arteries and the myocardium, while alpha-2, beta-1, and beta-2 receptors are expressed in all types of vessels and the myocardium. In the arteries and veins, alpha-receptor stimulation causes vasoconstriction, and beta-receptor stimulation results in vasodilatation. Both alpha- and beta-adrenoreceptors are frequently expressed in the membrane of the same cell. Therefore, the response of the given cell to epinephrine or norepinephrine depends on the relative abundance of the receptor types expressed.[23] Of clinical importance is the regulation of the expression of the cardiovascular adrenergic receptors by corticosteroids, the high incidence of relative adrenal insufficiency in preterm neonates and critically ill term infants (see Chapter 30), the role of glucocorticoids and mineralocorticoids in maintaining the sensitivity of the cardiovascular system to endogenous and exogenous catecholamines, and the downregulation of the cardiovascular adrenergic receptors in response to the increased release of endogenous catecholamines or the administration of exogenous catecholamines in critical illness.[24–26] Typically, arteries and arterioles of the skin, gut, and muscle constrict in response to increases in endogenous catecholamine production, whereas those of the heart and brain either do not constrict or even dilate (see later). The response also depends on the resting tone of the given vessel. Furthermore, the sensitivity of a vessel to circulating norepinephrine may be less than the sensitivity to norepinephrine produced by increased sympathetic nerve activity, since alpha-1 receptors may be particularly abundant in the membrane regions close to where the nerve secretes the transmitter. The signaling pathways of the adrenoreceptors are complex and dependent on the receptor subtype. Activation of alpha-adrenoreceptors generally results in vasoconstriction mediated by increased release of calcium from intracellular stores as a first step, while beta-receptor-induced vasodilation is mediated by increased cyclic adenosine monophosphate (AMP) generation. However, the system is far more complex and, among other mechanisms, receptor activation-associated changes in K^+ conductance and local NO synthesis are also involved. Finally, the sympathetic nervous system is activated during hypoxia, hypotension, or hypovolemia via the stimulation of different chemoreceptors and baroreceptors in the vessel walls and the vasomotor centers in the medulla. Activation of the sympathetic nervous system plays a central role in the cardiovascular response to stress and it is the mainstay of the diving reflex response during hypoxia-ischemia.

Humoral Factors in General Circulation

A large number of endogenous vasoactive factors, other than those mentioned earlier, also play a role in the extremely complex process of organ blood flow regulation, such as angiotensin II, arginine-vasopressin, vasointestinal peptide, neuropeptide gamma, and endothelin-1. However, none of these vasoactive factors has been shown to have a significant importance in isolation under normal conditions except for the role of angiotensin II in regulating renal microhemodynamics.

In conclusion, a great many factors have an input and interact to define the degree of contraction of the vascular smooth muscle cells and, hence, regulate arterial and arteriolar tone (see Fig. 2.4). Although many details are unknown, especially in the developing immature animal or human, the final common pathway appears to involve the smooth-cell membrane potential, cytoplasmic calcium concentration, and the calcium/calmodulin myosin light chain kinase-mediated phosphorylation of the regulatory light chains of myosin resulting in the interaction of actin and myosin (Fig. 2.5). However, the complexity of the known factors and their interplay as well as the differences in the response among the different organs are overwhelming, and no simple or unifying principle of vascular tone regulation has gained a foothold. Indeed, the complexity predicts that vascular tone and reactivity in a particular arterial segment in a particular tissue may differ markedly from that in other segments or other tissues. Unfortunately, the insights are as yet insufficient to allow any quantitative predictions for different organs or vascular tree segments.

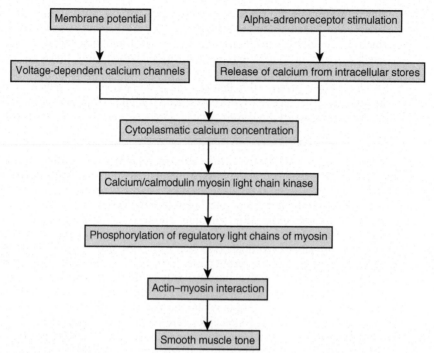

Fig. 2.5 A scheme of the pathway from smooth muscle cell membrane potential and alpha-adrenoreceptor stimulation to changes in smooth muscle tone.

Blood Flow to the Brain

Brain injury is common in newborn infants. It can occur rapidly, is frequently irreversible, and rarely, in itself, prevents survival. Injury to no other organs in the neonatal period has the same clinical importance, as the other organs have a better capacity to recover even from severe hypoxic-ischemic damage. Disturbances in blood flow and inflammation have been proposed as the major factors in the development of neonatal brain injury.

Autoregulation of Cerebral Blood Flow in the Immature Brain

Pressure-flow autoregulation has been widely investigated in the immature cerebral vasculature since the original observation of direct proportionality of CBF to systolic blood pressure in a group of neonates during stabilization after birth.[27]

An adequate autoregulatory plateau, shifted to the left to match the lower perinatal blood pressure, has been demonstrated in several animal species shortly after birth, including dogs, lambs, and rats.[28–32] In fetal lambs, autoregulation is not present at 0.6 weeks' gestation, but is functional at 0.9 weeks' gestation.[33] The lower threshold of the autoregulation is developmentally regulated and it is closer to the normal resting systemic mean blood pressure at 0.75 gestation compared with 0.9 gestation.[34] Thus, in the more immature subject there is less vasodilator reserve, which limits the effectiveness of CBF autoregulation at the earlier stages of development. In newborn lambs, autoregulation could be completely abolished for 4 to 7 hours by 20 minutes of hypoxemia with arterial oxygen saturations about 50%.[35]

Observational studies of global CBF in stable neonates without evidence of major brain injury suggest that autoregulation is intact.[36–44] In contrast, evidence of absent autoregulation has been found under pathologic conditions, such as following severe birth asphyxia in term infants, and in preterm infants in association with brain injury or death.[39,41,45–49]

Imaging of CBF during arterial hypotension suggested that CBF to the periventricular white matter may be selectively reduced at blood pressures less than 30 mm Hg,[50] supporting the notion that the periventricular white matter is a "watershed area." Another study also found some evidence for the lower threshold of the autoregulatory curve for the global CBF around 29 mm Hg.[51]

In conclusion, the lower threshold for CBF autoregulation may be around 30 mm Hg or somewhat below, and autoregulation can be assumed to operate in most newborn infants, even the most immature. When blood pressure falls below the threshold, CBF will fall proportionally more due to the elastic reduction in vascular diameter. However, significant blood flow is believed to be present until systemic mean blood pressure is less than 20 mm Hg, and it may in general be more appropriate to consider arterial blood pressure-CBF reactivity (i.e., autoregulation) as a degree of capacity, rather than an on-off phenomenon.[52] Finally, while poor clinical outcomes may be predicted by impaired autoregulation, it remains to be demonstrated that it has clinical value to estimate the state of the autoregulation.[53] One way could be to determine the level of arterial blood pressure, where the pressure-flow reactivity is lowest—the optimal blood pressure—and then to treat arterial hypotension using this individualized target.[54]

Effect of Carbon Dioxide on Cerebral Blood Flow

Changes in carbon dioxide tension (P_{CO_2}) have more pronounced effects on CBF than on blood flow in other organs due to the presence of the blood-brain barrier. The blood-brain barrier is an endothelium with tight junctions, which does not allow HCO_3^- to pass through readily. The restricted diffusion of HCO_3^- means that hypercapnia and hypocapnia decreases and increases, respectively, the pH in the perivascular space in the brain more readily than in blood where buffering is more effective due to the presence of hemoglobin. This response to a change in P_{CO_2} continues until HCO_3^- equilibrates over the course of hours.

In normocapnic adults, small acute changes in arterial P_{CO_2} (Pa_{CO_2}) result in a change in CBF by 30% per kPa (4% per mm Hg Pa_{CO_2}). Similar reactivity has been demonstrated in the normal human neonate by venous occlusion plethysmography and in stable preterm ventilated infants without major germinal layer hemorrhage by using the ^{133}Xe clearance technique.[38,55,56] However, Pa_{CO_2} reactivity is less than 30% per kPa during the first 24 hours.[39]

Contrary to the vasodilation induced by increases in the P_{CO_2}, a hyperventilation-related decrease in Pa_{CO_2} causes hypocapnic cerebral vasoconstriction and has been found to be associated with brain injury in preterm but not in term infants or adults.[38,57–59] It is an open question whether hypocapnia alone can cause ischemia, or if it works in combination with other factors, such as hypoxemia, hypoglycemia, the presence of high levels of cytokines, sympathetic activation, or seizures.

Metabolic Control of Blood Flow to the Brain

CBF in term infants, estimated by venous occlusion plethysmography, is greater during active sleep than during quiet sleep and, in preterm infants of 32 to 35 weeks' postmenstrual age, in the wake state compared with sleep.[60–63] Thus there is flow-metabolism coupling even before term gestation in the brain. This finding is further supported by the documented increase in CBF seen during seizure activity and by the strong relation between CBF and blood hemoglobin concentration.[36,40]

The cerebrovascular response to functional activation by sensory stimulation was found to be variable by initial studies using magnetic resonance imaging and near-infrared spectroscopy (NIRS).[64–68] More recently, a clear coupling between increases in local metabolic rate and blood flow has been demonstrated in preterm infants[69] and also between burst activity and cerebral oxygenation in term infants with neonatal encephalopathy.[70]

Cerebrovenous oxygen saturation was entirely normal (64% $\pm$ 5%) as estimated by NIRS and jugular occlusion technique in 11 healthy, term infants 3 days after birth.[71] In a simple way, this finding indicates that there is a balance between blood flow and cerebral oxygen consumption in the newborn.

Adrenergic Mechanisms Affecting Cerebral Blood Flow

Based on findings in animal studies, the sympathetic system appears to play a greater role affecting CBF and its autoregulation in the perinatal period than it does later in life.[72–76] This finding has been attributed to the relative immaturity of the NO-induced vasodilatory mechanisms during early development.[77] The adrenergic effect, at least in part, results in enhanced constriction of conduit arteries.

A rare study of human neonatal arteries in vitro (obtained postmortem from preterm neonates of 23 to 34 weeks' gestation) showed basal tone and a pressure-diameter relation quite similar to those seen in the adult pial arteries.[78] However, the neonatal arteries were significantly more sensitive to exogenous norepinephrine and electrical field activation of adventitial sympathetic nerve fibers, and had a much higher sympathetic nerve density compared with those in the adult pial arteries.[79,80]

Effect of Medications on Cerebral Blood Flow

Indomethacin reduces CBF in experimental animals, adults, and preterm neonates.[81] The concern has been whether it reduces CBF to ischemic levels resulting in injury in the developing brain. Interestingly, although indomethacin decreases the incidence of severe peri/intraventricular hemorrhage, this early effect does not seem to translate to better long-term neurodevelopmental outcomes.[82] Contrary to indomethacin, ibuprofen does not have significant cerebrovascular effects.[19,83] However, it is not known whether the long-term neurodevelopmental outcome in neonates exposed to ibuprofen is better than in those having been treated with indomethacin.

Among the methylxanthines, aminophylline reduces CBF and $Paco_2$ in experimental animals, adults, and preterm infants, but caffeine has less of an effect on CBF.[84,85] Methylxanthines are potent adenosine receptor antagonists. However, it is not entirely clear whether the reduction of CBF is the direct effect of methylxanthines on the adenosine receptors, a result of the associated decrease in $Paco_2$, or a combination.

Dopamine does not appear to have a selective (dilatory) effect on brain vasculature[86,87] and its administration has been found to be associated with impaired autoregulation.[49,88] Individual studies have varied regarding its effect on CBF,[86–90] but using a meta-analytic approach, dopamine administration results in increases in CBF in hypotensive neonates.[91]

Ischemic Thresholds in the Brain

In the newborn puppy, Svo_2 may decrease from 75% to 40% without provoking significant lactate production.[92] The exact minimum value of "normal" Svo_2 depends on, among other things, the oxygen dissociation curve. Therefore, it may be affected by changes in pH and the proportion of fetal hemoglobin present in the blood.

In the cerebral cortex of the adult baboon and man, the threshold of blood flow sufficient to maintain tissue integrity depends on the duration of the low flow. For instance, if the low flow lasts for a few hours, the limit of minimal CBF to maintain tissue integrity is around 10 mL/100 g/min.[93] In acute localized brain ischemia, blood flow may remain sufficient to maintain structural integrity but fail to sustain functional (electrical) activity, a phenomenon called "border zone" or "penumbra."[94] Indeed, in progressing ischemia, electrical failure is a warning for the impending development of permanent tissue injury. In the adult human brain cortex, electrical function ceases at about 20 mL/100 g/min of blood flow, while in the subcortical gray matter and brainstem of the adult baboon, the blood flow threshold is around 10 to 15 mL/100 g/min.[95]

In normal newborn infants at rest the global CBF is 15 to 20 mL/100 g/min (see Chapter 16). The ischaemic threshold values of CBF for neonates are not known. However, in view of the low resting levels of CBF and the comparatively longer survival in total ischemia or anoxia, neonatal CBF thresholds are likely to be considerably less than 10 mL/100 g/min. Indeed, in ventilated preterm infants visual evoked responses were unaffected at global CBF levels below 10 mL/100 g/min corresponding to a cerebral oxygen delivery of 50 μmol/100 g/min.[38,96]

Low CBF and cerebral oxygen delivery carry a risk of later death, cerebral atrophy, or neurodevelopmental deficit,[97–100] but it is unclear whether treatment aimed at increasing CBF (or its surrogate, cerebral oxygenation) can improve the outcome.[101]

Blood Flow to Other Organs

Based on studies on the distribution of cardiac output in term fetal lambs and newborn piglets, the typical abdominal organ blood flow appears to be around 100 to 350 mL/100 g/min.[102,103] In the fetus, abdominal organ blood flow is higher than in the newborn with the exception of the intestine.

Kidney

The adult kidneys constitute 0.5% of body weight but represent 25% of resting cardiac output, making them the most richly perfused organ of the body. In the newborn, although the kidneys are relatively larger, they receive less blood flow probably due to the immaturity of the renal function. Renal arteries display appropriate autoregulation with a lower threshold adjusted to the prevailing lower blood pressure.[104] In addition to structural immaturity, high levels of circulating vasoactive mediators, such as angiotensin II, vasopressin, and endogenous catecholamines, explain the relatively low renal blood flow in the immediate postnatal period. Indeed, after the alpha-adrenergic receptor blockade, renal nerve stimulation results in increased blood flow. To counterbalance the renal vasoconstriction and increased sodium reabsorption caused by the aforementioned hormones, the neonatal kidney is more dependent on the local production of vasodilatory prostaglandins compared to later in life. This explains why indomethacin, a cyclooxygenase (COX) inhibitor, readily reduces renal blood flow and urinary output in the neonate, but not in the euvolemic child or adult. Interestingly, the renal side effects of another COX inhibitor, ibuprofen, are less pronounced in the neonate.[105] Finally, dopamine selectively increases renal blood flow at a low dose with minimal effect on blood pressure.[86]

Liver

The liver is a large organ that has a dual blood supply with blood originating from the stomach and intestines through the portal system and also from the hepatic branch of the celiac artery through the hepatic artery. The proportion of blood flow from these sources in the normal adult is 3:1, respectively. Hepatic vessels are richly innervated with sympathetic and parasympathetic nerves. The hepatic artery constricts in response to sympathetic nerve stimulation and exogenous norepinephrine while the response of the portal vein is less well characterized. Angiotensin II is a potent vasoconstrictor of the hepatic vascular beds. During the first days after birth, a portion of the portal blood flow continues to be shunted past the liver through the ductus venosus until it closes. Portal liver blood flow in lambs is 100 to 150 mL/100 g/min during the first postnatal day and increases to over 200 mL/100 g/min by the end of the first week.[106]

Stomach and Intestines

The stomach and intestines are motile organs, and variation in intestinal wall tension influences vascular resistance.[107] For example, the stimulation of sympathetic nerves results in constriction of the intestinal arteries and arterioles and in the relaxation of the intestinal wall. Thus the sympathetic effects on vascular resistance and intestinal wall tension are opposite. Furthermore, a number of gastrointestinal hormones and paracrine substances, such as gastrin, glucagon, and cholecystokinin, dilate the intestinal vessels, which likely contributes to the increase in intestinal blood flow during digestion. Local metabolic coupling also contributes to the digestion-associated increase in intestinal blood flow. Intestinal blood flow also shows well-developed autoregulation, and responses to sympathetic nerve stimulation, exogenous catecholamines, and angiotensin II similar to that of the other abdominal organs in the immature animal.

Table 2.1   ORGAN WEIGHTS IN TERM AND EXTREMELY LOW BIRTH WEIGHT NEONATES

Organ or Tissue	Body and Organ Weight (g)	
	3500	1000
Brain	411 (12%)	143 (15%)
Heart	23 (1%)	8 (1%)
Liver	153 (4%)	47 (5%)
Kidney	28 (1%)	10 (1%)
Fat	23%[a]	<5%

[a]Data from Uthaya S, Bell J, Modi N: Adipose tissue magnetic resonance imaging in the newborn. *Horm Res* 62(Suppl 3):1430–1438, 2004.
Organ weight in percent of body weight (%).
Total body water is around 75% and 85% to 90% of body weight in term neonates and extremely low birth weight neonates, respectively.
Other data from Charles AD, Smith NM: Perinatal postmortem. In Rennie JM, editor: *Roberton's textbook of neonatology*, Beijing, 2005, Elsevier, pp 1207–1215.

Table 2.2   VOLUMETRIC BLOOD FLOW BY DOPPLER ULTRASOUND MEASUREMENT FOR THE UPPER PART OF THE BODY IN HEALTHY TERM INFANTS

Vessel	N	Age	Flow (mL/min)	Flow (mL/kg/min)	Reference
Vertebral arteries	42	39–42 (weeks)	22[a]		Kehrer[119]
Int. carotid arteries			56[a]		
Right com. carotid	21	Day 1–3	117[b]		Sinha[120]
Superior vena cava	14	Day 1	258	76	Kluckow[109]
Ascending aorta			500	147	

[a]Values for sum of right and left.
[b]Value multiplied by 2 for comparison.
Newborn infants born at term were mixed with former preterm infants reaching 39 to 40 postmenstrual weeks.[111]

Distribution of Cardiac Output in the Healthy Human Neonate

If the heart fails to increase cardiac output to maintain systemic blood pressure, a selective and marked increase in the flow to one organ can, in principle, compromise blood flow to other organs (the "steal" phenomenon). No single organ of critical importance is large in itself at birth (Table 2.1).

Blood Flow to the Upper Part of the Body

Blood flow to various organs differs considerably at the resting state. The data from recent Doppler flow volumetric studies allow some comparisons for the organs in the upper part of the body in healthy term infants. Blood flow to the brain, defined as the sum of the blood flowing through the two internal carotid and two vertebral arteries, corresponds to 18 mL/100 g/min using a mean brain weight of 385 g for the term infant (Table 2.2). This blood flow is close to what is expected from the data on CBF in the literature assessed by NIRS and ^{133}Xe clearance.

Blood Flow to the Lower Part of the Body

Lower body blood flows are less well studied in the human neonate. In a recent study in extremely low birth weight infants with no ductal shunt and a cardiac output of 200 mL/kg/min, aortic blood flow was found to be 90 mL/kg/min at the level of the diaphragm.[108] Although this finding is in agreement with the data by Kluckow and Evans showing that approximately 50% of left ventricular output returns through the superior vena cava (SVC) in preterm neonates, some caution is warranted because most preterm infants enrolled in the studies on SVC blood flow measurements had an open patent ductus arteriosus (PDA).[109]

The data on individual abdominal organ flows in neonates are less current but available with a renal blood flow (right + left) of 21 mL/kg/min, a superior mesenteric artery blood flow of 43 mL/kg/min, and a celiac artery blood flow of 70 mL/kg/min.[110–112] In the study by Agata and colleagues, the results were divided by 2 to account for the parabolic arterial flow profile.[112] However, since the sum of these abdominal organ blood flows exceeds the blood flow in the descending aorta and since blood flow from other organ systems in the lower body (e.g., bones, muscle, and skin) has not been taken into consideration, it is clear that blood flows to the abdominal organs have been overestimated in the neonate. The reasons for this discrepancy are unclear but they may, at least in part, be related to the use of less sophisticated Doppler equipment using lower ultrasound frequencies in the studies performed in the early 1990s. In terms of perfusion rate, the renal blood flow of 21 mL/min/kg body weight transforms to 210 mL/100 g kidney weight per minute. Again, this is higher than that expected from studies using hippuric acid clearance.[113] Taking all these findings into consideration, it is reasonable to conclude that normal organ flow in the human neonate is likely to be comparable to that in different animal species, and is around 100 to 300 mL/100 g/min. For comparison, lower limb blood flow in the human infant has been estimated by NIRS and the venous occlusion technique to be around 3.5 mL/100 g/min, only.[114]

In summary, cardiac output is distributed approximately equally to the upper and lower body in the normal healthy newborn infant at gestational ages from 28 to 40 weeks. It may come as a surprise to many readers that only 25% to 30% of the blood flow to the upper part of the body goes to the brain, whereas the abdominal organs can be assumed to account for the largest part of the blood flow to the lower part of the body. Although good estimates of abdominal organ perfusion rates are not available, they appear to be higher than the perfusion rate of the brain. Therefore, a relative hyperperfusion of the abdominal organs could result in a significant "steal" of cardiac output from the brain.

Mechanisms Governing the Redistribution of Cardiac Output in the Fetal "Diving" Reflex

Aerobic Diving

The diving reflex of sea mammals occurs within the "aerobic diving limit," that is, without hypoxia severe enough to lead to the production of lactic acid. The key components are reflex bradycardia mediated through the carotid chemoreceptors and the vagal nerve, reflex vasoconstriction of the vascular beds of "nonvital" organs, and recruitment of blood from the spleen. All of this results in a reduced cardiac output, a dramatically increased circulation time, and hence, a lag between tissue oxygen consumption and CO_2 production.[115]

Reactions to Hypoxia

Similarly, the immediate reaction to hypoxia in the perinatal mammal is bradycardia and peripheral vasoconstriction. Since the reaction to fetal distress is of great clinical interest, it has been extensively studied in the fetal lamb. The response to fetal distress is qualitatively similar but quantitatively different among the different modes of induction of fetal distress, such as maternal hypoxemia, graded reduction of umbilical blood flow, repeated or graded reduction or complete arrest of uterine blood flow, and reduction of fetal blood volume.[116] Among the vital organs, adrenal blood flow increases in all situations, whereas this is not the case when fetal distress is caused by the reduction of fetal blood volume (heart) or the arrest of uterine blood flow (brain). However, the fetal circulation is different, and its peculiar features may explain some of the aforementioned differences between fetal and postnatal hemodynamic responses to stress.

Modifying Effects

Preterm lambs appear less able to produce a strong epinephrine and norepinephrine response to stress and, accordingly, the blood pressure rise is less than at term.[116] Since carotid sinus denervation does not abolish the redistribution of cardiac output, supplementary mechanisms must be operational in the fetus.[117] Indeed, at least in the later phase (after 15 minutes) of the hemodynamic response, the renin-angiotensin system also seems to play an important role. Importantly, recent findings indicate that a systemic inflammatory response significantly interferes with the redistribution of cardiac output during the arrest of uterine blood flow in the fetal sheep, and compromises cardiac function and the chance of successful resuscitation.[118]

Distribution of Cardiac Output in the Shocked Newborn

The Term Neonate With Low Cardiac Output

The pale gray, yet awake term baby with congenital heart disease presenting with poor systemic perfusion due to decreased cardiac output (systemic blood flow) may be the best example for the operation of efficient cardiovascular centralization mechanisms in the human newborn. This baby may have very low central Svo$_2$, but will still produce urine, have bowel motility, and, at least in the initial phase of the cardiovascular compromise, have a normal blood lactate. There is little we may be able to do—short of the appropriate medical/pharmaceutical intervention in duct-dependent lesions, cardiac catheter-based therapy, and/or surgical procedure (see Chapter 32)—to help this baby improve the distribution of the limited systemic blood flow.

The Very Preterm Neonate During Immediate Postnatal Adaptation

In the very preterm neonate with poor systemic perfusion during the period of immediate postnatal transition with the fetal channels still open, the situation is likely to be different. This baby may present with a better color and capillary refill suggesting appropriate peripheral perfusion. Yet, motor activity is likely to be reduced, urinary output low, and blood lactate slightly high. Based on the findings discussed earlier, this baby may have immature and insufficient adrenergic mechanisms to rely on for maintaining sufficient perfusion pressure to the vital organs. In addition, owing to the immaturity of the myocardium, this patient may initially be unable to adapt to the sudden increase in the systemic vascular resistance following separation from the placenta, especially with immediate cord clamping. An impaired CBF autoregulation and possibly the endogenous sympathetic tone result in further reductions of CBF. Again, maintenance of both an appropriate systemic blood flow and perfusion pressure must be the goal of the intervention (see Chapters 1 and 26). In the future, direct monitoring of cerebral oxygen sufficiency may help to guide treatment.

Other Scenarios

Other scenarios relevant to the neonatologist are shock due to low peripheral vascular resistance in patients with specific (sepsis) and nonspecific inflammation and loss of blood volume. The effectiveness of available supportive treatment modalities of the critically ill septic neonate has not been systematically studied (see Chapters 27 and 29). In addition, microvascular pathophysiology (see Chapter 19), oxygen radical damage, and disturbances in the oxidative metabolism may affect systemic and organ blood flow and be as important as the issues of distribution of blood flow.

In contrast, the management of acute loss of circulating volume by hemorrhage or rapid fluid loss is relatively straightforward. Timely administration of adequate volumes of blood or saline, respectively, may be lifesaving for these patients. Importantly, repletion of circulating volume should not be delayed by concerns over specific peculiarities of the newborn.

Thus, clinical practice can be informed by pathophysiology. This is necessary since, unfortunately, there is very little evidence from randomized clinical trials with clinically relevant outcomes to guide therapy.

REFERENCES

1. Mortola JP: Implications of hypoxic hypometabolism during mammalian ontogenesis, *Respir Physiol Neurobiol* 141:345–356, 2004.
2. Heistad DD: What is new in cerebral microcirculation. Landis award lecture, *Microcirculation* 8:365–375, 2001.
3. Malcus P, Kjellmer I, Lingman G, et al.: Diameters of the common carotid artery and aorta change in different directions during acute asphyxia in the fetal lamb, *J Perinat Med* 19:259–267, 1991.
4. Lagaud G, Gaudreault N, Moore ED, et al.: Pressure-dependent myogenic constriction of cerebral arteries occurs independently of voltage-dependent activation, *Am J Physiol Heart Circ Physiol* 283:H2187–H2195, 2002.
5. Li Y, Baylie RL, Tavares MJ, et al.: TRPM4 channels couple purinergic receptor mechanoactivation and myogenic tone development in cerebral parenchymal arterioles, *J Cereb Blood Flow Metab* 34(10):1706–1714, 2014.
6. Hill MA, Zou H, Potocnik SJ, et al.: Invited review. Arteriolar smooth muscle mechanotransduction. Ca2 signaling pathways underlying myogenic reactivity, *J Appl Physiol* 91:973–983, 2001.
7. Gebremedin A, Lange AR, Lowry TF, et al.: Production of 20-HETE and its role in autoregulation of cerebral blood flow, *Circ Res* 87:60–65, 2000.
8. Dora KA: Does arterial myogenic tone determine blood distribution in vivo? *Am J Physiol Heart Circ Physiol* 289:1323–1325, 2005.
9. Pearce WJ, Harder DR: Cerebrovascular smooth muscle and endothelium. In Mraovitch S, Sercombe R, editors: *Neurophysiological Basis of Cerebral Blood Flow Control. An Introduction*, London, 1996, John Libbey, pp 153–158.
10. Pearce WJ: Hypoxic regulation of the fetal cerebral circulation, *J Appl Physiol* 100:731–738, 2006.
11. Liu Y, Harder DR, Lombard JH: Interaction of myogenic mechanisms and hypoxic dilation in rat middle cerebral arteries, *Am J Physiol Heart Circ Physiol* 283:H2276–H2281, 2002.
12. Aalkjær C, Poston L: Effects of pH on vascular tension. Which are the important mechanisms? *J Vasc Res* 33:347–359, 1996.
13. Wang Q, Pelligrino DA, Baughman VL, et al.: The role of neuronal nitric oxide synthetase in regulation of cerebral blood flow in normocapnia and hypercapnia in rats, *J Cereb Blood Flow Metab* 15:774–778, 1995.
14. Iadecola C, Zhang F: Permissive and obligatory roles of NO in cerebrovascular responses to hypercapnia and acetylcholine, *Am J Physiol* 271:R990–R1001, 1996.
15. Lindauer U, Vogt J, Schuh-Hofer S, et al.: Cerebrovascular vasodilation to extraluminal acidosis occurs via combined activation of ATP-sensitive and Ca2+-activated potassium channels, *J Cereb Blood Flow Metab* 23:1227–1238, 2003.
16. Wagerle LC, Mishra OP: Mechanism of CO2 response in cerebral arteries of the newborn pig: role of phospholipase, cyclooxygenase, and lipooxygenase pathways, *Circ Res* 62:1019–1026, 1988.
17. Rama GP, Parfenova H, Leffler CW: Protein kinase Cs and tyrosine kinases in permissive action of prostacyclin on cerebrovascular regulation in newborn pigs, *Pediatr Res* 41:83–89, 1996.
18. Edwards AD, Wyatt JS, Ricardsson C, et al.: Effects of indomethacin on cerebral haemodynamics in very preterm infants, *Lancet* i:1491–1495, 1992.
19. Patel J, Roberts I, Azzopardi D, et al.: Randomized double-blind controlled trial comparing the effects of ibuprofen with indomethacin on cerebral hemodynamics in preterm infants with patent ductus arteriosus, *Pediatr Res* 47:36–42, 2000.
20. Clifford PS, Hellsten Y: Vasodilatory mechanisms in contracting skeletal muscle, *J Appl Physiol* 97:393–403, 2004.
21. Koehler RC, Gebremedhin D, Harder DR: Role of astrocytes in cerebrovascular regulation, *J Appl Physiol* 100:307–317, 2006.
22. Phillis JW: Adenosine and adenine nucleotides as regulators of cerebral blood flow: roles of acidosis, cell swelling, and KATP channels, *Crit Rev Neurobiol* 16:237–270, 2004.
23. Guimaraes S, Moura D: Vascular adrenoreceptors. an update, *Pharm Rev* 53:319–356, 2001.
24. Seri I, Tan R, Evans J: The effect of hydrocortisone on blood pressure in preterm neonates with vasopressor-resistant hypotension, *Pediatrics* 107:1070–1074, 2001.
25. Watterberg KL: Adrenal insufficiency and cardiac dysfunction in the preterm infant, *Pediatr Res* 51:422–424, 2002.
26. Noori S, Seri I: Pathophysiology of newborn hypotension outside the transitional period, *Early Hum Dev* 81:399–404, 2005.
27. Lou HC, Lassen NA, Friis-Hansen B: Low cerebral blood flow in hypotensive perinatal distress, *Acta Neurol Scand* 56:343–352, 1977.
28. Hernandez MJ, Brennan RW, Bowman GS: Autoregulation of cerebral blood flow in the newborn dog, *Brain Res* 184:199–201, 1980.
29. Pasternak JF, Groothuis DR: Autoregulation of cerebral blood flow in the newborn beagle puppy, *Biol Neonate* 48:100–109, 1985.
30. Tweed WA, Cote J, Pash M, et al.: Arterial oxygenation determines autoregulation of cerebral blood flow in the fetal lamb, *Pediatr Res* 17:246–249, 1983.
31. Papile LA, Rudolph AM, Heyman MA: Autoregulation of cerebral blood flow in the preterm fetal lamb, *Pediatr Res* 19:59–161, 1985.
32. Pryds A, Pryds O, Greisen G: Cerebral pressure autoregulation and vasoreactivity in the newborn rat, *Pediatr Res* 57:294–298, 2005.

33. Helau S, Koehler RC, Gleason CA, et al.: Cerebrovascular autoregulation during fetal development in sheep, *Am J Physiol Heart Circ Physiol* 266:H1069–H1074, 1994.
34. Müller T, Löhle M, Schubert H, et al.: Developmental changes in cerebral autoregulatory capacity in the fetal sheep parietal cortex, *J Physiol* 539:957–967, 2002.
35. Tweed WA, Cote J, Lou H, et al.: Impairment of cerebral blood flow autoregulation in the newborn lamb by hypoxia, *Pediatr Res* 20:516–519, 1986.
36. Younkin DP, Reivich M, Jaggi JL, et al.: The effect of haematocrit and systolic blood pressure on cerebral blood flow in newborn infants, *J Cereb Blood Flow Metab* 7:295–299, 1987.
37. Greisen G: Cerebral blood flow in preterm infants during the first week of life, *Acta Paediatr Scand* 75:43–51, 1986.
38. Greisen G, Trojaborg W: Cerebral blood flow, PaCO2 changes, and visual evoked potentials in mechanically ventilated, preterm infants, *Acta Paediatr Scand* 76:394–400, 1987.
39. Pryds O, Greisen G, Lou H, et al.: Heterogeneity of cerebral vasoreactivity in preterm infants supported by mechanical ventilation, *J Pediatr* 115:638–645, 1989.
40. Pryds O, Andersen GE, Friis-Hansen B: Cerebral blood flow reactivity in spontaneously breathing, preterm infants shortly after birth, *Acta Paediatr Scand* 79:391–396, 1990.
41. Pryds O, Greisen G, Lou H, et al.: Vasoparalysis is associated with brain damage in asphyxiated term infants, *J Pediatr* 117:119–125, 1990.
42. Tyszczuk L, Meek J, Elwell C, et al.: Cerebral blood flow is independent of mean arterial blood pressure in preterm infants undergoing intensive care, *Pediatrics* 102:337–341, 1998.
43. Noone MA, Sellwood M, Meek JH, et al.: Postnatal adaptation of cerebral blood flow using near infrared spectroscopy in extremely preterm infants undergoing high-frequency oscillatory ventilation, *Acta Paediatr* 92:1079–1084, 2003.
44. Wardle SP, Yoxall CW, Weindling AM: Determinants of cerebral fractional oxygen extraction using near-infrared spectroscopy in preterm neonates, *J Cereb Blood Flow Metab* 20:272–279, 2000.
45. Milligan DWA: Failure of autoregulation and intraventricular haemorrhage in preterm infants, *Lancet* i:896–899, 1980.
46. Tsuji M, Saul JP, du Plessis A, et al.: Cerebral intravascular oxygenation correlates with mean arterial pressure in critically ill premature infants, *Pediatrics* 106:625–632, 2000.
47. Wong FY, Leung TS, Austin T, et al.: Impaired autoregulation in preterm infants identified by using spatially resolved spectroscopy, *Pediatrics* 121:e604–e611, 2008.
48. O'Leary H, Gregas MC, Limperopoulos C, et al.: Elevated cerebral pressure passivity is associated with prematurity-related intracranial hemorrhage, *Pediatrics* 124:302–309, 2009.
49. Howlett JA, Northington FJ, Gilmore MM, et al.: Cerebrovascular autoregulation and neurologic injury in neonatal hypoxic-ischemic encephalopathy, *Pediatr Res* 74(5):525–535, 2013.
50. Børch K, Lou HC, Greisen G: Cerebral white matter flow and arterial blood pressure in preterm infants, *Acta Paediatr* 99:1489–1492, 2010.
51. Munro MJ, Walker AM, Barfield CP: Hypotensive extremely low birth weight infants have reduced cerebral blood flow, *Pediatrics* 114:1591–1596, 2004.
52. Greisen G: To autoregulate or not to autoregulate–that is no longer the question, *Semin Pediatr Neurol* 16(4):207–215, 2009.
53. Greisen G: Cerebral autoregulation in preterm infants. How to measure it–and why care? *J Pediatr* 165(5):885–886, 2014.
54. da Costa CS, Greisen G, Austin T: Is near-infrared spectroscopy clinically useful in the preterm infant? *Arch Dis Child Fetal Neonatal Ed* 100(6):F558–561, 2015.
55. Leahy FAN, Cates D, MacCallum M, et al.: Effect of CO2 and 100% O2 on cerebral blood flow in preterm infants, *J Appl Physiol* 48:468–472, 1980.
56. Rahilly PM: Effects of 2% carbon dioxide, 0.5% carbon dioxide, and 100% oxygen on cranial blood flow of the human neonate, *Pediatrics* 66:685–689, 1980.
57. Calvert SA, Hoskins EM, Fong KW, et al.: Atiological factors associated with the development of periventricular leucomalacia, *Acta Paediatr Scand* 76:254–259, 1987.
58. Graziani LJ, Spitzer AR, Mitchell DG, et al.: Mechanical ventilation in preterm infants. Neurosonographic and developmental studies, *Pediatrics* 90:515–522, 1992.
59. Ferrara B, Johnson DE, Chang P-N, et al.: Efficacy and neurologic outcome of profound hypocapneic alkalosis for the treatment of persistent pulmonary hypertension in infancy, *J Pediatr* 105:457–461, 1984.
60. Milligan DWA: Cerebral blood flow and sleep state in the normal newborn infant, *Early Hum Develop* 3:321–328, 1979.
61. Rahilly PM: Effects of sleep state and feeding on cranial blood flow of the human neonate, *Arch Dis Child* 55:265–270, 1980.
62. Mukhtar AI, Cowan FM, Stothers JK: Cranial blood flow and blood pressure changes during sleep in the human neonate, *Early Hum Develop* 6:59–64, 1982.
63. Greisen G, Hellstrom-Westas L, Lou H, et al.: Sleep-waking shifts and cerebral blood flow in stable preterm infants, *Pediatr Res* 19:1156–1159, 1985.
64. Born P, Leth H, Miranda MJ, et al.: Visual activation in infants and young children studied by functional magnetic resonance imaging, *Pediatr Res* 44:578–583, 1998.
65. Martin E, Joeri P, Loenneker T, et al.: Visual processing in infants and children studied using functional MRI, *Pediatr Res* 46:135–140, 1999.
66. Meek JH, Firbank M, Elwell CE, et al.: Regional hemodynamic responses to visual stimulation in awake infants, *Pediatr Res* 43:840–843, 1998.

67. Erberich GS, Friedlich P, Seri I, et al.: Brain activation detected by functional MRI in preterm neonates using an integrated radiofrequency neonatal head coil and MR compatible incubator, *Neuroimage* 20:683–692, 2003.
68. Erberich SG, Panigrahy A, Friedlich P, et al.: Somatosensory lateralization in the newborn brain, *Neuroimage* 29:155–161, 2006.
69. Roche-Labarbe N, Fenoglio A, Radhakrishnan H, et al.: Somatosensory evoked changes in cerebral oxygen consumption measured non-invasively in premature neonates, *Neuroimage* 85(Pt 1): 279–286, 2014.
70. Chalia M, Lee CW, Dempsey LA, et al.: Hemodynamic response to burst-suppressed and discontinuous electroencephalography activity in infants with hypoxic ischemic encephalopathy, *Neurophotonics* 3(3):031408, 2016.
71. Buchvald FF, Keshe K, Greisen G: Measurement of cerebral oxyhaemoglobin saturation and jugular blood flow in term healthy newborn infants by near-infrared spectroscopy and jugular venous occlusion, *Biol Neonate* 75:97–103, 1999.
72. Hernandez MJ, Hawkins RA, Brennan RW: Sympathetic control of regional cerebral blood flow in the asphyxiated newborn dog. In Heistad DD, Marcus ML, editors: *Cerebral Blood Flow, Effects of Nerves and Neurotransmitters*, New York, 1982, Elsevier, pp 359–366.
73. Hayashi S, Park MK, Kuelh TJ: Higher sensitivity of cerebral arteries isolated from premature and newborn baboons to adrenergic and cholinergic stimulation, *Life Sciences* 35:253–260, 1984.
74. Wagerle LC, Kumar SP, Delivoria-Papadopoulos M: Effect of sympathetic nerve stimulation on cerebral blood flow in newborn piglets, *Pediatr Res* 20:131–135, 1986.
75. Kurth CD, Wagerle LC, Delivoria-Papadopoulos M: Sympathetic regulation of cerebral blood flow during seizures in newborn lambs, *Am J Physiol* 255:H563–H568, 1988.
76. Goplerud JM, Wagerle LC, Delivoria-Papadopoulos M: Sympathetic nerve modulation of regional cerebral blood flow during asphyxia in newborn piglets, *Am J Physiol* 260:H1575–H1580, 1991.
77. Wagerle LC, Moliken W, Russo P: Nitric oxide and alpha-adrenergic mechanisms modify contractile responses to norepinephrine in ovine fetal and newborn cerebral arteries, *Pediatr Res* 38: 237–242, 1995.
78. Bevan RD, Vijayakumaran E, Gentry A, et al.: Intrinsic tone of cerebral artery segments of human infants between 23 weeks of gestation and term, *Pediatr Res* 43:20–27, 1998.
79. Bevan R, Dodge J, Nichols P, et al.: Responsiveness of human infant cerebral arteries to sympathetic nerve stimulation and vasoactive agents, *Pediatr Res* 44:730–739, 1998.
80. Bevan RD, Dodge J, Nichols P, et al.: Weakness of sympathetic neural control of human pial compared with superficial temporal arteries reflects low innervation density and poor sympathetic responsiveness, *Stroke* 29:212–221, 1998.
81. Pryds O, Greisen G, Johansen K: Indomethacin and cerebral blood flow in preterm infants treated for patent ductus arteriosus, *Eur J Pediatr* 147:315–316, 1988.
82. Schmidt B, Davis P, Moddemann D, et al.: Trial of Indomethacin Prophylaxis in Preterms Investigators. Long-term effects of indomethacin prophylaxis in extremely-low-birth-weight infants, *N Engl J Med* 344:1966–1972, 2001.
83. Mosca F, Bray M, Lattanzio M, et al.: Comparative evaluation of the effects of indomethacin and ibuprofen on cerebral perfusion and oxygenation in preterm infants with patent ductus arteriosus, *J Pediatr* 131:549–554, 1997.
84. Pryds O, Schneider S: Aminophylline induces cerebral vasoconstriction in stable, preterm infants without affecting the visual evoked potential, *Eur J Pediatr* 150:366–369, 1991.
85. Lundstrøm KE, Larsen PB, Brendstrup L, et al.: Cerebral blood flow and left ventricular output in spontaneously breathing, newborn preterm infants treated with caffeine or aminophylline, *Acta Paediatr* 84:6–9, 1995.
86. Seri I, Abbasi S, Wood DC, et al.: Regional hemodynamic effects of dopamine in the sick preterm neonate, *J Pediatr* 133:728–734, 1998.
87. Zhang J, Penny DJ, Kim NS, et al.: Mechanisms of blood pressure increase induced by dopamine in hypotensive preterm neonates, *Arch Dis Child* 81:F99–F104, 1999.
88. Eriksen VR, Hahn GH, Greisen G: Dopamine therapy is associated with impaired cerebral autoregulation in preterm infants, *Acta Paediatr* 103(12):1221–1226, 2014.
89. Lundstrøm KE, Pryds O, Greisen G: The haemodynamic effect of dopamine and volume expansion in sick preterm infants, *Early Hum Develop* 57:157–163, 2000.
90. Jayasinghe D, Gill AB, Levene MI: CBF reactivity in hypotensive and normotensive preterm infants, *Pediatr Res* 54:848–853, 2003.
91. Sassano-Higgins S, Friedlich P, Seri I: A meta-analysis of dopamine use in hypotensive preterm infants: blood pressure and cerebral hemodynamics, *J Perinatol* 31(10):647–655, 2011.
92. Reuter JH, Disney TA: Regional cerebral blood flow and cerebral metabolic rate of oxygen during hyperventilation in the newborn dog, *Pediatr Res* 20:1102–1106, 1986.
93. Jones TH, Morawetz RB, Crowell RM, et al.: Thresholds of focal cerebral ischaemia in awake monkeys, *J Neurosurg* 54:773–782, 1981.
94. Astrup J: Energy-requiring cell functions in the ischaemic brain, *J Neurosurg* 56:482–497, 1982.
95. Branston NM, Ladds A, Symon L, et al.: Comparison of the effects of ischaemia on early components of somatosensory evoked potentials in brainstem, thalamus, and cerebral cortex, *J Cereb Blood Flow Metab* 4:68–81, 1984.
96. Pryds O, Greisen G: Preservation of single flash visual evoked potentials at very low cerebral oxygen delivery in sick, newborn, preterm infants, *Pediatr Neurol* 6:151–158, 1990.

97. Lou HC, Skov H: Low cerebral blood flow: a risk factor in the neonate, *J Pediatr* 95:606–609, 1979.
98. Ment RL, Scott DT, Lange RC, et al.: Postpartum perfusion of the preterm brain: relationship to neurodevelopmental outcome, *Childs Brain* 10:266–272, 1983.
99. Pryds O: Low neonatal cerebral oxygen delivery is associated with brain injury in preterm infants, *Acta Paediatr* 83:1233–1236, 1994.
100. Krageloh-Mann I, Toft P, Lunding J, et al.: Brain lesions in preterms: origin, consequences and compensation, *Acta Paediatrica* 88:897–908, 1999.
101. Hyttel-Sorensen S, Pellicer A, Alderliesten T, et al.: Cerebral near infrared spectroscopy oximetry in extremely preterm infants: phase II randomised clinical trial, *BMJ* 350:g7635, 2015.
102. Fujimori K, Honda S, Sanpei M, et al.: Effects of exogenous big endothelin-1 on regional blood flow in fetal lambs, *Obstet Gynecol* 106:818–823, 2005.
103. Powell RW, Dyess DL, Collins JN, et al.: Regional blood flow response to hypothermia in premature, newborn, and neonatal piglets, *J Pediatr Surg* 34:193–198, 1999.
104. Jose PA, Haramati A, Fildes RD: Postnatal maturation of renal blood flow. In Polin RA, Fox WW, editors: *Fetal and Neonatal Physiology*, Philadelphia, 1998, WB Saunders, pp 1573–1578.
105. Pezzati M, Vangi V, Biagiotti R, et al.: Effects of indomethacin and ibuprofen on mesenteric and renal blood flow in preterm infants with patent ductus arteriosus, *J Pediatr* 135:733–738, 1999.
106. Rudolph CD, Rudolph AM: Fetal and postnatal hepatic vasculature and blood flow. In Polin RA, Fox WW, editors: *Fetal and Neonatal Physiology*, Philadelphia, 1998, WB Saunders, pp 1442–1449.
107. Clark DA, Miller MJS: Development of the gastrointestinal circulation in the fetus and newborn. In Polin RA, Fox WW, editors: *Fetal and Neonatal Physiology*, Philadelphia, 1998, WB Saunders, pp 929–933.
108. Shimada S, Kasai T, Hoshi A, et al.: Cardiocirculatory effects of patent ductus arteriosus in extremely low-birth-weight infants with respiratory distress syndrome, *Pediatr Int* 45:255–262, 2003.
109. Kluckow M, Evans N: Superior vena cava flow. A novel marker of systemic blood flow, *Arch Dis Child* 82:F182–F187, 2000.
110. Visser MO, Leighton JO, van de Bor M, et al.: Renal blood flow in the neonate: quantitation with color and pulsed Doppler ultrasound, *Radiology* 183:441–444, 1992.
111. Van Bel F, van Zwieten PH, Guit GL, et al.: Superior mesenteric artery blood flow velocity and estimated volume flow. Duplex Doppler US study of preterm and term neonates, *Radiology* 174:165–169, 1990.
112. Agata Y, Hiraishi S, Misawa H, et al.: Regional blood flow distribution and left ventricular output during early neonatal life: a quantitative ultrasonographic assessment, *Pediatr Res* 36:805–810, 1994.
113. Yao LP, Jose PA: Developmental renal hemodynamics, *Pediatr Nephrol* 9:632–637, 1995.
114. Bay-Hansen R, Elfving B, Greisen G: Use of near infrared spectroscopy for estimation of peripheral venous saturation in newborns; comparison with co-oximetry of central venous blood, *Biol Neonate* 82:1–8, 2002.
115. Stephenson R: Physiological control of diving behaviour in the Weddell seal Leptonychotes weddelli; a model based on cardiorespiratory control theory, *J Exp Biol* 208:1971–1991, 2005.
116. Jensen A, Garnier Y, Berger R: Dynamics of fetal circulatory responses to hypoxia and asphyxia, *Eur J Obstet Gynecol Reprod Biol* 84:155–172, 1999.
117. Green LR, McGarrigle HHG, Bennet L, et al.: Angiotensin II and cardiovascular chemoreflex responses to acute hypoxia in late gestation fetal sheep, *J Physiol* 507:857–867, 1998.
118. Coumans ABC, Garnier Y, Supcun S, et al.: Nitric oxide and fetal organ blood flow during normoxia and hypoxemia in endotoxin-treated fetal sheep, *Obstet Gynecol* 105:145–155, 2005.
119. Kehrer M, Krägeloh-Mann L, Goelz R, et al.: The development of cerebral perfusion in healthy preterm and term neonates, *Neuropediatrics* 34:281–286, 2003.
120. Sinha AK, Cane C, Kempley ST: Blood flow in the common carotid artery in term and preterm infants: reproducibility and relation to cardiac output, *Arch Dis Child* 91:31–35, 2006.

CHAPTER 3

Definition of Normal Blood Pressure Range: The Elusive Target

Eugene Dempsey and Istvan Seri

- In the context of neonatal care, invasive or noninvasive measurement of blood pressure can be accomplished with acceptable precision.
- Gestational- and postnatal-age-dependent population-based normative blood pressure ranges are available. However, their usefulness in the assessment of hypotension, defined as a blood pressure value associated with low systemic and organ blood flow and inadequate tissue oxygen delivery requiring treatment, is limited.
- Definition of hypotension based on physiologic principles, such as maintenance of cerebral blood flow autoregulation, provides more insight into the individual patient's ability to effectively compensate for decreases in tissue oxygen delivery, However, the need for complex hemodynamic monitoring and data acquisition systems required for this approach has so far limited its clinical usefulness.
- Due to our inability to accurately diagnose hypotension, data on the association between blood pressure and short- and long-term outcomes have remained difficult to interpret.
- Thorough bedside clinical assessment and the use of sophisticated hemodynamic monitoring and data acquisition systems hold the promise of defining the individual patient's compensatory capacity to combat decreases of tissue oxygen delivery. These approaches also enable the accurate, real-time, and individual-patient–based diagnosis of hypotension as well as provide the opportunity to test and find the most appropriate therapeutic interventions.

Targeting blood pressure (BP) values, in particular the mean arterial BP, as a surrogate of cardiovascular well-being has been the norm in neonatal intensive care units (NICUs) across the world for the past 30 years. Despite significant advances in other areas of newborn care, little has changed in our approach to this problem. A number of recent surveys conducted in Europe,[1] Canada,[2] and Australia[3] have highlighted the continued reliance of clinicians on such an approach.

The reliance on BP as a surrogate of cardiovascular well-being remains problematic on a number of levels. There are different methods of obtaining BP measurements; there are many different normative BP ranges; there is a poor relationship between BP values and end organ blood flow; and there is an inconsistency in the relationship between BP values and subsequent clinical outcomes. In this chapter, we will explore these areas in further detail and provide insight into the complexities involved in newborn cardiovascular assessment at the bedside. These are set out as follows:

1. Measuring BP
2. Normative BP Ranges

3. Clinical Factors Affecting BP
4. BP and Short- and Long-Term Outcomes
5. Bedside Clinical Assessment and Hemodynamic Monitoring

Measuring Blood Pressure

There are two main methods of obtaining BP measurements in newborn infants, noninvasively or invasively. Both methods have their own inherent advantages and potential problems, but the standard of care for any sick newborn infant should be invasive BP monitoring where feasible. Detailed recent reviews of BP measurement and monitoring in the neonate are available.[4]

The noninvasive method is based on oscillometry. Marey first described this method in 1876. When a limb was placed in a pressure chamber, the pressure in the chamber would fluctuate, and the magnitude of these fluctuations was dependent on the pressure contained within the chamber. The oscillometric method is based on the principal that blood moving through an artery creates oscillations/vibrations of the arterial vessel wall. Thus, application of external pressure via an inflated cuff placed on the limb will allow determination of "arterial" BP parameters. These oscillations are transmitted to the cuff, converted into an electrical signal by the transducer, and ultimately display systolic, mean, and diastolic noninvasive BP measurements. Prior to the development of automated devices, values were obtained clinically by either palpation or auscultation. The palpation method relies on feeling a pulse, the auscultation method on listening for sounds of turbulence generated by flow in the partially compressed vessel. Korotkoff first described indirect measurements of BP by auscultation in 1905.[5]

The systolic component of the BP measurement is just less than the systolic pressure at which the oscillations begin. The pressure at which the oscillations are at their maximum amplitude is the mean arterial pressure (MAP). The pressure in the cuff when blood first starts to flow continuously without vibration is an estimate of diastolic BP component. Various devices incorporate different algorithms to estimate the systolic and diastolic measurements.

There are a number of important factors that need to be considered when noninvasively measuring BP. Incorrect cuff size is the principal factor that will cause inaccurate measurements. The location of measurement, either an upper limb or a lower limb, may result in an overestimate or an underestimate of the true value, respectively. Also, different devices may result in slightly different readings related to the particular algorithm used. These will be discussed later.

The invasive method uses a fluid-filled transducer directly attached to an indwelling arterial catheter placed either in the aorta or in a peripheral artery. The pressure transducer converts the energy into an electrical signal that is then processed, amplified, and converted by a microprocessor into a visual display on the bedside monitor. There are a number of technical challenges that can result in inaccurate measurements, due to either overdamping or underdamping of the signal.[6] One possible source of inaccuracy is the presence of small air bubbles introduced into the system. These can cause excessive damping of the pulse pressure waveform, causing an underreading of systolic BP and overreading of diastolic BP, although the mean BP is relatively unaffected. The absence or distortion of the dicrotic notch of the downward slope of the arterial waveform should suggest the presence of overdamping. Further sources of overdamping may occur if blood contaminates the tubing, if the tubing is too long or too compliant, or if the initial calibration process is inaccurate. Underdamping can occur with stiff noncompliant tubing or when there is hypothermia, characterized by excessively high systolic BP and low diastolic BP, as in a resonant signal.

A number of groups have compared different noninvasive devices and how they compare with invasive measurements.[6–13] One of the author's (ED) group has previously evaluated noninvasive measurements compared to invasive measurements with three different automated oscillometric devices: (1) Procare 300 Compact (Criticon Inc., Tampa, Florida), (2) GE Marquette Solar 8000 Patient Monitor

(Fairfield, Connecticut), and (3) GE Dash 4000 Patient Monitor with DINAMAP technology (Fairfield, Connecticut). We also assessed the variability between simultaneously obtained upper and lower limb measurements. Measurement of the mid-arm and mid-calf circumference was obtained for each baby prior to placement of the appropriate-sized cuff (mid-arm and mid-calf circumference 0.45 to 0.55).[14] This was consistent with the American Heart Association's recommendation that the cuff bladder width and length be 40% and 80%, respectively, of the mid-arm circumference.[15] Invasive measurements were recorded using a fluid coupled pressure transducer (Transtar R 19 Neonatal monitoring kit with Kids Kit Blood Sampling System; Medex Inc., Carlsbad, California). We found no significant difference between the noninvasive recordings simultaneously obtained from the upper or lower limbs. However, all three noninvasive recorders consistently overestimated invasive BP values. The average difference between mean invasive and noninvasive BP was 5.1 mm Hg overall and was device specific, 2.4, 4.5, 8.4 mm Hg for Dash, Dinamap, and Marquette monitors, respectively. These findings were similar to the findings of a number of other studies. Dannevig et al.[12] found that Dinamap overreads mean BP by approximately 7.6 mm Hg, particularly in smaller infants. Diprose et al.[16] also reported that Dinamap tends to overread mean BP in hypotensive infants—a finding subsequently confirmed by Chia et al.[17]

The site at which the noninvasive recording is obtained may be one reason for this difference. A number of other studies comparing BP measurements from upper versus lower limbs have produced conflicting results. In term neonates, Park and Lee observed no difference in BP measurements between arm and calf measurements.[18] Piazza and colleagues compared upper and lower limb systolic BP in term neonates in the first 24 hours and found that higher readings were generally present in the upper versus lower limb.[19] However, higher readings in the lower limb were also common (28%). Cowan and colleagues determined arm and calf BP in term neonates in active and quiet sleep in the first 5 postnatal days.[20] The increase in BP was greater in the arm than in the calf during these periods. Kunk and McCain studied 65 preterm neonates.[21] They found no significant differences in systolic BP, diastolic BP, and mean BP between arm and calf values in the first 5 postnatal days, although arm BP values were consistently slightly higher. In summary, noninvasive BP measurements are device specific, and upper and lower limb mean BP values are similar, whereas noninvasive BP measurements tend to overestimate invasive BP values, particular in immature hypotensive preterm infants.[22]

Blood Pressure Standards

Traditionally in medicine, treatment decisions are made when a particular parameter is outside a defined normative range. We believe these values represent levels that warrant intervention and are concerned that nonintervention might lead to an adverse outcome. Thus there is an accepted range above or below which intervention is warranted. However, in some areas of newborn care such clarity is often lacking. The management of hypoglycemia remains contentious. What is a low blood glucose level and its duration when one should worry? Is there a threshold level that warrants intervention? Similarly, BP ranges and management of low BP, primarily in preterm infants and especially during the transitional period, remain complex. When we investigate BP standards or normative ranges, the striking findings are first, the lack of consistency across these numerous ranges and second, the absolute number of ranges that exist. Ranges are often based on birth weight, gestational age, and postnatal age criteria.[23–28] Similar populations of babies with different reference ranges suggest methodologic differences or problems. These statistically determined values vary considerably, which is not surprising considering how many of these ranges were derived. These include retrospective data collection; the inclusion of small numbers of patients; the collection of only a few data points and summation over wide time ranges; the combination of invasive and noninvasive measurements; and the inclusion of small for dates and appropriate for gestational age infants. In some instances, newborns who received volume or were on vasopressor-inotrope or

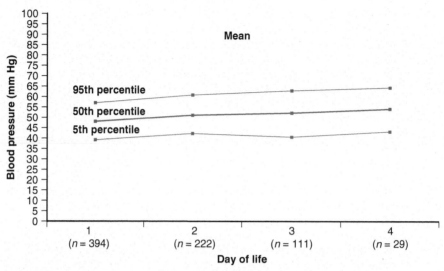

Fig. 3.1 Mean blood pressure values in well term newborns during the first postnatal days. These data serve as reference values for this population. (From Kent AL, Meskell S, Falk MC, Shadbolt B: Normative blood pressure data in non-ventilated premature neonates from 28-36 weeks gestation. *Pediatr Nephrol* 24:141–146, 2009. Used with permission from Elsevier Ltd.)

inotrope infusions are included in normative range development. Thus it makes interpretation of these values challenging, as they are unlikely to constitute population-based "normative ranges." However, they do provide very useful information to help inform clinicians at the bedside.

One of the first reference ranges developed was by Versmold et al. in 1981.[26] Data were obtained invasively on 16 infants less than 1000 g and were subsequently combined with data from 45 larger infants to develop new nomograms for BP values during the first 12 postnatal hours in infants weighing 610 to 4220 g. The authors concluded that they "hope that the new, extended nomograms for mean, systolic, and diastolic blood pressures ... will lead to more accurate assessment of the cardiovascular state in newborn infants, particularly in those born very prematurely." It is now more than 30 years since this statement was written. Other reference ranges were developed in the 1980s and 1990s, including those from Watkins et al.,[25] Spinazzola et al.,[24] and Hegyi et al.[28] While each study has some limitations, each provides important information. For example, Hegyi et al.[28] highlight lower BP values in preterm infants receiving mechanical ventilation.

Kent et al. measured BP values in 406 healthy term infants on the postnatal ward over the first 4 postnatal days.[29] The median systolic, diastolic, and mean BP values on the first postnatal day were 65, 45, and 48 mm Hg, respectively. On day 4, these values had increased to 70, 46, and 54 mm Hg. Fig. 3.1 depicts the mean BP values over the first days of postnatal life in well term newborns. These are useful reference guides when evaluating a term population of newborns. Kent and colleagues also evaluated noninvasive BP measurements in a group of stable preterm infants 28 to 36 weeks' gestation.[30] They measured BP on day 1, 2, 3, 4, 7, 14, 21, and 28 in a group of 147 infants. They found that premature neonates stabilize their mean BP after 14 days of postnatal life, and at this time they have a BP similar to that of term infants. Others have also shown an increase in BP over the first postnatal days.[23–25,27,31–34] Watkins et al. document the mean and 10th percentile BP over the first days after delivery based on birth weight (Table 3.1). Zubrow and colleagues reported the findings of a large multicenter study conducted by the Philadelphia Neonatal Blood Pressure Study Group.[34] In this investigation, systolic and diastolic BP was significantly correlated with birth weight, gestational age, and postconceptional age. In each of four gestational age groups, systolic and diastolic BP was significantly correlated with postnatal age over the first 5 postnatal days. Batton and colleagues[35] recently evaluated the change in BP over the first 24 hours after delivery in a population of extreme

Table 3.1   VARIATION OF MEAN BLOOD PRESSURE[a] WITH BIRTH WEIGHT AT 3 TO 96 HOURS OF POSTNATAL AGE

Birth Weight (g)	Time (h) Postnatal Age								
	3	12	24	36	48	60	72	84	96
500	35/23	36/24	37/25	38/26	39/28	41/29	42/30	43/31	44/33
600	35/24	36/25	37/26	39/27	40/28	41/29	42/31	44/32	45/33
700	36/24	37/25	38/26	39/28	42/29	42/30	43/31	44/32	45/34
800	36/25	37/26	39/27	40/28	41/29	42/31	44/32	45/33	46/34
900	37/25	38/26	39/27	40/29	42/30	43/31	44/32	45/34	47/35
1000	38/26	39/27	40/28	41/29	42/31	43/32	45/33	46/34	47/35
1100	38/27	39/27	40/29	42/30	43/31	44/32	45/34	46/35	48/36
1200	39/27	40/28	41/29	42/30	43/32	45/33	46/34	47/35	48/37
1300	39/28	40/29	41/30	43/31	44/32	45/33	46/35	48/36	49/37
1400	40/28	41/29	42/30	43/32	44/33	46/34	47/35	48/36	49/38
1500	40/29	42/30	43/31	44/32	45/33	46/35	48/36	49/37	50/38

[a]Numbers refer to average mean BP/10th percentile for mean blood pressure.
From Watkins AMC, West CR, Cooke RWI: Blood pressure and cerebral haemorrhage and ischaemia in very low birthweight infants. *Early Hum Dev* 19:103–110, 1989. Used with permission from Elsevier Ltd.

preterm infants. A drop in BP values characterized the first 4 postnatal hours. For the 164 untreated infants in this cohort, the systolic, diastolic, and mean arterial BP increased significantly ($P < .001$) at an estimated mean ± SD rate of 0.3 ± 0.5 (range: −2.15 to 1.50), 0.2 ± 0.4 (range: −1.10 to 1.10), and 0.2 ± 0.4 (range: −0.90 to 1.25) mm Hg/h thereafter. This equates to an approximately 5 mm Hg increase in mean BP over the first 24 postnatal hours in preterm infants born less than 26 weeks' gestation.

Another "normative range" often used to warrant intervention is a single absolute mean BP value chosen over a wide range of gestational ages. The most common is a mean BP less than 30 mm Hg.[36] This approach is based on findings suggesting that the lower limit of the BP autoregulatory curve is around 28 to 30 mm Hg in neonatal animal models as well as preterm neonates.[37,38] Munro and colleagues studied the relationship between mean arterial BP and cerebral blood flow assessed by near-infrared spectroscopy (NIRS) in 17 extremely preterm infants, 12 of whom were hypotensive and 5 were normotensive.[37] Patients who were hypotensive had lower cerebral blood flow compared with normotensive infants. When dopamine was commenced in the hypotensive infants, the mean BP and cerebral blood flow increased. Cerebral blood flow correlated with mean arterial BP in hypotensive infants before ($R = 0.62$) and during ($R = 0.67$) dopamine administration, but not in normotensive infants. Using complex statistical analysis, the authors suggested a "breakpoint" of mean arterial BP of 29 mm Hg in the untreated cohort of infants. These findings need to be interpreted cautiously considering the small number of patients included and the lack of inclusion of potential confounders, including the effect of gestational age and the partial pressure of carbon dioxide. An interesting finding was that once dopamine therapy was commenced, cerebral blood flow seemed to continue along a pressure-passive curve, suggesting a loss of autoregulatory capacity even when BP increased beyond the lower autoregulatory elbow of 29 mm Hg. Greisen and colleagues explored the relationship between white matter injury and blood flow in 13 preterm infants using single-photon emission computed tomography with ^{99}Tc labeled hexa-methylpropylenamide oxime as the tracer.[38] They found no statistically significant relationship between white matter blood flow percentage (WMBF%) and any of the variables studied, including mean arterial BP. However, using nonlinear regression assuming a plateau over a certain BP threshold and a positive slope below this threshold, the relation to WMBF% was statistically significant ($P = .02$) with a threshold identified at 29 mm Hg (95% confidence interval 26 to 33 mm Hg). They concluded that periventricular white matter is selectively vulnerable to ischemia during episodes of low BP. There were a number of limitations to this study as well, including the small number of infants included; two imaging studies were performed in only 3 of the 13 infants, while the relation between BP and WMBF% was statistically significant, two-thirds of the variance of WM% was still unexplained. Interestingly, these values approximate to data published almost 30 years ago by Miall-Allen et al.,[39] showing that in 33 infants of less than 31 weeks' gestation, a mean BP of less than 30 mm Hg for over an hour was significantly *associated with* severe intracranial hemorrhage, ischemic cerebral lesions, or death within 48 hours. No severe lesions developed in infants with a mean BP 30 mm Hg or greater. Accordingly, this value (30 mm Hg) is considered by some as a threshold to start intervention.[2] However, these data[37–39] need to be interpreted cautiously when applying this principle to those at greatest risk of brain injury, that is, the most immature preterm infants. Applying this principle to infants less than 26 weeks' gestation would essentially mean intervening for a significant majority in the first postnatal hours. Indeed Greisen and colleagues state that their "result should not be used for clinical decision making."[38] Therefore, routine intervention based solely on maintaining a BP greater than 30 mm Hg for extreme preterm infants should be avoided.

Another "range" commonly used is that of the Joint Working Group of the British Association of Perinatal Medicine. They recommended that the mean arterial BP in mm Hg should be maintained at or greater than the mean gestational age in weeks.[40] There is little published evidence to support this "rule," but it remains the most common criteria used to define hypotension.[1] Lee and colleagues identified that the lower limits of mean arterial BP for infants between 26 and 32 weeks' gestation were numerically similar to the gestational age.[23] The German Neonatal Network presented data recently on a very large cohort of preterm infants.[41] They showed the lowest mean arterial BP recorded on day 1 was similar to the gestational age in weeks (Table 3.2). However, there is growing evidence highlighting the inadequacy of this guideline. Cunningham et al. have shown a poor relationship between this rule and the incidence of intraventricular hemorrhage.[32] Data collected by the Canadian Neonatal Network (CNN) show that over 52% of preterm infants less than 28 weeks' gestation are "hypotensive" by this rule alone in the first postnatal day and, as such, may warrant intervention.[42] This simple rule also needs to be interpreted cautiously in light of the normal increase in BP over the first days, especially during the first 3 days after delivery. What is clear is that this rule is very easy to remember and is consistently used by many to guide intervention.[2,43]

In summary, numerous reference ranges exist. Many of these are problematic, especially because of the lack of a consistent relationship between low BP values and clinically relevant short- and long-term outcomes, and because there are very few data on the effectiveness of the commonly used treatment modalities to decrease the incidence of peri/intraventricular hemorrhage (P/IVH) and white matter injury. However, consistent observations are that BP in the first postnatal days is gestation specific, typically characterized by a drop in the first hours after delivery followed by an increase thereafter over the first 3 days. The timing of intervention for low BP

Table 3.2　LOWEST MEAN ARTERIAL BLOOD PRESSURE DURING THE FIRST 24 HOURS AND GESTATIONAL AGE (COMPLETED WEEKS)

Gestational Age Weeks	Number of Infants With Data	Lowest Mean Arterial Blood Pressure (mm Hg; Median [IQR])
22	25	21 (18–25)
23	178	21 (19–24)
24	339	22 (20–25)
25	431	24 (21–26)
26	583	24 (21–28)
27	666	26 (22–29)
28	725	27 (24–31)
29	725	29 (25–32)
30	709	30 (27–34)
31	526	31 (27–35)
All	4907	27 (23–31)

IQR, Interquartile range.

From Faust K, Härtel C, Preuß M, Rabe H, Roll C, Emeis M, Wieg C, Szabo M, Herting E, Göpel W; Neocirculation project and the German Neonatal Network (GNN): short-term outcome of very-low-birthweight infants with arterial hypotension in the first 24 hours of life. *Arch Dis Child Fetal Neonatal Ed* 100(5):F388–F392, 2015. Used with permission from BMJ Publishing Group.

in preterm infants occurs on day 1 in over 90% of cases, regardless of gestational age.[44] These factors need to be considered when evaluating BP values, whether one intervenes or not, and when designing future clinical trials in this area.

Clinical Factors Affecting Blood Pressure

Antenatal Steroids

Several investigators have reported that neonatal BP is higher in preterm infants whose mothers received antenatal steroids.[45–48] Moise and colleagues studied the amount of BP support received by extremely preterm infants (23 to 27 weeks' gestation) whose mothers did or did not receive antenatal steroids.[45] Infants not exposed to antenatal steroids had lower mean BP values from 16 to 48 hours postnatally. Furthermore, the use of dopamine was increased in infants not exposed to antenatal steroids. Demarini and colleagues reported that mean BP values during the first 24 postnatal hours were higher in very low birth weight (VLBW) infants whose mothers received antenatal steroids, and that volume expansion and vasopressor support were decreased in those infants.[46]

Elimian et al. evaluated whether incomplete courses of antenatal steroids were beneficial. After adjusting for gestational age, they found that one dose of betamethasone compared with none was associated with a significant reduction in the need for vasopressor-inotropes (odds ratio [OR], 0.35; 95% confidence interval [CI], 0.14, 0.85; $P < .02$) and the rate of P/IVH (OR, 0.42; 95% CI, 0.19, 0.92; $P < .03$).[47] In a subsequent randomized trial comparing betamethasone versus dexamethasone, they found no difference in the incidence of need for vasopressor-inotrope use between the two corticosteroid preparations.[49]

Placental Transfusion

A recent systematic review by Rabe et al.[50] found a lower mean BP and a greater need for vasopressor-inotrope support in those who received immediate cord clamping compared with those who had delayed clamping. There were no measures of cardiac output presented in this review but Somers et al., in a nested cohort study of 51 preterm infants, found an increase in superior vena cava (SVC) flow measurement over the first 4 postnatal days.[51] However, the results of the much larger Australian Placental Transfusion Study Echo Sub-Study[52] found no difference in the incidence of low BP using the gestational age–based rule for 15 minutes, in the use of vasopressor-inotropes, and in flow measurements between the groups. A recent meta-analysis of umbilical cord milking (UCM) identified two studies that reported BP data.[53] Systolic, diastolic, and mean BP were all significantly higher in the group who had UCM performed. However, there was significant heterogeneity in the studies. Katheria and colleagues found no significant difference in BP values between a group who received UCM versus immediate cord clamping,[54] but did identify a significant difference in SVC flow over the first 24 postnatal hours. However, this did not translate into a difference in the need for volume, vasopressor-inotrope, or hydrocortisone therapy. A recent meta-analysis of UCM found that while UCM was associated with some benefits and no adverse effects in the immediate postnatal period in preterm infants, further studies were warranted to assess the effect of UCM on short- and long-term outcomes.[55] Katheria and colleagues subsequently compared UCM with delayed cord clamping and found higher systemic blood flow with UCM compared with delayed cord clamping in preterm neonates delivered by cesarean section.[56] The best summary of this evidence to date is that placental transfusion is associated with higher BP values, but the effects on flow are not as clearly evident and it is not certain which approach (delayed cord clamping or UCM) is superior in improving postnatal hemodynamic transition (see Chapters 4 and 5).

Respiratory Support

Kluckow and Evans observed a highly significant negative influence of mean airway pressure on mean BP in preterm neonates requiring mechanical ventilation.[57,58] They subsequently highlighted the effects of an alteration of positive end expiratory pressure (PEEP) from 5 to 8 cm H_2O in ventilated preterm infants and showed a significant reduction in right ventricular output with increased PEEP.[59] Ventilation strategies that aim to avoid mechanical ventilation seem to have a lower incidence of low BP and low flow states.[60] De Waal and colleagues described the hemodynamic variables in infants who had the INtubation, SURfactant, Extubation (INSURE) procedure and found an incidence of hypotension of 16% and rates of intervention at 10%. Similar data are presented for the Avoidance of Mechanical Ventilation Trial[61] where 17% to 18% of patients had low BP overall. Although the evidence is primarily from cohort studies, it would appear that mechanical ventilation can have an adverse effect on cardiovascular status, likely by impeding venous return and thus cardiac filling, and should be a recognized potential cause of low BP and low systemic flow in preterm infants. There are two other potential effects associated with mechanical ventilation: tracheal suctioning and the use of sedation. Tracheal suctioning has been associated with alterations, predominantly increases, in mean BP. In addition, hypotension was associated with the use of morphine in the Neopain Trial.[62] Therefore, strategies to minimize mechanical ventilation should form a critical part of the assessment and management of low BP in preterm infants.

Blood Pressure and Short- and Long-Term Outcomes

This remains one of the most contentious areas of BP management, as it is unclear at present whether low BP is indeed associated with adverse outcome, whether the interventions for low BP improve outcome, and whether the treatment itself is detrimental to the developing brain. It is difficult to answer any of these questions retrospectively, but these are the best data that we currently have available, considering the paucity of adequately powered clinical trials in this area. Numerous studies have highlighted an adverse relationship between low BP and short- and long-term outcome.[25,36,39,63–79] We explored this relationship previously and highlighted some of the concerns in a systematic review of the literature at that time.[80] There were 18 studies identified, including cohort and case-controlled studies with small numbers of patients—none of which were powered for long-term neurodevelopmental follow-up. There were a number of problems identified in this review—the majority of which will not be surprising to the reader. The definition of hypotension varied substantially across the studies, as did the outcome assessment used. The overall conclusion of the data from this review was that there is some association between having a lower BP and a worse outcome but that there were several potentially confounding factors that precluded one from drawing any strong inference from this association.

A number of important studies have been published since this review and raise further questions in relation to this association. Logan et al. evaluated three indicators of hypotension: (1) lowest MAP in the lowest quartile for gestational age; (2) treatment with a vasopressor-inotrope; and (3) BP lability. They found no association between any of these definitions and adverse outcome defined as white matter abnormality on cranial ultrasound at discharge.[81] They found little evidence that these early postnatal hypotension indicators were associated with developmental delay at 24 months' corrected gestational age.[82] However, Batton and colleagues compared neurodevelopment in three cohorts of extremely preterm infants: those untreated with "normal" BP, untreated with "low" BP, and treated with low BP.[83] Low BP was defined as MAP of less than 25 mm Hg on more than three occasions in the first 72 hours after delivery. Infants with low BP—regardless of treatment—had worse neurodevelopmental outcomes than infants with normal BP. They concluded that early low BP may be independently associated with a poorer outcome. Data from the CNN showed that infants with hypotension defined as a lowest BP less than their gestational age, or a BP less than the 10th percentile using the criteria of Watkins et al.,[25] were statistically more likely to develop severe P/IVH. However, this association was no longer apparent when vasopressor-inotropes were included in the model.[42] A recent publication from the German Neonatal Network identified that hypotension during the first 24 postnatal hours was associated with adverse outcomes in VLBW infants.[41] This study examined the lowest mean BP on the first postnatal day in over 4900 preterm infants less than 32 weeks' gestation born in 47 centers throughout Germany. This retrospective study has many strengths, including a very large number of included infants and consistency in data entry and outcome definitions. On multivariate analysis, the minimum mean arterial BP during the first 24 postnatal hours was significantly associated with an increase in the odds of a P/IVH (OR, 0.97 mm Hg, CI, 0.95–0.99), suggesting again that low BP is associated with adverse outcome.

However, in a subsequent study, Batton et al. investigated the relationship between early BP changes, the receipt of antihypotensive therapy, and the outcomes for extreme preterm infants less than 27 weeks' gestation at 18 to 22 months' corrected age.[84] Of 367 infants, 203 (55%) received an antihypotensive therapy, 272 (74%) survived to discharge, and 331 (90%) had a known outcome at 18 to 22 months' corrected age. Early BP changes were defined by the expected rate of rise of 5 mm Hg over the first postnatal day. Accordingly, four groups of infants were identified: infants who did or did not receive antihypotensive therapy in whom BP did or did not rise at the expected rate. Interestingly, extremely preterm infants who received antihypotensive therapy in the first 24 hours after birth had a significantly higher rate of death or impaired neurodevelopment at 18 to 22 months' corrected age compared with untreated infants irrespective of early changes in the BP. Van Bel found no association between a mean arterial BP less than gestational age in weeks and lower neurodevelopmental outcome scores at 24 months.[85] However, they found that low regional cerebral oxygenation values were associated with lower neurodevelopmental outcome scores (see Chapter 18). This suggests that indirect assessment of end-organ blood flow and oxygen delivery (cerebral tissue oxygenation measure by NIRS) is important and might be more sensitive than mean BP values as a potential marker of long-term neurodisability (see Chapters 17 and 18). It is clear that the best approach would be to understand the status of both the systemic circulation (BP and cardiac output) and end-organ blood flow distribution (tissue oxygen delivery) to more appropriately evaluate the impact of transitional hemodynamics on short- and long-term outcomes (see Chapter 21).

While the issue of low BP and adverse outcome remains contentious, so too is the possibility that treatment (volume, vasopressor-inotropes, and/or inotropes) may be a contributing factor to adverse outcome.[86] Earlier neonatal animal work has shown an association between intervention and adverse outcome.[87] A number of recent publications exploring the relationship between hypotension and its treatment using retrospective data analysis have suggested that treatment itself may be detrimental. Fanaroff et al. found an association between "treated hypotension" and adverse outcome defined as delayed motor development, hearing loss, and death.[88] Limperopoulos et al. found an association between volume expansion on the second day of life and abnormal cranial ultrasound findings.[89] A study from the CNN published as an abstract also found no association between hypotension and adverse outcome when the use of vasoactive agents was included in the statistical model.[42] Another interesting finding from this dataset was that patients who were normotensive as per the authors' criteria, yet treated, had a worse outcome than infants who were hypotensive and not treated. There are two ways of interpreting this finding: treatment itself is detrimental or clinicians recognized other variables that warranted treatment, so a more global approach rather than reliance on BP targets directed the therapy received. Of course it is not possible to answer this question retrospectively. Batton et al. concluded that antihypotensive therapy exposure was associated with an increased risk of death/neurodevelopmental deficit at 18 to 22 months' corrected age when other risk factors known to affect survival and neurodevelopment were controlled for.[84] Although the German Neonatal Network study's findings also found an association between treatment with vasopressor-inotropes in the first 24 hours of postnatal life and P/IVH (OR, 1.86, CI [1.43 to 2.42]; $P < .001$) in a multilogistic regression model,[41] the authors emphasized that "vasoactive treatment might be due to complications, and is, therefore, not a completely independent cofactor." In addition, this study, like others in this area, did not factor in the timing of the injury and the timing of the intervention.

As the potential negative effects of treatment itself remain a concern, they need to be prospectively studied. However, due to the lack of prospectively collected data and the findings of other studies showing different results, no definitive conclusion can be drawn at present. The follow-up study to a randomized prospective trial[90] comparing the effectiveness of dopamine and epinephrine in increasing BP and cerebral blood flow in hypotensive VLBW neonates during the first postnatal day found that

A

neonates responding to treatment had long-term neurodevelopment outcomes comparable to age-matched normotensive controls, and that non-responders had worse long-term neurodevelopmental outcomes.[91] These findings suggest that treatment by careful, step-wise titration of vasopressor-inotropes may not be harmful. However, as the primary outcome measure of the original study was not long-term neurodevelopmental outcome, the follow-up study was not properly powered to address the concerns about vasoactive medication use and potential harm. A number of recent studies have also attempted to answer this question. Two ended early because of enrollment issues, namely the Hypotension in Preterms: Health Outcomes Protocol (HIPHOP) trial from Italy and the National Institute of Child Health and Human Development (NICHD) hypotension trial.[92] The NICHD trial enrolled 10 patients from an eligible population of 120 patients. Factors contributed to the low overall rate of enrollment included the inability to obtain consent in a timely manner and physicians' unwillingness to enroll. Informed consent for a trial of vasoactive medication use enrolling primarily in the first hours of postnatal life has many challenges. The Hypotension in Preterm Infants trial[93] is currently enrolling, and the NEOCIRC trial is about to begin enrollment. Of note is that, in addition to the harm vasoactive medications might potentially directly exert, inappropriate titration of the medications itself might cause sudden increases and/or decreases in BP and cerebral blood flow in patients without effective cerebral blood flow autoregulation (see Chapter 2), as suggested by Greisen above,[38] and thus might cause harm.[94,95] The understanding of the challenges associated with titration of vasoactive medications is critical to the safe delivery of continuous infusions of these medications in this vulnerable patient population. This includes long lag times before the agent actually reaches the patient, resulting in both a delay in delivery and, potentially, unpredictable effects.[96,97]

It is also interesting to note the wide variability in the incidence of hypotension and the incidence of intervention. Laughon and colleagues evaluated factors associated with intervention for hypotension in extremely low gestational age infants during the first postnatal week and found that neither the lowest MAP on the day of treatment nor other characteristics of the infants accounted for center differences in treatment.[44] This suggested that the decision to intervene was more strongly associated with the center where the care was provided than with the particular infant attributes. This may reflect institutional practices. Subsequently, Batton and colleagues showed similar variation among centers but also highlighted significant variability in intervention rates based on low BP values alone.[98] Antihypotensive therapy was often provided to infants without low BP and, paradoxically, not prescribed to infants with low BP. Antihypotensive therapy was administered to 28% to 41% of infants without BP values that most would consider low. In the study by Faust and colleagues,[4] the overall rate of a low BP, using the less than gestational age definition, was 52%, yet the overall vasopressor-inotrope treatment rate on the first postnatal day was 9.3% (433/4675). The Australian Placental Transfusion Study's Echo Sub-Study found an incidence of low BP also using the gestational age–based definition for at least a 15-minute duration, in greater than 30% of infants less than 30 weeks' gestational age.[52] However, the intervention rate was only around 11%. These three studies[41,52,98] suggest that other factors are taken into consideration when clinicians decide on whether to intervene, based on low BP values. Hence the concept of permissive hypotension[99] whereby one tolerates lower BP values if other parameters suggest that systemic and end-organ perfusion are appropriate. However, this approach carries the potential risk of delaying the initiation of treatment in patients whose perfusion may worsen to the point where it reaches the threshold of inadequate oxygen delivery. The most commonly used clinical criteria to evaluate end-organ perfusion are set out below, and other objective parameters are discussed in a later section.

Bedside Clinical Assessment and Hemodynamic Monitoring

Recent surveys of practice highlight the inclusion of clinical, biochemical, echocardiographic, and other methods to assist in decision making.[1,3] Three recent studies

Table 3.3 RELATIONSHIP BETWEEN CENTRAL-PERIPHERAL TEMPERATURE DIFFERENCE AND CAPILLARY REFILL TIME AND OTHER PARAMETERS AT 3 AND 10 HOURS POSTNATAL AGE

CPTd or CRT	Sn	Sp	PPV	NPV	LR+	LR−
CPTd ≥2°C						
3 h	29 (15–42)	78 (65–90)	20 (8–32)	85 (74–96)	1.29	0.92
10 h	41 (27–55)	66 (52–79)	41 (27–55)	66 (52–79)	1.19	0.90
All observations	40 (32–48)	69 (61–77)	23 (16–30)	83 (77–90)	1.30	0.87
CRT ≥3 sec						
3 h	54 (45–63)	79 (72–86)	23 (16–31)	93 (89–98)	2.55	0.58
10 h	59 (50–68)	75 (67–82)	51 (42–60)	80 (73–87)	2.33	0.55
All observations	55 (50–60)	80 (76–84)	33 (29–38)	91 (88–94)	2.78	0.56
CRT ≥4 sec						
3 h	38 (30–47)	93 (88–97)	38 (30–47)	93 (88–97)	5.24	0.66
10 h	26 (18–33)	97 (93–100)	77 (70–84)	74 (67–82)	7.44	0.77
All observations	29 (24–33)	96 (94–98)	55 (50–60)	88 (85–91)	6.84	0.75

Values in parentheses are 95% confidence intervals. *CPTd*, Central-peripheral temperature difference; *CRT*, capillary refill time; *LR+*, positive likelihood ratio; *LR−*, negative likelihood ratio; *NPV*, negative predictive value; *PPV*, positive predictive value; *Sn*, sensitivity; *Sp*, specificity.
From Osborn DA, Evans N, Kluckow M: Clinical detection of low upper body blood flow in very premature infants using blood pressure, capillary refill time, and central-peripheral temperature difference. *Arch Dis Child Fetal Neonatal Ed* 89:F168–F173, 2004. Used with permission from BMJ Publishing Group.

suggest that this is occurring in clinical practice.[41,52,98] Detail is not available on what criteria led to intervention in these retrospective studies, but one can assume that many babies had signs consistent with good perfusion and were not treated, and the contrary may also be true. There is no validated clinical scoring system available to diagnose shock in newborns, and assessment remains predominantly subjective. The assessment of capillary refill time (CRT), color, heart rate, BP, and urine output are readily made at the bedside. None of these parameters in isolation is specific in identifying poor perfusion. CRT values exist for the term neonate,[100–103] but there are limited data available for the preterm infant,[104–106] with some asking whether it is a useful parameter to be evaluated at all.[107,108] Osborn and colleagues studied the ability of CRT, central-peripheral temperature difference (CPTd) ≥ 2°C and BP to detect low SVC flow in neonates less than 30 weeks' gestation. Results for CPTd and CRT are listed in Table 3.3. The authors showed a statistically significant but weak association between CRT and systemic blood flow.[105] The sensitivity improved when mean BP values and central CRT ≥3 seconds were combined. Wodey and colleagues have shown a significant relationship between cardiac index (cardiac output/body surface area) and CRT in preterm neonates in a study using echocardiography in 100 preterm infants.[109] We previously also identified a weak relationship between CRT and simultaneously obtained SVC flow measurements in a preterm population.[104]

Assessment of color remains very subjective. More recently the relationship between skin color and illness severity in the newborn has been evaluated using an objective measurement tool.[110,111] Colorimeter values were found to be significantly different in the high illness severity group, particularly in the blue-yellow axis. However, no data on BP or cardiac function were provided in these studies. It seems that the next logical step would be to evaluate this parameter in further studies, specifically evaluating the relationship between colorimetry and cardiac output measurements. Heart rates are extremely variable; they vary with gestational and postnatal age and correlate with oxygen consumption. However, neither absolute heart rate nor trend analysis of heart rate has been validated as a way to assess cardiac function in term or preterm infants. In the first postnatal day, urine output is not a particularly useful parameter due to the perinatal surge of vasoconstrictive hormones and the complex transitional process of postnatal hemodynamics. Urine output is typically low and variable; however, an acceptable urine output (>1.5 to 2.0 mL/

kg/h) is somewhat reassuring to the clinician at the bedside deciding if one needs to initiate therapy for hypotension. While the positive predictive value of each of these individual parameters identifying poor perfusion is unknown and likely to be low, it does appear that clinical assessment using a combination of signs allows one to better identify patients with poor outcomes.[99] Combining clinical parameters along with BP values is clearly more logical than intervening based solely on BP values alone, unless the mean arterial BP is very low. Dempsey and colleagues have suggested using a BP value at least 5 mm Hg below the lower gestational age rule as the lowest acceptable BP during the first postnatal day.[93] This would equate to somewhere in the region of 18 to 20 mm Hg for babies delivered at 23 to 25 weeks' gestation, and this value is numerically similar to the critical closing pressure for cerebral blood flow in animal models (see Chapter 2). Evidence in very preterm neonates is not available as to whether this BP cutoff value is safe and effective to use when initiation of treatment is considered in a very preterm neonate. As it is close to the critical closing pressure, when cerebral blood flow ceases despite the presence of measurable systemic BP and cardiac output, studies are urgently needed to answer this clinically relevant and important question.

There are some potential objective parameters readily available at the bedside, but their usefulness in term and preterm newborns is debatable including central venous pressure (CVP) monitoring, mixed venous oxygen saturation, and plasma lactate levels.

CVP monitoring is commonly performed in adult and pediatric intensive care where it is often used to guide fluid management.[112,113] There are early reports of CVP measurements in newborns as well. Rudolph and colleagues recorded CVP in six babies with respiratory distress syndrome and found values between −6.5 and 0 mm Hg.[114] These patients were not ventilated and generated large negative intrathoracic pressures, hence the negative values. Siassi and colleagues reported a mean CVP of +1.6 mm Hg in healthy preterm neonates and negative values in babies with respiratory distress (−16 to +3 mm Hg).[115] A more recent study suggests normal values for CVP in preterm infants, which have a very wide range (2.8 to 13.9 mm Hg),[116] but there were numerous technical difficulties obtaining CVP measurements. It is unclear whether CVP correlates with circulating blood volume in the preterm infant[117] and, in any case, the majority of preterm infants with lower BP in the first few days are not significantly hypovolemic.[118,119] Thus CVP monitoring is probably of limited use in the NICU setting. Others have suggested noninvasive methods of assessing CVP, with subcostal estimates of the maximum and minimum diameter of the inferior vena cava (IVC) obtained by echocardiography.[120] The ratio of minimum to maximum diameter correlated with CVP in this study of 14 newborns. However, a previous study showed a poor correlation between similar noninvasive echocardiographic assessments of IVC diameter and CVP, especially in mechanically ventilated infants.[121] A recent meta-analysis of 37 studies concluded that the evidence does not support the measurement of IVC diameter by ultrasonography as an acceptable surrogate to determine CVP in critically ill patients.[122]

Mixed venous saturation monitoring is frequently used in adult and pediatric intensive care, but again the interatrial shunting and technical difficulties in obtaining a value limit its role, especially in the preterm neonate. There have been few studies in newborns, outside the setting of postoperative cardiac surgery, monitoring mixed venous saturation. O'Connor and colleagues studied 18 newborns in the first 3 postnatal days and obtained 100 paired values of arterial saturation and mixed venous saturation. They found that the mean mixed venous oxygen saturation was 83.3% and that there was a strong correlation with fractionated oxygen extraction.[123] Van der Hoeven and colleagues measured venous oxygen saturation continuously with a fiberoptic catheter placed in the right atrium via the IVC.[124] They found a central venous oxygen saturation ranging from 65% to 82% (5th and 95th percentile) during the first days after delivery in 10 stable preterm infants. More recently, Yapakci et al. measured IVC oxygen saturation in preterm infants as an indicator of mixed venous oxygenation in the first 3 days of life.[125] They identified a progressive decrease in venous oxygen saturation over the first few days with the highest mean IVC oxygen saturation of 79.9% on initial measurement and the lowest value of 64.8% for the final measurement performed at 72 hours postnatally. However, the usefulness of mixed venous saturation monitoring in assessing cardiovascular well-being, especially for the preterm infant, remains to be answered.

Lactate values have been analyzed in a number of clinical situations in the preterm infant, including the need for erythrocyte transfusion,[126,127] sepsis,[128] and necrotizing enterocolitis.[129,130] Initial elevated levels and subsequent increase in plasma lactate levels may predict progression of definite necrotizing enterocolitis (NEC) to surgery or death in preterm neonates with medical NEC.[130,131] Lactate values obtained in the first day of postnatal life have been used to predict outcome.[132,133] Deshpande and colleagues showed a worse outcome when plasma lactate concentrations remained persistently elevated in sick ventilated newborns of 23 to 40 weeks' gestation.[132] Mortality was 57% if two lactate values were above 5.6 mmol/L, highlighting the importance of serial lactate assessments. However, these measurements were obtained beyond the transitional period. Groenendaal and colleagues estimated the positive (PPV) and negative predictive value (NPV) of arterial lactate values obtained within 3 hours after birth and found that with a cutoff value of 5.7 mmol/L, the PPV was 0.47 and NPV 0.92 for a combined adverse outcome (death or poor neurodevelopmental outcome) in a cohort of preterm babies.[133] Recently we have shown that a single lactate value greater than 5.6 mmol/L obtained during the first postnatal day was associated with an increased risk of adverse outcome, defined as death or severe P/IVH.[134] Data are limited on the utilization of plasma lactate values specifically in hypotensive newborns. Wardle and colleagues found no difference in lactate levels between normotensive and hypotensive preterm infants.[135] In a cohort of VLBW infants, we previously identified a weak negative correlation between lactate values and SVC flow.[104] A combined lactate value of greater than 4 mmol and prolonged CRT greater than 4 seconds resulted in a positive predictive value of 80% and a negative predictive value of 88% for identifying low SVC flow, which highlights the value of combining clinical and biochemical parameters in the overall assessment. de Boode provides an excellent overview of the predictive value of the most commonly used indicators of circulatory failure, including BP, heart rate, urine output, CRT, and plasma lactate concentration.[136] In summary, combining different clinical hemodynamic and biochemical parameters enhances the predictive value in the overall detection of circulatory failure, but the accuracy is still limited.

In addition to obtaining clinical, biochemical, and echocardiographic hemodynamic information, a comprehensive, continuous, real-time hemodynamic monitoring and data acquisition system has recently been developed (see Chapter 21). In addition to monitoring heart rate, BP, arterial oxygen saturation, respiratory rate, and transcutaneous CO_2, this system employs available technologies, such as electrical impedance cardiometry and near infrared spectroscopy, and has the potential to include information collected by amplitude integrated electroencephalography. Using the traditionally collected data, along with the information provided by the nontraditional, more novel technologies on stroke volume, cardiac output, vital and nonvital organ perfusion, tissue oxygenation, and brain function, has the potential to also develop mathematical models predicting short- and long-term outcomes (Fig. 3.2; see Chapter 21). Using this approach, individualized medicine in neonatology will be established and, amongst others, the definition of hypotension in each patient at any given time point will become possible. Until then, the clinician needs to rely on the routinely available information when deciding whether a certain BP value or trend in a given patient represents tissue hypoperfusion, and thus, warrants intervention.

Conclusion

Despite its many limitations, mean BP values continue to be the mainstay of assessment and management of cardiovascular instability, particularly in preterm infants. Many normative ranges exist, but what is clear is that these should not be interpreted in isolation or considered generalizable for all patients born at the same gestational

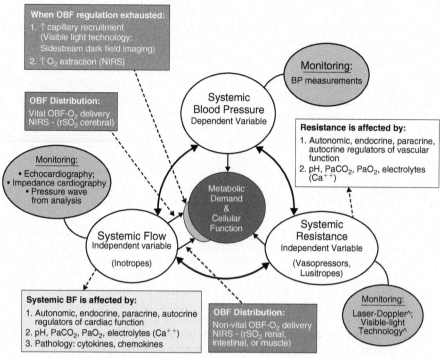

Fig. 3.2 Interaction among and monitoring of blood pressure (BP), blood flow, blood flow distribution, and vascular resistance. To satisfy cellular metabolic demand, an intricate interplay among blood flow, vascular resistance, and BP takes place. The regulation of organ blood flow distribution, capillary recruitment, and oxygen extraction is also essential for the maintenance of hemodynamic homeostasis. The monitoring methods depicted have been mostly used for clinical research purposes at this time. It is unknown whether laser Doppler and/or visible light technologies can reliably assess changes in systemic vascular resistance. *NIRS,* Near-infrared spectroscopy; *OBF,* organ blood flow; *rSO2,* regional tissue oxygen saturation. (From Soleymani S, Borzage M, Seri I: Hemodynamic monitoring in neonates: advances and challenges. *J Perinatol* 30:S38–S45, 2010. Used with permission from Nature Publishing Group.)

age, and at all times during transition. While more objective assessment methods are on the horizon, each has its own inherent limitations. Incorporating clinical and objective assessment tools provides the potential to overcome some of the disadvantages of each monitoring technique and ultimately to achieve a greater degree of accuracy in determining appropriate interventions. Current ongoing trials in this area may help to clarify some of the remaining uncertainties.

REFERENCES

1. Stranak Z, Semberova J, Barrington K, et al.: International survey on diagnosis and management of hypotension in extremely preterm babies, *Eur J Pediatr* 173:793–798, 2014.
2. Dempsey EM, Barrington KJ: Diagnostic criteria and therapeutic interventions for the hypotensive very low birth weight infant, *J Perinatol* 26:677–681, 2006.
3. Sehgal A, Osborn D, McNamara PJ: Cardiovascular support in preterm infants: a survey of practices in Australia and New Zealand, *J Paediatr Child Health* 48:317–323, 2012.
4. Darnall R: Blood-pressure monitoring. In Brans YHW, editor: *Physiological Monitoring and Instrument Diagnosis in Perinatal and Neonatal Medicine,* Cambridge, 1995, University Press, pp 246–266.
5. Korotkoff N: On methods of studying blood pressure [in Russian], *Bull Imperial Mil Med Acad* 11:365–367, 1905 (with discussions).
6. Cunningham S, Symon AG, McIntosh N: Changes in mean blood pressure caused by damping of the arterial pressure waveform, *Early Hum Dev* 36:27–30, 1994.
7. Shimokaze T, Akaba K, Saito E: Oscillometric and intra-arterial blood pressure in preterm and term infants: extent of discrepancy and factors associated with inaccuracy, *Am J Perinatol* 32:277–282, 2015.
8. Shimokaze T, Akaba K, Saito E: Oscillometric and intra-arterial blood pressure in preterm and term infants: extent of discrepancy and factors associated with inaccuracy, *Am J Perinatol*, 2014.
9. Lalan S, Blowey D: Comparison between oscillometric and intra-arterial blood pressure measurements in ill preterm and full-term neonates, *J Am Soc Hypertens* 8:36–44, 2014.

10. Holt TR, Withington DE, Mitchell E: Which pressure to believe? A comparison of direct arterial with indirect blood pressure measurement techniques in the pediatric intensive care unit, *Pediatr Crit Care Med* 12:e391–e394, 2011.

11. O'Shea J, Dempsey EM: A comparison of blood pressure measurements in newborns, *Am J Perinatol* 26:113–116, 2009.

12. Dannevig I, Dale HC, Liestol K, et al.: Blood pressure in the neonate: three non-invasive oscillometric pressure monitors compared with invasively measured blood pressure, *Acta Paediatr* 94:191–196, 2005.

13. Emery EF, Greenough A: Non-invasive blood pressure monitoring in preterm infants receiving intensive care, *Eur J Pediatr* 151:136–139, 1992.

14. Sonesson SE, Broberger U: Arterial blood pressure in the very low birthweight neonate. Evaluation of an automatic oscillometric technique, *Acta Paediatr Scand* 76:338–341, 1987.

15. Pickering TG, Hall JE, Appel LJ, et al.: Recommendations for blood pressure measurement in humans: an AHA scientific statement from the Council on High Blood Pressure Research Professional and Public Education Subcommittee, *J Clin Hypertens (Greenwich)* 7:102–109, 2005.

16. Diprose GK, Evans DH, Archer LN, et al.: Dinamap fails to detect hypotension in very low birthweight infants, *Arch Dis Child* 61:771–773, 1986.

17. Chia F, Ang AT, Wong TW, et al.: Reliability of the Dinamap non-invasive monitor in the measurement of blood pressure of ill Asian newborns, *Clin Pediatr (Phila)* 29:262–267, 1990.

18. Park MK, Lee DH: Normative arm and calf blood pressure values in the newborn, *Pediatrics* 83:240–243, 1989.

19. Piazza SF, Chandra M, Harper RG, et al.: Upper- vs lower-limb systolic blood pressure in full-term normal newborns, *Am J Dis Child* 139:797–799, 1985.

20. Cowan F, Thoresen M, Walloe L: Arm and leg blood pressures—are they really so different in newborns? *Early Hum Dev* 26:203–211, 1991.

21. Kunk R, McCain GC: Comparison of upper arm and calf oscillometric blood pressure measurement in preterm infants, *J Perinatol* 16:89–92, 1996.

22. Dasnadi S, Aliaga S, Laughon M, et al.: Factors influencing the accuracy of noninvasive blood pressure measurements in NICU infants, *Am J Perinatol* 32:639–644, 2015.

23. Lee J, Rajadurai VS, Tan KW: Blood pressure standards for very low birthweight infants during the first day of life, *Arch Dis Child Fetal Neonatal Ed* 81:F168–F170, 1999.

24. Spinazzola RM, Harper RG, de Soler M, et al.: Blood pressure values in 500- to 750-gram birthweight infants in the first week of life, *J Perinatol* 11:147–151, 1991.

25. Watkins AM, West CR, Cooke RW: Blood pressure and cerebral haemorrhage and ischaemia in very low birthweight infants, *Early Hum Dev* 19:103–110, 1989.

26. Versmold HT, Kitterman JA, Phibbs RH, et al.: Aortic blood pressure during the first 12 hours of life in infants with birth weight 610 to 4,220 grams, *Pediatrics* 67:607–613, 1981.

27. Hegyi T, Anwar M, Carbone MT, et al.: Blood pressure ranges in premature infants: II. The first week of life, *Pediatrics* 97:336–342, 1996.

28. Hegyi T, Carbone MT, Anwar M, et al.: Blood pressure ranges in premature infants. I. The first hours of life, *J Pediatr* 124:627–633, 1994.

29. Kent AL, Kecskes Z, Shadbolt B, et al.: Normative blood pressure data in the early neonatal period, *Pediat Nephrol* 22:1335–1341, 2007.

30. Kent AL, Meskell S, Falk MC, et al.: Normative blood pressure data in non-ventilated premature neonates from 28-36 weeks gestation, *Pediatr Nephrol* 24:141–146, 2009.

31. Batton B, Batton D, Riggs T: Blood pressure during the first 7 days in premature infants born at postmenstrual age 23 to 25 weeks, *Am J Perinatol* 24:107–115, 2007.

32. Cunningham S, Symon AG, Elton RA, et al.: Intra-arterial blood pressure reference ranges, death and morbidity in very low birthweight infants during the first seven days of life, *Early Hum Dev* 56:151–165, 1999.

33. Shortland DB, Evans DH, Levene MI: Blood pressure measurements in very low birth weight infants over the first week of life, *J Perinat Med* 16:93–97, 1988.

34. Zubrow AB, Hulman S, Kushner H, et al.: Determinants of blood pressure in infants admitted to neonatal intensive care units: a prospective multicenter study. Philadelphia Neonatal Blood Pressure Study Group, *J Perinatol* 15:470–479, 1995.

35. Batton B, Li L, Newman NS, et al.: Evolving blood pressure dynamics for extremely preterm infants, *J Perinatol* 34:301–305, 2014.

36. Bada HS, Korones SB, Perry EH, et al.: Mean arterial blood pressure changes in premature infants and those at risk for intraventricular hemorrhage, *J Pediatr* 117:607–614, 1990.

37. Munro MJ, Walker AM, Barfield CP: Hypotensive extremely low birth weight infants have reduced cerebral blood flow, *Pediatrics* 114:1591–1596, 2004.

38. Borch K, Lou HC, Greisen G: Cerebral white matter blood flow and arterial blood pressure in preterm infants, *Acta Paediatr* 99:1489–1492, 2010.

39. Miall-Allen VM, de Vries LS, Whitelaw AG: Mean arterial blood pressure and neonatal cerebral lesions, *Arch Dis Child* 62:1068–1069, 1987.

40. Report of working group of the British Association of Perinatal Medicine and Neonatal Nurses Association on categories of babies requiring neonatal care, *Arch Dis Child* 67:868–869, 1992.

41. Faust K, Hartel C, Preuss M, et al.: Short-term outcome of very-low-birthweight infants with arterial hypotension in the first 24 h of life, *Arch Dis Child Fetal Neonatal Ed* 100:F388–F392, 2015.

42. Barrington KJ, Stewart S, Lee S: Differing blood pressure thresholds in preterm infants, effects on frequency of diagnosis of hypotension and intraventricular haemorrhage, *Pediatr Res* 51:455A, 2002.

3

43. Stranak Z, Semberova J, Barrington K, et al.: International survey on diagnosis and management of hypotension in extremely preterm babies, *Eur J Pediatr*, 2014.

44. Laughon M, Bose C, Allred E, et al.: Factors associated with treatment for hypotension in extremely low gestational age newborns during the first postnatal week, *Pediatrics* 119:273–280, 2007.

45. Moise AA, Wearden ME, Kozinetz CA, et al.: Antenatal steroids are associated with less need for blood pressure support in extremely premature infants, *Pediatrics* 95:845–850, 1995.

46. Demarini S, Dollberg S, Hoath SB, et al.: Effects of antenatal corticosteroids on blood pressure in very low birth weight infants during the first 24 hours of life, *J Perinatol* 19:419–425, 1999.

47. Elimian A, Figueroa R, Spitzer AR, et al.: Antenatal corticosteroids: are incomplete courses beneficial? *Obstet Gynecol* 102:352–355, 2003.

48. Been JV, Kornelisse RF, Rours IG, et al.: Early postnatal blood pressure in preterm infants: effects of chorioamnionitis and timing of antenatal steroids, *Pediatr Res* 66:571–576, 2009.

49. Elimian A, Garry D, Figueroa R, et al.: Antenatal betamethasone compared with dexamethasone (betacode trial): a randomized controlled trial, *Obstet Gynecol* 110:26–30, 2007.

50. Rabe H, Diaz-Rossello JL, Duley L, et al.: Effect of timing of umbilical cord clamping and other strategies to influence placental transfusion at preterm birth on maternal and infant outcomes, *Cochrane Database Syst Rev* 8:CD003248, 2012.

51. Sommers R, Stonestreet BS, Oh W, et al.: Hemodynamic effects of delayed cord clamping in premature infants, *Pediatrics* 129:e667–e672, 2012.

52. Popat H, Robledo KP, Sebastian L, et al.: Effect of delayed cord clamping on systemic blood flow: a randomized controlled trial, *J Pediatr* 178:81.e2–86.e2, 2016.

53. Ghavam S, Batra D, Mercer J, et al.: Effects of placental transfusion in extremely low birthweight infants: meta-analysis of long- and short-term outcomes, *Transfusion* 54:1192–1198, 2014.

54. Katheria AC, Leone TA, Woelkers D, et al.: The effects of umbilical cord milking on hemodynamics and neonatal outcomes in premature neonates, *J Pediatr* 164:1045–1050 e1, 2014.

55. Al-Wassia H, Shah PS: Efficacy and safety of umbilical cord milking at birth: a systematic review and meta-analysis, *JAMA Pediatrics* 169:18–25, 2015.

56. Katheria AC, Truong G, Cousins L, et al.: Umbilical cord milking versus delayed cord clamping in preterm infants, *Pediatrics* 136:61–69, 2015.

57. Kluckow M, Evans N: Relationship between blood pressure and cardiac output in preterm infants requiring mechanical ventilation, *J Pediatr* 129:506–512, 1996.

58. Evans N, Kluckow M: Early determinants of right and left ventricular output in ventilated preterm infants, *Arch Dis Child Fetal Neonatal Ed* 74:F88–F94, 1996.

59. de Waal KA, Evans N, Osborn DA, et al.: Cardiorespiratory effects of changes in end expiratory pressure in ventilated newborns, *Arch Dis Child Fetal Neonatal Ed*, 2007.

60. Lakkundi A, Wright I, de Waal K: Transitional hemodynamics in preterm infants with a respiratory management strategy directed at avoidance of mechanical ventilation, *Early Hum Dev* 90:409–412, 2014.

61. Gopel W, Kribs A, Ziegler A, et al.: Avoidance of mechanical ventilation by surfactant treatment of spontaneously breathing preterm infants (AMV): an open-label, randomised, controlled trial, *Lancet* 378:1627–1634, 2011.

62. Hall RW, Kronsberg SS, Barton BA, et al.: Morphine, hypotension, and adverse outcomes among preterm neonates: who's to blame? Secondary results from the NEOPAIN trial, *Pediatrics* 115:1351–1359, 2005.

63. Perlman JM: Morphine, hypotension, and intraventricular hemorrhage in the ventilated premature infant, *Pediatrics* 115:1416–1418, 2005.

64. Osborn DA, Evans N, Kluckow M: Hemodynamic and antecedent risk factors of early and late periventricular/intraventricular hemorrhage in premature infants, *Pediatrics* 112:33–39, 2003.

65. Martens SE, Rijken M, Stoelhorst GM, et al.: Is hypotension a major risk factor for neurological morbidity at term age in very preterm infants? *Early Hum Dev* 75:79–89, 2003.

66. Koksal N, Baytan B, Bayram Y, et al.: Risk factors for intraventricular haemorrhage in very low birth weight infants, *Indian J Pediatr* 69:561–564, 2002.

67. Dammann O, Allred EN, Kuban KC, et al.: Systemic hypotension and white-matter damage in preterm infants, *Dev Med Child Neurol* 44:82–90, 2002.

68. Krageloh-Mann I, Toft P, Lunding J, et al.: Brain lesions in preterms: origin, consequences and compensation, *Acta Paediatr* 88:897–908, 1999.

69. Perlman JM: White matter injury in the preterm infant: an important determination of abnormal neurodevelopment outcome, *Early Hum Dev* 53:99–120, 1998.

70. Low JA, Froese AB, Galbraith RS, et al.: The association between preterm newborn hypotension and hypoxemia and outcome during the first year, *Acta Paediatr* 82:433–437, 1993.

71. Funato M, Tamai H, Noma K, et al.: Clinical events in association with timing of intraventricular hemorrhage in preterm infants, *J Pediatr* 121:614–619, 1992.

72. Kopelman AE: Blood pressure and cerebral ischemia in very low birth weight infants, *J Pediatr* 116:1000–1002, 1990.

73. Miall-Allen VM, de Vries LS, Dubowitz LM, et al.: Blood pressure fluctuation and intraventricular hemorrhage in the preterm infant of less than 31 weeks' gestation, *Pediatrics* 83:657–661, 1989.

74. Szymonowicz W, Yu VY, Wilson FE: Antecedents of periventricular haemorrhage in infants weighing 1250 g or less at birth, *Arch Dis Child* 59:13–17, 1984.

75. Ment LR, Duncan CC, Ehrenkranz RA, et al.: Intraventricular hemorrhage in the preterm neonate: timing and cerebral blood flow changes, *J Pediatr* 104:419–425, 1984.

76. Conner ES, Lorenzo AV, Welch K, et al.: The role of intracranial hypotension in neonatal intraventricular hemorrhage, *J Neurosurg* 58:204–209, 1983.
77. Mitchell W, O'Tuama L: Cerebral intraventricular hemorrhages in infants: a widening age spectrum, *Pediatrics* 65:35–39, 1980.
78. Fujimura M, Salisbury DM, Robinson RO, et al.: Clinical events relating to intraventricular haemorrhage in the newborn, *Arch Dis Child* 54:409–414, 1979.
79. Hambleton G, Wigglesworth JS: Origin of intraventricular haemorrhage in the preterm infant, *Arch Dis Child* 51:651–659, 1976.
80. Dempsey EM, Barrington KJ: Treating hypotension in the preterm infant: when and with what: a critical and systematic review, *J Perinatol* 27:469–478, 2007.
81. Logan JW, O'Shea TM, Allred EN, et al.: Early postnatal hypotension is not associated with indicators of white matter damage or cerebral palsy in extremely low gestational age newborns, *J Perinatol* 31:524–534, 2011.
82. Logan JW, O'Shea TM, Allred EN, et al.: Early postnatal hypotension and developmental delay at 24 months of age among extremely low gestational age newborns, *Arch Dis Child Fetal Neonatal Ed* 96:F321–F328, 2011.
83. Batton B, Zhu X, Fanaroff J, et al.: Blood pressure, anti-hypotensive therapy, and neurodevelopment in extremely preterm infants, *J Pediatr* 154:351.e1–357.7 e1, 2009.
84. Batton B, Li L, Newman NS, et al.: Early blood pressure, antihypotensive therapy and outcomes at 18-22 months' corrected age in extremely preterm infants, *Arch Dis Child Fetal Neonatal Ed* 101:F201–F206, 2016.
85. Alderliesten T, Lemmers PM, van Haastert IC, et al.: Hypotension in preterm neonates: low blood pressure alone does not affect neurodevelopmental outcome, *J Pediatr* 164:986–991, 2014.
86. Dempsey EM, Barrington KJ: Evaluation and treatment of hypotension in the preterm infant, *Clin Perinatol* 36:75–85, 2009.
87. Ment LR, Stewart WB, Duncan CC, et al.: Beagle puppy model of intraventricular hemorrhage, *J Neurosurg* 57:219–223, 1982.
88. Fanaroff JM, Wilson-Costello DE, Newman NS, et al.: Treated hypotension is associated with neonatal morbidity and hearing loss in extremely low birth weight infants, *Pediatrics* 117:1131–1135, 2006.
89. Limperopoulos C, Bassan H, Kalish LA, et al.: Current definitions of hypotension do not predict abnormal cranial ultrasound findings in preterm infants, *Pediatrics* 120:966–977, 2007.
90. Pellicer A, Valverde E, Elorza MD, et al.: Cardiovascular support for low birth weight infants and cerebral hemodynamics: a randomized, blinded, clinical trial, *Pediatrics* 115:1501–1512, 2005.
91. Pellicer A, Bravo MC, Madero R, et al.: Early systemic hypotension and vasopressor support in low birth weight infants: impact on neurodevelopment, *Pediatrics* 123:1369–1376, 2009.
92. Batton BJ, Li L, Newman NS, et al.: Feasibility study of early blood pressure management in extremely preterm infants, *J Pediatr* 161:65.e1–69.e1, 2012.
93. Dempsey EM, Barrington KJ, Marlow N, et al.: Management of hypotension in preterm infants (The HIP Trial): a randomised controlled trial of hypotension management in extremely low gestational age newborns, *Neonatology* 105:275–281, 2014.
94. Seri I, Rudas G, Bors ZS, et al.: The effect of dopamine on renal function, cerebral blood flow and plasma catecholamine levels in sick preterm neonates, *Pediatr Res* 34:742–749, 1993.
95. O'Leary H, Gregas MC, Limperopoulos C, et al.: Elevated cerebral pressure passivity is associated with prematurity-related intracranial hemorrhage, *Pediatrics* 124:302–309, 2009.
96. Schmidt N, Saez C, Seri I, et al.: Impact of syringe size on the performance of infusion pumps at low flow rates, *Pediatr Crit Care Med* 11:282–286, 2010.
97. Bartels K, Moss DR, Peterfreund RA: An analysis of drug delivery dynamics via a pediatric central venous infusion system: quantification of delays in achieving intended doses, *Anesth Analg* 109:1156–1161, 2009.
98. Batton B, Li L, Newman NS, et al.: Use of antihypotensive therapies in extremely preterm infants, *Pediatrics* 131:e1865–e1873, 2013.
99. Dempsey EM, Al Hazzani F, Barrington KJ: Permissive hypotension in the extremely low birth-weight infant with signs of good perfusion, *Arch Dis Child Fetal Neonatal Ed* 94:F241–F244, 2009.
100. Raichur DV, Aralihond AP, Kasturi AV, et al.: Capillary refill time in term neonates: bedside assessment, *Indian J Pediatr* 68:613–615, 2001.
101. Raju NV, Maisels MJ, Kring E, et al.: Capillary refill time in the hands and feet of normal newborn infants, *Clin Pediatr (Phila)* 38:139–144, 1999.
102. Strozik KS, Pieper CH, Cools F: Capillary refilling time in newborns–optimal pressing time, sites of testing and normal values, *Acta Paediatr* 87:310–312, 1998.
103. Strozik KS, Pieper CH, Roller J: Capillary refilling time in newborn babies: normal values, *Arch Dis Child Fetal Neonatal Ed* 76:F193–F196, 1997.
104. Miletin J, Pichova K, Dempsey EM: Bedside detection of low systemic flow in the very low birth weight infant on day 1 of life, *Eur J Pediatr* 168:809–813, 2009.
105. Osborn DA, Evans N, Kluckow M: Clinical detection of low upper body blood flow in very premature infants using blood pressure, capillary refill time, and central-peripheral temperature difference, *Arch Dis Child Fetal Neonatal Ed* 89:F168–F173, 2004.
106. Kluckow M, Evans N: Low systemic blood flow in the preterm infant, *Semin Neonatol* 6:75–84, 2001.

107. LeFlore JL, Engle WD: Capillary refill time is an unreliable indicator of cardiovascular status in term neonates, *Adv Neonatal Care* 5:147–154, 2005.
108. Leonard PA, Beattie TF: Is measurement of capillary refill time useful as part of the initial assessment of children? *Eur J Emerg Med* 11:158–163, 2004.
109. Wodey E, Pladys P, Betremieux P, et al.: Capillary refilling time and hemodynamics in neonates: a doppler echocardiographic evaluation, *Crit Care Med* 26:1437–1440, 1998.
110. De Felice C, Flori ML, Pellegrino M, et al.: Predictive value of skin color for illness severity in the high-risk newborn, *Pediatr Res* 51:100–105, 2002.
111. De Felice C, Mazzieri S, Pellegrino M, et al.: Skin reflectance changes in preterm infants with patent ductus arteriosus, *Early Hum Dev* 78:45–51, 2004.
112. Sivarajan VB, Bohn D: Monitoring of standard hemodynamic parameters: heart rate, systemic blood pressure, atrial pressure, pulse oximetry, and end-tidal CO2, *Pediatr Crit Care Med* 12:S2–S11, 2011.
113. Pittman JA, Ping JS, Mark JB: Arterial and central venous pressure monitoring, *Int Anesthesiol Clin* 42:13–30, 2004.
114. Rudolph AM, Drorbaugh JE, Auld PA, et al.: Studies on the circulation in the neonatal period. The circulation in the respiratory distress syndrome, *Pediatrics* 27:551–566, 1961.
115. Siassi B, Wu PY, Li RK, et al.: Central venous pressure in preterm infants, *Biol Neonate* 37:285–290, 1980.
116. Trevor Inglis GD, Dunster KR, Davies MW: Establishing normal values of central venous pressure in very low birth weight infants, *Physiol Meas* 28:1283–1291, 2007.
117. Choi YS, Lee BS, Chung SH, et al.: Central venous pressure and renal function in very low birth weight infants during the early neonatal period, *J Matern Fetal Neonatal Med* 29:430–434, 2016.
118. Bauer K, Linderkamp O, Versmold HT: Short-term effects of blood transfusion on blood volume and resting peripheral blood flow in preterm infants, *Acta Paediatr* 82:1029–1033, 1993.
119. Bauer K, Linderkamp O, Versmold HT: Systolic blood pressure and blood volume in preterm infants, *Arch Dis Child* 69:521–522, 1993.
120. Sato Y, Kawataki M, Hirakawa A, et al.: The diameter of the inferior vena cava provides a noninvasive way of calculating central venous pressure in neonates, *Acta Paediatr* 102:e241–e246, 2013.
121. Hruda J, Rothuis EG, van Elburg RM, et al.: Echocardiographic assessment of preload conditions does not help at the neonatal intensive care unit, *Am J Perinatol* 20:297–303, 2003.
122. Alavi-Moghaddam M, Kabir A, Shojaee M, et al.: Ultrasonography of inferior vena cava to determine central venous pressure: a meta-analysis and meta-regression, *Acta Radiol*, 2016.
123. O'Connor TA, Hall RT: Mixed venous oxygenation in critically ill neonates, *Crit Care Med* 22:343–346, 1994.
124. van der Hoeven MA, Maertzdorf WJ, Blanco CE: Continuous central venous oxygen saturation (ScvO2) measurement using a fibre optic catheter in newborn infants. *Arch Dis Child Fetal Neonatal Ed* 74:F177–F181, 1996.
125. Yapakci E, Ecevit A, Ince DA, et al.: Inferior vena cava oxygen saturation during the first three postnatal days in preterm newborns with and without patent ductus arteriosus, *Balkan Med J* 31:230–234, 2014.
126. Izraeli S, Ben-Sira L, Harell D, et al.: Lactic acid as a predictor for erythrocyte transfusion in healthy preterm infants with anemia of prematurity, *J Pediatr* 122:629–631, 1993.
127. Moller JC, Schwarz U, Schaible TF, et al.: Do cardiac output and serum lactate levels indicate blood transfusion requirements in anemia of prematurity? *Intensive Care Med* 22:472–476, 1996.
128. Nguyen HB, Rivers EP, Knoblich BP, et al.: Early lactate clearance is associated with improved outcome in severe sepsis and septic shock, *Crit Care Med* 32:1637–1642, 2004.
129. Abubacker M, Yoxall CW, Lamont G: Peri-operative blood lactate concentrations in pre-term babies with necrotising enterocolitis, *Eur J Pediatr Surg* 13:35–39, 2003.
130. Srinivasjois R, Nathan E, Doherty D, et al.: Prediction of progression of definite necrotising enterocolitis to need for surgery or death in preterm neonates, *J Matern Fetal Neonatal Med* 23:695–700, 2010.
131. Lei G, Zhang J, Wang X, et al.: Plasma D-lactate levels in necrotizing enterocolitis in premature infants, *Iran J Pediatr* 26:e4403, 2016.
132. Deshpande SA, Platt MP: Association between blood lactate and acid-base status and mortality in ventilated babies, *Arch Dis Child Fetal Neonatal Ed* 76:F15–F20, 1997.
133. Groenendaal F, Lindemans C, Uiterwaal CS, et al.: Early arterial lactate and prediction of outcome in preterm neonates admitted to a neonatal intensive care unit, *Biol Neonate* 83:171–176, 2003.
134. Nadeem M, Clarke A, Dempsey EM: Day 1 serum lactate values in preterm infants less than 32 weeks gestation, *Eur J Pediatr* 169:667–670, 2010.
135. Yoxall CWWA: Blood lactate concentrations in sick neonates: normal range and prognostic significance of hyperlactataemia, *Pediatr Res* 40:557, 1996.
136. de Boode WP: Clinical monitoring of systemic hemodynamics in critically ill newborns, *Early Hum Dev* 86:137–141, 2010.

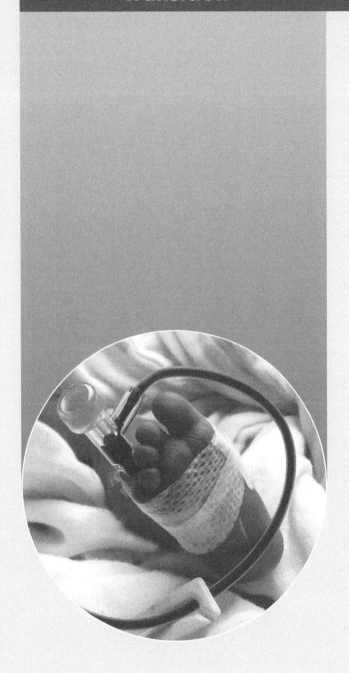

CHAPTER 4

Cardiorespiratory Effects of Delayed Cord Clamping

Stuart B. Hooper and Martin Kluckow

- There is a new and emerging understanding of the importance of the transitional circulation and the role that the timing of cord clamping plays in this.
- The cardiorespiratory transition at birth is a complex series of changes that begins with lung aeration and results in a chain of respiratory and cardiovascular events.
- The benefits of a delay in the clamping of the cord may be more than simply a placental transfusion, with time to transition also being a potential benefit.
- Placental transfusion volume is not just about time—there are other determinants including gravity, oxytocics, breathing, and crying.
- There are good animal data and a physiologic rationale that stabilization of the immediate postnatal hemodynamics is more likely with a deferral in cord clamping and initiation of breathing/lung inflation prior to clamping.
- A physiologic end point for determining cord clamping time is logical. This could be determined by either the onset of regular respirations or a particular volume of placental transfusion, which would require a specific way to quantitate the amount of transfusion, such as change in weight or real-time Doppler flow measurements.

The transition from intra- to extrauterine life involves a remarkable sequence of physiologic events that allow the fetus to survive after birth independent of the in utero milieu and a gaseous environment.[1,2] While these physiologic events are often studied and viewed independently, they are intimately linked and triggered by the one event that cannot occur in utero, lung aeration. Before birth, the developing lungs are liquid-filled and gas exchange occurs across the placenta.[3] At birth, the airways must be cleared of liquid to allow the entry of air and the onset of pulmonary ventilation so that the infant's site of gas exchange can transfer from the placenta to the lungs.[3] To facilitate the onset of pulmonary gas exchange, lung aeration also triggers a large decrease in pulmonary vascular resistance (PVR). As a result, right ventricular output is redirected through the lungs, rather than flowing through the ductus arteriosus (DA), causing a large increase in pulmonary blood flow (PBF).[4,5] In turn, the increase in PBF plays a vital role in sustaining the infant's cardiac output by replacing the venous return and ventricular preload lost due to clamping of the umbilical cord and removal of the placental blood flow. Before birth, as PBF is low, the majority of venous return and preload for the left ventricle is supplied by umbilical venous return which flows via the ductus venosus and foramen ovale directly into the left atrium.[6] As a result, at birth, clamping the umbilical cord before pulmonary ventilation has commenced and PBF has increased is potentially problematic, causing a large reduction (up to 50%) in cardiac output.[4]

Recognizing that the physiologic transition at birth is a sequence of interdependent events is vital to fully understand the consequences of clinical staff intervening in this process. In particular, umbilical cord clamping (UCC) at birth is the most common clinical intervention and is often viewed as an innocuous act. However, whether or not it is innocuous depends upon when it occurs during the progression through this physiologic sequence. For instance, if it occurs before the lung has aerated and PBF has increased, the infant is at increased risk of hypoxia and ischemia. Thus, it is important to understand the physiologic changes that occur at birth, as well as being able to recognize the stage within this transitional process that the infant has reached, in order to choose the correct timing for UCC after birth.

The Transition to Newborn Life

In utero, the fetus grows and develops in a liquid environment that is very different from the gaseous environment that it must survive in after birth. Gas exchange occurs across the placenta and the future airways are filled with a liquid that is produced by the lung and plays a vital role in stimulating fetal lung growth and development.[7] This liquid is actively retained within the airways by the fetus and keeps the lungs under a constant state of distension, resulting in a resting lung volume that is significantly larger than the functional residual capacity of the newborn lung.[7] This constant state of distension provides a mechanical stimulus for lung growth, which if absent, results in severe lung hypoplasia that is either lethal or causes significant morbidity in the newborn.[7,8] However, while airway liquid is essential for fetal lung growth, its presence is a major obstacle for the entry of air and the onset of pulmonary gas exchange after birth. As such it is important that the airways are cleared as rapidly as possible during the birth process to ensure that air can enter the terminal gas exchange regions of the lung and facilitate the onset of gas exchange.

Airway Liquid Clearance

Much interest has focused on the mechanisms of airway liquid clearance at birth, as reduced or heterogeneous airway liquid clearance is a major cause of perinatal morbidity, particularly in premature infants or term infants born by cesarean section.[9,10] Until recently, it was commonly thought that adrenaline-induced Na[+] reabsorption was the primary driver of airway liquid clearance at birth.[11] However, as this mechanism develops late in gestation and requires high circulating adrenaline levels to be activated, it doesn't readily explain how airway liquid is cleared in premature infants or in many of the infants born by cesarean section without the stress of labor.[2] Clearly, this is not the only mechanism and recent evidence even suggests that it is not the primary mechanism, accounting for less than 5% of airway liquid clearance in spontaneously breathing rabbits at birth.[12,13]

There are potentially three mechanisms that can contribute to airway liquid clearance at birth, which likely contribute to different degrees depending upon the timing and mode of delivery.[2] As the fetal respiratory system is highly compliant, any small increase in transthoracic pressure will greatly reduce the volume of airway liquid. It is well established that the loss of amniotic fluid and uterine contractions increase fetal spinal flexion which increases both abdominal and intrathoracic pressures resulting in lung liquid loss and a reduction in lung expansion.[14,15] Increased spinal flexion, caused by uterine contractions that force the fetal head through the cervix and vagina, likely explains the "gushes" of liquid from the nose and mouth that have been described following delivery of the head. While this mechanism can account for large reductions in airway liquid at birth, it does not explain how residual volumes of liquid are cleared from the airways after birth.

It has been proposed that increased circulating adrenaline levels during labor activate amiloride-sensitive Na[+] channels located on the apical surface of pulmonary epithelial cells.[11,16] The resulting uptake of Na[+] from the lung lumen and its transport across the epithelium into the pulmonary interstitium also increases the electropotential gradient for Cl⁻ ion flux in the same direction.[16] This reverses the osmotic gradient driving fetal lung liquid secretion, leading to liquid reabsorption from the airway lumen.[16] While this mechanism has been extensively studied and described, as indicated earlier, it only develops late in gestation, requires very high levels of circulating adrenaline, and at maximally stimulated rates (30 mL/h), it would take hours to clear all airway liquid.[2]

In a recent breakthrough, phase contrast x-ray imaging has allowed researchers to visualize the entry of air into the lungs at birth in both spontaneously breathing and mechanically ventilated term and preterm rabbits.[17–21] These studies clearly show that the air/liquid interface only moves distally during inspiration or during positive pressure inflations (Fig. 4.1). Between breaths or inflations, the air/liquid interface either remains stationary or moves proximally, indicating that some airway liquid reentry may occur between breaths.[12,13,21] Based on these results, it was concluded that after birth, airway liquid clearance primarily results from transepithelial hydrostatic pressures generated during inspiration/inflation.[2,13] That is, inspiration-induced hydrostatic pressure gradients between the airways and surrounding tissue drive the movement of liquid out of the airways across the pulmonary epithelium. This process was found to be extraordinarily rapid, with some newborn rabbits completely aerating their lungs in three to five breaths, generating an FRC of 15 to 20 mL/kg in that time (~30 seconds).[12,13]

Increase in Pulmonary Blood Flow at Birth in Response to Lung Aeration

At birth, lung aeration increases PBF 20- to 30-fold,[6] which not only enhances pulmonary gas exchange capacity but also plays a critical role in taking over the supply of preload for the left ventricle.[1,3] Numerous mechanisms are believed to mediate the pulmonary vasodilation in response to lung aeration, including increased oxygenation leading to the release of vasodilators such as nitric oxide, a reduction in lung distension caused by the formation of surface tension, and more recently, a vagally mediated vasodilation caused by the movement of liquid out of the airways into the surrounding tissue.[22] The latter mechanism was identified using simultaneous phase contrast x-ray imaging and angiography, designed to examine the spatial relationship between ventilation and perfusion during transition.[23] While the imaging was expected to show that partial lung aeration would increase PBF in only aerated lung regions, unexpectedly the imaging unequivocally demonstrated that

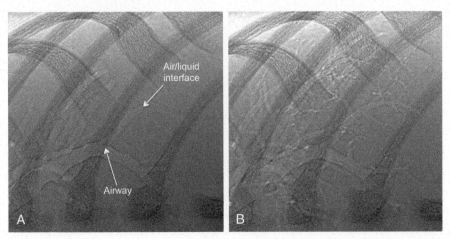

Fig. 4.1 High-resolution phase contrast x-ray images of a nondependent region of the lung shortly after the beginning of lung aeration. Images were acquired before (A) and after (B) a single breath in a spontaneously breathing near-term rabbit, demonstrating the amount of aeration that occurs with a single inspiration. Using this technique, liquid-filled airways are not visible and only become visible after they aerate. The air/liquid interface is clearly visible in (A) and, after one breath (B), at least another two generations of airways become visible.

partial lung aeration caused a global increase in PBF (Fig. 4.2). As ventilation with 100% nitrogen was able to produce a similar response as well as an increase in heart rate,[24] it appears that increased oxygenation is not a prerequisite for pulmonary vasodilation at birth, which is a consistently reported finding.[25,26] Nevertheless, ventilation with 100% oxygen enhanced the increase in PBF, but only in ventilated lung regions, indicating that the increase in PBF in response to lung aeration is multifactorial, with different mechanisms working independently.[24] As vagal nerve section abolished the increase in PBF induced by partial lung ventilation with 100% nitrogen, it was suggested that the movement of airway liquid into lung tissue activated receptors (possibly J receptors), which signaled via the vagus to stimulate a global increase in PBF.[27]

While the global increase in PBF that is stimulated by partial lung aeration causes a large ventilation/perfusion mismatch after birth, this is not necessarily problematic.[23] Indeed, as lung aeration is usually quite heterogeneous,[28] restricting the overall increase in PBF by only increasing PBF in aerated lung regions will reduce pulmonary venous return and may affect cardiac output. This is because, following UCC, pulmonary venous return becomes the primary source of preload for the left ventricle and restricting the increase in PBF restricts cardiac output.[4] As a result, the importance of clamping the umbilical cord at the appropriate time within this physiologic sequence (lung aeration followed by PBF increase) becomes self-evident.[3]

The Cardiovascular Transition at Birth: Effect of Umbilical Cord Clamping

The fetal circulatory system is very different from that of the newborn and is incompatible with independent life after birth. As such, the circulatory system must undergo substantial and rapid changes to transform from a fetal into a newborn phenotype.[3,6] Before birth, PBF is low and the majority of right ventricular output bypasses the lung and enters the descending thoracic aorta via the DA.[6] As a result, both left and right fetal ventricles pump in parallel, with both providing output for the systemic circulation; this circulation also includes perfusing an organ (the placenta) which at times during pregnancy is as big as, if not bigger than, the fetus.

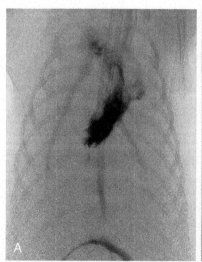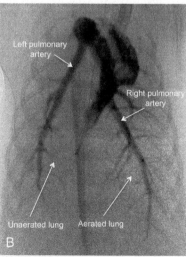

Fig. 4.2   Simultaneous phase contrast x-ray images and angiogram of a near-term newborn rabbit before (A) and after (B) partial lung aeration. An iodine solution is used as a contrast agent to highlight the blood vessels. Before lung aeration (A), pulmonary blood flow (PBF) is low, so very little iodine solution penetrates into the pulmonary arteries. However, after partial aeration of the right lung, PBF into both lungs greatly increases, irrespective of whether partial lung aeration occurs on the left or right side. This indicates that the increase in PBF at birth is not dependent upon total lung aeration and is not spatially related with aerated lung regions.

As the placenta receives a high percentage (30% to 50%) of fetal cardiac output, umbilical venous return must also provide a large proportion of venous return to the heart, which flows via the ductus venous and the liver via the IVC.[6] Of the umbilical venous return flowing through the ductus venosus, the majority of this blood bypasses the right atrium, right ventricle, and the lungs by flowing through the foramen ovale into the left atrium.[6] This has two important consequences. The first is that the relatively highly oxygenated umbilical venous blood can pass directly into the left side of the heart resulting in higher blood oxygen levels in preductal arteries perfusing the head and upper body.[6] The second, often overlooked consequence, is that umbilical venous blood provides a large percentage of the left ventricular preload in the fetus, particularly as PBF is low.[1,3]

The consequences of UCC at birth are multifactorial. The healthy placenta has a low-resistance, highly compliant vascular bed that receives a large percentage of fetal cardiac output. As a result, clamping the umbilical cord at birth not only separates the infant from its site of gas exchange, but also greatly increases systemic vascular resistance and therefore increases afterload on both the left and right ventricles.[4] This causes an instantaneous (within four heart beats) increase in arterial blood pressure (by ~30%), which results in an equally rapid increase in cerebral blood flow.[4] In addition, upon clamping the umbilical cord, umbilical venous return is lost, which significantly reduces left ventricular preload and, combined with the increase in afterload, greatly reduces cardiac output. The loss in cardiac output persists until the lung aerates and PBF increases to restore ventricular preload.[29] As such, if this period of reduced cardiac output at birth coincides with even a mild level of birth asphyxia, then the infant is at risk of further hypoxic/ischemic injury. This is because the fetus's primary defense against periods of hypoxia is to increase and redistribute cardiac output to increase blood flow to vital organs such as the brain.[30] However, if cardiac output is reduced, as occurs after cord clamping and before the onset of pulmonary ventilation, then the capacity of the fetus to defend itself from hypoxia is severely limited.

Neonatal Cardiovascular Responses to Umbilical Cord Clamping

Realization that the supply of left ventricular preload must switch from umbilical venous return to pulmonary venous return after birth underpins the rationale for delaying UCC until after the onset of pulmonary ventilation.[1,3,4] That is, if PBF increases before the umbilical cord is clamped, pulmonary venous return can immediately replace umbilical venous return as the primary source of preload for the left ventricle without any diminution in supply.[4] Under these circumstances, UCC does not result in a reduction in cardiac output. It is also important to recognize that the increase in pulmonary venous return following ventilation onset also increases right ventricular output, which increases rapidly with the increase in PBF.[4] For this to occur, blood flow through the foramen ovale (FO) must reverse to allow blood to flow from the left into the right atrium and contribute to right ventricular preload. While it has long been considered that the FO is a one-way valve, only flowing from right to left,[31] both experimental evidence and clinical observations indicate that this is not entirely accurate.[32]

Ventilating the lung and reducing PVR before clamping the umbilical cord also greatly mitigates the increase in arterial pressure caused by UCC, because the vasodilated lungs provide an additional low-resistance pathway for blood flow.[4] This initiates a competitive interplay between the pulmonary and placental circulations, whereby flow into either circulation depends upon the downstream resistance (or more precisely, impedance) in each vascular bed.[1,3] As such, following the reduction in PVR, the proportion of right ventricular output passing through the DA into the descending aorta is reduced and redirected into the pulmonary circulation. The result is a substantial reduction in umbilical blood flow entering and leaving the placenta.[33] It is interesting to speculate whether the decrease in PVR contributes to reduced flow and gradual closure of the umbilical vessels after birth. Indeed, anything that alters resistance in either vascular bed will alter the distribution of cardiac output between the two vascular beds and may contribute to umbilical vessel closure when flow into the pulmonary circulation is favored.[3] For instance, as uterine contractions increase placental vascular resistance and reduce umbilical blood flow, they increase the distribution of cardiac output into the pulmonary circulation. Similarly, the effect of gravity, caused by positioning the newborn above or below the placenta, induces the same response. That is, following ventilation onset, while umbilical artery flow is reduced as PBF increases, the reduction is much greater if the newborn is placed above the placenta compared with below the placenta.[33]

UCC following ventilation onset markedly alters the distribution of cardiac output within the newborn.[4] The loss of the low-resistance placental vascular bed causes a large increase in PBF, due to (1) the redirection of the entire right ventricular output into the lungs and (2) the very rapid reversal of blood flow through the DA, leading to a large left-to-right DA shunt.[4,5] As a result, both left and right ventricles contribute to PBF after birth, with the contribution of the left gradually diminishing as the DA closes.[5] It has been suggested that this ensures that pulmonary venous return and left ventricular preload are sufficient to maintain or increase (as needed) left ventricular output in the newborn period. It also allows the output of the two ventricles to gradually (over a few hours) come into balance before the two circulations separate, as at that time the outputs of the two ventricles must be equal.[3] Indeed, a continuing but gradually diminishing communication between the two atria (via the FO) and between the two arterial circulations (via the DA) should theoretically facilitate the gradual balancing of the two ventricular outputs.

Neonatal Cardiovascular Consequences of Umbilical Cord Milking

Many commentators have assumed that umbilical cord milking (UCM) equates to delayed UCC, mainly because they believe that the primary benefit of delayed UCC is placental to infant blood transfusion (see below).[34,35] However, this neglects the effect that total or intermittent occlusions of the umbilical cord has on the newborn's circulation. A variety of different UCM strategies have been proposed and include: (1) clamping the cord, but leaving a long segment open so that blood remaining in the cord can be "milked" into the infant and (2) leaving the cord intact and gradually "milking" blood into the infant, allowing the cord to refill with blood between milks.

Recent animal studies have clarified the physiologic consequences of UCM procedures. As expected, UCM necessitates that the cord is occluded during the milking procedure, which as previously described causes both a rapid increase in arterial pressure and cerebral blood flow and presumably a decrease in cardiac output,[36] similar to that seen after actual cord clamping.[4] As arterial pressures are quickly restored following release of the cord to allow it to refill, the resulting changes in arterial blood pressure and cerebral flow in subsequent "milks" are precisely replicated.[36] The net result is a concerning picture of several rapid increases and decreases in arterial pressure and cerebral blood flow, which resemble a "saw tooth" and are in stark contrast to the very stable pressures and flows that occur during delayed UCC. In a newborn infant with either an immature or inflamed cerebral vascular bed, these large "see-sawing" changes in arterial pressures and flows may be of even more concern (Fig. 4.3).

Whether or not UCM results in the net movement of blood from the cord into the infant likely depends on the method of UCM. Recent studies in sheep have shown that, following the "milk," if the cord is released at the newborn end, the cord will refill both from the infant and from the placenta, thereby losing any blood volume that was milked into the infant.[37] On the other hand, if the cord remains occluded at the infant end following the milk, blood refills the cord only from the placental end. This procedure results in net blood transfer into the newborn and has the added benefit of maintaining a relatively stable, albeit high, arterial blood pressure which is akin to normal UCC prior to ventilation onset.[37]

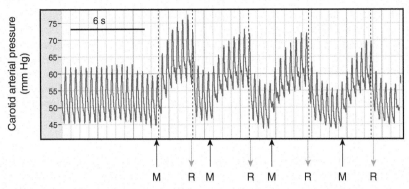

Fig. 4.3 Changes in carotid arterial pressure in response to four consecutive umbilical cord "milkings." Each cord milk is indicated *M*, whereas the cord release that occurred at the end of each milk is indicated by *R*. Note the large increases in arterial pressure that occurred with each milk.

Placental Transfusion During Delayed Umbilical Cord Clamping

The concept that blood volume will automatically shift from the placenta to the infant in a time-dependent manner after birth if UCC is delayed is complex and difficult to explain physiologically. This assumes that throughout the period of delayed UCC, umbilical venous flow will exceed umbilical artery flow, despite the vein being much more susceptible to reduced flow in response to external influences than the artery.[1] However, the fundamental principles of circulatory physiology dictate that flow into an organ will always equal flow out of an organ unless there is a major change in vascular compliance. While a large change in compliance will cause an imbalance in flow, the flow difference will always be transient. As such, blood volume will not automatically shift from the placenta to the infant unless the compliance of the vascular beds within either the infant or the placenta changes.[3,29] This is consistent with the fact that fetuses spend ~9 months in utero perfusing the placenta and during this time the distribution of blood volume between the fetus and placenta must be balanced to avoid a continuing net shift of blood from one compartment to the other.

Potential Mechanisms for Placental Blood Transfusion

Numerous mechanisms have been suggested to enhance placental-to-infant blood transfusion after birth, including gravity, uterine contractions, the increase in PBF, and thoracic pressure changes arising during inspiration.[3] On the other hand, an increase in thoracic and abdominal pressures arising from crying or grunting may lead to fetal-to-placental blood transfusion as would peripheral vasoconstriction possibly caused by birth asphyxia.[38] Doppler ultrasound measurements in the umbilical cords of human infants have revealed that breathing, particularly inspiration, and crying have a profound impact on blood flow in both the umbilical arteries and veins.[38] Large inspiratory efforts appeared to increase umbilical venous flow, whereas vigorous crying caused flow to cease in both vessels. As such it appears that breathing has a major influence on umbilical blood flows and more research is required to determine whether this mechanism could drive placental-to-infant blood transfusion.

Gravity and Uterine Contraction

While placing newborns below the placenta after birth reduces umbilical artery flow, it does not result in significant placental-to-newborn blood transfusion because umbilical venous flow is reduced by the same amount. On the other hand, placing the newborn above the placenta does not result in infant-to-placental blood transfusion as flows in both umbilical vessels are changed by this procedure.[33] These findings are consistent with a clinical trial showing no effect of placing infants above the mother on placental transfusion.[39]

Blood volume measurements in human infants suggest that uterine contractions facilitate blood transfusion into the infant after birth.[40] However, during labor, uterine contractions are known to increase placental vascular resistance and decrease umbilical blood flow, having differential effects on umbilical arteries and veins.[41] That is, as the veins are highly compliant low-pressure vessels, during contractions, the veins close earlier than arteries and then reopen after the arteries when the uterus relaxes.[41] This reasoning explains the fetal heart rate response to uterine contractions during labor, causing a transient increase in placental blood volume, which is released back into the infant following the contraction.[41] As such, uterine contractions do not readily explain placental-to-infant blood transfusion, but in particular do not "squeeze" blood out of the placenta and into the infant.

Increase in Pulmonary Blood Flow at Birth

A common explanation for placental-to-infant blood transfusion is the increase in PBF at birth which results in an increase in blood volume to accommodate the increased blood volume residing in the lung at any moment in time. However, while the increase in PBF after birth leads to a 40% increase in pulmonary blood volume, as the lung's blood volume is so small, this increase only accounts for a 2% overall increase in total blood volume (i.e., 2 mL/kg).[42] The mathematical explanation for this is simple. Dilation of a blood vessel increases its volume by the square of the radius change (r^2), whereas the resistance decreases by the change in radius to the fourth power (r^4). As such, the increase in PBF resulting from vasodilation is two orders of magnitude greater than the volume change, which explains why a large increase in organ blood flow does not necessarily translate into a large increase in organ blood volume.

Vaginal Birth

The early observations demonstrating a time-dependent increase in infant blood volume during delayed cord clamping only provide measurements made after birth in vaginally born infants.[40,43–45] The question therefore arises, what happens to an infant's blood volume during labor before birth? It is possible that during labor, the forces imposed on the infant increases abdominal and thoracic pressures, causing a net shift of blood from the infant into the placenta, which is then restored or "rebalanced" following delivery. As measurements have only been made after birth, this would appear as a placental transfusion. This concept may explain why delayed UCC is less effective in infants delivered by cesarean section without going through labor[46] and why multiple sheep experiments, where the lambs are delivered by cesarean section, have not been able to detect any placental transfusion.[33]

Recent studies in twins have shown that hemoglobin levels are significantly higher in the second born twin for the first 48 hours after birth if the infants are delivered vaginally, but not if the twins were delivered by cesarean section.[47,48] This effect was first observed in monochorionic twins, leading to the theory that labor induced the net movement of blood from the first-born twin into the second-born twin via anastomoses in the placenta.[48] However, as this effect was also present in dichorionic twins, it was suggested that earlier UCC in the first-born twin resulted in less placental blood transfusion compared with the second-born twin.[47] However, it is also possible that second-born twins are exposed to less compression than the first-born twin during delivery, resulting in less blood loss into the placenta during labor. Whatever the explanation, these studies indicate that the effects of labor and vaginal delivery are major determinants for whether increased hemoglobin content is observed postnatally. In any event, the term "placental transfusion" during delayed UCC is likely to be misleading and the concept of "blood volume restoration" or "rebalancing of the circulation" is probably more accurate.

Clinical Effects of Delayed/Deferred Umbilical Cord Clamping

Until recently, early UCC was performed on nearly every newborn baby in the developed world. The clinical reasons for introducing this medical procedure are unclear, although much attention has focused on early cord clamping to allow active management of the third stage of labor, with the perception that it reduces the risk of maternal postpartum hemorrhage. Systematic reviews, however, do not support this with no differences seen in the rates of postpartum hemorrhage between early and late cord clamping.[49] Other reasons for immediate clamping could include a response to the introduction of anesthetic and analgesic agents to mothers in labor, with the perception that a delay in clamping the cord would result in more transfer of these agents to the infant.

Deferral of cord clamping in term infants has long been practiced by midwives in low-risk settings. There is good evidence that deferral of cord clamping in the term infant with the possibility of some degree of placental transfusion/volume restoration results in both improved short-term[50] and longer-term outcomes including improved iron stores.[51] Consequently the majority of international professional bodies now advise deferral of cord clamping in *term infants* from 1 to 3 minutes. Deferral of cord clamping in the *preterm infant* has been more controversial with concerns being raised about the more frequent need for resuscitation at birth and whether deferral of cord clamping might lead to a delay in resuscitation with subsequent harm. However, there is mounting evidence that deferral of cord clamping is safe and likely of benefit in the preterm infant as well. Evidence from clinical trials and systematic reviews involving some 800 participants mainly show hemodynamic benefits: less hypotension and need for inotropes, less need for blood transfusion, and less severe intraventricular hemorrhage.[52] This benefit seems to hold even in the smallest of infants less than 1000 g,[53] but there is a paucity of evidence regarding long-term outcomes. This will be rectified soon as the follow-up results of the 1600 infant Australian Placental Transfusion Study become available (see conclusion for a summary of these results). The other main area of evidence for the benefits of a deferral of cord clamping in the preterm infant comes from a series of preterm sheep studies, which have explored the physiologic implications. In particular, these studies have emphasized the importance of the cardiorespiratory events at transition, with the concept that breathing and inflation of the lungs are key events—as described previously.[4,29] A delay in clamping of the cord, in addition to the potential hemodynamic benefits, also allows time for the lungs to aerate—either by spontaneous breaths or by inflation of the lungs as part of resuscitation. The subsequent increase in PBF and supplementation of the left ventricular preload is important in ensuring a stable transition.

Potential Mechanisms of Benefit: Transfusion Versus Timing

There are a number of possible mechanisms that may explain the apparent benefits of a deferral of cord clamping time in the preterm infant. The first and most accepted mechanism is that of allowing a placental transfusion—or a net flow of blood from the placenta to the infant.[45] However, as explained previously, the physiology of this is complex and there is little physiologic rationale for it, bearing in mind the fetus's ability to maintain euvolemia and the physics of blood supply to an organ where what goes in should come out again. The new concept of a restoration of blood lost to the placenta during labor discussed earlier also affects the way we understand placental transfusion. There are a number of suggested determinants of placental transfusion beyond that of time including relative position/gravity, uterine contractions and the role of oxytocin, mode of delivery, the role of breathing/crying, and the patency of the umbilical vessels with differential flow cessation times.[38] Another mechanism of benefit might include prevention of hypotension and low systemic blood flow,[54,55] both known associations with acute intraventricular hemorrhage (IVH)[56] and longer-term neurological injury.[57] The benefits of allowing some time for the infant to commence breathing or have the lungs aerated, while still receiving warm oxygenated blood from the placenta, increases the likelihood that increased PBF will have occurred prior to cord clamping—with the physiologic benefits described earlier—a process now termed *physiologically based cord clamping.*[58] Leading on from this benefit is the further development of a more hands-off, noninterventionist approach to preterm infant delivery—the concept of supporting the transition rather than "resuscitating" every infant. Potentially, supporting the transition while still attached to the placenta takes the pressure off the team to intervene with suction, occlusive masks, and attempted endotracheal intubation, all of which can be associated with vagal responses, hypoxia, and delay in establishing normal breathing. It is possible that a subsequent decrease in the need for mechanical ventilation and higher pressure/oxygen is one of the reasons for benefit seen in preterm infants who have a deferral in cord clamping time.

Determinants of the Placental Transfusion

Time

This is the most well-understood and most commonly cited determinant of the placental transfusion and is the basis of most of the recommendations for delay. However, there is little consistency between studies as to what the optimum time to UCC should be, with times ranging from 30 seconds to 3 minutes and more. Again, this most likely reflects our lack of understanding of the physiology and hemodynamics as well as our inability to accurately measure placental transfusion. The original time and gravity benefits in terms of volume of transfusion were described by Yao and colleagues in the late 1960s.[45] There are however some methodological concerns regarding these studies; in particular, they were performed only in vaginally born infants. Others have repeated this work using various methods of blood volume measurement and seen similar results.[59]

Position/Gravity

Intuitively, placing the infant below the level of the placenta should induce a gravity-based placental transfusion; however, there are a number of important caveats to this. The physiologic rationale for this is discussed earlier, but from a clinical viewpoint there has only been a single study addressing the relative position of the baby to the placenta and the effect on placental transfusion.[39] In this multicenter randomized controlled trial in 546 term healthy infants born vaginally, infants were weighed immediately at birth, then randomized to be held for 2 minutes at the level of the vaginal introitus or on the mother's abdomen or chest, the umbilical cord was then clamped and the infant reweighed. The main finding was that *both* groups of infants had a significant weight gain (56 vs. 53 g), equivalent to about a 50-mL transfusion. A difference in birthweight between early (60 seconds) and delayed cord clamp groups has been noted previously—with an average weight gain of about 100 g in the delayed group.[60] The implication from this large clinical study is that gravity is not the main driving factor for placental transfusion and that other factors (including lung inflation and breathing) may be more important. A recent study in preterm lambs, born by cesarean section, where a 10-cm change in height above/below the placenta was combined with the effect of initiation of ventilation prior to UCC, demonstrated that changing the body position had minimal and only transient effects on umbilical and cerebral blood flow, with no change in net blood volume recorded.[33]

Contractions/Oxytocics

The role of uterine contraction and the timing of oxytocic in relation to cord clamping time is surprisingly poorly studied. A single large clinical study did report the use of oxytocin with a univariate relationship between early (first minute) oxytocic and weight difference at 2 minutes, but once adjusted in a multivariate linear regression model, which included center, found no difference.[39] In an animal model, early oxytocin administration prior to clamping the cord resulted in a rapid decline in umbilical artery and vein blood flow and partly negated the benefits of delayed UCC seen in this model (manuscript submitted for publication). It was concluded that delaying oxytocin until after cord clamping would be optimal, if safe to do so. Clinical studies addressing the timing of oxytocic and cord clamping are under way.

Mode of Delivery

Several clinical studies have noted a difference between the amount of placental transfusion and change in hemoglobin level seen in elective cesarean delivery versus vaginal delivery.[46,59] The fundamental difference between vaginal delivery versus cesarean delivery is that the uterus is incised to deliver the infant and so the consequences of uterine contractions on the infant and placenta during delivery are mostly absent. While the role of uterine contractions enhancing placental transfusion is a convenient explanation, it is not supported by the science/physiology (see above). The novel concept that placental transfusion may actually be a homeostatic restoration of blood volume following fetal blood loss into the placenta during labor/delivery may also explain differences in mode of delivery. That is, the volume of placental transfusion is consistently greater following vaginal birth (i.e., following labor) than delivery via cesarean section without labor.[46,59] This may simply reflect the fact that vaginally delivered infants, who have all experienced labor and uterine contractions, lose more blood into the placenta during the labor and delivery process. Consequently, active transfer of blood via UCM may be more efficient at improving hemodynamic outcomes in cesarean section infants, although at the expense of other potential complications (see above and Chapter 5).

Umbilical Blood Vessel Patency

The equal flow of blood from fetus to placenta relies on both the umbilical artery and umbilical vein being patent. A cessation of flow in one of these vessels may result in differential transfer of blood from one side to the other. Studies examining blood flow in umbilical vessels during the third stage are few, although an early study has assessed flow indirectly,[44] whereas a more recent study[38] has measured flow in real time. The clinical study of 62 normal term deliveries by Yao and Lind[44] measured placental residual volume as the index of placental transfusion and compared clamping all blood vessels versus clamping arteries or veins differentially to estimate flow. They concluded that arterial flow was maintained for about 40 seconds after birth while umbilical venous flow continued for about 3 minutes and was influenced by uterine contractions. However, there are serious limitations with this study as they did not measure actual flow, but measured placental residual volumes, and compared these to expected volumes (from previous studies) to determine if there had been umbilical artery or venous flow.

Up until recently, the assumed net placental-to-infant transfusion has been measured indirectly: by measuring infant weight change,[39] placental residual volume,[45] or by measuring the change in total blood volume.[59] While the study of Yao and Lind suggested that umbilical arterial flow ceases within 30 to 40 seconds after birth,[44] no real explanation was provided as to how this could occur. It is also not consistent with the observations from commonly performed fetal surgery and the ExUtero intrapartum treatment (EXIT) procedure, which have demonstrated that if the fetal state is maintained, then umbilical arterial flow continues. Other physiologic events such as breathing and crying, as well as differential constriction of umbilical arteries and veins, may affect the volume of blood transfused. A recent clinical study by Boere et al. used Doppler ultrasound to measure umbilical blood flow and direction of flow in normally transitioning term infants who had their cord clamped at a time point determined by the midwife.[38] This study demonstrated that up to one third of babies still had umbilical venous flow when the cord was clamped (mean 05:13 minutes; 02:56 to 09:15) and 43% of infants had umbilical arterial flow at cord clamp time (mean 05:16 minutes; 03:32 to 10:10). Most importantly they found that flow ceased in the umbilical vein before the umbilical artery in over 50% of infants. Significant perturbations of blood flow were seen with breathing and crying; in particular, stopping or reversal of flow was often observed with crying and forced expirations.

Breathing/Crying

The effects of breathing and/or crying on the transitional circulation were reviewed earlier in this chapter. In addition to the direct effects on umbilical blood flow of crying and breathing seen in the study described earlier,[38] there is also a study from the 1960s which demonstrates the relationship of the onset of breathing to a change in residual placental volume.[61] In this study, normal-term infants who established respirations 10 seconds or more before UCC had less placental residual volume and by implication received more blood back from the placenta. The authors concluded that: "During delivery, cord-clamping should be delayed until spontaneous or induced breathing has begun."

Prevention of Hypotension/Low Systemic Blood Flow

An important beneficial mechanism strongly associated with delayed cord clamping is the prevention of low systemic blood flow and/or hypotension. The transitional circulation, particularly in very low birth weight (VLBW) infants, is vulnerable to impairment (see Chapter 1). The preterm myocardium is poorly adapted to the postnatal increase in systemic vascular resistance, the transitional circulation is affected by systemic to pulmonary shunts that move blood out of the systemic circulation, preload is affected by positive-pressure respiratory support, and the infant may be relatively hypovolemic due to failure of restoration of blood volume following labor and delivery as discussed earlier. All of these factors lead to a low-cardiac-output hemodynamic state that is associated with adverse outcomes such as cerebral injury including periventricular or intraventricular hemorrhage (P/IVH) and periventricular leukomalacia (PVL)[56] (see Chapters 6 and 26). Diagnosis of low cardiac output is not uniformly possible by simply measuring blood pressure,[62] and other measures of cardiovascular adequacy such as capillary refill time or lactic acidosis are more nonspecific in these patients.[63] The measure of superior vena cava (SVC) flow was first described over 15 years ago and has been correlated with both short- and long-term adverse events (see Chapter 11).[56,57] It is designed to be measurable in the transitional setting where other cardiac output measures such as the ventricular outputs are likely to be affected by the fetal shunts. It is therefore a useful measure to assess adequacy of systemic blood flow in a transitioning preterm infant. As such, SVC flow has been used as an outcome in a number of cord clamping time studies. Initially these were small observational or practice change studies, but more recently, results of larger randomized control studies have been published (Table 4.1).

Meyer et al. were the first to recognize an association between later clamping of the cord (30 to 45 seconds) and improved SVC flow in a small retrospective cohort study.[54] Subsequently, similar findings with improved SVC flow in the delayed clamping arm of a randomized control trial of immediate versus delayed (45 seconds) cord clamping in a group of less than 32 weeks' gestation infants were demonstrated.[55] More recently, UCM has also been shown to improve SVC flow (see Chapter 5).[64,65] The largest study to date of SVC flow in the setting of immediate versus delayed (60 seconds) cord clamping was published recently.[66] This trial demonstrated that there was no difference in SVC flow in a group of 266 infants less than 30 weeks' gestation randomized into the two arms, even though there was a small increase in the hematocrit in the delayed arm group. Additionally, the right ventricular output was found to be lower in the delayed arm, which may have reflected a higher hematocrit or an attenuated reduction in PVR with an adaptation of the cardiac output to the required oxygen carrying capacity. The causes of the discrepancy between the findings of the previous smaller studies and this study are unclear and

Table 4.1 SUMMARY OF STUDIES OF SYSTEMIC BLOOD FLOW CHANGES AFTER DIFFERENT TYPES OF UMBILICAL CORD MANAGEMENT

Study	N	Mean GA Weeks	Intervention	ICC Flow (mL/kg/min)	DCC/UCM Flow (mL/kg/min)	Age (h)
Meyer and Mildenhall, 2012[54]	30	26	DCC 30–40 s	52 (42–100)	91 (81–101)[a]	16
Sommers et al., 2012[55]	51	28	DCC 41 s versus 5 s	89 ± 24	112 ± 30[a]	6
Katheria et al., 2014[35]	28	<29	Intact UCM	66 ± 18	98 ± 27[a]	5
Popat et al., 2016[66]	266	28	DCC 60 s	92 ± 35	95 ± 41	3–6
Katheria et al., 2016[67]	125	28	DCC versus VDCC	86 ± 32[b]	83 ± 26[c]	<12

[a]P < .05 compared to ICC.
[b]Values for LSCS/DCC of 60 seconds.
[c]Values for LSCS/DCC and ventilation.
DCC, Delayed cord clamping; *GA,* gestational age; *ICC,* immediate cord clamping; *LSCS,* lower segment cesarean section; *UCM,* umbilical cord milking; *VDCC,* ventilated DCC.

the full results of the outcomes of this latter study, including neurodevelopment at 2 years of age, are awaited to allow correlation with the hemodynamic findings.

Low SVC flow has been associated with an increased incidence of P/IVH,[56] so prevention of low SVC flow by delayed cord clamping may be at least a partial reason as to why the systematic reviews of the outcomes of delayed cord clamping in preterm infants show a reduction in severe grade P/IVH.[52]

Less Intervention at Birth: Resuscitation Versus Transitioning

One of the unexpected outcomes of the introduction of deferral of the cord clamping time is the observation that many babies, including the smallest and most immature, have the opportunity to establish spontaneous breathing, while still supported by the placental circulation. A recent randomized trial of resuscitation with an intact cord[67] demonstrated that up to 90% of infants less than 32 weeks' gestation were able to establish breathing prior to clamping the cord at 60 seconds. Other trials of the frequency of small infants establishing breathing have also shown that up to 80% of extremely preterm infants spontaneously breathe at birth if left to transition spontaneously.[68] Spontaneous breathing has many advantages including making resuscitation easier, opening the glottis, and allowing transition to commence while the infant is still attached to the placenta. Other potential hemodynamic advantages include avoiding significant mechanical ventilation which has been closely associated with impairment of the cardiovascular system.[69] A large prospective observational study of a delay in cord clamping of 30 to 45 seconds versus 60 to 75 seconds showed that infants born during the period of the longer delay in cord clamping were *less likely to require delivery room intubation or in fact any intubation.*[70] Involvement in trials of deferral of cord clamping has led many neonatologists to reconsider the role of resuscitation—which often entails intervention with subsequent regression in transition process (suction, masks, positive pressure breaths) versus that of waiting and supporting the infant's transition. The fact that the newborn is still attached to the placenta and (assuming placental blood flow is still intact) receiving warmed, oxygenated blood makes waiting for transition to happen spontaneously potentially a more acceptable option. Trials to assess the validity of this approach are under way.[67,71]

Physiologically Based Cord Clamping

As with many things in medicine, the concept of arbitrarily picking a time interval to apply to a physiologic process such as time of cord clamping (45 seconds, 60 seconds, 3 minutes) is problematic. As discussed in this review, there are many factors to consider—immaturity, degree of prenatal asphyxia, distribution of the fetal-placental blood, position, uterine contractions and mode of delivery, facilitating the transition (breathing first, clamp later), or inhibiting the transition by intervention. There will not be a single time interval that suits all of these situations and consequently maximizes the cardiorespiratory outcomes of the given preterm infant. Research priorities should include trying to find ways to assess the progress of transition in real time. These may involve more accurate scales to measure change in weight due to blood redistribution, direct measurement of blood flow in umbilical vessels by Doppler ultrasound, or measuring other physiologic factors such as end-tidal carbon dioxide levels. Thus we have coined the term *physiologically based cord clamping* to underscore the importance of taking into account the stages in the cardiorespiratory transition and timing cord clamping to fit with the transition of an individual infant.

Conclusions

The act of early clamping of the umbilical cord (usually within 15 to 20 seconds) is probably the most frequently performed medical procedure since the 1950s. The procedure was introduced into obstetric care with no clinical trial and little understanding of the physiologic effects that it might have in term and particularly preterm infants. It is only in the past 5 to 10 years that the physiologic rationale and an understanding of the potential benefits of waiting before cord clamping have emerged. This has been led by a group of clinicians and midwives documenting the clinical benefits of deferral of clamping and by a group of scientists using physiology and an animal model to understand the physiologic consequences of early clamping—similar to the backgrounds of the authors of this chapter—one a physiologist, the other a neonatologist. Understanding the complex cardiorespiratory physiology of the transition has been key to this discussion. The findings of the largest RCT of early vs late cord clamping to date[72] and an updated systematic review[73] support the notion that a delay in clamping of the umbilical cord can reduce mortality in preterm infants without harm to either mother or baby. The importance of the respiratory transition (airway liquid absorption, lung aeration, and increase in PBF) and its very close relationship to the cardiovascular transition (left ventricle preload, maintenance of cardiac output, and stabilization of a potentially labile circulation) has been increasingly understood. New concepts discussed here include that of placental volume restoration, rather than placental transfusion, and the importance of a physiologic end point to determine when to clamp the umbilical cord rather than an arbitrary time point. Along the way, much has been learned about very preterm infants and what they are capable of, if left to transition on their own, while still supported by a placental circulation. The iatrogenic insults of suction, inadvertent airway occlusion by mask in a spontaneously breathing infant, and mechanical ventilation with the significant change in physiology that it entails have been increasingly under the spotlight as we understand the normal transition and what is required to support even our tiniest babies through this. Although there are neonates, especially among the very preterm, that will still require resuscitation in the traditional sense, most neonates appear to do better if supported in commencing the transition to extrauterine life with the umbilical cord unclamped.

REFERENCES

1. Hooper SB, Polglase GR, te Pas AB: A physiological approach to the timing of umbilical cord clamping at birth, *Arch Dis Child Fetal Neonatal Ed* 100(4):F355–F360, 2015.
2. Hooper SB, Te Pas AB, Kitchen MJ: Respiratory transition in the newborn: a three-phase process, *Arch Dis Child Fetal Neonatal Ed* 101(3):F266–F271, 2016.
3. Hooper SB, Te Pas AB, Lang J, et al.: Cardiovascular transition at birth: a physiological sequence, *Pediatr Res* 77(5):608–614, 2015.
4. Bhatt S, Alison BJ, Wallace EM, et al.: Delaying cord clamping until ventilation onset improves cardiovascular function at birth in preterm lambs, *J Physiol* 591(Pt 8):2113–2126, 2013.
5. Crossley KJ, Allison BJ, Polglase GR, et al.: Dynamic changes in the direction of blood flow through the ductus arteriosus at birth, *J Physiol* 587(Pt 19):4695–4704, 2009.
6. Rudolph AM: Fetal and neonatal pulmonary circulation, *Annu Rev Physiol* 41:383–395, 1979.
7. Harding R, Hooper SB: Regulation of lung expansion and lung growth before birth, *J Appl Physiol (1985)* 81(1):209–224, 1996.
8. Hooper SB, Harding R: Fetal lung liquid: a major determinant of the growth and functional development of the fetal lung, *Clin Exp Pharmacol Physiol* 22:235–247, 1995.
9. Jain L, Dudell GG: Respiratory transition in infants delivered by cesarean section, *Semin Perinatol* 30(5):296–304, 2006.
10. Jobe AH: The new bronchopulmonary dysplasia, *Curr Opin Pediatr* 23(2):167–172, 2011.
11. Olver RE, Walters DV, S MW: Developmental regulation of lung liquid transport, *Annu Rev Physiol* 66:77–101, 2004.
12. Hooper SB, Kitchen MJ, Wallace MJ, et al.: Imaging lung aeration and lung liquid clearance at birth, *FASEB J* 21:3329–3337, 2007.
13. Siew ML, Wallace MJ, Kitchen MJ, et al.: Inspiration regulates the rate and temporal pattern of lung liquid clearance and lung aeration at birth, *J Appl Physiol* 106(6):1888–1895, 2009.
14. Harding R, Hooper SB, Dickson KA: A mechanism leading to reduced lung expansion and lung hypoplasia in fetal sheep during oligohydramnios, *Am J Obstet Gynecol* 163(6 Pt 1):1904–1913, 1990.
15. Albuquerque CA, Smith KR, Saywers TE, et al.: Relation between oligohydramnios and spinal flexion in the human fetus, *Early Hum Dev* 68(2):119–126, 2002.
16. Olver RE, Ramsden CA, Strang LB, et al.: The role of amiloride-blockable sodium transport in adrenaline-induced lung liquid reabsorption in the fetal lamb, *J Physiol* 376:321–340, 1986.
17. Kitchen MJ, Siew ML, Wallace MJ, et al.: Changes in positive end-expiratory pressure alter the distribution of ventilation within the lung immediately after birth in newborn rabbits, *PLoS ONE* 9(4):e93391, 2014.
18. te Pas AB, Siew M, Wallace MJ, et al.: Effect of sustained inflation length on establishing functional residual capacity at birth in ventilated premature rabbits, *Pediatr Res* 66(3):295–300, 2009.
19. Siew ML, Te Pas AB, Wallace MJ, et al.: Positive end-expiratory pressure enhances development of a functional residual capacity in preterm rabbits ventilated from birth, *J Appl Physiol (1985)* 106(5):1487–1493, 2009.

20. te Pas AB, Siew M, Wallace MJ, et al.: Establishing functional residual capacity at birth: the effect of sustained inflation and positive end-expiratory pressure in a preterm rabbit model, *Pediatr Res* 65(5):537–541, 2009.

21. Siew ML, Wallace MJ, Allison BJ, et al.: The role of lung inflation and sodium transport in airway liquid clearance during lung aeration in newborn rabbits, *Pediatr Res* 73(4 Pt 1):443–449, 2013.

22. Gao Y, Raj JU: Regulation of the pulmonary circulation in the fetus and newborn, *Physiol Rev* 90(4):1291–1335, 2010.

23. Lang JA, Pearson JT, Te Pas AB, et al.: Ventilation/perfusion mismatch during lung aeration at birth, *J Appl Physiol* 117(5):535–543, 2014.

24. Lang JA, Pearson JT, Binder-Heschl C, et al.: Increase in pulmonary blood flow at birth: role of oxygen and lung aeration, *J Physiol* 594(5):1389–1398, 2016.

25. Teitel DF, Iwamoto HS, Rudolph AM: Changes in the pulmonary circulation during birth-related events, *Pediatr Res* 27(4):372–378, 1990.

26. Sobotka KS, Hooper SB, Allison BJ, et al.: An initial sustained inflation improves the respiratory and cardiovascular transition at birth in preterm lambs, *Pediatr Res* 70(1):56–60, 2011.

27. Lang JA, Pearson JT, Binder-Heschl C, et al.: Vagal denervation inhibits the increase in pulmonary blood flow during partial lung aeration at birth, *J Physiol* 595(5):1593–1606, 2017.

28. Siew ML, Te Pas AB, Wallace MJ, et al.: Surfactant increases the uniformity of lung aeration at birth in ventilated preterm rabbits, *Pediatr Res* 70(1):50–55, 2011.

29. Bhatt S, Polglase GR, Wallace EM, et al.: Ventilation before umbilical cord clamping improves the physiological transition at birth, *Front Pediatr* 2:113, 2014.

30. Cohn HE, Sacks EJ, Heymann MA, et al.: Cardiovascular responses to hypoxemia and acidemia in fetal lambs, *Am J Obstet Gynecol* 120(6):817–824, 1974.

31. Dawes GS, Mott JC, Widdicombe JG: Closure of the foramen ovale in newborn lambs, *J Physiol* 128(2):384–395, 1955.

32. Evans N, Iyer P: Incompetence of the foramen ovale in preterm infants supported by mechanical ventilation, *J Pediatr* 125(5 Pt 1):786–792, 1994.

33. Hooper SB, Crossley KJ, Zahra VA, et al.: Effect of body position and ventilation on umbilical artery and venous blood flows during delayed umbilical cord clamping in preterm lambs, *Arch Dis Child Fetal Neonatal Ed* 2016.

34. Mercer JS, Erickson-Owens DA: Rethinking placental transfusion and cord clamping issues, *J Perinat Neonatal Nurs* 26(3):202–217, 2012. quiz 218–219.

35. Katheria AC, Leone TA, Woelkers D, et al.: The effects of umbilical cord milking on hemodynamics and neonatal outcomes in premature neonates, *J Pediatr* 164(5):1045.e1–1050.e1, 2014.

36. Blank D, Polglase GR, Kluckow M, et al.: Physiologic based cord clamping improves hemodynamic stability vs umbilical cord milking in preterm newborn lambs, *Pediatr Acad Soc* 2016.

37. Blank D, Polglase GR, Kluckow M, et al.: Comparison of umbilical cord milking techniques in preterm lambs, *Pediatr Acad Soc* 2016.

38. Boere I, Roest AA, Wallace E, et al.: Umbilical blood flow patterns directly after birth before delayed cord clamping, *Arch Dis Child Fetal Neonatal Ed* 2014.

39. Vain NE, Satragno DS, Gorenstein AN, et al.: Effect of gravity on volume of placental transfusion: a multicentre, randomised, non-inferiority trial, *Lancet* 384(9939):235–240, 2014.

40. Yao AC, Hirvensalo M, Lind J: Placental transfusion-rate and uterine contraction, *Lancet* 1(7539):380–383, 1968.

41. Westgate JA, Wibbens B, Bennet L, et al.: The intrapartum deceleration in center stage: a physiologic approach to the interpretation of fetal heart rate changes in labor, *Am J Obstet Gynecol* 197(3):236. e231–e211, 2007.

42. Walker AM, Alcorn DG, Cannata JC, et al.: Effect of ventilation on pulmonary blood volume of the fetal lamb, *J Appl Physiol* 39(6):969–975, 1975.

43. Yao AC, Lind J: Effect of gravity on placental transfusion, *Lancet* 2(7619):505–508, 1969.

44. Yao AC, Lind J: Blood flow in the umbilical vessels during the third stage of labor, *Biol Neonate* 25(3-4):186–193, 1974.

45. Yao AC, Moinian M, Lind J: Distribution of blood between infant and placenta after birth, *Lancet* 2(7626):871–873, 1969.

46. Katheria AC, Truong G, Cousins L, et al.: Umbilical cord milking versus delayed cord clamping in preterm infants, *Pediatrics* 136(1):61–69, 2015.

47. Verbeek L, Zhao DP, Middeldorp JM, et al.: Haemoglobin discordances in twins: due to differences in timing of cord clamping? *Arch Dis Child Fetal Neonatal Ed* 2016.

48. Verbeek L, Zhao DP, Te Pas AB, et al.: Hemoglobin differences in uncomplicated monochorionic twins in relation to birth order and mode of delivery, *Twin Res Hum Genet* 19(3):241–245, 2016.

49. McDonald SJ, Middleton P, Dowswell T, et al.: Cochrane in context: effect of timing of umbilical cord clamping in term infants on maternal and neonatal outcomes, *Evid Based Child Health* 9(2):398–400, 2014.

50. McDonald SJ, Middleton P, Dowswell T, et al.: Effect of timing of umbilical cord clamping of term infants on maternal and neonatal outcomes, *Cochrane Database Syst Rev* 7:CD004074, 2013.

51. Gupta R, Ramji S: Effect of delayed cord clamping on iron stores in infants born to anemic mothers: a randomized controlled trial, *Indian Pediatr* 39(2):130–135, 2002.

52. Rabe H, Diaz-Rossello JL, Duley L, et al.: Effect of timing of umbilical cord clamping and other strategies to influence placental transfusion at preterm birth on maternal and infant outcomes, *Cochrane Database Syst Rev* 8:CD003248, 2012.

53. Ghavam S, Batra D, Mercer J, et al.: Effects of placental transfusion in extremely low birthweight infants: meta-analysis of long- and short-term outcomes, *Transfusion (Paris)* 54(4):1192–1198, 2014.

54. Meyer MP, Mildenhall L: Delayed cord clamping and blood flow in the superior vena cava in preterm infants: an observational study, *Arch Dis Child Fetal Neonatal Ed* 97(6):F484–F486, 2012.
55. Sommers R, Stonestreet BS, Oh W, et al.: Hemodynamic effects of delayed cord clamping in premature infants, *Pediatrics* 129(3):e667–e672, 2012.
56. Kluckow M, Evans N: Low superior vena cava flow and intraventricular haemorrhage in preterm infants, *Arch Dis Child Fetal Neonatal Ed* 82:188–194, 2000.
57. Hunt RW, Evans N, Rieger I, et al.: Low superior vena cava flow and neurodevelopment at 3 years in very preterm infants, *J Pediatr* 145(5):588–592, 2004.
58. Hooper SB, Binder-Heschl C, Polglase GR, et al.: The timing of umbilical cord clamping at birth: physiological considerations, *Matern Health Neonatol Perinatol* 2:4, 2016.
59. Aladangady N, McHugh S, Aitchison TC, et al.: Infants' blood volume in a controlled trial of placental transfusion at preterm delivery, *Pediatrics* 117(1):93–98, 2006.
60. McDonald SJ, Middleton P, Dowswell T, et al.: Effect of timing of umbilical cord clamping of term infants on maternal and neonatal outcomes, *Evid Based Child Health* 9(2):303–397, 2014.
61. Redmond A, Isana S, Ingall D: Relation of onset of respiration to placental transfusion, *Lancet* 1(7380):283–285, 1965.
62. Kluckow M, Evans N: Relationship between blood pressure and cardiac output in preterm infants requiring mechanical ventilation, *J Pediatr* 129(4):506–512, 1996.
63. Osborn DA, Evans N, Kluckow M: Clinical detection of low upper body blood flow in very premature infants using blood pressure, capillary refill time, and central-peripheral temperature difference, *Arch Dis Child Fetal Neonatal Ed* 89(2):F168–F173, 2004.
64. Katheria A, Blank D, Rich W, et al.: Umbilical cord milking improves transition in premature infants at birth, *PLoS ONE* 9(4):e94085, 2014.
65. Takami T, Suganami Y, Sunohara D, et al.: Umbilical cord milking stabilizes cerebral oxygenation and perfusion in infants born before 29 weeks of gestation, *J Pediatr* 161(4):742–747, 2012.
66. Popat H, Robledo KP, Sebastian L, et al.: Effect of delayed cord clamping on systemic blood flow: a randomized controlled trial, *J Pediatr* 178:81.e2–86.e2, 2016.
67. Katheria A, Poeltler D, Durham J, et al.: Neonatal resuscitation with an intact cord: a randomized clinical trial, *J Pediatr* 178:75.e3–80.e3, 2016.
68. O'Donnell CP, Kamlin CO, Davis PG, et al.: Crying and breathing by extremely preterm infants immediately after birth, *J Pediatr* 156(5):846–847, 2010.
69. Evans N, Kluckow M: Early determinants of right and left ventricular output in ventilated preterm infants, *Arch Dis Child Fetal Neonatal Ed* 74(2):F88–F94, 1996.
70. Song D, Jegatheesan P, DeSandre G, et al.: Duration of cord clamping and neonatal outcomes in very preterm infants, *PLoS ONE* 10(9):e0138829, 2015.
71. Winter J, Kattwinkel J, Chisholm C, et al.: Ventilation of preterm infants during delayed cord clamping (ventFirst): a pilot study of feasibility and safety, *Am J Perinatol* 34(2):111–116, 2017.
72. Tarnow-Mordi W, Morris J, Kirby A, for the Australian Placental Transfusion Study Collaborative Group: delayed versus immediate cord clamping in preterm infants, *N Engl J Med* Oct 29, 2017. doi: 10.1056/NEJMoa1711281.
73. Fogarty M, Osborn D, Askie L, et al.: Delayed versus early umbilical cord clamping for preterm Infants: a systematic review and meta-analysis, *Am J Obstet Gynecol* 2017. doi: 10.1016/j.ajog.2017.10.231.

CHAPTER 5

Hemodynamic Significance and Clinical Relevance of Delayed Cord Clamping and Umbilical Cord Milking

Anup C. Katheria and Douglas Blank

- Both delayed cord clamping and umbilical cord milking provide a placental transfusion at birth.
- An important benefit aside from volume may be the stabilization of the transitional circulation.
- There is a good physiologic rationale for delaying umbilical cord clamping until after the infant begins to breathe.
- Umbilical cord milking may be superior at providing a placental transfusion at cesarean section and may provide a transfusion more quickly in nonbreathing infants but this needs more study.

Delayed cord clamping (DCC) and umbilical cord milking (UCM) are two techniques that provide placental transfusion to the newborn infant. Increasing fetal hemoglobin and blood volume by placental transfusion is an extremely effective method of enhancing arterial oxygen content, increasing cardiac output, and improving oxygen delivery to the tissues. Placental transfusion is the transfer of residual placental blood to the infant during the first few minutes after delivery. DCC is the practice of waiting to clamp the umbilical cord after birth for at least 30 seconds or longer. Studies have shown that DCC benefits in preterm infants including improved hemodynamics, less blood transfusions, lower rates of intraventricular hemorrhage, and necrotizing enterocolitis, as well as improved motor function at 18 to 22 months of age.[1–3] Term infants receiving DCC have higher hemoglobin levels at 24 hours after birth and improved iron stores at 3 to 6 months without an increase in reported maternal morbidities.[4] In resource-limited settings, there is observational evidence to suggest that mortality is reduced if umbilical cord clamping (UCC) occurs after the initiation of spontaneous respiration.[5] International recommendations advocate for a delay in UCC for 30 seconds to more than 60 seconds after birth if the infant is vigorous.[6–10]

It is primarily believed that, after delivery, the major recipient of placental blood is the pulmonary bed. Normally, as the infant initiates spontaneous breathing and establishes lung aeration, the pulmonary blood vessels dilate and the infant will draw blood from the placenta into the dilated pulmonary blood vessels.[1,2,11,12] If infants do not breathe at birth, guidelines recommend immediately clamping the umbilical cord and moving the infant to a resuscitation platform in order to provide positive pressure ventilation (PPV).[13–15] In the largest randomized clinical trial investigating delivery room respiratory support in infants less than 29 weeks' gestation at birth, over 60% received PPV. This outcome suggested that many infants would receive immediate cord clamping prior to inflation of the lungs.[16]

UCM is a procedure in which the clinician milks or pushes the blood in the umbilical cord from the placenta to the infant. There are two established techniques of UCM that have been described in the literature. One method is "intact umbilical cord milking." In this technique, the clinician milks 20 cm of the umbilical cord over 1 to 2 seconds, and releases the umbilical cord after each milk to allow the cord to refill with blood. This process is repeated 2 to 4 times prior to UCC.[17–22] Another UCM technique, called "cut-umbilical cord milking," is clamping the umbilical cord close to the placenta and milking the residual volume of blood in the umbilical cord after cord clamping.[3,23–25] Due to insufficient evidence, international recommendations currently discourage the use of UCM outside of clinical studies.[6–10]

The primary advantage of UCM over DCC is the rapid blood transfer from the placenta to the infant immediately after birth without interfering with the evaluation and the resuscitation of the newborn. In several trials, authors have concluded that UCM appears to confer the same benefits as DCC.[1,18–20,26,27] In addition, UCM may be a more effective method to transfer blood during cesarean deliveries because the uterus is not vigorously contracting.[20]

In this chapter, we will review the relevant literature regarding the effects of DCC and UCM in the delivery room on hemodynamics measurements in the first hours after birth, and on blood volume measurements. Finally, we will discuss outstanding questions and future directions of DCC and UCM.

Transitional Physiology and Animal Studies of Delayed Cord Clamping and Umbilical Cord Milking

Human studies have a limited ability to accurately measure physiologic changes immediately after delivery. Animal models can use invasive monitoring prior to delivery to study the effects of umbilical cord management strategies, specifically to understand the effects on cerebral and pulmonary blood flow.

In the fetal phase, the placenta performs the function of gas exchange, providing the fetus with oxygen and eliminating carbon dioxide. The lungs are filled with liquid secreted by the lungs and pulmonary blood flow is low. The umbilical circulation, via the umbilical vein, ductus venosus, and foramen ovale, provides the majority of blood flow to the left ventricle. The placental circulation is a low-resistance pathway that receives up to 50% of the fetal cardiac output. UCC dramatically affects the neonatal circulation by increasing peripheral resistance (afterload), as the low resistance placenta pathway is removed, and by the loss of umbilical venous supply to the left ventricle (preload). As the infant initiates breathing and the lungs aerate, pulmonary blood flow increases, replacing the umbilical venous flow to supply the left ventricle and providing adequate preload. In theory, increasing pulmonary blood flow and ensuring a pathway for a sustained left ventricular preload *before* UCC would better prepare the infant for the hemodynamic changes of UCC (Fig. 5.1).[28,29]

Animal models have shown benefits of initiating ventilation to increase pulmonary blood flow prior to UCC in preterm, anesthetized newborn lambs.[30,31] Newborn lambs at 126 days' gestational age (equivalent to ~26 weeks in humans) with UCC prior to ventilation had dangerous swings in cerebral blood flow, arterial blood pressure, heart rate, and cerebral oxygenation. Lambs that received ventilation prior to UCC had a much smoother transition to ex utero life, including attenuated changes in cerebral perfusion and blood pressure and increased levels of oxygenation. A major limitation is that the fetal lambs in these studies were under anesthesia and paralyzed without the ability to breathe spontaneously. In addition, lambs had their lung fluid drained and in some cases received a 20-second sustained inflation breath prior to being placed on a ventilator. Whereas this model provides important information regarding hemodynamics during placental transfusion, the model does not provide answers in regards to whether ventilation is beneficial or even required during DCC in premature newborns.

Human studies have suggested that gravity affects the amount of placental transfusion at vaginal birth.[32] Holding the neonate high above the placenta (head 40 to 60 cm above) decreases placental transfusion similar to immediate cord clamping (ICC).

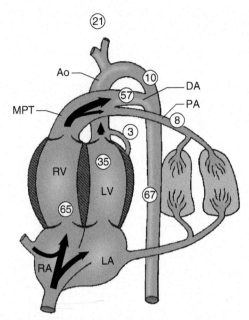

Fig. 5.1 Diagram of the fetal heart showing the percentages of combined ventricular output ejected by each ventricle and traversing the major vascular pathways. *Ao,* Aorta; *DA,* ductus arteriosus; *LA,* left atrium; *LV,* left ventricle; *MPT,* main pulmonary trunk; *PA,* pulmonary artery; *RA,* right atrium; *RV,* right ventricle. (From Rudolph AM: Distribution and regulation of blood flow in the fetal and neonatal lamb. *Circ Res* 57(6):811–821, 1985.)

A recent study found no difference in infant weights after DCC for 2 minutes with infants placed on the maternal abdomen versus at the introitus.[33] However, total weight gain was half of what was previously found,[34,35] indicating that 2 minutes may not be enough time for a full placental transfusion for the term infant. Mercer et al. found that term infants placed on the maternal abdomen immediately after birth who were assigned to DCC for 5 minutes received a significantly larger placental transfusion than those with a 2-minute delay.[36] However, the same may not be true for cesarean section (C/S). The effect of gravity on umbilical blood flow during DCC was investigated by measuring umbilical venous and arterial blood flow using ultrasonic flow probes and biotin labeled blood to measure placental transfusion volumes in preterm fetal lambs delivered by C/S.[37] Anesthetized fetal lambs were placed 10 cm above and 10 cm below the ewe during DCC and received subsequent mechanical ventilation prior to UCC. The onset of mechanical ventilation resulted in a decrease in both umbilical venous and arterial flow. The decrease in umbilical arterial and venous blood flow was proportional; therefore the net flow of blood to the fetal lamb did not change. There was no observed increase in blood volume during the period of DCC, therefore no placental transfusion was detected. In addition, the position of the fetal lamb in relation to the ewe did not affect the net flow of umbilical blood to the fetal lamb. Further animal studies are needed to explore physiologic changes during spontaneous breathing after birth and vaginal delivery.

Improved physiologic stability may play an important role in the benefits of DCC observed following C/S. In the animal model described earlier, ventilation prior to UCC increased pulmonary blood flow and resulted in less fluctuations in blood pressure, cerebral blood flow, and cerebral oxygenation; however, significant placental transfusion resulting in increased blood volume was not observed (Fig. 5.2). A possible explanation for these findings is the lack of spontaneous breathing in the anesthetized animals. Spontaneous breathing is commonly observed after delivery even in the most premature human infants. It may also stimulate placental transfusion by opening pulmonary capillary beds.[38] In a recent trial of premature infants randomized to assisted ventilation or tactile stimulation there was no difference in resuscitation interventions, transitional hemodynamics, or neonatal outcomes.[38] However, over 90% of premature infants had spontaneous ventilation whether they were provided with tactile stimulation alone or

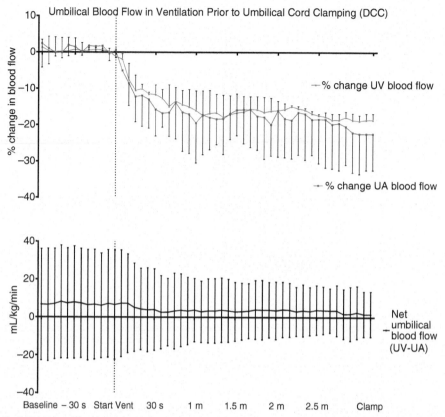

Fig. 5.2 Umbilical blood flow measured during ventilation prior to umbilical cord clamping in anesthetized preterm lambs. Umbilical venous and umbilical arterial blood flow were significantly reduced after initiation of ventilation ($P < .001$). However, net umbilical blood flow did not change during this time ($P = .99$), resulting in no placental transfusion. *UA,* Umbilical artery; *UV,* umbilical vein. (From Blank DA, Polglase GR, Kluckow M, et al.: Haemodynamic effects of umbilical cord milking in premature sheep during neonatal transition. *Arch Dis Child Fetal Neonatal Ed* Dec 5, 2017. doi 10.1136/archdischild-2017-314005.)

assisted ventilation (Fig. 5.3). It may be that a mechanism of benefit of DCC is allowing time for spontaneous breathing prior to the clamping of the cord and thus, by maintaining left ventricular preload, ensuring an unperturbed hemodynamic transition. Further clinical trials are needed to better determine whether assisted ventilation (with continuous positive airway pressure [CPAP] and positive pressure ventilation [PPV]) provides benefit during a placental transfusion.

Cardiovascular Effects of Delayed Cord Clamping and Umbilical Cord Milking in the Delivery Room

Despite the difficulties in obtaining accurate physiologic data immediately after birth of human infants, there are a few studies which have investigated the cardiovascular adaptation in newborns during DCC. In a cohort of healthy term, vaginally-delivered infants, arterial and venous umbilical blood flow was measured using Doppler ultrasound starting 30 seconds after birth until the umbilical cord was clamped.[39] Several different patterns of umbilical cord blood flow were observed, emphasizing that the physiology of umbilical cord blood flow is complex. The initiation of breathing appeared to promote venous flow to the newborn; however, crying often caused a reversal of flow. Arterial blood flow was observed to continue after umbilical cord pulsations ceased and umbilical arterial and venous blood flow often stopped at different times. The potential volume of the placental transfusion is increased if there is differential constriction of the umbilical arteries prior to the umbilical vein.[40] In another cohort of healthy term infants, continuously monitored cardiac output was measured via electrical impedance during DCC starting 90 seconds after birth. Every minute of postnatal life that the cord

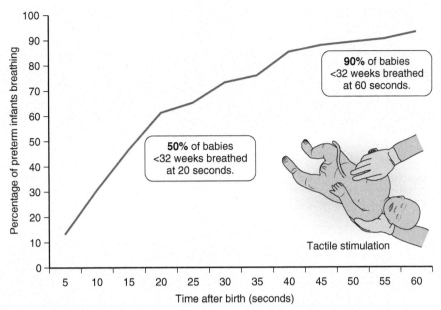

Fig. 5.3 Number of infants breathing at different time points with stimulation during delayed cord clamping. (Modified from Katheria AC, Lakshminrusimha S, Rabe H, McAdams R, Mercer JS. Placental transfusion: a review. *J Perinatol* 178:75–80, 2016, drawing by S. Lakshminrusimha.)

Table 5.1 HEART RATE COMPARISONS IN STUDIES COMPARING IMMEDIATE CORD CLAMPING AND DELAYED CORD CLAMPING. THE EXPECTED HEART RATE RANGE FOR INFANTS WHO BREATHE SPONTANEOUSLY AND RECEIVED IMMEDIATE CORD CLAMPING IS FROM DAWSON ET AL.[74]

Study	N	Time of Cord Clamping (s)	GA or BW	HR@1 min, BPM	SpO$_2$@ 1 min, %
Dawson, 2010[74,75]	468	<20	38 weeks (25–42)	96 (65–127)	66 (55–75)
Linde, 2016[76a]	55	44 (29–59)	3100 ± 428 g	149 ± 33	NA
Katheria, 2016[38]	150	64 ± 9	28 ± 2 weeks	115 ± 32	NA
Katheria, 2015[41]	20	318 ± 32	39 ± 1 weeks	176 ± 15	NA
Smit, 2014[77]	109	300 (180–420)	40 weeks (37–42)	61 (42–146)	78 (67–87)

[a]Gestational age was not reported in this study; heart rate reported at 40 seconds.
BW, Birth weight; *BPM,* beats per minute; *GA,* gestational age; *HR,* heart rate; *SpO$_2$,* saturation of oxygen.

was kept unclamped, the stroke volume increased and cardiac output increased 13% compared to baseline. The increase in stroke volume and cardiac output was observed even after umbilical cord pulsation ceased.[41] Again, these findings underscore the importance of allowing for a smooth change from placental to pulmonary blood flow supplying the left ventricular preload during the immediate transitional period.

In animal studies, DCC has been shown to improve oxygen saturations (SpO$_2$) and attenuate the swings in blood pressure and cerebral blood flow seen in ICC. After birth, if the infant is still connected to a functioning placenta that continues to provide gas exchange and left ventricular preload, one might expect infants with DCC to have higher heart rates and higher SpO$_2$. A few small studies have reported the heart rate and SpO$_2$ immediately after birth, in preterm and term infants who receive DCC. Compared with normative data, the studies have conflicting results of the effects of DCC (Table 5.1). Winter et al. reported all infants had a heart rate greater than 100 BPM at 60 seconds in a small pilot trial in which respiratory support could be provided during DCC in infants less than 32 weeks.[42] Finally, there is very little data on the effects of UCM on SpO$_2$ immediately after birth.

Table 5.2 COMPARISON OF ECHOCARDIOGRAPHIC FINDINGS IN STUDIES COMPARING IMMEDIATE CORD CLAMPING AND DELAYED CORD CLAMPING OR INTACT UMBILICAL CORD MILKING

Study	N	GA Weeks	Intervention	SVC ICC mL/kg/min	SVC Intervention mL/kg/min	Hours After Birth
Meyer, 2012[78]	30	26 (25–28)	DCC: 30–40s	52 (42–100)	91 (81–101)[a]	16
Sommers, 2012[49]	51	28 ± 1	DCC: 41 ± 9s	89 ± 24	112 ± 30[a]	6
Katheria, 2014[19]	60	28 ± 3	Intact UCM	69 ± 22	94 ± 27[a]	6
Popat, 2016[50]	266	28 ± 2	DCC: 60s (0–70)	92 ± 35	95 ± 41	3–6

[a]$P < .05$ compared to ICC.
DCC, Delayed cord clamping; *GA,* gestational age at birth; *ICC,* immediate cord clamping; *SVC,* superior vena cava flow; *UCM,* umbilical cord milking.

A small, randomized, controlled trial showed that heart rate and SpO_2 were higher immediately after birth, requiring lower amounts of inspired oxygen (FiO_2) and mean airway pressure, in preterm infants receiving intact UCM versus infants receiving ICC.[18] This suggests that cord milking may enhance early pulmonary blood flow and decrease pulmonary pressures. The decreased need for oxygen and mean airway pressure coincides with the finding that these infants also had a lower incidence of oxygen requirement at 36 weeks' postmenstrual age. There are no published results of the physiologic effects of cut-UCM in the delivery room.

Hemodynamic Measurements in the First Hours After Birth Following Delayed Cord Clamping and Umbilical Cord Milking

Studies have demonstrated that low systemic blood flow during the first 24 hours after birth increases the risk of peri/intraventricular hemorrhage (P/IVH), neurodevelopmental impairment, and death in extremely preterm infants.[43–45] Assessment of systemic blood flow, such as superior vena cava (SVC) flow, potentially provide a more accurate assessment of cardiovascular adequacy than blood pressure alone.[44,46] In trials, cardiovascular support with vasopressor-inotropes or inotropes and fluid boluses may increase low systemic blood flow but these interventions have not prevented adverse consequences such as the development of P/IVH nor have they improved neurodevelopmental outcomes (see Chapters 1, 3, 6 and 7).[47,48] As suggested earlier, DCC and UCM may aid in improving immediate hemodynamic transition and thus circulatory stability and also increase circulating blood volume after birth. Consequently, there is interest in studying umbilical cord management strategies and their role in prevention of low systemic blood flow states and subsequently decreasing the risk of P/IVH.

Recent studies measuring systemic blood flow by echocardiography that compare DCC to ICC have conflicting results (Table 5.2). In a small study by Sommers et al., DCC improved SVC flow compared to ICC.[49] However, in a much larger multicenter randomized controlled trial, DCC failed to show any improvement in SVC flow and infants randomized to DCC demonstrated lower right ventricular output.[50] Unfortunately, 22% of the infants allocated to the DCC arm had cord clamping prior to the targeted clamping at 1 minute mainly due to the obstetricians being uncomfortable with waiting when infants were less vigorous. However, it is in these very infants where DCC might be most advantageous. Several trials have shown that DCC in preterm infants leads to higher blood pressure in the first hours after birth and less treatment for low blood pressure, compared with infants receiving ICC.[51–54]

Cord milking may also be associated with improvements in hemodynamics particularly after C/S. UCM has been shown to improve systemic blood flow, cerebral oxygenation, and myocardial function compared to ICC.[19,26] Previous studies have suggested that placental transfusion may be impaired after C/S compared to vaginal birth.[4,55,56] In a comparison of intact UCM versus DCC for at least 45 seconds in 154 infants less than 32 weeks gestational age at birth delivered by cesarean section, SVC flow, right ventricular output, and blood pressure were all significantly higher in the infants receiving intact UCM than DCC in the first 12 hours after birth.[20] However, neither group had an excess of abnormal systemic flow and there were no differences in clinical outcomes. The hemodynamic changes of cut-UCM have not been studied. Finally, one study compared DCC for 60 seconds versus DCC for 60 seconds with respiratory support (mask ventilation/CPAP) if indicated in infants less than 32 weeks' gestation.[38] There were no differences in systemic blood flow measurements or cerebral oxygenation between the groups during the first 12 hours after birth.

Neonatal Blood Volume After Delayed Cord Clamping and Umbilical Cord Milking

In a randomized trial, Aladangady and colleagues used a biotin-labeled autologous red blood cell dilution method to compare red blood cell volume between very preterm infants receiving 30 to 90 seconds of DCC versus ICC.[56] At 4 hours after birth, the DCC infants had a significantly higher red blood cell volume than ICC (74 mL/kg vs. 63 mL/kg, $P < .001$). The difference was more pronounced in infants delivered vaginally. The authors found no difference in hematocrit levels at 1 hour after delivery despite measuring an increase in red blood cell volume. As the increased volume of blood providing the placental transfusion would be a proportionate transfer of red blood cells and plasma, no increase in hematocrit would be immediately detectable. A study by Strauss and colleagues also showed that despite an increase in red blood cell volume, initial hematocrit was not higher in preterm infants receiving DCC.[55] However, the infants receiving DCC had higher hematocrit levels at 7 days after birth. The higher hematocrit persisted during the first month after birth, and the authors speculated that this finding is potentially due to the increased blood volume coupled with improved hemodynamics leading to enhanced excretion of free water and less dilution from intravenous fluids in the DCC group.[55] However, a meta-analysis has found that preterm infants with DCC have higher hematocrit levels at 4 and 12 hours after birth, and a decreased need for red blood cell transfusions for either hypotension or anemia.

The total placento-fetal blood volume is reported to be 115 mL/kg at term of which 70 mL/kg is in the fetus and 45 mL/kg in the placenta.[57] Accordingly, the timing of cord clamping has the potential to influence neonatal blood volume in the term infant. If the umbilical cord is clamped immediately after delivery, the hematocrit in the newborn averages 48% to 51%.[57] However, waiting to clamp the cord 3 to 4 minutes after delivery increases the blood volume by 30%.[32] The hematocrit increases over the subsequent 30 minutes to 2 hours to average 59% to 62% at 6 hours of age and then decreases to 52% to 59% at 24 hours of age.[58]

A potential advantage of UCM over DCC for providing increased placental transfusion is that UCM is not dependent on uterine tone and thus UCM may be a more effective technique after cesarean delivery. The placental blood flow at 24 to 29 weeks' gestation is about 8 mL/s in the umbilical vein which increases to 10 mL/s at term.[59] Milking the preterm umbilical cord provides a blood volume of about 18 mL/kg over 2 seconds.[60] In a 1-kg infant this would provide a similar physiologic infusion of 9 mL/s. A recent study comparing UCM to DCC in premature infants born by C/S demonstrated an improved initial hematocrit, systemic blood flow, blood pressure, and urine output.[61] Milking the cord has also been shown to increase blood volume in term infants born via C/S. In one trial, performing UCM 5 times resulted in a mean hematocrit of 57% compared with 51% after ICC at 36 to 48 hours of age.[62]

Long-Term Outcomes and Mortality After Delayed Cord Clamping and Umbilical Cord Milking

There are a few studies reporting neurodevelopmental outcomes of DCC and UCM in preterm infants. Mercer and colleagues have published two studies finding that

DCC up to 45 seconds versus ICC improves motor function at 18 months as assessed by the Bayler Scales of Infant and Toddler Development in preterm infants less than 32 weeks' gestation.[2,63] Interestingly, improvement in motor function after DCC was more profound in male infants. In the only study reporting long-term outcomes comparing intact-UCM versus a 30-second delay in cord clamping, there was no difference in infants born at less than 33 weeks' gestation on Bayley III scores at 2 and 3.5 years.[22]

Andersson and colleagues conducted a randomized trial of over 380 healthy, term infants born in Sweden comparing DCC for ≥180 seconds to ICC (≤10 seconds).[64] Although neonatal hemoglobin and immunoglobulin G (IgG) levels and 4-month iron stores were higher in the DCC group, no differences in the iron status and neurodevelopment, assessed by the Ages and Stages Questionnaire (ASQ), were seen at 12 months. Male infants who received DCC had higher ASQ scores than male infants who received ICC, but female infants who received DCC had lower ASQ scores than female infants who received ICC. These intriguing gender differences have not been further evaluated. Finally, there are no published studies reporting long-term outcomes comparing UCM to ICC or after cut-UCM.

Two large, prospective, observational studies in resource-limited settings conducted by Ersdal and colleagues have investigated the relationship between DCC and death. In a cohort of over 12,000 spontaneously breathing term and late preterm infants, delaying UCC until after the initiation of spontaneous respirations reduced the risk of death and the combined risk of death and hospital admission at 24 hours after birth.[5] This happened despite the fact that the number of infants who died in this cohort was small (0.2% of the infants enrolled). A second observational study described the timing of UCC in over 1200 infants who received PPV for apnea after birth.[65] Initiating PPV prior to UCC did not significantly reduce the combined risk of death and admission at 24 hours after birth (18% if cord clamping occurred before initiating PPV vs. 14% if cord clamping occurred after initiating PPV, $P = .328$). The delay in the onset of PPV was significantly associated with the combined risk of death and admission at 24 hours. Of note, the timing of cord clamping was 39 ± 35 seconds in infants who received PPV. No significant difference in mortality has been observed between very preterm infants receiving DCC, UCM, or ICC.[4,54] However, as the incidence of death in very preterm infants was less than 5%, a larger cohort of infants is needed to appropriately address this question.

Conclusions and Future Directions

ICC was introduced with no prior evidence as an attempt to reduce the risk of postpartum hemorrhage. Both DCC and cord milking had been practiced and described centuries before the introduction of ICC. Aristotle described the cord milking procedure[66] in 350 BC: "It often happens that the child appears to have been born dead when it is merely weak, and when before the umbilical cord has been ligatured, the blood has run out into the cord and its surroundings. But experienced midwives have been shown to squeeze blood into the child's body from the cord, and immediately the child that a moment before was bloodless came back to life again." Improved short-term outcomes have already been demonstrated in several studies with UCM but long-term safety studies are lacking.[67] For DCC, there have never been any adverse maternal outcomes seen between the early and late cord clamping groups including severe postpartum hemorrhage, postpartum hemorrhage of 500 mL or more, mean blood loss, or maternal hemoglobin levels.[4] There has never been a trial published that demonstrates any benefit of ICC, and the majority of trials when compared to DCC and UCM suggest that it may actually be harmful.

Although a number of human studies suggest that the predominant benefit of DCC and UCM is the increase in blood volume, animal studies and one epidemiological study suggest that achieving lung aeration and pulmonary blood flow prior to cord clamping may be important.[13–15,68–73] Polglase and colleagues suggested the term "physiology-based cord clamping," in which a physiologic target indicating readiness for UCC is achieved prior to clamping the umbilical cord.[31] Delaying UCC until after the lungs are aerated, gas exchange is established, and pulmonary blood flow is increased could maintain physiologic stability by improving immediate hemodynamic transition and optimizing the potential for placental transfusion after birth. While promising, physiology-based cord clamping makes an appropriate target for the majority of clinicians challenging. A delay for perhaps 60 seconds in infants that demonstrate adequate breathing may be an appropriate starting point. Further studies are needed to determine whether cord milking is superior to DCC in neonates born via C/S, and whether it can be considered an alternative approach when DCC cannot be performed.

REFERENCES

1. Rabe H: Effect of timing of umbilical cord clamping and other strategies to influence placental transfusion at preterm birth on maternal and infant outcomes, *Cochrane Database Syst Rev* (8), 2012.
2. Mercer JS, Erickson-Owens DA, Vohr BR, et al.: Effects of placental transfusion on neonatal and 18 month outcomes in preterm infants: a randomized controlled trial, *J Pediatr* 168:50–55.e51, January 2016.
3. Katheria AC, Lakshminrusimha S, Rabe H, McAdams R, Mercer JS: Placental transfusion: a review, *J Perinatol*, September 22 2016.
4. McDonald SJ, Middleton P, Dowswell T, Morris PS: Effect of timing of umbilical cord clamping of term infants on maternal and neonatal outcomes, *Cochrane Database Syst Rev* (7):CD004074, July 11 2013.
5. Ersdal HL, Linde J, Mduma E, Auestad B, Perlman J: Neonatal outcome following cord clamping after onset of spontaneous respiration, *Pediatrics* 134(2):265–272, August 2014.
6. Perlman JM, Wyllie J, Kattwinkel J, et al.: Part 7: neonatal resuscitation: 2015 international consensus on cardiopulmonary resuscitation and emergency cardiovascular care science with treatment recommendations, *Circulation* 132(16 Suppl 1):S204–S241, October 20 2015.
7. Committee on obstetric practice ACoO, gynecologists: Committee Opinion No.543: timing of umbilical cord clamping after birth, *Obstet Gynecol* 120(6):1522–1526, December 2012.
8. Timing of umbilical cord clamping after birth, *Pediatrics* 131(4), e1323–e1323, 2013.
9. Committee WGAbtGR: *Guideline: delayed umbilical cord clamping for improved maternal and infant health and nutrition outcomes*, Geneva, 2014, World Health Organizationl.
10. Wyckoff MH, Aziz K, Escobedo MB, et al.: Part 13: neonatal resuscitation: 2015 american heart association guidelines update for cardiopulmonary resuscitation and emergency cardiovascular care, *Circulation* 132(18 Suppl 2):S543–S560, November 3 2015.
11. Ghavam S, Batra D, Mercer J, et al.: Effects of placental transfusion in extremely low birthweight infants: meta-analysis of long- and short-term outcomes, *Transfusion* 54(4):1192–1198, 2014.
12. Kaempf JW, Tomlinson MW, Kaempf AJ, et al.: Delayed umbilical cord clamping in premature neonates, *Obstet Gynecol* 120(2 Pt 1):325–330, August 2012.
13. Kattwinkel J, Perlman J: The Neonatal resuscitation program: the evidence evaluation process and anticipating edition 6, *NeoReviews* 11(12):e673–e680, 2010.
14. Perlman JM, Wyllie J, Kattwinkel J, et al.: Neonatal resuscitation: 2010 international consensus on cardiopulmonary resuscitation and emergency cardiovascular care science with treatment recommendations, *Pediatrics* 126(5):e1319–e1344, November 2010.
15. Singhal N, Lockyer J, Fidler H, et al.: Helping Babies Breathe: global neonatal resuscitation program development and formative educational evaluation, *Resuscitation* 83(1):90–96, January 2012.
16. Finer NN, Carlo WA, et al.: Early CPAP versus surfactant in extremely preterm infants, *N Engl J Med* 362(21):1970–1979, May 27 2010.
17. March MI, Hacker MR, Parson AW, Modest AM, de Veciana M: The effects of umbilical cord milking in extremely preterm infants: a randomized controlled trial, *J Perinatol* 33(10):763–767, October 2013.
18. Katheria A, Blank D, Rich W, Finer N: Umbilical cord milking improves transition in premature infants at birth, *PLoS One* 9(4):e94085, 2014.
19. Katheria AC, Leone TA, Woelkers D, Garey DM, Rich W, Finer NN: The effects of umbilical cord milking on hemodynamics and neonatal outcomes in premature neonates, *J Pediatr* 164(5):1045–1050.e1041, May 2014.
20. Katheria AC, Truong G, Cousins L, Oshiro B, Finer NN: Umbilical cord milking versus delayed cord clamping in preterm infants, *Pediatrics* 136(1):61–69, July 2015.
21. Rabe H, Jewison A, Alvarez RF, et al.: Milking compared with delayed cord clamping to increase placental transfusion in preterm neonates: a randomized controlled trial, *Obstet Gynecol* 117(2 Pt 1):205–211, February 2011.
22. Rabe H, Sawyer A, Amess P, Ayers S: Brighton Perinatal Study G. Neurodevelopmental outcomes at 2 and 3.5 years for very preterm babies enrolled in a randomized trial of milking the umbilical cord versus delayed cord clamping, *Neonatology* 109(2):113–119, 2016.
23. Hosono S, Mugishima H, Fujita H, et al.: Umbilical cord milking reduces the need for red cell transfusions and improves neonatal adaptation in infants born at less than 29 weeks' gestation: a randomised controlled trial, *Arch Dis Child Fetal Neonatal Ed* 93(1):F14–F19, January 2008.

24. Hosono S, Mugishima H, Takahashi S, et al.: One-time umbilical cord milking after cord cutting has same effectiveness as multiple-time umbilical cord milking in infants born at <29 weeks of gestation: a retrospective study, *J Perinatol* 35(8):590–594, August 2015.
25. Hosono S, Hine K, Nagano N, et al.: Residual blood volume in the umbilical cord of extremely premature infants, *Pediatr Int*, August 5 2014.
26. Takami T, Suganami Y, Sunohara D, et al.: Umbilical cord milking stabilizes cerebral oxygenation and perfusion in infants born before 29 weeks of gestation, *J Pediatr* 161(4):742–747, October 2012.
27. Upadhyay A, Gothwal S, Parihar R, et al.: Effect of umbilical cord milking in term and near term infants: randomized control trial, *Am J Obstet Gynecol* 208(2):120.e121–e126, February 2013.
28. Rudolph AM: Fetal and neonatal pulmonary circulation, *Annu Rev Physiol* 41:383–395, 1979.
29. Rudolph AM: Distribution and regulation of blood flow in the fetal and neonatal lamb, *Circ Res.* 57(6):811–821, Dec 1985.
30. Bhatt S, Alison BJ, Wallace EM, et al.: Delaying cord clamping until ventilation onset improves cardiovascular function at birth in preterm lambs, *J Physiol* 591(Pt 8):2113–2126, April 15 2013.
31. Polglase GR, Dawson JA, Kluckow M, et al.: Ventilation onset prior to umbilical cord clamping (physiological-based cord clamping) improves systemic and cerebral oxygenation in preterm lambs, *PLoS One* 10(2):e0117504, 2015.
32. Yao AC, Moinian M, Lind J: Distribution of blood between infant and placenta after birth, *Lancet* 2(7626):871–873, Oct 25 1969.
33. Vain NE, Satragno DS, Gorenstein AN, et al.: Effect of gravity on volume of placental transfusion: a multicentre, randomised, non-inferiority trial, *Lancet* 384(9939):235–240, July 19 2014.
34. Andersson O, Hellstrom-Westas L, Andersson D, Domellof M: Effect of delayed versus early umbilical cord clamping on neonatal outcomes and iron status at 4 months: a randomised controlled trial, *BMJ* 343:d7157, November 15 2011.
35. McDonald SJ, Middleton P, Dowswell T, Morris PS: Cochrane in context: effect of timing of umbilical cord clamping in term infants on maternal and neonatal outcomes, *Cochrane Database Syst Rev* 9(2):398–400, June 2014.
36. Mercer JS, Erickson-Owens DA: Rethinking placental transfusion and cord clamping issues, *J Perinat Neonatal Nurs* 26(3):202–217, July-September 2012. quiz 218–209.
37. Hooper SB, Crossley KJ, Zahra VA, et al.: Effect of body position and ventilation on umbilical artery and venous blood flows during delayed umbilical cord clamping in preterm lambs, *Arch Dis Child Fetal Neonatal Ed* 102(4):F312–F319, 2017.
38. Katheria A, Poeltler D, Durham J, et al.: Neonatal Resuscitation with an Intact Cord: A Randomized Clinical Trial, *J Pediatr* 178:75–80, 2016.
39. Boere I, Roest AA, Wallace E, et al.: Umbilical blood flow patterns directly after birth before delayed cord clamping, *Arch Dis Child Fetal Neonatal Ed* 100(2):F121–125, March 2015.
40. Yao AC, Lind J: Blood flow in the umbilical vessels during the third stage of labor, *Biol Neonate* 25(3-4): 186–193, 1974.
41. Katheria AC, Wozniak M, Harari D, Arnell K, Petruzzelli D, Finer NN: Measuring cardiac changes using electrical impedance during delayed cord clamping: a feasibility trial, *Matern Health Neonatol Perinatol* 1:15, 2015.
42. Winter J, Kattwinkel J, Chisholm C, Blackman A, Wilson S, Fairchild K: Ventilation of preterm infants during delayed cord clamping (VentFirst): a pilot study of feasibility and safety, *Am J Perinatol*, Jun 15 2016.
43. Hunt RW, Evans N, Rieger I, Kluckow M: Low superior vena cava flow and neurodevelopment at 3 years in very preterm infants, *J Pediatr* 145(5):588–592, Nov 2004.
44. Kluckow M: Low superior vena cava flow and intraventricular haemorrhage in preterm infants, *Arch Dis Child Fetal Neonatal Ed* 82(3):188F–194, 2000.
45. Kluckow M: Superior vena cava flow in newborn infants: a novel marker of systemic blood flow, *Arch Dis Child Fetal Neonatal Ed* 82(3):182F–187, 2000.
46. Evans N: Assessment and support of the preterm circulation, *Early Hum Dev* 82(12):803–810, Dec 2006.
47. Osborn D, Evans N, Kluckow M: Randomized trial of dobutamine versus dopamine in preterm infants with low systemic blood flow, *J Pediatr* 140(2):183–191, 2002.
48. Osborn DA, Evans N, Kluckow M, Bowen JR, Rieger I: Low superior vena cava flow and effect of inotropes on neurodevelopment to 3 years in preterm infants, *Pediatr* 120(2):372–380, August 2007.
49. Sommers R, Stonestreet BS, Oh W, et al.: Hemodynamic effects of delayed cord clamping in premature infants, *Pediatr* 129(3):e667–e672, March 2012.
50. Popat H, Robledo KP, Sebastian L, et al.: Effect of delayed cord clamping on systemic blood flow: a randomized controlled trial, *The Journal of Pediatrics* 178:81–86.e82, Nov 2016.
51. Backes CH, Rivera BK, Haque U, et al.: Placental transfusion strategies in very preterm neonates: a systematic review and meta-analysis, *Obstet Gynecol* 124(1):47–56, July 2014.
52. Ibrahim HM, Krouskop RW, Lewis DF, Dhanireddy R: Placental transfusion: umbilical cord clamping and preterm infants, *J Perinatol* 20(6):351–354, September 2000.
53. Mercer JS, McGrath MM, Hensman A, Silver H, Oh W: Immediate and delayed cord clamping in infants born between 24 and 32 weeks: a pilot randomized controlled trial, *J Perinatol* 23(6): 466–472, September 2003.
54. Rabe H, Diaz-Rosello JL, Duley L, Dowswell T: Effect of timing of umbilical cord clamping and other strategies to influence placental transfusion at preterm birth on maternal and infant outcomes, *Cochrane Database Syst Rev* (8):CD003248, August 15 2012.

55. Strauss RG, Mock DM, Johnson KJ, et al.: A randomized clinical trial comparing immediate versus delayed clamping of the umbilical cord in preterm infants: short-term clinical and laboratory endpoints, *Transfusion* 48(4):658–665, Apr 2008.
56. Aladangady N, McHugh S, Aitchison TC, Wardrop CA, Holland BM: Infants' blood volume in a controlled trial of placental transfusion at preterm delivery, *Pediatr* 117(1):93–98, January 2006.
57. Linderkamp O: Placental transfusion: determinants and effects, *Clin Perinatol* 9(3):559–592, October 1982.
58. Hutton EK, Hassan ES: Late vs early clamping of the umbilical cord in full-term neonates: systematic review and meta-analysis of controlled trials, *JAMA* 297(11):1241–1252, March 21 2007.
59. El Behery MM, Nouh AA, Alanwar AM, Diab AE: Effect of umbilical vein blood flow on perinatal outcome of fetuses with lean and/or hypo-coiled umbilical cord, *Arch Gynecol Obstet* 283(1):53–58, January 2011.
60. Hosono S, Hine K, Nagano N, et al.: Residual blood volume in the umbilical cord of extremely premature infants, *Pediatr Int* 57(1):68–71, 2015.
61. Katheria AC, Truong G, Cousins L, Oshiro B, Finer NN: Umbilical cord milking versus delayed cord clamping in preterm infants, *Pediatrics*, 2015.
62. Erickson-Owens DA, Mercer JS, Oh W: Umbilical cord milking in term infants delivered by cesarean section: a randomized controlled trial, *J Perinatol* 32(8):580–584, August 2012.
63. Mercer JS, Vohr BR, Erickson-Owens DA, Padbury JF, Oh W: Seven-month developmental outcomes of very low birth weight infants enrolled in a randomized controlled trial of delayed versus immediate cord clamping, *J Perinatol* 30(1):11–16, January 2010.
64. Andersson O, Domellof M, Andersson D, Hellstrom-Westas L: Effect of delayed vs early umbilical cord clamping on iron status and neurodevelopment at age 12 months: a randomized clinical trial, *JAMA Pediatr* 168(6):547–554, June 2014.
65. Ersdal HL, Linde J, Auestad B, et al.: Timing of cord clamping in relation to start of breathing or ventilation among depressed neonates-an observational study, *BJOG* 123(8):1370–1377, July 2016.
66. Dunn PM: Aristotle (384-322 BC): philosopher and scientist of ancient Greece, *Arch Dis Child Fetal Neonatal Ed* 91(1):F75–F77, January 2006.
67. Al-Wassia H, Shah PS: Efficacy and safety of umbilical cord milking at birth: a systematic review and meta-analysis, *JAMA Pediatric* 169(1):18–25, January 2015.
68. Hooper SB, Fouras A, Siew ML, et al.: Expired CO2 levels indicate degree of lung aeration at birth, *PLoS One* 8(8):e70895, 2013.
69. Hooper SB, Kitchen MJ, Wallace MJ, et al.: Imaging lung aeration and lung liquid clearance at birth, *FASEB* 21(12):3329–3337, October 2007.
70. Schmolzer GM, Hooper SB, Wong C, Kamlin CO, Davis PG: Exhaled carbon dioxide in healthy term infants immediately after birth, *J Pediatr*, January 13 2015.
71. te Pas AB, Davis PG, Hooper SB, Morley CJ: From liquid to air: breathing after birth, *J Pediatr* 152(5):607–611, May 2008.
72. van Vonderen JJ, Roest AA, Siew ML, Walther FJ, Hooper SB, te Pas AB: Measuring physiological changes during the transition to life after birth, *Neonatology* 105(3):230–242, 2014.
73. Blank D, Rich W, Leone T, Garey D, Finer N: Pedi-cap color change precedes a significant increase in heart rate during neonatal resuscitation, *Resuscitation* 85(11):1568–1572, Nov 2014.
74. Dawson JA, Kamlin CO, Wong C, et al.: Changes in heart rate in the first minutes after birth, *Arch Dis Child Fetal Neonatal Ed* 95(3):F177–F181, May 2010.
75. Dawson JA, Kamlin CO, Vento M, et al.: Defining the reference range for oxygen saturation for infants after birth, *Pediatr* 125(6):e1340–e1347, June 2010.
76. Linde JE, Schulz J, Perlman JM, et al.: Normal newborn heart rate in the first five minutes of life assessed by dry-electrode electrocardiography, *Neonatology* 110(3):231–237, 2016.
77. Smit M, Dawson JA, Ganzeboom A, Hooper SB, van Roosmalen J, te Pas AB: Pulse oximetry in newborns with delayed cord clamping and immediate skin-to-skin contact, *Arch Dis Child Fetal Neonatal Ed* 99(4):F309–F314, Jul 2014.
78. Meyer MP, Mildenhall L: Delayed cord clamping and blood flow in the superior vena cava in preterm infants: an observational study, *Arch Dis Child Fetal Neonatal Ed* 97(6):F484–F486, Nov 2012.

CHAPTER 6

Transitional Hemodynamics and Pathophysiology of Peri/Intraventricular Hemorrhage

Shahab Noori, Tai-Wei Wu, and Istvan Seri

- A period of systemic and cerebral hypoperfusion in the immediate postnatal period predisposes the extremely preterm infant to peri/intraventricular hemorrhage (P/IVH).
- Cardiovascular immaturity and maladaptation after birth contribute to the postnatal hypoperfusion.
- Ventilatory support, especially inappropriately high mean airway pressure, can accentuate the early postnatal hypoperfusion.
- Following the initial hypoperfusion, a period of improvement in systemic and cerebral perfusion precedes occurrence of P/IVH on the second or third postnatal day. Therefore ischemia-reperfusion is a major hemodynamic contributor to the pathogenesis of P/IVH.
- Hypercapnia especially $PaCO_2$ above 50 mm Hg may increase the risk of P/IVH by potentiating the reperfusion phase via increasing the cerebral blood flow and attenuating autoregulation.
- Delayed cord clamping and cord milking are associated with improved hemodynamic stability and appear to be beneficial in preventing P/IVH possibly by mitigating the risk of hypoperfusion

Peri/intraventricular hemorrhage (P/IVH) is a devastating complication of prematurity that affects about a third of extremely preterm infants (<28 weeks' gestation).[1] P/IVH is a major risk factor for poor neurodevelopmental outcome, hydrocephalus, and mortality among these patients.[2] Although the pathogenesis of P/IVH is complex and likely involves multiple different mechanisms, alteration in cerebral hemodynamics is thought to play a major role. Recent advances in noninvasive monitoring have highlighted the hemodynamic antecedents of P/IVH. This chapter reviews the inherent vulnerabilities of preterm infants during the transitional period and how the interaction between transitional hemodynamics and interventions aimed at supporting respiratory and cardiovascular function can increase the risk of P/IVH.

Fetal and Transitional Circulation

As the physiology of fetal circulation is discussed in Chapter 1 in detail, here we only provide a brief review of the main characteristics pertinent to the topic of this chapter. In utero, the most oxygenated blood with oxygen saturation around 75% to 85% flows from the umbilical vein through the ductus venosus to the inferior vena cava (IVC). Due to mixing with venous blood from the portal and hepatic circulations in the liver, and also due to some mixing with the venous blood flowing from the lower body in the IVC, oxygen saturation entering the heart is only about 70%. Of note is that the blood flowing in from the ductus venosus into the IVC is primarily diverted by the Eustachian valve toward the foramen ovale and into the left atrium.[3-5] The low flow of poorly oxygenated pulmonary venous return to the left atrium admixing with flow via the foramen ovale still ensures supply of relatively well-oxygenated blood to the heart and brain with an oxygen saturation around 60%. On the other hand, blood returning from the superior vena cava (SVC) and the stream in the IVC representing blood returning from the lower part of body are preferentially directed to the right ventricle. As most of right ventricular output (RVO) is diverted through the patent ductus arteriosus (PDA) toward the aorta, both ventricles contribute to the systemic circulation. Given the low blood flow to the lungs due to high pulmonary vascular resistance, left ventricular preload is relatively small. As such, during fetal life, the contribution of the right ventricle to systemic blood flow is greater than that of the left ventricle. In the fetus, the combined cardiac output is about 400 to 450 mL/kg/min with only about 11% to 25% constituting the pulmonary circulation.[3,6-9] This is in contrast to the postnatal circulation where the left and right cardiac outputs are equal and average about 200 mL/kg/min. The low resistance placental circulation facilitates the high cardiac output in the fetus by reducing the afterload. At birth, pulmonary vascular resistance drops precipitously as the newborn starts breathing and the lungs become the organ of gas exchange. This increases pulmonary blood flow and changes the ductal flow pattern in a way that progressively directs blood from the right ventricle to the pulmonary circulation.[10] The increased pulmonary blood flow in turn increases left-sided preload and promotes functional closure of the foramen ovale. This, along with the closure of the ductus arteriosus over the following 2 to 3 days, transforms the circulation to the adult-type (postnatal) circulation in which the pulmonary and systemic circuits are not functioning as parallel circulations anymore but as circulations in series. Despite its complexity, this transformation occurs smoothly in the vast majority of term infants. However, in preterm infants, especially those born before 28 weeks' gestation, this process is hindered by immaturity of the organ systems and is more likely to represent an abnormal cardiorespiratory transition. Accordingly, it is likely to be associated with circulatory compromise, as discussed in detail in this chapter.

Cerebral Blood Flow

Understanding the evolution of cerebral hemodynamics from the fetal circulation through the postnatal transition is critical in understanding the role of abnormal transition in the pathogenesis of P/IVH. However, measurement of cerebral blood flow (CBF) is challenging in neonates, especially in preterm infants and during the immediate postnatal period. CBF has been assessed using radioactive xenon clearance, positron emission tomography, Doppler ultrasonography, magnetic resonance imaging, and near-infrared spectroscopy (NIRS). Each of these methods has its own significant limitations. Due to their noninvasive nature and bedside availability, Doppler and NIRS are the most commonly used methods for the assessment of CBF. With Doppler ultrasonography, various surrogates of CBF, such as SVC blood flow and blood flow velocity in major cerebral arteries have been used to characterize intermittent changes in cerebral hemodynamics. On the other hand, NIRS allows for the continuous assessment of regional tissue oxygen saturation (rSO_2) or tissue oxygenation index (TOI). Although NIRS does not measure blood flow directly, by considering *cerebral* regional oxygen saturation ($CrSO_2$), clinical information, and certain other parameters, changes in CBF can be deduced. Taking into account arterial oxygen saturation (SPO_2), the index of cerebral fractional oxygen extraction (CFOE) can be calculated according to the following formula: $(SPO_2 - CrSO_2) / SPO_2$. $CrSO_2$ has a direct and CFOE has an inverse relationship with changes in CBF. In other words, a reduction in $CrSO_2$ or an increase in CFOE indicates a decrease in CBF, provided certain assumptions hold true. These assumptions include no significant changes in SPO_2 (with $CrSO_2$), organ metabolism, hemoglobin and/or the distribution of blood in tissue among arteries, veins, and capillaries.

Normal Changes in Cerebral Blood Flow

During fetal development, brain blood flow increases both as an absolute value and per gram of tissue.[11,12] Animal and human studies have shown a decrease in CBF at and immediately after birth.[13,14] The cause of this reduction is unclear, but in part may be related to an increase in tissue oxygenation at birth compared with fetal life.[10,13] Interestingly, the progressive change of PDA flow pattern from right-to-left to left-to-right during the first few minutes after birth strongly and inversely correlates with middle cerebral artery mean blood flow velocity (MCA-MV), a surrogate of CBF.[10] This suggests a possible role of the PDA immediately after birth in reduction of CBF. Alternatively, the changes in PDA flow pattern and reduction in CBF may be independent, and both reflective of the increasing oxygen tension following delivery. It is clear that more data are needed to elucidate the normal changes in cardiovascular function and cerebral hemodynamics at and immediately after birth, especially in preterm infants.

After the immediate postnatal period, CBF increases rather significantly over the following days and more gradually afterward in both preterm and term infants.[15-18] Despite the rise in CBF, it remains at only a fraction of the adult value.[19,20] Moreover, sick preterm infants have even lower CBF.[19] The low CBF in neonates may be explained by lower brain metabolism; however, cardiovascular maladaptation in preterm infants may also contribute to the observed low CBF.

Cerebral Blood Flow and Peri/Intraventricular Hemorrhage

Preterm infants who develop P/IVH have a lower CBF after birth. Studies using NIRS found higher CFOE on the first postnatal day in preterm infants who later develop P/IVH.[21] Serial measurements of SVC flow, a surrogate for CBF, also found that low SVC blood flow in the first few hours after birth is a risk factor for P/IVH.[22] However, caution needs to be exercised when using SVC flow as a surrogate for CBF since, in the preterm neonate, only around 30% of the blood flow in the SVC represents blood returning from the brain (see Chapter 2). The last two decades have seen an increased use of ultrasonography by neonatologists to elucidate the cardiovascular adaptation during the transitional period. In addition, advances in monitoring technology have brought NIRS to a more widespread use in research and also have facilitated its introduction into clinical care. The newer NIRS sensors have allowed for more continuous and prolonged monitoring of rSO_2 and for quick application of the sensors in situations when time is of the essence (e.g., in the delivery room). Therefore, despite the limitations mentioned earlier, increased application of the newer NIRS technology and ultrasonography have provided valuable insights into the cerebral hemodynamic changes that precede P/IVH.

A recent nested case-control study compared $CrSO_2$ and CFOE between preterm infants with and without P/IVH during the first 15 days after birth.[23] Measurements were done daily for 2 hours for 8 days and, then, on day 15.[23] The authors found lower $CrSO_2$ and higher CFOE in the P/IVH group suggestive of lower CBF throughout the first 8 days. While low CBF in the first postnatal day has consistently been reported, its persistence for a week has not.[17,21,22,24] In contrast, another nested case-control study monitoring cerebral oxygenation during first few postnatal days found higher $CrSO_2$ and lower CFOE during the 24 hours prior to detection of severe P/IVH.[25] In other words, this study suggests that higher rather than lower CBF precedes brain hemorrhage. This discrepancy may be explained by the differences in the timing and duration of monitoring between the two studies.[26] In a recent study, in addition to performing frequent and regularly timed head ultrasounds and echocardiography, we prospectively and continuously monitored extremely preterm infants (<28 weeks) during the first 3 postnatal days and found a unique pattern with identifiable phases of changes, among others, in the indices of CBF in patients who developed P/IVH (Fig. 6.1).[27] The $CrSO_2$ and CFOE were indicative of low CBF in the earlier hours of the first postnatal day, followed by a period of an increase in CBF before detection of P/IVH around 48 hours after birth and, thereafter, a subsequent decrease in CBF. These findings suggest that there are two distinct hemodynamic phases in the pathogenesis of P/IVH: an early hypoperfusion and a later reperfusion phase. The prospective, comprehensive, and continuous design of the study allowed for detection of the two phases. Given the dynamic changes in CBF over the first few days, an intermittent or short period of monitoring will miss either the hypoperfusion or reperfusion phase.[26]

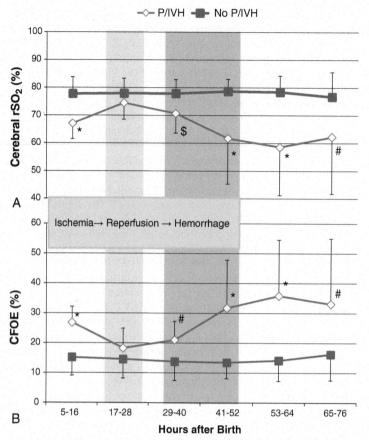

Fig. 6.1 Changes in cerebral regional oxygen saturation (rSO$_2$) and cerebral fractional oxygen extraction (CFOE) in two groups of very preterm neonates presenting with *(white diamonds)* and without *(red squares)* peri/intraventricular hemorrhage (PIVH) during first 3 postnatal days. The No-P/IVH group exhibited stable cerebral rSO$_2$ (A) and CFOE (B) values, while the P/IVH group presented with a characteristic pattern of changes. The P/IVH group had lower cerebral rSO$_2$ and higher CFOE during the first 12 hours of the study, followed by normalization of these parameters (highlighted in *light red*) just before the two study periods when P/IVH was detected (highlighted in *red*). These findings suggest that initial cerebral hypoperfusion is followed by a period of reperfusion before the occurrence of the P/IVH. After the second study period, cerebral rSO$_2$ decreased and CFOE increased suggesting a decrease in cerebral blood flow during and after the development of P/IVH. Statistically significant differences between the two groups: *$P <$ .005, #$P <$ .04 and $^\$ P <$ .05. The values represent the mean ±SD of the data obtained in each 12-hour data collection period. (From Noori S, McCoy M, Anderson MP, Ramji F, Seri I. Changes in cardiac function and cerebral blood flow in relation to peri/intraventricular hemorrhage in extremely preterm infants. J Pediatr 164:264–270.e1-e3, 2014.)

In the remainder of this chapter, we will discuss the vulnerabilities of preterm infants during the transitional period that increase the risk of P/IVH and focus on the causes and risk factors that lead to or potentiate the hypoperfusion and/or reperfusion phases.

Vulnerabilities of Preterm Infants During Transition

Inherent Vulnerability of the Immature Brain

The brain of a preterm infant is vulnerable to development of P/IVH due to both structural and functional immaturity. The germinal matrix is the site of active proliferation of future neuronal and glial cells, and as such is a highly vascularized and metabolically active tissue.[28] Its capillary network consisting of thin-walled fragile vessels is susceptible to rupture.[29] The germinal matrix involutes between 28 and 34 weeks.[28,30] Therefore, until its final involution, the germinal matrix is susceptible to bleeding, especially in preterm infants <28 weeks' gestation. In addition, the germinal matrix lies within an arterial end zone, which makes it particularly vulnerable to hypoperfusion-reperfusion injury.[31] The immature venous system is prone to congestion, which further increases the risk of hemorrhage in this population.[28,30]

The ability to maintain CBF relatively constant despite fluctuations in blood pressure (i.e., CBF autoregulation) is an important protective mechanism against ischemia and hyperperfusion (see Chapter 2). The correlation between mean blood pressure and TOI or rSO_2 using NIRS allows for continuous assessment of CBF autoregulation by analyzing coherence and transfer function gain. Coherence is a measure of linear correlation between blood pressure and an index of CBF (i.e., cerebral oxygenation), and therefore an arbitrary cutoff, usually 0.5, is used to define the presence or absence of autoregulation. On the other hand, transfer function gain assesses the degree of impairment by measuring the effects of changes in the amplitude of the blood pressure waveform on the amplitude of changes in cerebral tissue oxygenation. Both methods have their strengths and limitations and are not routinely used in clinical settings (see Chapter 2).[32]

The brain of preterm infants has immature CBF autoregulation.[33-35] In addition, the majority of very preterm neonates have mean blood pressures very close to the lower elbow of the blood pressure autoregulatory curve during the first 24 hours after delivery (see Chapter 2). Although CBF autoregulation is present even in the most immature preterm infant, the autoregulatory plateau is quite narrow. Moreover, immaturity per se and/or the interventions aiming to support these patients can result in systemic changes that alter CBF autoregulation (see the section on hypotension and permissive hypercapnia in Chapter 2). Given the role of CBF autoregulation in ensuring maintenance of adequate CBF and prevention of hyperperfusion, immature and impaired autoregulation has long been considered as a risk factor for P/IVH. Indeed, most but not all studies of CBF autoregulation in preterm infants have shown an association between impaired autoregulation and the occurrence P/IVH.[33-38]

Another vulnerability of the brain of the very preterm neonate ($\leq$28 weeks' gestation) is immaturity of the forebrain (including cortex, thalamus, hypothalamus, basal ganglia) vasculature, displaying characteristics of the blood flow regulation of a nonvital organ during the first postnatal days. In other words, the vessels of the forebrain respond with vasoconstriction to decreasing perfusion pressure or hypoxia, rather than with vasodilation, as expected for the vessels of a vital organ (brain, heart, and adrenal gland).[39] Several lines of evidence support this notion.[40-42] For example, beagle pups exposed to hypoxia exhibit vasodilation of the hindbrain (medulla, pons, cerebellum) but vasoconstriction of the forebrain.[40] In humans, CBF autoregulation appears in the brainstem first and in the forebrain only later in gestation.[41] Therefore vital organ assignment appears to be developmentally regulated, with the forebrain lagging behind the hindbrain in acquiring the properties of a high-priority vascular bed.

Immature Myocardium

The myocardium of a neonate, even at term, is immature and quite different from that of older children and adults. It has more water content and less contractile elements. In addition, the immature sarcoplasmic reticulum makes cytosolic calcium the primary source of second messenger calcium for myocardial function. These differences affect both systolic and diastolic function. Indeed, the neonatal myocardium is more sensitive to afterload, its lower compliance adversely affects ventricular filling, and it is dependent on extracellular calcium for its function. Preterm infants, especially during the transition, exhibit a cardiovascular response to acidosis that is different than that of adults. A recent study in hemodynamically stable very preterm infants during the transitional period showed that while acidic pH was not associated with a decrease in myocardial contractility, cardiac output failed to increase, presumably because the expected, acidosis-associated decrease in systemic vascular resistance did not take place.[43] It has been postulated that immaturity of the myocardium predisposes preterm infants to a low systemic flow state[22,44] and therefore contributes to the low CBF observed in a subset of very preterm neonates who later develop P/IVH. If we consider SVC flow as a surrogate for systemic flow, the finding of low SVC flow in P/IVH group represents low cardiac output in the immediate postnatal period with the fetal channels open.[22] Indeed, low left ventricular output (LVO) and RVO have been shown to be prevalent in those who later develop P/IVH (Fig. 6.2).[27] However, the underlying causes of this low cardiac output are unclear. Among others, a sudden *high afterload*

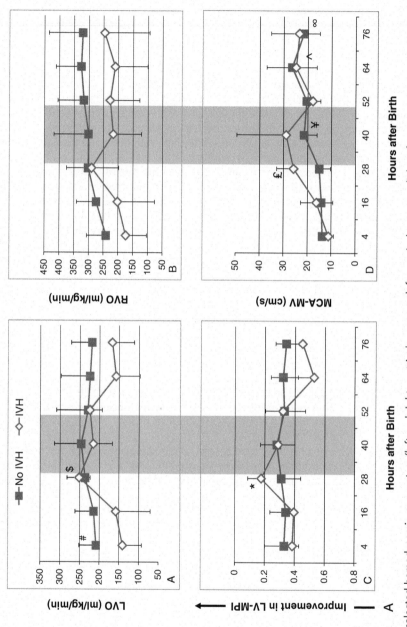

Fig. 6.2 Changes in selected hemodynamic parameters (left and right ventricular output, left ventricular myocardial performance index and middle cerebral artery mean flow velocity) during the first 76 hours in very preterm neonates with (white diamonds) and without (red squares) P/IVH. The changes+ in LVO (a), RVO (b), left ventricular myocardial performance index (LV-MPI) (c) and MCA-MV (d) in the two groups during the study are shown. There was a trend for a lower LVO in the P/IVH group at baseline with a trend for improvement before the occurrence of P/IVH (highlighted in pink). Lower MPI (i.e., better function) and higher MCA-MV in the P/IVH group also preceded occurrence of P/IVH. The pattern of changes in LVO between the two groups tended to be statistically significant (P = .068) while that in RVO, MPI and MCA-MV did not reach statistical significance. Statistically significant differences between groups: *P = .04 and £P =.016, No-P/IVH group; compared with baseline: ¥P = .02, ^P < .0001, ‾P = .044. Differences approaching statistical significance and suggesting a difference between the groups: #P < .055, and within the P/IVH group compared with baseline: $P = .07. The values represent the mean ±SD of the data obtained upon entry into the study and every 12 hours thereafter.

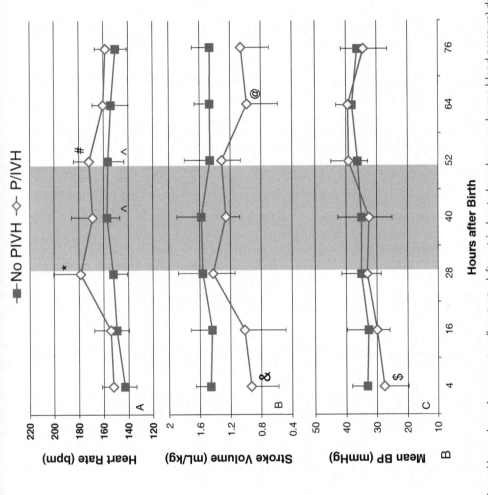

Fig. 6.2, cont'd (B) Changes in selected hemodynamic parameters (heart rate, left ventricular stroke volume, and mean blood pressure) during the first 76 hours in very preterm neonates with and without P/IVH. Changes in heart rate (a), left ventricular stroke volume (b), and mean blood pressure (c) in the two groups during the study are shown. Heart rate significantly increased in the No-P/IVH group (ANOVA $P = .004$), while there was a trend for an increase in the P/IVH group (ANOVA $P = .051$) during the study. Compared with the No-P/IVH group, left ventricular stroke volume in patients of the P/IVH group was lower at the baseline but similar before the occurrence of the P/IVH. Mean blood pressure (c) tended to increase in the P/IVH group (ANOVA $P = .052$), while it remained unchanged and relatively stable in the No-P/IVH group (ANOVA $P = .2$). In addition, mean blood pressure at baseline also tended to be lower in patients in the P/IVH group. The pattern of changes in heart rate and stroke volume, but not in mean blood pressure, was different between the two groups. No-P/IVH group; compared with baseline: $^\wedge P = .007$. Between groups: $^*P = .004$, $^\#P = .03$, $^\&P = .007$, $^@P = .048$, $^\$P = .085$. The values represent the mean $\pm$ SD of the data obtained upon entry into the study and every 12 hours thereafter. The area highlighted in *pink* represents the period when P/IVH occurred. *bpm*, Beat per minute; *LVO*, left ventricular output; *MCA*, middle cerebral artery mean flow velocity; *MPI*, myocardial performance index; *P/IVH*, peri/intraventricular hemorrhage; *RVO*, right ventricular output. (From Noori S, McCoy M, Anderson MP, Ramji F, Seri I. Changes in cardiac function and cerebral blood flow in relation to peri/intraventricular hemorrhage in extremely preterm infants. J Pediatr 164:264–270.e1–e3, 2014.)

following removal of the low resistance placental circulation in the setting of an immature myocardium has been postulated to be one of the underlying causes of this finding. Indeed, there is a difference in the inverse linear relationship of contractility and afterload among preterm infants with normal and low SVC flow, with patients having low SVC flow as a group exhibiting a steeper regression line suggestive of lower contractility in this group.[44] However, this is not a consistent finding, and a recent study found no difference in afterload or load-dependent and load-independent indices of contractility between patients who develop P/IVH and those who don't.[27] Whether *low preload* could explain the observed low cardiac output is not known, in part because of the difficulty in assessing preload using noninvasive techniques. However, recent studies of delayed cord clamping and cord milking suggest a possible role for low preload in the observed low cardiac output state (see below). Thus it is likely that the low cardiac output is multifactorial with abnormalities in preload, contractility, and afterload, and other factors such as ductal shunting contributing to a varying degree in different patients. Following the initial low flow state, cardiovascular function improves and cardiac output normalizes. This improvement in systemic flow is also associated with reperfusion of the brain and precedes occurrence of P/IVH (see Fig. 6.2).[27]

Hypovolemia and Timing of Cord Clamping

Recent studies of the timing of cord clamping show a better hemodynamic status and possible lower rate of P/IVH when clamping of the umbilical cord is delayed for 30 to 60 seconds.[45-48] These data suggest a smoother postnatal transition with delayed cord clamping. A more gradual separation from the low resistance placental circulation might facilitate the adaptation of the left ventricle to the postnatal increase in afterload. Prolonging the time of cord clamping also promotes placental transfusion. In the term neonate delivered vaginally, about 16 and 23 mL/kg of blood is transfused from the placenta to the neonate, with a 1- and 3-minute delay in the timing of cord clamping, respectively.[49] Importantly, the onset of breathing before cord clamping promotes earlier establishment of pulmonary blood flow, and thus better maintains left ventricular preload, and increases placental transfusion to the newborn.[50] Although all of the above mechanisms are likely contributory, increased intravascular volume due to placental transfusion has been speculated as the most important cause for the better transition in preterm infants with delayed or physiologic cord clamping. This speculation is based on the finding that similar cardiovascular benefits are seen with milking of the cord.[51-53] Preterm infants receiving placental transfusion by milking of the cord have higher cerebral oxygenation and SVC flow, cardiac output and urine output, and a decreased incidence of hypotension, and are less likely to receive vasopressor-inotropes or inotropes compared with those with immediate cord clamping.[51-53]

Historically, hypovolemia was thought not to be prevalent in the newborn, given the absent or weak relationship between measured blood volume and blood pressure. However, the finding of a more stable cardiovascular status in preterm infants with placental transfusion, either from delayed cord clamping or cord milking, indicates that hypovolemia may indeed play a role in hemodynamic instability during the immediate transition period and, as such, might contribute to pathogenesis of P/IVH. As mentioned earlier, preterm infants who develop P/IVH have lower CBF in the first hours after birth, as suggested by lower $CrSO_2$ and SVC flow. The findings of a higher $CrSO_2$ and SVC flow with delayed cord clamping and cord milking suggests that the incidence of low CBF after birth can be reduced and therefore might explain the observed reduction in the incidence of P/IVH associated with these approaches. However, the importance of the onset of breathing in delayed/physiological cord clamping also indicates that a gradual, smooth shift from placental blood flow to pulmonary blood as the source of left ventricular preload immediately after birth is among the key contributors to improved hemodynamic status in the very preterm neonate during early transition.

Patent Ductus Arteriosus

Although there is an association between PDA and P/IVH, the extent of contribution, if any, of PDA to the pathogenesis of P/IVH is unclear. As discussed in Chapters 2 and 22, the pattern of CBF is affected by a PDA. Moreover, with an inadequately compensated cardiac output for the degree of the left-to-right PDA shunt, CBF is also reduced. Most studies assessing cerebral oxygenation using NIRS have shown a lower $CrSO_2$ with a PDA and improvement after closure of the ductus arteriosus.[54-56] The increased stroke volume and, as a result, the increased LVO represent a compensatory mechanism to attenuate the effect of the shunt on systemic perfusion, especially preductally. This adaptive process may be limited in a subset of patients, especially during first the few hours after birth. As discussed earlier, this is the period when cerebral ischemia is prevalent in patients who later develop P/IVH. Indeed, there is a temporal relationship between a hemodynamically significant PDA and low indices of CBF during this critical period.[10,22] Authors of earlier studies showing a reduction in the incidence of P/IVH with indomethacin prophylaxis suggested that, in addition to a direct, cyclooxygenase inhibition, an independent, vasoconstrictive effect of indomethacin on the cerebral vasculature in infants with early PDA might have a role in the development of P/IVH. However, a lack of any effect of prophylactic ibuprofen on the incidence of P/IVH, despite a significant reduction in PDA rate, casts doubt on a role for early PDA in the development of P/IVH. Nevertheless, the strong relationship between a significant PDA and low CBF and $CrSO_2$ does suggest that PDA may be a contributing factor to the ischemic phase preceding the development of P/IVH.

Hypotension

Hypotension is common in preterm infants during transition. It is discussed in detail in Chapter 3, suffice to say that there are many reasons for a preterm infant to be hypotensive during the transitional period. These include postnatal maladaptation superimposed on immaturity of the cardiovascular system, inadequate compensation for a PDA shunt, prevalence of relative adrenal insufficiency, increased rate of sepsis, acidosis, and the detrimental impact of inappropriate ventilator support on neonatal hemodynamics. Hypotension has long been recognized as a risk factor for P/IVH.[57,58] Given the fact that hypotension is a hallmark of uncompensated shock, the association between hypotension and P/IVH is not surprising. However, the uncertainty about the definition of hypotension and the influence of other coexisting variables (see Chapter 3) make it difficult to propose a "safe" blood pressure range.

Over the past decade, there has been an increasing concern about the possible role of treatment of hypotension in the occurrence of P/IVH and poor neurodevelopmental outcome associated with hypotension.[59-61] This is indeed a possibility, at least theoretically. By definition, hypotensive preterm infants are outside the CBF autoregulatory range where cerebral perfusion is pressure passive.[62,63] Therefore, inappropriate titration of vasopressor-inotropes can increase blood pressure and brain blood flow[62,64] and thus, in theory, increase the risk of P/IVH (see Chapter 3). However, of note is that although careful, stepwise titration of vasopressor-inotropes for hypotension restores brain blood flow along with the blood pressure, CBF autoregulation does not regain its functionality for a period of time.[62,64] Yet there are data, although not conclusive, on the potential beneficial effects of careful titration of cardiovascular medications.[58,65,66] It is likely that the underlying pathophysiology of brain injury associated with hypotension is multifactorial and that low CBF due to low perfusion pressure, inappropriate treatment, and titration of vasopressor-inotropes resulting in intermittent cerebral hypo- and hyperperfusion and other coexisting factors independent of hypotension all contribute in varying degrees to the development of P/IVH. The fact that hypotension is almost always treated,[67] albeit at different thresholds, makes establishing causality for adverse outcomes and defining the extent of contribution of various aspects of clinical care to the development of P/IVH in response to hypotension nearly impossible. There are many challenges in designing a study to ascertain the impact of each of these factors in the pathogenesis of P/IVH and poor neurodevelopmental outcome. These include the inability to utilize a physiology-based and individualized definition of hypotension for each patient, the heterogeneous etiology and pathophysiology of hypotension (i.e., abnormality in preload, contractility, afterload and/or vascular tone dysregulation), and the complexity of selecting the appropriate treatment for the given pathophysiology and clinical presentation. In addition, given the strong belief among neonatologists of the harmful effect of hypotension, conducting randomized control trials with a no treatment arm appears not feasible.[67] However, several ongoing trials are investigating the effect of hypotension on outcome by using different thresholds for treatment or by incorporating advanced monitoring technology to enhance the identification of the threshold of hypotension (see Chapter 3).

Cardiorespiratory Interaction

The close anatomic and physiologic relationship between the respiratory and cardiovascular systems results in the notion that changes in the two systems mutually affect one another. Due to the vulnerability of the preterm infant, these interactions are particularly important during the early postnatal transitional period. The vast majority of very preterm infants require some level of respiratory support due to immaturity of the lungs and the respiratory center.

The impact of positive airway pressure and invasive or noninvasive ventilation has been studied in animals and to a lesser extent in humans. Animal studies demonstrate that with increasing positive end expiratory pressure, the pulmonary vascular resistance significantly increases, thereby raising right ventricular afterload resulting in reductions in RVO.[68,69] In addition, the increased intrathoracic pressure-driven decrease in systemic venous return further reduces RVO, and as a result, systemic blood flow also decreases. Studies in human neonates have reported inconsistent results, with some findings being similar to those obtained in animal models, albeit with a milder impact, while others show no effect.[70-73] The reason for this discrepancy is unclear but likely involves limitations of assessment tools and differences in lung compliance among the patients in the different studies. The latter reason could explain the significant hemodynamic alteration observed in animal models where lung compliance is normal and therefore intrathoracic pressure is more readily transmitted to the vasculature and the heart. Although the effect of positive airway pressure in the range commonly used in clinical practice appears to be relatively small, inappropriately high pressure for the degree of lung disease can significantly reduce systemic blood flow and also lead to increased cerebral venous pressure, both of which may contribute to pathogenesis of P/IVH. Given the prevalence of less effective or impaired CBF autoregulation in sick, extremely preterm infants, decreases in systemic perfusion can relatively easily lead to a drop in CBF. In addition, the fluctuation of CBF associated with mechanical ventilation, perhaps due to asynchrony, increases the risk of P/IVH.[74] While positive pressure ventilation increases central and cerebral venous pressure, tension pneumothorax can result in a significant, abrupt rise in these pressures and subsequently increases the risk of P/IVH.[75,76] Surfactant administration can also impact CBF initially by altering carbon dioxide levels and subsequently by the hemodynamic consequences of potential lung hyperinflation following rapid improvement in lung compliance, particularly if the ventilator support has not been weaned in a timely fashion.[77-79] Tracheal suction can also significantly alter cerebral hemodynamics by increasing both arterial and venous blood pressure. In addition to the direct effects of ventilatory support, treatment strategies such as permissive hypercapnia with the resultant acidosis can impact cardiovascular function and CBF (see below).

Hypocapnia and Hypercapnia

Carbon dioxide has a potent effect on the vascular system in general and brain in particular. Increases and decreases in partial pressure of CO_2 ($PaCO_2$) cause cerebral vasodilation and vasoconstriction, respectively. In fact, changes in $PaCO_2$ are more potent regulators of CBF than changes in blood pressure, even outside the autoregulatory blood pressure range (see Chapter 2). Therefore hypocapnia and hypercapnia may impact the hypoperfusion and reperfusion phases preceding P/IVH, respectively. Although hypocapnia is associated with ischemic brain injury and periventricular leukomalacia,[80,81] it does not appear to play a significant role in the pathogenesis of P/IVH.[82] This could be due to absent or low reactivity of CBF to changes in $PaCO_2$ during the first postnatal day, a period when hypoperfusion is commonly reported in this population. Indeed, there is an evolution of the CBF-CO_2 reactivity in preterm infants with higher responsiveness of the cerebral vasculature to changes in $PaCO_2$ with each passing day during the first few postnatal days.[83,84] In one study, the CBF reactivity per kPa (7.5 mm Hg) change in $PaCO_2$ was about 11% on the first postnatal day compared with 32% during the second day.[85] A weak relationship between $PaCO_2$ and CBF on first postnatal day has also been shown using NIRS.[86] We found no relationship between MCA-MV, a surrogate for CBF, and $PaCO_2$ in the first postnatal day, and a progressively stronger positive linear relationship on postnatal days 2 and 3 in preterm infants.[84]

On the other hand, hypercapnia has consistently been shown to be associated with P/IVH.[82,87-89] The highest $PaCO_2$ during the first 3 postnatal days has a dose-dependent relationship with odds of developing P/IVH.[87] Although a cause-and-effect relationship has not been established, the increase in CBF with hypercapnia can accentuate the reperfusion phase preceding the occurrence of P/IVH.[27] In addition, hypercapnia attenuates CBF autoregulation. A study of the correlation between blood pressure and MCA-MV demonstrated a steeper coefficient line with higher $PaCO_2$ values, suggesting a progressive impairment of CBF autoregulation with rising $PaCO_2$ above normal.[90] Similarly, we found no relationship between MCA-MV and blood pressure in normotensive preterm infants, but when adjusted for $PaCO_2$ levels, a significant positive relationship emerged, suggesting that higher $PaCO_2$ is associated with impairment of CBF autoregulation.[84] Furthermore, we found a breakpoint in the relationship between $PaCO_2$ and MCA-MV, with no relation below $PaCO_2$ values of 52 to 53 mm Hg and a strong positive linear relation above this cutoff (Fig. 6.3).

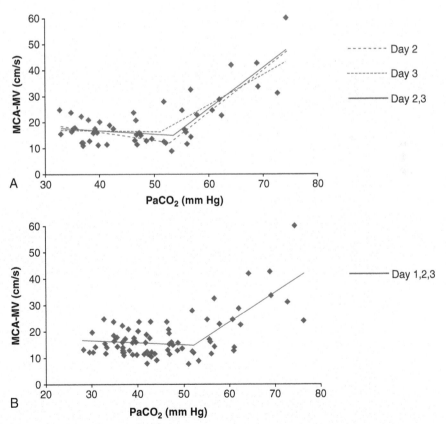

Fig. 6.3   Relationship between carbon dioxide and index of CBF. The graphs depict piecewise bi-linear regression identifying a breakpoint in the MCA-MV–$PaCO_2$ relationship. "Graph A" shows the breakpoints at a $PaCO_2$ value of 52.7 mm Hg for day #2 (broken line, R^2 = 0.74, P < .0001), 51.0 mm Hg for day #3 (dotted line, R^2 = 0.60, P < .034) and 53.2 mm Hg for days #2 and #3 combined (solid line, R^2 = 0.66, P < .0001). "Graph B" shows the breakpoint at $PaCO_2$ of 51.7 mm Hg (R^2 = 0.49, P < .0001) for all data points, including postnatal day #1. CBF, Cerebral blood flow; MCA-MV, middle cerebral artery mean flow velocity; $PaCO_2$ = partial pressure of arterial carbon dioxide.

Despite being used as a common treatment strategy during the first postnatal days and weeks, permissive hypercapnia is poorly defined, and the safe cutoff for a given gestational and chronological age is unknown. Several randomized controlled trials (RCTs) were unable to show any reduction in the rate of BPD with this strategy, and some have also raised the possibility of harm.[91-93] A recent RCT in Europe comparing mild permissive hypercapnia to a higher $PaCO_2$ strategy among extremely preterm infants on mechanical ventilation during the first postnatal day found no effect on the primary outcome of death or moderate to severe BPD, but found an increase in necrotizing enterocolitis in the higher $PaCO_2$ group.[93] Yet the 2-year follow-up of this study showed no difference in neurodevelopmental outcome, contrary to an earlier study finding worse outcomes in the permissive hypercapnia group.[92,94]

Conclusions

Pathogenesis of P/IVH is complex and involves different mechanisms. Most agree that disturbances in CBF play a major role in the development of P/IVH. Improved understanding of the physiology of the transitional circulation, especially in preterm infants during the past decade, has shed some light on the role of cardiovascular compromise and altered cerebral hemodynamics in the pathogenesis of P/IVH. The increased availability of more sophisticated, comprehensive monitoring technology and the more widespread application of these tools provide us with an opportunity to identify the subpopulation at greatest risk for circulatory compromise and development of P/IVH. This in turn can prove useful data for designing appropriate RCTs targeting the high-risk population and the underlying pathophysiology, rather than enrolling all patients in the same gestational age range and unnecessarily exposing many patients to intervention who are at minimal or no risk for the development of P/IVH.

REFERENCES

1. Stoll BJ, et al.: Neonatal outcomes of extremely preterm infants from the NICHD Neonatal Research Network, *Pediatrics* 126:443–456, 2010.
2. Mukerji A, Shah V, Shah PS: Periventricular/intraventricular hemorrhage and neurodevelopmental outcomes: a meta-analysis, *Pediatrics* 136:1132–1143, 2015.
3. Rudolph AM: Distribution and regulation of blood flow in the fetal and neonatal lamb, *Circ Res* 57:811–821, 1985.
4. Rothstein R, Longo L: In Cowett R, editor: *Principles of perinatal-neonatal metabolism*, 1998, Springer-Verlag, p 451.
5. Kiserud T, Acharya G: The fetal circulation, *Prenat Diagn* 24:1049–1059, 2004.
6. Sutton MS, Groves A, MacNeill A, et al.: Assessment of changes in blood flow through the lungs and foramen ovale in the normal human fetus with gestational age: a prospective Doppler echocardiographic study, *Br Heart J* 71:232–237, 1994.
7. Rasanen J, Wood DC, Weiner S, et al.: Role of the pulmonary circulation in the distribution of human fetal cardiac output during the second half of pregnancy, *Circulation.* 94:1068–1073, 1996.
8. Mielke G, Benda N: Cardiac output and central distribution of blood flow in the human fetus, *Circulation* 103:1662–1668, 2001.
9. Prsa M, et al.: Reference ranges of blood flow in the major vessels of the normal human fetal circulation at term by phase-contrast magnetic resonance imaging, *Circ Cardiovasc Imaging* 7:663–670, 2014.
10. Noori S, et al.: Transitional changes in cardiac and cerebral hemodynamics in term neonates at birth, *J Pediatr* 160:943–948, 2012.
11. Rudolph AM, Heymann MA: Circulatory changes during growth in the fetal lamb, *Circ Res* 26:289–299, 1970.
12. Meerman RJ, van Bel F, van Zwieten PH, et al.: Fetal and neonatal cerebral blood velocity in the normal fetus and neonate: a longitudinal Doppler ultrasound study, *Early Hum Dev* 24:209–217, 1990.
13. Iwamoto HS, Teitel D, Rudolph AM: Effects of birth-related events on blood flow distribution, *Pediatr Res* 22:634–640, 1987.
14. Kempley ST, Vyas S, Bower S, et al.: Cerebral and renal artery blood flow velocity before and after birth, *Early Hum Dev* 46:165–174, 1996.
15. Meek JH, Tyszczuk L, Elwell CE, Wyatt JS: Cerebral blood flow increases over the first three days of life in extremely preterm neonates, *Arch Dis Child Fetal Neonatal Ed* 78:F33–F37, 1998.
16. Kluckow M, Evans N: Superior vena cava flow in newborn infants: a novel marker of systemic blood flow, *Arch Dis Child Fetal Neonatal Ed* 82:F182–F187, 2000.
17. Kissack CM, Garr R, Wardle SP, Weindling AM: Postnatal changes in cerebral oxygen extraction in the preterm infant are associated with intraventricular hemorrhage and hemorrhagic parenchymal infarction but not periventricular leukomalacia, *Pediatr Res* 56:111–116, 2004.

18. Kehrer M, et al.: Development of cerebral blood flow volume in preterm neonates during the first two weeks of life, *Pediatr Res* 58:927–930, 2005.

19. Greisen G: Cerebral blood flow in preterm infants during the first week of life, *Acta Paediatr Scand* 75:43–51, 1986.

20. Altman DI, et al.: Cerebral blood flow requirement for brain viability in newborn infants is lower than in adults, *Ann Neurol* 24:218–226, 1988.

21. Meek JH, Tyszczuk L, Elwell CE, Wyatt JS: Low cerebral blood flow is a risk factor for severe intraventricular haemorrhage, *Arch Dis Child Fetal Neonatal Ed* 81:F15–F18, 1999.

22. Kluckow M, Evans N: Low superior vena cava flow and intraventricular haemorrhage in preterm infants, *Arch Child Fetal Neonatal Ed* 82:F188–F194, 2000.

23. Verhagen EA, et al.: Cerebral oxygenation in preterm infants with germinal matrix-intraventricular hemorrhages, *Stroke J Cereb Circ* 41:2901–2907, 2010.

24. Sorensen LC, Maroun LL, Borch K, et al.: Neonatal cerebral oxygenation is not linked to foetal vasculitis and predicts intraventricular haemorrhage in preterm infants, *Acta Paediatr Oslo Nor 1992* 97:1529–1534, 2008.

25. Alderliesten T, et al.: Cerebral oxygenation, extraction, and autoregulation in very preterm infants who develop peri-intraventricular hemorrhage, *J Pediatr* 162:698–704.e2, 2013.

26. Noori S, Seri I: Hemodynamic antecedents of peri/intraventricular hemorrhage in very preterm neonates, *Semin Fetal Neonatal Med* 20:232–237, 2015.

27. Noori S, McCoy M, Anderson MP, et al.: Changes in cardiac function and cerebral blood flow in relation to peri/intraventricular hemorrhage in extremely preterm infants, *J Pediatr* 164:264–270.e1–e3, 2014.

28. Bassan H: Intracranial hemorrhage in the preterm infant: understanding it, preventing it, *Clin Perinatol.* 36:737–762, v, 2009.

29. Ballabh P: Intraventricular hemorrhage in premature infants: mechanism of disease, *Pediatr Res* 67:1–8, 2010.

30. Hambleton G, Wigglesworth JS: Origin of intraventricular haemorrhage in the preterm infant, *Arch Dis Child* 51:651–659, 1976.

31. du Plessis AJ: Cerebrovascular injury in premature infants: current understanding and challenges for future prevention, *Clin Perinatol* 35:609–641, v, 2008.

32. Greisen G: Cerebral autoregulation in preterm infants. How to measure it-and why care? *J Pediatr* 165:885–886, 2014.

33. Soul JS, et al.: Fluctuating pressure-passivity is common in the cerebral circulation of sick premature infants, *Pediatr Res* 61:467–473, 2007.

34. Wong FY, et al.: Impaired autoregulation in preterm infants identified by using spatially resolved spectroscopy, *Pediatrics* 121:e604–e611, 2008.

35. Vesoulis ZA, Liao SM, Trivedi SB, et al.: A novel method for assessing cerebral autoregulation in preterm infants using transfer function analysis, *Pediatr Res* 79:453–459, 2016.

36. Tsuji M, et al.: Cerebral intravascular oxygenation correlates with mean arterial pressure in critically ill premature infants, *Pediatrics* 106:625–632, 2000.

37. O'Leary H, et al.: Elevated cerebral pressure passivity is associated with prematurity-related intracranial hemorrhage, *Pediatrics* 124:302–309, 2009.

38. Riera J, et al.: New time-frequency method for cerebral autoregulation in newborns: predictive capacity for clinical outcomes, *J Pediatr* 165:897–902.e1, 2014.

39. Noori S, Stavroudis TA, Seri I: Systemic and cerebral hemodynamics during the transitional period after premature birth, *Clin Perinatol* 36:723–736, v, 2009.

40. Hernandez M, Hawkins R, Brennan R: In Heistad D, Marcus M, editors: *Cerebral blood flow, effects of nerves and neurotransmitters*, 1982, Elsevier, pp 359–366.

41. Ashwal S, Dale PS, Longo LD: Regional cerebral blood flow: studies in the fetal lamb during hypoxia, hypercapnia, acidosis, and hypotension, *Pediatr Res* 18:1309–1316, 1984.

42. Victor S, Appleton RE, Beirne M, et al.: The relationship between cardiac output, cerebral electrical activity, cerebral fractional oxygen extraction and peripheral blood flow in premature newborn infants, *Pediatr Res* 60:456–460, 2006.

43. Noori S, Wu TW, Seri I: pH effects on cardiac function and systemic vascular resistance in preterm infants, *J Pediatr* 162:958–963.e1, 2013.

44. Osborn DA, Evans N, Kluckow M: Left ventricular contractility in extremely premature infants in the first day and response to inotropes, *Pediatr Res* 61:335–340, 2007.

45. Baenziger O, et al.: The influence of the timing of cord clamping on postnatal cerebral oxygenation in preterm neonates: a randomized, controlled trial, *Pediatrics* 119:455–459, 2007.

46. Sommers R, et al.: Hemodynamic effects of delayed cord clamping in premature infants, *Pediatrics* 129:e667–e672, 2012.

47. Rabe H, Reynolds G, Diaz-Rossello J: A systematic review and meta-analysis of a brief delay in clamping the umbilical cord of preterm infants, *Neonatology* 93:138–144, 2008.

48. Ghavam S, et al.: Effects of placental transfusion in extremely low birthweight infants: meta-analysis of long- and short-term outcomes, *Transfusion (Paris)* 54:1192–1198, 2014.

49. Yao AC, Moinian M, Lind J: Distribution of blood between infant and placenta after birth, *Lancet* 2:871–873, 1969.

50. Bhatt S, et al.: Delaying cord clamping until ventilation onset improves cardiovascular function at birth in preterm lambs, *J Physiol* 591:2113–2126, 2013.

51. Hosono S, et al.: Blood pressure and urine output during the first 120 h of life in infants born at less than 29 weeks' gestation related to umbilical cord milking, *Arch Dis Child Fetal Neonatal Ed* 94:F328–F331, 2009.

52. Takami T, et al.: Umbilical cord milking stabilizes cerebral oxygenation and perfusion in infants born before 29 weeks of gestation, *J Pediatr* 161:742–747, 2012.

53. Katheria AC, Truong G, Cousins L, et al.: Umbilical cord milking versus delayed cord clamping in preterm infants, *Pediatrics* 136:61–69, 2015.

54. Lemmers PMA, Toet MC, van Bel F: Impact of patent ductus arteriosus and subsequent therapy with indomethacin on cerebral oxygenation in preterm infants, *Pediatrics* 121:142–147, 2008.

55. Lemmers PMA, et al.: Patent ductus arteriosus and brain volume, *Pediatrics* 137, 2016.

56. Chock VY, Rose LA, Mante JV, Punn R: Near-infrared spectroscopy for detection of a significant patent ductus arteriosus, *Pediatr Res* 80:675–680, 2016.

57. Watkins AM, West CR, Cooke RW: Blood pressure and cerebral haemorrhage and ischaemia in very low birthweight infants, *Early Hum Dev* 19:103–110, 1989.

58. Pellicer A, et al.: Early systemic hypotension and vasopressor support in low birth weight infants: impact on neurodevelopment, *Pediatrics* 123:1369–1376, 2009.

59. Batton B, Batton D, Riggs T: Blood pressure during the first 7 days in premature infants born at post-menstrual age 23 to 25 weeks, *Am J Perinatol* 24:107–115, 2007.

60. Dempsey EM, Al Hazzani F, Barrington KJ: Permissive hypotension in the extremely low birth-weight infant with signs of good perfusion, *Arch Dis Child Fetal Neonatal Ed* 94:F241–F244, 2009.

61. Batton B, et al.: Blood pressure, anti-hypotensive therapy, and neurodevelopment in extremely pre-term infants, *J Pediatr* 154:351–357, 357.e1, 2009.

62. Munro MJ, Walker AM, Barfield CP: Hypotensive extremely low birth weight infants have reduced cerebral blood flow, *Pediatrics* 114:1591–1596, 2004.

63. Lightburn MH, Gauss CH, Williams DK, Kaiser JR: Observational study of cerebral hemodynamics during dopamine treatment in hypotensive ELBW infants on the first day of life, *J Perinatol Off J Calif Perinat Assoc* 33:698–702, 2013.

64. Seri I, Rudas G, Bors Z, et al.: Effects of low-dose dopamine infusion on cardiovascular and renal functions, cerebral blood flow, and plasma catecholamine levels in sick preterm neonates, *Pediatr Res* 34:742–749, 1993.

65. Pellicer A, et al.: Cardiovascular support for low birth weight infants and cerebral hemodynamics: a randomized, blinded, clinical trial, *Pediatrics* 115:1501–1512, 2005.

66. Vesoulis ZA, et al.: Response to dopamine in prematurity: a biomarker for brain injury? *J Perinatol Off J Calif Perinat Assoc*, 2016. https://doi.org/10.1038/jp.2016.5.

67. Batton BJ, et al.: Feasibility study of early blood pressure management in extremely preterm infants, *J Pediatr.* 161:65–69.e1, 2012.

68. Cheifetz IM, et al.: Increasing tidal volumes and pulmonary overdistention adversely affect pulmo-nary vascular mechanics and cardiac output in a pediatric swine model, *Crit Care Med* 26:710–716, 1998.

69. Polglase GR, et al.: Positive end-expiratory pressure differentially alters pulmonary hemodynamics and oxygenation in ventilated, very premature lambs, *J Appl Physiol Bethesda Md 1985* 99:1453–1461, 2005.

70. Hausdorf G, Hellwege HH: Influence of positive end-expiratory pressure on cardiac performance in premature infants: a Doppler-echocardiographic study, *Crit Care Med* 15:661–664, 1987.

71. de Waal KA, Evans N, Osborn DA, Kluckow M: Cardiorespiratory effects of changes in end expira-tory pressure in ventilated newborns, *Arch Dis Child Fetal Neonatal Ed* 92:F444–F448, 2007.

72. Abdel-Hady H, Matter M, Hammad A, et al.: Hemodynamic changes during weaning from nasal continuous positive airway pressure, *Pediatrics* 122:e1086–e1090, 2008.

73. Beker F, Rogerson SR, Hooper SB, et al.: The effects of nasal continuous positive airway pressure on cardiac function in premature infants with minimal lung disease: a crossover randomized trial, *J Pediatr* 164:726–729, 2014.

74. Perlman JM, McMenamin JB, Volpe JJ: Fluctuating cerebral blood-flow velocity in respiratory-dis-tress syndrome. Relation to the development of intraventricular hemorrhage, *N Engl J Med* 309:204–209, 1983.

75. Cowan F, Thoresen M: The effects of intermittent positive pressure ventilation on cerebral arterial and venous blood velocities in the newborn infant, *Acta Paediatr Scand* 76:239–247, 1987.

76. Skinner JR, Milligan DW, Hunter S, Hey EN: Central venous pressure in the ventilated neonate, *Arch Dis Child* 67:374–377, 1992.

77. Kaiser JR, Gauss CH, Williams DK: Surfactant administration acutely affects cerebral and systemic hemodynamics and gas exchange in very-low-birth-weight infants, *J Pediatr* 144:809–814, 2004.

78. Saliba E, Nashashibi M, Vaillant MC, et al.: Instillation rate effects of Exosurf on cerebral and car-diovascular haemodynamics in preterm neonates, *Arch Dis Child Fetal Neonatal Ed* 71:F174–F178, 1994.

79. Roll C, Knief J, Horsch S, Hanssler L: Effect of surfactant administration on cerebral haemodynamics and oxygenation in premature infants–a near infrared spectroscopy study, *Neuropediatrics* 31:16–23, 2000.

80. Wiswell TE, et al.: Effects of hypocarbia on the development of cystic periventricular leukomalacia in premature infants treated with high-frequency jet ventilation, *Pediatrics* 98:918–924, 1996.

81. Shankaran S, et al.: Cumulative index of exposure to hypocarbia and hyperoxia as risk factors for periventricular leukomalacia in low birth weight infants, *Pediatrics* 118:1654–1659, 2006.

82. Ambalavanan N, et al.: $PaCO_2$ in surfactant, positive pressure, and oxygenation randomised trial (SUPPORT), *Arch Dis Child Fetal Neonatal Ed* 100:F145–F149, 2015.

83. Levene MI, Shortland D, Gibson N, Evans DH: Carbon dioxide reactivity of the cerebral circulation in extremely premature infants: effects of postnatal age and indomethacin, *Pediatr Res* 24:175–179, 1988.

84. Noori S, Anderson M, Soleymani S, Evans DH: Effect of carbon dioxide on cerebral blood flow velocity in preterm infants during postnatal transition, *Acta Paediatr Oslo Nor.1992* 103:e334–e339, 2014.

85. Pryds O, Greisen G, Lou H, Friis-Hansen B: Heterogeneity of cerebral vasoreactivity in preterm infants supported by mechanical ventilation, *J Pediatr* 115:638–645, 1989.

86. Tyszczuk L, Meek J, Elwell C, Wyatt JS: Cerebral blood flow is independent of mean arterial blood pressure in preterm infants undergoing intensive care, *Pediatrics* 102:337–341, 1998.

87. Kaiser JR, Gauss CH, Pont MM, Williams DK: Hypercapnia during the first 3 days of life is associated with severe intraventricular hemorrhage in very low birth weight infants, *J Perinatol Off J Calif Perinat Assoc* 26:279–285, 2006.

88. Fabres J, Carlo WA, Phillips V, et al.: Both extremes of arterial carbon dioxide pressure and the magnitude of fluctuations in arterial carbon dioxide pressure are associated with severe intraventricular hemorrhage in preterm infants, *Pediatrics* 119:299–305, 2007.

89. McKee LA, et al.: PaCO$_2$ and neurodevelopment in extremely low birth weight infants, *J Pediatr* 155:217–221.e1, 2009.

90. Kaiser JR, Gauss CH, Williams DK: The effects of hypercapnia on cerebral autoregulation in ventilated very low birth weight infants, *Pediatr Res* 58:931–935, 2005.

91. Carlo WA, et al.: Minimal ventilation to prevent bronchopulmonary dysplasia in extremely-low-birth-weight infants, *J Pediatr* 141:370–374, 2002.

92. Thome UH, et al.: Outcome of extremely preterm infants randomized at birth to different PaCO$_2$ targets during the first seven days of life, *Biol Neonate* 90:218–225, 2006.

93. Thome UH, et al.: Permissive hypercapnia in extremely low birthweight infants (PHELBI): a randomised controlled multicentre trial, *Lancet Respir Med* 3:534–543, 2015.

94. Thome UH, et al.: Neurodevelopmental outcomes of extremely low birthweight infants randomised to different PCO$_2$ targets: the PHELBI follow-up study, *Arch Dis Child Fetal Neonatal Ed*, 2017. https://doi.org/10.1136/archdischild-2016-311581.

6

The Immature Autonomic Nervous System, Hemodynamic Regulation, and Brain Injury in the Preterm Neonate

Sarah B. Mulkey and Adré J. du Plessis

7

- The premature infant has an immature cardiovascular and intrinsic cerebral autoregulatory system.
- The autonomic nervous system (ANS) is immature in premature newborns, particularly the parasympathetic division which is relatively underdeveloped compared with the sympathetic division at the time of premature birth.
- Autonomic dysmaturation may result when the ANS develops in the nonphysiologic conditions of premature ex utero life. Such autonomic dysmaturation of prematurity may have long-term health (e.g., adult hypertension) and psychoaffective consequences.
- Knowledge about cerebral hemodynamics in premature newborns is limited by a lack of bedside continuous clinical monitoring technologies.
- Cerebral blood flow (CBF) can be measured by the techniques of arterial spin labeling (ASL) magnetic resonance imaging (MRI) and diffuse correlation spectroscopy (DCS). These techniques confirm increasing CBF with advancing gestational age (GA) in premature newborns.
- The incidence of severe intraventricular hemorrhage (IVH) and of cystic periventricular leukomalacia has declined in recent decades.

Regulation of brain perfusion and oxygen/substrate delivery is, broadly speaking, dependent upon two partially overlapping systems. These are cardiovascular-respiratory regulation by the brainstem autonomic nervous system (ANS) centers and intrinsic cerebral autoregulatory systems (with a relatively minor contribution from the ANS). The period of transition from the relatively protected and supported intrauterine environment to the complexities of the external world requires the coordination of the newborn's cardiovascular and respiratory systems.

The ANS plays a central role in maintaining homeostasis for the infant under fluctuating external conditions. In infants born prematurely, these vital body systems are immature and unprepared to provide reliable support for the infant in the ex utero environment, exposing the infant to the risks of respiratory and hemodynamic instability. Importantly, immature ANS regulation and impaired hemodynamics may lead to brain injury, but may also result in a spectrum of more subtle neurodevelopmental changes whose effects may not become evident until later in childhood.

Significant advances in obstetric and neonatal intensive care, ventilation strategies, and management of neonatal hemodynamics have led to a decline in the earlier, often devastating, forms of brain injury seen in the premature newborn, for example, periventricular leukomalacia (PVL) and grade IV intraventricular hemorrhage

(IVH). Survival of premature newborns has greatly improved, as has the prevalence of motor impairment and epilepsy among survivors. Unfortunately, this enhanced survival and a reduction in severe motor disabilities have unmasked psychoaffective and behavioral disorders that may be equally limiting in quality of life. Thus, the spectrum of neurologic morbidity remains prevalent in survivors of premature birth. In this chapter we explore the immature hemodynamic system of the premature newborn and its relation to brain injury, seek to understand the influence of the immature ANS on brainstem responses and how this may affect higher cortical functions, and review how these immature systems may relate to prematurity-related brain injury.

Magnitude of the Problem

Prematurity-related brain injury remains a major public health concern.[1,2] Survivors of prematurity are at risk for long-term motor, cognitive, and psychoaffective disorders (Fig. 7.1).[3–5] Both the incidence and severity of brain injury in premature infants are inversely related to gestational age (GA).[5] Because advances in survival have been greatest among the sickest, smallest, most immature infants, that is, those at greatest risk for cerebral circulatory instability and brain injury,[6] it is perhaps not surprising that survivors of extreme prematurity have the highest risk for the

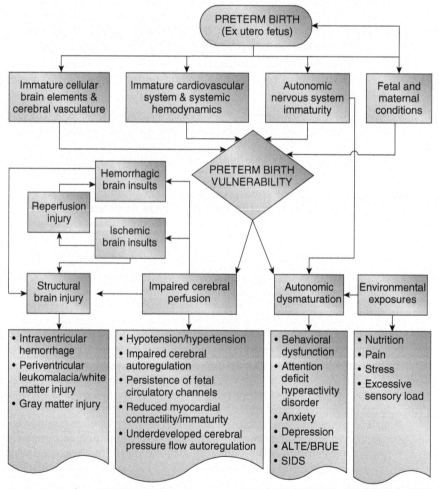

Fig. 7.1 **Preterm brain vulnerability.** There is a complex interplay of multiple factors that affect the preterm newborn's brain. The immature cardiovascular, hemodynamic, and autonomic nervous systems, as well as fetal and maternal conditions and environmental exposures, contribute to preterm brain vulnerability. Structural brain injury and autonomic dysmaturation may occur which can impact long-term neurologic, cognitive, and behavioral outcomes. *ALTE*, Apparent life-threatening events; *BRUE*, brief resolved unexplained events; *SIDS*, sudden infant death syndrome.

development of cerebral palsy.[7] Of major concern are the 25% to 50% of ex-preterm children who demonstrate potentially debilitating behavioral or learning problems by school age,[3,4,8,9] with moderate to severe impairment in academic achievement.[10] Children born very preterm are also at increased risk for autism spectrum disorder.[5,11]

Cerebrovascular insults leading to both hemorrhagic and hypoxic-ischemic injury have long been considered a leading cause of acute and long-term neurologic morbidity in this population (see Fig. 7.1).[12–17] Hypoxia-ischemia/reperfusion injury has been implicated in the causal pathway of prematurity-related brain injury. Systemic hemodynamic impairment is commonly diagnosed and treated in the premature infant and is related inversely to GA at birth. This maturational association in premature infants between disturbed systemic hemodynamics and cerebrovascular injury has led to the notion that the relationship is causative. However, despite plausible extrapolations from human adult and supporting animal studies,[18–21] establishing a causal link in the premature infant has many challenges, which in turn continues to impede development of rational, safe, and effective interventions.

The principal forms of prematurity-related brain injury are germinal matrix-intraventricular hemorrhage (GM-IVH) and injury to the parenchyma, particularly to the immature white matter. Both anatomic and physiologic features of the premature brain predispose it to cerebrovascular injury (see Fig. 7.1). The germinal matrices in the periventricular regions of the developing brain are supported by a profuse but transient vascular system of fragile thin-walled vessels with a deficient basal lamina, no muscularis layer,[22,23] and a predisposition to hypoxia-ischemia/reperfusion injury increasing their vulnerability to rupture.[24] These germinal matrices are also vulnerable to ischemic insults during hypoperfusion and to rupture during fluctuations in perfusion pressure, the so-called "water-hammer" effect.[25] Over the past two decades, the incidence of GM-IVH in premature newborns has decreased; however, not in infants born below 26 weeks' gestation where the incidence has remained at about 27%.[6,26] Both the acute and long-term complications of GM-IVH are more serious in the smallest, sickest infants.[27,28] The most serious complications of GM-IVH are periventricular hemorrhagic infarction, with an adverse long-term outcome rate exceeding 85%,[29,30] and posthemorrhagic hydrocephalus,[31] which has an adverse long-term outcome in up to 75% of patients.[27,32] Fortunately, the incidence of this type of white matter injury has also shown a decline.[6]

Undervascularized end zones in the premature cerebral white matter are susceptible to hypoxic-ischemic injury during periods of decreased perfusion pressure due to incomplete arterial in-growth during prematurity.[33–39] White matter damage, seen on cranial ultrasound (US) as either hyper- or hypoechoic areas, with IVH in extremely preterm infants, increases the risk of long-term neurologic impairment.[40] Although the severe form of white matter injury, termed as cystic PVL that can be easily appreciated on US now has a very low prevalence, magnetic resonance imaging (MRI) studies[41] describe a high prevalence of diffuse noncystic white matter injury[42,43] to which cranial US is insensitive.[44] This diffuse form of white matter injury can be detected by MRI in more than 50% of very premature infants.[41,43]

While parenchymal brain injury in the premature infant has a predilection for the developing white matter, there is increasing recognition of injury and impaired development of gray matter structure and volumes.[45,46] Neuroimaging and pathology studies have expanded the spectrum of parenchymal lesions in survivors of prematurity by highlighting developmental disruption in both cortical and subcortical gray matter.[47] Brain volume changes can be appreciated in children born prematurely. For example, parietal and temporal lobe brain volumes are smaller in children born in the late preterm period and these findings seem to relate to increased symptoms of anxiety.[46] Differences in early brain structure and volume in premature newborns persist into adulthood with a few areas showing higher volumes (i.e., medial/anterior frontal gyrus gray matter volume), while other areas show reduced volumes (i.e., basal ganglia, thalamus, temporal, frontal, insular, and occipital gray matter).[48] In this same study, similar reductions were seen in the subcortical white matter.[48] These altered brain volumes provide a measure of the structural brain changes that are associated with impaired neurologic outcome, including cognitive and psychoaffective functions in survivors of prematurity.

Hemodynamic Vulnerability in Premature Infants

Immature ANS responses likely contribute to hemodynamic and cardiovascular instability in premature newborns.[49,50] The prevailing paradigm for hemodynamically mediated brain injury in the premature infant is centered on a confluence of insults emanating from the unstable immature cardiovascular system and immature intrinsic cerebral autoregulation acting on the fragile cerebral vasculature. The brain's cellular elements are also vulnerable, in particular immature oligodendrocytes, enhancing the risk for brain injury from hemodynamic instability.

The Premature Autonomic Nervous System

The ANS consists of the sympathetic and parasympathetic divisions and has integral control functions on many physiologic aspects of the human body. In addition, the ANS might also provide key input to the development of higher cortical structures involved in emotion, behavior, and thought processing. This important component of our nervous system matures during fetal development and into infancy.[51,52] Measurement of ANS function is challenging and somewhat limited in the fragile premature newborn. Heart rate variability (HRV), the fluctuation in the length of time between heart beats (R-R intervals), can be analyzed non-invasively to assess sympathetic and parasympathetic tone, providing a window to the ANS in newborns.[51,53] High-frequency variability reflects parasympathetic function and is influenced by the respiratory rate (respiratory sinus arrhythmia), while low-frequency variability reflects a combination of sympathetic and parasympathetic inputs, and is responsible for baroreflex-induced changes in heart rate (HR).[54] HRV is also influenced by the newborn's sleep state with active sleep having more sympathetic tone (low-frequency variability) compared with quiet sleep.[51]

Studies have evaluated the relative maturation of the sympathetic and parasympathetic divisions of the ANS using the HRV technique. In these studies, the sympathetic division develops earlier than the parasympathetic division, which shows accelerated maturation at 25 to 30 weeks' gestation, a time period when many prematurely born newborns may be undergoing transition.[49,50,55] Therefore, preterm newborns are born with underdeveloped ANS, especially of the parasympathetic division.[56] The premature engagement of the ANS under the condition of preterm birth may result in "*dysmaturation*," or a shift in the temporal program of ANS maturation due to aberrant programming.[57]

In addition to prematurity itself, there are a multitude of "unexpected" stimuli in the ex utero environment, which the premature newborn's ANS may be unprepared to experience and process. The sensory experience in the neonatal intensive care unit (NICU) environment is far harsher than that experienced in the muted intrauterine milieu. Depending on the GA and morbidity of the infant, the extraordinary experiences may include oxygenation disturbances and positive pressure ventilation forces on the premature lungs, hemodynamic instability which is increased by the patent ductus arteriosus, infections, painful procedures, light, and air and temperature changes on the delicate skin, among others. All of these unexpected stimuli can create a challenging environment for maturation of the ANS. Under these conditions, dysmaturation of the ANS may result when the normal programming is disturbed. Importantly, ANS dysmaturation may increase the risk for IVH in premature newborns[58] and for subsequent sudden infant death syndrome and brief resolved unexplained events (BRUE, formerly "apparent life threatening events" [ALTE]).[59–61] These consequences will be discussed later in the chapter.

Key ANS centers within the brainstem, namely the nucleus tractus solitarius and dorsal motor nucleus of the vagus, receive input from peripheral sensory receptors and exert autonomic control to regulate HR and other critical body functions. In addition, supratentorial ANS centers including the anterior thalamus, anterior cingulate gyrus, and the amygdala integrate the more primitive functions of the ANS with higher cortical processes, a major evolutionary advantage for humans. It is the impaired influence on these higher order cortical structures that likely contributes to the high rate of psychoaffective disorders in children and young adults born prematurely.[62]

The Premature Cardiovascular System

The early period of transition to extrauterine life in the premature newborn is a particularly challenging time for the immature cardiovascular system (see Chapter 1), as well as the ANS, as described above. In the premature infant, the normal postnatal closure of fetal circulatory channels, such as the ductus arteriosus and foramen ovale, may be delayed for days or even weeks, compromising cardiovascular efficiency. In addition, the myocardium is also immature, which may compromise systemic blood flow. In certain pathophysiologic conditions, including extreme prematurity, the relationship between systemic blood pressure (BP) and blood flow becomes complex. After normal birth, the term infant experiences a brisk increase in cardiac output, which is determined by HR and myocardial contractility.[63] In the extremely premature infant, this early increase in cardiac output tends to be delayed;[64-68] in fact, one-third of these infants may experience periods of low cardiac output during the first 24 hours after birth,[64] when the risk for brain injury is particularly high.[69,70] These low systemic blood flow states are mediated by several mechanisms. First, as detailed previously, the maturation of the fetal sympathetic nervous system precedes that of the parasympathetic system, which remains underdeveloped in the premature infant.[55] This autonomic immaturity leaves the baroreflex and chemoreflex systems underdeveloped prior to term.[71,72] During periods of low cardiac output, the premature infant becomes particularly dependent on HR; however, with baseline sympathetic activity already close to maximal, the ability to increase cardiac output by increasing HR alone is limited. Second, the immature myocardium has fewer mitochondria and lower energy stores, and its contractility at baseline is close to maximal, with a limited ability to increase stroke volume. The positive pressure ventilation frequently required by extremely premature infants may further reduce cardiac output by decreasing venous return and compressing the cardiac chambers. Third, the premature cardiovascular system is confronted at birth by a sudden and significant increase in afterload during the transition from a low-resistance placental bed to the higher postnatal peripheral resistance.[64-68] Systemic vascular resistance increases in the postnatal period because of increased release of catecholamines into the circulation. In addition, fluctuations in resistance may result from episodic sympathetic activation during oxyhemoglobin desaturation, suctioning, handling, and hypercarbia, events common in neonatal critical care.

Although cardiac output is the critical measure of overall systemic blood flow, it is not easily measured in the premature infant. Conversely, continuous intraarterial BP monitoring is widely used to manage hemodynamics in critically ill premature newborns. Hemodynamic management is thus largely pressure based in premature infants. Normal arterial BP may be defined broadly as the range of BP required to maintain perfusion appropriate for the functional and structural integrity of the tissues. In the extremely premature infant, the combination of increased peripheral resistance and myocardial immaturity may translate into decreased tissue blood flow. The above definition of "normal BP" can fail in this situation (see Chapter 3).

There have been a number of attempts to define normal BP in premature infants (see Chapter 3). Population-based studies have described statistical norms for BP in premature infants without evidence of significant brain injury.[73-76] In these studies, BP increases with GA at birth as well as with postnatal age during the first week.[73,74,76–78] Other studies have tried to define the limits of normal BP by comparing BP in premature infants with and without brain injury.[79–82] Despite these studies, the range of "normal BP" remains largely unknown for premature infants, and BP management continues to differ markedly between, and even within, centers.[83] The lack of established normative data for BP notwithstanding, "hypotension" remains commonly diagnosed and treated, especially in smaller and sicker premature infants.[83,84] Furthermore, there is very little evidence that treatment of hypotension improves neurodevelopmental outcome.[84,85]

Cerebral Hemodynamic Control in Premature Infants

The hemodynamic physiology of the immature brain increases its vulnerability to injury. Unlike the mature brain where CBF exceeds the ischemic injury threshold by fivefold,[86] the premature brain has significantly lower global and regional CBF,[87] especially in the white matter where there is a much lower ischemic injury threshold.[88,89] This suggests a reduced margin of safety for cerebral perfusion, but has to be considered in the context of reduced oxygen metabolism in the premature brain (see Chapter 2). Monitoring of cerebral tissue oxygenation is an emerging and likely very important monitoring approach during transition of the premature newborn during the first few hours after birth (see Chapters 17 and 18).[90]

Under normal conditions, cerebral perfusion is maintained by a background perfusion pressure provided by the cardiovascular system, which is then "fine-tuned" within the cerebral vasculature by complex intrinsic autoregulatory mechanisms (see Chapter 2). However, if cerebral insults are sustained, these responses eventually fail, leading to irreversible brain injury.[91] Cerebral pressure autoregulation maintains CBF relatively constant across a range of cerebral perfusion pressure called the autoregulatory plateau.[92] In addition to these upper and lower pressure bounds, cerebral pressure autoregulation also has a limited impulse-response time, of the order of 5 to 15 seconds.[93] Outside of these pressure and temporal bounds, CBF is pressure passive, with an increased risk of cerebrovascular injury.

Cerebral pressure-flow autoregulation emerges during fetal life but is underdeveloped in the immature brain. With decreasing GA, the autoregulatory plateau is narrower and lower,[94,95] and normal resting BP is closer to the lower threshold of autoregulation.[96] Although cerebral pressure-flow autoregulation is well characterized in children and adults, this is not the case for the newborn,[96] least of all the sick premature infant.[98–105] Some studies in stable preterm infants have suggested a lower autoregulatory limit around 25 to 30 mm Hg;[100,106,107] however, in the sick premature infant, the existence and limits of cerebral pressure autoregulation remain controversial.[98,99,104,108–112]

Evidence for an Association Between Systemic Hemodynamic Disturbances and Prematurity-Related Brain Injury

A variety of BP disturbances have been implicated in prematurity-related brain injury, including arterial hypotension,[81,113–119] hypertension,[120,121] cerebral venous hypertension,[122–124] and/or fluctuating BP.[125–127] Different mechanisms have been proposed for the role of "hypotension" in GM-IVH. With intact pressure autoregulation, hypotension triggers cerebral vasodilation, with the increased cerebral blood volume potentially leading to the rupture of fragile vessels. Conversely, with disrupted cerebral pressure autoregulation, or with BPs below the autoregulatory plateau, there is greater variability in CBF. During hypotension, hypoxic-ischemic injury to the vessel walls may further disrupt cerebral pressure autoregulation,[97,128–134] and vessels may rupture during reperfusion. In addition to GM-IVH, systemic hypotension has also been implicated in the development of white matter injury in premature infants.[79,81,82,113,135] However, other studies have shown no such relationship.[117,120,136,137] The diastolic closing margin, the difference between the diastolic arterial BP and the critical closing pressure (the arterial BP at which CBF stops), is higher in premature infants that develop GM-IVH.[138,139] Critical closing pressure, however, increases during the second and third trimesters which may be why some premature newborns show a better ability to handle hypotension without resulting brain injury.[140] Unlike hypotension, sustained hypertension is not commonly diagnosed in premature humans, although it may also result in the development of GM-IVH.[120,121] Fluctuating BP in premature infants, particularly during positive pressure ventilation, has been associated with GM-IVH in a number of reports, presumably through a "water-hammer" effect of fluctuations in perfusion of the fragile germinal matrix vessels.* However, the role of fluctuating cerebral perfusion in prematurity-related brain injury remains controversial, since several studies found no such association.[99,127] In summary, the role of systemic BP disturbances and impaired cerebral pressure-flow autoregulation in prematurity-related brain injury is unclear and further studies are needed to more appropriately address this important question.

Doppler US and functional echocardiography studies have identified periods of low cardiac output and low "cerebral" perfusion in premature infants during the early hours after birth. In these studies, the authors observed that these low-flow states are not reliably detected by systemic BP measurements[65–68,144] and do not always respond to vasopressor inotropes.[68] In addition, these low cardiac output states are associated with low superior vena cava (SVC) flow, suggesting decreased cerebral perfusion.[65,66,145–148] Up to 80% of premature infants have their lowest SVC flow between 5 and 12 hours after birth. Periods of low SVC flow are associated with disturbed cerebral oxygenation by near-infrared spectroscopy (NIRS).[149,150] Both the nadir and duration of low SVC flow are associated with severe GM-IVH,[148,150,151] and later adverse neurologic outcomes.[65,66] In summary, the association between systemic BP disturbances, as currently measured and interpreted, and prematurity-related brain injury remains somewhat controversial (see Chapter 6).

Resolving the Relationship Between Systemic Hemodynamics and Prematurity-Related Brain Injury: Obstacles to Progress

Several fundamental and interrelated challenges continue to impede our understanding of the relationship between changes in systemic hemodynamics, the immature response of the ANS, and brain injury in the premature infant. Advancing the field will require insight into the interaction between the immature systemic and cerebral hemodynamic systems, the ANS, and how this mediates injury to the immature brain.

Measurement of Relevant Hemodynamic and Metabolic Indices

Currently there are no established techniques for making continuous, *quantitative* measurements of systemic or CBF in the fragile newborn infant (see Chapter 21). Arterial BP, the only continuous systemic hemodynamic signal available in the premature infant, has several important limitations. First, there are no widely accepted noninvasive techniques for acquiring continuous BP in the premature infant.[60,152–154] Second, the relationship between BP and systemic blood flow is not constant, particularly during periods of critical physiologic instability. Arterial BP is often used as a surrogate for cerebral perfusion pressure because the effect of venous pressure is disregarded in many clinical situations. However, in premature infants requiring positive pressure ventilatory support, the effect of increased intrathoracic pressure may have a significant impact on cerebral perfusion. At present, techniques for monitoring cerebral perfusion pressure are not available.[103,113,115,121,126,127,141–143]

Cardiac output is considered the gold standard measure of systemic blood flow (see Chapter 14). However, there are currently no well-accepted techniques for the measurement of *continuous* cardiac output in the premature infant. Similar challenges confront the measurement of continuous CBF volume. Transcranial Doppler US measures cerebral hemodynamics and CBF velocity,[93,111,126,155–158] but not actual CBF. In the absence of reliable techniques for *continuous* CBF measurement, a number of intermittent, so-called static approaches have been used to measure quantitative CBF in the premature infant.[65,66,110,145–147,159–163] These techniques are largely based on the Fick principle, using tracers ranging from Xe^{133} to oxyhemoglobin measured by NIRS. Another approach has been the use of intermittent measurement of SVC flow by Doppler US as a surrogate for CBF. These studies have also demonstrated the association between abnormally low SVC flow and neurologic morbidity.[65,66,145–147] However, these measurements of SVC flow are not continuous and, in the very preterm infant, less than 50% of the blood in the SVC represents the blood coming from the brain (see Chapter 2).[164] Thus, all of the so-called static measurements of CBF suffer from the inability to capture the dynamic nature of cerebral hemodynamics during the period of major physiologic change associated with transition to premature postnatal life.

The ability to measure the relationship between cerebral oxygen demand and supply would provide major insights into the mechanisms of brain injury in premature infants. This is important because it is clear that not only cerebral oxygen deficiency but also excessive cerebral oxygenation may be harmful to the immature brain.[165,166] In stable premature infants, the premature brain might be "hyper-oxygenated" at baseline compared with the mature brain.[167] NIRS devices measure continuous cerebral tissue hemoglobin saturation as a surrogate measure of the adequacy of cerebral oxygen delivery (see Chapters 17 and 18). The rationale behind this approach is that normal autoregulatory mechanisms maintain appropriate cerebral oxygen delivery and cerebral oxygen extraction;[91] conversely, increasing cerebral oxygen extraction is interpreted as decreased oxygen delivery, presumably due to decreasing CBF. However, this approach assumes that neurovascular coupling is intact in sick premature infants. Furthermore, cerebral oxygen extraction may actually decrease after significant brain insults. For these reasons, measures of cerebral tissue hemoglobin oxygenation may be misleading when considered in isolation.

Understanding CBF in the premature infant has been limited by the lack of bedside techniques capable of measuring *regional* blood flow within the brain. Not only is global CBF lower in these infants, but blood flow is also particularly low in the most vulnerable white matter regions.[87,168] Arterial spin labeling (ASL) perfusion MRI at 3 Tesla can measure regional cerebral perfusion noninvasively and without the need for contrast.[169] In a study using pseudo-continuous ASL, frontal brain regions showed a faster increase in CBF with increasing GA compared with the occipital regions.[87] In another study using ASL, neonates born prematurely were found to have higher perfusion at term GA compared with term newborns, indicating a potential effect of ex utero development on brain perfusion.[170] The ASL technique does have some technical challenges in the high-risk preterm neonate, and similar to many other imaging techniques, it is not portable to the bedside and does not allow for a true continuous measurement. Diffuse correlation spectroscopy (DCS) is an emerging technique to monitor CBF in premature newborns. Advantages are that it is noninvasive, portable to the bedside, and provides continuous monitoring of cerebral microvascular blood flow. DCS measures a CBF index, which correlates with CBF as measured by the ASL-MRI technique.[171] In a study using frequency domain-NIRS and DCS, higher indices of CBF, cerebral blood volume, and cerebral hemoglobin oxygenation were found in the temporal and parietal regions compared with the frontal lobe in both premature and term newborns, and this increased with increasing GA.[172] These hemodynamic parameters were also greater in the right hemisphere compared with the left and were higher in male than in female infants.[172] The finding of hemodynamic differences between the hemispheres may be related to different developmental time courses between the right and left forebrain. The etiology of the difference in development between the hemispheres is still being explored and may relate to ductal effects in addition to other factors. DCS and NIRS can be combined to yield quantification of regional cerebral oxygen metabolism ($CMRO_2$).[173] DCS also has limitations with depth of penetration and is sensitive to motion artifacts.[173] Increased use of these newer techniques will hopefully enhance understanding of CBF in premature infants.

Potential for "Dysmaturation" of the Autonomic Nervous System in Premature Newborns

As discussed earlier, at the time of premature birth, the newborn has an immature ANS, with greater sympathetic than parasympathetic influence.[56] The premature engagement of the ANS under ex utero conditions of preterm birth may result in *dysmaturation*, or a shift in the temporal program of ANS maturation due to aberrant programming.[57] Premature newborns have an increased risk for sudden infant death syndrome and for BRUE/ALTE[59] after discharge from the NICU, which may be due to reduced cardiorespiratory system control from ANS dysmaturation.[60] In a study of premature newborns that developed BRUE/ALTE, there was a paradoxical increase in parasympathetic tone and lower sympathetic tone at 36 weeks' postmenstrual age, likely restricting the ability of these infants to autoresuscitate by increasing HR and BP during a cardiovascular or respiratory-induced event.[61] Immature ANS function may also increase risk for IVH in premature newborns.[58] Measures of HRV were different in very low birth weight infants who developed IVH compared with infants who did not develop IVH, indicating that impaired ANS function may be an antecedent risk factor for the development of IVH.[58] Brain injury in preterm newborns may alter the trajectory of ANS development which can have long-term consequences on neurologic and psychoaffective development into childhood and adulthood.[62]

Fetal oxygen and nutrient deprivation may have similar dysmaturational influences on ANS development. Two examples of such hypoxemic and potentially nutrient-deprived conditions are complex congenital heart disease and fetal growth restriction with placental insufficiency. The fetal brain, in the third trimester, undergoes rapid growth, maturation, and enhanced complexity of its neuronal connections.[174] Complex forms of congenital heart disease, such as hypoplastic left heart syndrome, are complicated by in utero hypoxemia and hypoperfusion.[175] Fetuses with hypoplastic left heart syndrome have reduced HR and reduced HRV compared with healthy control fetuses at similar GA, suggesting that ANS maturation may be delayed even prior to birth in these fetuses.[176] Similarly, fetal growth restriction is associated with placental insufficiency/failure, nutrient deprivation, and hypoxemia and a recent study found reduced HRV in fetuses affected by fetal growth restriction compared with healthy controls.[177,178] ANS immaturity under these circumstances may increase the need for early neonatal vasopressor support and mechanical ventilation and may prolong duration of intensive care. Infants who experience suboptimal fetal oxygen and nutrient environments may continue to have reduced HRV, which can be associated with lifelong cardiovascular morbidities.[179]

Characterizing "Significant" Systemic Hemodynamic Insults and Establishing a Temporal Relationship Between Hemodynamic Changes and Brain Insults Is Difficult in Sick Premature Infants

Understanding the role of systemic hemodynamic factors in prematurity-related brain injury has been impeded by a fundamental lack of understanding of the "dose" of hemodynamic insult required to injure the premature brain. Insults capable of causing injury to the premature brain are likely distinctly different from those injuring the mature brain. In the extremely premature infant, the risk period for hypoxic-ischemic brain insults may extend for weeks or months during the prolonged NICU stay. Presumably, injury thresholds exist for brief but severe, mild but prolonged, and repetitive hemodynamic insults, as well as for the cumulative impact of these insults. The prolonged risk period for, and variety of, hemodynamic insults that might theoretically cause brain injury in the premature infant have made it difficult to design appropriate experimental models or to monitor the human premature brain appropriately.

Establishing a temporal association between systemic hemodynamic disturbances and brain insult is particularly challenging in the sick premature infant because the exact onset of brain injury is often unknown and brain injury may be cumulative.[180] Premature infants rarely demonstrate acute signs at the onset of brain dysfunction and therefore may provide little or no clue to the timing of brain insult. Furthermore, neurodevelopmental deficits may only become evident months to years after the initial injury, sometimes as late as school age,[5,181] or beyond. During this interval, multiple factors such as socioeconomic status and maternal education that are unrelated to the initial insult may significantly influence long-term outcome.[182] In the premature infant, brain injury precedes critical third-trimester events in brain development and neuronal migration is still very active into early infancy.[183] The unfolding of these events after brain injury may have implications for long-term outcomes in infants that are as, or more, important than the primary cerebral injury. On the one hand, normal third trimester developmental events may be derailed by acute injury resulting in acquired brain malformations (disruptions).[184] Conversely, the ameliorating effect of brain plasticity may play an important role in outcome.[185] In addition, other potentially injurious mechanisms may operate before (e.g., fetal inflammation), during (e.g., blood gas disturbances), and after (e.g., apnea and bradycardia) the immediate period of postnatal hemodynamic instability. Of particular importance is the role of infection and inflammation, known to be associated with prematurity-related white matter injury,[186–188] which may act in concert with hemodynamic insults.

Establishing a causal link between early hemodynamic insults and brain injury is also challenging; specifically identifying *acute structural injury* during periods of critical illness has been limited by the lack of sensitive portable neuroimaging. Infants are usually too ill to be transported to MRI scanners, especially early in their hospitalization. Cranial US, although sensitive to hemorrhage, is insensitive to and delayed in its detection of diffuse white matter injury. This has been confirmed at autopsy[189,190] but also in MRI studies that indicate that the majority of white matter injury is undetected by neonatal cranial US.[41,191] MRI-compatible incubators allow for safer transport of critically ill premature infants to MRI scanners which can advance detection of hyperacute brain injury.

Measures of *acute changes in brain function* have similarly been difficult in the premature infant, in whom even severe injury may remain clinically silent. The use of the electroencephalogram (EEG) as a monitor of brain function has the advantage of being continuous and noninvasive, especially when using limited-lead amplitude-integrated EEG techniques.[192] Some EEG studies in sick premature infants showed a decrease in EEG amplitude during hypotension.[193–195] Victor and colleagues[75] found that in infants less than 30 weeks' gestation, EEG and cerebral oxygen extraction remained normal despite systemic BP levels as low as 23 mm Hg, and suggested that cerebral pressure autoregulation is maintained above this systemic BP level. Indeed, this level of hypotension might represent the "functional threshold" of BP, where cellular function is affected and it is below the documented CBF autoregulatory elbow of 28 to 30 mm Hg (see Chapters 2 and 3). In extremely premature infants, EEG may be less useful as a measure of brain function since the EEG background has a limited range of features at early GAs.

Intrinsic cerebrovascular systems aim to maintain brain oxygen/substrate delivery when systemic delivery fails.[91] These compensatory mechanisms are temporizing at best and, if systemic delivery does not recover, these mechanisms will collapse, elevating the risk for irreversible brain injury. For these reasons, a definition of systemic hypotension, using as a threshold the BP below which cerebral pressure-flow autoregulation begins to fail, appears logical. Because the onset of cerebral pressure autoregulatory failure heralds an elevated risk for cerebrovascular injury at a point prior to irreversible injury, detection of cerebral pressure passivity might provide a sensitive cerebrovascular biomarker to relate to systemic BP changes. However, the presence and characteristics of pressure autoregulation in the sick premature infant remain controversial, in part due to the ongoing lack of established techniques for detecting cerebral pressure passivity. The NIRS hemoglobin difference (HbD) signal, which can be measured continuously, can be time-locked to measurements of systemic BP and applied to the study of cerebral pressure-flow autoregulation in premature infants.[98,196–198] This approach can identify periods of pressure passivity using coherence function analysis to identify significant concordance between systemic BP and cerebral HbD changes.[197] The magnitude of pressure passivity during these periods can then be measured using transfer gain analysis.[99] Using this approach, an association between cerebral pressure-passivity and brain injury has been described,[98] as well as between the magnitude of pressure passivity and GM-IVH,[198] and in the term newborn, hypoxic-ischemic encephalopathy.[199] This approach highlighted the prevalence and dynamic nature of cerebral pressure flow autoregulation, with periods of pressure passivity interspersed with apparent autoregulation in most extremely premature infants.[99] Pressure autoregulation is not only affected by BP, but by other influences as well.[99]

There are several limitations, in addition to technical difficulties discussed above, in using the onset of cerebral pressure passivity to define hypotension. Despite constant BP, this threshold may fluctuate, presumably due to other vasoactive factors such as hypoxemia, hypercarbia, and inflammation, among others. Of note is that, among factors affecting CBF, including the BP outside the autoregulatory range, changes in arterial carbon dioxide tension cause the most significant CBF alterations (see Chapter 2). Furthermore, preceding insults (e.g., an intrapartum event) may temporarily abolish pressure autoregulation, making it unreliable as a criterion for "normative" definitions of hypotension. Continuous monitoring for cerebral pressure passivity is clearly much needed; however predictable gestational/postnatal age-related BP bounds, between which cerebral perfusion is maintained constant, is a spurious concept.

Conclusion

The transition of the fetus to the extrauterine world presents a complex time in human cardiovascular physiology; for premature newborns, this period of transition may be suboptimal due to, amongst other things immaturity of the vital systems necessary for the proper regulation of HR, BP, and CBF. Brain injury may result due to impaired regulation of these systems, which can yield a long-term neurologic burden of neurodevelopmental delay, epilepsy, cerebral palsy, and psychoaffective disorders that can last into adulthood. This chapter has explored the fundamental challenges in our understanding of systemic and cerebral hemodynamics and the immature ANS, as well as the potentials and constraints of current techniques for addressing these complex but critically important questions. The etiology of brain injury in premature newborns is multifactorial and the insult is likely chronic and cumulative. The ANS is an integral driver in brainstem control of HR and BP, but more importantly, at least for the long-term neurologic health of survivors of prematurity, it is emerging as an important brain system for promoting affect, mood, stress responses, and behavior through its linkages to higher order cortical centers.[62,200] New quantitative brain imaging techniques are enabling better assessment of brain structure, function, and cerebral metabolism. Future studies in premature newborns should be aimed at finding methods to detect risk for brain injury in a timely enough way to prevent brain injury or before irreversible changes occur. We therefore must seek to develop better methods to continuously monitor the health of the immature brain and protect this vital structure.

REFERENCES

1. Behrman R, Stith Butler A: *Institute of Medicine Committee on Understanding Premature Birth and Assuring Healthy Outcomes Board on Health Sciences Outcomes: Preterm Birth: Causes, Consequences, and Prevention*, Washington, DC, 2007, National Academies Press.
2. Martin JA, Kung HC, Mathews TJ, et al.: Annual summary of vital statistics: 2006, *Pediatrics* 121:788–801, 2008.
3. Schendel DE, Stockbauer JW, Hoffman HJ, et al.: Relation between very low birth weight and developmental delay among preschool children without disabilities, *Am J Epidemiol* 146:740–749, 1997.

4. Piecuch RE, Leonard CH, Cooper BA, et al.: Outcome of extremely low birth weight infants (500 to 999 grams) over a 12-year period, *Pediatrics* 100:633–639, 1997.
5. Bhutta AT, Cleves MA, Casey PH, et al.: Cognitive and behavioral outcomes of school-aged children who were born preterm: a meta-analysis, *JAMA* 288:728–737, 2002.
6. Stoll BJ, Hansen NI, Bell EF, et al.: Trends in care practices, morbidity, and mortality of extremely preterm neonates, 1993-2012, *JAMA* 314:1039–1051, 2015.
7. Hagberg B, Hagberg G, Beckung E, et al.: Changing panorama of cerebral palsy in Sweden. VIII. Prevalence and origin in the birth year period 1991-94, *Acta Paediatr* 90:271–277, 2001.
8. Leonard CH, Piecuch RE: School age outcome in low birth weight preterm infants, *Semin Perinatol* 21:240–253, 1997.
9. O'Shea TM, Klinepeter KL, Goldstein DJ, et al.: Survival and developmental disability in infants with birth weights of 501 to 800 grams, born between 1979 and 1994, *Pediatrics* 100:982–986, 1997.
10. Aarnoudse-Moens CS, Weisglas-Kuperus N, van Goudoever JB, et al.: Meta-analysis of neurobehavioral outcomes in very preterm and/or very low birth weight children, *Pediatrics* 124:717–728, 2009.
11. Limperopoulos C, Bassan H, Sullivan NR, et al.: Positive screening for autism in ex-preterm infants: prevalence and risk factors, *Pediatrics* 121:758–765, 2008.
12. Shalak L, Perlman JM: Hemorrhagic-ischemic cerebral injury in the preterm infant: current concepts, *Clin Perinatol* 29:745–763, 2002.
13. Khwaja O, Volpe JJ: Pathogenesis of cerebral white matter injury of prematurity, *Arch Dis Child Fetal Neonatal Ed* 93:F153–F161, 2008.
14. Volpe JJ: Brain injury in the premature infant—current concepts, *Preven Med* 23:638–645, 1994.
15. Volpe JJ: Brain injury in the premature infant: overview of clinical aspects, neuropathology, and pathogenesis, *Semin Pediatr Neurol* 5:135–151, 1998.
16. du Plessis AJ, Volpe JJ: Intracranial hemorrhage in the newborn infant. In Burg FD, Ingelfinger JR, Wald ER, et al.: *Gellis & Kagan's Current Pediatric Therapy 16*, Philadelphia, 1999, Saunders Company, pp 304–308.
17. du Plessis AJ, Volpe JJ: Perinatal brain injury in the preterm and term newborn, *Curr Opin Neurol* 15:151–157, 2002.
18. Back SA, Riddle A, Hohimer AR: Role of instrumented fetal sheep preparations in defining the pathogenesis of human periventricular white-matter injury, *J Child Neurol* 21:582–589, 2006.
19. Ment LR, Stewart WB, Duncan CC, et al.: Beagle puppy model of intraventricular hemorrhage, *J Neurosurg* 57:219–223, 1982.
20. Goddard J, Lewis RM, Alcala H, et al.: Intraventricular hemorrhage–an animal model, *Biol Neonate* 37:39–52, 1980.
21. Goddard-Finegold J, Michael LH: Cerebral blood flow and experimental intraventricular hemorrhage, *Pediatr Res* 18:7–11, 1984.
22. Anstrom JA, Brown WR, Moody DM, et al.: Subependymal veins in premature neonates: implications for hemorrhage, *Pediatr Neurol* 30:46–53, 2004.
23. Ghazi-Birry HS, Brown WR, Moody DM, et al.: Human germinal matrix: venous origin of hemorrhage and vascular characteristics, *Am J Neuroradiol* 18:219–229, 1997.
24. Grunnet ML: Morphometry of blood vessels in the cortex and germinal plate of premature neonates, *Pediatr Neurol* 5:12–16, 1989.
25. Hambleton G, Wigglesworth JS: Origin of intraventricular haemorrhage in the preterm infant, *Arch Dis Child* 51:651–659, 1976.
26. Hefti MM, Trachtenberg FL, Haynes RL, et al.: A century of germinal matrix intraventricular hemorrhage in autopsied premature infants: a historical account, *Pediatr Dev Pathol* 19:108–114, 2016.
27. du Plessis AJ: Posthemorrhagic hydrocephalus and brain injury in the preterm infant: dilemmas in diagnosis and management, *Semin Pediatr Neurol* 5:161–179, 1998.
28. Ment LR, Scott DT, Ehrenkranz RA, et al.: Neurodevelopmental assessment of very low birth weight neonates: effect of germinal matrix and intraventricular hemorrhage, *Pediatr Neurol* 1:164–168, 1985.
29. Bassan H, Feldman HA, Limperopoulos C, et al.: Periventricular hemorrhagic infarction: risk factors and neonatal outcome, *Pediatr Neurol* 35:85–92, 2006.
30. Bassan H, Benson CB, Limperopoulos C, et al.: Ultrasonographic features and severity scoring of periventricular hemorrhagic infarction in relation to risk factors and outcome, *Pediatrics* 117:2111–2118, 2006.
31. Volpe JJ: *Intracranial Hemorrhage: Germinal Matrix-Intraventricular Hemorrhage of the Premature Infant. Neurology of the Newborn*, ed 5, Philadelphia, 2008, Saunders Elsevier, pp 517–588.
32. Ventriculomegaly Trial Group: Randomised trial of early tapping in neonatal posthaemorrhagic ventricular dilatation: results at 30 months, *Arch Dis Child Fetal Neonatal Ed* 70:F129–F136, 1994.
33. De Reuck JL: Cerebral angioarchitecture and perinatal brain lesions in premature and full-term infants. *Acta Neurol Scand* 70:391–395, 1984.
34. Takashima S, Armstrong DL, Becker LE: Subcortical leukomalacia. Relationship to development of the cerebral sulcus and its vascular supply, *Arch Neurol* 35:470–472, 1978.
35. De Reuck J: The human periventricular arterial blood supply and the anatomy of cerebral infarctions, *Eur Neurol* 5:321–334, 1971.
36. De Reuck J: The cortico-subcortical arterial angio-architecture in the human brain, *Acta Neurol Belg* 72:323–329, 1972.

37. Rorke LB: Anatomical features of the developing brain implicated in pathogenesis of hypoxic-ischemic injury, *Brain Pathol* 2:211–221, 1992.
38. Takashima S, Tanaka K: Development of cerebrovascular architecture and its relationship to periventricular leukomalacia, *Arch Neurol* 35:11–16, 1978.
39. Nakamura Y, Okudera T, Hashimoto T: Vascular architecture in white matter of neonates: its relationship to periventricular leukomalacia, *J Neuropathol Exp Neurol* 53:582–589, 1994.
40. O'Shea TM, Allred EN, Kuban KC, et al.: Intraventricular hemorrhage and developmental outcomes at 24 months of age in extremely preterm infants, *J Child Neurol* 27:22–29, 2012.
41. Maalouf EF, Duggan PJ, Counsell SJ, et al.: Comparison of findings on cranial ultrasound and magnetic resonance imaging in preterm infants, *Pediatrics* 107:719–727, 2001.
42. Volpe JJ: Cerebral white matter injury of the premature infant—more common than you think, *Pediatrics* 112:176–180, 2003.
43. Dyet LE, Kennea N, Counsell SJ, et al.: Natural history of brain lesions in extremely preterm infants studied with serial magnetic resonance imaging from birth and neurodevelopmental assessment, *Pediatrics* 118:536–548, 2006.
44. De Vries LS, Wigglesworth JS, Regev R, et al.: Evolution of periventricular leukomalacia during the neonatal period and infancy: correlation of imaging and postmortem findings, *Early Hum Dev* 17:205–219, 1988.
45. Volpe JJ: Encephalopathy of prematurity includes neuronal abnormalities, *Pediatrics* 116:221–225, 2005.
46. Rogers CE, Barch DM, Sylvester CM, et al.: Altered gray matter volume and school age anxiety in children born late preterm, *J Pediatr* 165:928–935, 2014.
47. Pierson CR, Folkerth RD, Billiards SS, et al.: Gray matter injury associated with periventricular leukomalacia in the premature infant, *Acta Neuropathol* 114:619–631, 2007.
48. Nosarti C, Nam KW, Walshe M, et al.: Preterm birth and structural brain alterations in early adulthood, *Neuroimage Clin* 6:180–191, 2014.
49. Longin E, Gerstner T, Schaible T, et al.: Maturation of the autonomic nervous system: differences in heart rate variability in premature vs. term infants, *J Perinat Med* 34:303–308, 2006.
50. Patural H, Barthelemey JC, Pichot V, et al.: Birth prematurity determines prolonged autonomic nervous system immaturity, *Clin Auton Res* 14:391–395, 2004.
51. Fyfe KL, Yiallourou SR, Wong FY, et al.: The effect of gestational age at birth on post-term maturation of heart rate variability, *Sleep* 38:1635–1644, 2015.
52. Karin J, Hirsch M, Akselrod S: An estimate of fetal autonomic state by spectral analysis of fetal heart rate fluctuations, *Pediatr Res* 34:134–138, 1993.
53. Electrophysiology TFotESoCtNASoP: Heart rate variability. Standards of measurement, physiological interpretation, and clinical use, *Circulation* 93:1043–1065, 1996.
54. Malliani A, Lombardi F, Pagani M: Power spectrum analysis of heart rate variability: a tool to explore neural regulatory mechanisms, *Br Heart J* 71:1–2, 1994.
55. Chatow U, Davidson S, Reichman BL, et al.: Development and maturation of the autonomic nervous system in premature and full-term infants using spectral analysis of heart rate fluctuations, *Pediatr Res* 37:294–302, 1995.
56. Yiallourou SR, Witcombe NB, Sands SA, et al.: The development of autonomic cardiovascular control is altered by preterm birth, *Early Hum Dev* 89:145–152, 2013.
57. Zouikr I, Bartholomeusz MD, Hodgson DM: Early life programming of pain: focus on neuroimmune to endocrine communication, *J Transl Med* 14:123, 2016.
58. Tuzcu V, Nas S, Ulusar U, et al.: Altered heart rhythm dynamics in very low birth weight infants with impending intraventricular hemorrhage, *Pediatrics* 123:810–815, 2009.
59. Tieder JS, Bonkowsky JL, Etzel RA, et al.: Brief resolved unexplained events (formerly apparent life-threatening events) and evaluation of lower-risk infants: executive summary, *Pediatrics*137, 2016.
60. Fyfe K, Odoi A, Yiallourou SR, et al.: Preterm infants exhibit greater variability in cerebrovascular control than term infants, *Sleep* 38:1411–1421, 2015.
61. Nino G, Govindan RB, Al-Shargabi T, et al.: Premature infants rehospitalized because of an apparent life-threatening event had distinctive autonomic developmental trajectories, *Am J Resp Crit Care Med* 194:379–381, 2016.
62. Porges SW, Furman SA: The early development of the autonomic nervous system provides a neural platform for social behavior: a polyvagal perspective, *Infant Child Dev* 20:106–118, 2011.
63. Agata Y, Hiraishi S, Oguchi K, et al.: Changes in left ventricular output from fetal to early neonatal life, *J Pediatr* 119:441–445, 1991.
64. Evans N, Osborn D, Kluckow M: Preterm circulatory support is more complex than just blood pressure, *Pediatrics* 115:1114–1115, 2005. author reply 1115–1116.
65. Kluckow M, Evans N: Low superior vena cava flow and intraventricular haemorrhage in preterm infants, *Arch Dis Child Fetal Neonatal Ed* 82:F188–F194, 2000.
66. Hunt RW, Evans N, Rieger I, et al.: Low superior vena cava flow and neurodevelopment at 3 years in very preterm infants, *J Pediatr* 145:588–592, 2004.
67. Kluckow M, Evans N: Low systemic blood flow and hyperkalemia in preterm infants, *J Pediatr* 139:227–232, 2001.
68. Osborn D, Evans N, Kluckow M: Randomized trial of dobutamine versus dopamine in preterm infants with low systemic blood flow, *J Pediatr* 140:183–191, 2002.

7

69. Paneth N, Pinto-Martin J, Gardiner J, et al.: Incidence and timing of germinal matrix/intraventricular hemorrhage in low birth weight infants, *Am J Epidemiol* 137:1167–1176, 1993.

70. Perlman JM, Volpe JJ: Intraventricular hemorrhage in extremely small premature infants, *Am J Dis Child* 140:1122–1124, 1986.

71. Drouin E, Gournay V, Calamel J, et al.: Assessment of spontaneous baroreflex sensitivity in neonates, *Arch Dis Child Fetal Neonatal Ed* 76:F108–F112, 1997.

72. Andriessen P, Koolen AMP, Berendsen RCM, et al.: Cardiovascular fluctuations and transfer function analysis in stable preterm infants, *Pediatr Res* 2003(53):89–97, 2003.

73. Nuntnarumit P, Yang W, Bada-Ellzey HS: Blood pressure measurements in the newborn, *Clin Perinatol* 26:981–996, 1999.

74. Cunningham S, Symon AG, Elton RA, et al.: Intra-arterial blood pressure reference ranges, death and morbidity in very low birthweight infants during the first seven days of life, *Early Hum Dev* 56:151–165, 1999.

75. Victor S, Marson AG, Appleton RE, et al.: Relationship between blood pressure, cerebral electrical activity, cerebral fractional oxygen extraction, and peripheral blood flow in very low birth weight newborn infants, *Pediatr Res* 59:314–319, 2006.

76. Batton B, Batton D, Riggs T: Blood pressure during the first 7 days in premature infants born at postmenstrual age 23 to 25 weeks, *Am J Perinatol* 24:107–115, 2007.

77. Lee JM, Zipfel GJ, Choi DW: The changing landscape of ischaemic brain injury mechanisms, *Nature* 399(6738 Suppl):A7–A14, 1999.

78. Northern Neonatal Nursing Initiative: Systolic blood pressure in babies of less than 32 weeks gestation in the first year of life, *Arch Dis Child Fetal Neonatal Ed* 80:F38–F42, 1999.

79. de Vries LS, Regev R, Dubowitz LM, et al.: Perinatal risk factors for the development of extensive cystic leukomalacia, *Am J Dis Child* 142:732–735, 1988.

80. Limperopoulos C, Bassan H, Kalish LA, et al.: Current definitions of hypotension do not predict abnormal cranial ultrasound findings in preterm infants, *Pediatrics* 120:966–977, 2007.

81. Watkins AM, West CR, Cooke RW: Blood pressure and cerebral haemorrhage and ischaemia in very low birthweight infants, *Early Hum Dev* 19:103–110, 1989.

82. Weindling AM, Wilkinson AR, Cook J, et al.: Perinatal events which precede periventricular haemorrhage and leukomalacia in the newborn, *Br J Obstet Gynaecol* 92:1218–1223, 1985.

83. Al-Aweel I, Pursley DM, Rubin LP, et al.: Variations in prevalence of hypotension, hypertension, and vasopressor use in NICUs, *J Perinatol* 21:272–278, 2001.

84. Batton B, Li L, Newman NS, et al.: Early blood pressure, antihypotensive therapy and outcomes at 18-22 months' corrected age in extremely preterm infants, *Arch Dis Child Fetal Neonatal Ed* 101:F201–F206, 2016.

85. Pellicer A, Bravo MC, Madero R, et al.: Early systemic hypotension and vasopressor support in low birth weight infants: impact on neurodevelopment, *Pediatrics* 123:1369–1376, 2009.

86. Powers WJ, Grubb Jr RL, Darriet D, et al.: Cerebral blood flow and cerebral metabolic rate of oxygen requirements for cerebral function and viability in humans, *J Cereb Blood Flow Metab* 5:600–608, 1985.

87. Ouyang M, Liu P, Jeon T, et al.: Heterogeneous increases of regional cerebral blood flow during preterm brain development: preliminary assessment with pseudo-continuous arterial spin labeled perfusion MRI, *NeuroImage* 147:233–242, 2016.

88. Altman DI, Powers WJ, Perlman JM, et al.: Cerebral blood flow requirement for brain viability in newborn infants is lower than in adults, *Ann Neurol* 24:218–226, 1988.

89. Borch K, Greisen G: Blood flow distribution in the normal human preterm brain, *Pediatr Res* 43:28–33, 1998.

90. Pichler G, Binder C, Avian A, et al.: Reference ranges for regional cerebral tissue oxygen saturation and fractional oxygen extraction in neonates during immediate transition after birth, *J Pediatr* 163:1558–1563, 2013.

91. du Plessis AJ: Cerebrovascular injury in premature infants: current understanding and challenges for future prevention, *Clin Perinatol* 35:609–641, 2008.

92. Lassen NA, Christensen MS: Physiology of cerebral blood flow, *Br J Anaesth* 48:719–734, 1976.

93. Panerai RB, Kelsall AW, Rennie JM, et al.: Cerebral autoregulation dynamics in premature newborns, *Stroke* 26:74–80, 1995.

94. van Os S, Liem D, Hopman J, et al.: Cerebral O2 supply thresholds for the preservation of electrocortical brain activity during hypotension in near-term-born lambs, *Pediatr Res* 57:358–362, 2005.

95. Van Os S, Klaessens J, Hopman J, et al.: Cerebral oxygen supply during hypotension in near-term lambs: a near-infrared spectroscopy study, *Brain Dev* 28:115–121, 2006.

96. Szymonowicz W, Walker AM, Yu VY, et al.: Regional cerebral blood flow after hemorrhagic hypotension in the preterm, near-term, and newborn lamb, *Pediatr Res* 28:361–366, 1990.

97. Lou HC, Lassen NA, Friis-Hansen B: Impaired autoregulation of cerebral blood flow in the distressed newborn infant, *J Pediatr* 94:118–121, 1979.

98. Tsuji M, Saul JP, du Plessis A, et al.: Cerebral intravascular oxygenation correlates with mean arterial pressure in critically ill premature infants, *Pediatrics* 106:625–632, 2000.

99. Soul JS, Hammer PE, Tsuji M, et al.: Fluctuating pressure-passivity is common in the cerebral circulation of sick premature infants, *Pediatr Res* 61:467–473, 2007.

100. Pryds O, Andersen GE, Friis-Hansen B: Cerebral blood flow reactivity in spontaneously breathing, preterm infants shortly after birth, *Acta Paediatr Scand* 79:391–396, 1990.

101. Pryds O: Control of cerebral circulation in the high-risk neonate, *Ann Neurol* 30:321–329, 1991.

102. Milligan DW: Failure of autoregulation and intraventricular haemorrhage in preterm infants, *Lancet* 1:896–898, 1980.

103. Miall-Allen VM, de Vries LS, Dubowitz LM, et al.: Blood pressure fluctuation and intraventricular hemorrhage in the preterm infant of less than 31 weeks' gestation, *Pediatrics* 83:657–661, 1989.

104. Ramaekers VT, Casaer P, Daniels H, et al.: Upper limits of brain blood flow autoregulation in stable infants of various conceptional age, *Early Hum Dev* 24:249–258, 1990.

105. Verma PK, Panerai RB, Rennie JM, et al.: Grading of cerebral autoregulation in preterm and term neonates, *Pediatr Neurol* 23:236–242, 2000.

106. van de Bor M, Walther FJ: Cerebral blood flow velocity regulation in preterm infants, *Biol Neonate* 59:329–335, 1991.

107. Munro MJ, Walker AM, Barfield CP: Hypotensive extremely low birth weight infants have reduced cerebral blood flow, *Pediatrics* 114:1591–1596, 2004.

108. Lou HC, Lassen NA, Friis-Hansen B: Low cerebral blood flow in the hypotensive distressed newborn, *Acta Neurol Scand Suppl* 64:428–429, 1977.

109. Lou HC, Skov H, Pedersen H: Low cerebral blood flow: a risk factor in the neonate, *J Pediatr* 95:606–609, 1979.

110. Younkin DP, Reivich M, Jaggi J, et al.: Noninvasive method of estimating human newborn regional cerebral blood flow, *J Cereb Blood Flow Metab* 2:415–420, 1982.

111. Boylan GB, Young K, Panerai RB, et al.: Dynamic cerebral autoregulation in sick newborn infants, *Pediatr Res* 48:12–17, 2000.

112. Anthony MY, Evans DH, Levene MI: Neonatal cerebral blood flow velocity responses to changes in posture, *Arch Dis Child* 69(3 Spec No):304–308, 1993.

113. Miall-Allen VM, de Vries LS, Whitelaw AG: Mean arterial blood pressure and neonatal cerebral lesions, *Arch Dis Child* 62:1068–1069, 1987.

114. Bada HS, Korones SB, Perry EH, et al.: Frequent handling in the neonatal intensive care unit and intraventricular hemorrhage, *J Pediatr* 117:126–131, 1990.

115. Bada HS, Korones SB, Perry EH, et al.: Mean arterial blood pressure changes in premature infants and those at risk for intraventricular hemorrhage, *J Pediatr* 117:607–614, 1990.

116. Low JA, Froese AB, Smith JT, et al.: Hypotension and hypoxemia in the preterm newborn during the four days following delivery identify infants at risk of echosonographically demonstrable cerebral lesions, *Clin Invest Med* 15:60–65, 1992.

117. Perlman JM, Risser R, Broyles RS: Bilateral cystic periventricular leukomalacia in the premature infant: associated risk factors, *Pediatrics* 97:822–827, 1996.

118. Murphy DJ, Hope PL, Johnson A: Neonatal risk factors for cerebral palsy in very preterm babies: case-control study, *BMJ* 314:404–408, 1997.

119. Fanaroff JM, Wilson-Costello DE, Newman NS, et al.: Treated hypotension is associated with neonatal morbidity and hearing loss in extremely low birth weight infants, *Pediatrics* 117:1131–1135, 2006.

120. Trounce JQ, Shaw DE, Levene MI, et al.: Clinical risk factors and periventricular leucomalacia, *Arch Dis Child* 63:17–22, 1988.

121. Gronlund JU, Korvenranta H, Kero P, et al.: Elevated arterial blood pressure is associated with peri-intraventricular haemorrhage, *Eur J Pediatr* 153:836–841, 1994.

122. Cowan F, Thoresen M: The effects of intermittent positive pressure ventilation on cerebral arterial and venous blood velocities in the newborn infant, *Acta Paediatr Scand* 76:239–247, 1987.

123. Svenningsen L, Lindemann R, Eidal K: Measurements of fetal head compression pressure during bearing down and their relationship to the condition of the newborn, *Acta Obstet Gynecol Scand* 67:129–133, 1988.

124. Skinner JR, Milligan DWA, Hunter S, et al.: Central venous pressure in the ventilated neonate, *Arch Dis Child* 67:374–377, 1992.

125. Hambleton G, Wigglesworth JS: Origin of intraventricular haemorrhage in the preterm infant, *Arch Dis Child* 51:651–659, 1976.

126. Perlman JM, McMenamin JB, Volpe JJ: Fluctuating cerebral blood-flow velocity in respiratory-distress syndrome: relation to the development of intraventricular hemorrhage, *N Engl J Med* 309:204–209, 1983.

127. van Bel F, Van de Bor M, Stijnen T, et al.: Aetiological role of cerebral blood-flow alterations in development and extension of peri-intraventricular haemorrhage, *Dev Med Child Neurol* 29:601–614, 1987.

128. Lou H: The "lost autoregulation hypothesis" and brain lesions in the newborn: an update, *Brain Dev* 10:143–146, 1988.

129. Leffler CW, Busija DW, Beasley DG, et al.: Postischemic cerebral microvascular responses to norepinephrine and hypotension in newborn pigs, *Stroke* 20:541–546, 1989.

130. Leffler CW, Busija DW, Mirro R, et al.: Effects of ischemia on brain blood flow and oxygen consumption of newborn pigs, *Am J Physiol* 257:H1917–H1926, 1989.

131. Pryds O, Christensen NJ, Friis HB: Increased cerebral blood flow and plasma epinephrine in hypoglycemic, preterm neonates, *Pediatrics* 85:172–176, 1990.

132. Laptook A, Corbett R, Ruley J, et al.: Blood flow and metabolism during and after repeated partial brain ischemia in neonatal piglets, *Stroke* 23:380–387, 1992.

133. Conger J, Weil J: Abnormal vascular function following ischemia-reperfusion injury, *J Investig Med* 43:431–432, 1995.

134. Blankenberg FG, Loh NN, Norbash AM, et al.: Impaired cerebrovascular autoregulation after hypoxic-ischemic injury in extremely low-birth-weight neonates: detection with power and pulsed wave Doppler US, *Radiology* 205:563–568, 1997.

135. Low JA, Froese AB, Galbraith RS, et al.: The association between preterm newborn hypotension and hypoxemia and outcome during the first year, *Acta Paediatr* 82:433–437, 1993.

136. Dammann O, Allred EN, Kuban KC, et al.: Systemic hypotension and white-matter damage in preterm infants, *Dev Med Child Neurol* 44:82–90, 2002.

137. Bejar RF, Vaucher YE, Benirschke K, et al.: Postnatal white matter necrosis in preterm infants, *J Perinatol* 12:3–8, 1992.

138. Rhee CJ, Kibler KK, Easley RB, et al.: The diastolic closing margin is associated with intraventricular hemorrhage in premature infants, *Acta Neurochir Suppl* 122:147–150, 2016.

139. Rhee CJ, Kaiser JR, Rios DR, et al.: Elevated diastolic closing margin is associated with intraventricular hemorrhage in premature infants, *J Pediatr* 174:52–56, 2016.

140. Rhee CJ, Fraser 3rd CD, Kibler K, et al.: The ontogeny of cerebrovascular critical closing pressure, *Acta Neurochir Suppl* 122:249–253, 2016.

141. Fujimura M, Salisbury DM, Robinson RO, et al.: Clinical events relating to intraventricular haemorrhage in the newborn, *Arch Dis Child* 54:409–414, 1979.

142. McDonald MM, Koops BL, Johnson ML, et al.: Timing and antecedents of intracranial hemorrhage in the newborn, *Pediatrics* 74:32–36, 1984.

143. Perlman J, Thach B: Respiratory origin of fluctuations in arterial blood pressure in premature infants with respiratory distress syndrome, *Pediatrics* 81:399–403, 1988.

144. Kluckow M, Evans N: Relationship between blood pressure and cardiac output in preterm infants requiring mechanical ventilation, *J Pediatr* 129:506–512, 1996.

145. Kluckow M, Evans N: Superior vena cava flow in newborn infants: a novel marker of systemic blood flow, *Arch Dis Child Fetal Neonatal Ed* 82:F182–F187, 2000.

146. Kluckow M, Evans N: Low systemic blood flow in the preterm infant, *Semin Neonatol* 6:75–84, 2001.

147. Miletin J, Dempsey EM: Low superior vena cava flow on day 1 and adverse outcome in the very low birthweight infant, *Arch Dis Child Fetal Neonatal Ed* 93:F368–F371, 2008.

148. Evans N, Kluckow M, Simmons M, et al.: Which to measure, systemic or organ blood flow? Middle cerebral artery and superior vena cava flow in very preterm infants, *Arch Dis Child Fetal Neonatal Ed* 87:F181–F184, 2002.

149. Moran M, Miletin J, Pichova K, et al.: Cerebral tissue oxygenation index and superior vena cava blood flow in the very low birth weight infant, *Acta Paediatr* 98:43–46, 2009.

150. Kissack CM, Garr R, Wardle SP, et al.: Cerebral fractional oxygen extraction in very low birth weight infants is high when there is low left ventricular output and hypocarbia but is unaffected by hypotension, *Pediatr Res* 55:400–405, 2004.

151. Osborn DA, Evans N, Kluckow M: Hemodynamic and antecedent risk factors of early and late periventricular/intraventricular hemorrhage in premature infants, *Pediatrics* 112:33–39, 2003.

152. Fyfe KL, Yiallourou SR, Wong FY, et al.: Gestational age at birth affects maturation of baroreflex control, *J Pediatr* 166:559–565, 2015.

153. Witcombe NB, Yiallourou SR, Sands SA, et al.: Preterm birth alters the maturation of baroreflex sensitivity in sleeping infants, *Pediatrics* 129:e89–e96, 2012.

154. Andriessen P, Schoffelen RL, Berendsen RC, et al.: Noninvasive assessment of blood pressure variability in preterm infants, *Pediatr Res* 55:220–223, 2004.

155. Perlman JM, Volpe JJ: Cerebral blood flow velocity in relation to intraventricular hemorrhage in the premature newborn infant, *J Pediatr* 100:956–959, 1982.

156. Rennie JM, South M, Morley CJ: Cerebral blood flow velocity variability in infants receiving assisted ventilation, *Arch Dis Child* 62:1247–1251, 1987.

157. van Bel F, de Winter PJ, Wijnands HBG, et al.: Cerebral and aortic blood flow velocity patterns in preterm infants receiving prophylactic surfactant treatment, *Acta Paediat* 81:504–510, 1992.

158. O'Brien NF: Reference values for cerebral blood flow velocities in critically ill, sedated children, *Childs Nerv Syst* 31:2269–2276, 2015.

159. Edwards A, Richardson C, Cope M, et al.: Cotside measurement of cerebral blood flow in ill newborn infants by near infrared spectroscopy, *Lancet* ii:770–771, 1988.

160. Tyszczuk L, Meek J, Elwell C, et al.: Cerebral blood flow is independent of mean arterial blood pressure in preterm infants undergoing intensive care, *Pediatrics* 102:337–341, 1998.

161. Meek JH, Tyszczuk L, Elwell CE, et al.: Cerebral blood flow increases over the first three days of life in extremely preterm neonates, *Arch Dis Child Fetal Neonatal Ed* 78:F33–F37, 1998.

162. Lassen NA: Control of cerebral circulation in health and disease, *Circ Res* 34:749–760, 1974.

163. Greisen G, Pryds O: Intravenous 133Xe clearance in preterm neonates with respiratory distress. Internal validation of CBF infinity as a measure of global cerebral blood flow, *Scand J Clin Lab Invest* 48:673–678, 1988.

164. Drayton MR, Skidmore R: Vasoactivity of the major intracranial arteries in newborn infants, *Arch Dis Child* 62:236–240, 1987.

165. Cerbo RM, Scudeller L, Maragliano R, et al.: Cerebral oxygenation, superior vena cava flow, severe intraventricular hemorrhage and mortality in 60 very low birth weight infants, *Neonatology* 108:246–252, 2015.

166. Verhagen EA, Van Braeckel KN, van der Veere CN, et al.: Cerebral oxygenation is associated with neurodevelopmental outcome of preterm children at age 2 to 3 years, *Dev Med Child Neurol* 57:449–455, 2015.

167. Sorensen LC, Greisen G: The brains of very preterm newborns in clinically stable condition may be hyperoxygenated, *Pediatrics* 124:e958–e963, 2009.

168. Borch K, Lou HC, Greisen G: Cerebral white matter blood flow and arterial blood pressure in preterm infants, *Acta Paediatr* 99:1489–1492, 2010.

169. Goff DA, Buckley EM, Durduran T, et al.: Noninvasive cerebral perfusion imaging in high-risk neonates, *Semin Perinatol* 34:46–56, 2010.

170. Miranda MJ, Olofsson K, Sidaros K: Noninvasive measurements of regional cerebral perfusion in preterm and term neonates by magnetic resonance arterial spin labeling, *Pediatr Res* 60:359–363, 2006.

171. Durduran T, Yodh AG: Diffuse correlation spectroscopy for non-invasive, micro-vascular cerebral blood flow measurement, *NeuroImage* 85(Pt 1):51–63, 2014.

172. Lin PY, Roche-Labarbe N, Dehaes M, et al.: Regional and hemispheric asymmetries of cerebral hemodynamic and oxygen metabolism in newborns, *Cereb Cortex* 23:339–348, 2013.

173. Buckley EM, Parthasarathy AB, Grant PE, et al.: Diffuse correlation spectroscopy for measurement of cerebral blood flow: future prospects. *Neurophotonics* 1(1):2014.

174. Clouchoux C, Guizard N, Evans AC, et al.: Normative fetal brain growth by quantitative in vivo magnetic resonance imaging, *Am J Obstet Gynecol* 206:173:e171–e178, 2012.

175. Petit CJ, Rome JJ, Wernovsky G, et al.: Preoperative brain injury in transposition of the great arteries is associated with oxygenation and time to surgery, not balloon atrial septostomy, *Circulation* 119:709–716, 2009.

176. Siddiqui S, Wilpers A, Myers M, et al.: Autonomic regulation in fetuses with congenital heart disease, *Early Hum Dev* 91:195–198, 2015.

177. Stampalija T, Casati D, Monasta L, et al.: Brain sparing effect in growth-restricted fetuses is associated with decreased cardiac acceleration and deceleration capacities: a case-control study, *BJOG* 123:1947–1954, 2016.

178. Stampalija T, Casati D, Montico M, et al.: Parameters influence on acceleration and deceleration capacity based on trans-abdominal ECG in early fetal growth restriction at different gestational age epochs, *Eur J Obstet Gynecol Reprod Biol* 188:104–112, 2015.

179. Cohen E, Wong FY, Horne RS, et al.: Intrauterine growth restriction: impact on cardiovascular development and function throughout infancy, *Pediatr Res* 79:821–830, 2016.

180. Noori S, McCoy M, Anderson MP, et al.: Changes in cardiac function and cerebral blood flow in relation to peri/intraventricular hemorrhage in extremely preterm infants, *J Pediatr* 164: 264.e3–270.e3, 2014.

181. Msall ME, Tremont MR: Measuring functional outcomes after prematurity: developmental impact of very low birth weight and extremely low birth weight status on childhood disability, *Ment Retard Dev Disabil Res Rev* 8:258–272, 2002.

182. Gross SJ, Mettelman BB, Dye TD, et al.: Impact of family structure and stability on academic outcome in preterm children at 10 years of age, *J Pediatr* 138:169–175, 2001.

183. Paredes MF, James D, Gil-Perotin S, et al.: Extensive migration of young neurons into the infant human frontal lobe, *Science* 354(6308), 2016.

184. Messerschmidt A, Brugger PC, Boltshauser E, et al.: Disruption of cerebellar development: potential complication of extreme prematurity, *AJNR Am J Neuroradiol* 26:1659–1667, 2005.

185. Karolis VR, Froudist-Walsh S, Brittain PJ, et al.: Reinforcement of the brain's rich-club architecture following early neurodevelopmental disruption caused by very preterm birth, *Cereb Cortex* 26:1322–1335, 2016.

186. Kadhim H, Tabarki B, Verellen G, et al.: Inflammatory cytokines in the pathogenesis of periventricular leukomalacia, *Neurology* 56:1278–1284, 2001.

187. Volpe JJ: Neurobiology of periventricular leukomalacia in the premature infant, *Pediatr Res* 50: 553–562, 2001.

188. Yoon BH, Romero R, Yang SH, et al.: Interleukin-6 concentrations in umbilical cord plasma are elevated in neonates with white matter lesions associated with periventricular leukomalacia, *Am J Obstet Gynecol* 174:1433–1440, 1996.

189. Hope PL, Gould SJ, Howard S, et al.: Precision of ultrasound diagnosis of pathologically verified lesions in the brains of very preterm newborn infants, *Dev Med Child Neurol* 30:457–471, 1988.

190. Paneth N, Rudelli R, Monte W, et al.: White matter necrosis in very low birth weight infants: neuropathologic and ultrasonographic findings in infants surviving six days or longer, *J Pediatr* 116:975–984, 1990.

191. Ou X, Glasier CM, Ramakrishnaiah RH, et al.: Impaired white matter development in extremely low-birth-weight infants with previous brain hemorrhage, *AJNR Am J Neuroradiol* 35:1983–1989, October 2014.

192. Hellstrom-Westas L, de Vries L, Rosen I: *An Atlas of Amplitude-Integrated EEG's in the Newborn*, ed 1, New York, 2003, Parthenon Publishing.

193. Greisen G, Pryds O, Low CBF: discontinuous EEG activity, and periventricular brain injury in ill, preterm neonates, *Brain Dev* 11:164–168, 1989.

194. Greisen G, Pryds O, Rosen I, et al.: Poor reversibility of EEG abnormality in hypotensive, preterm neonates, *Acta Paediatr Scand* 77:785–790, 1988.

195. Shah D, Paradisis M, Bowen JR: Relationship between systemic blood flow, blood pressure, inotropes, and aEEG in the first 48 h of life in extremely preterm infants, *Pediatr Res* 74:314–320, 2013.

196. Soul JS, du Plessis AJ, Walter GL, et al.: Near-infrared spectroscopy monitoring detects changes in cerebral blood flow in an animal model of acute hydrocephalus (abstr), *Ann Neurol* 44:535, 1998.

197. Bassan H, Gauvreau K, Newburger JW, et al.: Identification of pressure passive cerebral perfusion and its mediators after infant cardiac surgery, *Pediatr Res* 57:35–41, 2005.

198. O'Leary H, Gregas MC, Limperopoulos C, et al.: Elevated cerebral pressure passivity is associated with prematurity-related intracranial hemorrhage, *Pediatrics* 124:302–309, 2009.

199. Massaro AN, Govindan RB, Vezina G, et al.: Impaired cerebral autoregulation and brain injury in newborns with hypoxic-ischemic encephalopathy treated with hypothermia, *J Neurophysiol* 114:818–824, 2015.

200. Montagna A, Nosarti C: Socio-emotional development following very preterm birth: pathways to psychopathology, *Front Psychol* 7:80, 2016.

CHAPTER 8

Pathophysiology of Persistent Pulmonary Hypertension of the Newborn—Cellular Basis and Lessons from Animal Studies

Bobby Mathew and Satyan Lakshminrusimha

8

- The fetal circulation is characterized by high pulmonary vascular resistance (PVR) and low placental vascular resistance.
- Following birth, with ventilation of the lungs and umbilical cord clamping, PVR decreases and systemic vascular resistance increases.
- Mechanical factors (lung liquid, cuboidal endothelium), high levels of endothelin (ET), low oxygen, and various arachidonic acid metabolites contribute to the high PVR in utero.
- Ventilation of the lungs and improved oxygenation results in release of nitric oxide (NO) and prostacyclin (PGI_2) from the pulmonary vascular endothelium leading to reduction of pulmonary arterial pressure, reversal of the ductal shunt, and increased pulmonary blood flow after delivery.
- Chronic hypoxia, monocrotaline, prenatal ductal ligation, prenatal aortopulmonary shunt placement, prenatal nitrofen ingestion, and surgical creation of diaphragmatic hernia can induce pulmonary hypertension in animal models.
- Inhaled nitric oxide (iNO) stimulates soluble guanylate cyclase (sGC) and increases cyclic guanosine monophosphate (cGMP) resulting in smooth muscle cell relaxation.
- Inactivation by superoxide anions, reduced activity of sGC, and increased activity of phosphodiesterase 5 can reduce the efficacy of inhaled NO.
- Limiting formation of and/or scavenging superoxide anions, stimulators and activators of sGC, inhibitors of PDE 3 and 5 enzymes, and ET receptor blockers are potential therapeutic strategies in PPHN.
- Future therapeutic options include L-citrulline, Rho-kinase inhibitors and stem-cell-based therapies.

Persistent pulmonary hypertension of the newborn (PPHN) is a syndrome of failed circulatory adaptation at birth due to the delay in or impairment of the normal fall in pulmonary vascular resistance (PVR) that occurs following delivery. The incidence of PPHN is about 1.8 to 2.0 per 1000 births[1,2] and has not significantly changed over the last two decades. It occurs in about 2% of premature infants with respiratory distress syndrome (RDS). It is the final common pathway of a number of etiologic factors leading to persistent elevation of PVR resulting in hypoxemia and respiratory failure. The adult counterpart of this condition, idiopathic pulmonary arterial hypertension, differs substantially from an etiologic standpoint but shares many commonalities in pathophysiology and treatment. However, due to physiological and developmental differences between the fetus, the newborn in transition, the infant, and the adult, studies have to be performed in age-appropriate animal models and clinical trials in neonates prior to routine clinical use of different treatment modalities in the neonatal intensive care unit. Inhaled nitric oxide (iNO) remains the only therapy for PPHN currently approved by the Food and Drug Administration (FDA). Although this therapy is commonly used in late preterm and term infants, approximately 40% to 50% of patients fail to have a sustained response to this therapy.[3] This chapter highlights the biochemical, physiological, and cellular changes during normal and abnormal cardiovascular transition at birth using information from human studies and various animal models of PPHN. The clinical relevance of these findings, applied physiology, and therapeutic strategies to correct these abnormalities are also discussed.

Physiology of the Fetal Circulation

In all mammalian species, the organ of gas exchange receives approximately 50% of the combined ventricular output. In the fetus, with the placenta being the site of gas exchange, the majority of the right ventricular output is diverted through the ductus arteriosus and aorta to the placenta. The fetal circulation is characterized by high-resistance, low-flow pulmonary circulation and low-resistance, high-flow placental circulation (Fig. 8.1, see Chapter 1).

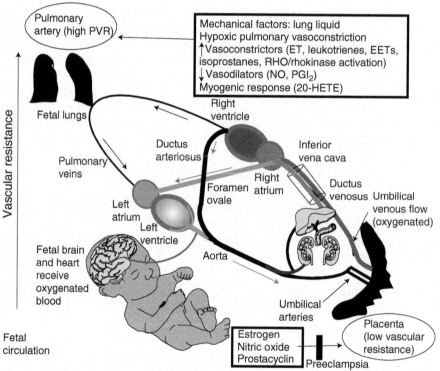

Fig. 8.1   Fetal circulation. Blood flow is governed by the presence of high pulmonary vascular resistance (PVR) and low placental vascular resistance. Oxygenated blood from the placenta reaches the fetus through the umbilical vein and enters the right atrium bypassing the liver through the ductus venosus. The umbilical venous blood with a higher oxygen content is preferentially streamed in the left atrium through the foramen ovale and reaches the left ventricle. High pulmonary vascular resistance limits the blood entering the pulmonary circulation and diverts it toward the placenta through the ductus arteriosus. The coronary and carotid arteries receive blood with higher oxygen content proximal to the right-to-left shunt across the ductus arteriosus. Factors maintaining pulmonary and placental vascular resistance are shown in boxes. Disruption of these factors can be associated with preeclampsia. See text for details. *EETs*, Epoxyeicosatrienoic acids; *ET*, endothelin; *NO*, nitric oxide; *PGI$_2$*, prostacyclin. (Copyright Satyan Lakshminrusimha [modified from Kline MW, Blaney MS, Giarding AP, et al.: *Rudolph's textbook of pediatrics*, ed 23, McGraw Hill, in press 2018].)

Low Placental Vascular Resistance

Low placental vascular resistance is secondary to high estrogen levels and an abundant production of nitric oxide (NO) and prostaglandins by the placental vascular endothelium.[4] In pregnant mothers with preeclampsia, increased oxidative stress impairs NO and prostacyclin (PGI_2) function resulting in elevated placental vascular resistance and growth restriction[4] and interestingly, preeclampsia is also associated with an increased risk of pulmonary hypertension in the offspring.[5]

High Fetal Pulmonary Vascular Resistance

At-term gestation (141 to 150 days gestation—near term), the lungs in fetal lambs receive about 7% to 8% of the combined ventricular cardiac output.[6] In human fetuses at 20 weeks' gestation, 13% of combined ventricular cardiac output perfuses the lung which increases to 25% at 30 weeks' gestation. At close-to-term gestation (38 weeks), 20% to 21% of combined ventricular output enters the lungs based on Doppler studies.[7] Factors responsible for high fetal PVR include:

1. Hypoxic pulmonary vasoconstriction (HPV): During fetal life, the PVR and pulmonary blood flow (Qp) change with the stages of lung maturation and with advancing gestation, become responsive to the various mediators that control the balance of vasoconstriction and vasodilation (Fig. 8.2). In the canalicular stage (at 20 weeks' gestation), about 13% of the combined ventricular output circulates through the lungs. The cross-sectional area of the pulmonary vascular network is low at this stage resulting in elevated PVR. With the rapid growth of the pulmonary vascular network during the saccular stage, PVR decreases and the Qp increases to 25% to 30% of combined ventricular output. As the fetus reaches near term in the alveolar stage, the sensitivity of the pulmonary vasculature to oxygen and various other mediators increases and the PVR is elevated in part due to HPV. In fetal lambs, pulmonary vasodilation in response to endothelium-independent mediators such as NO precedes the response to endothelium-dependent mediators such as acetylcholine and oxygen.[8] In the extremely preterm ovine fetus (<0.65 gestation or <101 days' gestation), there is no pulmonary vasodilator response to maternal hyperoxygenation. In contrast, a marked increase in Qp is observed with increase in fetal oxygenation near term (see Fig. 8.2).[9] Response to NO is dependent on the activity of its target enzyme, soluble guanylate cyclase (sGC), in the smooth muscle cell (Fig. 8.3). In the ovine fetus, sGC mRNA levels are low during early preterm (126 days) gestation and markedly increase during late preterm and early term gestation (137 days).[10] Low levels of pulmonary arterial sGC activity during late canalicular and early saccular stages of lung development could partly explain the poor response to iNO observed in some extremely preterm infants.[11]

2. Mechanical forces such as fetal lung liquid contribute to fetal PVR: An infusion of saline increases, and withdrawal of fetal lung liquid decreases, PVR.[12] Tracheal occlusion and hyperexpansion of the alveoli with lung liquid decreases Qp in lambs.[13] Fetal lung expansion with air, nitrogen, or oxygen (but not saline) decreases PVR.[14] Remodeling of the vascular walls occurs with a change in shape of the smooth muscle cell from cuboidal in the fetus to spindle shape and flattening of the endothelial cells, all of which lead to an increase in the caliber of the vessel lumen.

3. Myogenic response: Increases and decreases in intravascular pressure cause constriction and vasodilation, respectively. Following constriction of the ductus arteriosus (see animal models below), the increase in intravascular pressure in the pulmonary circulation transiently increases Qp (flow-mediated vasodilation). However, Qp decreases subsequently due to the myogenic response. This myogenic response is normally masked by endothelium-dependent vasodilation mediated via the nitric oxide synthase (NOS) enzymes. In the presence of endothelial dysfunction (as in some patients with PPHN or with the use of NOS inhibitors in an experimental setting), myogenic response may become the predominant regulatory mechanism of PVR.[15] Arachidonic acid metabolites such as 20-hydroxyeicosatetraenoic acid (20-HETE) may be one of the mediators of the myogenic response.[16]

8

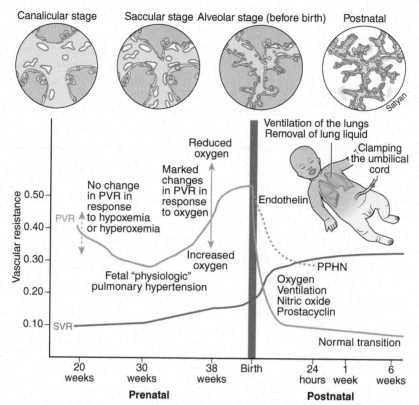

Fig. 8.2 Changes in pulmonary (PVR) and systemic (SVR) vascular resistance during human gestation. In the canalicular stage of lung development pulmonary vascular resistance (PVR) is elevated due to the paucity of pulmonary blood vessels. The PVR decreases in the saccular stage with extension of the vascular network. With advancing gestation, the pulmonary vasculature develops sensitivity to hypoxia and the increase in PVR at this stage is attributed to hypoxic pulmonary vasoconstriction and endothelin. Ventilation of the lungs and clamping of the umbilical cord at birth are associated with a rapid decline in PVR mediated by oxygen, ventilation, nitric oxide, and prostacyclin. Systemic vascular resistance (SVR) increases following clamping of the umbilical cord and removal of the low-resistance placenta. Impaired transition can lead to sustained elevation of PVR and present as persistent pulmonary hypertension of the newborn (PPHN). See text for details. (Copyright Satyan Lakshminrusimha [modified from Polin RA, Abman S, Fox WW, et al.: *Fetal and neonatal physiology*, ed 5 Philadelphia, 2017, Elsevier].)

4. Arachidonic acid metabolites: Leukotrienes (products of the 5′lipoxygenase pathway of arachidonic acid metabolism), thromboxane (cyclooxygenase—COX pathway), cytochrome P450 metabolites of arachidonic acid (epoxyeicosatrienoic acids, dihydroxyeicosatetraenoic acids and hydroxyeicosatetraenoic acids), and isoprostanes potentially play a role in maintaining pulmonary vasoconstriction during the fetal period.[17]

5. ETs are a family of vasoactive peptides with at least three different isoforms: ET-1, ET-2, and ET-3. Infusion of ET-1 to fetal lambs causes a transient pulmonary vasodilation due to stimulation of the ET_B receptor, which stimulates endothelial NO production (see Fig. 8.3), followed by a sustained vasoconstriction due to stimulation of ET_A receptors on the smooth muscle cell.[18] ET_A receptor-mediated vasoconstriction increases from 120 days to 140 days of gestation (term 145 to 150 days) in fetal lambs and could be one of the mechanisms responsible for the increased PVR in late gestation in spite of increased pulmonary vascular surface area (see Fig. 8.2). Blockade of ET_B does not alter fetal PVR suggesting that endogenous ET-1 predominantly mediates vasoconstriction through ET_A during fetal life.[19]

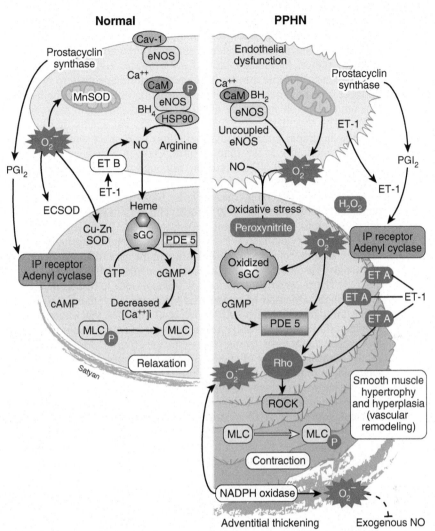

Fig. 8.3 Cellular and biochemical pathways in normal *(left)* and pulmonary arteries from subjects with PPHN *(right)*. Nitric oxide (NO) is produced by the vascular endothelial cell from arginine in the presence of endothelial nitric oxide synthase enzyme (eNOS) coupled to heat shock protein 90 (HSP90) and cofactor tetrahydrobiopterin (BH$_4$). The eNOS protein is bound to caveolin-1 (Cav 1) prior to its release by a calcium–calmodulin (CaM) dependent process. Manganese superoxide dismutase (MnSOD, present in the mitochondria), Cu, ZnSOD in the cytosol, and extracellular superoxide dismutase (ECSOD) scavenge superoxide anions and attenuate oxidative stress induced inactivation/uncoupling of eNOS. Endothelin-1 (ET-1) binding to endothelin B (ET$_B$) receptors stimulates NO production. NO binds to the reduced soluble guanylate cyclase (sGC) enzyme and catalyzes the conversion GTP to cGMP in the smooth muscle cells. cGMP decreases the cytosolic concentration of ionized calcium and leads to dephosphorylation of the myosin light chains (MLC) resulting in smooth muscle relaxation and vasodilation. In PPHN, endothelial dysfunction leads to uncoupling of eNOS. Decreased levels of antioxidants MnSOD and ECSOD increase oxidative stress and formation of superoxide anions. Superoxide inactivates NO by enhancing the formation of toxic peroxynitrite. Oxidized sGC is incapable of increasing cGMP in presence of NO. Phosphodiesterase (PDE) enzyme activation occurs in presence of superoxide anions leading to enhanced breakdown of cGMP further decreasing cGMP levels. Pulmonary arterial endothelial cells in PPHN pulmonary arteries produce increased levels of ET-1, a potent vasoconstrictor. ET-1 acts through ET$_A$ receptor and stimulates the Rho A Rho-kinase (ROCK) pathway leading to MLC phosphorylation and smooth muscle contraction. The pulmonary arterial endothelial cells in PPHN have low ET$_B$ receptors. The net effect is a shift to increased vasoconstrictor tone with decreased level of cGMP and increased sensitization of the smooth muscle to ionized calcium. Pulmonary arteries in PPHN demonstrate thickening of the muscle layer, and the adventitia could be an additional source of superoxide anions. See text for details. (Copyright Satyan Lakshminrusimha [modified from Polin RA, Abman S, Fox WW, et al. *Fetal and Neonatal Physiology*, ed 5, Philadelphia, 2017, Elsevier].)

Transition at Birth

After birth and following initiation of air breathing, Qp markedly increases,[20,21] resolving the fetal "physiologic pulmonary hypertension." Clamping of the umbilical cord removes the low resistance placental circulation and increases systemic vascular resistance. Pulmonary blood flow increases eightfold following initiation of air breathing. Multiple mechanisms operate simultaneously to rapidly increase Qp. Of these, the most important are the ventilation of the lungs, the increase in oxygen tension, and the change in the direction of the ductal shunt to predominantly left to right.[22] The vascular endothelium releases several agents that play a critical role in achieving rapid pulmonary vasodilation. Pulmonary endothelial NO production increases markedly at the time of birth. Oxygen is believed to play an important role in the increased NO production, although the precise mechanism is not clear. In term lambs, ventilation alone without change in the partial pressure of oxygen in arterial blood (PaO_2) increases Qp by four- to fivefold—an effect mediated predominantly by NO and possibly prostacyclin.[23] In near-term fetal lambs (132 to 146 days' gestation), increasing fetal PaO_2 from 25 to 55 mm Hg by maternal inhalation of hyperbaric oxygen increases the proportion of right ventricular output distributed to the fetal lung from 8% to 59%.[9] Unlike in the case of ventilation, oxygen-induced pulmonary vasodilation is predominantly mediated by NO and not by prostacyclin.[24,25] The sheer stress associated with increased Qp further increases NO production through activation of endothelial nitric oxide synthase (eNOS). NO exerts its action through sGC and cGMP. Bloch et al. reported that expression of sGC peaks in late gestation in rats, which might, at least in part, explain the better response to NO in neonates at birth compared to other age groups.[26] Phosphodiesterase 5 (PDE5) catalyzes the breakdown of cGMP. Similar to that of sGC, expression of PDE5 in the lungs peaks in the immediate newborn period in sheep and rats.[27] The arachidonic acid-prostacyclin pathway also plays an important role in the transition at birth. The COX enzyme acts on arachidonic acid to produce prostaglandin endoperoxides. Prostaglandins activate adenylate cyclase and thus increase cAMP concentrations in vascular smooth muscle cells. Phosphodiesterase 3A (PDE3A) catalyzes the breakdown of cAMP.[28] In some infants with adverse in utero events or with abnormalities of pulmonary transition at birth, pulmonary hypertension persists into the newborn period resulting in PPHN and hypoxemic respiratory failure (HRF). The cellular basis for failed cardiopulmonary transition at birth and PPHN is well studied in various animal models of pulmonary hypertension.

Animal Models of Pulmonary Hypertension in the Newborn

Antenatal Ductal Ligation Model in Sheep With Reduced Pulmonary Blood Flow

In this popular model of PPHN, antenatal ductal ligation or constriction results in forcing of the right ventricular output through an immature and constricted pulmonary circuit.[29–31] The increased sheer stress, myogenic response, endothelial dysfunction, and subsequent smooth muscle thickening and extension lead to decreased pulmonary blood flow and elevated PVR (Fig. 8.4). Fetal ductal ligation is performed through hysterotomy usually at 125 to 127 days' gestation (term ~145 to 150 days) and the lamb is placed back in the uterus for 8 to 9 days and delivered by C/S. Distal muscularization of the pulmonary vasculature results in increased PVR and causes pressure overload of the right ventricle.[32] This leads to right ventricular and septal hypertrophy and subendocardial ischemic changes. At birth, the newborn lamb has severe pulmonary hypertension with hypoxia and occasionally a degree of right ventricular failure.

Cellular and Biochemical Changes

Biochemically, increased markers of oxidative stress due to uncoupling of eNOS, reduced expression and activity of eNOS, prostacyclin synthase, and IP receptor, increased activity of phosphodiesterase 5 (PDE5) with preserved PDE3, and adenylyl

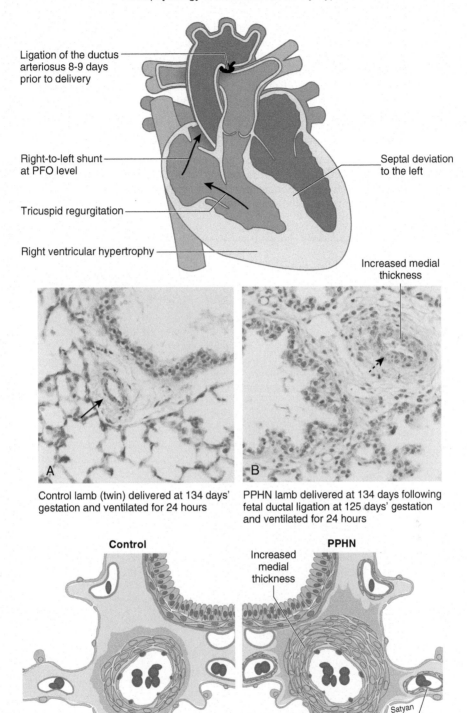

Fig. 8.4 Ductal ligation model of persistent pulmonary hypertension of the newborn (PPHN) in fetal lambs. Newborn lambs develop severe pulmonary hypertension and hypoxemic respiratory failure. There is right ventricular hypertrophy with interventricular septal deviation to the left, right-to-left shunting across the foramen ovale, and tricuspid regurgitation. There is increased medial and adventitial thickening in the pulmonary arteries and extension of muscularization into the intraacinar arterioles. See text for details. *PFO*, Patent foramen ovale. (Copyright Satyan Lakshminrusimha.)

cyclase activity are seen in this model (see Fig. 8.3). This profile most closely represents the idiopathic/black lung PPHN. However, ligation prevents right to left shunting of the blood across the PDA, which is one of the pathophysiologic hallmarks of PPHN in human neonates presenting with differential cyanosis. This model benefits from the consistency of the phenotype as it pertains to the severity of pulmonary hypertension and degree of hypoxemia. Preclinical studies of iNO for PPHN were conducted in this model.[33,34]

Aortopulmonary Graft With Pulmonary Overcirculation

This is a model that recapitulates pulmonary hypertension in congenital heart disease (CHD) with increased Qp. Fetal surgery is performed at 137 to 141 days' gestation. Through a left lateral thoracotomy, an 8-mm vascular graft is placed between the ascending aorta and the main pulmonary artery (Fig. 8.5). The left-to-right shunt

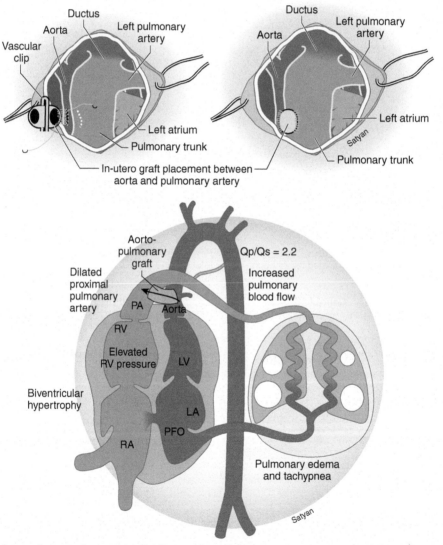

Fig. 8.5 Aortopulmonary shunt model of pulmonary hypertension. In utero surgery is performed and a 2 cm long 8 mm Gore-Tex graft is sutured into place. The posterior aspect of the pulmonary artery (PA) is then clamped, an arteriotomy incision is made, and the other end of the graft is sutured to the PA. The vascular clip is removed to establish graft patency. Newborn lambs have evidence of heart failure with tachypnea and are given furosemide and supplemental iron. Newborn lambs develop increasing pulmonary blood flow with Qp to Qs ratio of 2.2 by one month of age. See text for details. *LA*, Left atrium; *LV*, left ventricle; *PFO*, patent foramen ovale; *Qp*, pulmonary blood flow; *Qs*, systemic blood flow; *RA*, right atrium; *RV*, right ventricle. (Copyright Satyan Lakshminrusimha.)

is present at birth, during the period of rapid decrease in PVR, and thus this model truly mimics the characteristics of CHD. Following spontaneous delivery at term, the lambs stay with the ewe and are maintained on a regular diet, diuretics (furosemide during periods of tachypnea), and iron supplementation. The lambs with shunt have a continuous murmur on auscultation. The Qp is increased and the Qp/Qs (pulmonary to systemic blood flow ratio) is 2.2 ± 1.2. At 4 weeks of age, these lambs have elevated pulmonary arterial pressure compared to controls (44.8 ± 11.7 vs. 16.2 ± 2.9 mm Hg). However, the calculated PVR is not increased compared to controls. The number of pulmonary blood vessels are increased per unit area with increased medial thickness and extension of the muscularization into the walls of the intraacinar arteries. The shunted animals have biventricular hypertrophy with an increase in the size of the proximal portion of the pulmonary artery. The vascular response to hypoxia and to vasoconstrictor U46619 (9, 11 dideoxy 11α 9α–epoxymethanoprostaglandin $F_{2\alpha}$—a thromboxane analog) is increased in the shunted lambs compared to controls.[35]

Cellular and Biochemical Changes

Unlike the ductal ligation model of PPHN, eNOS expression is increased in the pulmonary arteries with impaired endothelium-dependent pulmonary vasodilation.[36] Pretreatment with superoxide dismutase (SOD) and catalase enhanced relaxation to the calcium ionophore, A 23187 (a stimulant of eNOS), suggesting oxidative stress and increased superoxide generation leading to decreased eNOS activity. Impaired constriction to norepinephrine following pretreatment with N-nitro L-arginine, suggestive of decreased endogenous NO production, is also observed in isolated pulmonary arterial rings from "shunt" lambs. Relaxation responses to exogenous NO donor, S-nitroso N-acetyl-penicillamine (through sGC pathway) and atrial natriuretic peptide (through particulate guanylate cyclase—pGC pathway) were preserved in this model resulting in elevation of tissue and plasma cGMP levels.[37,38]

Drug Induced Pulmonary Hypertension

Infusion of the thromboxane analog, U 46619, increases pulmonary artery pressure 160% to 200% above baseline.[39] Infusion of NOS antagonists can also elevate PVR.[40] These models are minimally invasive and reversible on discontinuation of the infusion. However, U46619 may cause both systemic and coronary vasoconstriction that can lead to negative inotropy.[41] Unlike the previous two models, this model has no histological, cellular, or biochemical changes associated with pulmonary hypertension.

Meconium Aspiration Model

A new model of perinatal asphyxia and spontaneous aspiration of meconium during gasping was developed as a modification to the previous postnatal intratracheal meconium instillation model of PPHN. This is a model of secondary PPHN that combines both acute asphyxia and parenchymal lung disease. A slurry of 20% meconium in warm, fresh amniotic fluid (~5 mL/kg) is poured into a syringe and connected to the tracheal tube (Fig. 8.6). The umbilical cord is occluded intermittently to induce asphyxia and gasping. With each gasp, meconium is aspirated by the generated negative pressure into the fluid-filled lung resulting in uniform distribution. In this model, there is a better deposition of meconium into the distal airspaces (see Fig. 8.6—*inset*) and a more consistent degree of pulmonary hypertension as compared to postnatal tracheal instillation. This model has been used to evaluate the effect of suctioning of meconium at delivery, determination of optimal oxygenation and capnography during resuscitation.[42–44] However, the elevation of PVR is only modest compared to the ductal ligation model and no histological changes are observed in the pulmonary vasculature.

Chronic Hypoxia

One- to three-day-old piglets are placed in normobaric hypoxic chambers for 3 to 5 (short exposure) or 10 days (chronic exposure). Oxygen concentration in the chamber

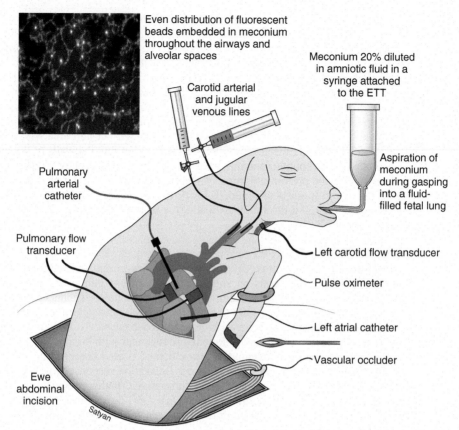

Even distribution of fluorescent beads embedded in meconium throughout the airways and alveolar spaces

Meconium 20% diluted in amniotic fluid in a syringe attached to the ETT

Carotid arterial and jugular venous lines

Aspiration of meconium during gasping into a fluid-filled fetal lung

Pulmonary arterial catheter

Pulmonary flow transducer

Left carotid flow transducer

Pulse oximeter

Left atrial catheter

Vascular occluder

Ewe abdominal incision

Fig. 8.6 The perinatal meconium aspiration and asphyxia model of secondary persistent pulmonary hypertension of the newborn. The pregnant ewe is placed under general anesthesia and, following hysterotomy (at 140 to 142 days' gestation), the fetal lamb is partially exteriorized, and intubated. A syringe containing a 20% slurry of meconium in amniotic fluid is attached to the endotracheal tube. Following instrumentation and a period of recovery, asphyxia is induced by cord occlusion twice for 5 minutes with a 5-minute recovery period of cord release. During cord occlusion, the meconium is aspirated by spontaneous gasping allowing distribution of the meconium into the fluid-filled distal airways. The inset shows the uniform distribution of fluorescent beads mixed with meconium in the alveoli in this model. See text for details. *ETT*, Endotracheal tube. (Copyright Satyan Lakshminrusimha.)

is maintained between 10% and 12% and CO_2 between 3 and 6 mm Hg. Pulmonary hypertension develops within 3 days of hypoxia with progressive increase in medial thickening of the pulmonary blood vessels with increasing duration of exposure to hypoxia.[45] In piglets exposed to chronic hypoxia, pulmonary vascular response to acetylcholine (NOS stimulant) and L-NAME (NOS inhibitor) are blunted.[46] NO production is downregulated as evidenced by decreased exhaled NO, plasma nitrates and nitrites, and decreased eNOS levels in lung homogenates.[47] Similar to the piglet model, in a neonatal rat pup model of chronic hypoxia induced pulmonary hypertension (13% O_2 from birth until 14 days of age), elevated PVR, right ventricular hypertrophy, and arterial medial thickening is observed. In this model, Rho A and Rho-kinase (ROCK) expression is increased in the pulmonary arteries and treatment with fasudil or Y-27632 (a Rho-kinase inhibitor) attenuates structural and hemodynamic changes of PPHN.[48]

Monocrotaline-Induced Pulmonary Hypertension in Rats

Monocrotaline is a pyrrolizidine alkaloid that causes pulmonary arterial hypertension in rats.[49,50] A single subcutaneous injection of 60 mg/kg results in pulmonary hypertension within 2 to 3 weeks. It causes pulmonary mononuclear vasculitis, pulmonary arterial medial hypertrophy, and dysregulation of NO signaling and right ventricular hypertrophy. Advantages of this model are its technical simplicity, reproducibility, and low cost. However, the injury from monocrotaline is not limited to the pulmonary arterial vasculature but also causes alveolar edema, interstitial fibrosis, pulmonary venous occlusion, and myocarditis. The right ventricular hypertrophy in this model is likely due to myocarditis rather than pressure overload from pulmonary hypertension. This model mimics pediatric and adult-onset pulmonary hypertension and is extensively used in studies evaluating the cellular mechanisms and new therapies.

Intrauterine Growth Restriction

Intrauterine growth restriction (IUGR) is an independent risk factor for developing pulmonary hypertension. Check et al., in a retrospective study of infants ≤28 weeks' gestation with moderate to severe bronchopulmonary dysplasia (BPD) and an echocardiogram performed, found that a birthweight below the 25th percentile was an independent risk factor for pulmonary hypertension.[51] IUGR, induced by different mechanisms in animal models, has been shown to have pulmonary arterial and cardiac dysfunction leading to pulmonary hypertension. Studies in a model of IUGR by maternal exposure to hyperthermia during the pregnancy have shown decreased pulmonary alveolar and vascular growth and endothelial dysfunction as the underlying mechanisms of pulmonary hypertension in IUGR.[52] In a model of maternal hypoxia-induced fetal IUGR in rats, ageing was associated with pulmonary hypertension and left ventricular diastolic dysfunction.[53] In a maternal undernutrition model of IUGR, Rexhaj et al. have shown that hypoxia increased pulmonary artery pressure and RV to LV + septal weight ratio, and was associated with poor relaxation of pulmonary arterial rings to acetylcholine and decreased DNA methylation in lung tissue.[54] These changes were reversed by administration of histone deacetylase inhibitors. Xu et al. studied the epigenetic changes associated with pulmonary hypertension developing following exposure to hypoxic conditions in IUGR rats (maternal undernutrition model).[55] Pulmonary vascular endothelial cells isolated from IUGR rats had increased histone acetylation as the promoter of ET-1 contributing to higher sensitivity of the IUGR rats to pulmonary vascular remodeling and PH following exposure to hypoxia. These models and clinical data demonstrate the association between IUGR and pulmonary hypertension.

Congenital Diaphragmatic Hernia

Three different approaches have been used to develop models of CDH: (1) a surgically created model, which has been reported mostly in lambs but also in rabbits, (2) a teratogen-induced model reported in rats and mice, and (3) a congenital model which is present in a specific pig herd.[56] The first two models are described in this chapter.

Fetal Surgical Model in Lambs

In 1967, Delorimier created the surgical model of CDH in lambs.[57] The timing of surgery is variable but typically is performed at 72 to 75 days' gestation (equivalent of 10 weeks of gestation in humans) in the pseudoglandular stage of lung development. The lungs are hypoplastic with a markedly reduced number of alveoli but the alveolar-to-arterial ratio is normal.[58] In addition, reduced cross-sectional area of the pulmonary vascular bed and pulmonary arterial medial hypertrophy is evident with signs of pulmonary hypertension.[59] This model is suitable for investigation of interventional strategies (such as iNO, surfactant, and tracheal occlusion). The lung compliance, total phospholipids, and percentage of phosphatidyl choline are decreased in this lamb model of CDH.[60]

Cellular and Biochemical Changes

Relaxation of pulmonary arteries in response to the endothelium-dependent vasodilator, acetylcholine, and phosphodiesterase inhibitors (such as zaprinast) are normal in the lamb model of CDH.[61] Some studies have demonstrated impaired vasorelaxation to PDE5 inhibitors in this model.[62,63] However, relaxation to sodium nitroprusside (an endothelium-independent vasodilator) is impaired with reduced sGC activity and normal PDE5 activity.[61] Poor response to iNO in the clinical trial of

PPHN associated with CDH could potentially be secondary to inadequate sGC activity.[64] Increased contractile response to catecholamines[63] and upregulation of ET_A receptor activity (suggested by a more profound relaxation to ET_A receptor blockade) implies an imbalance favoring vasoconstriction.[65] The clinical observation that infants with CDH who have poor outcomes have higher plasma ET-1 levels emphasizes the importance of vasoconstrictor mediators in CDH.[66]

Nitrofen Model in Rats

Nitrofen (2, 4 dichlorophenyl-p-nitrophenyl ether) is a teratogenic agent, which, when administered on day 9 or 11 of gestation to rats, leads to CDH in about 60% to 70% of the offspring. This teratogenic effect is likely mediated through the retinoid signaling pathway. The condition in the rats is very similar to the human form of the disease as to the location of the hernia, pulmonary hypoplasia, pulmonary hypertension, and associated anomalies in the cardiovascular and skeletal systems.[67] The disadvantages of this model are that the size of the animal precludes any in vivo physiological studies and only a relatively limited amount of samples are available to evaluate cellular mechanisms.

Cellular and Biochemical Abnormalities

Similar to the lamb CDH model, impaired sGC activity and normal PDE5 activity are observed in rats with CDH induced by maternal nitrofen.[64] As PDE5 activity is preserved in this model, antenatal sildenafil therapy increases fetal lung cGMP, improves lung structure, increases pulmonary vessel density, reduces right ventricular hypertrophy, and improves NO donor-induced pulmonary arterial relaxation.[68] In contrast, prenatal dexamethasone decreases the number of arteries and arterioles with a marked increase in percent medial wall thickness.[69]

Medications in Pregnancy and Persistent Pulmonary Hypertension of the Newborn: Cellular Basis

Selective Serotonin Reuptake Inhibitors

Maternal intake of selective serotonin reuptake inhibitors (SSRI) is identified as a risk factor for PPHN in the offspring.[70–72] Serotonin increases PVR and serotonin antagonists cause pulmonary vasodilation. Infusion of SSRI increases PVR in fetal lambs.[73] Pulmonary vasoconstriction is mediated by stimulation of 5-HT 2A receptors and Rho-kinase activation. Exposure of pregnant rats to fluoxetine leads to pulmonary hypertension and increased mortality in the pups.[74] Mice overexpressing the 5-HT plasma membrane transporter (5HTT) also develop pulmonary hypertension[75] and mice lacking 5HTT have attenuated hypoxic pulmonary vascular constrictor response.[76] Anorexigens (such as fenfluramine) may contribute to pulmonary hypertension by boosting 5-HT levels in the bloodstream and thus directly stimulating smooth muscle cell growth, or altering the 5HTT expression.[77,78]

Nonsteroidal Antiinflammatory Drugs

Prostaglandin E2 (PGE_2) plays a major role in maintaining ductal patency in utero. In addition, prostacyclin (PGI_2) is an important pulmonary vasodilator. NSAIDs such as aspirin used in the third trimester can block COX-mediated production of PGE_2 and PGI_2 and lead to premature closure of the ductus arteriosus and PPHN. Meconium analysis in neonates has demonstrated the presence of NSAIDs—aspirin, ibuprofen, and naproxen—in infants with PPHN.[79] However, epidemiological studies have not been able to establish an association between maternal NSAIDs and neonatal PPHN.[80]

Antenatal Betamethasone

Antenatal betamethasone decreases oxidative stress and improves relaxation response to ATP and NO donors in fetal lambs with PPHN induced by ductal ligation.[81] This also increases pulmonary blood flow and facilitates postnatal transition in PPHN lambs.[82] The beneficial effects of antenatal steroids in animal models of

CDH are variable. Vascular deterioration is observed in the nitrofen-rat model with dexamethasone[69] but improved compliance and vascular morphometry is observed in the lamb model of CDH.[83–85] In human neonates with CDH, antenatal glucocorticoid use is associated with suppression of the hypothalamic-pituitary-adrenal axis[86] without any difference in survival, length of stay, or oxygen use at 30 days of postnatal age.[87]

Free Radicals in Persistent Pulmonary Hypertension of the Newborn

Oxidative Stress

Oxidative stress occurs when the delicate balance between the production of reactive oxygen species (ROS) exceeds the capacity of host antioxidant defenses. Free radicals are chemical species that have a single unpaired electron in their outer orbit. They are unstable and highly reactive molecules due to the tendency of the unpaired electrons to pair with other electrons. Stepwise reduction of oxygen leads to the formation of superoxide, hydrogen peroxide, and hydroxyl radical. Exposure of the tissues to high oxygen tension or hypoxia can both trigger oxidative stress. In the tissues, the major source of ROS is the mitochondrial respiratory chain. In the process of oxidative phosphorylation, about 1% to 2% of oxygen entering the respiratory chain is released as superoxide anions. Extramitochondrial sources of ROS include uncoupled NOS, NADPH oxidases, xanthine oxidase, and reactions involving metals such as the Fenton reaction (Fig. 8.7). Furthermore, with increasing oxygen tension as with hyperoxia there is an increase in superoxide production as well.

Uncoupled Endothelial Nitric Oxide Synthase as a Source of Reactive Oxygen Species

Endothelial NOS requires a molecular chaperone such as heat shock protein-90, tetrahydrobiopterin (BH_4), and L-arginine to produce NO. Uncoupling of eNOS can occur under suboptimal conditions (such as the absence of the above factors and endothelial dysfunction in PPHN) and is evident in the ductal ligation model of PPHN.[88–90] Uncoupled NOS can produce superoxide anions and contribute to oxidative stress (see Fig. 8.7).

Reactive Nitrogen Species

In the pulmonary vasculature, NO is produced by the endothelial cells and diffuses to the smooth muscle cell to activate sGC (see Fig. 8.7). NO is a free radical and has a very short half-life in biologic systems.[91] NO combines with oxygen and is converted to nitrogen dioxide (NO_2). However, this reaction is too slow to be significant at physiological concentrations. NO binds avidly to other free radicals such as superoxide anions to form peroxynitrite, and this reaction occurs at the near-diffusion-limited rate of $6.7 \pm 0.9 \times 10^9/M/s$.[91] This rate is 3 to 6 times faster than the dismutation (partitioning) of superoxide by Cu,Zn SOD. In other words, every collision between superoxide and NO results in the irreversible formation of peroxynitrite. Superoxide reacts with NO 7000 times faster than with cytochrome c. In fact, SOD, by scavenging superoxide anions, doubles the half-life of NO in biological systems. Although the concentration of superoxide is kept low by SOD, a large flux of superoxide is produced by aerobic metabolism, and this flux may be enhanced further by exposure to excessive supplemental oxygen and hyperoxemia.[92,93]

The nitration of tyrosine residues to give 3-nitrotyrosine (3-NT) is a footprint left by peroxynitrite in vivo and is a marker of reactive nitrogen-centered oxidants being produced.[91] Administration of 20 ppm iNO and mechanical ventilation with 100% oxygen (without weaning in spite of supraphysiological PaO_2) markedly increases 3-NT in the pulmonary vasculature in lambs with PPHN. This increase is abolished by intratracheal SOD.[92] Similar to findings in animal models, exposure to iNO for 24 to 48 hours significantly increases serum 3-NT levels in term infants with PPHN/HRF.[94]

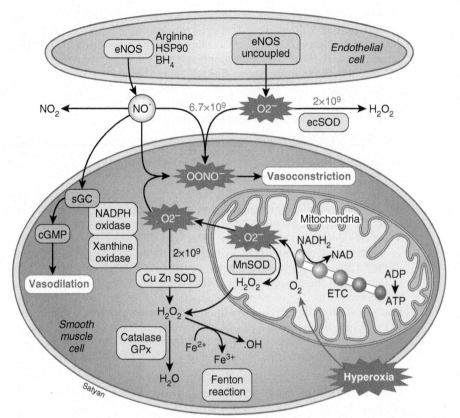

Fig. 8.7 Reactive oxygen and nitrogen species in persistent pulmonary hypertension of the newborn. Reactive oxygen species such as superoxide anions can be produced by the electron transport chain (ETC) in the mitochondria, due to exposure to hyperoxia or from enzymes such as uncoupled nitric oxide synthase (NOS), NADPH oxidase, and xanthine oxidase or the Fenton reaction. Nitric oxide (NO) is a free radical and avidly binds to superoxide anion (O_2^-) to form peroxynitrite (OONO$^-$) at the rate of 6.7/M/s. This rate is considerably faster than the rate of dismutation of superoxide anions by superoxide dismutase (SOD) to form hydrogen peroxide (H_2O_2). Hydrogen peroxide is then broken down by catalase and glutathione peroxidase (GPx) to water. NO and oxygen are vasodilators but peroxynitrite is a potent vasoconstrictor. See text for details. *ADP*, Adenosine diphosphate; *ATP*, adenosine triphosphate; *BH₄*, tetrahydrobiopterin; *ecSOD*, extracellular superoxide dismutase; *eNOS*, endothelial nitric oxide synthase; *HSP90*, heat shock protein 90; *MnSOD*, manganese superoxide dismutase; *NAD*, nicotinamide adenine dinucleotide; *NADH*, nicotinamide adenine dinucleotide (reduced); *NO₂*, nitrogen dioxide; *sGC*, soluble guanylate cyclase. (Copyright Satyan Lakshminrusimha.)

Pathological Vascular Remodeling in Persistent Pulmonary Hypertension of the Newborn

The structural changes in the pulmonary vasculature in subjects with PPHN include (a) fibroblastic infiltration of intima, (b) increased/abnormal smooth muscle proliferation in the media, and (c) increased extracellular matrix of the adventitia with deposition of collagen and elastin.

(a) Endothelial cells in PPHN are exposed to hypoxia, oxidative stress, inflammation, shear stress, and increased levels of mediators such as transforming growth factor β, interleukin 1β, and tumor necrosis factor α (TNFα). These factors induce the endothelial cells to lose the characteristic endothelial markers such as von Willebrand factor, vascular endothelial cadherin, and CD31. Endothelial cells possess plasticity to transition to mesenchymal cells or myofibroblasts with loss of endothelial markers and expression of α smooth muscle actin, type 1 collagen, and vimentin.[95] These cells secrete proinflammatory cytokines interleukin (IL)-4, IL-6, IL-8, IL-13, and TNF α, leading to loss of tight gap junctions, separation from basement membrane, and migration into the medial layer.[96]

(b) Increased muscular layer thickness decreases the caliber of the arterial lumen and causes obstruction to blood flow with concomitant increase in pulmonary arterial pressure. Pulmonary vascular remodeling depends on the balance of mediators that promote smooth muscle cell proliferation such as ET, platelet activating factor, and ROCK pathways and inhibitors of proliferation such as mediators acting via NO-cGMP and prostaglandin-cAMP pathways, pro-apoptotic pathways, and matrix metalloproteinases (MMP).[97] Hypoxia causes upregulation of Krüppel-like factor (KLF4) leading to dedifferentiation and migration and extension of muscularization to distal pulmonary blood vessels.[98] The fetal pulmonary arteries are approximately twice as thick as adult vessels and become thinner after birth. This change is brought about by enzymes including MMPs. Alterations in the balance between extracellular matrix production and its degradation brought about through MMPs and tissue inhibitors of metalloproteinases contribute to pathological vascular remodeling.

(c) Thickening of adventitial layer is commonly seen in vascular remodeling associated with PPHN. Following exposure to hypoxia, resident adventitial fibroblasts exhibit early and sustained proliferation. Early upregulation of collagen, fibronectin, and tropoelastin genes is followed by production and deposition of these proteins. The fibroblasts from the adventitia exert significant paracrine effect on other cell types and contribute to the vascular remodeling process.[99]

Cellular and Biochemical Basis of Various Persistent Pulmonary Hypertension of the Newborn Therapies

Oxygen

Supplemental oxygen is the mainstay of therapy for PPHN and HRF. The exact mechanism of HPV and normoxic (or oxygen-induced) pulmonary vasodilation is not known. HPV is intrinsic to the lung and is probably modulated upstream by the endothelium and downstream by calcium sensitization of the contractile apparatus (Rho kinase). The core mechanism of HPV involves a redox-based oxygen sensor (likely the mitochondria) that generates a diffusible redox mediator (likely H_2O_2) that is withdrawn during hypoxia, leading to hypoxic inhibition of certain voltage-gated K channels (Kv) in pulmonary arterial smooth muscle cells (PASMC).[100]

Human Data on Hypoxic Pulmonary Vasoconstriction

Clinical documentation of HPV by cardiac catheterization is not available in neonates with PPHN. Data from children with BPD (median age 5 years) undergoing cardiac catheterization for evaluation of pulmonary hypertension shows that a reduction in PaO_2 from 78.5 ± 4.9 to 46.9 ± 2.2 mm Hg results in an increase in pulmonary arterial pressure from 34.1 ± 2.6 to 45.2 ± 4.4 mm Hg. An increase in PaO_2 to 239 ± 30.7 mm Hg, however, did not significantly decrease pulmonary arterial pressure (34.1 ± 2.6 to 28.2 ± 2.6 mm Hg) compared to normoxia.[101]

Animal Data on Hypoxic Pulmonary Vasoconstriction and Persistent Pulmonary Hypertension of the Newborn

Data from neonatal animal models have demonstrated that alveolar hypoxia and hypoxemia increase PVR and contribute to the pathophysiology of PPHN.[102] PVR is regulated predominantly by PASMCs in the small-resistance precapillary pulmonary arterioles.[103] The oxygen tension in these PASMCs is determined by alveolar oxygen tension (PAO_2) and pulmonary arterial (or mixed venous) PO_2, although the partial pressure of oxygen in the alveolus (PAO_2) is considered to be the more important factor (Fig. 8.8).[100]

"Change Point"—Alveolar Versus Arterial Partial Pressure of Oxygen (PO_2) and Hypoxic Pulmonary Vasoconstriction

In clinical practice, arterial PaO_2 (either postductal, often from an umbilical arterial line, or preductal) is measured and is used to calculate alveolar PAO_2 (see Fig. 8.8). In subjects with heterogeneous lung disease, it is difficult to estimate regional alveolar PAO_2. Pulse oximetry or arterial blood gas PaO_2 are clinically used instead of alveolar PAO_2 to determine the optimal "change point"—the cut-off value below which PVR increases due to HPV.[104] The relationship between PVR and PaO_2 was first

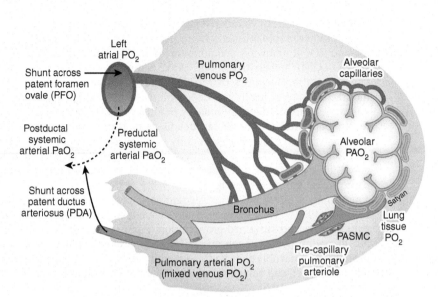

Fig. 8.8 Site of pulmonary vascular resistance (PVR) and oxygen tension. The precise site of PVR is debated but is thought by most to be the precapillary pulmonary arteriole in the lung. The pulmonary arterial smooth muscle cells (PASMC) are exposed to lung tissue PO_2, alveolar PAO_2, and pulmonary arterial (mixed venous) PO_2. It is thought that the rapid diffusion from alveolar PAO_2 is the predominant determinant of oxygen tension in PASMC. In infants with persistent pulmonary hypertension of the newborn (PPHN), PAO_2 can be approximately calculated using preductal PaO_2 values. The presence of a right-to-left shunt at the atrial level or ductal level can reduce PaO_2 levels in PPHN. See text for details. (Copyright Satyan Lakshminrusimha.)

described in a study of healthy newborn calves, which found a precipitous increase in PVR as the PaO_2 fell below 45 to 50 mm Hg.[102] A similar relationship between PaO_2 and PVR was later described in an ovine model of PPHN.[104] Healthy control lambs had an acute increase in PVR with preductal $PaO_2 < 52.5$ mm Hg. Similar change points were observed in acute PPHN induced by perinatal asphyxia and meconium aspiration syndrome (~45 mm Hg). In PPHN lambs, hypoxic vasoconstriction was greatly exaggerated with two PVR change points: severe hypoxemia with $PaO_2 < 13.9$ mm Hg resulted in a steep increase in PVR (up to 6 mm Hg/mL/kg/min—normal values in term control lambs are 0.2 to 0.3 mm Hg/mL/kg/min), whereas resistance declined more gradually when $PaO_2 > 59.6$ mm Hg. Within clinically relevant ranges of preductal oxygen saturations (SpO^2) (80% to 100%), PVR increased below SpO_2 of 85%.[105] In this model, PVR is low with preductal SpO_2 in the 90% to 97% range with preductal PaO_2 between 60 and 80 mm Hg.

With appropriate considerations, the findings from these ovine models have clinical relevance to the management of PPHN, as traditional practice often involves hyperoxic ventilation during the acute phase. However, such an approach has not been shown to produce persistent clinical benefit in PVR, and the animal studies suggest that this approach paradoxically impairs the subsequent response to iNO.[105] Lower fraction of inspired oxygen (FiO_2; <0.45 vs. >0.8) during initial management of PPHN with iNO has also been associated with lower serum interleukin concentrations (IL-6, IL-8, TNF-α).[106] Meta-analysis of oxygen saturation target studies in preterm infants have shown increased mortality with lower target range (85% to 89%) compared to higher target range (91% to 95%).[107] Interestingly, posthoc analysis of one of these studies (SUPPORT) suggests that increased mortality in the 85% to 89% target group may be due to respiratory causes (RDS and BPD) in small for gestational age infants,[108] a group at risk for pulmonary hypertension.[109]

The mechanisms underlying the hemodynamic effects of hyperoxia reflect, in part, an increased oxidative stress (see Fig. 8.7). Ventilation with 100% oxygen promotes formation of ROS such as superoxide anions that enhance vasoconstriction in the neonatal pulmonary circulation,[110–112] and inactivate NO through formation of peroxynitrite.[113,114] In addition, ROS decrease eNOS activity and sGC activity resulting in reduced cGMP levels[115,116] with consequent shift to vasoconstriction. Decreased responsiveness to iNO is reflected in a decreased intracellular cGMP response as well as increased PDE5 cGMP-hydrolytic activity.

Overall, the evidence from animal models indicates that hypoxia causes pulmonary vasoconstriction, and normoxia results in pulmonary vasodilation. However, hyperoxia (especially when the FiO_2 exceeds 0.5 *and* PaO_2 exceeds 80 to 100 mm Hg) does not cause further pulmonary vasodilation. Therefore avoiding hyperoxia is potentially as important as avoiding hypoxia in the management of PPHN. Clinicians should recognize that oxygen is also a drug and as such is a toxin at high doses, and should be used accordingly in the therapeutic context taking into account its potential benefits and side effects.[104,117]

Inhaled Nitric Oxide

The therapeutic potential of iNO in PPHN is discussed in Chapter 9. An important effect of prolonged therapy with iNO is the suppression of endogenous NOS activity, and thus the potential risk for rebound pulmonary hypertension.[118,119] Because of this reason, it may be important to wean NO stepwise titrating to the clinical response. Approximately 40% to 50% of term infants fail to show a sustained response to iNO.[3] From a cellular and biochemical standpoint, potential causes of poor or ill-sustained pulmonary vasodilator response to iNO include: (a) inactivation of iNO by superoxide anions and formation of peroxynitrite as discussed previously, (b) inactivation of sGC, and (c) increased activity of PDE5 and PDE3. In the ensuing paragraphs, we will discuss the cellular basis for management strategies to enhance vasodilatory effect of iNO.

Attenuating Inactivation of Inhaled Nitric Oxide by Superoxide

This can be achieved by avoiding hyperoxia,[93] inhibiting enzymes contributing to ROS formation,[120] and/or by scavenging superoxide anions by recombination human superoxide dismutase (rhSOD).[92] In lambs with PPHN and ventilated with 100% oxygen, treatment with intratracheal rhSOD (Fig. 8.9) improved oxygenation, decreased PDE5 expression and activity,[121] increased cGMP levels, decreased ROS, restored eNOS activity, and increased levels of BH_4 and GTP cyclohydrolase (cofactors in the conversion of L-arginine to NO).[92,116] However, clinical trials using this compound are limited to preterm infants with RDS[122,123] and this therapy has not been evaluated in term infants with PPHN.

Soluble Guanylate Cyclase Stimulators and Activators (see Fig. 8.9)

Nitric oxide produced by the endothelial cells affects pulmonary vasodilation by stimulating sGC to produce the second messenger, cGMP. sGC has a heme moiety that is essential for binding NO, and oxidation of the heme moiety impairs NO binding to sGC. NO independent activation of sGC is achieved through direct activators of sGC. Cinaciguat, a sGC activator, has been shown to enhance the levels of cGMP in fetal PASMC from both normal and PPHN-afflicted lambs.[124] The effect of cinaciguat on cGMP levels in isolated PASMC was also demonstrated following exposure to an sGC oxidizer (ODQ), hyperoxia, or H_2O_2.[124] In the partial ductal ligation model of PPHN, cinaciguat increased Qp and decreased pulmonary arterial pressure.[124] sGC stimulators act by directly stimulating the native, reduced heme form of the enzyme and rendering it more sensitive to endogenous or exogenous NO.[125] These agents have the potential to be effective in iNO-resistant PPHN.

Inhibition of Phosphodiesterase 5

Oxidative stress increases PDE5 expression and activity.[115] In patients with PPHN with prolonged hyperoxic exposure, increased PDE5 activity can potentially limit the pulmonary vasodilatory response to iNO. Use of PDE5 inhibitors such as sildenafil by the oral[126] or intravenous route[127] improves oxygenation in PPHN. In addition to vasodilation, sildenafil may have beneficial effects on angiogenesis[128] and alveolarization, especially in preterm infants with BPD.[129] In animal models of CDH, preservation of

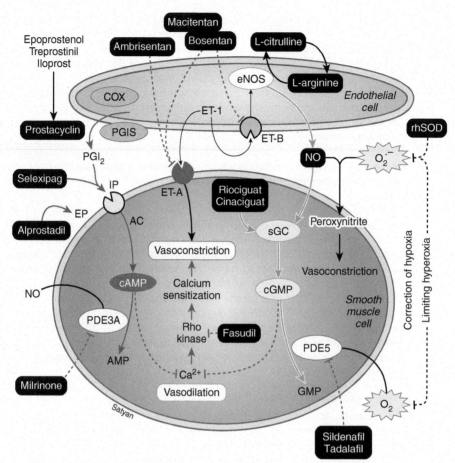

Fig. 8.9 Medical therapies, current and emerging, in the management of pulmonary arterial hypertension acting through the prostaglandin, endothelin (ET-1), nitric oxide (NO) and superoxide pathways. *COX*, Cyclooxygenase; *eNOS*, endothelial nitric oxide synthase; *EP*, prostaglandin E receptor; *ET-A* and *ET-B*, endothelin receptors; *IP*, prostacyclin receptor; *PDE*, phosphodiesterase; *PGI₂*, prostacyclin; *PGIS*, prostacyclin synthase; *rhSOD*, recombinant human superoxide dismutase; *selexipag*, IP receptor agonist; *sGC*, soluble guanylate cyclase. Please see text for details. (Copyright Satyan Lakshminrusimha.)

PDE5 activity suggests that sildenafil may be a potentially useful therapy in managing acute and chronic pulmonary hypertension in infants with CDH.[130–132]

Hydrocortisone

Hydrocortisone is occasionally used in the acute phase of PPHN to achieve hemodynamic stability in patients who develop systemic hypotension. In addition to its anti-inflammatory and blood pressure stabilizing effects, hydrocortisone has been shown to decrease oxidative stress, increase the levels of ECSOD, decrease PDE5 activity, and NFkB in fetal pulmonary artery smooth muscle cells of PPHN lambs exposed to 95% oxygen for 24 hours.[133] In neonatal lambs with PPHN ventilated with 100% oxygen, hydrocortisone treatment improved oxygenation, normalized PDE5 activity, and decreased oxidative stress.[134]

Inhibition of Phosphodiesterase 3

Infants with PPHN and on mechanical ventilation are often managed with a high fraction of inspired oxygen and iNO. Upregulation of PDE3 activity has been demonstrated in animal models of pulmonary hypertension[135] and studies in lambs and rats suggest that exposure to a combination of hyperoxia and NO further stimulates PDE3 activity.[28,136] This finding may explain, at least in part, the efficacy of milrinone, a PDE3 inhibitor and an inotrope in the management of PPHN resistant to iNO.[137] Milrinone can be synergistic with agents that increase cAMP such as prostacyclin analogs (see Fig. 8.9).[40,138,139]

Cellular Basis for Emerging Therapies

L-citrulline

Nitric oxide is synthesized from L-arginine by the NO synthase enzyme (see Fig. 8.9). Decreased bioavailability of L-arginine has been shown to contribute to vascular dysfunction in chronic pulmonary hypertension. Administration of L-arginine has been found to improve NO production in a newborn piglet model of chronic hypoxia-induced pulmonary hypertension.[140] However, studies of L-arginine supplementation have yielded inconsistent results. Bioavailability of L-arginine is poor following oral administration as it is catabolized to ornithine and urea by the arginase enzyme present in gut bacteria, intestinal epithelial cells, and hepatocytes. L-citrulline is a metabolic intermediary in the urea cycle and it is a substrate and the end product when arginine is converted to NO. L-citrulline is well absorbed and high plasma levels are achieved following oral therapy.[141] In pulmonary arterial endothelial cells cultured under hypoxic conditions, treatment with L-citrulline was shown to improve eNOS recoupling as evidenced by decreased superoxide generation and increased NO production.[142] Of note is that L-citrulline has been used as replacement therapy in urea cycle disorders and has been found to be safe for long-term use.

Rho-kinase inhibitors

Rho A is a small GTPase protein. Rho kinases (Rho associated protein kinase, ROCK) are serine or threonine kinases that determine the calcium sensitivity in smooth muscle cells (see Fig. 8.9) and contribute to the regulation of a variety of functions including smooth muscle contraction, gene expression, proliferation, and apoptosis. Accordingly, Rho A and Rho kinase are highly expressed in the vasculature and play a key role in regulation of PVR.[143] Rho-kinase activation inhibits MLC phosphatase leading to phosphorylation of MLC and augments smooth muscle contraction. Activation of ROCK plays a central role in HPV and in maintenance of high fetal pulmonary vascular tone.[143] Rho-kinase inhibitors increase eNOS expression and decrease vascular remodeling in lambs with PPHN.[144] Fasudil and Y 27632 are potent inhibitors of ROCK and are being evaluated in adults with pulmonary hypertension.[145–148] Concerns regarding potential for somatic growth restriction in animal studies have, however, reduced the enthusiasm for their use in newborns.[48]

Stem Cell Therapies

Pulmonary hypertension in ex-preterm infants with BPD remains a challenging clinical scenario with no effective therapies. Recent studies on stem-cell-based therapies may offer new avenues for its treatment that can reverse the pathophysiological changes and restore the disordered angiogenesis and alveolarization associated with BPD and pulmonary hypertension.[149] Six-week-old rats with monocrotaline-induced pulmonary hypertension were given a transfusion of human umbilical cord blood mesenchymal cells (3×10^6 cells) 1 week after the injury. The animals showed improvement in both clinical and histologic markers of pulmonary hypertension including a decrease in right ventricular pressure, reduced medial wall thickness in the pulmonary arterioles, and reduction in the number of muscularized intraacinar pulmonary arteries. These changes were associated with a decrease in the expression of ET-1, ET_A receptor, eNOS, and MMP 2.[150] Intratracheal administration of rat mesenchymal stem cells in another monocrotaline-induced pulmonary hypertension model resulted in decrease in right ventricular pressure, PVR, right ventricular hypertrophy, and demonstrated improved endothelium-dependent relaxation.[151] Finally, delayed cord clamping may offer an additional benefit to the pulmonary circulation by providing a natural source of stem cells for repair and regeneration (see Chapters 4 and 5).[152,153]

Conclusion

Animal studies have greatly enhanced our understanding of the pathophysiology of PPHN and aided in the identification of multiple biochemical pathways for the treatment of PPHN. Inhaled NO remains the only FDA approved therapy for pulmonary hypertension in neonates but approximately 40% to 50% of patients with PPHN have poor or ill-sustained response to iNO. Understanding the cellular and biochemical basis of pulmonary hypertension in various disease models will undoubtedly enhance our ability to develop new therapeutic strategies for the management of PPHN. Current treatment for infants is, however, limited to iNO and off-label use of agents approved for pulmonary hypertension in adults (see Fig. 8.9). Hence, there is a dire need to develop evidence-based strategies to evaluate new medications and approaches for the treatment of PPHN.

Founding Sources

Funded by: National Institutes of Health (National Institute of Child Health and Human Development) HD072929 and Women and Children's Hospital of Buffalo Foundation.

REFERENCES

1. Walsh-Sukys MC, Tyson JE, Wright LL, et al.: Persistent pulmonary hypertension of the newborn in the era before nitric oxide: practice variation and outcomes, *Pediatrics* 105(1 Pt 1):14–20, 2000.
2. Steurer MA, Jelliffe-Pawlowski LL, Baer RJ, et al.: Persistent pulmonary hypertension of the newborn in late preterm and term infants in california, *Pediatrics* 139(1), 2017.
3. Barrington KJ, Finer N, Pennaforte T, et al.: Nitric oxide for respiratory failure in infants born at or near term, *Cochrane Database Syst Rev* 1:CD000399, 2017.
4. Matsubara K, Higaki T, Matsubara Y, et al.: Nitric oxide and reactive oxygen species in the pathogenesis of preeclampsia, *Int J Mol Sci* 16(3):4600–4614, 2015.
5. Maron BA, Abman SH: Focusing on developmental origins and disease inception for the prevention of pulmonary hypertension, *Am J Respir Crit Care Med*, 2016.
6. Rudolph AM, Heymann MA: Circulatory changes during growth in the fetal lamb, *Circ Res* 26(3):289–299, 1970.
7. Rasanen J, Wood DC, Weiner S, et al.: Role of the pulmonary circulation in the distribution of human fetal cardiac output during the second half of pregnancy, *Circulation* 94(5):1068–1073, 1996.
8. Kinsella JP, McQueston JA, Rosenberg AA, et al.: Hemodynamic effects of exogenous nitric oxide in ovine transitional pulmonary circulation, *Am J Physiol* 263(3 Pt 2):H875–H880, 1992.
9. Morin 3rd FC, Egan EA, Ferguson W, et al.: Development of pulmonary vascular response to oxygen, *Am J Physiol* 254(3 Pt 2):H542–H546, 1988.
10. Mensah E, Morin 3rd FC, Russell JA, et al.: Soluble guanylate cyclase mRNA expression change during ovine lung development, *Pediatric Res* 43:290, 1998.
11. Kumar VH, Hutchison AA, Lakshminrusimha S, et al.: Characteristics of pulmonary hypertension in preterm neonates, *J Perinatol* 27(4):214–219, 2007.
12. Walker AM, Ritchie BC, Adamson TM, et al.: Effect of changing lung liquid volume on the pulmonary circulation of fetal lambs, *J Appl Physiol (1985)* 64(1):61–67, 1988.
13. Polglase GR, Wallace MJ, Morgan DL, et al.: Increases in lung expansion alter pulmonary hemodynamics in fetal sheep, *J Appl Physiol (1985)* 101(1):273–282, 2006.
14. Dawes GS, Mott JC, Widdicombe JG, et al.: Changes in the lungs of the new-born lamb, *J Physiol* 121(1):141–162, 1953.
15. Storme L, Rairigh RL, Parker TA, et al.: In vivo evidence for a myogenic response in the fetal pulmonary circulation, *Pediatric Res* 45(3):425–431, 1999.
16. Parker TA, Grover TR, Kinsella JP, et al.: Inhibition of 20-HETE abolishes the myogenic response during NOS antagonism in the ovine fetal pulmonary circulation, *Am J Physiol Lung Cell Mol Physiol* 289(2):L261–L267, 2005.
17. Aschner JL, Fike CD: New developments in the pathogenesis and management of neonatal pulmonary hypertension. In Bancalari E, editor: *The Newborn Lung. Neonatology questions and controversies*, Philadelphia, 2008, Saunders Elsevier, pp 241–299.
18. Chatfield BA, McMurtry IF, Hall SL, et al.: Hemodynamic effects of endothelin-1 on ovine fetal pulmonary circulation, *Am J Physiol* 261(1 Pt 2):R182–R187, 1991.
19. Ivy DD, le Cras TD, Parker TA, et al.: Developmental changes in endothelin expression and activity in the ovine fetal lung, *Am J Physiol Lung Cell Mol Physiol* 278(4):L785–L793, 2000.
20. Teitel DF, Iwamoto HS, Rudolph AM: Changes in the pulmonary circulation during birth-related events, *Pediatric Res* 27(4 Pt 1):372–378, 1990.
21. Lakshminrusimha S, Steinhorn RH: Pulmonary vascular biology during neonatal transition, *Clin Perinatol* 26(3):601–619, 1999.
22. Crossley KJ, Allison BJ, Polglase GR, et al.: Dynamic changes in the direction of blood flow through the ductus arteriosus at birth, *J Physiol* 587(Pt 19):4695–4704, 2009.
23. Cornfield DN, Chatfield BA, McQueston JA, et al.: Effects of birth-related stimuli on L-arginine-dependent pulmonary vasodilation in ovine fetus, *Am J Physiol* 262(5 Pt 2):H1474–H1481, 1992.
24. Morin 3rd FC, Egan EA, Lundgren CE, et al.: Prostacyclin does not change during an oxygen induced increase in pulmonary blood flow in the fetal lamb, *Prostaglandins Leukot Essent Fatty Acids* 32(3):139–144, 1988.
25. Morin 3rd FC, Egan EA, Norfleet WT: Indomethacin does not diminish the pulmonary vascular response of the fetus to increased oxygen tension, *Pediatric Res* 24(6):696–700, 1988.

26. Bloch KD, Filippov G, Sanchez LS, et al.: Pulmonary soluble guanylate cyclase, a nitric oxide receptor, is increased during the perinatal period, *Am J Physiol* 272(3 Pt 1):L400–L406, 1997.
27. Sanchez LS, de la Monte SM, Filippov G, et al.: Cyclic-GMP-binding, cyclic-GMP-specific phosphodiesterase (PDE5) gene expression is regulated during rat pulmonary development, *Pediatric Res* 43(2):163–168, 1998.
28. Busch CJ, Graveline AR, Jiramongkolchai K, et al.: Phosphodiesterase 3A expression is modulated by nitric oxide in rat pulmonary artery smooth muscle cells, *J Physiol Pharmacol* 61(6):663–669, 2010.
29. Abman SH, Accurso FJ: Acute effects of partial compression of ductus arteriosus on fetal pulmonary circulation, *Am J Physiol* 257(2 Pt 2):H626–H634, 1989.
30. Morin 3rd FC, Egan EA: The effect of closing the ductus arteriosus on the pulmonary circulation of the fetal sheep, *J Dev Physiol* 11(5):283–287, 1989.
31. Wild LM, Nickerson PA, Morin 3rd FC: Ligating the ductus arteriosus before birth remodels the pulmonary vasculature of the lamb, *Pediatric Res* 25(3):251–257, 1989.
32. Agger P, Lakshminrusimha S, Laustsen C, et al.: The myocardial architecture changes in persistent pulmonary hypertension of the newborn in an ovine animal model, *Pediatric Res* 79(4):565–574, 2016.
33. Zayek M, Cleveland D, Morin 3rd FC: Treatment of persistent pulmonary hypertension in the newborn lamb by inhaled nitric oxide.[comment], *J Pediatr* 122(5 Pt 1):743–750, 1993.
34. Zayek M, Wild L, Roberts JD, et al.: Effect of nitric oxide on the survival rate and incidence of lung injury in newborn lambs with persistent pulmonary hypertension, *J Pediatr* 123(6):947–952, 1993.
35. Reddy VM, Meyrick B, Wong J, et al.: In utero placement of aortopulmonary shunts. A model of postnatal pulmonary hypertension with increased pulmonary blood flow in lambs, *Circulation* 92(3):606–613, 1995.
36. Black SM, Fineman JR, Steinhorn RH, et al.: Increased endothelial NOS in lambs with increased pulmonary blood flow and pulmonary hypertension, *Am J Physiol* 275(5 Pt 2):H1643–H1651, 1998.
37. Steinhorn RH, Russell JA, Lakshminrusimha S, et al.: Altered endothelium-dependent relaxations in lambs with high pulmonary blood flow and pulmonary hypertension, *Am J Physiol Heart Circ Physiol* 280(1):H311–H317, 2001.
38. Lakshminrusimha S, Wiseman D, Black SM, et al.: The role of nitric oxide synthase-derived reactive oxygen species in the altered relaxation of pulmonary arteries from lambs with increased pulmonary blood flow, *Am J Physiol Heart Circ Physiol* 293(3):H1491–H1497, 2007.
39. Obaid L, Johnson ST, Bigam DL, et al.: Intratracheal administration of sildenafil and surfactant alleviates the pulmonary hypertension in newborn piglets, *Resuscitation* 69(2):287–294, 2006.
40. Kumar VH, Swartz DD, Rashid N, et al.: Prostacyclin and milrinone by aerosolization improve pulmonary hemodynamics in newborn lambs with experimental pulmonary hypertension, *J Appl Physiol (1985)* 109(3):677–684, 2010.
41. Holzgrefe HH, Buchanan LV, Bunting S: In vivo characterization of synthetic thromboxane A2 in canine myocardium, *Circ Res* 60(2):290–296, 1987.
42. Lakshminrusimha S, Mathew B, Nair J, et al.: Tracheal suctioning improves gas exchange but not hemodynamics in asphyxiated lambs with meconium aspiration, *Pediat Res* 77(2):347–355, 2015.
43. Rawat M, Chandrasekharan PK, Williams A, et al.: Oxygen saturation index and severity of hypoxic respiratory failure, *Neonatol* 107(3):161–166, 2015.
44. Rawat M, Chandrasekharan PK, Swartz DD, et al.: Neonatal resuscitation adhering to oxygen saturation guidelines in asphyxiated lambs with meconium aspiration, *Pediatr Res* 79(4):583–588, 2016.
45. Fike CD, Kaplowitz MR: Effect of chronic hypoxia on pulmonary vascular pressures in isolated lungs of newborn pigs, *J Appl Physiol (1985)* 77(6):2853–2862, 1994.
46. Fike CD, Kaplowitz MR: Chronic hypoxia alters nitric oxide-dependent pulmonary vascular responses in lungs of newborn pigs, *J Appl Physiol (1985)* 81(5):2078–2087, 1996.
47. Fike CD, Kaplowitz MR, Thomas CJ, et al.: Chronic hypoxia decreases nitric oxide production and endothelial nitric oxide synthase in newborn pig lungs, *Am J Physiol* 274(4 Pt 1):L517–L526, 1998.
48. Ziino AJ, Ivanovska J, Belcastro R, et al.: Effects of rho-kinase inhibition on pulmonary hypertension, lung growth, and structure in neonatal rats chronically exposed to hypoxia, *Pediatr Res* 67(2):177–182, 2010.
49. Todorovich-Hunter L, Dodo H, Ye C, et al.: Increased pulmonary artery elastolytic activity in adult rats with monocrotaline-induced progressive hypertensive pulmonary vascular disease compared with infant rats with nonprogressive disease, *Am Rev Resp Dis* 146(1):213–223, 1992.
50. Prie S, Stewart DJ, Dupuis J: EndothelinA receptor blockade improves nitric oxide-mediated vasodilation in monocrotaline-induced pulmonary hypertension, *Circulation* 97(21):2169–2174, 1998.
51. Check J, Gotteiner N, Liu X, et al.: Fetal growth restriction and pulmonary hypertension in premature infants with bronchopulmonary dysplasia, *J Perinatol* 33(7):553–557, 2013.
52. Rozance PJ, Seedorf GJ, Brown A, et al.: Intrauterine growth restriction decreases pulmonary alveolar and vessel growth and causes pulmonary artery endothelial cell dysfunction in vitro in fetal sheep, *Am J Physiol Lung Cell Mol Physiol* 301(6):L860–L871, 2011.
53. Rueda-Clausen CF, Morton JS, et al.: Effects of hypoxia-induced intrauterine growth restriction on cardiopulmonary structure and function during adulthood, *Cardiovasc Res* 81(4):713–722, 2009.
54. Rexhaj E, Bloch J, Jayet PY, et al.: Fetal programming of pulmonary vascular dysfunction in mice: role of epigenetic mechanisms, *Am J Physiol Heart Circ Physiol* 301(1):H247–H252, 2011.

8

55. Xu XF, Lv Y, Gu WZ, et al.: Epigenetics of hypoxic pulmonary arterial hypertension following intrauterine growth retardation rat: epigenetics in PAH following IUGR, *Respir Res* 14:20, 2013.
56. Wilcox DT, Irish MS, Holm BA, et al.: Animal models in congenital diaphragmatic hernia, *Clin Perinatol* 23(4):813–822, 1996.
57. Adzick NS, Outwater KM, Harrison MR, et al.: Correction of congenital diaphragmatic hernia in utero. IV. An early gestational fetal lamb model for pulmonary vascular morphometric analysis, *J Pediatr Surg* 20(6):673–680, 1985.
58. Ting A, Glick PL, Wilcox DT, et al.: Alveolar vascularization of the lung in a lamb model of congenital diaphragmatic hernia, *Am J Respir Critic Care Med* 157(1):31–34, 1998.
59. O'Toole SJ, Irish MS, Holm BA, et al.: Pulmonary vascular abnormalities in congenital diaphragmatic hernia, *Clin Perinatol* 23(4):781–794, 1996.
60. Glick PL, Stannard VA, Leach CL, et al.: Pathophysiology of congenital diaphragmatic hernia II: the fetal lamb CDH model is surfactant deficient, *J Pediatr Surg* 27(3):382–387, 1992. discussion 7–8.
61. Thebaud B, Petit T, De Lagausie P, et al.: Altered guanylyl-cyclase activity in vitro of pulmonary arteries from fetal lambs with congenital diaphragmatic hernia, *Am J Respir Cell Mol Biol* 27(1):42–47, 2002.
62. de Buys Roessingh A, Fouquet V, Aigrain Y, et al.: Nitric oxide activity through guanylate cyclase and phosphodiesterase modulation is impaired in fetal lambs with congenital diaphragmatic hernia, *J Pediatr Surg* 46(8):1516–1522, 2011.
63. Irish MS, Glick PL, Russell J, et al.: Contractile properties of intralobar pulmonary arteries and veins in the fetal lamb model of congenital diaphragmatic hernia, *J Pediatr Surg* 33(6):921–928, 1998.
64. The Neonatal Inhaled Nitric Oxide Study Group N: Inhaled nitric oxide and hypoxic respiratory failure in infants with congenital diaphragmatic hernia. The Neonatal Inhaled Nitric Oxide Study Group (NINOS), *Pediatrics* 99(6):838–845, 1997.
65. Thebaud B, de Lagausie P, Forgues D, et al.: ET(A)-receptor blockade and ET(B)-receptor stimulation in experimental congenital diaphragmatic hernia, *Am J Physiol Lung Cell Mol Physiol* 278(5):L923–L932, 2000.
66. Keller RL, Tacy TA, Hendricks-Munoz K, et al.: Congenital diaphragmatic hernia: endothelin-1, pulmonary hypertension, and disease severity, *Am J Respir Critic Care Med* 182(4):555–561, 2010.
67. van Loenhout RB, Tibboel D, Post M, et al.: Congenital diaphragmatic hernia: comparison of animal models and relevance to the human situation, *Neonatology* 96(3):137–149, 2009.
68. Luong C, Rey-Perra J, Vadivel A, et al.: Antenatal sildenafil treatment attenuates pulmonary hypertension in experimental congenital diaphragmatic hernia, *Circulation* 123(19):2120–2131, 2011.
69. Kattan J, Cespedes C, Gonzalez A, et al.: Sildenafil stimulates and dexamethasone inhibits pulmonary vascular development in congenital diaphragmatic hernia rat lungs, *Neonatology* 106(1):74–80, 2014.
70. Chambers CD, Hernandez-Diaz S, Van Marter LJ, et al.: Selective serotonin-reuptake inhibitors and risk of persistent pulmonary hypertension of the newborn, *New Eng J Med* 354(6):579–587, 2006.
71. Belik J: Fetal and neonatal effects of maternal drug treatment for depression, *Semin Perinatol* 32(5):350–354, 2008.
72. Kieler H, Artama M, Engeland A, et al.: Selective serotonin reuptake inhibitors during pregnancy and risk of persistent pulmonary hypertension in the newborn: population based cohort study from the five Nordic countries, *BMJ* 344:d8012, 2012.
73. Delaney C, Gien J, Grover TR, et al.: Pulmonary vascular effects of serotonin and selective serotonin reuptake inhibitors in the late-gestation ovine fetus, *Am J Physiol Lung Cell Mol Physiol* 301(6):L937–L944, 2011.
74. Fornaro E, Li D, Pan J, et al.: Prenatal exposure to fluoxetine induces fetal pulmonary hypertension in the rat, *Am J Respir Critic Care Med* 176(10):1035–1040, 2007.
75. Eddahibi S, Humbert M, Fadel E, et al.: Serotonin transporter overexpression is responsible for pulmonary artery smooth muscle hyperplasia in primary pulmonary hypertension, *J Clinic Invest* 108(8):1141–1150, 2001.
76. Eddahibi S, Hanoun N, Lanfumey L, et al.: Attenuated hypoxic pulmonary hypertension in mice lacking the 5-hydroxytryptamine transporter gene, *J Clinic Invest* 105(11):1555–1562, 2000.
77. Eddahibi S, Adnot S, Frisdal E, et al.: Dexfenfluramine-associated changes in 5-hydroxytryptamine transporter expression and development of hypoxic pulmonary hypertension in rats, *J Pharmacol Exp Ther* 297(1):148–154, 2001.
78. Eddahibi S, Adnot S: Anorexigen-induced pulmonary hypertension and the serotonin (5-HT) hypothesis: lessons for the future in pathogenesis, *Respir Res* 3:9, 2002.
79. Alano MA, Ngougmna E, Ostrea Jr EM, et al.: Analysis of nonsteroidal antiinflammatory drugs in meconium and its relation to persistent pulmonary hypertension of the newborn, *Pediatrics* 107(3):519–523, 2001.
80. Van Marter LJ, Hernandez-Diaz S, Werler MM, et al.: Nonsteroidal antiinflammatory drugs in late pregnancy and persistent pulmonary hypertension of the newborn, *Pediatrics* 131(1):79–87, 2013.
81. Chandrasekar I, Eis A, Konduri GG: Betamethasone attenuates oxidant stress in endothelial cells from fetal lambs with persistent pulmonary hypertension, *Pediatr Res* 63(1):67–72, 2008.
82. Konduri GG, Bakhutashvili I, Eis A, et al.: Antenatal betamethasone improves postnatal transition in late preterm lambs with persistent pulmonary hypertension of the newborn, *Pediatr Res* 73(5):621–629, 2013.
83. Kapur P, Holm BA, Irish MS, et al.: Lung physiological and metabolic changes in lambs with congenital diaphragmatic hernia after administration of prenatal maternal corticosteroids, *J Pediatr Surg* 34(2):354–356, 1999.

84. Davey MG, Danzer E, Schwarz U, et al.: Prenatal glucocorticoids and exogenous surfactant therapy improve respiratory function in lambs with severe diaphragmatic hernia following fetal tracheal occlusion, *Pediatr Res* 60(2):131–135, 2006.

85. Davey MG, Danzer E, Schwarz U, et al.: Prenatal glucocorticoids improve lung morphology and partially restores surfactant mRNA expression in lambs with diaphragmatic hernia undergoing fetal tracheal occlusion, *Pediatr Pulmonol* 41(12):1188–1196, 2006.

86. Paddock H, Beierle EA, Chen MK, et al.: Administration of prenatal betamethasone suppresses the adrenal-hypophyseal axis in newborns with congenital diaphragmatic hernia, *J Pediatr Surg* 39(8):1176–1182, 2004.

87. Lally KP, Bagolan P, Hosie S, et al.: Corticosteroids for fetuses with congenital diaphragmatic hernia: can we show benefit? *J Pediatr Surg* 41(4):668–674, 2006. discussion -74.

88. Konduri GG, Ou J, Shi Y, et al.: Decreased association of HSP90 impairs endothelial nitric oxide synthase in fetal lambs with persistent pulmonary hypertension, *Am J Physiol Heart Circ Physiol* 285(1):H204–H211, 2003.

89. Mata-Greenwood E, Jenkins C, Farrow KN, et al.: eNOS function is developmentally regulated: uncoupling of eNOS occurs postnatally, *Am J Physiol Lung Cell Mol Physiol* 290(2):L232–L241, 2006.

90. Konduri GG, Bakhutashvili I, Eis A, et al.: Oxidant stress from uncoupled nitric oxide synthase impairs vasodilation in fetal lambs with persistent pulmonary hypertension, *Am J Physiol Heart Circ Physiol* 292(4):H1812–H1820, 2007.

91. Beckman JS, Koppenol WH: Nitric oxide, superoxide, and peroxynitrite: the good, the bad, and ugly, *Am J Physiol* 271(5 Pt 1):C1424–C1437, 1996.

92. Lakshminrusimha S, Russell JA, Wedgwood S, et al.: Superoxide dismutase improves oxygenation and reduces oxidation in neonatal pulmonary hypertension, *Am J Respir Critic Care Med* 174(12):1370–1377, 2006.

93. Lakshminrusimha S, Steinhorn RH, Wedgwood S, et al.: Pulmonary hemodynamics and vascular reactivity in asphyxiated term lambs resuscitated with 21 and 100% oxygen, *J Appl Physiol (1985)* 111(5):1441–1447, 2011.

94. Van Meurs KP, Cohen TL, Yang G, et al.: Inhaled NO and markers of oxidant injury in infants with respiratory failure, *J Perinatol* 25(7):463–469, 2005.

95. Frid MG, Kale VA, Stenmark KR: Mature vascular endothelium can give rise to smooth muscle cells via endothelial-mesenchymal transdifferentiation: in vitro analysis, *Circ Res* 90(11):1189–1196, 2002.

96. Good RB, Gilbane AJ, Trinder SL, et al.: Endothelial to mesenchymal transition contributes to endothelial dysfunction in pulmonary arterial hypertension, *Am J Pathol* 185(7):1850–1858, 2015.

97. Stenmark KR, Fagan KA, Frid MG: Hypoxia-induced pulmonary vascular remodeling: cellular and molecular mechanisms, *Circ Res* 99(7):675–691, 2006.

98. Sheikh AQ, Misra A, Rosas IO, et al.: Smooth muscle cell progenitors are primed to muscularize in pulmonary hypertension, *Sci Transl Med* 7(308):308ra159, 2015.

99. Stenmark KR, Davie N, Frid M, et al.: Role of the adventitia in pulmonary vascular remodeling, *Physiology (Bethesda)* 21:134–145, 2006.

100. Moudgil R, Michelakis ED, Archer SL: Hypoxic pulmonary vasoconstriction, *J Appl Physiol* 98(1):390–403, 2005.

101. Mourani PM, Ivy DD, Gao D, et al.: Pulmonary vascular effects of inhaled nitric oxide and oxygen tension in bronchopulmonary dysplasia, *Am J Respir Critic Care Med* 170(9):1006–1013, 2004.

102. Rudolph AM, Yuan S: Response of the pulmonary vasculature to hypoxia and H+ ion concentration changes, *J Clinic Invest* 45(3):399–411, 1966.

103. Kato M, Staub NC: Response of small pulmonary arteries to unilobar hypoxia and hypercapnia, *Circ Res* 19(2):426–440, 1966.

104. Lakshminrusimha S, Konduri GG, Steinhorn RH: Considerations in the management of hypoxemic respiratory failure and persistent pulmonary hypertension in term and late preterm neonates, *J Perinatol* 36(Suppl 2):S12–S19, 2016.

105. Lakshminrusimha S, Swartz DD, Gugino SF, et al.: Oxygen concentration and pulmonary hemodynamics in newborn lambs with pulmonary hypertension, *Pediatr Res* 66(5):539–544, 2009.

106. Gitto E, Pellegrino S, Aversa S, et al.: Oxidative stress and persistent pulmonary hypertension of the newborn treated with inhaled nitric oxide and different oxygen concentrations, *J Matern Fetal Neonatal Med*, 2012.

107. Manja V, Saugstad OD, Lakshminrusimha S: Oxygen saturation targets in preterm infants and outcomes at 18-24 months: a systematic review, *Pediatrics* 139(1), 2017.

108. Walsh MC, Di Fiore JM, Martin RJ, et al.: Association of oxygen target and growth status with increased mortality in small for gestational age infants: further analysis of the surfactant, positive pressure and pulse oximetry randomized trial, *JAMA Pediatri* 170(3):292–294, 2016.

109. Lakshminrusimha S, Manja V, Steinhorn RH: Interaction of target oxygen saturation, bronchopulmonary dysplasia, and pulmonary hypertension in small for gestational age preterm neonates, *JAMA Pediatri*, 2016. in press.

110. Sanderud J, Norstein J, Saugstad OD: Reactive oxygen metabolites produce pulmonary vasoconstriction in young pigs, *Pediatr Res* 29(6):543–547, 1991.

111. Sanderud J, Bjoro K, Saugstad OD: Oxygen radicals stimulate thromboxane and prostacyclin synthesis and induce vasoconstriction in pig lungs, *Scand J Clinic Lab Invest* 53(5):447–455, 1993.

112. Sanderud J, Saugstad OD: Oxygen radicals induce pulmonary vasoconstriction in pigs without activating plasma proteolytic cascade systems, *Eur Surg Res* 25(3):137–145, 1993.

113. Belik J, Jankov RP, Pan J, et al.: Chronic O2 exposure in the newborn rat results in decreased pulmonary arterial nitric oxide release and altered smooth muscle response to isoprostane, *J Appl Physiol* 96(2):725–730, 2004.

114. Faraci FM, Didion SP: Vascular protection: superoxide dismutase isoforms in the vessel wall, *Arterioscler Thromb Vasc Biol* 24(8):1367–1373, 2004.

115. Farrow KN, Groh BS, Schumacker PT, et al.: Hyperoxia increases phosphodiesterase 5 expression and activity in ovine fetal pulmonary artery smooth muscle cells, *Circ Res* 102(2):226–233, 2008.

116. Farrow KN, Lakshminrusimha S, Reda WJ, et al.: Superoxide dismutase restores eNOS expression and function in resistance pulmonary arteries from neonatal lambs with persistent pulmonary hypertension, *Am J Physiol Lung Cell Mol Physiol* 295(6):L979–L987, 2008.

117. Lakshminrusimha S, Saugstad OD: The fetal circulation, pathophysiology of hypoxemic respiratory failure and pulmonary hypertension in neonates, and the role of oxygen therapy, *J Perinatol* 36(Suppl 2):S3–S11, 2016.

118. Sheehy AM, Burson MA, Black SM: Nitric oxide exposure inhibits endothelial NOS activity but not gene expression: a role for superoxide, *Am J Physiol* 274(5 Pt 1):L833–L841, 1998.

119. Black SM, Heidersbach RS, McMullan DM, et al.: Inhaled nitric oxide inhibits NOS activity in lambs: potential mechanism for rebound pulmonary hypertension, *Am J Physiol* 277(5 Pt 2):H1849–H1856, 1999.

120. Wedgwood S, Lakshminrusimha S, Farrow KN, et al.: Apocynin improves oxygenation and increases eNOS in persistent pulmonary hypertension of the newborn, *Am J Physiol Lung Cell Mol Physiol* 302(6):L616–L626, 2012.

121. Farrow KN, Lakshminrusimha S, Czech L, et al.: Superoxide dismutase and inhaled nitric oxide normalize phosphodiesterase 5 expression and activity in neonatal lambs with persistent pulmonary hypertension, *Am J Physiol Lung Cell Mol Physiol* 299(1):L109–L116, 2010.

122. Davis JM, Parad RB, Michele T, et al.: Pulmonary outcome at 1 year corrected age in premature infants treated at birth with recombinant human CuZn superoxide dismutase, *Pediatrics* 111(3):469–476, 2003.

123. Davis JM, Rosenfeld WN, Richter SE, et al.: Safety and pharmacokinetics of multiple doses of recombinant human CuZn superoxide dismutase administered intratracheally to premature neonates with respiratory distress syndrome, *Pediatrics* 100(1):24–30, 1997.

124. Chester M, Seedorf G, Tourneux P, et al.: Cinaciguat, a soluble guanylate cyclase activator, augments cGMP after oxidative stress and causes pulmonary vasodilation in neonatal pulmonary hypertension, *Am J Physiol Lung Cell Mol Physiol* 301(5):L755–L764, 2011.

125. Belik J: Riociguat, an oral soluble guanylate cyclase stimulator for the treatment of pulmonary hypertension, *Curr Opin Investig Drugs* 10(9):971–979, 2009.

126. Baquero H, Soliz A, Neira F, et al.: Oral sildenafil in infants with persistent pulmonary hypertension of the newborn: a pilot randomized blinded study, *Pediatrics* 117(4):1077–1083, 2006.

127. Steinhorn RH, Kinsella JP, Pierce C, et al.: Intravenous sildenafil in the treatment of neonates with persistent pulmonary hypertension, *J Pediatr* 155(6):841–847 e1, 2009.

128. Ladha F, Bonnet S, Eaton F, et al.: Sildenafil improves alveolar growth and pulmonary hypertension in hyperoxia-induced lung injury, *Am Journal of Respir Critic Care Med* 172(6):750–756, 2005.

129. Steinhorn RH, Kinsella JP, Abman SH: Beyond pulmonary hypertension: sildenafil for chronic lung disease of prematurity, *Am J Respir Cell Mol Biol* 48(2):iii–v, 2013.

130. Keller RL, Hamrick SE, Kitterman JA, et al.: Treatment of rebound and chronic pulmonary hypertension with oral sildenafil in an infant with congenital diaphragmatic hernia, *Pediatr Critic Care Med* 5(2):184–187, 2004.

131. Behrsin J, Cheung M, Patel N: Sildenafil weaning after discharge in infants with congenital diaphragmatic hernia, *Pediatr Cardiol* 34(8):1844–1847, 2013.

132. Zhang YH, Wang J, Zhu Y, et al.: Effectiveness of nitric oxide inhalation combined with oral sildenafil for the treatment of serious congenital diaphragmatic hernia, *Zhongguo Dang Dai Er Ke Za Zhi* 16(9):944–946, 2014.

133. Perez M, Wedgwood S, Lakshminrusimha S, et al.: Hydrocortisone normalizes phosphodiesterase-5 activity in pulmonary artery smooth muscle cells from lambs with persistent pulmonary hypertension of the newborn, *Pulm Circ* 4(1):71–81, 2014.

134. Perez M, Lakshminrusimha S, Wedgwood S, et al.: Hydrocortisone normalizes oxygenation and cGMP regulation in lambs with persistent pulmonary hypertension of the newborn, *Am J Physiol Lung Cell Mol Physiol*, 2011.

135. Murray F, MacLean MR, Pyne NJ: Increased expression of the cGMP-inhibited cAMP-specific (PDE3) and cGMP binding cGMP-specific (PDE5) phosphodiesterases in models of pulmonary hypertension, *Br J Pharmacol* 137(8):1187–1194, 2002.

136. Chen B, Lakshminrusimha S, Czech L, et al.: Regulation of phosphodiesterase 3 in the pulmonary arteries during the perinatal period in sheep, *Pediatr Res* 66(6):682–687, 2009.

137. McNamara PJ, Shivananda SP, Sahni M, et al.: Pharmacology of milrinone in neonates with persistent pulmonary hypertension of the newborn and suboptimal response to inhaled nitric oxide, *Pediatr Critic Care Med* 14(1):74–84, 2013.

138. Lakshminrusimha S, Porta NF, Farrow KN, et al.: Milrinone enhances relaxation to prostacyclin and iloprost in pulmonary arteries isolated from lambs with persistent pulmonary hypertension of the newborn, *Pediatr Critic Care Med* 10(1):106–112, 2009.

139. Rashid N, Morin 3rd FC, Swartz DD, et al.: Effects of prostacyclin and milrinone on pulmonary hemodynamics in newborn lambs with persistent pulmonary hypertension induced by ductal ligation, *Pediatr Res* 60(5):624–669, 2006.

140. Fike CD, Kaplowitz MR, Rehorst-Paea LA, et al.: L-Arginine increases nitric oxide production in isolated lungs of chronically hypoxic newborn pigs, *J Appl Physiol (1985)* 88(5):1797–1803, 2000.

141. Rouge C, Des Robert C, Robins A, et al.: Manipulation of citrulline availability in humans, *Am J Physiol Gastrointest Liver Physiol* 293(5):G1061–G1067, 2007.

142. Dikalova A, Fagiana A, Aschner JL, et al.: Sodium-coupled neutral amino acid transporter 1 (SNAT1) modulates L-citrulline transport and nitric oxide (NO) signaling in piglet pulmonary arterial endothelial cells, *PloS One* 9(1):e85730, 2014.

143. Parker TA, Roe G, Grover TR, et al.: Rho kinase activation maintains high pulmonary vascular resistance in the ovine fetal lung, *Am J Physiol Lung Cell Mol Physiol* 291(5):L976–L982, 2006.

144. Gien J, Seedorf GJ, Balasubramaniam V, et al.: Chronic intrauterine pulmonary hypertension increases endothelial cell Rho kinase activity and impairs angiogenesis in vitro, *Am J Physiol Lung Cell Mol Physiol* 295(4):L680–L687, 2008.

145. Odagiri K, Watanabe H: Effects of the Rho-kinase inhibitor, fasudil, on pulmonary hypertension, *Circ J* 79(6):1213–1214, 2015.

146. Liu P, Zhang HM, Tang YJ, et al.: Influence of Rho kinase inhibitor fasudil on late endothelial progenitor cells in peripheral blood of COPD patients with pulmonary artery hypertension, *Bratisl Lek Listy* 116(3):150–153, 2015.

147. Xiao JW, Zhu XY, Wang QG, et al.: Acute effects of Rho-kinase inhibitor fasudil on pulmonary arterial hypertension in patients with congenital heart defects, *Circ J* 79(6):1342–1348, 2015.

148. Jiang R, Ai ZS, Jiang X, et al.: Intravenous fasudil improves in-hospital mortality of patients with right heart failure in severe pulmonary hypertension, *Hypertens Res* 38(8):539–544, 2015.

149. O'Reilly M, Thebaud B: Cell-based therapies for neonatal lung disease, *Cell Tissue Res*, 2016.

150. Lee H, Lee JC, Kwon JH, et al.: The effect of umbilical cord blood derived mesenchymal stem cells in monocrotaline-induced pulmonary artery hypertension rats, *J Kor Med Sci* 30(5):576–585, 2015.

151. Baber SR, Deng W, Master RG, et al.: Intratracheal mesenchymal stem cell administration attenuates monocrotaline-induced pulmonary hypertension and endothelial dysfunction, *Am J Physiol Heart Circ Physiol* 292(2):H1120–H1128, 2007.

152. Katheria AC, Lakshminrusimha S, Rabe H, et al.: Placental transfusion: a review, *J Perinatol*, 2016.

153. Totapally B, Raju N, Perlman M: Decreased placental transfusion may lead to persistent pulmonary hypertension of the newborn (PPHN) - abstract PAS, *Pediatr Res* 43(S4):198, 1998.

8

CHAPTER 9

Pathophysiologically Based Management of Persistent Pulmonary Hypertension of the Newborn

Chandra Rath and Martin Kluckow

- The primary pathophysiologic event in persistent pulmonary hypertension of the newborn (PPHN) occurs when the pulmonary vascular resistance fails to appropriately decrease at birth.
- PPHN is made up of a number of underlying pathophysiological subgroups with the clinical presentation dependent on the emphasis of each of these elements.
- There are multiple treatment modalities available for PPHN and a logical treatment strategy requires an understanding of the underlying pathophysiology.
- Appropriate management will include care of the underlying condition, respiratory management, treatment of myocardial impairment, use of inotrope/vasopressors, and use of pulmonary vasodilators.
- Cardiac ultrasound is an important assessment tool, allowing understanding of the underlying physiology, targeting of treatment, documentation of response to treatment, and identification of when to wean therapy.

The primary pathophysiologic event in persistent pulmonary hypertension of the newborn (PPHN) occurs when the pulmonary vascular resistance (PVR) fails to appropriately decrease at birth. The resultant low oxygen saturation is poorly tolerated after birth and affected neonates may develop multi-organ dysfunction/failure because of hypoxemia. The clinical manifestations of raised pulmonary pressure will depend on the severity of pulmonary vasoconstriction, the presence and magnitude of, or absence of, shunting through the patent ductus arteriosus (PDA) and foramen ovale, the relative pressure/impedance at each end of the ductus arteriosus, the contractility and efficacy of each of the ventricles, and the presence of associated morbidities.

The severity of PPHN can run the full clinical spectrum from respiratory distress with mild hypoxemia to severe hypoxemia and cardiopulmonary instability necessitating advanced intensive care support. Treatment requirements vary according to the severity of the pathophysiology and the individual components of the condition. Consequently, a good understanding of the pathophysiology is essential to allow targeting of the many different treatment modalities available.

Pathophysiology, Hemodynamics and Treatment Targets

The primary underlying pathophysiological abnormality in PPHN is raised PVR or a failure of the normally high in utero pulmonary pressures to appropriately fall in the postnatal period. Initiating factors include hypoxemia and the associated metabolic acidosis in the perinatal and/or immediate postnatal period, as both of these conditions are potent pulmonary vasoconstrictors. The clinical manifestations of raised PVR will depend on other factors including whether the fetal shunts are patent, the status of left and right ventricular function, the systemic blood pressure, the additional impact of mechanical ventilation on pulmonary blood flow, and the volume status. In many cases there will be sustained or advancing hypoxemia, ventilation perfusion (VQ) mismatch, and acidosis, which contribute to, or further enhance, the increased PVR. In addition, high PVR in association with mechanical ventilation can impair oxygenation and reduce the preload to the left ventricle, resulting in inadequate left ventricular function, and reduced systemic perfusion. Finally, sustained mild/moderate in utero hypoxia may result in remodeling of the pulmonary vasculature with smooth muscle cell migration into the more distal pulmonary vessels, making the condition, at least initially, less responsive to the administration of pulmonary vasodilators.

Understanding the contribution of the individual pathophysiological elements potentially allows a more targeted approach to care. For example, if the presentation is due to asphyxia with associated myocardial impairment, in addition to administering pulmonary vasodilators, cautious volume administration, early institution of inotropic support and optimization of ventilation to improve cardiorespiratory function are priorities. Alternatively, if the patient presents with open fetal channels with right to left shunting and adequate myocardial function, using pulmonary vasodilators and careful supportive care may be most useful.

In PPHN, there are generally two treatment targets: relaxation of the pulmonary vasculature, and addressing myocardial dysfunction and the abnormalities of peripheral vascular regulation. The hemodynamic derangements are most frequently secondary to increased pulmonary vascular pressure and, if present, to myocardial dysfunction. The use of drugs with inotropic, vasopressor, and/or lusitropic effects may alter the hemodynamic presentation during management. Therefore, it is imperative to understand the cardiovascular disturbances in PPHN in order to identify and address them in a timely manner. Following the performance of an echocardiographic study to rule out congenital heart disease, repeated bedside cardiac ultrasound examinations by the neonatologist caring for the patient play an indispensable role in recognizing the underlying elements of PPHN, and in assessing the hemodynamic response to treatment. Severe pulmonary hypertension increases right ventricular afterload, which may result in right ventricular failure unless the right ventricle can offload via a nonrestricting PDA. In addition, the elevated right ventricular pressure often causes right-to-left shunting through the patent foramen ovale (PFO) as well, and right-to-left shunting through both fetal channels worsens hypoxemia. Because of a high degree of interdependence between the right and the left ventricles, changes in right ventricle size and geometry often impacts left ventricular geometry and function. Thus, in addition to decreased left ventricular preload, compromised left ventricular geometry and function contribute to lower systemic blood pressure and low cardiac output necessitating the use of cardiovascular support.

Understanding the role of the PDA in this setting is of great importance. Increased right-to-left shunting through the PDA worsens the hypoxemia and acidosis in the organs supplied by the post-ductal circulation, which in turn results in further pulmonary vasoconstriction. On the other hand, shunting through the fetal channels may support cardiac output and maintain cerebral perfusion when the preload to the left heart is severely compromised. Finally, right ventricle failure can occur when the ductus arteriosus is closed or restricted, and re-opening of the ductus arteriosus with prostaglandins can be a life-saving immediate supportive measure in these cases.

The hemodynamic presentation in PPHN is complex and variable as it is affected by cardiovascular, pulmonary, and other factors, as well as by the treatment and the individual patient's response. Understanding these factors, their interdependence, and their impact on treatment is of great importance and likely affects patient outcomes. Therefore, the clinician needs access to reliable, longitudinal bedside information on the cardiorespiratory status and the hemodynamic changes during the course of the disease in each patient. The use of point-of-care ultrasound (POCU) significantly improves the clinician's ability to obtain the required information (see Chapter 10). By using POCU, the physician will have an understanding of the hemodynamic status of each infant and the response to treatment rather than only relying on standardized algorithms for management of these often critically ill neonates.

Principles of Management of Persistent Pulmonary Hypertension of the Newborn

The primary therapeutic goals are to lower the PVR while supporting the cardiovascular and respiratory function. Management of PPHN is accomplished by utilizing a careful, stepwise approach with progressive escalation of treatment if necessary. Some infants who present with mild clinical features of PPHN are candidates for close observation initially with careful, comprehensive cardiorespiratory monitoring, as the presentation may evolve into a more severe form of PPHN. The overall approach focuses on normalizing the cardiopulmonary adaptation while avoiding/minimizing lung injury and the potential adverse effects of ventilator support on the systemic perfusion. Variations in severity, and thus the clinical presentation of PPHN, result in a wide range of variation in management of PPHN in clinical practice.[1,2]

Supportive Care

When PPHN is associated with parenchymal lung disease or systemic illness, the treatment should also target the accompanying morbidities. Exposure to environmental factors, like noxious stimuli, tracheal suctioning, heel pricks, and excessive noise may augment pulmonary vasoconstriction and increase the frequency and severity of hypoxemic episodes, the hallmarks of unstable pulmonary vasoregulation. Maintenance of normothermia and correction of metabolic, electrolyte, and hematologic abnormalities (e.g., acidosis, hypoglycemia, hypocalcemia, and polycythemia) are clearly of importance. However, pH, partial pressure of O_2 (PaO$_2$), and CO_2 (PaCO$_2$) are to be kept in the normal range as overcorrection of these parameters may be more harmful than beneficial.

Sedation, usually with opioids and benzodiazepines, is widely used to minimize fluctuation in oxygenation and to facilitate ventilation, but it is not evidence-based nor is it without side effects. In addition to the potential for the development of systemic hypotension, generalized edema, reduced cerebral blood flow, and deterioration of lung function with the prolonged use of sedation, the usefulness of sedative agents in the setting of PPHN has not been subjected to well-designed studies. Therefore, sedation should be used with appropriate caution in neonates with PPHN. Neuromuscular blockade has also been commonly used as an adjunctive therapy to limit fluctuations of oxygenation due to patient interference with mechanical ventilation. Commencement of muscle relaxation can suddenly change preload and afterload, resulting in rapid cardiovascular changes. If an infant is dependent on systemic blood pressure to limit right-to-left ductal shunting, this can cause a sudden decrease in oxygen saturation. Of note is that the use of neuromuscular blockers has been linked to an increased incidence of hearing impairment in survivors of PPHN; however, the mechanism of this association is unclear.[3] According to studies performed before the routine use of inhaled nitric oxide (iNO), this treatment was also associated with increased mortality.[4] Short-term administration of neuromuscular blockers may be considered in infants with severe and unstable clinical presentation of PPHN despite the appropriate use of sedation. Finally, neuromuscular blockers should never be administered without provision of appropriate sedation.

Mechanical Ventilation and Surfactant

Many infants with severe PPHN require invasive ventilatory support. The primary goal of mechanical ventilation is to ensure adequate lung inflation and thus enhance the effectiveness of inhaled vasodilators (oxygen and iNO). Indeed, in patients with significant parenchymal lung disease, administration of inhaled pulmonary vasodilators without lung recruitment results in a suboptimal vasodilatory effect.[5] In addition, as parenchymal lung significantly contributes to hypoxia in PPHN, appropriate ventilator management is clearly warranted.[6] However, the use of inappropriately high mean airway pressure, especially after surfactant administration, can reduce cardiac output and therefore worsen hypoxia. Consequently, a role for noninvasive ventilation in the management of PPHN in neonates with less severe presentation has been suggested and the advent of the possibility of delivering iNO noninvasively has further facilitated this strategy.[7] The incidence of lung disease associated with PPHN has changed over the years. The overall incidence of meconium aspiration syndrome has declined, coinciding with a decrease in the number of post-term pregnancies.[8,9] In contrast, respiratory distress syndrome (RDS) in late preterm neonates delivered by elective or indicated Cesarean section at 34 to 36 weeks of gestation and pneumonia/sepsis have become more frequent preludes to PPHN.

Vasodilator Therapy in Persistent Pulmonary Hypertension of the Newborn

Oxygen and Carbon Dioxide

The primary goal of PPHN treatment is to improve oxygen delivery to the tissues and decrease PVR by selective pulmonary vasodilation without compromising systemic hemodynamics. Oxygen itself can potentially help achieve both these goals. However, oxygen is a toxin at higher doses, and it may be harmful when administered in excess. Oxygen is a potent and selective pulmonary vasodilator; thus increased oxygen tension results in a reduction of PVR. Among other effects, O_2 stimulates endothelial NO synthase and NO production and contributes to pulmonary vasodilatation at birth.[10] However exposure to hyperoxia results in the formation of oxygen free radicals, such as peroxides, superoxide, hydroxyl radical, and singlet oxygen, which all can cause lung injury.[11,12]

In animal studies, an arterial PaO_2 of less than 45 to 50 mm Hg results in increased PVR in newborn calves and lambs. In contrast, maintaining PaO_2 greater than 70 to 80 mm Hg does not result in any additional decrease in PVR in both control lambs and lambs with PPHN.[12,13] In lambs with PPHN, PVR increases substantially in severe hypoxemia with a PaO_2 of less than 13.9 mm Hg, whereas vascular resistance declines more gradually at PaO_2 levels greater than 59.6 mm Hg. Similarly, PVR increases below an oxygen saturation of 85%. Therefore, a pre-ductal PaO_2 of 60 to 80 mm Hg and a pre-ductal oxygen saturation of 90% to 97% would seem to be reasonable targets during the treatment of neonates with PPHN.

Carbon-dioxide-related changes to the pulmonary vascular tone differ between the normal and injured lung, and they also vary depending on pulmonary pressures and the presence of endogenous NO. Of importance, the effect of hypoxia on the pulmonary vasculature is more pronounced than any effect of pH and/or CO_2.[14] It is also important to consider the acid-base status in the context of O_2 administration and its effect on pulmonary vessels. Animal studies have shown that lower pH exaggerates the vasoconstrictive response of the pulmonary vessels to hypoxia. Accordingly, the acceptable PaO_2 range devoid of the hypoxic pulmonary vasoconstrictor response, is not absolute, as it is affected by the acid-base status. Therefore, avoiding acidosis offers some protection against pulmonary vasoconstriction in response to hypoxia.[15]

In a stepwise approach to the management of PPHN, the optimization of O_2 administration and appropriate ventilation to target SpO_2 and CO_2 levels to maximize pulmonary vasodilation is the first step preceding the initiation of more lung-specific therapies, such as surfactant and iNO administration. POCU allows identification of infants who have early evidence of elevated pulmonary pressure and cardiac dysfunction, flagging those who should have blood gases and O_2 saturation carefully monitored, and in whom avoidance of sudden decreases in O_2 saturation and/or hypercapnia encourages normalization of circulatory transition.

Inhaled Nitric Oxide

NO is a potent endothelium-derived factor that has diverse effects on the pulmonary circulation, including vasodilation, pro-angiogenic, anti-inflammatory, and anti-oxidant properties.[16] Treatment with iNO is one of the cornerstones of PPHN management. Inhaled NO reaches the alveolar space and diffuses into the vascular smooth muscle of the adjacent pulmonary arteries, where it causes a cyclic guanosine monophosphate (cGMP)-mediated vasodilation. In the pulmonary arteries, it is rapidly bound to hemoglobin, restricting its effect to the pulmonary circulation, without any clinically relevant effect on the systemic circulation. Inhaled NO is preferentially distributed to the ventilated segments of the lungs underscoring the importance of optimal lung recruitment prior to the initiation of iNO administration. Accordingly, iNO administration results in an improved ventilation/perfusion ratio, decreased intra-alveolar shunting and improved oxygenation. Infants who have evidence of raised PVR with decreased pulmonary blood flow and an open PDA with predominantly right-to-left shunting are most likely to have a dramatic response to iNO. Importantly, infants with low systemic blood pressure, often with accompanying myocardial impairment and a significant respiratory component contributing to the increased FiO_2 requirements, are less likely to respond well to iNO, and require more extensive cardiovascular and respiratory support.

The role of iNO in term and near-term infants with oxygenation failure is well known. Although iNO reduces the need for extracorporeal membrane oxygenation (ECMO), mortality without the use of ECMO is not reduced.[17] Oxygenation improves in approximately 50% of infants receiving iNO and the response is dependent on the underlying pathophysiology of the particular infant. Targeting iNO to infants with responsive physiology will significantly increase the response rate. If a patient responds, the oxygenation index (OI) decreases within 30 to 60 minutes after commencing therapy and PaO_2 rapidly increases. The apparent lack of benefit of iNO on the survival of term neonates with PPHN is most likely due to the fact that term neonates would not be allowed to die of hypoxic respiratory failure without a trial of ECMO in developed countries where these trials were conducted. ECMO is very effective in reducing mortality in term infants with PPHN.[17]

Early Introduction of Inhaled Nitric Oxide in Persistent Pulmonary Hypertension of the Newborn Management

The severity of PPHN is commonly assessed by calculating the OI, which reflects a combination of the ventilator support applied and oxygenation.

$$OI = MAP \times FiO_2 \times 100/PaO_2$$

(*MAP*, Mean airway pressure; *FiO$_2$*, fraction of Inspired O_2; *PaO$_2$*, partial pressure of O_2)

Hypoxemic respiratory failure has been classified as mild (OI $\leq$ 15), moderate (OI > 15 to 25), severe (OI > 25 to 40) and very severe (OI > 40).[18] Introduction of iNO therapy at a lower OI and thus usually earlier in the course of the disease may be beneficial in the management of PPHN. Initiating therapy before alveolar atelectasis from lung disease or ventilator-induced barotrauma or O_2 toxicity occurs, could potentially lessen lung injury with a consequent reduction in the duration of respiratory support and/or length of hospital stay. However, it should be emphasized that adequate alveolar recruitment is a prerequisite for effective iNO delivery as the response to iNO in PPHN is more effective when lung recruitment is optimal.[5] The initial notion that starting iNO for respiratory failure in the earlier stages of disease evolution (targeted to an OI of 15 to 25) does not decrease the incidence of ECMO or death or improve other patient outcomes has been changing with the addition of the findings from more recent studies. In most of the initial studies of iNO use, ECMO, in combination with mortality, served as a primary composite endpoint.[17] As noted earlier, iNO significantly decreases the need for ECMO support in newborns with PPHN. However, data indicate that up to 40% of infants do not improve oxygenation or maintain a response to iNO. There are two schools of thought pertaining to this issue. One suggests that early iNO does not decrease the incidence of death or the need for ECMO or improve other patient outcomes. The other group hypothesizes that the relatively poor response is likely due to the "early" introduction of iNO to patients with prior lung damage secondary to iatrogenic hyperoxia and ventilation. An alternative explanation is that clinicians are not targeting therapies to the appropriate pathophysiological targets. In this case, gaining more relevant information from investigations using real-time cardiorespiratory monitoring (see Chapter 21) and cardiac ultrasound (see Chapter 10) could improve targeting. Few of the recent studies have addressed this question. Yet the field of precision or personalized medicine, targeting individual patient characteristics, is rapidly expanding (see Chapter 21).[19]

On the basis of available evidence, a recent systematic review has concluded that it appears reasonable to use iNO at an initial concentration of 20 ppm for term and near-term infants with hypoxic respiratory failure who do not have a diaphragmatic hernia.[20] Due to the rapid onset of action of iNO, a response, if present, can be seen quickly (within 1 hour). Evidence is lacking for the benefit of continuing iNO therapy in patients who do not respond with improved oxygenation. In selected cases, the use of noninvasive ventilation might be a good option to decrease ventilator-associated lung injury. Indeed, there have been case reports and case series describing iNO delivered through continuous positive airway pressure to newborn infants as part of a treatment strategy without adverse effects.[7,21-24]

Role of Inhaled Nitric Oxide in Preterm Oxygenation Failure

The role of iNO in the management of hypoxic respiratory failure in preterm neonates is less straight forward. In preterm neonates, an increased pulmonary arterial pressure may be associated with pneumonia, RDS, bronchopulmonary dysplasia (BPD), premature prolonged rupture of membranes (PPROM), and oligohydramnios-associated pulmonary hypoplasia.[25-28] Addressing the basic etiology is often the first step in selecting the most appropriate management strategy of preterm hypoxic failure. Furthermore, preterm neonates are at much higher risk of complications such as BPD, peri/intraventricular hemorrhage (P/IVH), and long-term neurodevelopment abnormalities. In addition to selective pulmonary vasodilatation, many studies have found that iNO might decrease lung inflammation, reduce oxidant stress, and enhance alveolarization and lung growth.[16] Most of the trials of iNO undertaken in the preterm population have been focused on preterm hypoxic respiratory failure with ventilator dependence. In these trials, very few infants had documentation of cardiac ultrasound findings pretreatment, so the incidence of the potentially responsive pathophysiology of raised pulmonary pressures and right-to-left ductal shunt is unknown. There have been at least 16 randomized control trials (RCTs) evaluating the role of iNO in prevention of BPD. However, a Cochrane meta-analysis concluded that iNO as rescue therapy for the preterm infant does not appear to be effective.[29] In addition, early routine use of iNO in preterm infants with respiratory disease does not affect serious brain injury or improve survival without BPD.[30] Importantly in the systematic review, there is no clear effect of iNO on the frequency of all grades of P/IVH or of severe P/IVH, nor was there any effect on the incidence of neurodevelopmental impairment found. The initial concerns of P/IVH and poor neurodevelopmental outcome associated with iNO administration to preterm infants appear to be unfounded.[31]

The focus in preterm infants has been on the role of iNO in BPD prevention.[29] However, there is a subset of preterm infants who present with raised PVR that might benefit from iNO. This subset includes preterm neonates in whom the presentation of PPHN is associated with PPROM, oligohydramnios, and presumed pulmonary hypoplasia. As this is a relatively rare condition, only a few case series, small studies, and retrospective data analyses have been published. In many of these studies, a favorable response to iNO therapy in preterm infants born after PPROM and oligohydramnios has been reported.[32-34] In the most recent case series, infants with a history of PPROM, pulmonary hypoplasia, and PPHN who were treated with iNO had a survival rate of 86%.[35]

Specific cardiac ultrasound markers, such as pure right-to-left shunting at ductal level or a low left pulmonary artery blood flow velocity, may allow prediction of iNO response in the preterm infant[36] and it is important to identify the target preterm population who may benefit from iNO treatment[37] It seems that preterm infants with elevated PVR, decreased pulmonary blood flow (diagnosed by reduced left pulmonary artery velocity on cardiac ultrasound), and an open PDA with predominantly right-to-left flow are most likely to have a dramatic response to iNO.

Weaning Inhaled Nitric Oxide

Identifying the right time to wean iNO is crucial to reduce unnecessary exposure to a treatment with potential side effects in unresponsive infants. Identifying the optimal time to wean iNO in the clinical setting can be challenging as FiO_2 requirement and SpO_2/pCO_2 lability can persist, even though the underlying pathophysiology has changed. Waiting for a clear clinical improvement may take several days. Once the PVR has reduced and, in particular, once the lability of an open PDA with changing proportions of right-to-left shunt has resolved, it is our experience that iNO may be weaned. Longitudinal cardiac ultrasound assessment (1 to 2 times daily) allows tracking of hemodynamic improvement and often helps identify the time to commence weaning iNO administration and, if the patient remains stable, hemodynamic support. This may be as early as 24 to 48 hours after commencing therapy.

However, rebound vasoconstriction following abrupt withdrawal of iNO is a real concern, and weaning iNO from 20 ppm gradually over a period of time before its discontinuation has been shown to be a safer approach that minimizes the chance of occurrence of the rebound effect.[38,39] Of note is that, even in infants who show no response to iNO, sudden discontinuation of the gas can precipitate pulmonary vasoconstriction and rapid deterioration.[40] Secondary analysis of a large blinded study reported that decreases in PaO_2 were observed only at the final step of withdrawal around iNO discontinuation.[41] iNO reduction should be started when PaO_2 is above 60 mm Hg or when the OI is less than 10. A reduction to 1 ppm before discontinuation seems to minimize rebound hypoxemia. In one study it was reported that withdrawing iNO in nonresponders did not result in rebound hypoxemia when NO exposure was limited to 30 minutes.[42] This finding supports the approach to discontinue iNO following a very short trial in nonresponders.[42]

Other Pulmonary/Systemic Vasodilators

Administration of O_2 at appropriate concentrations, normalization of the acid-base status, and administering iNO are the mainstays of vasodilator therapy in infants with PPHN. However, about one third of cases fail to respond to iNO or only have a transient treatment effect. In addition, there are many centers, particularly in the developing world, who do not have access to iNO. Fortunately, there are a number of adjunct and/or alternate pulmonary vasodilator options available. However, their efficacy and safety have not been tested in large randomized trials comparable to those with iNO, nor have the long-term outcomes been carefully examined. Moreover, as some of these vasodilatory agents also have systemic effects, systemic hypotension might occur and can worsen right-to-left shunting and tissue O_2 delivery in some clinical settings.

Phosphodiesterase-5 Inhibitors

Endogenous NO stimulates cGMP generation in the smooth muscle cells of the pulmonary vessels, which leads to the relaxation of the smooth muscle. In addition, iNO-induced direct activation of K^+ channels and modulation of angiotensin II receptor expression and activity contribute to the pulmonary vasodilatory effects of iNO. cGMP is primarily metabolized by phosphodiesterase-5 (PDE-5), an enzyme also expressed in the vessels of the lungs, and its downregulation enhances NO-mediated vascular relaxation during normal pulmonary vascular transition after birth.[43] Thus, inhibition of PDE-5 will increase cGMP concentrations in pulmonary smooth muscle cells and facilitate endogenous or iNO-induced vasodilatation in the pulmonary vasculature. In addition, PDE-5 inhibition may also result in a decrement in medial muscular hypertrophy in neonates with exposure to intra-uterine hypoxia and remodeled pulmonary vasculature. Sildenafil, vardenafil, and tadalafil belong to the class of PDE-5 inhibitors, with sildenafil being the most widely studied drug of this class in neonatal pulmonary hypertension.

Based on the available evidence, the use of sildenafil has several potential indications in neonatal intensive care. It can be used as an acute adjuvant to iNO, given in iNO-resistant PPHN, or to facilitate weaning of iNO. Sildenafil can also be used as a primary drug in the treatment of PPHN if iNO is not available or is contraindicated. Furthermore, it may be used for chronic treatment of pulmonary hypertension in conditions, such as BPD or congenital diaphragmatic hernia (CDH).[44]

Sildenafil maybe given enterally or intravenously[45] usually without clinically significant side effects. However, the development of systemic hypotension is a potential problem, especially if a loading dose is used and it is administered over less than 30 minutes. Administration of sildenafil in combination with iNO was also not associated with a significant decrease in systemic blood pressure and it improved oxygenation. In two recently published studies, there were also no significant adverse events.[46,47]

Phosphodiesterase-3 Inhibitors

Another class of vasodilators are the phosphodiesterase-3 (PDE-3) inhibitors such as milrinone which act by inhibiting the breakdown of cyclic adenosine monophosphate (cAMP). Milrinone plays two important roles in the context of PPHN management. First, via its inotropic and lusitropic effects, it has a role in improving ventricular function. Second, by increasing the concentration of cAMP in both pulmonary arterial smooth muscle cells and cardiomyocytes, it improves ventricular diastolic function and induces further pulmonary vasodilation. PDE-3 expression and activity increase dramatically in spontaneously breathing lambs by 24 hours after birth.[48] Accordingly, milrinone may not be as effective as a pulmonary vasodilator or an inotrope immediately after birth, but it may be increasingly useful after the first postnatal day. Ventilation with 21% O_2 or 100% O_2 attenuates the postnatal upregulation of PDE-3, while exposure to iNO plus 100% O_2 markedly increases PDE-3 expression.[48] Therefore, milrinone may be a potentially useful adjunct treatment modality when iNO and high O_2 concentrations are used in neonates with PPHN.

Based on animal, and human pediatric, adult, and scarce neonatal data, there are several clinical situations where milrinone may particularly be of use in the management of neonatal PPHN. When perinatal asphyxia- or sepsis-associated PPHN presents with ventricular dysfunction and high pulmonary venous pressure, there may be a left-to-right shunt through the PFO instead of the expected bidirectional or right-to-left shunt characteristic of pulmonary arterial hypertension. In this situation, milrinone may have a definite, even preferred role, as iNO may worsen the hemodynamic presentation by dilating the pulmonary vasculature and thus aggravating the myocardial dysfunction-associated pulmonary venous congestion. As mentioned earlier, milrinone also may be used as an adjuvant to iNO especially in infants only partially responsive to iNO. Similarly, milrinone may have a role in iNO-unresponsive PPHN. Indeed, there have been several case series in term neonates with iNO-refractory PPHN demonstrating effectiveness of milrinone in reducing the pulmonary pressure.[49-51] In addition, a retrospective case review reported improved myocardial performance and pulmonary hypertension after treatment with milrinone in less than 32 weeks' gestation preterm neonates.[52]

A loading dose of 50 mcg/kg over 30 to 60 minutes followed by a maintenance dose of 0.33 mcg/kg/min and escalated to 0.66 and then to 1 mcg/kg/min based on response, is commonly used. However, the loading dose is not recommended in the presence of systemic hypotension or prematurity; therefore, in some centers milrinone is used without a loading dose in all patients.[53] There have been reports of systemic hypotension after milrinone use in the adult intensive care unit. In a recent retrospective data analysis, the authors identified 322 neonates who were exposed to milrinone in their study period of 13 years and reported 40% of the infants experienced clinical or laboratory adverse effects. Surprisingly PPHN (40%) was the most commonly reported diagnosis at the start of milrinone administration. Hypotension requiring vasopressors (20%) and PDA requiring treatment (13%) were the most commonly reported clinical adverse events during milrinone therapy.[54]

Prostaglandins

Prostaglandin-E1 (PGE1) is usually used as a bridging therapy to keep the ductus arteriosus patent in neonates with duct-dependent congenital cardiac conditions before undertaking corrective surgical therapy. A study in near-term and term infants with PPHN found that the ductus arteriosus was patent in 72% of the infants compared to 34% in the control group without PPHN.[53] The PDA functions as a pressure pop-off valve to release the high right ventricular pressure from raised PVR, thereby improving overall cardiac function and alleviating the need for PGE1 infusion in many infants.[55] By augmenting endogenous production of cAMP, PGE1 also causes nonselective pulmonary vasodilatation. Although one group of investigators[55] reported encouraging results with the use of PGE1 in two small pilot trials, PGE1 use is generally recommended in infants with PPHN with a closed duct and evidence of right ventricular dysfunction as an adjunctive treatment to O_2 and iNO and the other pulmonary vasodilators discussed earlier.

Prostacyclin (PGI2) is another endogenously produced arachidonic acid metabolite that also causes vasodilatation via the cAMP pathway. PGI2 production appears to increase in late gestation and early postnatal life, suggestive of its involvement in promoting neonatal pulmonary vascular dilatation at birth.[56,57] In neonates and children with PPHN there is a decrease in the biosynthesis of PGI2 accompanied by increased synthesis of the vasoconstrictor thromboxane-A2.[58] PGI2 vasodilates both the pulmonary and systemic vascular bed. However, PGI2 mostly induces vasodilation in the pulmonary venous system and thus its use may result in pulmonary congestion and edema formation. Intravenous PGI2 is one of the more commonly used therapies in adult pulmonary hypertension management. However, there have been only case series and case reports pertaining to newborn intravenous PGI2 use. Although it might be beneficial in the management of PPHN, systemic hypotension has been reported in almost all the case series and reports, significantly limiting its use in acute pulmonary hypertension.[59] Investigators have used PGI2 by inhalation with some success both in term and preterm neonates.[60-63] Because of its very short half-life (~6 minutes), epoprostenol must be administered continuously and unplanned interruptions in drug delivery may rapidly lead to rebound pulmonary hypertension. Inhaled Iloprost, a stable PGI2 analogue, has been used successfully in preterm and term infants with both idiopathic PPHN and BPD- and CDH-associated PPHN without major side effects. However, the studies are mainly case series or case reports and thus the findings must be viewed with caution.[64-69]

Endothelin Receptor Antagonists

Endothelin-1 (ET-1), synthesized by the vascular endothelial cells, is a potent vasoconstrictor and acts through two receptors (ETA and ETB). ETA primarily mediates vasoconstriction while ETB promotes vasodilation mediated by endothelium-derived NO. Elevated plasma ET-1 levels are observed in infants with CDH and PPHN, and they have been used as a marker of disease severity and poor prognosis.[70,71] Endothelin receptor antagonists are categorized according to their selectivity for ETA or ETB receptors. Bosentan is a nonselective ET receptor antagonist and has been principally used to treat pulmonary hypertension in adults. There have also been case reports and case series on the use of bosentan in the management of pediatric pulmonary hypertension. Use of bosentan as a stand-alone therapy or an adjuvant to iNO and sildenafil in term and preterm neonates with pulmonary hypertension has also been reported.[72-74] In an RCT in term and near-term neonates with PPHN[74a] and an OI of greater than 40, bosentan, at an enteral dose of 1 mg/kg twice a day induced significant improvement in the OI and SpO_2 in the majority (87.5%) of the neonates within 6 hours after initiation of treatment. There was no rebound hypoxemia after drug discontinuation, and the duration of mechanical ventilation was decreased. At the 6-month follow-up evaluation, major sequelae, including neurological sequelae, were significantly lower in infants treated with bosentan compared to the controls. However, in another recent, although smaller RCT of oral bosentan given at a dose of 2 mg/kg twice daily as an adjunctive therapy to iNO in neonates with PPHN and respiratory failure, there were no clinical benefits.[75] Thus, due to the limited neonatal data, routine use of bosentan cannot be recommended, although the drug may have a role in the management of PPHN not responding to conventional vasodilators, optimized ventilation, and supportive therapy.

Magnesium Sulfate

Magnesium sulfate ($MgSO_4$) is a nonselective vasodilator and acts by antagonizing the entry of calcium ions into the smooth muscle cells. Beside its vasodilatory properties, magnesium has other effects including sedation, muscle relaxation, bronchodilation, and neuroprotection, which might make it potentially useful in certain presentations of PPHN.

The role of $MgSO_4$ in newborn PPHN has never been tested in an RCT trial. There have been small case studies in term and preterm neonates with some positive results[76-80] In the absence of safety data and RCTs, $MgSO_4$ should be a last line of therapy when other effective pulmonary vasodilator-treatment and ECMO support are not available.

Utilizing Pathophysiology to Guide the Use of Vasodilators in Persistent Pulmonary Hypertension of the Newborn

As discussed, there are several vasodilators available in addition to O_2 and iNO. The key advantage of iNO is its ability to be delivered via gaseous inhalation, thus allowing optimization of VQ matching by primarily delivering the vasodilatory effect to aerated lung fields. As iNO is rapidly deactivated by hemoglobin in the blood, there is little systemic vasodilation with an associated drop in systemic blood pressure. As for the other vasodilators, the actual clinical and hemodynamic scenario can serve as guidance when deciding what medication(s) and when to use. For instance, without appreciation of the underlying pathophysiology, commencement of a nonspecific vasodilator may result in the development of systemic hypotension and worsening hypoxemia. Furthermore, in infants presenting with a wide-open ductus arteriosus and predominant right-to-left shunting, good right ventricular function, and indirect evidence of relative systemic vasoconstriction, perfusion and oxygenation may worsen when a medication with a systemic vasodilatory effect, such as milrinone, systemic PGI2, or $MgSO_4$, is added. On the other hand, infants with a small and/or constricting ductus arteriosus, predominantly left-to-right ductal shunting and an "obstructed" right ventricle with reduced right ventricular function may benefit from a drug with both inotropic effect and vasodilatory effect, such as milrinone. Indeed, with this latter hemodynamic presentation, the infant is less likely to develop worsening oxygenation if systemic blood pressure decreases (up to a certain point) with the introduction of a vasodilator/lusitropic agent.

Vasopressor Therapy in Persistent Pulmonary Hypertension of the Newborn

Pulmonary vasoconstriction is the pathophysiological pivot in PPHN, which results in hypoxic respiratory failure by causing severe ventilation-perfusion mismatch even if there is no parenchymal pathology. Other secondary hemodynamic compromises are not absolute but often accompany pulmonary vasoconstriction. The hemodynamics and potential pathophysiological targets have been discussed earlier and are depicted in Figs. 9.1 and 9.2 and discussed further in Chapters 26, 27 and 29 when PPHN is a comorbidity in patients with different primary conditions.

Right ventricular and/or left ventricular dysfunction is an important pathophysiological aspect of PPHN—yet it is not a constant feature. In a retrospective study, around two thirds of infants with PPHN had evidence of low ventricular output.[55,81-83] Of note is that, when the preload to the left ventricle is decreased due to severe pulmonary vasoconstriction-associated decreases in pulmonary blood flow, cardiac output will be compromised even in the presence of normal ventricle function. As with

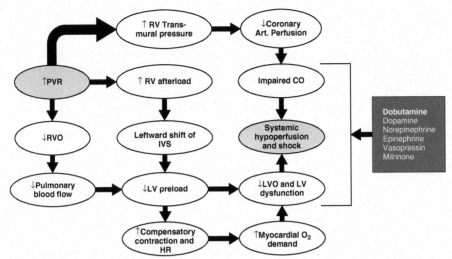

Fig. 9.1 Increased pulmonary vascular resistance plays a direct role in biventricular cardiac failure. Judicious use of cardiovascular agents (inotropes, vasopressors, vasopressor-inotropes, lusitropes) has been recommended in specific clinical situations. *Square box* shows the potential drugs that can be used to improve cardiac function. *CO*, Cardiac output; *HR*, heart rate; *IVS*, interventricular septum; *LV*, left ventricle; *LVO*, left ventricular output; *PVR*, pulmonary vascular resistance; *RV*, right ventricle; *RVO*, right ventricular output.

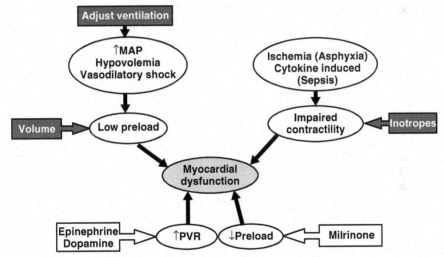

Fig. 9.2 Cardiac compromise due to causes other than a primary increase in pulmonary vascular resistance *(PVR)*. Judicious use of fluid, ventilation, and cardiovascular agents tailored to the specific clinical situation has been recommended *(colored boxes)*. Note that some treatment choices may result in myocardial dysfunction in some circumstances *(white boxes)*. *MAP*, Mean airway pressure.

other aspects of PPHN therapy, inotropic treatment (dobutamine) and vasopressor-inotrope use (dopamine, epinephrine, norepinephrine)[84] need to be individualized depending on the underlying hemodynamic physiology (Table 9.1).

   There are two additional vasopressor agents with a dose-dependent and presumably selective pulmonary vasodilatory action.

1. *Norepinephrine* has been proposed as a potentially effective vasopressor-inotrope due to its dose-dependent pulmonary vasodilatory action.[85] After starting norepinephrine and despite a rise in both pulmonary artery pressure (PAP) and systemic artery pressure (SAP), the PAP/SAP ratio and oxygen requirement decreased.[85] In addition, in a recent retrospective cohort study in preterm infants with cardiovascular compromise, where 23% of the patients also presented with pulmonary hypertension, normotension and improved systemic oxygenation were achieved in all but one infant at a median dose of 0.5 mcg/kg/min within a median of 1 hour.[86]

Table 9.1 CARDIOVASCULAR SUPPORTIVE MEDICATIONS, THEIR MECHANISM(S) OF ACTION, AND THE POSSIBLE CLINICAL AND PATHOPHYSIOLOGICAL SCENARIOS WHERE THEIR USE IS MOST APPROPRIATE

Cardiovascular Support Agents	Expected Actions	Comments	Pathophysiologic Target
Volume	Improves cardiac preload (input)	Judicious use is recommended in presence of affected myocardial contractility	Low preload, collapsed systemic veins
Dopamine[a]	Vasopressor/Inotrope	Increases afterload May increase PAP/SAP	Systemic hypotension, but with normal or high cardiac output
Dobutamine	Inotrope	Tachycardia May decrease SAP but also increases PAP[97]	Poor contractility, low blood flow/cardiac output
Epinephrine[a]	Vasopressor/Inotrope	Tachycardia Beta2-adrenergic receptor stimulation causing hyperglycemia and increased lactate May decrease PAP/SAP	Poor contractility, Systemic vasodilation, Low blood flow/cardiac output, systemic hypotension
Norepinephrine[a]	Vasopressor/Inotrope	Increases afterload Decreases PAP/SAP	Poor contractility, Systemic vasodilation Systemic hypotension
Milrinone[a]	Inodilator/Lusitrope/Pulmonary vasodilator	Reduces afterload Pulmonary vasodilation, Tachycardia, systemic hypotension May exacerbate right-to-left shunting	Poor contractility, low blood flow/cardiac output, High afterload, normal blood pressure Small/closing PDA
Vasopressin[a]	Vasopressor/Pulmonary vasodilator	Improves systemic blood pressure/coronary perfusion Can decrease PAP/SAP	Refractory systemic hypotension
Steroid[b]	Enhances cardiovascular responsiveness to catecholamines	Hemodynamic stability Cardiovascular actions via genomic and nongenomic steroidal effects	As an add-on therapy in PPHN with unresponsive systemic hypotension

[a]Particularly dose-dependent hemodynamic effects.[84]
[b]See Chapter 30 for details.
PAP, Pulmonary artery pressure; *PDA*, patent ductus arteriosus; *PPHN*, persistent pulmonary hypertension of the newborn; *SAP*, systemic artery pressure.
Adopted and modified with permission from de Waal K, Kluckow M: Prolonged rupture of membranes and pulmonary hypoplasia in very preterm infants: pathophysiology and guided treatment. *J Pediatr.* 2015;166(5):1113–1120.

2. *Vasopressin* acts through the V1a and V2 receptors, which induce vasoconstriction and vasodilation, respectively. The V1a and V2 receptors are coupled to phospholipase-C and adenylyl cyclase, respectively and thus exert their cellular actions via the inositol triphosphate and cAMP pathways. In animal models, low dose vasopressin causes selective vasodilatation in the pulmonary, renal, coronary, and cerebral vasculature under hypoxic conditions while causing vasoconstriction in the other vascular beds.[87-89] Vasopressin has been used in vasodilatory shock caused by specific (sepsis) or nonspecific (post bypass following cardiac surgery) inflammation, and vasopressor-resistant shock. A drug-induced decrease in pulmonary artery pressure and the positive effect on systemic blood pressure are desirable properties when used in PPHN. In a retrospective PPHN chart review, administration of vasopressin to infants receiving iNO was associated with a significant improvement in the OI by 6 hours after the start of the drug infusion and a reduction in the dose of iNO.[90] Although there is little high-quality evidence from neonatal trials, vasopressin may be an appropriate adjunct medication with a favorable hemodynamic profile to be considered in neonates with PPHN presenting with systemic vasodilation and hypotension with poor response to conventional vasopressor-inotropes.

Using Pathophysiology to Guide Use of Vasopressors in Persistent Pulmonary Hypertension of the Newborn

Systemic hypotension is common in PPHN and is usually associated with ventricular dysfunction caused by decreased ventricular preload, poor myocardial function, or both. It potentially exacerbates right-to-left ductal shunting and worsens hypoxemia in PPHN. Cardiac output and systemic blood pressure may not correlate well, and thus, an increase in systemic pressure does not necessarily reflect an improvement in cardiac output.[91] It is important to ascertain the cause of hypotension and address it accordingly. For example, if the hypotension is primarily caused by cardiac dysfunction secondary to PPHN-associated decreased left ventricle preload, then addressing PPHN itself with the use of selective pulmonary vasodilator(s) (iNO with or without milrinone) will likely alleviate hypotension. If hypotension is due to hypovolemia or fluid redistribution, an appropriate fluid bolus may be helpful. However, if sepsis is a primary or associated morbidity, in addition to antibiotics, vasopressor-inotrope treatment would be the first choice of drugs to address systemic hypotension. In all scenarios, using a ventilation strategy appropriate for the pulmonary status is important, as inappropriately high ventilator settings in a patient with compliant lungs can compromise cardiac preload and thus reduce systemic blood flow and O_2 delivery.

Furthermore, the relationship between systemic blood pressure and ductal shunting in PPHN is a complex one, and a full understanding of the hemodynamic status is imperative for selecting the most appropriate treatment strategy. As alluded to earlier, there is a particular hemodynamic scenario where the interplay between systemic blood pressure and ductal shunting is of particular importance. This occurs in patients with severe PPHN, where the open ductus arteriosus acts as a pop-off valve for the struggling right ventricle. In this presentation, administration of a vasopressor-inotrope to increase systemic blood pressure may decrease right-to-left shunting and thus might worsen right ventricular strain and further decrease cardiac output, systemic blood pressure, and oxygenation. In this situation, the pathophysiologically appropriate treatment should be directed to providing the most effective means of selective pulmonary vasodilatation while maintaining blood pressure in the low-normal range. Following serum lactate levels might aid in the definition of the "low-normal" blood pressure range in a given patient. In summary, by acting as a pressure relief valve, ductal shunting may be useful in the acute phase of the disease, although at the expense of postductal oxygenation. However, when PPHN resolves and the shunt through the ductus arteriosus becomes predominantly left-to-right, there is a theoretical possibility of the now dilated pulmonary vessels being flooded. This might cause volume-induced pulmonary hypertension, especially if the ductus arteriosus is large and systemic blood pressure is high. As PPHN is a dynamic condition, appropriate bedside cardiopulmonary monitoring and hemodynamic evaluation using cardiac ultrasound is important to understand the changing pathophysiology and guide the management strategy accordingly.

In patients with PPHN, cardiovascular support should be individualized with the best possible medication or combination of medications based on information obtained from cardiorespiratory monitoring, ultrasonography, and blood pressure measurement. The ideal treatment strategy aims to improve pulmonary perfusion by decreasing PVR, appropriately increasing systemic blood pressure, and supporting cardiac function. The effect of most vasopressor-inotropes on PAP seems to be influenced by the state of pulmonary blood flow with a more pronounced drug-induced increase with high underlying pulmonary flow.[92] Yet, most of these drugs increase both the systemic and pulmonary pressure, and thus their use must be monitored to avoid inducing an unwanted increase in the PAP/SAP ratio. Similarly, vasodilators/lusitropes can cause systemic hypotension in patients with PPHN exacerbating the right-to-left ductal shunting already present and increasing postductal and potentially systemic hypoxemia. Table 9.1 summarizes medications supporting cardiovascular function, their mechanisms of action and possible clinical and physiological situations where their use may be considered in the context of PPHN. More extensive discussions of the pharmacology and role of each medication in PPHN can be found in Chapters 1, 9, 26 and 29.

The choice of vasopressor-inotrope is also of importance in patients with PPHN and should be targeted to the individual infant's pathophysiology. There are some clinical/hemodynamic scenarios where improving the systemic blood pressure from low to normal or, sometimes even from normal to high normal, may be warranted. Such a scenario is when the patient presents with significant right-to-left ductal shunting, and normal right ventricular function and pulmonary blood flow. A vasopressor-inotrope, such as dopamine or epinephrine, is best suited for this purpose. In other situations, with impaired myocardial function and low pulmonary blood flow, a pure inotrope, such as dobutamine is most useful. Although milrinone also can be used in this latter scenario, in the setting of significant right-to-left ductal shunting and associated lability in systemic oxygenation, the risk of systemic hypotension and worsening oxygenation needs to be considered when milrinone is administered. Milrinone is best suited to a setting where there is a small or mainly left-to-right ductal shunt with poor pulmonary blood flow and thus compromised pulmonary venous return. In this setting, the right ventricle often will appear obstructed with significant dilation. On the other hand, infants with PPHN, sepsis, and low systemic blood pressure resulting in a more pronounced right-to-left ductal shunt may respond well to vasopressin. It is also obvious that assessment of atrial- and ductal-level shunts provides essential information when managing a newborn with PPHN. For example, left-to-right shunting at the foramen ovale and ductus arteriosus with marked hypoxemia suggests the presence of predominant intrapulmonary shunting, and interventions should be directed at optimizing lung inflation. Pulmonary vasodilator therapy with iNO may also not be effective in improving oxygenation in the presence of severe left ventricular dysfunction. Indeed, increased left atrial pressure secondary to left ventricular failure results in pulmonary venous hypertension. Administration of iNO to a patient with pulmonary venous hypertension can result in potential further flooding of the pulmonary capillary bed with worsening pulmonary edema and clinical deterioration.

As stressed across the chapter, cardiac ultrasound performed longitudinally has a significant role in the management of PPHN. Bedside ultrasound should be used to rule out cyanotic congenital heart disease (best done by a pediatric cardiologist), measure pulmonary pressures, evaluate shunt and assess right and left ventricular function, filling, and output during the initial phase of the management. Ultrasound is also useful in determining the likely hemodynamic response to the interventions. Beside the traditional ultrasound measurements, newer Doppler parameters such as myocardial performance index, systolic-to-diastolic duration ratio, and tissue Doppler may also have a role in the assessment and management of PPHN (see Chapters 11 to 13).

Table 9.2 describes some of the commonly occurring clinical scenarios and suggested treatment options based on the underlying pathophysiology.

Table 9.2 COMMONLY OCCURRING CLINICAL SCENARIOS AND SUGGESTED TREATMENT OPTIONS BASED ON THE UNDERLYING PATHOPHYSIOLOGY

Clinical Scenario With PPHN	Systemic Blood Pressure	Choice of Cardiovascular Drug
Asphyxia with myocardial depression	Normal	Dobutamine Milrinone (if afterload remains high)
Septic shock with myocardial depression	Low	Fluid bolus as required, dopamine or epinephrine Add vasopressin or norepinephrine if poor response
Septic shock with normal cardiac function	Low	Fluid bolus as required, Vasopressin/noradrenaline
Shock refractory to catecholamines	Low	Steroid ± vasopressin
Compromised cardiac function with diastolic dysfunction/RV dysfunction		Dobutamine or milrinone

PPHN, Persistent pulmonary hypertension of the newborn; *RV*, right ventricular.

Extracorporeal Membrane Oxygenation

ECMO provides primarily respiratory (veno-venous ECMO) or both respiratory and cardiac (veno-arterial ECMO) support in patients with a high chance of not surviving without this intervention, and facilitates and provides time for postnatal adaptation to occur while allowing the potentially remodeled pulmonary circulation and/or the lungs to recover. ECMO is generally undertaken in term and near-term infants if the OI is greater than 40 or the alveolar-arterial O_2 difference is greater than 600 with the presence of cardiovascular instability. ECMO is not recommended in premature infants less than 34 weeks' gestation in most centers because of the very high risk of P/IVH. A retrospective analysis of all patients with PPHN supported with ECMO from 2000 to 2010 involving 1569 neonates showed encouraging results with 81% survival.[93] Use of ECMO in the management of PPHN decreased from the late 1980s to 2000 as the result of advancements in the medical management of PPHN, specifically the use of high-frequency ventilation, iNO, and surfactant.[94-96] A decision to treat a newborn with ECMO should be taken at the appropriate time, which is one of the more difficult decisions a neonatologist faces. Patients should not be put on the circuit early in the course of the disease; however, infants also should not be exposed to the adverse effects of conventional treatment for too long, as studies have shown adverse outcomes in patients with prolonged periods of profound hypoxemia and acidosis.

In many countries, including even the more developed ones like Australia, neonatal ECMO for respiratory failure is not easily available. In Australia for instance, there is a general consensus that early transfer to a tertiary center, early targeted treatment interventions, and iNO along with surfactant in the presence of associated parenchymal lung disease seems to have significantly decreased the need for ECMO in patients without pulmonary hypoplasia. However, infants with PPHN secondary to pulmonary hypoplasia caused by severe CDH for instance, continue to benefit from early ECMO treatment.

Conclusions

PPHN presents as a heterogeneous group of pathophysiological scenarios that together form the syndrome of hypoxic respiratory failure in infants at any gestational age. It is crucial to understand the underlying pathophysiology in each case to allow appropriate therapy to be utilized. Although the pivotal pathophysiological feature is raised PVR as the name implies, there are a number of additional important factors that may be present in an infant that will influence the clinical presentation. These factors include abnormalities of the lungs with significant V/Q mismatch, asphyxial injury to the myocardium and other organs, the presence of an open ductus arteriosus, the relative pressures/impedances at either end of the ductus arteriosus determining shunt direction, the volume/filling state of the circulation, and the interdependence between the two cardiac ventricles at multiple levels. Different combinations of these factors will be present in each infant, and as a result there is not a single treatment algorithm that will suit every baby.

In managing infants with high oxygen requirements, the first step is to identify the respiratory pathology and to optimize the respiratory support. Indeed, in some patients, the ensuing improvement in oxygenation and control of the acid-base status may be enough to reverse the process and encourage pulmonary vasodilation. The next step is to identify the underlying cardiovascular pathology, including the status of the function of the heart, by studying preload, contractility, and afterload, as well as the status of peripheral vasoregulation. Using the information obtained, and targeting the cardiovascular management accordingly, has a high chance of normalizing systemic blood pressure and cardiac output, and of improving systemic oxygenation. It is important to assess volume status and filling by visual review of the heart and systemic veins followed by titration of volume to the clinical state. The direction of ductal shunt is determined by the relative systemic and pulmonary pressures/impedances, so attention to improving the systemic blood pressure is one way to potentially

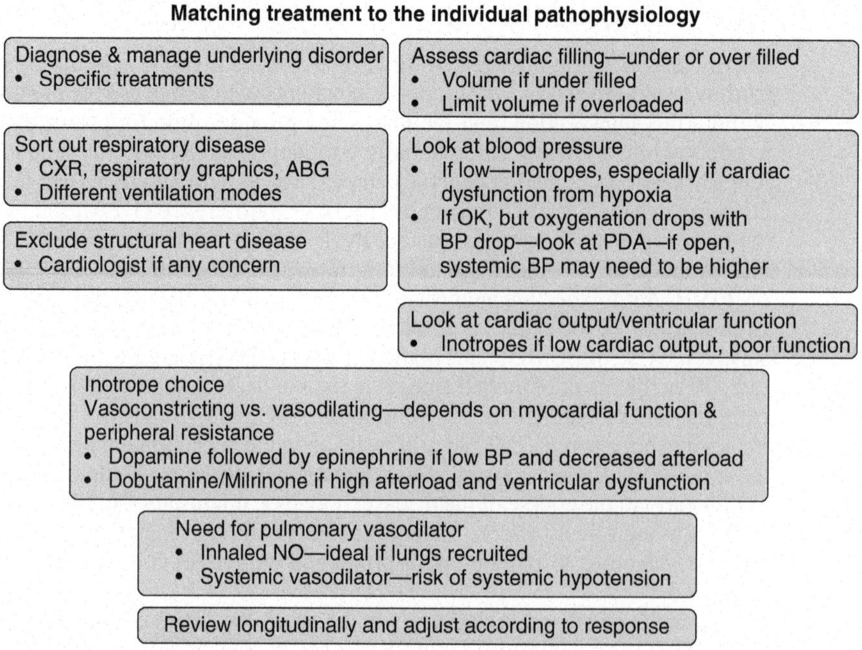

Matching treatment to the individual pathophysiology

Diagnose & manage underlying disorder • Specific treatments	Assess cardiac filling—under or over filled • Volume if under filled • Limit volume if overloaded

Sort out respiratory disease
• CXR, respiratory graphics, ABG
• Different ventilation modes
	Look at blood pressure
	• If low—inotropes, especially if cardiac
	   dysfunction from hypoxia
	• If OK, but oxygenation drops with
	   BP drop—look at PDA—if open,
	   systemic BP may need to be higher

Exclude structural heart disease • Cardiologist if any concern	

Look at cardiac output/ventricular function
• Inotropes if low cardiac output, poor function

Inotrope choice
Vasoconstricting vs. vasodilating—depends on myocardial function &
peripheral resistance
• Dopamine followed by epinephrine if low BP and decreased afterload
• Dobutamine/Milrinone if high afterload and ventricular dysfunction

Need for pulmonary vasodilator
• Inhaled NO—ideal if lungs recruited
• Systemic vasodilator—risk of systemic hypotension

Review longitudinally and adjust according to response

Fig. 9.3 Diagrammatic representation of the stepwise clinical approach to persistent pulmonary hypertension of the newborn management using pathophysiological information obtained from bedside ultrasound. *ABG*, Arterial blood gas; *BP*, blood pressure; *CXR*, chest x-ray; *NO*, nitric oxide; *PDA*, patent ductus arteriosus.

improve systemic oxygenation. Improving right ventricular output is just as important, as systemic preload is dependent on adequate pulmonary blood flow, and this can be impacted by not only the increases in PVR but also by the mean airway pressure and the contractility of the right ventricle. Excessive peripheral vasoconstriction can increase afterload and impair ventricular outputs, so a decision to use an inotrope with vasodilatory properties can be useful in this setting. Once myocardial function and systemic vascular resistance have been stabilized and optimized, respectively, the final target is the pulmonary vasculature. Selective pulmonary vasodilation, usually by the administration of iNO, commences immediately after the exclusion of congenital heart disease and the establishment of the diagnosis of PPHN or, in patients with very severe hypoxic respiratory failure, it might be started even before this diagnostic step. There is a range of systemic and specific pulmonary vasodilators available, and the most appropriate choice will be determined by the underlying pathophysiology. Infants with primary respiratory disease might not respond well to iNO initially, but likely will after administration of surfactant and appropriate lung recruitment. Patients with ultrasound evidence of high pulmonary pressure, such as reduced right ventricle output, altered right ventricle output waveform, a measurable tricuspid jet, and predominantly right-to-left ductal shunt, are most likely to respond well and rapidly to iNO. Infants with high afterload on the right and/or left side, and an obstructed right ventricle with a closing or small ductus arteriosus are more likely to respond to systemic vasodilators such as milrinone or PGI2. Finally, regular reassessment of the cardiovascular pathophysiology will allow identification of the resolution of the abnormal pathophysiology and, subsequently, the most appropriate sequence of weaning the pulmonary vasodilatory and systemic hemodynamic support to reduce iNO use, lung injury, and neonatal intensive care unit (NICU) stay (Fig. 9.3).

Optimal management of the infant with hypoxic respiratory failure and PPHN depends on obtaining early, accurate, and repeated information about the underlying pathophysiology in the individual infant. Establishing the most appropriate treatment strategy for the particular infant can be guided by the use of bedside cardiac ultrasound to assess the pathophysiology and the response to the particular therapy. This individualization/personalization of the treatment approach is increasingly common in all areas of medicine, and is particularly suited to this hemodynamic scenario.

REFERENCES

1. Shivananda S, Ahliwahlia L, Kluckow M, et al.: Variation in the management of persistent pulmonary hypertension of the newborn: a survey of physicians in Canada, Australia, and New Zealand, *Am J Perinatol* 29(7):519–526, 2012.
2. Alapati D, Jassar R, Shaffer TH: Management of supplemental oxygen for infants with persistent pulmonary hypertension of newborn: a Survey, *Am J Perinatol* 2016.
3. Cheung PY, Tyebkhan JM, Peliowski A, et al.: Prolonged use of pancuronium bromide and sensorineural hearing loss in childhood survivors of congenital diaphragmatic hernia, *J Pediatr* 135(2 Pt 1):233–239, 1999.
4. Walsh-Sukys MC, Tyson JE, Wright LL, et al.: Persistent pulmonary hypertension of the newborn in the era before nitric oxide: practice variation and outcomes, *Pediatrics* 105(1 Pt 1):14–20, 2000.
5. Kinsella JP, Truog WE, Walsh WF, et al.: Randomized, multicenter trial of inhaled nitric oxide and high-frequency oscillatory ventilation in severe, persistent pulmonary hypertension of the newborn, *J Pediatr* 131(1 Pt 1):55–62, 1997.
6. Konduri GG, Solimano A, Sokol GM, et al.: A randomized trial of early versus standard inhaled nitric oxide therapy in term and near-term newborn infants with hypoxic respiratory failure, *Pediatrics* 113(3 Pt 1):559–564, 2004.
7. Sahni R, Ameer X, Ohira-Kist K, Wung JT: Non-invasive inhaled nitric oxide in the treatment of hypoxemic respiratory failure in term and preterm infants, *J Perinatol* 37(1):54–60, 2017.
8. Fischer C, Rybakowski C, Ferdynus C, et al.: A population-based study of meconium aspiration syndrome in neonates born between 37 and 43 weeks of gestation, *Int J Pediatr* 2012:321545, 2012.
9. Yoder BA, Kirsch EA, Barth WH, Gordon MC: Changing obstetric practices associated with decreasing incidence of meconium aspiration syndrome, *Obstet Gynecol* 99(5 Pt 1):731–739, 2002.
10. Cornfield DN, Chatfield BA, McQueston JA, et al.: Effects of birth-related stimuli on L-arginine-dependent pulmonary vasodilation in ovine fetus, *Am J Physiol* 262(5 Pt 2):H1474–H1481, 1992.
11. Lakshminrusimha S, Russell JA, Steinhorn RH, et al.: Pulmonary arterial contractility in neonatal lambs increases with 100% oxygen resuscitation, *Pediatr Res* 59(1):137–141, 2006.
12. Lakshminrusimha S, Swartz DD, Gugino SF, et al.: Oxygen concentration and pulmonary hemodynamics in newborn lambs with pulmonary hypertension, *Pediatr Res* 66(5):539–544, 2009.
13. Rudolph AM, Yuan S: Response of the pulmonary vasculature to hypoxia and H+ ion concentration changes, *J Clin Invest* 45(3):399–411, 1966.
14. Kregenow DA, Swenson ER: The lung and carbon dioxide: implications for permissive and therapeutic hypercapnia, *Eur Respir J* 20(1):6–11, 2002.
15. Afolayan AJ, Eis A, Alexander M, et al.: Decreased endothelial nitric oxide synthase expression and function contribute to impaired mitochondrial biogenesis and oxidative stress in fetal lambs with persistent pulmonary hypertension, *Am J Physiol Lung Cell Mol Physiol* 310(1):L40–L49, 2016.
16. Klinger JR, Abman SH, Gladwin MT: Nitric oxide deficiency and endothelial dysfunction in pulmonary arterial hypertension, *Am J Respir Crit Care Med* 188(6):639–646, 2013.
17. Barrington KJ, Finer N, Pennaforte T, Altit G: Nitric oxide for respiratory failure in infants born at or near term, *Cochrane Database Syst Rev* 1:CD000399, 2017.
18. Golombek SG, Young JN: Efficacy of inhaled nitric oxide for hypoxic respiratory failure in term and late preterm infants by baseline severity of illness: a pooled analysis of three clinical trials, *Clin Ther* 32(5):939–948, 2010.
19. Cahan A, Cimino JJ: Improving precision medicine using individual patient data from trials, *CMAJ* 2016.
20. Finer NN, Barrington KJ: Nitric oxide for respiratory failure in infants born at or near term, *Cochrane Database Syst Rev* (4)CD000399, 2006.
21. Kinsella JP, Parker TA, Ivy DD, Abman SH: Noninvasive delivery of inhaled nitric oxide therapy for late pulmonary hypertension in newborn infants with congenital diaphragmatic hernia, *J Pediatr* 142(4):397–401, 2003.
22. Welzing L, Bagci S, Abramian A, et al.: CPAP combined with inhaled nitric oxide for treatment of lung hypoplasia and persistent foetal circulation due to prolonged PPROM, *Early Hum Dev* 87(1):17–20, 2011.
23. Lindwall R, Blennow M, Svensson M, et al.: A pilot study of inhaled nitric oxide in preterm infants treated with nasal continuous positive airway pressure for respiratory distress syndrome, *Intensive Care Med* 31(7):959–964, 2005.
24. Trevisanuto D, Doglioni N, Micaglio M, Zanardo V: Feasibility of nitric oxide administration by neonatal helmet-CPAP: a bench study, *Paediatr Anaesth* 17(9):851–855, 2007.
25. Skinner JR, Boys RJ, Hunter S, Hey EN: Pulmonary and systemic arterial pressure in hyaline membrane disease, *Arch Dis Child* 67(4):366–373, 1992.
26. Bhat R, Salas AA, Foster C, et al.: Prospective analysis of pulmonary hypertension in extremely low birth weight infants, *Pediatrics* 129(3):e682–e689, 2012.
27. Mourani PM, Sontag MK, Younoszai A, et al.: Early pulmonary vascular disease in preterm infants at risk for bronchopulmonary dysplasia, *Am J Respir Crit Care Med* 191(1):87–95, 2015.
28. Kilbride HW, Thibeault DW: Neonatal complications of preterm premature rupture of membranes. Pathophysiology and management, *Clin Perinatol* 28(4):761–785, 2001.
29. Barrington KJ, Finer N, Pennaforte T: Inhaled nitric oxide for respiratory failure in preterm infants, *Cochrane Database Syst Rev* 1:CD000509, 2017.
30. Barrington KJ, Finer N: Inhaled nitric oxide for respiratory failure in preterm infants, [Update of Cochrane Database Syst Rev. 2007;(3):CD000509; PMID: 17636641], *Cochrane Database Syst Rev* (12)CD000509, 2010.

31. Allen MC, Donohue P, Gilmore M, et al.: Inhaled nitric oxide in preterm infants, *Evid Rep Technol Assess (Full Rep)* 195:1–315, 2010.

32. Peliowski A, Finer NN, Etches PC, et al.: Inhaled nitric oxide for premature infants after prolonged rupture of the membranes, *J Pediatr* 126(3):450–453, 1995.

33. Chock VY, Van Meurs KP, Hintz SR, et al.: Inhaled nitric oxide for preterm premature rupture of membranes, oligohydramnios, and pulmonary hypoplasia, *Am J Perinatol* 26(4):317–322, 2009.

34. Shah DM, Kluckow M: Early functional echocardiogram and inhaled nitric oxide: usefulness in managing neonates born following extreme preterm premature rupture of membranes (PPROM), *J Paediatr Child Health* 47(6):340–345, 2011.

35. Semberova J, O'Donnell SM, Franta J, Miletin J: Inhaled nitric oxide in preterm infants with prolonged preterm rupture of the membranes: a case series, *J Perinatol* 35(4):304–306, 2015.

36. Desandes R, Desandes E, Droulle P, et al.: Inhaled nitric oxide improves oxygenation in very premature infants with low pulmonary blood flow, *Acta Paediatr* 93(1):66–69, 2004.

37. Cheng DR, Peart S, Tan K, Sehgal A: Nitric therapy in preterm infants: rationalised approach based on functional neonatal echocardiography, *Acta Paediatr* 105(2):165–171, 2016.

38. Aly H, Sahni R, Wung JT: Weaning strategy with inhaled nitric oxide treatment in persistent pulmonary hypertension of the newborn, *Arch Dis Child Fetal Neonatal Ed* 76(2):F118–F122, 1997.

39. Sokol GM, Fineberg NS, Wright LL, Ehrenkranz RA: Changes in arterial oxygen tension when weaning neonates from inhaled nitric oxide, *Pediatr Pulmonol* 32(1):14–19, 2001.

40. Davidson D, Barefield ES, Kattwinkel J, et al.: Safety of withdrawing inhaled nitric oxide therapy in persistent pulmonary hypertension of the newborn, *Pediatrics* 104(2 Pt 1):231–236, 1999.

41. Day RW, Allen EM, Witte MK: A randomized, controlled study of the 1-hour and 24-hour effects of inhaled nitric oxide therapy in children with acute hypoxemic respiratory failure, *Chest* 112(5):1324–1331, 1997.

42. Carriedo H, Rhine W: Withdrawal of inhaled nitric oxide from nonresponders after short exposure, *J Perinatol* 23(7):556–558, 2003.

43. Farrow KN, Steinhorn RH: Phosphodiesterases: emerging therapeutic targets for neonatal pulmonary hypertension, *Handb Exp Pharmacol* 204:251–277, 2011.

44. Lakshminrusimha S, Mathew B, Leach CL: Pharmacologic strategies in neonatal pulmonary hypertension other than nitric oxide, *Semin Perinatol* 40(3):160–173, 2016.

45. Steinhorn RH, Kinsella JP, Pierce C, et al.: Intravenous sildenafil in the treatment of neonates with persistent pulmonary hypertension, *J Pediatr* 155(6):841–847.e841, 2009.

46. Al Omar S, Salama H, Al Hail M, et al.: Effect of early adjunctive use of oral sildenafil and inhaled nitric oxide on the outcome of pulmonary hypertension in newborn infants. A feasibility study, *J Neonatal Perinatal Med* 9(3):251–259, 2016.

47. Limjoco J, Paquette L, Ramanathan R, et al.: Changes in mean arterial blood pressure during sildenafil use in neonates with meconium aspiration syndrome or sepsis, *Am J Ther* 22(2):125–131, 2015.

48. Chen B, Lakshminrusimha S, Czech L, et al.: Regulation of phosphodiesterase 3 in the pulmonary arteries during the perinatal period in sheep, *Pediatr Res* 66(6):682–687, 2009.

49. McNamara PJ, Shivananda SP, Sahni M, et al.: Pharmacology of milrinone in neonates with persistent pulmonary hypertension of the newborn and suboptimal response to inhaled nitric oxide, *Pediatr Crit Care Med* 14(1):74–84, 2013.

50. Bassler D, Choong K, McNamara P, Kirpalani H: Neonatal persistent pulmonary hypertension treated with milrinone: four case reports, *Biol Neonate* 89(1):1–5, 2006.

51. McNamara PJ, Laique F, Muang-In S, Whyte HE: Milrinone improves oxygenation in neonates with severe persistent pulmonary hypertension of the newborn, *J Crit Care* 21(2):217–222, 2006.

52. James AT, Bee C, Corcoran JD, et al.: Treatment of premature infants with pulmonary hypertension and right ventricular dysfunction with milrinone: a case series, *J Perinatol* 35(4):268–273, 2015.

53. James AT, Corcoran JD, McNamara PJ, et al.: The effect of milrinone on right and left ventricular function when used as a rescue therapy for term infants with pulmonary hypertension, *Cardiol Young* 26(1):90–99, 2016.

54. Samiee-Zafarghandy S, Raman SR, van den Anker JN, et al.: Safety of milrinone use in neonatal intensive care units, *Early Hum Dev* 91(1):31–35, 2015.

55. Aggarwal S, Natarajan G: Echocardiographic correlates of persistent pulmonary hypertension of the newborn, *Early Hum Dev* 91(4):285–289, 2015.

56. Brannon TS, MacRitchie AN, Jaramillo MA, et al.: Ontogeny of cyclooxygenase-1 and cyclooxygenase-2 gene expression in ovine lung, *Am J Physiol* 274(1 Pt 1):L66–L71, 1998.

57. Brannon TS, North AJ, Wells LB, Shaul PW: Prostacyclin synthesis in ovine pulmonary artery is developmentally regulated by changes in cyclooxygenase-1 gene expression, *J Clin Invest* 93(5):2230–2235, 1994.

58. Christman BW, McPherson CD, Newman JH, et al.: An imbalance between the excretion of thromboxane and prostacyclin metabolites in pulmonary hypertension, *N Engl J Med* 327(2):70–75, 1992.

59. Rao S, Bartle D, Patole S: Current and future therapeutic options for persistent pulmonary hypertension in the newborn, *Expert Rev Cardiovasc Ther* 8(6):845–862, 2010.

60. Bindl L, Fahnenstich H, Peukert U: Aerosolised prostacyclin for pulmonary hypertension in neonates, *Arch Dis Child Fetal Neonatal Ed* 71(3):F214–F216, 1994.

61. Soditt V, Aring C, Groneck P: Improvement of oxygenation induced by aerosolized prostacyclin in a preterm infant with persistent pulmonary hypertension of the newborn, *Intensive Care Med* 23(12):1275–1278, 1997.

62. Olmsted K, Oluola O, Parthiban A, Raghuveer T: Can inhaled prostacyclin stimulate surfactant in ELBW infants? *J Perinatol* 27(11):724–726, 2007.

63. Kelly LK, Porta NF, Goodman DM, et al.: Inhaled prostacyclin for term infants with persistent pulmonary hypertension refractory to inhaled nitric oxide, *J Pediatr* 141(6):830–832, 2002.

64. Ehlen M, Wiebe B: Iloprost in persistent pulmonary hypertension of the newborn, *Cardiol Young* 13(4):361–363, 2003.

65. Kahveci H, Yilmaz O, Avsar UZ, et al.: Oral sildenafil and inhaled iloprost in the treatment of pulmonary hypertension of the newborn, *Pediatr Pulmonol* 49(12):1205–1213, 2014.

66. Lambert V, Serraf A, Durand P, Losay J: Aerosolized iloprost therapy in an infant with chronic pulmonary hypertension after a neonatal arterial switch operation, *Arch Pediatr* 8(11):1218–1221, 2001.

67. Chotigeat U, Jaratwashirakul S: Inhaled iloprost for severe persistent pulmonary hypertension of the newborn, *J Med Assoc Thai* 90(1):167–170, 2007.

68. Hwang SK, O YC, Kim NS, et al.: Use of inhaled iloprost in an infant with bronchopulmonary dysplasia and pulmonary artery hypertension, *Korean Circ J* 39(8):343–345, 2009.

69. Yilmaz O, Kahveci H, Zeybek C, et al.: Inhaled iloprost in preterm infants with severe respiratory distress syndrome and pulmonary hypertension, *Am J Perinatol* 31(4):321–326, 2014.

70. Keller RL, Tacy TA, Hendricks-Munoz K, et al.: Congenital diaphragmatic hernia: endothelin-1, pulmonary hypertension, and disease severity, *Am J Respir Crit Care Med* 182(4):555–561, 2010.

71. Kumar P, Kazzi NJ, Shankaran S: Plasma immunoreactive endothelin-1 concentrations in infants with persistent pulmonary hypertension of the newborn, *Am J Perinatol* 13(6):335–341, 1996.

72. Nakwan N, Choksuchat D, Saksawad R, et al.: Successful treatment of persistent pulmonary hypertension of the newborn with bosentan, *Acta Paediatr* 98(10):1683–1685, 2009.

73. Goissen C, Ghyselen L, Tourneux P, et al.: Persistent pulmonary hypertension of the newborn with transposition of the great arteries: successful treatment with bosentan, *Eur J Pediatr* 167(4):437–440, 2008.

74. Radicioni M, Bruni A, Camerini P: Combination therapy for life-threatening pulmonary hypertension in a premature infant: first report on bosentan use, *Eur J Pediatr* 170(8):1075–1078, 2011.

74a. Mohamed WA, Ismail M: A randomized, double-blind, placebo-controlled, prospective study of bosentan for the treatment of persistent pulmonary hypertension of the newborn, *J Perinatol* 32(8):608–613, 2012.

75. Steinhorn RH, Fineman J, Kusic-Pajic A, et al.: Bosentan as adjunctive therapy for persistent pulmonary hypertension of the newborn: results of the randomized multicenter placebo-controlled exploratory trial, *J Pediatr* 177:90–96.e93, 2016.

76. Wu TJ, Teng RJ, Tsou KI: Persistent pulmonary hypertension of the newborn treated with magnesium sulfate in premature neonates, *Pediatrics* 96(3 Pt 1):472–474, 1995.

77. Daffa SH, Milaat WA: Role of magnesium sulphate in treatment of severe persistent pulmonary hypertension of the neoborn, *Saudi Med J* 23(10):1266–1269, 2002.

78. Chandran S, Haqueb ME, Wickramasinghe HT, Wint Z: Use of magnesium sulphate in severe persistent pulmonary hypertension of the newborn, *J Trop Pediatr* 50(4):219–223, 2004.

79. Tolsa JF, Cotting J, Sekarski N, et al.: Magnesium sulphate as an alternative and safe treatment for severe persistent pulmonary hypertension of the newborn, *Arch Dis Child Fetal Neonatal Ed* 72(3):F184–F187, 1995.

80. Raimondi F, Migliaro F, Capasso L, et al.: Intravenous magnesium sulphate vs. inhaled nitric oxide for moderate, persistent pulmonary hypertension of the newborn. A multicentre, retrospective study, *J Trop Pediatr* 54(3):196–199, 2008.

81. Sehgal A, Athikarisamy SE, Adamopoulos M: Global myocardial function is compromised in infants with pulmonary hypertension, *Acta Paediatr* 101(4):410–413, 2012.

82. Skinner JR, Hunter S, Hey EN: Haemodynamic features at presentation in persistent pulmonary hypertension of the newborn and outcome, *Arch Dis Child Fetal Neonatal Ed* 74(1):F26–F32, 1996.

83. Fraisse A, Geva T, Gaudart J, Wessel DL: Doppler echocardiographic predictors of outcome in newborns with persistent pulmonary hypertension, *Cardiol Young* 14(3):277–283, 2004.

84. Noori S, Seri I: Neonatal blood pressure support: the use of inotropes, lusitropes, and other vasopressor agents, *Clin Perinatol* 39(1):221–238, 2012.

85. Tourneux P, Rakza T, Bouissou A, et al.: Pulmonary circulatory effects of norepinephrine in newborn infants with persistent pulmonary hypertension, *J Pediatr* 153(3):345–349, 2008.

86. Rowcliff K, de Waal K, Mohamed AL, Chaudhari T: Noradrenaline in preterm infants with cardiovascular compromise, *Eur J Pediatr* 2016.

87. Tamaki T, Kiyomoto K, He H, et al.: Vasodilation induced by vasopressin V2 receptor stimulation in afferent arterioles, *Kidney Int* 49(3):722–729, 1996.

88. Evora PR, Pearson PJ, Schaff HV: Arginine vasopressin induces endothelium-dependent vasodilatation of the pulmonary artery. V1-receptor-mediated production of nitric oxide, *Chest* 103(4):1241–1245, 1993.

89. Sai Y, Okamura T, Amakata Y, Toda N: Comparison of responses of canine pulmonary artery and vein to angiotensin II, bradykinin and vasopressin, *Eur J Pharmacol* 282(1-3):235–241, 1995.

90. Mohamed A, Nasef N, Shah V, McNamara PJ: Vasopressin as a rescue therapy for refractory pulmonary hypertension in neonates: case series, *Pediatr Crit Care Med* 15(2):148–154, 2014.

91. Kluckow M, Evans N: Relationship between blood pressure and cardiac output in preterm infants requiring mechanical ventilation, *J Pediatr* 129(4):506–512, 1996.

92. Bouissou A, Rakza T, Klosowski S, et al.: Hypotension in preterm infants with significant patent ductus arteriosus: effects of dopamine, *J Pediatr* 153(6):790–794, 2008.

93. Lazar DA, Cass DL, Olutoye OO, et al.: The use of ECMO for persistent pulmonary hypertension of the newborn: a decade of experience, *J Surg Res* 177(2):263–267, 2012.

94. Hintz SR, Suttner DM, Sheehan AM, et al.: Decreased use of neonatal extracorporeal membrane oxygenation (ECMO): how new treatment modalities have affected ECMO utilization, *Pediatrics* 106(6):1339–1343, 2000.
95. Christou H, Van Marter LJ, Wessel DL, et al.: Inhaled nitric oxide reduces the need for extracorporeal membrane oxygenation in infants with persistent pulmonary hypertension of the newborn, *Crit Care Med* 28(11):3722–3727, 2000.
96. Roy BJ, Rycus P, Conrad SA, Clark RH: The changing demographics of neonatal extracorporeal membrane oxygenation patients reported to the Extracorporeal Life Support Organization (ELSO) Registry, *Pediatrics* 106(6):1334–1338, 2000.
97. Cheung PY, Barrington KJ, Bigam D: The hemodynamic effects of dobutamine infusion in the chronically instrumented newborn piglet, *Crit Care Med* 27(3):558–564, 1999.

B

Assessment of Systemic Blood Flow and Cardiac Function: Ultrasound

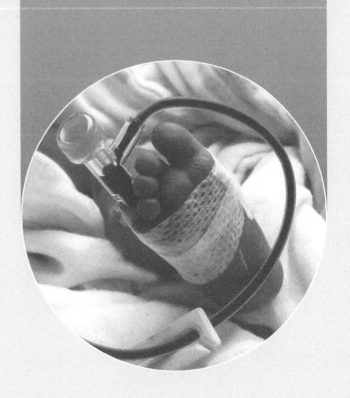

CHAPTER 10

Point of Care Ultrasound in the Assessment of the Neonatal Cardiovascular System

Nicholas Evans and Martin Kluckow

- The use of point of care ultrasound (POCU) in the care of sick and preterm neonates is rapidly expanding.
- The benefits of a portable, bedside technique that is able to provide real time, longitudinal data regarding the physiology of individual patients allowing more targeted treatment is being progressively recognized as we move towards the era of personalized medicine in neonatology.
- POCU has an important role in managing the transitioning term or preterm infant, the septic/asphyxiated infant, the shocked or hypotensive infant and infants with suspected PPHN or congenital heart disease.
- POCU is usually a predominantly 'rule in' diagnostic modality and does not aim to 'rule out' all diagnoses whereas consultative ultrasound should also be a 'rule out' diagnostic modality.
- With the acceptance of the usefulness of ultrasound in the clinical setting, the need for appropriate training programs and accreditation increases.
- Approaches to training and accreditation vary across different countries.

It is a limitation in the intensive care of the newborn infant that we have few tools with which to monitor cardiovascular and hemodynamic function. There is usually the ability to continuously monitor invasive blood pressure and heart rate and that's about it. Beyond that, reliance is placed on rather inaccurate measures of contemporaneous hemodynamic well-being such as skin capillary refill time and urine output and measures that do not reflect the changes in the hemodynamic status in real time, such as the acid-base status. Near-infrared spectroscopy (NIRS) is evolving as a potentially useful monitoring tool[1] for the real-time assessment of tissue oxygenation of the organ interrogated (brain, kidney, muscle, or intestines; see Chapters 16 to 18). As for measuring cardiac output, there is little outcome-based validation for tools designed to measure cardiac output (see Chapters 14 and 21). The difficulties of small patient size and a smaller commercial market limit neonatology access to a range of tools for monitoring cardiac output which are available for the intensive care of the older subject, such as thermodilution, electrical impedance velocimetry, continuous Doppler methodologies, and derivations from blood pressure waveforms.

Doppler cardiac ultrasound provides a noninvasive, albeit noncontinuous, technique from which it is possible to derive estimates of a wide range of hemodynamic parameters as well as information on structure and function of the organ that drives the circulation, the heart. Integration of cardiac ultrasound into routine neonatal intensive care has been limited by the concentration of the necessary skills in specialist groups who work predominantly outside the neonatal intensive care unit (NICU). This results in information that is often neither timely nor particularly well focused on hemodynamics. From a research perspective, it meant that there were assumptions derived from a limited number of snapshots rather than serial studies to document natural history.

Neonatology, like many acute care specialties, has recognized the limitations of an external consultative ultrasound model and neonatologists are increasingly developing cardiac ultrasound skills themselves so they can be applied at the acute point of care.[2] This has allowed more systematic serial studies, which in turn is facilitating the development of the research and clinical monitoring potential of these methodologies. It should be emphasized that acute point of care ultrasound (POCU) does not replace the need for consultative ultrasound. Rather it addresses different questions and complements consultative ultrasound. The best outcomes are achieved when the two models work collaboratively alongside each other.

This chapter will provide an overview on the use of cardiac ultrasound to assess the neonatal circulation (details of the individual techniques will be outlined in other chapters), as well as discussing issues of training, accreditation, and interaction with other imaging specialists.

Politics of Ultrasound

The evolution of ultrasound into the area of acute care has its political problems and this has not been confined to neonatology. On one side of the argument, acute care specialists have recognized the rapid diagnostic potential of ultrasound, a potential that is difficult to fulfill within a consultative model of ultrasound.[3] The improvement in quality of imaging and portability of equipment has made ultrasound accessible to anyone with a good understanding of anatomy and access to training. On the other side of the argument, some consultative imaging specialists have resisted this on the basis of concerns about lack of accredited training and the risk of diagnostic error.[4] Importantly, a recent review of medico-legal cases involving neonatal/pediatric POCU in the United States found no evidence of this risk.[5] Like all political divides, there are merits to both arguments. Consultative ultrasound specialists have neither the ability nor often the desire to be available 24/7 for the rapid diagnostic situations facing acute care specialists. POCU, particularly in neonatology, has often evolved with a lack of good training and accreditation structures. Many of the early adopters of POCU were largely self-taught, or taught by a cardiologist with a balanced perspective of the usefulness of functional ultrasound in the NICU. While this is changing, as will be described later, there is a risk that this may lead to diagnostic error. As always, the answer lies in the middle with a system that takes advantage of the strengths of both systems and minimizes the risks. POCU is usually a predominantly "rule in" diagnostic modality and does not aim to "rule out" all diagnoses, whereas consultative ultrasound should also be a "rule out" diagnostic modality. For example, a neonatologist, when faced with a baby with possible pulmonary hypertension at 2:00 a.m., wants to assess pulmonary artery pressure, direction of shunts through the fetal channels, and estimate systemic and pulmonary blood flow. He or she would hope to recognize congenital heart disease (CHD), but would not be able to rule it out. That would be a job for the cardiologist who would come the next day. So, the baby benefits from the timely use of ultrasound to guide appropriate intensive care intervention and also benefits from the expertise of the cardiologist in being able to confirm structural normality or otherwise. Such collaborative care should not be a source of interdisciplinary conflict. Rather, it strengthens collaboration and has the potential to significantly improve patient care.

It is our experience that much of the resistance to establishing a POCU program is based on a lack of understanding of the goals. Resolution comes from reassurance about training and quality issues and education about purpose, most importantly, that the intent is *to complement, not replace, the role of those consultative specialties.*

What's in a Name?

The biggest risk of cardiac ultrasound performed by non-cardiologists is that it is recorded that a baby has had an echocardiogram and so it is assumed by subsequent health care providers that CHD has been excluded. Recognizing this risk, there has been a range of terminology applied including functional echocardiography[6] and targeted echocardiography.[7] Our opinion on terminology has evolved from these terms, understanding that the communication risk comes, at least in part, from the use of the word echocardiography. Because this term grew up within the specialty of cardiology, if it is applied to a study, whatever the prefix, there is a risk of assumption that it has been performed by a cardiologist. Because of this risk, in this chapter, we refer to "cardiac ultrasound" with a prefix that communicates that the study was not performed by a cardiologist but by an acute care physician. This could be "point of care," "clinician-performed," or, more specifically, neonatologist-performed cardiac ultrasound. This also has the advantage that it does not confine the terminology to the heart, recognizing that neonatal POCU has many uses beyond the heart.

Training and Accreditation in Point of Care Ultrasound

It is the nature of the evolution of any procedure or technology that the early adopters are often self-taught. Development of training and accreditation structures follows when the need is identified and there is enough of a critical mass of early adopters to provide the necessary support. There are good examples of training structures in POCU such as that developed by the American College of Emergency Physicians;[8,9] however, there is a long way to go in neonatal POCU. Internationally, there is difference of opinion in the relative weight that should be given to training provided by those outside neonatology compared with those within. In Australia and New Zealand, we have developed a training program which is based on the philosophy that training for POCU in the NICU is best undertaken in the NICU under supervision of appropriately trained and accredited neonatologists while also recognizing the need for support from the consultative imaging specialists.[3] The program was developed in 2007 under the auspices of the Australasian Society of Ultrasound in Medicine (ASUM) who, having recognized the inevitable evolution of ultrasound into acute care areas, had developed a qualification called the Certificate in Clinician Performed Ultrasound (CCPU). There were already modules for several acute care specialties and neonatology was developed as another module. The program was developed by a steering committee consisting of mainly neonatologists from around Australia and New Zealand, which included a radiologist and a pediatric cardiologist. The qualification is based on course attendance and supervised logbooks of ultrasound scans. The trainees have to complete an on-line physics course, then the ultrasound training is in two stages, basic and advanced. Basic training is aimed at normal image acquisition of the heart and brain, while advanced training is aimed at interpretation of abnormal hemodynamic and cerebral findings, as well as learning some other aspects of neonatal POCU such as basic abdominal organ imaging and central line localization. The core part of training is undertaken within the neonatal unit under the supervision of a qualified POCU clinician who can also teach the skills of integration of the ultrasound and clinical findings. The advanced module includes training in recognition of common CHD with the understanding that the ability to exclude CHD will require further training under the supervision of pediatric cardiology. The expectation is that only a few neonatologists undertake this extra training and others will continue to consult with pediatric cardiology colleagues to exclude structural cardiac abnormalities. This program has been running since 2007, and there are more than 60 graduates with the CCPU (neonatal) and 40 trainees currently undertaking training. The Australasian CCPU was the first and, to the best of our knowledge, is still the only dedicated and functioning neonatal point of care training and accreditation program.[10]

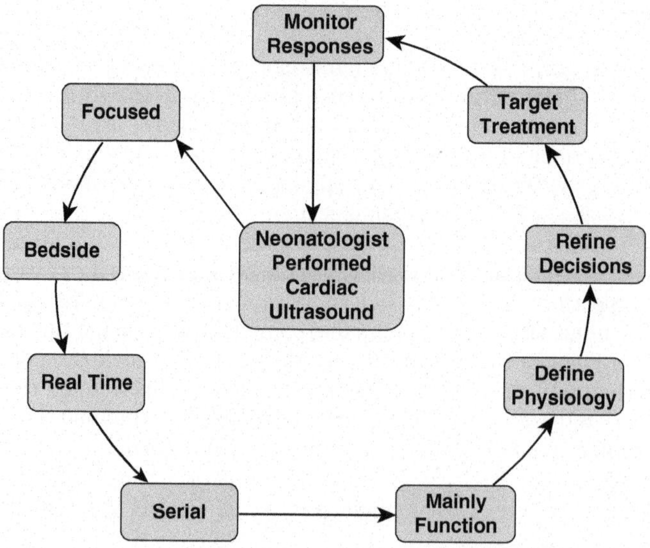

Fig. 10.1 Diagrammatic representation of the process of use of point of care ultrasound, diagnosing physiology, integrating into the clinical decision making, and obtaining longitudinal feedback to validate treatment decisions made. (Modified from Kluckow 2015 *Arch Dis Child* 99(4):F332-F337, 2014.)

Consensus statements on neonatal cardiac ultrasound training have been published from North America and Europe and the United Kingdom.[7,11] Both of these statements take a different focus with an emphasis on training within pediatric cardiology. Neither of these statements addresses the wider role for neonatal POCU beyond the heart. The development of national or regional administered structured training programs under these guidelines is still in progress.

It is our view that to achieve the goal of quality assurance in standards of neonatal POCU, a training program needs to be both relevant and workable. For this to happen, the practical component of the training needs to occur mainly within the NICU and the training needs to be mainly provided by neonatologists. A core component of training is understanding how to integrate imaging skills into the other clinical information available for a particular patient. Further, the training program needs to embrace the fact that POCU in any acute care specialty embraces more than one organ.

Using Physiology to Target Treatment

A key use of POCU in the clinical setting is to help understand the underlying physiology and subsequently to more accurately decide on what treatment is most useful for the individual patient. An illustration of the process of identifying individual physiology in a focused ultrasound, applying this information, and assessing the outcome of treatment choices is shown in Fig. 10.1. This targeting of treatment with the ability to longitudinally monitor response is the way we most often use POCU and is best demonstrated by some case presentations.

CASE STUDY 1

Thirty-eight-week gestation, emergency lower segment caesarean section (LSCS) for maternal pre-eclampsia. Clear amniotic fluid. Respiratory distress from birth with increasing oxygen requirement requiring CPAP at 7–8 cm H_2O. By 6 hours of age, requiring 0.75 FiO_2 to maintain arterial O_2 saturation of >85%. At 6.5 hours, sudden deterioration with arterial O_2 saturations below 80% in FIO_2 1.0. Chest x-ray (CXR) showed some centralized opacification in both

CASE STUDY 1—cont'd

lung fields and a small right-sided pneumothorax. Options considered include mechanical ventilation, needle drainage of pneumothorax, and use of inhaled nitric oxide (iNO). As oxygen requirements were out of proportion to CXR and labile clinical state, iNO was the favored clinical option. Prior to commencement of iNO, a POCU was performed.

Findings: See Fig. 10.2.

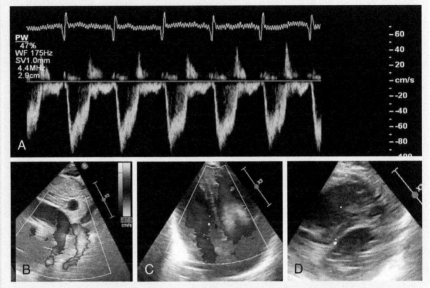

Fig. 10.2 **Findings for case study 1.** (A) Parasternal view—Normal right ventricular output. (B) Ductal view—No patent ductus arteriosus. (C) Subcostal view—Good contractility and no evidence of tricuspid incompetence. (D) Parasternal short axis—normal right ventricle. Normal cardiac anatomy—later confirmed by cardiology.

OUTCOME CASE STUDY 1

Cardiac POCU showed no evidence of raised pulmonary pressures with normal cardiovascular function. Consequently, no iNO was administered. There was an attempted needle aspiration of pneumothorax—no air recovered. Mechanical ventilation was transitioned to high-frequency ventilation, given surfactant, a lung recruitment strategy was used and CO_2 controlled with a gradual improvement in FIO_2 requirements. Rapid recovery in 12–18 hours. Case illustrates that sometimes POCU supports a clinical decision to not introduce specific therapies such as iNO.

CASE STUDY 2

Twenty-five-week gestation, incomplete antenatal steroid coverage. Initial CPAP at 6 cm H_2O. Intubated and given surfactant at 2 hours of age due to increasing oxygen requirements (0.35 FIO_2). Given intravenous antibiotics. Rapidly extubated back to CPAP 6 cm H_2O in air. Now 10 hours old and increasing FIO_2 to >0.40 with borderline blood pressure (mean BP = 25 mm Hg). CPAP increased to 7 cm H_2O with transient improvement. CXR shows well-expanded lungs. Options considered were to re-ventilate and give further surfactant, wait for further improvement, or gain more clinical information from a POCU.

CASE STUDY 2—cont'd

Findings: See Fig. 10.3.

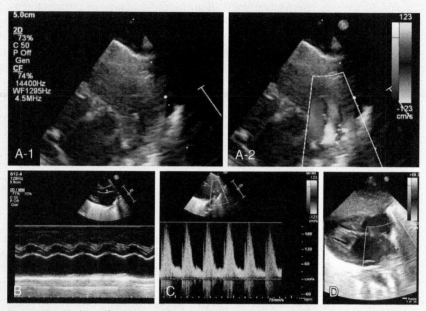

Fig. 10.3 Findings for case study 2. (A-1) 2D Ductal view. (A-2) Color Doppler ductal view—Large patent ductus arteriosus measuring 2.5 mm, unconstricted. Left to right shunt. (B) Dilated left atrium (LA: Aortic ratio = 1:2.2). (C) Ductal view Doppler—High velocity pulsatile pattern. (D) Parasternal views—Large left to right shunt at patent foramen ovale. In addition, there was reverse flow in diastole in the descending aorta and increased diastolic flow in the left pulmonary artery.

OUTCOME CASE STUDY 2

Cardiac POCU showed evidence of an unconstricted large left-to-right ductal shunt with added left-to-right shunt at the patent foramen ovale (PFO). There were also signs of increased pulmonary blood flow and impairment of systemic blood flow (SBF). Early targeted treatment with indomethacin at 0.2 mg/kg was started to attempt patent ductus arteriosus (PDA) closure. Cardiac POCU 24 hours later showed a closed PDA and return of the hemodynamic state to normal. There was concurrent improvement in ventilation requirements with decreasing FIO_2 and CPAP pressure requirements. Case illustrates that a small number of infants (particularly <26 weeks, incomplete steroid cover) still have early symptomatic PDA that has the potential to respond well to early treatment.

CASE STUDY 3

Term baby born in perinatal center by elective cesarean section admitted at 2 hours with persisting mild tachypnea. Normal cardiovascular examination and CXR shows normal heart size and changes consistent with transient tachypnea of the newborn. Cultured, started on antibiotics, and nursed in 25% oxygen. At 48 hours, still tachypneic with mild increased work of breathing. CXR unchanged and normal cardiac examination. Decision to perform a POCU. Performed by fellow in training with POCU certified neonatologist to review.

Findings: See Fig. 10.4.

CASE STUDY 3—cont'd

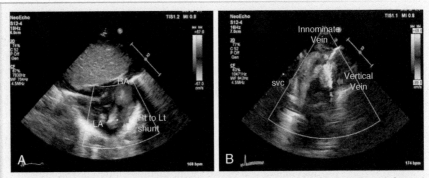

Fig. 10.4 **Findings for case study 3.** (A) Subcostal four-chamber view—Right to left atrial shunt noted by fellow. (B) Suprasternal coronal posterior view—Ascending vertical vein to innominate vein consistent with supra-diaphragmatic total anomalous pulmonary venous drainage (unobstructed) confirmed by a cardiologist. *LA,* Left atrial; *RA,* right atrial; *SVC,* superior vena cava.

OUTCOME CASE STUDY 3

Fellow confirmed a structurally normal heart but unsure of pulmonary veins and found a pure right-to-left shunt across the PFO. Knowing the latter could be a marker of CHD, requested early review by neonatologist who confirmed total anomalous venous drainage. Immediate consult and transfer to pediatric cardiology center where diagnosis confirmed and successful surgery undertaken. Case highlights the importance of nonspecific ultrasound markers in recognizing CHD and potential of POCU in early diagnosis of clinically unsuspected CHD.

CASE STUDY 4

Known case of prolonged oligohydramnios due to premature rupture of membranes at 20 weeks' gestation. Presented in labor at 30 weeks' gestation, delivery by cesarean section due to breech position. Baby born with limb contractures and lungs very stiff at resuscitation. Just adequate oxygenation achieved with surfactant, 100% oxygen, and high-pressure conventional ventilation at 35/5 cm H_2O of PIP/PEEP. Transfer to NICU. Rapid POCU of lungs (to exclude pneumothorax) and heart performed by neonatologist while awaiting CXR.

Findings: See Fig. 10.5.

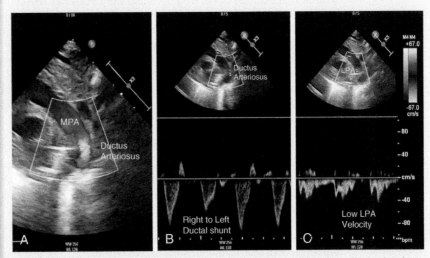

Fig. 10.5 **Findings for case study 4.** (A) Ductal view color Doppler—Showed right to left ductal shunt. (B) Ductal view pulsed Doppler—Showed right to left ductal shunt. (C) Ductal view left pulmonary artery (LPA)—Showed very low velocity consistent with low pulmonary blood flow. *MPA,* Main pulmonary artery.

CASE STUDY 4—cont'd

> OUTCOME CASE STUDY 4
>
> Ultrasound of lungs confirmed no pneumothorax. Cardiac ultrasound showed low pulmonary blood flow and pulmonary hypertension with pure right-to-left ductal shunt and mainly right-to-left atrial shunt. Inhaled NO started by 45 minutes of age. Oxygen requirements and ventilator pressures fell over next 30 minutes to 25% oxygen and pressures of 20/5. Repeat cardiac ultrasound showed bidirectional ductal shunt and increased left pulmonary artery (LPA) velocities. Baby extubated to CPAP by 48 hours. Case highlights that POCU is not just about the heart and the use of POCU to define persistent pulmonary hypertension of the newborn (PPHN) as the primary problem, allowing very early treatment targeted at actual rather than presumed physiology.

Uses of Point of Care Ultrasound in the Neonatal Intensive Care Unit

While the focus of this book (and so this chapter) is on the cardiovascular system, it must be emphasized that the value of POCU extends well beyond the heart to include many organ systems as well as procedural uses such as long line placement. Therefore, a brief review of these other uses is included.

M-mode and two-dimensional (2D) imaging results from ultrasound waves reflecting off solid or liquid interfaces of different density to allow definition of a structure. In the heart, this is the interface between muscle, fiber, and blood. Projection of these structures against time allows definition of movement within the cardiac cycle, both of the structures themselves, but also relative to other structures. The Doppler principle can be applied to ultrasound waves because they change frequency as they reflect off moving objects; in the case of the heart and blood vessels, these are the red blood cells. From this change of frequency, both the direction and the velocity of the blood can be derived. Color Doppler maps this direction and the velocity of blood onto the 2D image. Measurement of movement from 2D and M-mode is the basis of most myocardial function tests. Doppler allows identification of the presence of shunts as well as the direction and velocity of shunt flow. Measurement of velocity also allows estimation of pressure gradient using the modified Bernoulli equation ($dP = 4V^2$). Measuring these pressure gradients across the tricuspid valve or a PDA allows estimation of pulmonary artery pressure. Flow measurements, such as ventricular outputs, can be derived by integrating vessel cross-sectional area (using 2D or M-mode), mean velocity, and heart rate. By putting all this together, cardiac ultrasound allows understanding of the complete hemodynamic presentation and allows treatment targeted at that hemodynamic pattern.

In general terms, the traditional clinical pointers to circulatory failure are limited in their accuracy and often only become reliably abnormal when the hemodynamic pathology is well established.[12] In other words, the problem will often be identified late. Because of this, the best use of cardiac ultrasound is proactively in defined high-risk clinical situations.

The immediate postnatal period

Babies with signs of circulatory failure in the immediate postresuscitation period are usually asphyxiated, hypovolemic, or, occasionally, both. This is often, but not exclusively, seen in term babies. These two main pathologies can be difficult to differentiate on clinical grounds.

Asphyxia is diagnosed on the basis of the usual markers: fetal distress, low Apgar scores, need for resuscitation, and lactic acidosis seen in measurement of the umbilical cord arterial blood. Such babies will appear pale and shutdown in the immediate postresuscitation period and, in many, this will improve in time with resolution of the acidosis. However, some of these babies remain at risk of circulatory failure due to compromised myocardial function and abnormal peripheral vasoregulation.[13] While recognizing the importance of initially attending to respiratory, metabolic, and neurological homeostasis and neuroprotection, an early cardiac ultrasound to assess myocardial function and SBF with measurement of superior vena cava (SVC) flow and right ventricular (RV) output may allow early direction of appropriate circulatory support (see Chapters 28 and 29). This postresuscitation pallor needs to be differentiated from hypovolemia, which is rare, but the immediate postnatal period is the most likely time when there can be life-threatening hypovolemia. The causes of perinatal hypovolemia are often clinically occult at the time of resuscitation and include vasa previa, feto-placental hemorrhage, and acute feto-fetal and feto-maternal hemorrhage. All these can be acute or chronic and, when chronic, the problem is anemia, not hypovolemia. Cardiac ultrasound allows immediate differentiation of the well-filled poorly contractile asphyxiated heart from the poorly filled hypovolemic heart, which, in turn, can be differentiated from the dilated hyperdynamic heart which results from chronic fetal anemia. Appropriate treatment can then be provided.

Circulatory transition in the very preterm baby

The early transitional period is one of exquisite circulatory vulnerability for the very preterm infant and 10% to 20% of babies born before 30 weeks' gestation will have a period of low SBF.[14] The causes of this are complex and relate to many factors including immaturity, nonspecific or specific inflammatory responses, positive pressure ventilation, and shunts out of the systemic circulation through the fetal channels, mainly the ductus arteriosus (see Chapters 1, 6, 26, and 29). Low SBF is predictive of mortality and a range of morbidities.[15] Low SBF develops during the first 12 hours and then improves spontaneously in almost all babies by 24 hours. Early detection depends on prospective measures of SBF (most frequently by cardiac ultrasound) during the high-risk period of the first 12 hours because low SBF is poorly predicted by clinical parameters including blood pressure (see Chapter 26). In our own services, we perform prospective cardiac ultrasound from 3 to 6 hours of age with a focus on measures of SBF using SVC flow and RV output in all preterm neonates born before 28 weeks' gestation. In addition, we screen preterm neonates born after 27 weeks' gestation with higher risk for low SBF, for example, limited exposure to antenatal steroids and/or with RDS requiring significant ventilator support. We would also use reactive cardiac ultrasound in any baby with severely or persistently low blood pressure or other clinical signs of circulatory compromise. With the latter group, it is important to highlight that low SBF is uncommon in preterm babies after 24 hours unless critically unwell and most hypotension after this time is vasodilatory, for example, low blood pressure presents with normal or high SBF. This highlights the illogicality of a standard treatment for all preterm hypotension, as the correct treatment for pump failure will often be the wrong treatment for loss of vascular tone, and vice versa (see Chapters 26 and 29).

These cardiac ultrasound examinations should also include the common assessments used for pulmonary hypertension (described later). Severe pulmonary hypertension is uncommon as a primary pathology in preterm babies, but can occur in certain subgroups, in particular it is almost universal in babies born after premature prolonged rupture of membranes and oligohydramnios.[16,17]

Assessment for PDA

Assessment of the ductus arteriosus should be a part of all preterm neonatal cardiac ultrasound whether it be proactive during circulatory transition or reactive in response to clinical signs. Ultrasound allows estimation of the two main factors determining the significance of a PDA: that is, the diameter (or degree of constriction) using color Doppler and/or 2D imaging as well as the pressure gradient across the ductus from the Doppler-derived flow direction and velocity. Additional information on shunt significance can be derived from the change in diastolic flow at either side of the ductus in the descending aorta and the LPA. A significant left-to-right ductal shunt causes reversed diastolic flow in the former and exaggerated forward diastolic flow in the latter. How to use this information to determine whether to treat a PDA is another whole topic and is addressed in Chapters 22 to 25. However, it is important to highlight here that early postnatal constriction of the ductus arteriosus predicts early spontaneous closure and may be a useful guide to the need for early treatment.[18]

The septic baby

Cardiac ultrasound is useful for determining the hemodynamics in suspected or proven sepsis with measures of SBF and assessment for pulmonary hypertension. The hemodynamic compromise of late-onset sepsis is almost always vasodilatory (low BP but normal or high SBF) in the newborn.[19,20] In advanced septic shock, evidence of tissue ischemia can persist despite normalization of systemic hemodynamics. Although little studied in the newborn, this may be due to the microvascular dysfunction described in older subjects with sepsis (see Chapter 19). The hemodynamics of early-onset sepsis is more variable. It can be vasodilatory, but pulmonary hypertension can be a significant factor particularly in early-onset group B streptococcal pneumonia. Assessment and management of neonatal sepsis and shock is discussed in Chapter 27.

Suspected PPHN

This is usually a term or late preterm baby with high ventilator/oxygen requirements. Not all babies with high ventilator/oxygen requirements have pulmonary hypertension. The hemodynamics are as varied as the underlying pathologies and need to be assessed individually with cardiac ultrasound. It is particularly important that CHD is excluded immediately upon presentation in these babies, and this may require cardiology consultation. Transposition of the great arteries and total anomalous pulmonary venous drainage can both masquerade as pulmonary hypertension. Pulmonary artery pressure can be estimated from the pressure gradient across the tricuspid valve or, if patent, the ductus arteriosus. The direction of shunting across the ductus arteriosus and foramen ovale can be assessed. These babies are at high risk for low SBF particularly during the first 24 hours.[21] In some, the low SBF probably results, at least in part, from the negative circulatory effect of high positive intrathoracic pressure during the period of circulatory transition. In most babies with low pulmonary blood flow PPHN, the systemic compromise is the consequence of the restricted pulmonary blood flow and will improve if the pulmonary vascular resistance can be reduced with iNO or other vasodilators. Pulmonary blood flow can be estimated using Doppler velocity in the LPA. Babies with primary PPHN often have low LPA velocities reflecting the fact that blood is bypassing the lungs. This low pulmonary blood flow hemodynamic predicts the oxygenation response to iNO.[22,23] Assessment and management of the infant with PPHN is discussed in more detail in Chapter 9.

Babies presenting with collapse/shock

Babies with primary cardiac problems can also present as circulatory failure. This presentation is not common, but must be considered in any baby presenting with shock. Because neonatologists using cardiac POCU spend most of their time examining structurally normal hearts, the ability to spot a heart that is not structurally normal and which needs an expert opinion comes quite early in the learning process. So, the reality is that in a hospital without an on-site pediatric cardiology service, cardiac POCU can be useful for rapid/early diagnosis of primary cardiac conditions such as ductal dependent CHD, cardiomyopathies, or myocarditis. It can be lifesaving in patients without CHD; for example, babies have died from central venous long line tips misplaced in the heart, perforating the atrial wall and causing tamponade.[24] These babies die because this is a clinically occult diagnosis, often made at autopsy. With ultrasound, it is an obvious diagnosis, even to an inexpert eye, and needs an immediate pericardiocentesis and line removal or repositioning.

In newborn transport

Many of the above issues are brought into focus in babies who need retrieval from smaller hospitals to a center with a NICU. These are a particularly high-risk group.

Preterm babies needing ex utero transfer tend to be born after precipitate delivery, without full antenatal steroid cover, and might have received inexperienced resuscitation and early management. Their high risk reflects in worse outcome. More mature babies often present with unexpected respiratory failure/PPHN, asphyxia, or both. Sometimes these babies have acute presentations, which may be cardiac in origin. Increasing portability of ultrasound equipment creates the opportunity to take imaging equipment on transport. Our group has recently completed a prospective observational study of point of care cardiac and cerebral ultrasound in the transport of about 100 sick newborns across New South Wales, Australia.[25] We showed that POCU in newborn transport is feasible and, in the late preterm/term group of babies, we confirmed a high incidence of clinically unsuspected hemodynamic compromise as well as several patients with CHD who had been diagnosed clinically as PPHN, and in whom transport was re-directed to a cardiac center. In preterm neonates, there was an even higher incidence of hemodynamic abnormalities, particularly low SBF. There are clearly challenges to implementing this practice on a wider basis, most specifically with having equipment and skills available for the transport. The portability of ultrasound equipment continues to improve with tablet-sized machines available with adequate resolution and more neonatologists are learning ultrasound skills, particularly those now in training. It is now unusual for neonatologists in Australia and New Zealand to qualify without appropriate ultrasound skills. It would seem inevitable that neonatal retrieval is another area where POCU will become commonplace in the not too distant future.

Avoiding Inappropriate Therapy and Weaning

Much research time and energy has been spent on developing guidelines for commencing extra therapy in response to hemodynamic complications and abnormal physiology. However, one of the very important uses of POCU is to allow the physician to decide when expensive and potentially harmful therapies may not be required. Case study 1 illustrates a common scenario we observe where there is what appears to be clinical evidence of PPHN with high oxygen requirements and lability, but without ultrasound evidence of raised pulmonary pressures or right-to-left ductal shunting (the duct may often be closed).[21] Inhaled NO in this setting has a high chance of being ineffective and may cause harm by changing the vascular resistance in a baby with balanced physiology. Other examples might include excessive use of volume in an infant who already has adequate cardiac filling/preload or use of vasopressor-inotropes in a baby with a low blood pressure but normal cardiac output.[26] Similarly deciding when to wean an infant with significant hemodynamic support can be assisted by POCU. Key information, such as identifying when the cardiac function has improved to start weaning inotropes or when the pulmonary pressures have dropped and the PDA shunt direction is becoming predominantly left-to-right to allow weaning of iNO or when the PDA has closed to limit exposure to nonsteroidal anti-inflammatory drugs (NSAID),[27] is available in real time to the clinician. This new way of managing the individual infant now has a name—precision or personalized medicine.[28]

Other uses of neonatal POCU

Neonatal ultrasound tends to be focused on the heart and brain but the point of care possibilities extend to many other organ systems. Even with cerebral ultrasound, which is often not considered an acute imaging area, there are important rapid diagnoses in the acutely deteriorated infant that can be made with POCU, particularly with large symptomatic intraventricular or subdural hemorrhages. There is an increasing interest in lung ultrasound where the absence of the normal airspace ultrasound artifact allows diagnosis of pulmonary edema or collapse.[29] Ultrasound can be used to localize endotracheal tube tip position as well as to diagnose pneumothorax.[30,31] It is invaluable in diagnosing pleural effusions and also in monitoring the effectiveness of drainage of effusions, particularly in congenital chylothoraces where maintenance of effective drainage can be difficult.

Abdominal ultrasound also has a range of point of care possibilities from something as simple as identifying that there is urine in the bladder prior to performing suprapubic urine sampling to diagnosis of necrotizing enterocolitis (NEC). With ultrasound, it is possible to identify free peritoneal fluid, to assess bowel motility, and to see gas in the bowel wall in NEC.[32] Liver ultrasound is useful to ensure that the umbilical venous catheter (UVC) tip has advanced beyond the liver, as well as observing portal venous gas in NEC and diagnosing the rare but serious complication of intrahepatic UVC extravasation. Ultrasound is also a useful addition to x-ray in PICC line tip localization; most specifically, one can ultrasound the appropriate cavo-atrial junction to ensure that the tip is not in the heart and avoid the tamponade risk described previously.[33] In addition, line insertion time, number of manipulations, time to XR confirmation of placement, and radiation exposure can be significantly reduced if real-time POCU is used.[34]

In older subjects, POCU is widely used in procedures such as venous access for long line placement. This use has not had as much penetration, particularly in preterm neonatology, but visualizing the small vessels of a preterm baby becomes possible with the resolution achievable with the high-frequency transducers now available.

Does Point of Care Ultrasound Make a Difference?

Introduction of a new diagnostic imaging technology is often accompanied by calls for validation and justification of the cost.[4] Ultrasound machines are large and costly, though in the past few years there has been reduction both in size and in cost, such that portable tablet-sized machines are now affordable to most NICUs. Training in ultrasound also entails a significant time commitment. The introduction of POCU is different from introducing a new, high-level diagnostic imaging modality. It is the additive improvement in care that comes from having ultrasound easily available to help with treatment choices which needs to be measured. There are several randomized trials that have used POCU in the decision making within the protocol and demonstrated improved outcomes. These include indomethacin dose minimization during PDA treatment,[27] identification of infants at high risk of pulmonary hemorrhage and reducing risk by early PDA treatment,[35] prevention of postoperative cardiorespiratory lability following PDA ligation,[36] and others who have used PDA treatment targeted to improve short-term outcomes.[37] In addition, there are a number of services which have published the results of auditing the introduction of this practice—generally these audits have shown benefits ranging from discovery of unexpected findings to avoidance of planned interventions.[38,39]

Other medical craft groups (anesthetists, intensivists, emergency physicians) have adopted POCU as part of clinical practice and there is a significant body of literature supporting use in children and adults in the intensive care setting. The approach in this setting has been on a focused assessment with specific aims or goals specified.[40] This is similar to the way that POCU is taught in Australia/New Zealand.

Conclusions

The use of POCU in the care of sick and preterm neonates is rapidly expanding. The benefits of a portable, bedside technique that is able to provide real-time, longitudinal data regarding the physiology of individual patients are being progressively recognized. The role of POCU in managing the transitioning term or preterm infant, the septic/asphyxiated infant, the shocked or hypotensive infant, and infants with suspected PPHN or CHD is increasingly recognized. With the acceptance of the usefulness of ultrasound in the clinical setting, the need for appropriate training programs and accreditation increases. Internationally, countries have adopted different approaches to these needs. In Australia/New Zealand, a training program based on modular education with periods of self-directed learning under the supervision of an accredited and experienced neonatologist has been adopted. This has led to an almost universal take-up of ultrasound training in neonatal trainees with a subsequent wide distribution of ultrasound skills in most NICUs in Australia/New Zealand.

10

REFERENCES

1. Plomgaard AM, van Oeveren W, Petersen TH, et al.: The SafeBoosC II randomized trial: treatment guided by near-infrared spectroscopy reduces cerebral hypoxia without changing early biomarkers of brain injury, *Pediatr Res* 79(4):528–535, 2016.
2. Kluckow M, Seri I, Evans N, et al.: Echocardiography and the neonatologist, *Pediatr Cardiol* 29(6):1043–1047, 2008.
3. Kluckow M, Evans N: Point of care ultrasound in the NICU-training, accreditation and ownership, *Eur J Pediatr* 175(2):289–290, 2016.
4. Mertens L: Neonatologist performed echocardiography-hype, hope or nope, *Eur J Pediatr* 175(2):291–293, 2016.
5. Nguyen J, Cascione M, Noori S: Analysis of lawsuits related to point-of-care ultrasonography in neonatology and pediatric subspecialties, *J Perinatol* 36(9):784–786, 2016.
6. Evans NJ: Functional echocardiography in the neonatal intensive care unit. In Kleinman CS, Seri I, editors: *Hemodynamics and Cardiology*, vol. 2, Philadelphia, 2012, Elsevier, pp 95–123.
7. Mertens L, Seri I, Marek J, et al.: Targeted neonatal echocardiography in the neonatal intensive care unit: practice guidelines and recommendations for training, *Eur J Echocardiogr* 12(10):715–736, 2011.
8. Marin JR, Lewiss RE: American Academy of Pediatrics CoPEM, Society for Academic Emergency Medicine AoEU, American College of Emergency Physicians PEMC, World Interactive Network Focused on Critical U. Point-of-care ultrasonography by pediatric emergency medicine physicians, *Pediatrics* 135(4):e1113–e1122, 2015.
9. Marin JR, Lewiss RE, American Academy of Pediatrics CoPEM, et al.: Point-of-care ultrasonography by pediatric emergency physicians. Policy statement, *Ann Emerg Med* 65(4):472–478, 2015.
10. *Australasian Society for ultrasound in medicine: certificate in clinician performed ultrasound*, 2013.
11. Singh Y, Gupta S, Groves AM, et al.: Expert consensus statement "Neonatologist-performed Echocardiography (NoPE)"-training and accreditation in UK, *Eur J Pediatr* 175(2):281–287, 2016.
12. Osborn DA, Evans N, Kluckow M: Clinical detection of low upper body blood flow in very premature infants using blood pressure, capillary refill time, and central-peripheral temperature difference, *Arch Dis Child Fetal Neonatal Ed* 89(2):F168–F173, 2004.
13. Cetin I, Kantar A, Unal S, et al.: The assessment of time-dependent myocardial changes in infants with perinatal hypoxia, *J Matern Fetal Neonatal Med* 25(9):1564–1568, 2012.
14. Kluckow M, Evans N: Low systemic blood flow in the preterm infant, *Semin Neonatol* 6(1):75–84, 2001.
15. Osborn DA, Evans N, Kluckow M: Hemodynamic and antecedent risk factors of early and late peri-ventricular/intraventricular hemorrhage in premature infants, *Pediatrics* 112(1 Pt 1):33–39, 2003.
16. Semberova J, O'Donnell SM, Franta J, et al.: Inhaled nitric oxide in preterm infants with prolonged preterm rupture of the membranes: a case series, *J Perinatol* 35(4):304–306, 2015.
17. Shah DM, Kluckow M: Early functional echocardiogram and inhaled nitric oxide: usefulness in managing neonates born following extreme preterm premature rupture of membranes (PPROM), *J Paediatr Child Health* 47(6):340–345, 2011.
18. Kluckow M, Evans N: Early echocardiographic prediction of symptomatic patent ductus arteriosus in preterm infants undergoing mechanical ventilation, *J Pediatr* 127(5):774–779, 1995.
19. de Waal K, Evans N: Hemodynamics in preterm infants with late-onset sepsis, *J Pediatr* 156(6): 918.e1–922.e1, 2010.
20. Saini SS, Kumar P, Kumar RM: Hemodynamic changes in preterm neonates with septic shock: a prospective observational study, *Pediatr Crit Care Med* 15(5):443–450, 2014.
21. Evans N, Kluckow M, Currie A: Range of echocardiographic findings in term neonates with high oxygen requirements, *Arch Dis Child Fetal Neonatal Ed* 78(2):F105–F111, 1998.
22. Roze JC, Storme L, Zupan V, et al.: Echocardiographic investigation of inhaled nitric oxide in new-born babies with severe hypoxaemia, *Lancet* 344(8918):303–305, 1994.
23. Desandes R, Desandes E, Droulle P, et al.: Inhaled nitric oxide improves oxygenation in very prema-ture infants with low pulmonary blood flow, *Acta Paediatr* 93(1):66–69, 2004.
24. Kabra NS, Kluckow MR: Survival after an acute pericardial tamponade as a result of percutaneously inserted central venous catheter in a preterm neonate, *Indian J Pediatr* 68(7):677–680, 2001.
25. Browning Carmo K, Lutz T, Berry A, et al.: Feasibility and utility of portable ultrasound during retrieval of sick term and late preterm infants, *Acta Paediatr* 2016.
26. Kluckow M, Evans N: Relationship between blood pressure and cardiac output in preterm infants requiring mechanical ventilation, *J Pediatr* 129(4):506–512, 1996.
27. Carmo KB, Evans N, Paradisis M: Duration of indomethacin treatment of the preterm patent ductus arteriosus as directed by echocardiography, *J Pediatr* 155(6):819–822, 2009.
28. Cahan A, Cimino JJ: Improving precision medicine using individual patient data from trials, *CMAJ* 2016.
29. Cattarossi L: Lung ultrasound: its role in neonatology and pediatrics, *Early Hum Dev* 89(Suppl 1):S17–S19, 2013.
30. Skinner JR: Detection of pneumothorax in the preterm infant with ultrasound, *J Paediatr Child Health* 52(12):1122, 2016.
31. Raimondi F, Rodriguez Fanjul J, Aversa S, et al.: Lung ultrasound for diagnosing pneumothorax in the critically ill neonate, *J Pediatr* 175:74.e1–78.e1, 2016.
32. Aliev MM, Dekhqonboev AA, Yuldashev RZ: Advantages of abdominal ultrasound in the manage-ment of infants with necrotizing enterocolitis, *Pediatr Surg Int* 2016.

33. Jain A, McNamara PJ, Ng E, et al.: The use of targeted neonatal echocardiography to confirm placement of peripherally inserted central catheters in neonates, *Am J Perinatol* 29(2):101–106, 2012.
34. Katheria AC, Fleming SE, Kim JH: A randomized controlled trial of ultrasound-guided peripherally inserted central catheters compared with standard radiograph in neonates, *J Perinatol* 33(10):791–794, 2013.
35. Kluckow M, Jeffery M, Gill A, et al.: A randomised placebo-controlled trial of early treatment of the patent ductus arteriosus, *Arch Dis Child Fetal Neonatal Ed* 99(2):F99–F104, 2014.
36. Jain A, Sahni M, El-Khuffash A, et al.: Use of targeted neonatal echocardiography to prevent postoperative cardiorespiratory instability after patent ductus arteriosus ligation, *J Pediatr* 160(4):584–589, 2012.
37. O'Rourke DJ, El-Khuffash A, Moody C, et al.: Patent ductus arteriosus evaluation by serial echocardiography in preterm infants, *Acta Paediatr* 97(5):574–578, 2008.
38. El-Khuffash A, Herbozo C, Jain A, et al.: Targeted neonatal echocardiography (TnECHO) service in a Canadian neonatal intensive care unit: a 4-year experience, *J Perinatol* 33(9):687–690, 2013.
39. Harabor A, Soraisham AS: Utility of targeted neonatal echocardiography in the management of neonatal illness, *J Ultrasound Med* 34(7):1259–1263, 2015.
40. Via G, Hussain A, Wells M, et al.: International evidence-based recommendations for focused cardiac ultrasound, *J Am Soc Echocardiogr* 27(7):683.e1–683.e33, 2014.

CHAPTER 11

Assessment of Systemic Blood Flow and Myocardial Function in the Neonatal Period Using Ultrasound

Eirik Nestaas, Drude Fugelseth, and Beate Horsberg Eriksen

11

- Echocardiography is useful for the assessment of systemic blood flow and myocardial function.
- Systemic blood flow is a dynamic, complex variable.
- Blood flow through persistent fetal shunts influences cardiac output measurements of systemic blood flow from both ventricles.
- Superior vena cava flow can be used as a surrogate measure of systemic blood flow in neonates with persistent fetal shunts.
- Fractional shortening and ejection fraction are the most commonly used indices of left ventricular cavity function.
- The assessment of right ventricular size, volumes, and function by echocardiography is controversial because of the complex geometric structure of the ventricle.
- Mitral and tricuspid annular plane systolic excursions assess the motion of the atrioventricular plane relative to the apex and are, respectively, indices of left and right ventricular systolic function.
- None of these indices of heart function are independent of load.
- It is important to interpret any (conventional) echocardiographic index of heart function in context with the clinical situation, loading conditions, and other echocardiographic indices.

Although monitoring itself cannot directly improve outcomes, it helps the intensivist to assess a patient's hemodynamic status. Reliable methods to monitor cardiovascular and hemodynamic function are important for assessing circulatory disturbances and guiding optimal therapy.[1] In clinical practice as well as in clinical research, echocardiography has been useful for this assessment. A complex integration of different echocardiographic modalities is necessary for the assessment of structure and dimension, blood flow, myocardial function, and loading conditions. Basic knowledge of physical and technical principles of the different modalities, sufficient operator skills, and experience measuring relevant echocardiographic indices—as well as a comprehensive understanding of normal physiologic and pathologic processes—are essential for the optimal use of echocardiography.[2]

Traditionally echocardiography has been used to diagnose and monitor congenital heart disease and to screen for patent ductus arteriosus (PDA), primarily in preterm neonates. It is also useful for assessment of the hemodynamic status of newborns with abnormal cardiovascular adaptation, circulatory disturbances, myocardial dysfunction, pericardial or pleural effusion, thrombosis, and for assistance with the placement of central lines.[3]

An understanding of the physiology of cardiovascular adaptation and the effect of different diseases and degrees of prematurity is a key factor for the interpretation of findings. The complex cardiorespiratory changes that take place during the transitional period from the fetal to neonatal circulation phenotype may be critical in both preterm and sick term infants. The onset of breathing promotes a rapid decrease in pulmonary vascular resistance, with a subsequent increase in pulmonary blood flow.[4] The increased pulmonary venous return increases the left heart preload and enables the left heart to handle the raised afterload following cord clamping and disconnection of the low-resistance placental circuit.[5–7] The impact of the timing of cord clamping on cardiovascular transition is discussed in Chapters 4 and 5. Although the right ventricle (RV) plays the dominant role in fetal life, the left ventricle (LV) takes over after delivery.

Closure of the fetal shunts normally starts with functional closure of the foramen ovale due to the altered pressure difference between the two sides of the heart. However, a small left-to-right shunt across the foramen ovale may persist for a while after birth. The inverted pressure difference between the aorta and the pulmonary artery after birth reverses the shunting of blood through the ductus arteriosus from right to left to left to right.[8] In term neonates, the functional closure of the ductus arteriosus normally takes place within the first 2 to 3 days of postnatal life, while the ductus venosus may persist for several days after birth.[9–11]

A variety of conditions in the perinatal period—such as asphyxia, respiratory distress, sepsis, and metabolic and hematologic diseases—can disturb the transitional phase and affect the cardiovascular system. Persistent pulmonary hypertension of the newborn (PPHN) with persistent high pulmonary vascular resistance may be due to fetal and/or perinatal hypoxia, resulting in abnormal pulmonary vascular development, responsiveness to local vascular mediators, and/or to hypoxia caused by lung disease or apnea.[12] PPHN is characterized by right-to-left shunting across the foramen ovale and ductus arteriosus and increased RV afterload, especially when ductal flow is restrictive. The latter may affect coronary blood flow and subsequently myocardial function; as a result, the decreased left ventricular filling further affects myocardial function. If left untreated, systemic circulatory failure (shock) may develop due to low systemic blood flow.[13]

Preterm infants are especially vulnerable in the transitional circulatory phase (see Chapters 1 and 26). The fetal myocardium has a higher water content and is less organized than it is later in life. The immature myocardium is dominated by mononucleated myocytes, fewer sarcomeres, and different isoforms of contractile proteins.[14–16] Consequently it is less compliant, has less contractile ability, and is less tolerant of the abrupt changes in preload and afterload at birth than the mature heart.[17–19] In preterm neonates with a PDA, the effect of the gradually increasing left-to-right ductal shunting on cardiac performance has opposite effects on the pulmonary and systemic circulation. It contributes to the increased pulmonary blood flow immediately after birth,[20] but a significant left-to-right shunt may impair systemic blood flow and cause a deterioration in cardiac performance and organ perfusion.[21]

Assessment of Systemic Blood Flow by Ultrasound

Systemic blood flow is a complex dynamic variable with rapid fluctuations caused by changes in the functional activity and metabolic demand of the different organs. Doppler echocardiography offers direct and indirect measures of systemic and organ blood flow.[22,23]

Blood flow by Doppler echocardiography is calculated as the product of the displacement of the velocity profile, called the velocity-time integral (VTI) of blood flow velocity; the cross-sectional area of the vessel at the site of the measurement; and the heart rate. VTI is measured by tracing the pulsed Doppler velocity signal and the cross-sectional area by measuring the diameter (D) and calculating the area as $\pi \times$ radius $(D/2)^2$.[24] Assuming a circular vessel with a constant cross-sectional area, blood flow (volume per time, usually mL/min) is calculated as VTI (for one heartbeat) $\times \pi \times (D/2)^2 \times$ heart rate.[25,26] A prerequisite for this calculation is a laminar parabolic flow profile representative of long, straight blood vessels under steady flow conditions. Blood flow in neonates is usually indexed by weight (mL/kg/min). In obtaining the VTI, it is important to minimize the angle of insonation and to assess the diameter with the ultrasound beam perpendicular to the vessel at the true (maximal) diameter. An inappropriate angle will underestimate the VTI and overestimate the diameter. Owing to the squaring of the radius in the formula, inaccurate measures of the diameter may have considerable influence. It is recommended to average the measurements from a minimum of five cardiac cycles in order to minimize measurement error.[27] Flow measurements are hampered by significant intra- and interobserver variability.[28]

Left Ventricular Output

Left ventricular output (LVO) reflects the systemic blood flow in the absence of ductus arteriosus shunt. LVO velocity is usually measured at the aortic valve or in the ascending aorta from an apical or suprasternal window (Fig. 11.1). The angle of insonation may be a challenge in neonates because the aorta exits the heart more horizontally in infants than in adults. A reproducible left outflow diameter is easier to achieve. There are different opinions about where to measure the diameter; from the low parasternal window at the hinge of the aortic valve cusps, at the systolic leaflet separation, or just beyond the sinus of Valsalva in the ascending aorta.[29] It is important to perform serial measures in a consistent way. Accurate measures require assessment of the VTI and cross-sectional area at the same position within the heart. Several studies have validated flow measurements by VTI and cross-sectional area against other techniques.[25,27,30,31] Importantly, LVO will overestimate systemic blood flow if there is left-to-right shunting across the ductus arteriosus; this is especially relevant in preterm infants with a large ductal flow.[26] In PPHN with a large amount of right-to-left shunting, LVO may underestimate the systemic blood flow.

Right Ventricular Output

Right ventricular output (RVO) may be a more feasible index for systemic blood flow in neonates and especially in preterm babies.[32] Even though RVO may be confounded by shunting across the foramen ovale, the atrial shunting is usually less than the ductal shunting[26]; impaired systemic blood flow is therefore extremely rare when

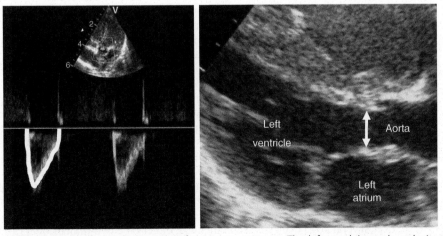

Fig. 11.1 Assessment of left ventricular output from a term neonate. The *left panel* shows the velocity time integral (VTI) of the aortic flow velocity for two heartbeats at the aortic valve's hinges from the apical four-chamber view. The *white envelope* denotes tracing the VTI of the first heartbeat. The *right panel* shows a magnified parasternal long-axis view of the left ventricle. The *white arrow* denotes the diameter of the aortic valve's "ring."

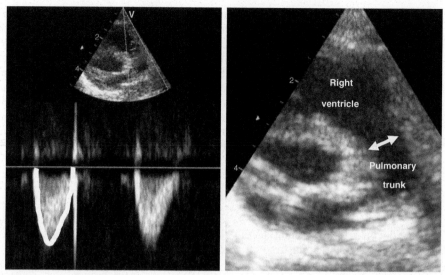

Fig. 11.2   Assessment of right ventricular output from a term neonate. The *left panel* shows the velocity time integral (VTI) of the pulmonic flow velocity for two heartbeats at the pulmonary valve from the parasternal short-axis view. The *white envelope* denotes tracing the VTI of the first heartbeat. The *right panel* shows a parasternal short-axis view of the outflow tract of the right ventricle. The *white arrow* denotes the diameter at the pulmonary valve.

the RVO is normal. Because the main pulmonary artery is directed in a posterior direction, it is usually possible to obtain an optimal insonation angle for velocity measurements from the parasternal view (Fig. 11.2). The diameter measurement of the pulmonary artery is challenging. It is best obtained at the valve leaflet insertion from a parasternal short-axis or long-axis view.[33]

The normal cardiac output from both the left and right ventricles in neonates is in the range of 150 to 300 mL/kg/min.[26]

Superior Vena Cava Flow

Due to the influence of fetal shunts on cardiac output from both ventricles, assessment of superior vena cava (SVC) blood flow can be used as a substitute for or an additional measure of systemic blood flow.[34] As the brain is one of the main target organs for adequate perfusion, a focus on the return of blood from the upper body and brain may be justified. However, one must use caution in using SVC flow to assess brain blood flow because, contrary to the adult, only around 30% of the blood in the SVC of a preterm neonate represents blood returning from the brain (see Chapter 2). A desirable angle of insonation for Doppler velocity measurement can be obtained from the low subcostal window (Fig. 11.3). The SVC VTI often exhibits three peaks per heart cycle; one positive peak in systole, one positive peak in early diastole, and one (usually negative) peak in late diastole (during atrial systole). The original description of the technique recommends subtracting the significant negative peaks in assessing the VTI and averaging the VTI from 10 cardiac cycles because of the impact of respiration and the cardiac variations on the velocity profile (see Fig. 11.3).[34] As for the other estimates of blood flow, it is important to assess the VTI and the cross-sectional area of the vessel from the same place. The diameter is best measured at the entrance into the right atrium—just prior to the "funneling" or opening up of the vessel into the right atrium—from a long-axis low- to midparasternal view at the inlet into the right atrium (see Fig. 11.3). SVC diameter varies more in size than the great arteries and an average of the maximum and minimum diameter over several heart cycles is recommended, either on a two-dimensional (2-D) image or by use of M-mode.[34] Mean SVC flow increases from about 70 to 90 mL/kg/min from 5 to 48 hours postnatally; the normal range is suggested to be between 40 and 120 mL/kg/min.[34]

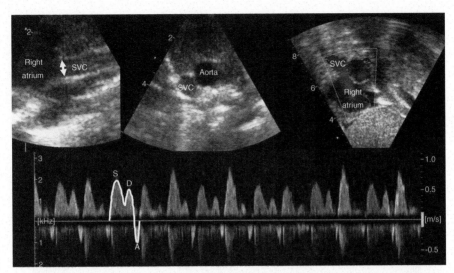

Fig. 11.3 Assessment of superior vena cava (SVC) flow. The *left upper panel* shows a modified parasternal view with a longitudinal view of the SVC entering the right atrium. The *middle panel* shows a modified parasternal view with cross-sections of the SVC and aorta. Note the ellipsoid cross-sectional shape of the SVC. The *right upper panel* shows a subcostal short-axis view of blood *(red)* entering the right atrium from the SVC. The *lower panel* shows the SVC VTI over several heart cycles. The S and D peaks denote velocity peaks of flow into the right atrium during systole *(S)* and early diastole *(D)*. The negative A wave denotes reversal of flow in the SVC during atrial systole. The *white envelope* denotes tracing the VTI of one heartbeat. *VTI,* Velocity time integral.

The technique for measuring SVC flow by ultrasound has limitations. Although Doppler measures of arterial blood flow in the central circulation have good reproducibility and correlate well with invasive measures of blood flow, it is debated whether this is also the case for venous flow. The most important methodologic problems with the assessment of SVC flow relate to the uncertainty associated with calculating the cross-sectional area of the vein. The formula presupposes a perfectly round vessel and uses the square of the vessel diameter to calculate a static cross-sectional area. These geometric presuppositions and the squaring of linear data amplify measurement errors. A modification of the technique for measuring SVC flow was recently published.[27] By interrogating SVC Doppler flow from a suprasternal window and measuring the cross-sectional area from a short-axis view where the maximum and minimum cross-sectional areas are directly traced, agreement with the magnetic resonance imaging (MRI)–derived SVC flow is better. Additionally, the measure has less inter-user variation. The middle panel of Fig. 11.3 shows the SVC in cross-section, where a direct area tracing may be measured.

No study has yet compared RVO or SVC flow by echocardiography against invasive measures in neonates. One MRI study found the SVC method to be inaccurate,[35] but others have criticized the study for not fulfilling standard criteria for repeated measurement validations.[36] Most guidelines for functional echocardiography in neonates do recommend the use of SVC flow, and it has been validated against longer-term outcomes.[2,37,38]

Cavity Measures

Calculation of cavity function indices involves assessment of changes between the largest and smallest cavity measurements in the cardiac cycle (usually systole and diastole). Indices based on percentage change between measurements or sizes describe heart function relatively independent of heart size. More geometric assumptions are a prerequisite for the estimation of cavity sizes from unidimensional measurements compared with using two-dimensional measurements.

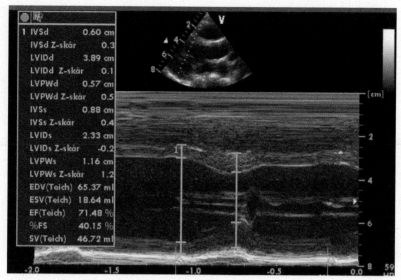

Fig. 11.4   Fractional shortening of the left ventricle assessed by M-mode from a parasternal long-axis view. The image shows assessment of the septum, internal diameter of the left ventricle, and posterior wall. The fractional shortening is the change in diameter of the left ventricular diameter relative to the diameter at end-diastole. (LVIDd-LVIDs)/LVIDd x 100. *LVIDd*, Left ventricular internal diameter in diastole; *LVIDs*, left ventricular internal diameter in systole.

Cavity Measures of the Left Ventricle

LV function indices are the most frequently used indices of heart function in neonates. Despite growing evidence of its shortcomings and low ability for detecting pathology and maturational changes,[39–44] the most frequently used cavity index in neonates is fractional shortening (FS). FS is assessed as the relative change in the internal diameter of the LV during the cardiac cycle. Diameters in systole and diastole relate closely to weight, whereas normal FS values are often 30% to 45% and exhibit little variation by weight.[39–42,45] FS can be obtained from the parasternal or subcostal views[33,46] using M-mode or two-dimensional images (Fig. 11.4). Measurements from two-dimensional recordings enable the interrogation of lines crossing the ultrasound beams (Fig. 11.5), but this also has lower time-resolution than M-mode images. The diameter is assessed perpendicular to the cavity at the tip of the mitral valve leaflets.[33] Its use as a cavity measure has, as a prerequisite, normal LV geometry and symmetric contraction, including normal septal motion.[33,46]

Ejection fraction (EF) is the fraction of end-diastolic volume ejected during systole. Guidelines[33,47] acknowledge the estimation of EF by LV cavity areas from apical four-chamber and two-chamber views at end-systole and end-diastole by the Simpson biplane method. Biplane EF has shown better discriminating capabilities than FS in neonates.[42,43] The Teich formula estimates the EF from the FS.[48] The geometric assumptions for this formula are seldom met in pathologic states, and guidelines today do not recommend reporting EF estimates from FS.[47]

Older assessment methods of EF, rarely used nowadays, include area-length methods and fractional change of LV area from apical four-chamber views.

Cavity Measures of the Right Ventricle

There are still controversies on how to assess RV size, volume, and function because of the RV's complex geometric structure, and no accepted echocardiographic gold standard is available at present.[33] Cavity measurements of the RV using ultrasound underestimate measurements by MRI, and the two modalities correlate poorly, especially in situations with volume overload.[49,50] The fractional area change assesses the relative change in RV area during contraction; it is usually obtained from an RV-focused apical four-chamber recording by counterclockwise rotation from the standard four-chamber view to expand the RV cavity to its maximum area.[47]

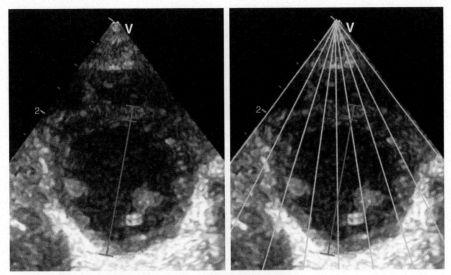

11

Fig. 11.5   Assessment of left ventricular diameter by direct measurement from a gray-scale image. The *red line* shows end-diastolic measurements from the septum, left ventricle, and posterior wall assessed in a parasternal two-dimensional short-axis image. The *green lines* illustrate how the ultrasound beams spread out in the sector from the probe. Note that assessment by two-dimensional images enables the measurement of interrogation lines crossing the ultrasound beams, as illustrated by the *red line* crossing the *green lines*.

Use of Cavity Measures

Cavity measures assess the myocardial function relative to the loading conditions and are not per se indices of the contractile properties of the myocardium. Preload has a direct impact on most diastolic cavity sizes. A high preload tends to increase diastolic sizes. The diastolic cavity sizes are the denominators in the formulas and, if isolated, this would decrease the cavity functional indices. However, high preload also increases contraction due to the Frank-Starling effect,[51] and the net effect of the increased preload is increased cavity functional indices in most clinical situations. Increased afterload tends to increase end-systolic sizes and hence to reduce the cavity functional indices. Factors within the myocardial wall can affect cavity measurements, as hypertrophic walls lead to smaller cavity measurements. The relative impact on the measurements could be higher in systole, leading to higher cavity functional indices.

Severe preload and afterload alterations will influence the measurements in different hemodynamic scenarios. A premature neonate with normal LV contractility for maturity and gestational age and with a large persistent ductus arteriosus might have LV function indices indicating normal or higher-than-normal function because of the high preload and low afterload. A neonate with normal RV contractility and PPHN might have reduced RV indices due to high afterload and possibly reduced LV indices due to low preload. In situations of reduced intrinsic myocardial contractility, cavity measures can be low in severe cases.[40] Other studies have shown that cavity measures are relatively insensitive as heart function indices in clinical situations with reduced contractility, especially for unidimensional measurements.[39,40,44,52–55]

Mitral and Tricuspid Annular Plane Systolic Excursion

The LV has a complex myocardial architecture. Fibers are principally longitudinally oriented in the subendocardial and subepicardial layers and mostly circumferentially oriented in the midmyocardial layer.[56] The intraventricular septum has a mixture of both longitudinal and circulatory fibers.[57] The longitudinal shortening of the LV relates closely to the LV stroke volume (SV) and the EF.[58–60] In the RV, longitudinal muscle fibers predominate in the free wall[57] and longitudinal shortening contributes more than circumferential shortening to overall RV function.[61,62] Thus the long-axis functions of the ventricles are important measures of global ventricular function.

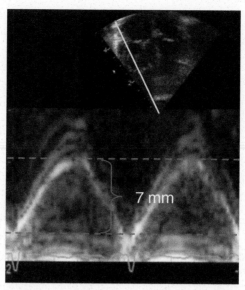

Fig. 11.6 Postprocessed M-mode tracing of tricuspid annular plane excursion in a term neonate. The *upper panel* shows the gray-scale image, with the *green line* denoting the direction of the M-mode line. The *white line* in the *lower panel* is the signal from the right lateral hinge of the atrioventricular plane in two heart cycles. The *red lines* denote the positions at end-diastole and end-systole. The distance between systolic and diastolic positions is the excursion, which is 7 mm in this example.

The base of the heart descends toward the apex in systole because of longitudinal shortening and ascends to its former position in diastole while the apex is stationary. The use of ultrasound to measure the motion of the mitral plane was first described in 1967,[63] and mitral annular plane systolic excursion (MAPSE) is now an accepted method for quantifying LV long-axis systolic function.[56,64] Reference values for MAPSE have been published for term infants.[65]

Similarly, tricuspid annular plane systolic excursion (TAPSE) reflects the longitudinal systolic function of the RV.[66] TAPSE correlates well with EF as measured by 2-D echocardiography and radionuclide angiography in adults.[67] Cross-sectional studies providing reference values for term infants have also been published.[68]

The sonographer can assess AV annular excursions using the standard M-mode technique with the interrogation line crossing the attachments of the MV (left lateral and septal MAPSE) and at the lateral attachment of the TV (TAPSE) from the four-chamber view. It is also possible to obtain the M-mode images by postprocessing two-dimensional B-mode recordings. The measurement at each hinge is the distance between the maximal backward excursion from the apex in diastole and the maximal systolic excursion in systole (Fig. 11.6). Tables 11.1 and 11.2 show reference values for MAPSE and TAPSE, respectively, in neonates.

It is important to align the M-mode cursor parallel to the motion of the annulus. Contrary to the effect on velocity using Doppler measurements, angle deviation will tend to overestimate M-mode measurements (Fig. 11.7). Because M-mode images assess excursion along the hypotenuse, the excursion will be overestimated depending on the cosine of the angle between the motion direction and the ultrasound beam. In general, angle deviation will be less in septal than in lateral recordings in apical four-chamber views due to better septal alignment with the ultrasound beam. TAPSE increases linearly with gestational age and with weight.[69]

Apart from reference values, there are also some data on TAPSE and MAPSE in pathologic conditions in neonates. TAPSE improved and MAPSE was unchanged in premature neonates with RV afterload reduction after administration of surfactant.[70] TAPSE improved following the postnatal reduction in pulmonary vascular resistance.[42,71] Finally, TAPSE was lower in term neonates with PPHN than in controls.[71]

Table 11.1 MEASUREMENTS OF MAPSE (CM) FROM THE LATERAL HINGE OF THE ATRIOVENTRICULAR PLANE BY GESTATIONAL AGE

GA	Mean − 2 SD	Mean	Mean + 2 SD
26	0.26	0.36	0.46
27	0.28	0.38	0.48
23	0.25	0.4	0.55
29	0.29	0.42	0.54
30	0.26	0.42	0.58
31	0.32	0.45	0.58
32	0.27	0.43	0.59
33	0.24	0.44	0.64
34	0.36	0.48	0.6
35	0.34	0.49	0.64
36	0.33	0.48	0.63
37	0.31	0.5	0.68
38	0.41	0.53	0.65
39	0.32	0.52	0.71
40	0.40	0.56	0.73

GA, Gestational age; *Mean − 2 SD*, mean value minus 2 standard deviations; *Mean*, mean value; *Mean + 2 SD*, mean value plus 2 standard deviations.
From Koestenberger M, Nagel B, Ravekes W, et al: Longitudinal systolic left ventricular function in preterm and term neonates: reference values of the mitral annular plane systolic excursion (MAPSE) and calculation of z-scores. *Pediatr Cardiol* 36(1):20–26, 2015.

Table 11.2 MEASUREMENTS OF TAPSE (CM) BY GESTATIONAL AGE

GA	Mean − 2 SD	Mean	Mean + 2 SD
26	0.30	0.44	0.59
27	0.36	0.48	0.61
28	0.37	0.52	0.68
29	0.41	0.57	0.73
30	0.48	0.60	0.71
31	0.53	0.63	0.74
32	0.51	0.68	0.85
33	0.58	0.70	0.83
34	0.60	0.73	0.87
35	0.61	0.74	0.88
36	0.65	0.78	0.92
37	0.68	0.82	0.96
38	0.75	0.86	0.97
39	0.77	0.90	1.02
40	0.81	0.95	1.10

GA, Gestational age; *Mean − 2 SD*, mean value minus 2 standard deviations; *Mean*, mean value; *Mean + 2 SD*, mean value plus 2 standard deviations.
From Koestenberger M, Nagel B, Ravekes W, et al: Systolic right ventricular function in preterm and term neonates: reference values of the tricuspid annular plane systolic excursion (TAPSE) in 258 patients and calculation of Z-score values. *Neonatology* 100(1):85–92, 2011.

Conclusions

The most evident scenarios for recommending the use of functional echocardiography in neonates are (1) the transitional circulation period in very premature infants, (2) the assessment of PDA beyond the early transitional period, (3) an exploration of the reasons for circulatory compromise and hypotension, and (4) the diagnosis of PPHN and its follow-up treatment. In all situations the exclusion of congenital heart defects is of considerable importance.

Transitional Period in the Very Preterm Baby

The very preterm baby is especially vulnerable to low systemic blood flow. The assessment of blood flow, left ventricular myocardial function, and signs of early ductal constriction may be helpful in guiding therapy. Because of the persistence

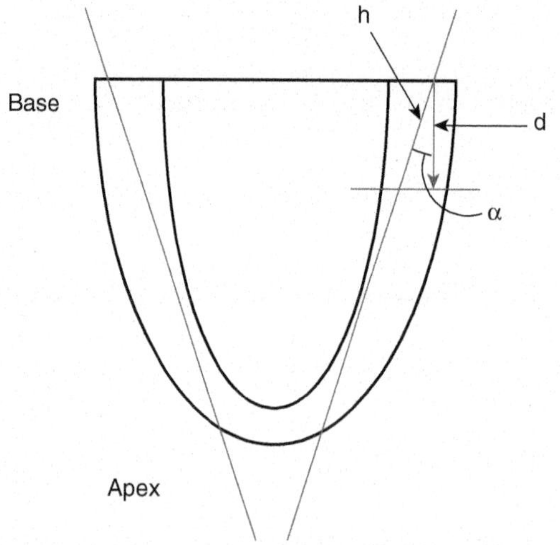

Fig. 11.7   The effect of angle error on the measured atrioventricular plane excursion. *Gray line*; direction of the ultrasound beam. *d,* True excursion; *h,* measured excursion (hypotenuse of the triangle, falsely high excursion); α, the angle error. In measurements from an M-mode image, the excursion is the hypotenuse of the triangle (h) measured along the direction of the ultrasound beam. The true excursion is the distance (d) that the AV-plane moves during systole. α is the angle between the direction of the atrioventricular plane excursion and ultrasound beam, i.e., between the vector for the true excursion (d) and the vector for the ultrasound beam (h). The excursion assessed by M-mode (h in the figure) will overestimate the true excursion (d in the figure), with a factor of $1/\cos(\alpha)$ (α = angle error); the measured excursion (h) = true excursion (d)/cos (α).

of fetal shunts that interfere with LVO measurement, sequential measurements of RVO as well as SVC flow measurements may be useful in this setting. The degree of ductal shunting may be assessed by measuring the minimum diameter from the color Doppler image and the systolic and diastolic velocity patterns of the ductal shunt signal. Cavity indices of heart function are dependent on load; they can be reduced in cases where normal circulatory adaption fails, leaving the neonate with a high pulmonary vascular resistance.

Suspected PDA Beyond the Early Transitional Period

It is always important to interpret echocardiographic indices in relation to the loading conditions. Shunting between the atria is usually smaller than shunting across the PDA. Large left-to-right ductal flow reduces right heart preload and left heart afterload and increases right heart afterload and left heart preload. The FS and aortic flow can both be normal or supranormal due to the high preload, low afterload, and (usually) high contractile state of the LV, even in cases when the shunting is so large that the systemic blood flow is impaired. Reduced aortic flow, FS, and MAPSE in combination with left-to-right PDA flow can be markers of low systemic blood flow. The situation for the right heart is the opposite. As preload becomes low and afterload increases in the presence of significant left-to-right PDA shunting, normal or subnormal pulmonary blood flow and right heart function indices are markers of normal systemic blood flow. Subnormal values are not necessarily markers of reduced systemic blood flow and reduced heart function; they might just be due to the altered loading conditions.

Circulatory Compromise in Neonates

The main determinants of heart function are preload, afterload, and intrinsic myocardial function (contractility). The task of the heart is to provide sufficient blood supply to the body to ensure adequate delivery of oxygen. When the blood flow decreases, compensatory mechanisms redistribute the blood supply to vital organs by selective vasodilatation and vasoconstriction. In this compensatory phase of shock, the blood pressure can remain normal although the blood supply to the body is low. As long as the net systemic vascular resistance is higher than normal, the blood pressure can remain normal despite reduced systemic blood flow. Assessment of systemic blood flow and the other indices discussed in this chapter can help the intensivist to identify shock in this compensatory phase, enabling intervention at an early stage. The indices discussed can also show the effects of the interventions applied, allowing feedback to the clinician as to the results of treatment decisions.

In other situations, intrinsic myocardial function is reduced. Examples include perinatal hypoxic ischemic insults, myocarditis, and cardiomyopathies. In these cases, all myocardial function indices might be reduced, and the reduction might not be due to loading conditions. In these cases, studies have shown FS to be less sensitive than other indices of left myocardial function, probably because the shape of the LV changes. Longitudinal function indices are more sensitive than FS, showing the limitations of FS as a cavity index of heart function.[40,52,54]

Persistent Pulmonary Hypertension in the Neonate

In severe cases of PPHN, the preload for the LV is low and the afterload for the RV is high, and shunting through the foramen ovale and ductus arteriosus is right to left. Systemic blood flow is usually low. FS is often normal, as the small end-diastolic size is the denominator in the estimation of FS. There are often signs of high systolic pressure in the right heart and pulmonary arteries; the RV is often dilated and the septum flattened, especially in systole.[13] Congenital heart defects (CHDs) with duct-dependent systemic circulation and PPHN share many echocardiographic findings, but treatment strategies are different. Therapies aimed at decreasing pulmonary vascular resistance are indeed adequate if PPHN is present but will reduce the systemic perfusion pressure in patients with a duct-dependent systemic circulation, with possible devastating effects on the systemic blood flow. Similarly, treatment to maintain and increase the ductal flow is adequate in patients with a duct-dependent systemic circulation but can decrease the pulmonary perfusion pressure and hence pulmonary perfusion in PPHN.

This chapter describes different indirect conventional echocardiographic methods for the assessment of heart size and function; systemic blood flow, ventricular size, and myocardial function in newborns. In line with most diagnostic tools, there is no specific single gold standard echocardiographic method or index. Evidence that functional echocardiography improves neonatal outcome is emerging in the form of audits showing changes in care and reduced use of medications such as indomethacin for PDA treatment and inotropes for borderline hypotension with normal systemic blood flow. The neonatologist must always interpret an echocardiographic index in context with other indices and the clinical situation. A combination of the different methods and indices can provide useful information about the hemodynamic situation in sick newborn infants and may help to guide management.[72]

It is important to interpret individual conventional echocardiographic indices of heart function in context with the clinical situation, loading conditions, and other echocardiographic indices. Systemic blood flow is best assessed from the aortic or pulmonary blood flow when the fetal shunts are closed. If there is a significant left-to-right shunt over either of the fetal shunts, the systemic blood flow is usually sufficient if the right heart output is within the normal range. Cavity measures of left heart function are highly dependent on load. Longitudinal indices (MAPSE and TAPSE) are promising indices of left and right heart function that await further exploration.

REFERENCES

1. Vincent JL, Rhodes A, Perel A, et al.: Clinical review: update on hemodynamic monitoring—a consensus of 16, *Crit Care* 15(4):229, 2011.
2. Mertens L, Seri I, Marek J, et al.: Targeted neonatal echocardiography in the neonatal intensive care unit: practice guidelines and recommendations for training, *Eur J Echocardiogr* 12(10):715–736, 2011.
3. Kluckow M: Use of ultrasound in the haemodynamic assessment of the sick neonate, *Arch Dis Child Fetal Neonatal Ed* 99(4):F332–337, 2014.

4. Teitel DF, Iwamoto HS, Rudolph AM: Changes in the pulmonary circulation during birth-related events, *Pediatr Res* 27(4 Pt 1):372–378, 1990.
5. Agata Y, Hiraishi S, Oguchi K, et al.: Changes in left ventricular output from fetal to early neonatal life, *J Pediatr* 119(3):441–445, 1991.
6. Bhatt S, Alison BJ, Wallace EM, et al.: Delaying cord clamping until ventilation onset improves cardiovascular function at birth in preterm lambs, *J Physiol* 591(8):2113–2126, 2013.
7. Hooper SB, Te Pas AB, Lang J, et al.: Cardiovascular transition at birth: a physiological sequence, *Pediatr Res* 77(5):608–614, 2015.
8. Mott JC: Control of the foetal circulation, *J Exp Biol* 100:129–146, 1982.
9. Fugelseth D, Lindemann R, Liestol K, et al.: Ultrasonographic study of ductus venosus in healthy neonates, *Arch Dis Child Fetal Neonatal Ed* 77(2):F131–F134, 1997.
10. Fugelseth D, Lindemann R, Liestol K, et al.: Postnatal closure of ductus venosus in preterm infants < or = 32 weeks. An ultrasonographic study, *Early Hum Dev* 53(2):163–169, 1998.
11. Kondo M, Itoh S, Kunikata T, et al.: Time of closure of ductus venosus in term and preterm neonates, *Arch Dis Child Fetal Neonatal Ed* 85(1):F57–F59, 2001.
12. Steinhorn RH: Neonatal pulmonary hypertension, *Pediatr Crit Care Med* 11(2 Suppl):S79–S84, 2010.
13. Jain A, McNamara PJ: Persistent pulmonary hypertension of the newborn: advances in diagnosis and treatment, *Semin Fetal Neonatal Med* 20(4):262–271, 2015.
14. Paradis AN, Gay MS, Zhang L: Binucleation of cardiomyocytes: the transition from a proliferative to a terminally differentiated state, *Drug Discov Today* 19(5):602–609, 2014.
15. Morrison JL, Botting KJ, Dyer JL, et al.: Restriction of placental function alters heart development in the sheep fetus, *Am J Physiol Regul Integr Comp Physiol* 293(1):R306–R313, 2007.
16. Iruretagoyena JI, Gonzalez-Tendero A, Garcia-Canadilla P, et al.: Cardiac dysfunction is associated with altered sarcomere ultrastructure in intrauterine growth restriction, *Am J Obstet Gynecol* 210(6):550, e551–e557, 2014.
17. Noori S, Friedlich P, Seri I, et al.: Changes in myocardial function and hemodynamics after ligation of the ductus arteriosus in preterm infants, *J Pediatr* 150(6):597–602, 2007.
18. Eiby YA, Lumbers ER, Headrick JP, et al.: Left ventricular output and aortic blood flow in response to changes in preload and afterload in the preterm piglet heart, *Am J Physiol Regul Integr Comp Physiol* 303(7):R769–R777, 2012.
19. Lee A, Nestaas E, Liestol K, et al.: Tissue Doppler imaging in very preterm infants during the first 24 h of life: an observational study, *Arch Dis Child Fetal Neonatal Ed* 99(1):F64–F69, 2014.
20. Noori S, Wlodaver A, Gottipati V, et al.: Transitional changes in cardiac and cerebral hemodynamics in term neonates at birth, *J Pediatr* 160(6):943–948, 2012.
21. Evans N, Moorcraft J: Effect of patency of the ductus arteriosus on blood pressure in very preterm infants, *Arch Dis Child* 67(10 Spec No):1169–1173, 1992.
22. Nishimura RA, Tajik AJ: Quantitative hemodynamics by Doppler echocardiography: a noninvasive alternative to cardiac catheterization, *Prog Cardiovasc Dis* 36(4):309–342, 1994.
23. Anavekar NS, Oh JK: Doppler echocardiography: a contemporary review, *J Cardiol* 54(3):347–358, 2009.
24. Ihlen H, Amlie JP, Dale J, et al.: Determination of cardiac output by Doppler echocardiography, *Br Heart J* 51(1):54–60, 1984.
25. Alverson DC, Eldridge M, Dillon T, et al.: Noninvasive pulsed Doppler determination of cardiac output in neonates and children, *J Pediatr* 101(1):46–50, 1982.
26. Evans N, Kluckow M: Early determinants of right and left ventricular output in ventilated preterm infants, *Arch Dis Child Fetal Neonatal Ed* 74(2):F88–F94, 1996.
27. Ficial B, Bonafiglia E, Padovani EM, et al.: A modified echocardiographic approach improves reliability of superior vena caval flow quantification, *Arch Dis Child Fetal Neonatal Ed* 102(1):F7–F11, 2017.
28. Lee A, Liestol K, Nestaas E, et al.: Superior vena cava flow: feasibility and reliability of the off-line analyses, *Arch Dis Child Fetal Neonatal Ed* 95(2):F121–F125, 2010.
29. Roman MJ, Devereux RB, Kramer-Fox R, et al.: Two-dimensional echocardiographic aortic root dimensions in normal children and adults, *Am J Cardiol* 64(8):507–512, 1989.
30. Pugsley J, Lerner AB: Cardiac output monitoring: is there a gold standard and how do the newer technologies compare? *Semin Cardiothorac Vasc Anesth* 14(4):274–282, 2010.
31. Mellander M, Sabel KG, Caidahl K, et al.: Doppler determination of cardiac output in infants and children: comparison with simultaneous thermodilution, *Pediatr Cardiol* 8(4):241–246, 1987.
32. Evans N: Which inotrope for which baby? *Arch Dis Child Fetal Neonatal Ed* 91(3):F213–F220, 2006.
33. Lopez L, Colan SD, Frommelt PC, et al.: Recommendations for quantification methods during the performance of a pediatric echocardiogram: a report from the Pediatric Measurements Writing Group of the American Society of Echocardiography Pediatric and Congenital Heart Disease Council, *J Am Soc Echocardiogr* 23(5):465–495, 2010.
34. Kluckow M, Evans N: Superior vena cava flow in newborn infants: a novel marker of systemic blood flow, *Arch Dis Child Fetal Neonatal Ed* 82(3):F182–F187, 2000.
35. Ficial B, Finnemore AE, Cox DJ, et al.: Validation study of the accuracy of echocardiographic measurements of systemic blood flow volume in newborn infants, *J Am Soc Echocardiogr* 26(12):1365–1371, 2013.
36. Kluckow MR, Evans NJ: Superior vena cava flow is a clinically valid measurement in the preterm newborn, *J Am Soc Echocardiogr* 27(7):794, 2014.
37. Singh Y, Gupta S, Groves AM, et al.: Expert consensus statement 'Neonatologist-performed Echocardiography (NoPE)'-training and accreditation in UK, *Eur J Pediatr* 175(2):281–287, 2016.
38. de Boode WP, Singh Y, Gupta S, et al.: Recommendations for neonatologist performed echocardiography in Europe: consensus statement endorsed by European Society for Paediatric Research (ESPR) and European Society for Neonatology (ESN), *Pediatr Res* 80(4):465–471, 2016.

39. Nestaas E, Stoylen A, Brunvand L, et al.: Longitudinal strain and strain rate by tissue Doppler are more sensitive indices than fractional shortening for assessing the reduced myocardial function in asphyxiated neonates, *Cardiol Young* 21(1):1–7, 2011.

40. Wei Y, Xu J, Xu T, et al.: Left ventricular systolic function of newborns with asphyxia evaluated by tissue Doppler imaging, *Pediatr Cardiol* 30(6):741–746, 2009.

41. Abdel-Hady HE, Matter MK, El-Arman MM: Myocardial dysfunction in neonatal sepsis: a tissue Doppler imaging study, *Pediatr Crit Care Med* 13(3):318–323, 2012.

42. James AT, Corcoran JD, Jain A, et al.: Assessment of myocardial performance in preterm infants less than 29 weeks gestation during the transitional period, *Early Hum Dev* 90(12):829–835, 2014.

43. Hirose A, Khoo NS, Aziz K, et al.: Evolution of left ventricular function in the preterm infant, *J Am Soc Echocardiogr* 28(3):302–308, 2015.

44. Malowitz JR, Forsha DE, Smith PB, et al.: Right ventricular echocardiographic indices predict poor outcomes in infants with persistent pulmonary hypertension of the newborn, *Eur Heart J Cardiovasc Imaging* 16(11):1224–1231, 2015.

45. Walther FJ, Siassi B, King J, et al.: Echocardiographic measurements in normal preterm and term neonates, *Acta Paediatr Scand* 75(4):563–568, 1986.

46. Lai WW, Geva T, Shirali GS, et al.: Guidelines and standards for performance of a pediatric echocardiogram: a report from the Task Force of the Pediatric Council of the American Society of Echocardiography, *J Am Soc Echocardiogr* 19(12):1413–1430, 2006.

47. Lang RM, Badano LP, Mor-Avi V, et al.: Recommendations for cardiac chamber quantification by echocardiography in adults: an update from the American Society of Echocardiography and the European Association of Cardiovascular Imaging, *Eur Heart J Cardiovasc Imaging* 16(3):233–270, 2015.

48. Teichholz LE, Kreulen T, Herman MV, et al.: Problems in echocardiographic volume determinations: echocardiographic-angiographic correlations in the presence of absence of asynergy, *Am J Cardiol* 37(1):7–11, 1976.

49. Helbing WA, Bosch HG, Maliepaard C, et al.: Comparison of echocardiographic methods with magnetic resonance imaging for assessment of right ventricular function in children, *Am J Cardiol* 76(8):589–594, 1995.

50. Lai WW, Gauvreau K, Rivera ES, et al.: Accuracy of guideline recommendations for two-dimensional quantification of the right ventricle by echocardiography, *Int J Cardiovasc Imaging* 24(7):691–698, 2008.

51. Patterson SW, Starling EH: On the mechanical factors which determine the output of the ventricles, *J Physiol* 48(5):357–379, 1914.

52. Nestaas E, Skranes JH, Stoylen A, et al.: The myocardial function during and after whole-body therapeutic hypothermia for hypoxic-ischemic encephalopathy, a cohort study, *Early Hum Dev* 90(5): 247–252, 2014.

53. Nestaas E, Stoylen A, Fugelseth D: Myocardial performance assessment in neonates by one-segment strain and strain rate analysis by tissue Doppler—a quality improvement cohort study, *BMJ Open* 2(4), 2012.

54. Czernik C, Rhode S, Helfer S, et al.: Left ventricular longitudinal strain and strain rate measured by 2-D speckle tracking echocardiography in neonates during whole-body hypothermia, *Ultrasound Med Biol* 39(8):1343–1349, 2013.

55. Molicki J, Dekker I: de GY, van BF. Cerebral blood flow velocity wave form as an indicator of neonatal left ventricular heart function, *Eur J Ultrasound* 12(1):31–41, 2000.

56. Henein MY, Gibson DG: Normal long axis function, *Heart* 81(2):111–113, 1999.

57. Naito H, Arisawa J, Harada K, et al.: Assessment of right ventricular regional contraction and comparison with the left ventricle in normal humans: a cine magnetic resonance study with presaturation myocardial tagging, *Br Heart J* 74(2):186–191, 1995.

58. Simonson JS, Schiller NB: Descent of the base of the left ventricle: an echocardiographic index of left ventricular function, *J Am Soc Echocardiogr* 2(1):25–35, 1989.

59. Jones CJ, Raposo L, Gibson DG: Functional importance of the long axis dynamics of the human left ventricle, *Br Heart J* 63(4):215–220, 1990.

60. Pai RG, Bodenheimer MM, Pai SM, et al.: Usefulness of systolic excursion of the mitral anulus as an index of left-ventricular systolic function, *Am J Cardiol* 67(2):222–224, 1991.

61. Brown SB, Raina A, Katz D, et al.: Longitudinal shortening accounts for the majority of right ventricular contraction and improves after pulmonary vasodilator therapy in normal subjects and patients with pulmonary arterial hypertension, *Chest* 140(1):27–33, 2011.

62. Kukulski T, Hubbert L, Arnold M, et al.: Normal regional right ventricular function and its change with age: a Doppler myocardial imaging study, *J Am Soc Echocardiogr* 13(3):194–204, 2000.

63. Zaky A, Grabhorn L, Feigenbaum H: Movement of the mitral ring: a study in ultrasoundcardiography, *Cardiovasc Res* 1(2):121–131, 1967.

64. Lundback S: Cardiac pumping and function of the ventricular septum, *Acta Physiol Scand Suppl* 550:1–101, 1986.

65. Koestenberger M, Nagel B, Ravekes W, et al.: Left ventricular long-axis function: reference values of the mitral annular plane systolic excursion in 558 healthy children and calculation of z-score values, *Am Heart J* 164(1):125–131, 2012.

66. Rudski LG, Lai WW, Afilalo J, et al.: Guidelines for the echocardiographic assessment of the right heart in adults: a report from the American Society of Echocardiography endorsed by the European Association of Echocardiography, a registered branch of the European Society of Cardiology, and the Canadian Society of Echocardiography, *J Am Soc Echocardiogr* 23(7):685–713, 2010.

67. Kaul S, Tei C, Hopkins JM, et al.: Assessment of right ventricular-function using two-dimensional echocardiography, *Am Heart J* 107(3):526–531, 1984.

11

68. Koestenberger M, Ravekes W, Everett AD, et al.: Right ventricular function in infants, children and adolescents: reference values of the tricuspid annular plane systolic excursion (TAPSE) in 640 healthy patients and calculation of z score values, *J Am Soc Echocardiogr* 22(6):715–719, 2009.
69. Koestenberger M, Nagel B, Ravekes W, et al.: Systolic right ventricular function in preterm and term neonates: reference values of the tricuspid annular plane systolic excursion (TAPSE) in 258 patients and calculation of Z-score values, *Neonatology* 100(1):85–92, 2011.
70. Vitali F, Galletti S, Aceti A, et al.: Pilot observational study on haemodynamic changes after surfactant administration in preterm newborns with respiratory distress syndrome, *Ital J Pediatr* 40(1):26, 2014.
71. Zakaria D, Sachdeva R, Gossett JM, et al.: Tricuspid annular plane systolic excursion is reduced in infants with pulmonary hypertension, *Echocardiography* 32(5):834–838, 2015.
72. El-Khuffash A, Herbozo C, Jain A, et al.: Targeted neonatal echocardiography (TnECHO) service in a Canadian neonatal intensive care unit: a 4-year experience, *J Perinatol* 33(9):687–690, 2013.
73. Deleted in review.

CHAPTER 12

Tissue Doppler Imaging

Afif Faisal El-Khuffash, Colm Riobard Breatnach, and Amish Jain

- Tissue Doppler imaging (TDI) is a modality that employs the Doppler effect to assess muscle wall characteristics throughout the cardiac cycle including velocity, displacement, deformation, and event timings.
- TDI is feasible and reliable in the neonatal population with recent literature describing the normative and maturation values of the various measurements in a wide range of gestational ages.
- Those measurements can be used to assess myocardial performance in various disease states, monitor treatment response, and provide important prognostic information.
- TDI velocity and deformation assessment measure myocardial performance rather than intrinsic contractility, and as such, the values are highly influenced by loading conditions (in addition to intrinsic contractility). Increased preload increases systolic tissue Doppler velocities while increased afterload reduces those velocities.

The Doppler effect is the term given to the change in frequency of a wave reflected by an acoustic source when there is relative movement between the source and the wave transmitter. It was first described by Christian Doppler, an Austrian physicist, born in Salzburg in 1803. He observed that the frequency of a wave depended on the relative speed of both the source and the observer. This became known as the Doppler effect. The difference between the transmitted and received frequencies can be used to measure the velocity of the moving acoustic source. The use of color flow Doppler in echocardiography was first described by engineers in Washington, although its clinical applicability was soon demonstrated in Japan in 1984 when Doppler waves were used to assess the velocity of blood through the heart.[1]

Traditionally, Doppler-based echocardiography is used in clinical practice to evaluate the velocity of blood flow. The stationary ultrasound probe emits high-frequency waves, which are reflected by moving blood and received by the probe again. The frequency of the emitted waves is different from that reflected back to the receiver within the probe. Each moving cell generates its own Doppler signal, which is scattered in all directions. Signals are reflected back to the ultrasound probe by millions of blood cells. The difference in frequencies is then expressed as both an audible pitch and velocity on the screen. The clinical applications of Doppler include pulse-wave, continuous-wave, and color flow Doppler methods.

More recently, the use of the Doppler effect has expanded to the assessment of heart muscle (tissue) characteristics. This was first demonstrated by Isaaz et al. in their assessment of the left ventricular wall using a pulse wave frequency signal.[2] Tissue Doppler imaging (TDI) captures information using high frame rates (typically greater than 200 frames per second). The high temporal resolution achieved using

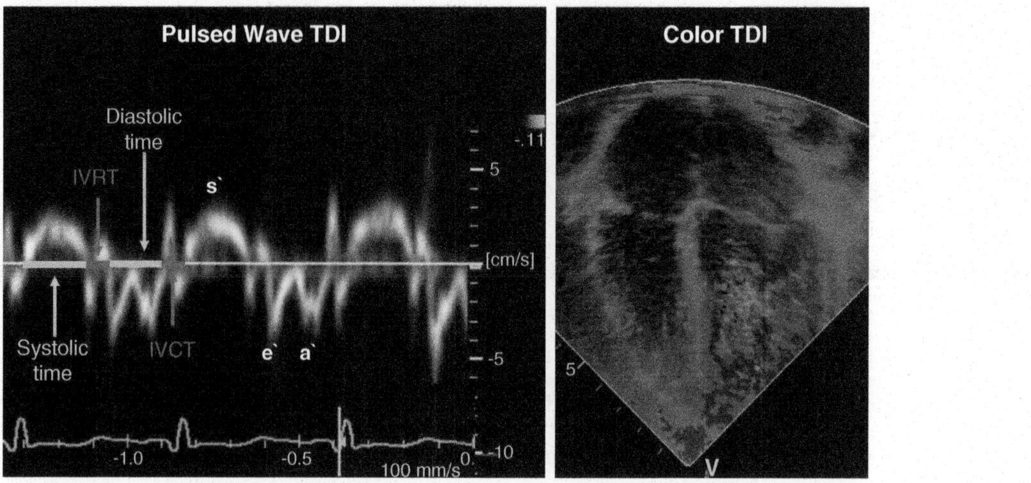

Fig. 12.1   Pulsed wave tissue Doppler imaging (TDI) and color tissue Doppler imaging (cTDI). Pulsed wave tissue Doppler imaging can be used to derive myocardial velocity during systole (s`) and diastole (e` and a`), in addition to event timings (see text for further details) including isovolumic relaxation time (IVRT) and isovolumic contraction time (IVCT). Movement toward the probe is depicted as positive, and movement away from the probe is depicted as negative. cTDI can be used to derive velocity and deformation values. Conventionally in color TDI, the muscle is colored *red* when traveling toward the probe and *blue* when traveling away from the probe.

this technique facilitates the measurements of a wide array of myocardial muscle characteristics, including the velocity of muscle movement during systole and diastole, deformation measurements (also known as strain and strain rate [SR] measurements), in addition to the measurements of the timing of events within the cardiac cycle (systolic and diastolic times/isovolumic contraction and relaxation times). Those measurements can now be derived by pulsed wave tissue Doppler imaging (pwTDI) and color tissue Doppler imaging (cTDI; Fig. 12.1).

Unlike conventional methods of functional assessment, which mainly assess changes in cavity dimension and blood flow velocity; namely, shortening fraction, ejection fraction, and blood pool analysis, this modality directly assesses muscle wall characteristics, such as velocity and deformation. In addition, it has shown improved sensitivity over older methods as an intensive care monitoring tool for myocardial dysfunction in critically ill term and preterm infants in conditions such as congenital diaphragmatic hernia and neonatal sepsis.[3–6] This provides the physician with valuable data on myocardial performance and has the ability to assist in outcome prediction.[7–10] Unfortunately, like other echocardiography modes, TDI is influenced by loading conditions and, therefore, is not a true surrogate for intrinsic myocardial function (see below).[4,11]

Principles of Cardiac Function

To understand the relative strengths and weaknesses of all the measurements obtained using TDI, a thorough understanding of the mechanics of ventricular pump performance is required. It is important to distinguish between intrinsic myocardial function (termed contractility) and ventricular pump function (termed myocardial performance). Contractility refers to the crosslinking of the actin and myosin filaments resulting in active myofiber force development and the shortening of sarcomeres. Myocardial performance or pump function describes the overall ventricular pressure development and deformation resulting in the ejection of blood from the ventricular cavity. Myocardial performance is therefore dependent on important physiologic factors: (1) *Preload:* defined as the amount of blood present in the ventricle at end-diastole before contraction begins. Up to a certain point, higher preload results in greater force generation and improved function (Frank-Starling relationship). Left and right ventricular preloads are dependent primarily on pulmonary blood flow/pulmonary venous return and

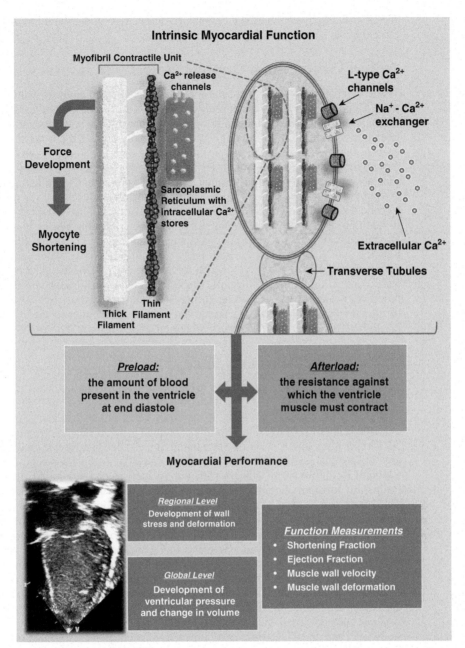

Fig. 12.2 **Overview of cardiac function mechanics.** Cellular calcium *(white circles)* enters the cell via L-type calcium channels. This, in turn, activates the release of large amounts of intracellular calcium stored in the sarcoplasmic reticulum into the cytosol. This results in contraction of the myofilament. The interaction between intrinsic function, preload, and afterload determines myocardial performance.

systemic venous return, respectively. Hydration and diastolic function are the two other important determinants. (2) *Afterload:* also known as wall stress is defined as the resistance against which the ventricle muscle must contract. This is primarily dependent on vascular resistance, blood viscosity, ventricular muscle wall thickness, and ventricular outflow tract obstructions. Higher afterload results in a reduction in deformation and myocardial performance, particularly in the preterm infant. (3) *Contractility:* is the intrinsic ability of the myocardial fibers to shorten as described above. This is determined by the efficiency of calcium-dependent crosslinking on the thick and thin filaments within the muscle fiber (Fig. 12.2).[12,13] The functional measurements obtained using TDI predominantly assess myocardial performance rather than intrinsic function, and as such, interpretation of values obtained during assessment should be done in the context of the clinical situation and loading conditions.

Pulsed Wave Tissue Doppler Velocity Measurements

Tissue Doppler (TD) velocities can be acquired by spectral analysis using a pulsed wave Doppler technique. The muscle tissue wall moves at a significantly slower velocity and a higher decibel amplitude range than blood, thus facilitating a high temporal resolution with minimal artifact from blood.[14] Recent advances have enabled the distinction between the faster moving blood (>50 cm/s) and the slower moving muscle tissue (<25 cm/s). PwTDI assesses longitudinal velocity of a ventricular wall segment from base to apex, providing a measure of systolic function that is recorded as the peak systolic velocity of the myocardial muscle (s` wave).[15–17] The systolic wave is usually preceded by a short upstroke during isovolumic contraction. In addition, a measure of diastolic performance can be obtained as the ventricular wall moves away from the apex in the opposite direction. The diastolic wave is biphasic and is recorded as the peak early diastolic velocity (e` wave) and the late diastolic peak velocity (a` wave), which reflects the active ventricular relaxation and atrial contraction phases of diastole, respectively. The diastolic waves are usually preceded by another short upstroke during isovolumic relaxation time. The duration of the isovolumic relation and contraction phases, in addition to the systolic and diastolic times, also can be accurately obtained using this modality (see Fig. 12.1).

Color Tissue Doppler Velocity

cTDI uses phase shift analysis to capture atrioventricular annular excursions. Compared with pwTDI, cTDI provides the ability to visualize multiple segments of the heart from one single view. It measures mean rather than peak systolic and diastolic velocities. As a result, velocities obtained using this technique are generally 20% lower in systole and diastole compared to pwTDI. Therefore, the two methods are not interchangeable.[16,18] cTDI does have the advantage of combining the high temporal resolution seen with pwTDI, with a high spatial resolution. In addition to this, myocardial velocities recorded at the left and right ventricular bases, and septal wall, can be obtained from a single image for offline analysis. A comparison between left and right ventricular function can therefore be performed. Muscle tissue at the base moves at a higher velocity than that closer to the apex. cTDI can be used to assess this velocity gradient across the wall of interest (Fig. 12.3). As with other TDI modalities, images are obtained from the apical four-chamber view. Eriksen et al. compared cTDI with tricuspid and mitral annular plane systolic excursions in a cohort of preterm infants. They found that the values obtained from cTDI were lower and more dependent on image quality than excursions by gray-scale M-mode.[19] Another potential disadvantage to cTDI is poor reproducibility as reported in some studies.[20] Data on cTDI values and clinical applicability in the neonatal setting are limited. This is likely due to the need for offline analysis to obtain those values when compared with pwTDI, where data can be acquired at the bedside. The data presented below relate only to pwTDI.

Measurement of Tissue Doppler Imaging Velocities

Accurate TDI velocity measurements are highly dependent on obtaining good quality images. This may be challenging in the neonatal setting, particularly in premature infants where lung artifact can interfere with obtaining clear images of the walls of interest. Images are usually obtained from an apical four-chamber view. The sector width of the field of view is usually narrowed to only include the wall of interest. This ensures that the temporal resolution is enhanced and a frame rate of over 200 frames per second is obtained. A pulsed wave Doppler sample is placed at the base of the left ventricular free wall, the base of the septum, and at the base of the right ventricular free wall. The sample gate is narrowed to only capture the velocity of the area of

12

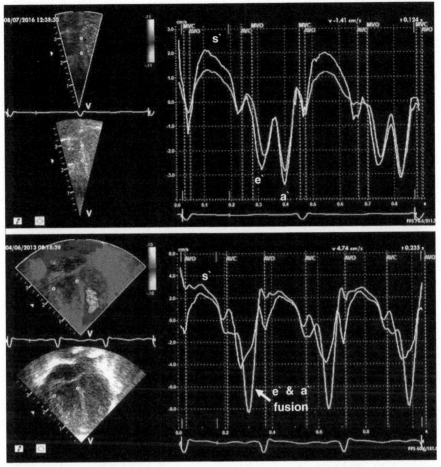

Fig. 12.3 **Color tissue Doppler imaging.** The top demonstrates an assessment of the velocity gradients of the septal wall in a term infant. Note that the velocities measured at the base (*yellow*) are higher in systole and diastole than those measured in the mid-segment of the wall (*green*). The bottom panel demonstrates the assessment of the septal wall and the right ventricular free wall in a preterm infant. Right ventricular velocities (*green*) are higher than septal velocities (*yellow*). Note the fusion of the e` and a` occurring due to the higher heart rate seen in preterm infants.

interest (usually 1 to 2 mm). It is crucial to maintain an angle of insonation of less than 20 degrees to prevent underestimation of velocities. TDI velocity measurement modality will only assess muscle movement parallel to the probe beam (Fig. 12.4). This is a limitation of this modality as muscle movement perpendicular to the line of interrogation will not be assessed and as a result, TDI velocity measurements are reserved for longitudinal (base to apex) muscle tissue movement.

As outlined earlier, TDI velocity assessment measures myocardial performance rather than intrinsic contractility, and as such, the values are highly influenced by loading conditions (in addition to intrinsic contractility). Increased preload increases systolic TD velocities, while increased afterload reduces those velocities.[4,11] Therefore interpretation of those measurements must take into account made the loading conditions likely to be present in the clinical situation. This has important implications for therapeutic interventions where, in some instances, it may be more beneficial to improve preload (using volume support) or reduce afterload (using lusitropic medication) rather than targeting an improvement in intrinsic contractility (Fig. 12.5). In addition, it is important to recognize that TD velocity imaging cannot distinguish between active muscle movement and translational wall motion (a nondeforming segment tethered to a functioning segment). TD velocities may be falsely elevated as they interrogate motion at a single point in the muscle wall with reference to the

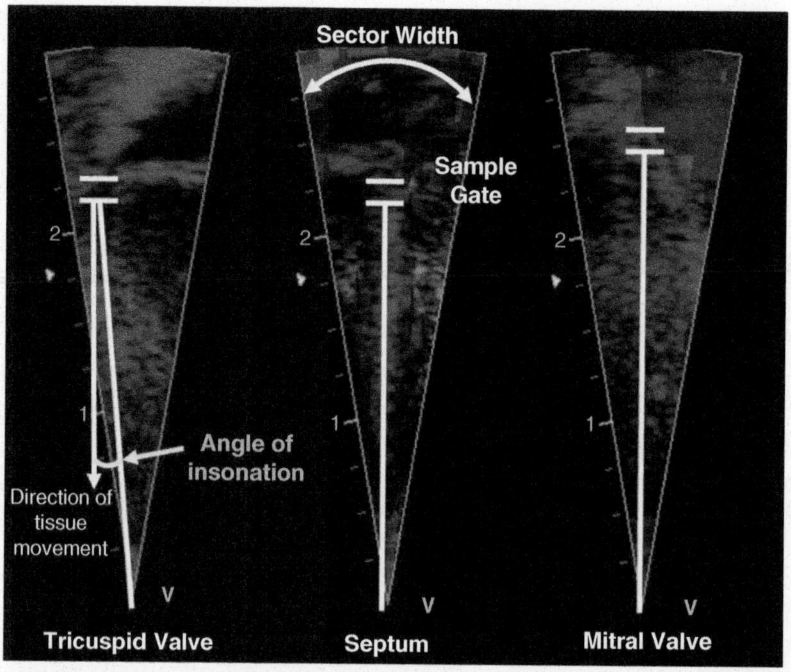

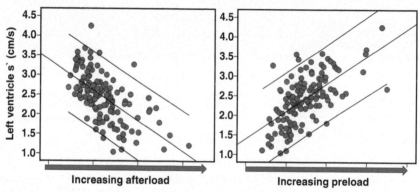

Fig. 12.4 **Measurement of tissue Doppler imaging velocities.** Narrowing the sector width and reducing the sample gate increases the frame rate and improves the temporal resolution. This enables easier identification of the various events throughout the cardiac cycle. The angle of insonation should be less than 20° to avoid underestimating the velocity values.

Fig. 12.5 **Effect of loading conditions on tissue Doppler imaging systolic velocities.** Increasing afterload reduces systolic velocities. Increasing preload increases systolic velocities. (Data modified from a cohort of 141 preterm infants <29 weeks' gestation on the first postnatal day.)

ultrasound transducer. Therefore this movement can be influenced by translational motion.[21] Deformation imaging (see later) can easily differentiate between the two.

Clinical Application of Tissue Doppler Imaging Velocity Measurements

The use of TDI in the neonatal setting has significantly expanded in recent years. TDI assessment is very feasible in small infants and has been validated in term and premature neonatal populations[22,23] as well as in fetuses.[11] Reference values for both term and preterm infants are shown in Table 12.1.[24–27] Several studies have documented serial changes in those functional measurements over the first day of life and up to 36 weeks' postmenstrual age.[24,25,28] TD velocity imaging is dependent on the gestational age, with lower gestations exhibiting lower myocardial velocities in

Table 12.1 TISSUE DOPPLER IMAGING VELOCITIES AND EVENT TIMES IN PRETERM AND TERM INFANTS OVER THE TRANSITIONAL PERIOD

	Preterm Cohort		Term Cohort	
	Day 1	Day 2	Day 1	Day 2
Left Ventricle Free Wall				
s`	2.8 (0.9)	3.3 (0.7)	4.9 (0.8)	4.6 (0.6)
e`	3.6 (1.4)	4.2 (1.3)	6.7 (1.4)	6.5 (1.2)
a`	4.0 (1.5)	4.8 (1.4)	5.5 (1.3)	5.4 (1.3)
e`/a`	0.95 (0.36)	0.91 (0.25)	1.3 (0.4)	1.3 (0.4)
Septum				
s`	2.4 (0.6)	3.0 (0.6)	3.6 (0.6)	3.5 (0.5)
e`	2.8 (0.8)	3.6 (1.1)	4.7 (1.1)	4.8 (0.9)
a`	3.9 (1.1)	4.7 (1.4)	4.2 (0.8)	4.4 (0.8)
e`/a`	0.76 (0.21)	0.91 (0.25)	1.1 (0.23)	1.1 (0.23)
Right Ventricle Free Wall				
s`	3.6 (0.9)	4.4 (1.0)	6.6 (1.1)	6.5 (1.1)
e`	3.9 (1.3)	4.5 (1.1)	8.0 (1.6)	7.3 (1.2)
a`	6.7 (1.8)	8.6 (2.6)	8.3 (1.6)	8.0 (1.3)
Left Ventricle Event Times				
Heart rate	154 (14)	160 (12)	119 (15)	125 (18)
Isovolumic relaxation time	58 (13)	52 (12)	53 (12)	52 (10)
Isovolumic contraction time	56 (13)	46 (11)	65 (14)	65 (12)
Systolic time	147 (20)	150 (18)	188 (23)	184 (16)
Diastolic time	131 (22)	126 (22)	199 (43)	195 (44)

The preterm cohort comprised 66 infants less than 29 weeks' gestation free of inotropes. The term cohort comprised 50 infants between 37 and 42 weeks' gestation, appropriately grown and free of significant maternal illness. Modified from Jain A, El-Khuffash AF, Kuipers BC, et al.: Left ventricular function in healthy term neonates during the transitional period, *J Pediatr* 182:197–203, 2017; Jain A, Mohamed A, El-Khuffash A, Connelly KA, et al.: A comprehensive echocardiographic protocol for assessing neonatal right ventricular dimensions and function in the transitional period: normative data and z scores, *J Am Soc Echocardiogr* 27(12):1293–1304, 2014; and James AT, Corcoran JD, Jain A, et al.: Assessment of myocardial performance in preterm infants less than 29 weeks gestation during the transitional period, *Early Hum Dev* 90(12):829–835, 2014.

both systole and diastole.[25,28,29] Reduced myocardial velocity is also present during the transitional period from the fetal to the neonatal circulation and increases over the first few postnatal weeks. This is likely due to the changing loading conditions seen during this period, which become more favorable. In premature infants, TDI velocities have been used to predict clinical deterioration following patent ductus arteriosus (PDA) ligation and as a guide to institute targeted therapy. In addition, they can be used to assess treatment response in this scenario[3] when conventional measures of function, including shortening and ejection fraction, are not sensitive enough. Incorporating TDI for the assessment of myocardial performance in the setting of a PDA during the first few days of age may facilitate a more targeted approach to PDA treatment[30] and facilitate the development of prediction markers for adverse outcomes. Of note is that there is also an emerging association between lower diastolic function measured using TDI and chronic lung disease in premature infants.[30]

In term infants, TDI can be used to assess right ventricle (RV) function to provide important clinical prognostic information in infants with congenital diaphragmatic hernia[31] and may be used to monitor treatment response in infants with persistent pulmonary hypertension of the newborn (PPHN).[32] The superior sensitivity of TDI to subtle myocardial dysfunction when compared with shortening and ejection fraction in term infants was recently demonstrated. In infants born to mothers with diabetes mellitus (of any cause), left and right systolic function measured using TDI velocity is lower than for control term infants. This occurs without differences in shortening fraction between the two groups.[33]

In summary, muscle tissue velocities obtained using TDI are a feasible, reliable, and valid modality for the assessment of myocardial performance in the premature

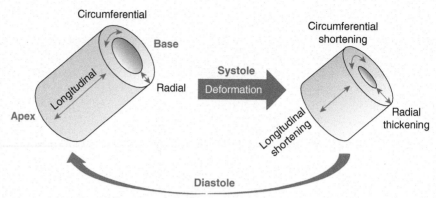

Fig. 12.6   **Deformation of the left ventricle.**

and term neonatal population. Those measurements are highly influenced by loading conditions; therefore, they do not represent intrinsic function (contractility). Reference ranges across a wide variety of gestations have emerged; and their use in detecting myocardial dysfunction, guiding therapeutic interventions, predicting important clinical outcomes, and monitoring response to treatment is expanding in the neonatal population.

Tissue Doppler-Derived Deformation Measurements

Principles of Deformation Imaging

Myocardial deformation at the ventricular level refers to the change in shape of the myocardium in several planes from its baseline shape in diastole to its deformed shape in systole. This occurs as a consequence of myofibril shortening described earlier. As the myocyte unit is not compressible, deformation of the ventricles occurs while maintaining the overall muscle volume while resulting in a reduction of the ventricular cavity volume. The left ventricle (LV) deforms in three planes including longitudinal (base to apex), radial, and circumferential. The LV shortens longitudinally and circumferentially, but thickens in the radial plane. This facilitates the maintenance of muscle volume while reducing the volume of the ventricular cavity to facilitate the ejection of blood during systole. During diastole, the ventricle returns to its baseline undeformed shape (Fig. 12.6).[34] The RV predominantly deforms in the longitudinal plane.[35]

The term used to describe deformation (change in shape) is "strain," which is expressed as a percentage of the original baseline length. Negative strain is used to express shortening (in the longitudinal and circumferential planes), and positive strain is used to express radial thickening. Peak systolic strain occurs at the end of systole at aortic valve closure. Strain rate (SR) is used to describe the speed at which the strain occurs in systole (systolic SR) and the speed at which the ventricles shape returns to baseline (diastolic SR). Like TD velocities, diastolic SR is biphasic with an early and a late phase. SR is expressed as 1/s. Peak systolic SR occurs in mid-systole and returns to baseline (zero velocity) at aortic valve closure when no deformation occurs (Fig. 12.7).

Deformation imaging has the advantage over velocity imaging in distinguishing between movement due to tethering and true deformation. Velocity imaging will register a displacement velocity of this nondeforming segment as it may be tethered by an adjacent functioning segment. However, an infarcted segment of the myocardium will not deform and its strain values will be close to zero. Strain can be used to assess regional and global myocardial performance. Strain is analogous to ejection fraction and, as a result, it will be dependent on loading conditions as well as intrinsic contractility. SR, on the other hand, is thought to be less dependent on preload and afterload, and as a result, it may represent a more accurate reflection of intrinsic contractile function. Therefore, deformation imaging may be used to distinguish

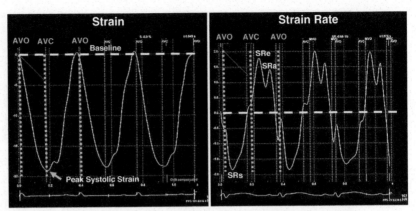

Fig. 12.7 **Tissue Doppler-derived strain and strain rate (SR) of three cardiac cycles.** Strain peaks at the end of systole at aortic valve closure (AVC) and returns to baseline at the end of diastole at aortic valve opening (AVO). Negative strain depicts shortening. Systolic SRs peaks in mid-systole. Diastolic SR is biphasic (SRe and SRa).

between reduced performance resulting from loading conditions (which will affect strain but not SR) and reduced performance resulting from intrinsic contractile dysfunction (which will affect both strain and SR).[36–39]

Tissue Doppler Derived Deformation Imaging

There are two methods available for the measurement and calculation of strain and SR: TD-derived deformation imaging and two-dimensional gray scale speckle tracking echocardiography (2DSTE). 2DSTE is considered in Chapter 13. TD-derived deformation imaging uses the velocity gradient, which is present in the longitudinal plane described earlier (see Fig. 12.3—*top panel*), to derive deformation values. TD-derived longitudinal deformation imaging calculates SR by measuring the differences in velocity between small segments of the myocardium along the longitudinal plane and deriving SR. Strain values are then derived from the SR calculation by integrating it with time. TD-derived strain will only obtain deformation values from velocities directly parallel to the ultrasound beam; therefore, minimizing the angle of insonation between the plane of interest and the ultrasound probe is of paramount importance. In addition, clear views of the myocardial region of interest (ROI) are required for reliable measurements. Due to this limitation, strain measurement using TDI is usually only applied in the longitudinal plane in the neonatal population (usually from the base of the heart). TDI is more suited in neonates for measuring SR values due to the high temporal resolution of this technique (>200 frames per second).[39,40]

TD-derived deformation is not interchangeable with 2DSTE as it measures Eulerian strain rather than natural (or Lagrangian) strain. Eulerian strain calculates the frame-by-frame instantaneous strain values, where the change in length is divided by the instantaneous length at each frame and not by the length at end diastole. The sum of all those measurements constitutes Eulerian strain. The denominator in the fraction becomes smaller during contraction for longitudinal strain. Therefore, Eulerian strain measurements are usually larger than Lagrangian strain.

The same principles of image acquisition also apply to TD-derived deformation imaging as described above for TDI. However, currently, deformation values using TD can only be measured offline. An ROI along the longitudinal plane of the wall of interest is defined by the operator by setting the length and width. The width of the ROI should not project outside the borders of the wall of interest, and the length of the ROI should not include any atrial tissue (Fig. 12.8).

Clinical Applications in the Neonatal Population

The use of TD-derived deformation imaging in the neonatal population is gaining interest, and recent studies have demonstrated that it is feasible, reproducible, and

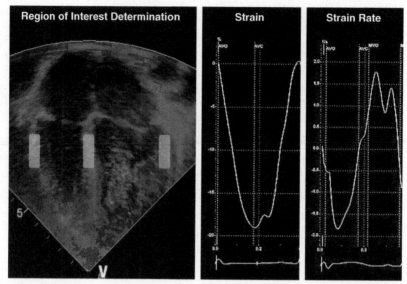

Fig. 12.8 Tissue Doppler-derived deformation measurement. The sector width should be narrowed to increase the frame rate. The basal segment of the wall is usually interrogated to obtain strain rate (SR) and strain values. The region of interest (ROI) dimensions *(yellow rectangle)* are set by the operator. The ROI can be moved slightly along the wall to obtain a clean and noise-free SR, and the strain curves are illustrated. *AVC,* Aortic valve closure; *AVO,* aortic valve opening; *MVO,* mitral valve opening .

Table 12.2 TISSUE DOPPLER-DERIVED DEFORMATION VALUES

	Preterm		Term
	Day 1	Day 2	20 h
Left Ventricle Free Wall			
S	−12.2 (2.8)	−12.8 (2.8)	−24.5 (3.8)
SRs	−1.5 (0.5)	−1.7 (0.6)	−1.8 (0.4)
SRe	1.6 (0.8)	2.1 (0.6)	3.2 (1.5)
SRa	2.6 (0.8)	2.7 (1.0)	2.1 (1.3)
Septum			
S	−15.5 (3.0)	−17.4 (3.5)	−25.9 (4.8)
SRs	−1.6 (0.3)	−1.9 (0.4)	−1.9 (0.6)
SRe	1.7 (0.6)	2.1 (0.6)	3.2 (1.6)
SRa	2.3 (0.8)	2.7 (1.0)	2.4 (0.9)
Right Ventricle Free Wall			
S	−22.8 (4.8)	−24.3 (4.7)	−28.3 (4.9)
SRs	−2.1 (0.5)	−2.5 (0.7)	−1.9 (0.5)
SRe	2.4 (0.8)	2.6 (0.7)	2.8 (0.8)
SRa	3.6 (1.0)	4.4 (1.3)	2.1 (0.9)

The preterm cohort comprised 105 infants less than 29 weeks' gestation free of inotropes. The term cohort comprised 55 infants between 37 and 42 weeks' gestation, appropriately grown and free of significant maternal illness.
Modified from James AT, Corcoran JD, Breatnach CR, Franklin O, Mertens L, El-Khuffash A: Longitudinal assessment of left and right myocardial function in preterm infants using strain and strain rate imaging. *Neonatology* 109(1):69–75, 2016; Pena JL, da Silva MG, Faria SC, Salemi VM, Mady C, Baltabaeva A, Sutherland GR: Quantification of regional left and right ventricular deformation indices in healthy neonates by using strain rate and strain imaging. *J Am Soc Echocardiogr* 22(4):369–375, 2009.

valid in both preterm and term infants.[41–47] Reference ranges across a variety of gestational ages for basal deformation measurements of the LVs and RVs, as well as the septum, have been published (Table 12.2). Their potential clinical utility in the premature and term neonatal population is emerging. In term infants, TD-derived deformation can identify poor myocardial performance in infants undergoing therapeutic hypothermia for neonatal encephalopathy by demonstrating lower strain and SR values compared with healthy controls. This difference occurs in spite of a lack of difference in shortening fraction.[46] This dysfunction is apparent in infants with neonatal encephalopathy irrespective of whether or not they are cooled. The lower SR values obtained in this population suggest that the poor performance can be due to poor intrinsic contractility and not just a consequence of adverse loading conditions.[48] In term infants with severe PPHN who are not responsive to inhaled nitric oxide, strain measurements can be utilized to monitor treatment response when additional therapeutic interventions are used.[32]

Preterm infants have lower strain and SR values than term infants during the transitional period (see Table 12.2). The adverse loading conditions experienced by preterm infants, in addition to the inefficient contractile mechanism, can explain those differences. In the preterm population, LV strain values appear to remain stable over the first week of age before increasing closer to term. In contrast, septal and RV free wall strain show a more steady increase over the first week of age.[39,49] Finally, preterm infants with bronchopulmonary dysplasia (BPD) have a lower RV strain and RV SR at 36 weeks' postmenstrual age when compared with preterm infants without BPD. BPD is associated with increased pulmonary arterial pressure, which may explain this association.[39,49]

Conclusion

The assessment of TD-derived velocity and deformation measurements in neonates continues to gain considerable interest. The emerging literature has clearly demonstrated their feasibility and reproducibility in the neonatal population and the relative advantages of those techniques when compared with conventional measures. With reference ranges and normative data continuing to emerge, in addition to studies assessing their diagnostic and prognostic values and their ability to monitor treatment response, their routine clinical use is likely to become more common.

REFERENCES

1. Omoto R, Yokote Y, Takamoto S, et al.: The development of real-time two-dimensional Doppler echocardiography and its clinical significance in acquired valvular diseases. With special reference to the evaluation of valvular regurgitation, *Jpn Heart J* 25(3):325–340, 1984.
2. Isaaz K, Thompson A, Ethevenot G, et al.: Doppler echocardiographic measurement of low velocity motion of the left ventricular posterior wall, *Am J Cardiol* 64(1):66–75, 1989.
3. El-Khuffash AF, Jain A, Weisz D, et al.: Assessment and treatment of post patent ductus arteriosus ligation syndrome, *J Pediatr* 165(1):46–52, 2014.
4. El-Khuffash AF, Jain A, Dragulescu A, et al.: Acute changes in myocardial systolic function in preterm infants undergoing patent ductus arteriosus ligation: a tissue Doppler and myocardial deformation study, *J Am Soc Echocardiogr* 25(10):1058–1067, 2012.
5. Saleemi MS, Bruton K, El-Khuffash A, et al.: Myocardial assessment using tissue Doppler imaging in preterm very low-birth weight infants before and after red blood cell transfusion, *J Perinatol* 33(9):681–686, 2013.
6. Saleemi MS, El-Khuffash A, Franklin O, et al.: Serial changes in myocardial function in preterm infants over a four week period: the effect of gestational age at birth, *Early Hum Dev* 90(7):349–352, 2014.
7. Moenkemeyer F, Patel N: Right ventricular diastolic function measured by tissue Doppler imaging predicts early outcome in congenital diaphragmatic hernia, *Pediatr Crit Care Med* 15(1):49–55, 2014.
8. Matter M, Abdel-Hady H, Attia G, et al.: Myocardial performance in asphyxiated full-term infants assessed by Doppler tissue imaging, *Pediatr Cardiol* 31(5):634–642, 2010.
9. Murase M, Ishida A, Momota T: Serial pulsed Doppler assessment of early left ventricular output in critically ill very low-birth-weight infants, *Pediatr Cardiol* 23(4):442–448, 2002.
10. Abdel-Hady HE, Matter MK, El-Arman MM: Myocardial dysfunction in neonatal sepsis: a tissue Doppler imaging study, *Pediatr Crit Care Med* 13(3):318–323, 2012.
11. Iwashima S, Sekii K, Ishikawa T, et al.: Serial change in myocardial tissue Doppler imaging from fetus to neonate, *Early Hum Dev* 89(9):687–692, 2013.
12. Kluckow M: Low systemic blood flow and pathophysiology of the preterm transitional circulation, *Early Hum Dev* 81(5):429–437, 2005.
13. Evans N, Osborn D, Kluckow M: Preterm circulatory support is more complex than just blood pressure, *Pediatrics* 115(4):1114–1115, 2005.
14. Weidemann F, Eyskens B, Sutherland GR: New ultrasound methods to quantify regional myocardial function in children with heart disease, *Pediatr Cardiol* 23(3):292–306, 2002.
15. Hiarada K, Orino T, Yasuoka K, et al.: Tissue Doppler imaging of left and right ventricles in normal children, *Tohoku J Exp Med* 191(1):21–29, 2000.

12

16. Nagueh SF, Middleton KJ, Kopelen HA, et al.: Doppler tissue imaging: a noninvasive technique for evaluation of left ventricular relaxation and estimation of filling pressures, *J Am Coll Cardiol* 30(6):1527–1533, 1997.

17. Yu CM, Sanderson JE, Marwick TH, et al.: Tissue Doppler imaging a new prognosticator for cardiovascular diseases, *J Am Coll Cardiol* 49(19):1903–1914, 2007.

18. Frommelt PC, Ballweg JA, Whitstone BN, et al.: Usefulness of Doppler tissue imaging analysis of tricuspid annular motion for determination of right ventricular function in normal infants and children, *Am J Cardiol* 89(5):610–613, 2002.

19. Eriksen BH, Nestaas E, Hole T, et al.: Longitudinal assessment of atrioventricular annulus excursion by grey-scale m-mode and colour tissue Doppler imaging in premature infants, *Early Hum Dev* 89(12):977–982, 2013.

20. Mandysova E, Mraz T, Taborsky M, et al.: Reproducibility of tissue Doppler parameters of asynchrony in patients with advanced LV dysfunction, *Eur J Echocardiogr* 9(4):509–515, 2008.

21. James AT, Corcoran JD, Franklin O, et al.: Clinical utility of right ventricular fractional area change in preterm infants, *Early Hum Dev* 92:19–23, 2016.

22. Negrine RJ, Chikermane A, Wright JG, et al.: Assessment of myocardial function in neonates using tissue Doppler imaging, *Arch Dis Child Fetal Neonatal Ed* 97(4):F304–F306, 2012.

23. Alp H, Karaarslan S, Baysal T, et al.: Normal values of left and right ventricular function measured by M-mode, pulsed Doppler and Doppler tissue imaging in healthy term neonates during a 1-year period, *Early Hum Dev* 88(11):853–859, 2012.

24. Murase M, Morisawa T, Ishida A: Serial assessment of right ventricular function using tissue Doppler imaging in preterm infants within 7 days of life, *Early Hum Dev* 91(2):125–130, 2015.

25. Murase M, Morisawa T, Ishida A: Serial assessment of left-ventricular function using tissue Doppler imaging in premature infants within 7 days of life, *Pediatr Cardiol* 34(6):1491–1498, 2013.

26. James A, Corcoran JD, Mertens L, et al.: Left ventricular rotational mechanics in preterm infants less than 29 weeks' gestation over the first week after birth, *J Am Soc Echocardiogr* 2015.

27. Jain A, Mohamed A, El-Khuffash A, et al.: A comprehensive echocardiographic protocol for assessing neonatal right ventricular dimensions and function in the transitional period: normative data and z scores, *J Am Soc Echocardiogr* 27(12):1293–1304, 2014.

28. Eriksen BH, Nestaas E, Hole T, et al.: Myocardial function in term and preterm infants. Influence of heart size, gestational age and postnatal maturation, *Early Hum Dev* 90(7):359–364, 2014.

29. Lee A, Nestaas E, Liestol K, et al.: Tissue Doppler imaging in very preterm infants during the first 24 h of life: an observational study, *Arch Dis Child Fetal Neonatal Ed* 99(1):F64–F69, 2014.

30. El-Khuffash A, James AT, Corcoran JD, et al.: A patent ductus arteriosus severity score predicts chronic lung disease or death before discharge, *J Pediatr* 167(6):1354–1361.e1352, 2015.

31. Patel N, Mills JF, Cheung MM: Assessment of right ventricular function using tissue Doppler imaging in infants with pulmonary hypertension, *Neonatology* 96(3):193–199, 2009.

32. James AT, Corcoran JD, McNamara PJ, et al.: The effect of milrinone on right and left ventricular function when used as a rescue therapy for term infants with pulmonary hypertension, *Cardiol Young* 26(1):90–99, 2016.

33. Al-Biltagi M, Tolba OA, Rowisha MA, et al.: Speckle tracking and myocardial tissue imaging in infant of diabetic mother with gestational and pregestational diabetes, *Pediatr Cardiol* 36(2):445–453, 2015.

34. Greenbaum RA, Ho SY, Gibson DG, et al.: Left ventricular fibre architecture in man, *Br Heart J* 45(3):248–263, 1981.

35. de Waal K, Lakkundi A, Othman F: Speckle tracking echocardiography in very preterm infants: feasibility and reference values, *Early Hum Dev* 90(6):275–279, 2014.

36. Weidemann F, Jamal F, Sutherland GR, et al.: Myocardial function defined by strain rate and strain during alterations in inotropic states and heart rate, *Am J Physiol Heart Circ Physiol* 283(2):H792–H799, 2002.

37. Greenberg NL, Firstenberg MS, Castro PL, et al.: Doppler-derived myocardial systolic strain rate is a strong index of left ventricular contractility, *Circulation* 105(1):99–105, 2002.

38. Ferferieva V, Van den Bergh A, Claus P, et al.: The relative value of strain and strain rate for defining intrinsic myocardial function, *Am J Physiol Heart Circ Physiol* 302(1):H188–H195, 2012.

39. James AT, Corcoran JD, Breatnach CR, et al.: Longitudinal assessment of left and right myocardial function in preterm infants using strain and strain rate imaging, *Neonatology* 109(1):69–75, 2016.

40. de WK, Lakkundi A, Othman F: Speckle tracking echocardiography in very preterm infants: feasibility and reference values, *Early Hum Dev* 90(6):275–279, 2014.

41. James AT, Corcoran JD, Jain A, et al.: Assessment of myocardial performance in preterm infants less than 29 weeks gestation during the transitional period, *Early Hum Dev* 90(12):829–835, 2014.

42. Nestaas E, Stoylen A, Sandvik L, et al.: Feasibility and reliability of strain and strain rate measurement in neonates by optimizing the analysis parameters settings, *Ultrasound Med Biol* 33(2):270–278, 2007.

43. Nestaas E, Stoylen A, Fugelseth D: Optimal types of probe, and tissue Doppler frame rates, for use during tissue Doppler recording and off-line analysis of strain and strain rate in neonates at term, *Cardiol Young* 18(5):502–511, 2008.

44. Poon CY, Edwards JM, Joshi S, et al.: Optimization of myocardial deformation imaging in term and preterm infants, *Eur J Echocardiogr* 12(3):247–254, 2011.

45. Joshi S, Edwards JM, Wilson DG, et al.: Reproducibility of myocardial velocity and deformation imaging in term and preterm infants, *Eur J Echocardiogr* 11(1):44–50, 2010.

46. Nestaas E, Stoylen A, Fugelseth D: Myocardial performance assessment in neonates by one-segment strain and strain rate analysis by tissue Doppler—a quality improvement cohort study, *BMJ Open* 2(4), 2012.
47. Helfer S, Schmitz L, Buhrer C, et al.: Reproducibility and optimization of analysis parameters of tissue Doppler-derived strain and strain rate measurements for very low birth weight infants, *Echocardiography* 30(10):1219–1226, 2013.
48. Nestaas E, Skranes JH, Stoylen A, et al.: The myocardial function during and after whole-body therapeutic hypothermia for hypoxic-ischemic encephalopathy, a cohort study, *Early Hum Dev* 90(5):247–252, 2014.
49. Helfer S, Schmitz L, Buhrer C, et al.: Tissue Doppler-derived strain and strain rate during the first 28 days of life in very low birth weight infants, *Echocardiography* 31(6):765–772, 2013.

12

CHAPTER 13

Speckle Tracking Echocardiography in Newborns

Koert de Waal and Nilkant Phad

- Two-dimensional speckle tracking echocardiography (2DSTE) is a non-Doppler technique that applies computer software analysis of images generated by conventional ultrasound techniques.
- 2DSTE calculates parameters of motion (displacement, velocity) and deformation (strain, strain rate) in all three axes.
- Advantages of 2DSTE are its relative angle independency, the option for retrospective analysis, and most parameters of interest are provided from a few selected views.
- As with any ultrasound technique, image quality is the most important aspect to optimize feasibility and reliability.
- Reliability is superior compared with current conventional parameters, and reference values have been established in the term and preterm population.
- 2DSTE and tissue Doppler studies have significantly increased our knowledge of systolic and diastolic function and its development in preterm infants.
- Deformation parameters are more sensitive in detecting abnormalities in specific newborn populations, such as severe growth restriction, maternal diabetes, hypoxic ischemic encephalopathy, and congenital heart disease.
- Intervendor and intravendor variation in algorithms used in the 2DSTE software limits direct comparison of results.

Echocardiography is the most commonly used diagnostic modality for cardiovascular assessment in the newborn. It is a noninvasive bedside method to study cardiac structure and provide an estimate of cardiac function. However, measuring the true nature of cardiac mechanics is difficult due to the complex myocardial geometry and how the determinants of cardiac function (i.e., preload, contractility, afterload) interact with each other.

The developing heart starts out as an isotropic tissue built of cardiomyocytes and supportive tissues and gradually develops into an anisotropic tissue where groups of cardiomyocytes are structured as laminar sheets of fibers.[1] In the subendocardial region the fibers are longitudinally oriented along the axis of the heart, with an angle to the right (right-handed helix), in the midwall the fibers are circumferentially orientated, and in the subepicardial region they are longitudinal again but with an angle to the left (left-handed helix; Fig. 13.1).[2,3] This double helical structure of the heart is important for its function. Being able to shorten in longitudinal and circumferential directions simultaneously and thus creating a twisting motion greatly improves energy efficiency and the ability to empty and fill the heart with blood. In the adult heart a 60% ejection fraction (EF) can be achieved with only 15% fiber shortening.[4]

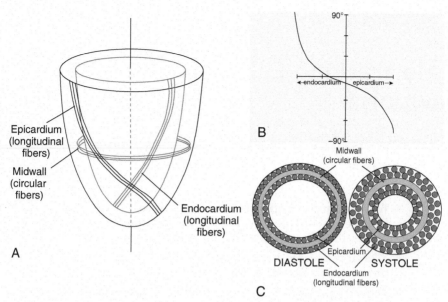

Fig. 13.1 (A) Schematic representation of the left ventricle showing the longitudinal endocardial and epicardial fibers and the circular midwall fibers. (B) The angle of the cardiac fibers according to the cardiac short axis changes from the endocardium to the epicardium. (C) Variable fiber angles help to produce a shortening and twisting motion during systole and a lengthening and untwisting motion during diastole. Wall thickening consists of thickening and inward shift of cardiac fibers.

Ventricular motion thus consists of narrowing, shortening, lengthening, widening, and twisting. Furthermore, as the myocardium moves and changes its position, it will undergo deformation and change its shape because not all parts move with the same velocity. Because the myocardial fibers are not compressible, any shortening in one direction leads to expansion in other directions. Part of this will be actual deformation, but wall thickening is greater than the sum of the individual fiber thickenings due to longitudinal fibers shifting inward (shearing).[5]

Not all aspects of cardiac mechanics can be captured using conventional echocardiography techniques. It is difficult to capture the twisting motion or to capture wall thickening for the whole ventricle. Furthermore, wall motion measurements cannot differentiate between active and passive movement of a myocardial segment. On conventional echocardiography, a myocardial segment which has lost its function will still show movement due to the tethering effect of adjacent segments. Deformation analysis is an approach in which the limitations of conventional techniques are minimized. Deformation analysis is possible using invasive sonomicrometry, magnetic resonance imaging (MRI), tissue Doppler imaging (TDI), and a novel technique called speckle tracking echocardiography. This chapter will introduce the reader to two-dimensional speckle tracking echocardiography (2DSTE) of the left ventricle (LV) and right ventricle (RV). We will discuss some basic concepts, terminology, the practicalities of hardware setup and image acquisition, and its current status in newborn infants. For in-depth technical aspects of ultrasound in general and deformation imaging with 2DSTE in adults, we recommend the following website: http://folk.ntnu.no/stoylen/strainrate/.

Basic Concepts and Terminology

Speckle tracking echocardiography is a non-Doppler technique that applies computer software analysis of images generated by conventional ultrasound techniques. The Doppler ultrasound signal generates artifacts due to random reflections, called speckles. These speckles stay stable during the cardiac cycle and can act as natural acoustic markers. Speckle tracking software can define and follow a cluster of speckles from frame to frame to calculate parameters of motion (displacement

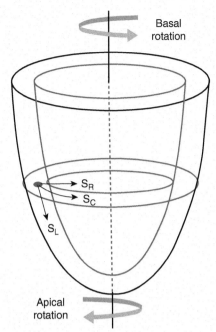

Fig. 13.2 Schematic representation of the left ventricle, showing the longitudinal (S$_L$), circumferential (S$_C$), and radial (S$_R$) axis, and basal and apical rotation.

and velocity) and parameters of deformation (referred to as strain and strain rate [SR]).[3,6,7] Strain is the percentage of change from its original length, with negative values describing narrowing or shortening and positive values lengthening or thickening. SR is the average change in strain per unit of time and is expressed as 1/s. Motion and deformation are three dimensional (3D) and described along the three cardiac axes. The nomenclature is longitudinal for base-to-apex, circumferential for rotational, and radial or transverse for inward motion and deformation (Fig. 13.2). The difference in the rotation of the myocardium between the apical and basal short axis plane is commonly referred to as twist and reported in degrees. If rotation is normalized to the distance between the respective image planes, it is referred to as torsion and reported in degrees per centimeter. Normalizing twist to LV length facilitates comparison of LV rotational mechanics across differing age groups, but this can only be done accurately with 3D imaging.

Recommended nomenclature, units, and abbreviations for 2DSTE-derived parameters are provided in an important consensus report.[8] The report also provides consensus on timing of mechanical events, essential for standardization of almost all derived parameters of motion and deformation. To be able to report on Lagrangian strain (where the original length is known), the software would need a reference point in time (the beginning of the cardiac cycle) and an end point where deformation is determined according to its reference point. End diastole is commonly taken at the beginning of the cardiac cycle, either determined from the four-chamber images as the frame before the mitral valve completely closes or using surrogates such as the R peak of the electrocardiogram (ECG) or the largest volume of the LV. End systole is the usual end point and coincides with aorta valve closure, determined from apical long axis views or using surrogates such as the end of the T wave of the ECG, the end of the negative spike after ejection on the 2DSTE-derived velocity trace, or the minimum volume of the LV.[9,10] The current consensus in adult cardiology is to report on end systolic strain, with other parameters reported in addition (Fig. 13.3).

Most studies of newborns reported on peak systolic strain (the first peak strain value found) or maximum systolic strain (the highest strain value found). Postsystolic strain has not been reported in newborns but could prove to be an important parameter in fetal growth restriction.[11]

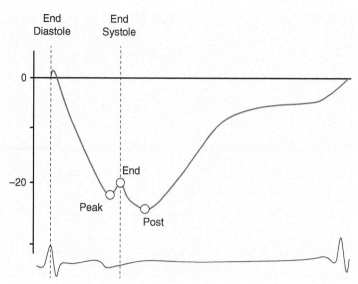

Fig. 13.3   Representative curve showing cardiac time and the ECG trace on the x-axis and strain on the y-axis. End diastole is determined from the R wave of the ECG. End systole is marked in this example to show the difference between peak systolic strain, end systolic strain, and postsystolic strain.

Because the heart contains layers of fibers in different directions, motion and deformation can vary depending on where in the myocardial wall they are measured (i.e., at the endocardium, midwall, or averaged over the entire cardiac wall).[12] Whether this also plays a role in the analysis of the thin walled and immature myocardium of newborn infants is unclear. Older software versions generally report on endocardial deformation, whereas newer versions report on (the lower) global or midwall deformation with separate reporting for each wall area.

To help interpret the data, it is important to understand the difference between global and segmental motion and deformation. The term global deformation should be reserved for the combined findings from the four chamber, two chamber, and long axis apical views or from the basal level of the papillary muscle and apical short axis views. Segmental deformation can be vendor specific because the segmental model used could describe 16, 17, or 18 segments. Most software packages would divide the ventricular wall into six equidistant segments termed basal, mid, and apical segments for the apical views and anatomically for the short axis views (i.e., anteroseptal, anterior, lateral, posterior, inferior, and septal wall segment). Data can be reported as global (all segments of all views), for the four chamber view alone (six segments), per ventricular wall (three segments of respectively the LV free wall, RV free wall, and the septum), or per individual segments (i.e., basal segments only for 2DSTE-derived myocardial velocities). Most 2DSTE data to date in newborns have been determined from the apical four-chamber view alone or per free wall because not all software can calculate global parameters when heart rate varies too much between the different views.

Image Acquisition

Speckle tracking analysis can be performed on normal 2D gray-scale images but does require some adjustments to optimize feasibility of successful analysis. As mentioned earlier, 2DSTE tracks artifacts that are there because of random reflections of the Doppler signal; hence the optimal image should contain a combination of a perfect 2D gray-scale image with enough artifacts (speckles) within the myocardial wall. This is not always easy to achieve. The feasibility of 2DSTE analysis in newborns has been reported between 70% and 95% of the images acquired, with the highest feasibility in the more recent studies. As with any ultrasound imaging, the

Table 13.1   IMAGE QUALITY SCORING SHEET FOR TWO-DIMENSIONAL SPECKLE TRACKING
ECHOCARDIOGRAPHY IMAGE ANALYSIS

Quality Item	Description
Ventricle shape	No chamber foreshortening (apical views)
	Symmetry of the basal segments and valve (apical views)
	Contains circular images, not oblique cuts with ellipsoid shape (short axis views)
Endocardial and epicardial borders	Enough speckles within each segment of interest
	Clear view of the endocardial and epicardial borders of all segments throughout the cardiac cycle
Gain settings	Overall gain and image settings
	Distribution of gain over the myocardial segments
Artifacts	Reverberation, drop outs, breathing motion
Frame rate	Optimized to 0.7–0.9 frames/sec/bpm
ECG signal	Clear R wave

13

poorer the image quality, the less useful is the analysis. Images selected for analysis should be reviewed for image quality before analysis is attempted. Using a subjective or objective image quality scoring sheet can assist in increasing the feasibility of 2DSTE analysis.[13] Quality items include completeness of the ventricle, how the endocardial and epicardial borders appear, the presence of artifacts, the ECG trace, and frame rate used (Table 13.1).

For optimal clarity of the endocardial borders, the overall gain setting and time-gain compensation should be adjusted to produce images that appear brighter than those typically used in conventional echocardiography. Newborns are often not sedated for image acquisition, so motion and breathing can cause some segments to move in and out of the plane of view.

Reproducibility of newborn deformation parameters were most robust when images were obtained with a frame rate to heart rate ratio between 0.7 and 0.9.[14] Low frame rate can cause undersampling and thus underestimate peak systolic SR values. Strain is less frame rate sensitive because the rate of change is lowest at end systole. The operator can adjust depth and sector width to optimize frame rate, but reaching optimal frame rates might still be a challenge in newborns with very high heart rate and will require high-end ultrasound machines.

A clear ECG signal is important for the speckle tracking software to allow proper gating of the images (i.e., capture two to four cardiac beats triggered by the R wave). On most modern equipment, the ECG trace can easily be obtained by connecting the ultrasound machine to the neonatal monitor without the need for machine-specific ECG leads.

Although 2DSTE as a technique is angle independent, the angle of insonation can still make a small difference in strain and SR.[15] This could be explained by differences in image quality and the appearance of the speckles under different angles. Parallel insonification of some segments of the apical views or the anterior and inferior-septal segments of the short axes images can lead to a significant reduction of speckles due to the fiber orientation (Fig. 13.4).

Sending and Storage of Acquired Images

After image acquisition, most operators would send and store selected images for offline analysis on a dedicated workstation. It is crucial to check the send and storage settings on the ultrasound machine before deformation imaging is started. The default setting for most commercial ultrasound machines is to send all images in compressed format Digital Imaging and Communications in Medicine (DICOM) at a frame rate of 30 Hz. Some ultrasound machines now include a separate acquire button to send selected images in RAW format, but these images can only be analyzed using vendor-specific software. For vendor-independent software that uses DICOM images, the send and storage setting of the machine should be changed to "acquired frame rate." This setting will significantly increase the need for server storage space and might cause network congestion, depending on your local situation.

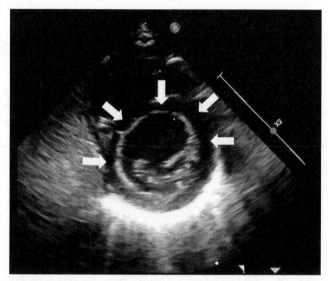

Fig. 13.4 Short axis image at the basal level of a 28 weeks' gestation preterm infant. The endocardial wall is clearly seen, but limited speckles can be appreciated within the midwall (*arrows*).

Image Processing

Postprocessing or the actual speckle tracking analysis is a semiautomated process of selecting a clip with optimal image quality and tracing the myocardial wall slightly within the endocardial border (or other areas of interest) as a sequence of points on a single frame. The software then generates a region of interest (ROI) to include the entire myocardial thickness. It is important to standardize settings for the width of the ROI, if available. There is a learning curve for operators new to the technique to optimize imaging of the entire endocardial wall throughout the cardiac cycle and provide reproducible point selection for tracing.

The software will track and trace the sequence of points from frame to frame throughout the cardiac cycle and renders a volume curve and segmental, average, and global curves for velocity, displacement, strain, and SR (Fig. 13.5). After the first analysis, the operator should perform a visual frame-by-frame analysis of tracking accuracy by reviewing the underlying image loop with the superimposed tracking results. Some analysis software offers an automated measure of tracking accuracy, but it is recommended to always perform an operator check, and if needed, adjust the ROI.

Interpretation of the Results

Most software will have the option to present many parameters of interest, but this chapter will focus on the deformation parameters. Strain is measured at end systole and thus at the end of ventricular contractile performance and is closely related to stroke volume (SV) in healthy hearts.[16,17] SR is recorded earlier in the cardiac cycle and thus will not be subject to load during the entirety of systole. SR is measured at peak ventricular performance and less load dependent, and thus SR is considered to be closely related to myocardial contractility.[18,19]

The vendor's software package will determine how the results are presented, but most packages would show the data as color-coded parametric images, systolic numerical values, and as time curves (see Fig. 13.5B). The patterns of strain should be reviewed by exploring base-to-apex and left-to-right gradients. In newborns, LV apical strain and SR are usually higher compared with the mid and the basal segments, and the reverse is true for displacement and velocity. Deformation in the septum is usually lower compared with both the RV and LV free wall. Segmental abnormalities, as seen after myocardial infarcts, are rare in newborns.

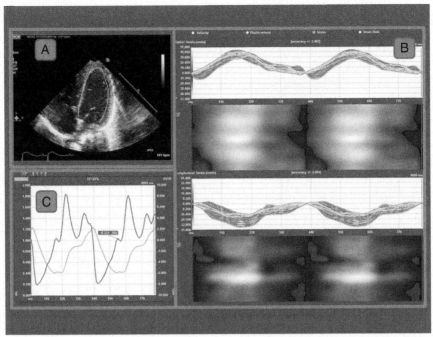

Fig. 13.5 Screen capture of speckle tracking analysis (Tomtec Cardiac Performance Analysis software version 1.1) of a four-chamber clip with two cardiac beats. (A) Shows the four-chamber clip with added tracking line *(green line)* placed along the endocardial border. (B) Shows radial *(top)* and longitudinal *(bottom)* motion and deformation data for each segment and as global average. Strain data are shown in this example. (C) Shows the data for volume *(orange line)* and rate of volume changes dVdt *(blue line)*.

The curves should also be reviewed for diastolic events, best appreciated in the basal segments for 2DSTE-derived myocardial velocities and in the apex for strain and SR. The reliability of diastolic 2DSTE parameters is not optimal, possibly due to the relative low frame rate per heart beat as compared with TDI. Another issue with diastolic events in newborns is that fusion of the early and late diastolic events (EA fusion) commonly occurs at high heart rates (>170/min). Such images would have to be omitted from analysis, prompting much data to be lost. It is not always clear how newborn investigators handled this issue. One study in preterm infants reported all fusion events as late diastolic events instead of omitting the data.[20]

Circumferential motion and deformation and rotational mechanics are derived from the short axis images. Cardiac mechanical dysfunction is usually present in all directions in newborns, but under certain circumstances rotational deformation can be a compensatory mechanism and provide clues for early detection of disease.[21,22]

All software also reports on radial and transverse deformation. The reliability for these parameters in newborns has been poor, possibly due to the small area changes, and is not routinely reported in newborn studies.

Cantinotti et al. suggested that deformation parameters should be normalized to age and body size.[23] We, and others, do not think that this is necessary for strain and SR.[24] Deformation parameters are fractional changes in length of a cardiac segment relative to its original length, and thus values are already normalized for cardiac size. In adult hearts, there is a clear relationship between cardiac size, SV, and deformation parameters, with a dilated heart able to generate a larger SV with the same contractile force. Only when the observed changes deviate from the predicted changes is myocardial contractility then reduced.[25] We could replicate some of these findings in a cohort of preterm infants with volume load due to a patent ductus arteriosus (PDA), suggesting that cardiac remodeling and subsequent mechanical changes are already present from very early cardiac developmental stages.[26]

Deformation parameters are load dependent and should be interpreted in the context of existing or changing loading conditions. Strain and SR are positively influenced by preload and negatively by afterload.[27,28] In a meta-analysis of normal ranges of longitudinal strain (S_L) in adult studies, systolic blood pressure (an important determinant of LV afterload) at the time of the study was associated with normal variation and should be considered in the interpretation of strain.[29]

Advantages of Two-Dimensional Speckle Tracking Echocardiography

In an expert consensus paper, Mor-Avi et al. described 2DSTE as "a significant contribution to the much needed process of the transformation of echocardiography from a subjective art of image interpretation to a set of objective diagnostic tools."[3] When a good-quality image is acquired, the process of 2DSTE is fairly easy and reproducible with postprocessing times reduced to acceptable levels with the ever-increasing advancements in computer processing. As the process is computerized, it takes away some of the subjective human components of analysis. 2DSTE can obtain most parameters of interest (motion, deformation, volume) from a few selected views, with SR being the closest echocardiographic parameter to measure actual contractility. As such, 2DSTE provides incremental value in the assessment of cardiac mechanics and cardiac function.

2DSTE offers minimal angle dependency, as opposed to TDI or conventional measurements. Aligning the probe to reduce the angle of insonation to less than 30 degrees can be difficult under specific situations. For example, preterm infants with volume overload have a more spherical shape of the LV, thus increasing the angle between the probe and the basal segment of the LV free wall. The same can occur in the RV in infants with severe pulmonary hypertension.

2DSTE allows for retrospective analysis of acquired images during specific unexpected events. Our group recently analyzed cardiac mechanics during bradycardia events in preterm infants and was able to retrospectively provide a full set of cardiac function parameters from beat to beat.[30] Systolic function and SV were maintained but cardiac output reduced proportionally to the decrease in heart rate.

Although not its primary purpose, 2DSTE can semiautomatically determine LV volumes.[31] SV is the most common parameter used in newborn echocardiography to describe cardiovascular function. We assessed the agreement between manual biplane SV, semiautomated biplane SV using 2DSTE, and SV using the velocity time integral (Vti) method in 50 preterm infants. Manual and semiautomated SV showed good agreement, but both were significantly lower compared with SV using the Vti method.[31a] Further development of this application has the potential to increase the reliability of SV measurements in newborn infants.

Limitations and Pitfalls of Two-Dimensional Speckle Tracking Echocardiography

Although 2DSTE is a relatively easy process, this can also be its problem. The software will render curves and output, sometimes irrespective of basic image issues such as foreshortening or Doppler artifacts, and it remains up to the experience of the operator to determine if the output is valid. Because true cardiac motion is 3D, speckles might move out of the 2D plane and can thus not always be tracked correctly using a 2D technique.

2DSTE has been validated in animal and human studies against sonomicrometry and tagged MRI.[32,33] However, in newborns and particularly in preterm infants, there is no clear noninvasive gold standard, as even MRI struggles with acquiring images in high resolution at very short time intervals.[34] Hence, the true accuracy of the technique has not been established in newborns.

Currently the most important issue with 2DSTE is the fact that each vendor has its own software algorithm to calculate motion and deformation parameters.

This has led to significant intervendor variation and is thus limiting the establishment of 2DSTE as a technique for everyday practice.[35,36] However, in a joint venture with the industry, further standardizations and upgrades of existing software algorithms were able to improve interobserver and intraobserver reproducibility of global S_L in adults. The reliability of 2DSTE is now comparable with or superior to that of EF and other conventional echocardiographic parameters.[37] We are not sure if these findings can be extrapolated to the analysis of the small hearts of preterm infants because the most recent versions of Qlab and Tomtec still showed significant differences in S_L.[31a]

Normal Two-Dimensional Speckle Tracking Echocardiography Values in Newborns

In the healthy developing fetus, 2DSTE-derived strain remains relatively stable and SR decreases from the second to the third trimester.[38–40] Absolute SR values were relatively high compared with newborn values, which can be explained by the intrinsic properties of the heart and the expected changes in preload and afterload. Small, poorly compliant hearts with high heart rates will need fast wall shortening. Fetal cardiac growth throughout the pregnancy ensured that SV increased for any given wall shortening.

Table 13.2 presents all clinical studies reported to date in term newborn infants in the first days or weeks after birth.[41–49] Most investigators reported on S_L, but data on circumferential strain, radial strain (S_R), twist, or RV S_L in healthy term infants were available from only one or two studies with only a few participants. Overall, the average S_L reported in the studies was around -20%, ranging from -18% to -22%, and it remained relatively stable throughout the neonatal period.

There are three recent published systematic reviews evaluating normal systolic deformation values in the pediatric population. Jashari et al. reported an average S_L of -21.0% (95% CI, -17.3 and -24.7) for healthy term newborn infants.[50] Global S_L and the more commonly performed S_L from the apical four-chamber view (average of six segments) were reported interchangeably in this review. Levy et al. reported a lower mean S_L of -19.4% (95% CI, -16.6 to -22.2) and analyzed separately for global S_L and S_L from the four-chamber view.[51] However, this review included a paper by Elkiran et al.[42] The findings of this study were irregular, possibly due to the use of alternative hardware and software. Segmental and average S_L values were significantly lower compared with any other newborn study and showed an unexpected and somewhat unphysiologic decreasing base-to-apex gradient. Cantinotti et al. argued that meta-analysis of 2DSTE data of small studies using variable hardware and methodology would not reveal valid results and reported studies individually.[23]

The reports of 2DSTE in preterm infants are listed in Table 13.3.[14,26,42,52–64] The average reported S_L was -21%, and with a wider range of findings between -15% and -28%. The wider variation is probably explained not only by the differences in hardware settings and software package used, but also by the inclusion of unstable preterm infants. In most cohorts a large portion of infants had a significant PDA and/or were mechanically ventilated at the time of the investigation. We found a slightly lower S_L compared with earlier reference S_L values using the same hardware and software in a cohort of very preterm infants who did not experience significant antenatal or postnatal complications and treatments.[62,64]

It seems that large population-based studies are still desirable in healthy or stable newborns. To help establish 2DSTE in local practice, we suggest collecting data of a local control group using the same hardware, software, and analysis methods. Because deformation parameters are relatively stable among different gestational age groups and postnatal ages, a large sample will not be required. We would recommend excluding infants for whom altered cardiac development is expected (fetal growth restriction, maternal diabetes, postnatal steroids) and excluding infants with significantly altered preload and afterload conditions (pulmonary hypertension, PDA and its treatments, use of vasopressor-inotropes and inotropes, mechanical ventilation). Ideally, local reference data of commonly used conventional parameters should be collected simultaneously.

Table 13.2 STUDIES TO DATE EXPLORING TWO-DIMENSIONAL SPECKLE TRACKING ECHOCARDIOGRAPHY IN TERM NEWBORN INFANTS

Study	Year	N	PNA (days)	Software	Frame Rate (/s)	S_L (%)	SR_L (1/s)	S_C (%)	S_R (%)	Twist (°)	RV S_L (%)	RV SR_L (1/s)
Zhang[41]	2010	29	15–28	EchoPAC	>50					1.9 (1.2)		
Elkiran[42]	2014	32	1–3	XStrain	50–75							
Sehgal[43]	2013	20	0–2	EchoPAC	>80	-11.2 (2.5)	-1.76 (0.2)	-13.7 (2.9)				
Schubert[44]	2013	30	7	EchoPAC	187	-21.5 (2.7)	-2.37 (0.8)					
Klitsie[45]	2013	28	1–3	EchoPAC	>80	-19.5 (2.1)	-1.75 (0.2)				-21.5 (4.2)	-2.56 (1.2)
Sehgal[46]	2014	21	3–4	EchoPAC	>80	-18.8 (3.5)		-19.7 (4.3)	29.4 (12.2)			
Jain[47]	2014	50	1–2	EchoPAC	80–100	-21.3 (2.8)					-21.2 (3.9)	
Al-Biltagi[48]	2015	45	0–2	EchoPAC	65	-19.0 (2.1)				5.4 (2.4)		
Jain[49]	2017	50	0–1	EchoPAC	80–100	-21.7 (1.9)	-2.05 (0.15)					

The data for healthy term newborns within the studies are presented. When segmental deformation was reported, the average deformation of the intraventricular septum and each respective free wall was calculated.

PNA, Postnatal age in days; *RV S_L*, longitudinal strain of the right ventricle; *S_C*, circumferential strain; *S_L*, longitudinal strain; *S_R*, radial strain; *SR_L*, longitudinal strain rate.

Table 13.3 STUDIES TO DATE EXPLORING TWO-DIMENSIONAL SPECKLE TRACKING ECHOCARDIOGRAPHY IN PRETERM NEWBORN INFANTS

Study	Year	N	GA (weeks)	PNA (days)	Software	Frame Rate (/s)	S_L (%)	SR_L (1/s)	S_C (%)	S_R (%)	Twist (°)	RV S_L (%)
El-Khuffash[52]	2012	19	23–26	28–42	EchoPAC	80–100	-19.7 (3.8)					
Elkiran[42]	2014	32	36–37	1–3	Xstrain	50–75	-10.4 (2.8)	-1.11 (0.2)	-13.4 (3.5)			
Levy[53]	2013	80	<30	28–56	EchoPAC	90–120	-19.1 (2.4)					
Sehgal[54]	2014	18	<30	4–17	EchoPAC	80–115	-18.7 (2.6)	-1.73 (0.3)	-19.5 (3.7)	32.1 (14.4)		
de Waal[55]	2014	51	<32	0–44	Tomtec	30	-15.1 (2.0)	1.55 (0.2)				
Czernik[56]	2014	96	<30	0–28	EchoPAC	115	-17.5 (5.3)					
James[57]	2015	38	<29	0–2	EchoPAC	110	-22.8 (4.0)					
Sanchez[14]	2015	20	<29	28–56	EchoPAC	90–160	-16.0 (3.3)	-1.63 (0.3)	-19.8 (3.5)		7.3 (3.5)	
Hirose[58]	2015	30	<30	28	EchoPAC		-24.2 (3.5)					
Nasu[59]	2015	21	28–36	0–3	Qlab	64–192						-19.5 (2.5)
James[60]	2015	51	<29	0–7	EchoPAC	125					10.2 (8.0)	-19.8 (4.6)
Schubert[61]	2016	25	<31	0–28	EchoPAC	187	-18.5 (3.0)	-2.22 (0.4)				
de Waal[62]	2016	54	<30	0–28	Tomtec	90–110	-23.2 (2.5)	-2.63 (0.4)				
de Waal[30]	2016	14	<30	3–41	Tomtec	90–110	-22.2 (2.3)	-2.71 (0.8)				
Hecker[63]	2016	26	23–36		Qlab	95	-28.1 (2.4)					
de Waal[64]	2016	25	<30	0–28	Tomtec	90–110	-21.9 (2.1)	-2.51 (0.4)				-28.7 (4.9)
de Waal[26]	2017	77	<30	3–70	Tomtec	99–110	-21.2 (2.1)	-2.44 (0.4)				-19.8 (4.1)

The data presented are from stable preterm infants where possible, or otherwise from all preterm newborns reported in the paper (stable or unwell). Where no global values were reported, an average was calculated from the segmental or free wall values.

GA, Gestational age in weeks; *PNA*, postnatal age in days; *RV S_L*, longitudinal strain of the right ventricle; *S_C*, circumferential strain; *S_L*, longitudinal strain; *S_R*, radial strain; *SR_L*, longitudinal strain rate.

Clinical Applications of Two-Dimensional Speckle Tracking Echocardiography

The possibility of segmental analysis with high sensitivity in detecting abnormal myocardium helped to establish 2DSTE as a diagnostic modality in detecting and quantifying myocardial ischemia and reperfusion viability in adult cardiology.[3,65] Global SL by 2DSTE is more sensitive than EF as a marker of LV dysfunction in adults, and it has become a useful marker in cardiomyopathies, cardiotoxicity during chemotherapy, heart failure, and valvular disease.[66]

In newborns the clinical role of 2DSTE has been tested in infants with birth asphyxia. Deformation parameters, either obtained via 2DSTE or TDI, were more sensitive as markers of cardiac dysfunction compared with the commonly used fractional shortening.[43,67–69] The effects of whole body therapeutic hypothermia on S_L were minimal, and no segmental abnormalities suggestive of myocardial infarcts were reported in any of the studies.

2DSTE has been shown to be more sensitive compared with conventional echocardiography in infants with morphologic changes and cardiac remodeling due to high fetal insulin levels (infants of diabetic mothers) or chronic hypoxia (often the cause of fetal growth restriction). 2DSTE was able to detect early cardiac dysfunction in infants of diabetic mothers in utero and postnatally.[48,70] Decreased myocardial deformation was seen in all directions and the characteristics of torsion were changed, indicating a diffuse pattern of myocardial involvement as has been reported for cardiomyopathies. In some newborns, 2DSTE could detect cardiac dysfunction even in the absence of morphologic cardiac changes.

In term infants with severe growth restriction due to placental dysfunction, impairment in myocardial deformation was noted in the presence of altered arterial biophysical properties.[46] Cardiac dysfunction was mostly subclinical, and further studies are needed to determine how these changes are related to long-term cardiovascular risk factors and the development of metabolic disease.[71]

In relatively uncomplicated preterm infants, S_L remained stable during the transition from fetus to preterm life, despite significant hemodynamic changes that occurred during this period.[59] Most conventional parameters, such as SV, increase after birth, suggesting that S_L might be a potential marker of cardiac well-being that is easy to interpret. Antenatal medications such as magnesium sulfate and steroids improved S_L and twist function on the first day of postnatal life after preterm birth.[60]

Czernik et al. explored myocardial deformation in the first 28 days after preterm birth and found an increased longitudinal SR in the first postnatal week in infants who developed bronchopulmonary dysplasia (BPD) versus those who did not.[56] This might be explained by the fact that most infants who developed BDP also had a PDA, thus increasing preload and reducing afterload. Our group studied a similar group of preterm babies and found similar associations between load changes and deformation.[55,62] In infants with a PDA the LV showed adaptive remodeling and consistently higher systolic deformation parameters and confirmed that increased preload of the PDA was not a common cause of LV dysfunction in preterm infants.[26] Further studies are needed to explore possible causes of PDA-associated cardiac dysfunction. Nonsteroidal antiinflammatory drugs and surgical ligation significantly reduce S_L, and it is unclear if it is the treatments themselves, the change in loading conditions, or both that are responsible for those changes.[52,54]

Hirose et al. studied preterm infants after 28 days of life to avoid the period of acute hemodynamic changes related to the presence of a PDA, acute respiratory pathology, and changing pulmonary vascular resistance.[58] Systolic function was stable throughout this neonatal period, but with altered diastolic function with a greater dependence on atrial contraction. The maturational changes in diastolic function occurred relatively independent of the timing of birth, but some of the diastolic abnormalities persisted near term gestation. Schubert et al. reported similar findings, with reduced systolic and diastolic parameters 6 months after preterm birth.[61] Both studies showed that 2DSTE can detect early signs of altered cardiac function after preterm birth. Preterm birth has been associated with significant changes to cardiac morphology and function in early adult life and could contribute to later cardiovascular risk factors.[72,73]

2DSTE is becoming an important tool in the functional assessment of newborns and infants with congenital heart disease.[74,75] Unlike most conventional parameters, 2DSTE is not based on geometric assumptions and can be applied on various shaped ROIs. Longitudinal assessments before and after surgical correction have enhanced insight into the cardiac remodeling process with congenital heart disease including shunts, detailed how the RV functions as a systemic ventricle and how atrial function changes with congenital heart disease, and showed the persistent changes in LV function after correction of aortic stenosis.[21,76–78]

Future Directions of Two-Dimensional Speckle Tracking Echocardiography

The role of 2DSTE in clinical practice has not been fully established in newborn care. 2DSTE has provided valuable insight in aspects of cardiac mechanics and cardiac function previously not detailed. Systolic deformation parameters are very robust at any gestation, and, throughout the neonatal intensive care period, they describe the cardiac mechanical response to changes in loading conditions and have the diagnostic ability to detect subclinical disease. Its predictive value for major cardiovascular events is superior to conventional measurements. Improved reliability, ease of use, and industry standardization of software will further help to establish 2DSTE in newborn clinical practice. We expect to see further clinical studies in newborns with sepsis for whom 2DSTE could be used to select patients for early treatments or inclusion into clinical trials.[79,80] Patients might be selected for long-term follow-up based on 2DSTE parameters at discharge from the neonatal intensive care unit.[61,81] New information on the clinical relevance of left atrial deformation analysis is constantly emerging in adult cardiology, and our group is currently exploring the feasibility of left atrial deformation in preterm infants.[82] Interesting new developments are forthcoming using 2DSTE on plane wave imaging to improve the measurement of peak velocities for the evaluation of shunt flow in atrial and ventricular septal defects in newborns.[83,84]

The ultimate goal would be working toward real-time 3DSTE, where all aspects of cardiac mechanics and myocardial function can be captured and analyzed from one perfect view. 3DSTE is gaining interest in adult cardiology, but experiences are limited in the pediatric population due to technical limitations and availability of hardware to accommodate measurements at high frame rates in newborn infants.[85]

Echocardiography in newborns has come a long way since the initial M-mode echocardiography to estimate LV function and left atrium size.[86] Not many standard M-mode measurements remain in adult echocardiography, but they are still the backbone of neonatal echocardiography.[87,88] The most recent practice guideline for neonatal echocardiography was published in 2011, just before the development of 2DSTE and other novel echocardiography parameters in newborns.[88] 2DSTE has been thoroughly tested in term and preterm infants, is often better compared with commonly used conventional parameters, and is expected to find a place in the updated recommendations for clinical practice.

REFERENCES

1. Mekkaoui C, Porayette P, Jackowski MP, et al.: Diffusion MRI tractography of the developing human fetal heart, *PLoS One* 8(8):e72795, 2013.
2. Geyer H, Caracciolo G, Abe H, et al.: Assessment of myocardial mechanics using speckle tracking echocardiography: fundamentals and clinical applications, *J Am Soc Echocardiogr* 23(4):351–369, 2010.
3. Mor-Avi V, Lang RM, Badano LP, et al.: Current and evolving echocardiographic techniques for the quantitative evaluation of cardiac mechanics: ASE/EAE consensus statement on methodology and indications endorsed by the Japanese Society of Echocardiography, *Eur J Echocardiogr* 12(3):167–205, 2011.
4. Buckberg G, Hoffman JI, Mahajan A, et al.: Cardiac mechanics revisited: the relationship of cardiac architecture to ventricular function, *Circulation* 118(24):2571–2587, 2008.

5. Greenbaum RA, Ho SY, Gibson DG, et al.: Left ventricular fibre architecture in man, *Br Heart J* 45(3):248–263, 1981.
6. Blessberger H, Binder T: Non-invasive imaging: Two dimensional speckle tracking echocardiography: basic principles, *Heart* 96(9):716–722, 2010.
7. Uematsu M: Speckle tracking echocardiography—Quo Vadis? *Circ J* 79(4):735–741, 2015.
8. Voigt JU, Pedrizzetti G, Lysyansky P, et al.: Definitions for a common standard for 2D speckle tracking echocardiography: consensus document of the EACVI/ASE/Industry task force to standardize deformation imaging, *Eur Heart J Cardiovasc Imaging* 16(1):1–11, 2015.
9. Mada RO, Lysyansky P, Daraban AM, et al.: How to define end-diastole and end-systole?: impact of timing on strain measurements, *JACC Cardiovasc Imaging* 8(2):148–157, 2015.
10. Aase SA, Torp H, Støylen A: Aortic valve closure: relation to tissue velocities by Doppler and speckle tracking in normal subjects, *Eur J Echocardiogr* 9(4):555–559, 2008.
11. Crispi F, Bijnens B, Sepulveda-Swatson E, et al.: Postsystolic shortening by myocardial deformation imaging as a sign of cardiac adaptation to pressure overload in fetal growth restriction, *Circ Cardiovasc Imaging* 7(5):781–787, 2014.
12. Shi J, Pan C, Kong D, et al.: Left ventricular longitudinal and circumferential layer-specific myocardial strains and their determinants in healthy subjects, *Echocardiography* 33(4):510–518, 2016.
13. Colan SD, Shirali G, Margossian R, et al.: Pediatric Heart Network Investigators. The ventricular volume variability study of the Pediatric Heart Network: study design and impact of beat averaging and variable type on the reproducibility of echocardiographic measurements in children with chronic dilated cardiomyopathy, *J Am Soc Echocardiogr* 25(8):842–854, 2012.
14. Sanchez AA, Levy PT, Sekarski TJ, et al.: Effects of frame rate on two-dimensional speckle tracking-derived measurements of myocardial deformation in premature infants, *Echocardiography* 32(5):839–847, 2015.
15. Forsha D, Risum N, Rajagopal S, et al.: The influence of angle of insonation and target depth on speckle-tracking strain, *J Am Soc Echocardiogr* 28(5):580–586, 2015.
16. Pedrizzetti G, Mangual J, Tonti G: On the geometrical relationship between global longitudinal strain and ejection fraction in the evaluation of cardiac contraction, *J Biomech* 47(3):746–749, 2014.
17. Thorstensen A, Dalen H, Amundsen BH, et al.: Peak systolic velocity indices are more sensitive than end-systolic indices in detecting contraction changes assessed by echocardiography in young healthy humans, *Eur J Echocardiogr* 12(12):924–930, 2011.
18. Weidemann F, Jamal F, Sutherland GR, et al.: Myocardial function defined by strain rate and strain during alterations in inotropic states and heart rate, *Am J Physiol Heart Circ Physiol* 283(2):H792–H799, 2002.
19. Greenberg NL, Firstenberg MS, Castro PL, et al.: Doppler-derived myocardial systolic strain rate is a strong index of left ventricular contractility, *Circulation* 105(1):99–105, 2002.
20. El-Khuffash A, James AT, Corcoran JD, et al.: A patent ductus arteriosus severity score predicts chronic lung disease or death before discharge, *J Pediatr* 167(6):1354–1361, 2015.
21. Laser KT, Haas NA, Fischer M, et al.: Left ventricular rotation and right-left ventricular interaction in congenital heart disease: the acute effects of interventional closure of patent arterial ducts and atrial septal defects, *Cardiol Young* 24(4):661–674, 2014.
22. Forsey J, Benson L, Rozenblyum E, et al.: Early changes in apical rotation in genotype positive children with hypertrophic cardiomyopathy mutations without hypertrophic changes on two-dimensional imaging, *J Am Soc Echocardiogr* 27(2):215–221, 2014.
23. Cantinotti M, Kutty S, Giordano R, et al.: Review and status report of pediatric left ventricular systolic strain and strain rate nomograms, *Heart Fail Rev* 20(5):601–612, 2015.
24. Oxborough D, Batterham AM, Shave R, et al.: Interpretation of two-dimensional and tissue Doppler-derived strain (epsilon) and strain rate data: is there a need to normalize for individual variability in left ventricular morphology? *Eur J Echocardiogr* 10(5):677–682, 2009.
25. Marciniak A, Claus P, Sutherland GR, et al.: Changes in systolic left ventricular function in isolated mitral regurgitation. A strain rate imaging study, *Eur Heart J* 28(21):2627–2636, 2007.
26. de Waal K, Phad N, Collins N, et al.: Cardiac remodeling in preterm infants with prolonged exposure to a patent ductus arteriosus, *Congenit Heart Dis* 12(3):364–372, 2017.
27. Becker M, Kramann R, Dohmen G, et al.: Impact of left ventricular loading conditions on myocardial deformation parameters: analysis of early and late changes of myocardial deformation parameters after aortic valve replacement, *J Am Soc Echocardiogr* 20(6):681–689, 2007.
28. Burns AT, La Gerche A, D'hooge J, et al.: Left ventricular strain and strain rate: characterization of the effect of load in human subjects, *Eur J Echocardiogr* 11(3):283–289, 2010.
29. Yingchoncharoen T, Agarwal S, Popović ZB, et al.: Normal ranges of left ventricular strain: a meta-analysis, *J Am Soc Echocardiogr* 26(2):185–191, 2013.
30. de Waal K, Phad N, Collins N, et al.: Myocardial function during bradycardia events in preterm infants, *Early Hum Dev.* 98:17–21, 2016.
31. Nishikage T, Nakai H, Mor-Avi V, et al.: Quantitative assessment of left ventricular volume and ejection fraction using two-dimensional speckle tracking echocardiography, *Eur J Echocardiogr* 10(1):82–88, 2009.
31a. de Waal K: unpublished data.
32. Amundsen BH, Helle-Valle T, Edvardsen T, et al.: Noninvasive myocardial strain measurement by speckle tracking echocardiography: validation against sonomicrometry and tagged magnetic resonance imaging, *J Am Coll Cardiol* 47(4):789–793, 2006.
33. Korinek J, Kjaergaard J, Sengupta PP, et al.: High spatial resolution speckle tracking improves accuracy of 2-dimensional strain measurements: an update on a new method in functional echocardiography, *J Am Soc Echocardiogr* 20(2):165–170, 2007.

13

34. Singh GK, Cupps B, Pasque M, et al.: Accuracy and reproducibility of strain by speckle tracking in pediatric subjects with normal heart and single ventricular physiology: a two-dimensional speckle-tracking echocardiography and magnetic resonance imaging correlative study, *J Am Soc Echocardiogr* 23(11):1143–1152, 2010.

35. Koopman LP, Slorach C, Manlhiot C, et al.: Assessment of myocardial deformation in children using Digital Imaging and Communications in Medicine (DICOM) data and vendor independent speckle tracking software, *J Am Soc Echocardiogr* 24(1):37–44, 2011.

36. Takigiku K, Takeuchi M, Izumi C, et al.: JUSTICE investigators. Normal range of left ventricular 2-dimensional strain: Japanese Ultrasound Speckle Tracking of the Left Ventricle (JUSTICE) study, *Circ J* 76(11):2623–2632, 2012.

37. Farsalinos KE, Daraban AM, Ünlü S, et al.: Head-to-head comparison of global longitudinal strain measurements among nine different vendors: the EACVI/ASE Inter-Vendor Comparison Study, *J Am Soc Echocardiogr* 28(10):1171–1181, 2015.

38. Willruth AM, Geipel AK, Berg CT, et al.: Comparison of global and regional right and left ventricular longitudinal peak systolic strain, strain rate and velocity in healthy fetuses using a novel feature tracking technique, *J Perinat Med* 39(5):549–556, 2011.

39. Kapusta L, Mainzer G, Weiner Z, et al.: Changes in fetal left and right ventricular strain mechanics during normal pregnancy, *J Am Soc Echocardiogr* 26(10):1193–1200, 2013.

40. Maskatia SA, Pignatelli RH, Ayres NA, et al.: Longitudinal changes and interobserver variability of systolic myocardial deformation values in a prospective cohort of healthy fetuses across gestation and after delivery, *J Am Soc Echocardiogr* 29(4):341–349, 2016.

41. Zhang Y, Zhou QC, Pu DR, et al.: Differences in left ventricular twist related to age: speckle tracking echocardiographic data for healthy volunteers from neonate to age 70 years, *Echocardiography* 27(10):1205–1210, 2010.

42. Elkiran O, Karakurt C, Kocak G, et al.: Tissue Doppler, strain, and strain rate measurements assessed by two-dimensional speckle-tracking echocardiography in healthy newborns and infants, *Cardiol Young* 24(2):201–211, 2014.

43. Sehgal A, Wong F, Menahem S: Speckle tracking derived strain in infants with severe perinatal asphyxia: a comparative case control study, *Cardiovasc Ultrasound* 11:34, 2013.

44. Schubert U, Müller M, Norman M, et al.: Transition from fetal to neonatal life: changes in cardiac function assessed by speckle-tracking echocardiography, *Early Hum Dev* 89(10):803–808, 2013.

45. Klitsie LM, Roest AA, Haak MC, et al.: Longitudinal follow-up of ventricular performance in healthy neonates, *Early Hum Dev* 89(12):993–997, 2013.

46. Sehgal A, Doctor T, Menahem S: Cardiac function and arterial indices in infants born small for gestational age: analysis by speckle tracking, *Acta Paediatr* 103(2):e49–e54, 2014.

47. Jain A, Mohamed A, El-Khuffash A, et al.: A comprehensive echocardiographic protocol for assessing neonatal right ventricular dimensions and function in the transitional period: normative data and z scores, *J Am Soc Echocardiogr* 27(12):1293–1304, 2014.

48. Al-Biltagi M, Tolba OA, Rowisha MA, et al.: Speckle tracking and myocardial tissue imaging in infant of diabetic mother with gestational and pregestational diabetes, *Pediatr Cardiol* 36(2):445–453, 2015.

49. Jain A, El-Khuffash AF, Kuipers BC, et al.: Left ventricular function in healthy term neonates during the transitional period, *J Pediatr* 182:197–203, 2017.

50. Jashari H, Rydberg A, Ibrahimi P, et al.: Normal ranges of left ventricular strain in children: a meta-analysis, *Cardiovasc Ultrasound* 13:37, 2015.

51. Levy PT, Machefsky A, Sanchez AA, et al.: Reference ranges of left ventricular strain measures by two-dimensional speckle-tracking echocardiography in children: a systematic review and meta-analysis, *J Am Soc Echocardiogr* 29(3):209–225, 2016.

52. El-Khuffash AF, Jain A, Dragulescu A, et al.: Acute changes in myocardial systolic function in preterm infants undergoing patent ductus arteriosus ligation: a tissue Doppler and myocardial deformation study, *J Am Soc Echocardiogr* 25(10):1058–1067, 2012.

53. Levy PT, Holland MR, Sekarski TJ, et al.: Feasibility and reproducibility of systolic right ventricular strain measurement by speckle-tracking echocardiography in premature infants, *J Am Soc Echocardiogr* 26(10):1201–1213, 2013.

54. Sehgal A, Doctor T, Menahem S: Cyclooxygenase inhibitors in preterm infants with patent ductus arteriosus: effects on cardiac and vascular indices, *Pediatr Cardiol* 35(8):1429–1436, 2014.

55. de Waal K, Lakkundi A, Othman F: Speckle tracking echocardiography in very preterm infants: feasibility and reference values, *Early Hum Dev* 90(6):275–279, 2014.

56. Czernik C, Rhode S, Helfer S, et al.: Development of left ventricular longitudinal speckle tracking echocardiography in very low birth weight infants with and without bronchopulmonary dysplasia during the neonatal period, *PLoS One* 9(9):e106504, 2014.

57. James AT, Corcoran JD, Hayes B, et al.: The effect of antenatal magnesium sulfate on left ventricular afterload and myocardial function measured using deformation and rotational mechanics imaging, *J Perinatol* 35(11):913–918, 2015.

58. Hirose A, Khoo NS, Aziz K, et al.: Evolution of left ventricular function in the preterm infant, *J Am Soc Echocardiogr* 28(3):302–308, 2015.

59. Nasu Y, Oyama K, Nakano S, et al.: Longitudinal systolic strain of the bilayered ventricular septum during the first 72 hours of life in preterm infants, *J Echocardiogr* 13(3):90–99, 2015.

60. James A, Corcoran JD, Mertens L, et al.: Left ventricular rotational mechanics in preterm infants less than 29 weeks' gestation over the first week after birth, *J Am Soc Echocardiogr* 28(7):808–817, 2015.

61. Schubert U, Müller M, Abdul-Khaliq H, et al.: Preterm birth is associated with altered myocardial function in infancy, *J Am Soc Echocardiogr* 29(7):670–678, 2016.
62. de Waal K, Phad N, Lakkundi A, et al.: Cardiac function after the immediate transitional period in very preterm infants using speckle tracking analysis, *Pediatr Cardiol* 37(2):295–303, 2016.
63. Hecker T, Swan A, McLeod A, et al.: Feasibility and reproducibility of left ventricular longitudinal strain measurements in pre-term babies using two dimensional speckle tracking echocardiography, *Heart Lung Circ* 25(2):S231–S232, 2016.
64. de Waal K, Phad N, Lakkundi A, et al.: Post-transitional adaptation of the left heart in uncomplicated, very preterm infants, *Cardiol Young* 27(6):1167–1173, 2017.
65. Hoit BD: Strain and strain rate echocardiography and coronary artery disease, *Circ Cardiovasc Imaging* 4(2):179–190, 2011.
66. Smiseth OA, Torp H, Opdahl A, et al.: Myocardial strain imaging: how useful is it in clinical decision making? *Eur Heart J* 37(15):1196–1207, 2016.
67. Nestaas E, Støylen A, Brunvand L, et al.: Longitudinal strain and strain rate by tissue Doppler are more sensitive indices than fractional shortening for assessing the reduced myocardial function in asphyxiated neonates, *Cardiol Young* 21(1):1–7, 2011.
68. Czernik C, Rhode S, Helfer S, et al.: Left ventricular longitudinal strain and strain rate measured by 2-D speckle tracking echocardiography in neonates during whole-body hypothermia, *Ultrasound Med Biol.* 39(8):1343–1349, 2013.
69. Nestaas E, Skranes JH, Støylen A, et al.: The myocardial function during and after whole-body therapeutic hypothermia for hypoxic-ischemic encephalopathy, a cohort study, *Early Hum Dev.* 90(5):247–252, 2014.
70. Kulkarni A, Li L, Craft M, et al.: Fetal myocardial deformation in maternal diabetes mellitus and obesity, *Ultrasound Obstet Gynecol* 49(5):630–636, 2017.
71. Belbasis L, Savvidou MD, Kanu C, et al.: Birth weight in relation to health and disease in later life: an umbrella review of systematic reviews and meta-analyses, *BMC Med* 14(1):147, 2016.
72. Lewandowski AJ, Augustine D, Lamata P, et al.: Preterm heart in adult life: cardiovascular magnetic resonance reveals distinct differences in left ventricular mass, geometry, and function, *Circulation* 127(2):197–206, 2013.
73. Parkinson JR, Hyde MJ, Gale C, et al.: Preterm birth and the metabolic syndrome in adult life: a systematic review and meta-analysis, *Pediatrics* 131(4):e1240–e1263, 2013.
74. Forsey J, Friedberg MK, Mertens L: Speckle tracking echocardiography in pediatric and congenital heart disease, *Echocardiography* 30(4):447–459, 2013.
75. Colquitt JL, Pignatelli RH: Strain imaging: the emergence of speckle tracking echocardiography into clinical pediatric cardiology, *Congenit Heart Dis* 11(2):199–207, 2016.
76. Tham EB, Smallhorn JF, Kaneko S, et al.: Insights into the evolution of myocardial dysfunction in the functionally single right ventricle between staged palliations using speckle-tracking echocardiography, *J Am Soc Echocardiogr* 27(3):314–322, 2014.
77. Khoo NS, Smallhorn JF, Kaneko S, et al.: The assessment of atrial function in single ventricle hearts from birth to Fontan: a speckle-tracking study by using strain and strain rate, *J Am Soc Echocardiogr* 26(7):756–764, 2013.
78. Marcus KA, de Korte CL, Feuth T, et al.: Persistent reduction in left ventricular strain using two-dimensional speckle-tracking echocardiography after balloon valvuloplasty in children with congenital valvular aortic stenosis, *J Am Soc Echocardiogr* 25(5):473–485, 2012.
79. Basu S, Frank LH, Fenton KE, et al.: Two-dimensional speckle tracking imaging detects impaired myocardial performance in children with septic shock, not recognized by conventional echocardiography, *Pediatr Crit Care Med* 13(3):259–264, 2012.
80. Chang WT, Lee WH, Lee WT, et al.: Left ventricular global longitudinal strain is independently associated with mortality in septic shock patients, *Intensive Care Med* 41(10):1791–1799, 2015.
81. Levy PT, El-Khuffash A, Patel MD, et al.: Maturational patterns of systolic ventricular deformation mechanics by two-dimensional speckle-tracking echocardiography in preterm infants over the first year of age, *J Am Soc Echocardiogr* 30(7):685–698, 2017.
82. Vieira MJ, Teixeira R, Gonçalves L, et al.: Left atrial mechanics: echocardiographic assessment and clinical implications, *J Am Soc Echocardiogr* 27(5):463–478, 2014.
83. Fadnes S, Nyrnes SA, Torp H, et al.: Shunt flow evaluation in congenital heart disease based on two-dimensional speckle tracking, *Ultrasound Med Biol* 40(10):2379–2391, 2014.
84. Van Cauwenberge J, Lovstakken L, Fadnes S, et al.: Assessing the performance of ultrafast vector flow imaging in the neonatal heart via multiphysics modeling and in vitro experiments, *IEEE Trans Ultrason Ferroelectr Freq Control* 63(11):1772–1785, 2016.
85. Zhang L, Gao J, Xie M, et al.: Left ventricular three-dimensional global systolic strain by real-time three-dimensional speckle-tracking in children: feasibility, reproducibility, maturational changes, and normal ranges, *J Am Soc Echocardiogr* 26(8):853–859, 2013.
86. Silverman NH, Lewis AB, Heymann MA, et al.: Echocardiographic assessment of ductus arteriosus shunt in premature infants, *Circulation* 50(4):821–825, 1974.
87. Feigenbaum H: Role of M-mode technique in today's echocardiography, *J Am Soc Echocardiogr* 23(3):240–257, 2010.
88. Mertens L, Seri I, Marek J, et al.: Writing Group of the American Society of Echocardiography; European Association of Echocardiography; Association for European Pediatric Cardiologists. Targeted neonatal echocardiography in the neonatal intensive care unit: practice guidelines and recommendations for training. Writing Group of the American Society of Echocardiography (ASE) in collaboration with the European Association of Echocardiography (EAE) and the Association for European Pediatric Cardiologists (AEPC), *J Am Soc Echocardiogr* 24(10):1057–1078, 2011.

13

Assessment of Systemic Blood Flow and Cardiac Function: Other Methods

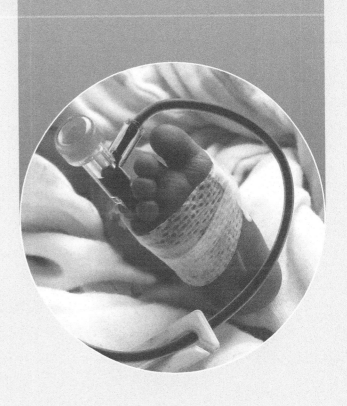

CHAPTER 14

Assessment of Cardiac Output in Neonates

TECHNIQUES USING THE FICK PRINCIPLE, INDICATOR DILUTION TECHNOLOGY, DOPPLER ULTRASOUND, THORACIC ELECTRICAL IMPEDANCE, AND ARTERIAL PULSE CONTOUR ANALYSIS

Willem-Pieter de Boode, Markus Osypka, Sadaf Soleymani, and Shahab Noori

- Cardiac output monitoring in preterm and term neonates is feasible but remains challenging despite the availability of different technologies.
- The best systems to monitor cardiac output in the clinical setting in neonatal intensive care at present are transthoracic echocardiography, transpulmonary indicator dilution, thoracic electrical bioimpedance, and arterial pulse contour analysis.
- Non-invasiveness of cardiac output monitoring is inversely related to accuracy; hence there will always be a compromise between these two characteristics.
- A normal cardiac output does not imply adequate perfusion of all tissues; cardiac output assessment will only provide information about global blood flow.
- Advanced hemodynamic monitoring in itself will not improve outcome; it is the correct interpretation of the acquired variables and the resultant, appropriately tested hemodynamic management approaches that may result in better outcomes.

As discussed in Chapters 1, 10, and 21, appropriate monitoring of the cardiovascular system and thus the treatment of critically ill neonates with cardiovascular compromise hinges on the ability to monitor at least two of the three interdependent cardiovascular parameters (blood pressure, cardiac output, and systemic vascular resistance), determining systemic blood flow and thus systemic oxygen delivery.

In the following equation, the Hagen-Poiseuille law is applied to systemic blood flow (similar to Ohm's law in electrical circuits):

$$SVR = \frac{SABP - RAP}{CO} \tag{14.1}$$

where CO = cardiac output (i.e., systemic blood flow), (SABP − RAP) = pressure difference between systolic arterial blood pressure (SABP) and right atrial pressure (RAP), and SVR = systemic vascular resistance.

Oxygen delivery can be calculated when cardiac output and arterial oxygen content are known:

$$DO_2 = CO \times CaO_2 \tag{14.2}$$

where DO_2 = oxygen delivery to the tissues, CO = cardiac output, and CaO_2 = arterial oxygen content.

At present, only blood pressure can be monitored continuously in absolute numbers in real time, albeit only invasively (see Chapter 3). Since monitoring SVR is not possible at present, continuous, noninvasive real-time assessment of beat-to-beat cardiac output has become the "holy grail" of modern-day neonatal intensive care. This is even more relevant considering the limited ability to clinically assess cardiac output using indirect parameters of systemic blood flow irrespective of the experience level of the clinician.[1-3] With the ability to continuously monitor both blood pressure and cardiac output in real time, the neonatologist is able to more accurately diagnose and perhaps treat neonatal shock (see Chapters 1, 21, 22, and 27).

Several methods of cardiac output measurement are available. However, not all technologies are feasible in neonates due to size restraints, potential indicator toxicity, risk of fluid overload, difficulties in vascular access, and the presence of shunts during the transitional phase and in patients with congenital heart defects. A classification of the different methods used for cardiac output measurement is depicted in Box 14.1.

An ideal method for the assessment of cardiac output is expected to include appropriate validation for accuracy and precision in real-time and absolute numbers, as well as that the method is continuous, reliable, practical, affordable, and easy to use and document. In addition, its ability to assess systemic blood flow in neonates with extra- and intracardiac shunting is an important requirement. Currently none of the available and routinely used methods come even close to fulfilling these requirements.

The Importance of Validation

It is of the upmost importance to pay attention to the validation of cardiac output monitoring systems prior to the introduction into clinical practice. Validation studies, especially in preterm neonates, are scarce and generally include only small numbers of patients. A new technology for cardiac output measurement must be validated against a gold standard reference method that is known to be accurate and precise and does not affect the technology being tested. Ideally this means

---

Box 14.1   CLASSIFICATION OF METHODS FOR CARDIAC OUTPUT ASSESSMENT

Fick principle based methods
  Oxygen Fick (O_2-Fick)
  Carbon dioxide Fick (CO_2-Fick)
  • Modified carbon dioxide Fick method (mCO_2F)
  • Carbon dioxide re-breathing technology (CO_2-R)
Indicator dilution techniques
  Pulmonary artery thermodilution (PATD)
  Transpulmonary thermodilution (TPTD)
  Transpulmonary lithium dilution (TPLiD)
  Transpulmonary ultrasound dilution (TPUD)
  Pulse dye densitometry (PDD)
Doppler ultrasound
  Transesophageal echocardiography/Doppler (TEE/TED)
  Transcutaneous Doppler (TCD)
  Transthoracic echocardiography (TTE)
Thoracic electrical impedance
  Electrical velocimetry (EV)
  Bioreactance (BR)
Arterial pulse contour analysis (APCA)
  As an adjunct to and calibrated by indicator dilution methods
  Modelflow method
  Pressure recording analytical method (PRAM)
Cardiac magnetic resonance imaging (MRI)

In this box different methods used for cardiac output measurement are summarized, divided into six categories.

validation against transit time flow probes, since this is considered the optimal in vivo reference method with a variability of less than 10%.[4–6] The flow probe should be positioned around the pulmonary artery, since this will represent true systemic blood flow in the absence of shunts. Placing the flow probe around the ascending aorta will underestimate systemic blood flow, because coronary blood flow is not taken into account.[7] Given the invasiveness of this reference method, its use is generally limited to animal studies. The Fick technology and the trans-pulmonary thermodilution (TPTD) cardiac output measurement are considered the clinical gold standard methods in pediatric critical care.[8–10] However, these technologies are not feasible in newborn infants.

Bland and Altman analysis is the most appropriate statistical method for comparing cardiac output measurements using two different technologies.[11] Correlation and regression analysis are not sufficient for this purpose. With Bland and Altman analysis the difference between the two methods (bias) is plotted against their mean. The accuracy is expressed as the mean bias, while the precision is defined as the limits of agreement (LOA). The LOA can be calculated from the standard deviation (SD) of the mean bias (LOA = ± 1.96 × SD). The LOA provides us with a range of the difference in cardiac output between two methods for 95% of the study population. It is recommended to express both accuracy and precision as a percentage of mean cardiac output instead of an absolute value.[12] Bias percentage (bias%) is defined as the mean bias divided by mean cardiac output multiplied by 100 (%), while the error percentage (error%) is calculated as 100% × LOA/mean cardiac output. The difference between accuracy and precision is further explained in Fig. 14.1.[13]

For acceptance of a new technology, the accuracy (bias%) and precision (error%) should at least be comparable with the reference method. This stresses the importance of the use of a valid, preferably gold standard technique for reference. A new technology is generally accepted when the error% is ±30 or less.[12] However, this cutoff value is based on the assumption that the precision of the reference method is ±10% to 20% with the acceptance of a new technology when the error% is no more than ±20. When using a reference method with an error% more than 20%, the cutoff value for acceptance of the tested technique should be adjusted.[12,13] The combined error% can be calculated using the following formula:

$$error\%_{COMP+REF} = \sqrt{(error\%_{COMP})^2 + (error\%_{REF})^2}, \tag{14.3}$$

where error%$_{COMP+REF}$ is the combined error%, error%$_{COMP}$ is the error% of the comparator (new method), and error%$_{REF}$ is the error% of the reference method.

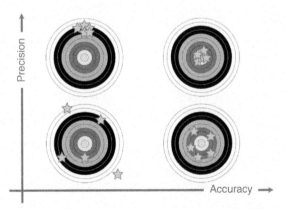

Fig. 14.1 Validation of the new method of cardiac output measurement expressed as accuracy and precision. The closer every measurement with the new technique (comparator) is to the bull's-eye (gold standard reference technology), the more accurate the comparator is; the more the spread between multiple measurements, the more imprecise the comparator is. (Modified from Cecconi M, Rhodes A, Poloniecki J, Della Rocca G, Grounds RM: Bench-to-bedside review: the importance of the precision of the reference technique in method comparison studies—with specific reference to the measurement of cardiac output. *Crit Care* 13(1):201, 2009.)

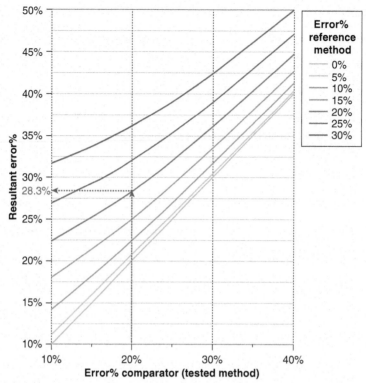

Fig. 14.2   Resultant error% as function of the error-percentages of the used reference method and tested comparator (errorgram). *X*-axis: error% of the tested method (comparator). *Y*-axis: resultant error% dependent on the precision of the used reference method (isolines).[12] For example, when the limits of agreement of the comparator are ±20%, and the used reference method has an error% of 20% *(red line)*, the resultant error% is 28.3% *(red arrows)*.

The resultant error percentage as a function of the error percentage of the tested method (comparator) and the reference method, respectively, is displayed as an errorgram as shown in Fig. 14.2.[12]

In addition, the agreement in monitoring temporal changes in cardiac output should be analyzed, for example by polar plot methodology.[14]

This chapter will provide an overview of all available technologies for the assessment of cardiac output, with emphasis on their applicability in (preterm) newborn infants. A summary of the characteristics, the advantages, and limitations for each method is presented in Table 14.1. When available, the results of neonatal validation studies are shown in tables within the appropriate paragraphs.

Fick Principle

Methods using the Fick principle might utilize the direct Fick method or one of its modifications to render the technique more clinically applicable. However, the modifications often come at the expense of accuracy.

In 1870 the German physiologist Adolf Eugen Fick stated that the volume of blood flow in a given period (cardiac output) equals the amount of a substance entering the bloodstream in the same period divided by the difference in concentrations of the substance upstream and downstream, respectively.[15]

Oxygen Fick

Determination of cardiac output according to the original or direct Fick method requires the application of a face mask (or some means of assessing oxygen consumption) and consideration of arterial and venous oxygen concentration, which is usually obtained by taking blood samples for laboratory analysis. The direct Fick

Table 14.1 OVERVIEW OF DIFFERENT METHODS OF CARDIAC OUTPUT MONITORING

Method	Invasive?	Continuous (C) or Intermittent (I)	Equipment	Feasible in Neonates?	Validated in Neonates?	Advantages	Limitations
Fick Principle							
O_2-Fick	+	I	AC, CVC	+	−	Accurate, especially in low flow state	Need for multiple, multisite blood sampling; accuracy limited in the presence of cardiopulmonary disease, air leakage, and enhanced pulmonary oxygen consumption (as in preterms with bronchopulmonary dysplasia); affected by shunts; less reliable in high flow state
mCO_2F	+	I	AC, CVC	+	−	No specific additional equipment required; reliable in the presence of significant left-to-right shunt; use of regular arterial and central venous catheters	Need for multiple, multisite blood sampling; inaccuracy related to calculation error of carbon dioxide concentration in blood
CO_2-R	−	I	ET	−	−	Easy to use; noninvasive	Not feasible/accurate in children with BSA <0.6 m² and tidal volume <300 mL; only applicable in intubated patients; contraindicated in patients susceptible to fluctuating arterial carbon dioxide levels
Indicator Dilution							
PATD	+++	I (& C)	PAC	−	−	Clinical gold standard of cardiac output monitoring in adults; ancillary hemodynamic variables provided	Very invasive; not feasible in small children; relatively high complication rate; transient bradycardia in response to fast injection of cold saline; results affected by shunt
TPTD	++	I (& C)	Dedicated AC, CVC	−	−	Clinical gold standard in pediatric patients; continuous monitoring when used to calibrate APCA; ancillary hemodynamic variables provided; reliable in presence of significant LtR-shunt	Dedicated thermistor-tipped arterial catheter required; catheterization of femoral, brachial, or axillary artery needed; repetitive measurements affect fluid balance
TPLiD	++	I (& C)	AC, CVC	−	−	Regular catheters used; continuous monitoring when used to calibrate APCA; ancillary hemodynamic variables provided	Lithium toxicity; need to withdraw blood; limited repeated measurements possible; not compatible with nondepolarizing muscle relaxants; influenced by hyponatremia; results affected by shunts

Continued

14

Table 14.1 OVERVIEW OF DIFFERENT METHODS OF CARDIAC OUTPUT MONITORING—cont'd

Method	Invasive?	Continuous (C) or Intermittent (I)	Equipment	Feasible in Neonates?	Validated in Neonates?	Advantages	Limitations
TPUD	++	I (& C)	AC, CVC	+	−	Nontoxic indicator; small indicator volume; ancillary hemodynamic variables provided; safe with regard to cerebral and systemic oxygenation and circulation; reliable in presence of significant LtR-shunt or heterogeneous lung injury	Repetitive measurements affect fluid balance; necessity to use extracorporeal loop
PDD	+	I	CVC	+	−	Noninvasive detection of indocyanine green; intravascular volume measurement possible	Limited repeated measurements possible; inaccuracy due to poor peripheral perfusion, motion artifact or excess light; rarely side effects; difficulty in the acquisition of reliable pulse waveforms in small children and newborns
Doppler Ultrasound							
TEE	+	I	Esophageal probe	±	−	Less invasive; evaluation of cardiac function and structure	Significant training required; highly operator-dependent; inaccuracy due to errors in the calculation of velocity time integral, cross-sectional area and angle of insonation; not feasible in infants <3 kg; small risk of complications; not tolerated by conscious patients
TED	+	I	Esophageal probe	±	−	Less invasive; continuous monitoring	Inaccuracy due to errors in the calculation of velocity time integral, cross-sectional area and angle of insonation; not feasible in infants <3 kg; small risk of complications; not tolerated by conscious patients
TCD	−	I	External probe	+	+	Noninvasive; easy to use	Blind aiming of transducer for signal acquisition; error due to insonation angle deviation; no real measurement of cross-sectional area of outflow tract; large interobserver variability

C

Table 14.1 OVERVIEW OF DIFFERENT METHODS OF CARDIAC OUTPUT MONITORING—cont'd

Method	Invasive?	Continuous (C) or Intermittent (I)	Equipment	Feasible in Neonates?	Validated in Neonates?	Advantages	Limitations
TTE	−	I	Echocardiograph	+	+	Noninvasive; evaluation in detail of cardiac function and structure; additional information about potential intra- and extracardiac shunting; most used method of cardiac output monitoring in neonatal clinical care	Significant training required; highly operator-dependent; not an easy, bedside method; high intra- and interobserver variability; inaccuracy due to errors in the calculation of velocity time integral, cross-sectional area and angle of insonation
Thoracic Electrical Impedance							
EC/BR	−	C	Surface electrodes	+	+	Only real noninvasive technology; continuous monitoring; user-independent; ancillary hemodynamic variables provided; easy to apply	Sensitive to motion artifact; inaccuracy due to alteration in position or contact of the electrodes, irregular heart rates, and acute changes in tissue water content; compromised reliability on high frequency ventilation
Arterial Pulse Contour Analysis							
PulseCO	++	C	AC, CVC	−	−	Less invasive; continuous monitoring	Repeated calibration required; use of small arterial catheters can cause distortion of the shape of the pressure wave and overdamped curves; accuracy influenced by changes in arterial compliance, changes in vasomotor tone, and irregular heart rate
PiCCO	++	C	Dedicated AC, CVC	−	−	Less invasive; continuous monitoring	Repeated calibration required; accuracy influenced by changes in arterial compliance, changes in vasomotor tone, and irregular heart rate
PRAM	+	C	AC	+	+	Less invasive; continuous monitoring; no calibration required	Use of small arterial catheters can cause distortion of the shape of the pressure wave and overdamped curves; accuracy influenced by changes in arterial compliance, changes in vasomotor tone, and irregular heart rate

AC, Arterial catheter; *APCA*, arterial pulse contour analysis; *BR*, bioreactance; *BSA*, body surface area; *CO₂-R*, CO₂ rebreathing; *CVC*, central venous catheter; *EC*, electrical cardiometry; *ET*, endotracheal tube; *LtR*, left-to-right; *mCO₂F*, modified CO₂ Fick method; *O₂-Fick*, oxygen Fick; *PAC*, pulmonary artery catheter; *PATD*, pulmonary artery thermodilution; *PDD*, pulse dye densitometry; *PiCCO*, APCA calibrated by TPTD; *PRAM*, pressure recording analytical method; *PulseCO*, APCA calibrated by TCD; *TCD*, transcutaneous Doppler; *TED*, transesophageal Doppler; *TEE*, transesophageal echocardiography; *TPLiD*, transpulmonary lithium dilution; *TPTD*, transpulmonary thermodilution; *TPUD*, transpulmonary ultrasound dilution; *TTE*, transthoracic echocardiography.

14

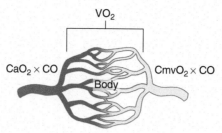

Fig. 14.3   Fick principle. See text for details. *CaO$_2$*, Arterial oxygen concentration; *CmvO$_2$*, mixed venous oxygen concentration; *CO*, cardiac output; *VO$_2$*, pulmonary oxygen uptake (O$_2$ consumption)

method employing a measurement of pulmonary oxygen uptake (discussed later) is considered the gold standard for assessing cardiac output, despite several disadvantages. It is of note though that recent advances in magnetic resonance imaging (MRI) technology have initiated a shift in our thinking, and cardiac output measurement by MRI is now considered by many as the gold standard for the measurement of cardiac output. However, MRI-based cardiac output measurement is only feasible in stable patients fit enough to undergo MRI scanning (see Chapter 15). According to the direct Fick principle, cardiac output is calculated by dividing oxygen consumption (VO$_2$) by the difference in the oxygen content of the aortic blood (CaO$_2$) and the mixed venous blood (CmvO$_2$).

The applicability in its original form, measuring VO$_2$ instead of assuming it, is limited by the fact that in nonintubated patients a face mask must be used. With respect to the application in neonates, a further limitation is that multiple and multi-site blood sampling is required. With oxygen being the substance for this method, the Fick principle states that during steady state, the oxygen taken up in the pulmonary system (pulmonary oxygen uptake) equals the oxygen consumption in the tissues (Fig. 14.3). Cardiac output (pulmonary blood flow) can be calculated by dividing the pulmonary oxygen uptake by the oxygen concentration gradient (difference) between arterial blood (CaO$_2$) and CmvO$_2$. Under steady-state condition, tissue oxygen consumption is equal to pulmonary oxygen uptake (VO$_2$). Hence,

$$CO = \frac{VO_2}{CaO_2 - CmvO_2} \tag{14.4}$$

where CO = cardiac output in L/min, VO$_2$ = pulmonary oxygen uptake in mL O$_2$/min, CaO$_2$ = oxygen concentration of arterial blood in mL O$_2$/L, and CmvO$_2$ = oxygen concentration of mixed venous blood (preferably determined in the pulmonary artery) in mL O$_2$/L.

Pediatric and adult patients differ significantly in oxygen consumption. Cardiac index is higher in neonates and infants by 30% to 60% to help meet their increased oxygen consumption. Fetal hemoglobin, present in fetal life and, in decreasing concentration, up to 3 to 6 months following birth, has higher oxygen affinity and thus does not deliver oxygen to the tissues as effectively as does adult hemoglobin when arterial oxygen saturation increases from the fetal levels of 75% in the ascending aorta to 98% to 100% after birth. In neonates, the combination of a higher hemoglobin concentration (16 to 19 g/dL compared with 13.5 to 17.5 g/dL in men and 12 to 16 g/dL in women), higher blood volume per kilogram of body weight, and increased cardiac output compensate for the decreased release of oxygen from hemoglobin to the tissues.

Pulmonary Oxygen Uptake

Pulmonary oxygen uptake (VO$_2$), or oxygen consumption, can be measured via a Douglas bag, by mass spectrometry, spirometry, or metabolic monitors (indirect calorimetry).[16] Table 14.2 depicts VO$_2$ measurements obtained in different patient populations and under different clinical conditions.[17–19]

Table 14.2 PULMONARY OXYGEN UPTAKE OR OXYGEN CONSUMPTION (VO_2) IN DIFFERENT PATIENT POPULATIONS

Group	VO_2 (Mean ± SD)	Notes
Adults	125 mL O_2/min/m^2	Indexed for body surface area
Healthy newborns (Bauer, 2002)[18]	6.7 ± 0.6 to 7.1 ± 0.4 mL O_2/min/kg	Indexed for body weight (n = 7)
Neonates with sepsis (Bauer, 2002)[18]	7.0 ± 0.3 to 8.2 ± 0.4 mL O_2/min/kg	n = 10
Mechanically ventilated preterm infants (Shiao, 2006)[19]	8.0 ± 3.73 mL O_2/min/kg	<8 h after blood drawn (n = 202)
	11.3 ± 5.65 mL O_2/min/kg	≥8 h after blood drawn (n = 65)
Preterm and term infants before and 1 hour after feeding (Stothers and Warner, 1979)[17]	4.8 mL O_2/min/kg (estimated from Fig. 6.1)	n = 9 preterm infants n = 9 term infants
Term infants during sleep	5.97 mL O_2/min/kg during REM sleep 5.72 mL O_2/min/kg during non-REM sleep	n = 30

Pulmonary oxygen uptake in adults, healthy term newborns, neonates with sepsis, mechanically ventilated preterm neonates, and preterm and term neonates before and after feeding.[17–19]
See text for details.
REM, Rapid eye movement.

Instead of actually measuring pulmonary oxygen uptake, this can also be estimated with the use of different regression equations.[20,21] However, the estimation of VO_2, which is also referred to as the indirect Fick method, is subject to errors for the determination of cardiac output potentially exceeding 50%. Because of the potential errors and its questionable adaptability to neonates, the cardiac output obtained by the indirect Fick method may be used in neonates for orientation purposes only.

Oxygen Concentration Gradient

Oxygen concentration (cO_2) is calculated by determining hemoglobin concentration (Hb) and oxygen saturation (sO_2), which traditionally is obtained by blood gas analysis:

$$cO_2 = (Hb \times sO_2 \times 1.36) + (pO_2 \times 0.0032) \qquad (14.5)$$

where Hb = hemoglobin in g/dL, sO_2 = oxygen saturation as gradient, 1.36 = oxygen binding capacity of hemoglobin in mL O_2/g, 0.0032 = solubility coefficient of oxygen in mL O_2/mm Hg, and pO_2 = partial pressure of oxygen in mm Hg.

Note that the aforementioned equation obtains oxygen content (cO_2) in mL O_2/dL. To obtain oxygen concentration (cO_2) in mL O_2/L, one needs to multiply the result by 10 (1 L = 10 dL).

Because in the normal range of pO_2, dissolved oxygen contributes very little to the total oxygen-carrying capacity, oxygen content can be approximated by

$$cO_2 = Hb \times sO_2 \times 1.36 \qquad (14.6)$$

and the gradient by

$$cO_2 = Hb \times 1.36 \times (SaO_2 - SmvO_2) \qquad (14.7)$$

where Hb = hemoglobin in g/dL, SaO_2 = arterial (pulmonary vein) oxygen saturation as gradient, and $SmvO_2$ = mixed venous (pulmonary artery) oxygen saturation as gradient.

Alternative to blood gas analysis, SaO_2 and SvO_2 may be obtained via catheters (e.g., Opticath catheter in combination with Oximetric-3 monitors, Abbott Critical Care Systems, Abbott Laboratories, Abbott Park, Illinois). The limitation is, however, that not mixed venous but central venous blood is sampled, and these are not interchangeable regarding oxygen saturation or oxygen content. Arterial oxygen saturation (SaO_2) may be approximated noninvasively by SpO_2 obtained via pulse oximetry.

Cardiac Output (Calculation Examples)

Assuming a neonate with VO_2 of 7 mL O_2/min/kg, Hb of 17 g/dL, SaO_2 of 99%, and $SmvO_2$ of 75%,

$$cO_2 = Hb \times 1.36 \times (SaO_2 - SmvO_2)$$

$$= 17 \left(\frac{g}{dL}\right) \times 1.36 \left(\frac{mLO_2}{g}\right) \times (99 - 75)\%$$

$$= 5.55 \frac{mLO_2}{dL}$$

With VO_2 normalized for weight, the cardiac output is

$$CI = \frac{VO_2}{CaO_2 - CmvO_2} = \frac{7.0 \left(\frac{mLO_2}{min \cdot kg}\right)}{5.55 \left(\frac{mLO_2}{dL}\right)} = 1.26 \left(\frac{dL}{min \cdot kg}\right) = 0.126 \frac{L}{min \cdot kg}$$

According to this calculation, cardiac output is 126 mL/kg/min in a neonate under physiologic circumstances. In a study by Tibby and colleagues, in five neonates with birth weights of 3.2 kg or less, the median CO following surgical correction of their congenital heart disease was 138 mL/kg/min.[8] However, CO measured by echocardiography in neonates averages around 200 mL/kg/min. There are several reasons why our calculation suggests lower cardiac output compared with the CO assessed by echocardiography. While the Hb concentration assumed in the equation is normal for term neonates in the transitional period, it is likely too high for neonates who underwent cardiac catheterization for clinical reasons and had their CO determined using the Fick principle. These patients' oxygen consumption is also likely to be higher than that of a healthy term neonate. In addition, the methods using the direct Fick principle yield a lower CO compared with that assessed by echocardiography because of the approximately 20% physiologic shunting present in the lungs. Indeed, if we change the Hb concentration and the VO_2 to 15 g/dL and 8 mL O_2/min/kg, respectively, and add 20% to compensate for the physiologic shunting in the lungs, we get a CO of 196 mL/kg/min, which is the same as the estimated 200 mL/kg/min of average CO determined by echocardiography.

Carbon Dioxide Fick

With the CO_2-Fick method, instead of using oxygen as a marker, the exchange of carbon dioxide may be used. This principle is used in the *modified carbon dioxide Fick method* (mCO_2F) and the *carbon dioxide rebreathing technology* (CO_2R).

Modified Carbon Dioxide Fick Method

The mCO_2F is based on the principle that steady-state carbon dioxide production in the tissue is equal to pulmonary carbon dioxide exchange (VCO_2):

$$CO = \frac{VCO_2}{CvCO_2 - CaCO_2} \tag{14.8}$$

where CO = cardiac output in L/min, VCO_2 = pulmonary carbon dioxide exchange in mL CO_2/min, $CaCO_2$ = carbon dioxide concentration in arterial blood in mL CO_2/min, and $CvCO_2$ = carbon dioxide concentration of venous blood (preferably determined in the pulmonary artery), measured in mL CO_2/L.

Pulmonary carbon dioxide exchange (VCO_2) may be measured using volumetric capnography. In a ventilated patient, VCO_2 can be determined by analysis of the expiratory airflow (Q_{exp}) and carbon dioxide fraction in the expiratory air ($FeCO_2$):

$$VCO_2 = \left\{\int_0^T Q_{exp(t)} \cdot FeCO_2(t) \cdot dt\right\} \cdot T^{-1} \tag{14.9}$$

where Q_{exp} = expiratory airflow in L/min, $FeCO_2$ = carbon dioxide fraction in expiratory air in mL CO_2/L, and T = time in minutes.

Carbon dioxide in an arterial or venous blood sample ($CbCO_2$) can be measured by the Douglas equation.[22] The amount of both pulmonary CO_2 exchange and systemic CO_2 production must be converted to *standard temperature pressure, dry conditions*. This method has been validated in an animal model, and the site of venous blood sampling has been shown to be of minor importance.[23] Interestingly, the presence of a significant left-to-right shunt through an artificial ductus arteriosus did not influence the accuracy of the mCO_2F method in another study using a juvenile animal model.[24] No studies in newborn infants have been published, probably related to the limitation of the need for frequent and multisite blood sampling.

Carbon Dioxide Rebreathing Technology

In the rebreathing method, mixed venous CO_2 concentration is estimated from exhaled gas and in this way obviates the need for direct measurement.

The change in CO_2 exchange and resultant change in arterial CO_2 concentration secondary to an end-expiratory hold or an addition of dead space is used in the CO_2-Fick equation:

$$Q_{PCBF} = \frac{VCO_2n}{CmvCO_2n - CaCO_2n} = \frac{VCO_2r}{CmvCO_2r - CaCO_2r} \tag{14.10}$$

where Q_{PCBF} = pulmonary capillary blood flow in L/min, VCO_2 = pulmonary carbon dioxide exchange in mL CO_2/min, n = in normal situation, r = rebreathing, $CaCO_2$ = carbon dioxide concentration in arterial blood in mL CO_2/min, and $CmvCO_2$ = carbon dioxide concentration of mixed venous blood in ml CO_2/L.

Pulmonary blood flow is considered constant during the measurements. Another assumption is that $CmvCO_2$ is not significantly changed throughout the period of rebreathing and nonrebreathing, implying that

$$CmvCO_2n \cong CmvCO_2r. \tag{14.11}$$

Therefore,

$$Q_{PCBF} = \frac{VCO_2n - VCO_2r}{(CmvCO_2n - CaCO_2n) - (CmvCO_2r - CaCO_2r)} = \frac{\Delta VCO_2}{\Delta CaCO_2} \tag{14.12}$$

where ΔVCO_2 = change in pulmonary CO_2 exchange, and $\Delta CaCO_2$ = change in arterial carbon dioxide concentration.

Pulmonary capillary blood flow only yields an estimate of the nonshunted blood flow participating in gas exchange. The blood bypassing the lung (shunted blood flow) may be estimated and added to Q_{PCBF} to determine overall cardiac output as follows:[25]

$$CO = Q_{PCBF} + Q_{SHUNT}. \tag{14.13}$$

Moreover, it is not the change in $CaCO_2$ that is measured in clinical practice, but the change in the partial pressure of carbon dioxide (pCO_2) at the endotracheal tube, assuming that endotracheal ΔpCO_2, alveolar ΔpCO_2, and arterial $\Delta CaCO_2$ are interchangeable. This may lead to errors in cardiac output calculation, especially in situations with large dead space ventilation.

The NICO system (Philips Respironics, Pittsburgh, Pennsylvania) is an example of a monitor incorporating the carbon dioxide rebreathing method. However, this device is not feasible in small children because of the large dead space of the rebreathing valve. In newborn infants, particularly in premature infants, partial rebreathing is contraindicated, since the technology is based on changes in arterial carbon dioxide concentrations causing significant changes in cerebral blood flow. Indeed, significant alterations in $PaCO_2$ have been shown to be associated with an increased risk of intraventricular hemorrhage, periventricular leukomalacia, and impaired neurodevelopmental outcome (see Chapters 1, 2, and 6).[26–28]

14

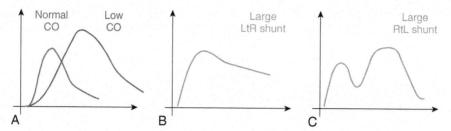

Fig. 14.4   Indicator dilution curves. Several configurations of transpulmonary indicator dilution curves. (A) Cardiac output (CO) is inversely proportional to the area under the dilution curve. (B) Large left-to-right (LtR) shunt will lead to early recirculation and therefore a prolonged detection of the indicator. (C) Large right-to-left (RtL) shunt will in fact lead to two dilution curves. The first curve is caused by the indicator that is bypassing the pulmonary circulation and detected very soon; the nonshunted, transpulmonary passage of the indicator is detected as a second curve.

Indicator Dilution Techniques

In 1761 Haller reported a new methodology to measure pulmonary circulation time with the use of a colored dye in an animal model.[29] This principle was adopted and modified initially by Stewart[30,31] and later by Hamilton,[32,33] and it's now known as the indicator dilution technique. An indicator dilution curve can be obtained by measuring the change in time of the concentration of a known quantity of indicator that is injected proximal to the point of measurement. With the use of the Stewart-Hamilton equation, blood flow (cardiac output) can be derived from the dilution curve:

$$CO = \frac{60 \cdot i}{\int C(t)\, dt},$$
(14.14)

where CO = cardiac output in L/min, i = injected quantity of indicator in mg, C = concentration of indicator in mg/L (area under the indicator dilution curve), and t = time in seconds.

Cardiac output is inversely proportional to the area under the dilution curve. The lower the blood flow, the higher the measured indicator concentration—hence the larger the area under the dilution curve (Fig. 14.4A).

Different indicators are used to obtain dilution curves, such as indocyanine green (ICG), Evans blue and brilliant red in dye dilution, cold solutions in thermodilution, lithium in lithium dilution, and isotonic saline in ultrasound dilution.

The following prerequisites need to be met for a reliable interpretation of the indicator dilution technique: fast, instantaneous injection of a small volume of indicator; fast and complete mixing of indicator and blood; no indicator loss between site of injection and detection; no changes in blood volume; uniform volume flow; no shunting; minimal valve regurgitation; flow of indicator must be identical to blood flow; blood flow should not be influenced by the volume of injected indicator; steady-state status; and stable hemodynamics during the measurement.[16] Potential limitations of this technology include the lack of indicator stability, inaccuracy in indicator measurement, and accumulation of indicator. The influence of a left-to-right shunt and right-to-left shunt on the indicator dilution curve is shown in Fig. 14.4B and C, respectively.

Pulmonary Artery Thermodilution

A specific thermistor-tipped pulmonary artery catheter, also known as a Swan-Ganz catheter, is used to measure the change in blood temperature downstream after the injection of a cold solution in the right atrium. This change in blood temperature is used to obtain an indicator dilution curve from which the cardiac output is calculated. Despite many sources of potential errors, pulmonary artery thermodilution (PATD) is regarded as one of the clinical gold standard technologies in adult critical care. For obvious reasons, the insertion of a flow-directed pulmonary catheter is not feasible in small infants.

Transpulmonary Indicator Dilution and Thermodilution

The technique of *transpulmonary indicator dilution* (TPID) has been developed in order to avoid the potential complications associated with the insertion and use of a pulmonary artery catheter. In this method, the indicator is injected into a central vein and detected after passing the pulmonary circulation in a systemic artery. However, the increased path length between the sites of injection and detection implies a higher risk of indicator loss, but also less variation in cardiac output measurements induced by cardiopulmonary interaction.

Cardiac output assessment with *transpulmonary thermodilution* is done by the injection of 3 to 5 mL of isotonic saline (cold or at body temperature) via a central venous catheter, which is subsequently detected by a dedicated, thermistor-tipped catheter positioned in the femoral, brachial, or axillary artery. Cardiac output is calculated by using blood temperature, temperature and volume of injected saline, area under the thermodilution curve, and a "correction factor" in the modified Stewart-Hamilton equation. TPTD has been validated in animal studies[9,34] and in children in the pediatric intensive care setting.[8,35,36] The central venous catheter should not be placed in close proximity to the arterial catheter—for example, in the femoral vein and artery on the same side. This is due to cross-talk phenomenon causing possible direct interference and erroneous cardiac output calculation.[37] TPTD is regarded the clinical gold standard for pediatric cardiac output measurement.[10] TPTD can be used to calibrate software for continuous cardiac output monitoring using arterial pulse contour analysis (APCA; PiCCO, Pulsion Medical Systems, Feldkirchen, Germany). Validation studies in newborn infants are lacking, but the use of TPTD has been described in newborn infants (3.0 to 4.9 kg) undergoing arterial switch surgery.[38] Because of the preferred position of a dedicated arterial catheter, this technique is not safely applicable in smaller infants.

Transpulmonary Lithium Dilution

The use of lithium as an indicator to obtain a dilution curve for cardiac output calculations was first described in 1993.[39] The choice of lithium was based on the minimal loss of this substance during the first passage and the rapid distribution, which enables multiple measurements.[40,41] Lithium is injected intravenously in a known quantity and detected by a lithium ion sensitive electrode that is attached to a peripheral arterial catheter. Blood is drawn through this sensor at a specific rate by a roller pump. For an accurate calculation of cardiac output, a correction is needed for blood sodium concentration, since sodium is the main determinant of the potential difference across the sensor in the absence of lithium, and therefore it determines the baseline voltage. Since lithium is only distributed in plasma, a correction is also needed for hematocrit.

The first feasibility study of transpulmonary lithium dilution (TPLiD) in 17 children receiving intensive care (2.6 to 28.2 kg) was performed by Linton et al. and validated against TPTD (Table 14.3).[42] TPLiD can be used to calibrate software for continuous cardiac output monitoring using APCA (LiDCOplus, LiDCO Ltd., London, United Kingdom). The potential toxicity of lithium in newborns is of major concern, especially after repeated measurements, and therefore this technology is not feasible in newborn infants.

Table 14.3 VALIDATION STUDY OF TRANSPULMONARY LITHIUM DILUTION IN NEONATES AND CHILDREN

Subjects	Comparison	CO, Mean	Mean Bias (Absolute)	LOA (Absolute)	Bias%	Error%
17 patients (3 weeks–9 years; 2.6 ± 34 kg); PICU; 48 paired measurements	TPLiD vs. TPTD	1.9 L/min	−0.1 L/min	±0.61 L/min	5%	32%

CO, Cardiac output; *LOA,* limits of agreement; *PICU,* pediatric intensive care unit; *TPLiD,* transpulmonary lithium dilution; *TPTD,* transpulmonary thermodilution.
From Linton RA, Jonas MM, Tibby SM, et al: Cardiac output measured by lithium dilution and transpulmonary thermodilution in patients in a paediatric intensive care unit. *Intensive Care Med* 26(10):1507–1511, 2000.

Transpulmonary Ultrasound Dilution

Since ultrasound travels slower through normal saline (1533 m/s) in comparison with blood (1560 to 1585 m/s), injection of isotonic saline via a central vein will lead to a decrease in ultrasound velocity in blood that can be detected in a systemic artery. Sensors have to be placed on both the arterial and venous sides of the circulation for measurement of flow and ultrasound dilution by means of an extracorporeal circuit. This is constructed by connecting a disposable, arteriovenous (AV) loop in between regular arterial and central venous catheters. Isotonic saline at body temperature is rapidly injected in a volume of 0.5 to 1.0 mL/kg into the venous limb of the AV loop. The decrease in ultrasound velocity is detected after transpulmonary passage through the body in the arterial limb of the AV loop, from which an ultrasound dilution curve is obtained. With the use of the Stewart-Hamilton equation, the cardiac output is calculated. Transpulmonary ultrasound dilution (TPUD) has been validated in vitro[43] and in animal models.[44–48] In an animal model, the interventions needed to measure cardiac output using TPUD, such as starting and stopping blood flow through the AV loop and the fast injection of isotonic saline at body temperature, did not cause clinically relevant changes in cerebral and systemic circulation and oxygenation.[49] The accuracy of cardiac output calculation by TPUD is not influenced by the presence of a significant left-to-right shunt[50] or heterogeneous lung injury.[45] TPUD has also been shown to accurately detect a left-to-right shunt.[48,51] Hemodynamic volumetry by TPUD is a promising technique for monitoring changes in active circulating blood volume, central blood volume, and total end-diastolic volume.[47] Validation studies have been published in children, and the first clinical neonatal studies are also in progress.[51–53]

Pulse Dye Densitometry

The original dye dilution technology requires direct, continuous, and invasive blood sampling through a cuvette for measurement of the injected indicator (e.g., ICG) in arterial blood for the acquisition of a dye dilution curve. Consequently this cannot be regarded as a clinical method of cardiac output estimation, especially in small children.

Interestingly, the problem of unacceptable blood withdrawal has been overcome with the use of a new technology, *pulse dye densitometry* (PDD). The injected ICG is noninvasively detected in this method via a fingertip sensor by analyzing the pulsatile changes in ICG concentration. However, PDD for cardiac output calculation has not been validated in newborn infants, most probably because of the difficulty in the acquisition of reliable pulse waveforms in small children and newborns.[54]

Doppler Ultrasound

The principle underlying ultrasonic measurement of stroke volume (SV) is quite simple: if the distance (d, measured in cm) traversed by a cylindrical column of blood is measured over its ejection interval (t, measured in seconds) and multiplied by the measured cross-sectional area conduit (CSA, measured in cm²) through which it flows, then SV (measured in mL) can be calculated as

$$SV = CSA \cdot d \tag{14.15}$$

where CSA of the right or left ventricular outflow tract (pulmonary or aortic valve) is calculated via diameter measurements employing ultrasonic echo imaging. The distance (d) is calculated using the Doppler envelope of blood velocity extracted from ultrasonic Doppler velocimetry (see Chapter 11).

According to the Doppler principle, when an emitted ultrasonic wave of constant magnitude is reflected (backscattered) from a moving object (red blood cell), the frequency of the reflected ultrasound is altered. The frequency difference between the ultrasound emitted (f_0) and that received (f_R) by the Doppler transducer is called frequency shift $\Delta f = f_R - f_0$. This instantaneous frequency shift depends upon the magnitude of the instantaneous velocity of the reflecting targets, their direction with respect to the Doppler transducer, and the cosine of angle at which the emitted ultrasound intersects these targets[55]:

$$\Delta f = \frac{2f_0 \cdot v_i \cdot \cos\theta}{C} \tag{14.16}$$

where Δf is the instantaneous frequency shift; f_0 the emitted constant magnitude ultrasonic frequency; C is the speed (propagation velocity) of ultrasound in tissue (blood); θ is the incident angle formed by the axial flow of red blood cells and the emitted ultrasonic signal; and v_i is the instantaneous velocity of red cells within the scope of the interrogating ultrasound perimeter or target volume.

By algebraic rearrangement,

$$v_i = \frac{C}{2f_0} \cdot \frac{\Delta f}{\cos\theta}. \tag{14.17}$$

Since C and f_0 are constants, then

$$v_i = K \cdot \frac{\Delta f}{\cos\theta}. \tag{14.18}$$

If the angle of incidence between the axial flow of blood and the ultrasonic beam is $0°$ (i.e., $\theta = 0°$), then cosine θ equals 1, and thus

$$v_i = K \cdot \Delta f \tag{14.19}$$
$$v_i \propto \Delta f$$

The opening of the ventriculo-arterial (VA) valve velocity rapidly accelerates from zero to reach a maximum (peak velocity) during the first one-third or one-half of the ejection phase of systole and a more gradual deceleration phase back to zero velocity occurs with the closure of the VA valve, v_i is not constant. Thus in order to obtain the distance d traversed by the cylindrical column of blood according to the model described earlier, v_i has to be integrated over time—that is, from the point in time t_0 representing the opening of the valve to t_1 representing the closure of the valve:

$$d(t) = \int_{t_0}^{t_1} v_i(t)\, dt = VTI \tag{14.20}$$

where this integral is called the velocity time integral (VTI) and defines the stroke distance in centimeters.

SV is then calculated as

$$SV = CSA \cdot VTI. \tag{14.21}$$

Cardiac output is subsequently calculated by multiplying SV by heart rate (HR):

$$CO = SV \cdot HR. \tag{14.22}$$

A number of assumptions are made when developing Eq. 14.21. A first assumption is that the blood flows through the ventricular outflow tract in an undisturbed laminar flow. Because under certain conditions the flow can be turbulent, this assumption has questionable validity.

Another important problem is that the assumption of a circular vessel of constant internal diameter is only fulfilled superficially in a largely undetermined patient population. In fact, aortas of patients can be, for example, oval or have the shape of an irregular circle. Furthermore, the ascending aorta is not rigid, as assumed, since it pulsates during systolic ejection, producing 5% to 17% changes in the CSA from its diastolic to systolic pressure extremes.[56]

Moreover, even if the aorta were circular, the accuracy of any echocardiographic method is limited by spatial resolution. Indeed, poor correlation has been found between aortic diameters measured intraoperatively and those measured by a commercially available A-mode echo device preoperatively.[57] In addition, errors in

Table 14.4   AORTIC RADIUS/DIAMETER AND CORRESPONDING CROSS-SECTIONAL AREA, ASSUMING A CIRCULAR SHAPED AORTA

Radius (r) (mm)	Diameter (d) (mm)	CSA mm²	Relative	Change of CSA
2.5	5.0	19.6		
3.0	6.0	28.3	44%	Larger than when r = 2.5 mm
3.5	7.0	38.5	36%	Larger than when r = 3.0 mm
4.0	8.0	50.3	31%	Larger than when r = 3.5 mm
4.5	9.0	63.6	27%	Larger than when r = 4.0 mm

Relatively small errors in determining the true diameter of the aorta result in significant errors when calculating the CSA, and in turn stroke volume and cardiac output.
CSA, Cross-sectional area.

Table 14.5   UNDERESTIMATION OF VELOCITY PER ANGLE OF INSONATION

Angle of Insonation (θ)	Cos θ	Underestimation of Velocity
0	1	0
10	0.98	2%
20	0.94	6%
30	0.87	13%
40	0.77	23%

Cos, Cosine.

echocardiographic diameter (D) are magnified to the second power ($CSA = \pi \cdot D^2/4$). This becomes more of an issue with the smaller diameter of the aorta in the neonate. Table 14.4 presents a range of aortic radiuses and diameters and for each range the corresponding CSA. The last column refers to the relative change of CSA if the diameter of the aorta were assessed to be larger by 1 mm. (At the 5-mm aortic diameter of neonates, especially preterm neonates, the echocardiographically "measured" CSA would indeed be 44% larger than the actual value.)

Errors in the velocity measurement are increased by interrogating the axial blood flow at an angle greater than 0° by the emitted ultrasonic signal. However, because the cosine of θ < 20° is close to 1 (Table 14.5), determining velocity with an acceptable accuracy is still possible. With the increase in angle of insonation (θ) beyond 20°, the velocity is progressively underestimated and therefore angle correction is needed.

Transthoracic Echocardiography

Echocardiography has its first and foremost use as an imaging technique to evaluate the mechanical function of the neonate's heart. The use of echocardiography for Doppler velocimetry and determination of SV and cardiac output is a readily available and frequently utilized option at the bedside. The accuracy of SV and cardiac output measurements using echocardiography, however, depend on the skills of the operator, and the various sources of errors must be taken into account when utilizing this method. Transthoracic echocardiography (TTE)–derived cardiac output measurements have been validated against several reference techniques, such as dye dilution, direct Fick, and thermodilution, and yielded a bias of less than 10% with a relatively wide range (−37% to +16%) and a precision (±1.96 SD) of ±30%.[58] The intra- and interobserver variability have been reported in the range of 2.1% to 22% and 3.1% to 21.7%, respectively. The use of TTE for neonatal hemodynamic assessment is beyond the scope of this chapter and extensively described in Chapters 10 to 13.

Transesophageal Echocardiography

Real-time imaging of the heart can be acquired by transesophageal echocardiography (TEE) from which both the VTI in the left and/or right ventricular outflow tract and the CSA of the aortic and/or pulmonary valve can be measured. Besides cardiac output calculation, the cardiac anatomy, preload status, and myocardial performance can be assessed. TEE is mainly used perioperatively for functional and structural imaging in children with congenital heart defects. Although anecdotal cases have been

Table 14.6 VALIDATION STUDIES OF TRANSCUTANEOUS DOPPLER IN NEWBORNS

Reference	Subjects	Comparison	CO, Mean	Mean Bias (Absolute)	LOA (Absolute)	Bias%	Error%
Phillips, 2006	37 Preterm infants (1.13 ± 0.47 kg); 66 paired measurements	TCD vs. TTE (LVO)	0.37 L/min	0.00 L/min	±0.16 L/min	0%	43%
Patel, 2011	56 (Pre)term infants; median (range) 39 (31–41) weeks, 3.4 (1.4–4.9 kg); 56 paired measurements	TCD vs. TTE (LVO) TCD vs. TTE (RVO)	251 mL/kg/min 279 mL/kg/min	14 mL/kg/min −59 mL/kg/min	±108 mL/kg/min ±160 mL/kg/min	6% 21%	43% 57%

CO, Cardiac output; *LOA*, limits of agreement; *LVO*, left ventricular output; *RVO*, right ventricular output; *TCD*, transcutaneous Doppler; *TTE*, transthoracic echocardiography.
See references 65 and 67.

14

described where intraoperative TEE has been successfully used in low birth weight infants less than 1.6 kg,[59,60] it is advised to only consider TEE in children weighing 3 kg or more, since the smallest patients have an increased risk of complications, such as esophageal perforation, tracheal and bronchial compression, inadvertent endotracheal tube dislodgment, and compression of the aorta or left atrium.

Transesophageal Doppler

With transesophageal Doppler (TED), the blood flow velocity in the descending aorta is measured with the use of an ultrasound probe that is positioned in the esophagus. An essential difference with TEE is that no direct imaging of cardiovascular structures is acquired, so the ultrasound beam has to be aimed toward the aorta without direct visualization of the vessel by checking the signal quality. This also implies that the CSA of the aorta has to be acquired separately by M-mode echocardiography, although it is usually estimated using a nomogram based on age, sex, height, weight, or body surface area. However, it is understood that the aortic diameter is not a static value, since it varies with changes in blood pressure.[61] TED is mainly used intraoperatively to assess fluid responsiveness in children.[62,63] As with TEE, this method is mainly applicable in infants greater than 3 kg.

Transcutaneous Doppler

Transcutaneous Doppler (TCD) technology (USCOM 1A, USCOM Ltd, Sydney, Australia) uses the conventional Doppler method of acquiring a Doppler velocity time flow profile across the semilunar valves. This signal can be acquired from the suprasternal window angling down into the mediastinum perpendicular to the aortic valve and parallel to the transaortic blood flow. In addition, the Doppler beam can be angled perpendicular to the pulmonary valve and parallel to the transvalvular blood flow through the parasternal acoustic access in the third to fifth anterior intercostal spaces. This allows the acquisition of a simple Doppler velocity time flow profile for both the transaortic and transpulmonary blood flow, and from each flow profile the VTI can be calculated. Since there is no direct visualization of the semilunar valve, the correct position of the ultrasound beam must be assumed based on the acquired signal quality, and the cross-sectional area of the aortic and pulmonary valve is derived from an anthropometric algorithm, based on weight, height, and age.

The intraobserver variability ranges from 4% to 11%.[64–66] A limited number of validation studies in newborn infants of TCD have been published, which show an error-percentage above 40% (Table 14.6). This is in agreement with the conclusions from a systematic review of clinical studies comparing TCD with thermodilution as a reference method in adult patients finding an error-percentage of 43%.

Thoracic Electrical Bioimpedance

Thoracic electrical bioimpedance (TEB) technology is currently probably the only true noninvasive method of continuous cardiac output assessment. The development of this technique, aiming to analyze the effect of weightlessness on cardiac output, was published in 1966.[68]

The noninvasive and easy-to-apply impedance-based methods for determining cardiac output extract the changes in thoracic electrical impedance caused by the cardiac cycle. The methods differ in which component of bioimpedance is utilized to create the impedance cardiogram and in the interpretation of the waveform. Examples are electrical cardiometry (EC; ICON, AESCULON; Osypka Medical GmbH, Berlin, Germany) and the bioreactance method (BR; Starling, NICOM; Cheetah Medical Inc., Vancouver, WA).

Bioimpedance has two orthogonal components, bioresistance and bioreactance, the value of which depends on the frequency of the current or voltage applied. Bioimpedance is a property of the particular tissue. Each tissue in the thoracic compartment, such as blood, tissue of the different organs, or bone, has specific bioimpedance—that is, specific bioresistance and specific *bioreactance*. Blood has very low bioresistance and thus bioimpedance in contrast with bone tissue or compartments filled with air, such as the lungs at peak inspiration. Accordingly, one possible embodiment of bioimpedance measurement is to obtain the respiration rate.

In order to obtain hemodynamic parameters (i.e., parameters related to blood flow), bioimpedance measurement must encompass a major artery such as the aorta or even the brachial artery. If the intention is to derive SV or cardiac output from the blood flow in the aorta, then sensors for applying an electrical field are generally placed between a patient's neck and lower thorax (thus encompassing the aorta).

Obtaining hemodynamic parameters from bioimpedance measurements is a two-step process. In the first step, signal acquisition and processing have to acquire and record the portion of the change of bioimpedance specifically related to cardiac activity, referred to as the *impedance cardiogram*. The surface electrocardiogram (ECG), which is usually recorded in parallel, can serve as a reference for specific landmarks occurring in the course of the impedance cardiogram. The second step is to apply a model providing a translation of the measured bioimpedance into a meaningful hemodynamic variable.

Therefore a model and related assumptions are applied to derive from the measured bioimpedance a hemodynamic parameter. The same applies to the impedance cardiogram, no matter how it was derived and which component of bioimpedance (bioresistance or bioreactance) was pursued.

The estimation of SV and cardiac output by means of TEB requires the application of a low magnitude (~2 mA), high frequency (30 to 100 KHz) alternating current (AC) to the thorax. Bioimpedance is calculated as the ratio of the measured voltage U(t) and the applied current I(t):

$$Z(t) = \frac{U(t)}{I(t)} \ (Ohm \ Law). \quad (14.23)$$

If the current I(t) is of constant amplitude, the bioimpedance Z(t) is proportional to the measured voltage U(t):

$$Z(t) \approx U(t). \quad (14.24)$$

Upon application of an AC, in contrast to a direct current (DC), such as provided by a battery, the bioimpedance (Z) of tissue comprises not only a resistive component but also a reactive component. The reactive component causes a shift in phase between the AC applied and the alternating voltage measured. This occurs because biologic tissue can be modeled as a network of electrical resistances (e.g., blood plasma) and capacitors (e.g., cell membranes). As stated before, bioimpedance and its components are dependent on the frequency of the current applied. Imagine a cell membrane that cannot be "crossed" by an AC of low frequency but becomes more and more "permeable" to a current with increasing frequency. This applies to electrical impedance and is one of the reasons why bioimpedance-based methods use an electrical current, usually in the range of 30 to 100 KHz and not much higher or lower.

TEB is usually measured in the longitudinal direction of the human body, with surface electrodes (or sometimes electrodes on an esophageal catheter) placed in such a way that the electrical field established by the application of an AC encompasses the heart and, more preferably, the ascending aorta and a portion of the descending aorta. The reason for the focus on the aorta rather than the heart is that the most significant rapid change in bioimpedance related to the blood circulation occurs shortly (50 to 70 ms) after aortic valve opening, and thus this change is considered to be a phenomenon related to the aorta. This rapid change in bioimpedance with time t can be observed in both of its components, bioresistance $R(t)$ and bioreactance $X(t)$, which can also be expressed in magnitude $|Z(t)|$ and phase $\theta(t)$:

$$|Z(t)| = \sqrt{\left(R(t)^2\right) + \left(X(t)^2\right)} \tag{14.25}$$

$$\theta(t) = \arctan\left(\frac{X(t)}{R(t)}\right). \tag{14.26}$$

EC measures bioresistance $R(t)$ and bioreactance $X(t)$ and employs the temporal course of magnitude of impedance $|Z(t)|$ for determination of SV. In contrast, the BR focuses on the temporal course of the phase $\theta(t)$ of bioimpedance. Both methods reveal an impedance cardiogram that is to some extent similar to an arterial pressure waveform.

Validation studies of TEB are listed in Table 14.7.

Electrical Cardiometry

When measuring the temporal course of bioimpedance of the thorax, $Z(t)$, the result is the sum of the arrangement of tissue impedances in series and in parallel to each other. Most prevalent are the static and quasistatic impedances, referred to as Z_0, followed by a fairly significant dynamic change in bioimpedance corresponding to the respiratory cycle, $\Delta Z_R(t)$, and, to a lesser degree, a change in bioimpedance corresponding to the cardiac cycle, $\Delta Z_C(t)$, all of which are superimposed:

$$Z(t) = Z_0 + \Delta Z_R(t) + \Delta Z_C(t). \tag{14.27}$$

Because the determination of SV and cardiac output is of interest, the respiratory component of thoracic bioimpedance is omitted (practically by applying high-pass filters), and thus reducing bioimpedance to

$$Z(t) = Z_0 + \Delta Z_C(t). \tag{14.28}$$

Thoracic fluid content (TFC) is calculated from base impedance Z_0,

$$TFC = \frac{1000}{Z_0}, \tag{14.29}$$

and is indicative of excess fluids in the thorax such as pulmonary edema, pleural effusion, and pericardial effusion.

EC is based on the phenomenon that the conductivity of the blood in the aorta changes during the cardiac cycle.

Prior to opening of the aortic valve, the red blood cells (erythrocytes) assume a random orientation—there is no blood flow in the ascending aorta (Fig. 14.5). The electrical current applied must circumvent the red blood cells for passing through the aorta, which results in a higher voltage measurement and thus lower conductivity.

Table 14.7   VALIDATION STUDIES OF THORACIC ELECTRICAL BIOIMPEDANCE IN NEWBORNS

Reference	Subjects	Comparison	CO, Mean	Mean Bias (Absolute)	LOA (Absolute)	Bias%	Error%
Noori, 2012	20 healthy newborns (39.2 ± 1.1 weeks; 3094 ± 338 g); PNA < 48 h; PDA included 115 paired measurements	EC vs. TTE (LVO)	538 mL/min	–4 mL/min	±238 mL/min	1%	44%
Weisz, 2012	10 term neonates (median 37 weeks; 2.72 kg); 97 paired measurements	BR vs. TTE (LVO)	559 mL/min	153 mL/min	±155 mL/min	27%	28%
Song, 2014	40 preterms (mean 27 weeks); 108 paired measurements	EC vs. TTE (LVO)	218 mL/kg/min				
	• *Overall*			–18.8 mL/kg/min	±133 mL/kg/min	9%	61%
	• *Nonventilated*			–20.4 mL/kg/min	±105 mL/kg/min	9%	48%
	• *Room air*			–25.0 mL/kg/min	±44.6 mL/kg/min	11%	20%
	• *nCPAP*			–18.2 mL/kg/min	±125 mL/kg/min	8%	57%
	• *Ventilated*			–17.5 mL/kg/min	±156 mL/kg/min	8%	72%
	• *SIMV*			–30.2 mL/kg/min	±145 mL/kg/min	14%	67%
	• *HFJV*			–10.9 mL/kg/min	±160 mL/kg/min	5%	73%
	• *HFOV*			38.2 mL/kg/min	±179 mL/kg/min	18%	82%
Weisz, 2014	25 preterm infants (median 25 week) post-PDA ligation; 78 paired measurements	BR vs. TTE (LVO)	227 mL/kg/min	NA	NA	39%	32%
Grollmuss, 2014	28 preterms (mean 31.7 weeks); 228 paired measurements	EC vs. TTE (LVO)	256 mL/kg/min				
	• *All*			8.9 mL/kg/min	±63 mL/kg/min	3%	24%
	• *LBW (<2500 g)*			10.4 mL/kg/min	±61 mL/kg/min	4%	24%
	• *VLBW (<1500 g)*			5.3 mL/kg/min	±59 mL/kg/min	2%	23%
Torigoe, 2015	28 preterms (median 32 weeks); 81 paired measurements	EC vs. TTE (LVO)	317 mL/min				
	• *Overall*			–6 mL/min	±92 mL/min	2%	29%
	• *No hsPDA*			6 mL/min	±67 mL/min	2%	21%
	• *hsPDA*			–36 mL/min	±120 mL/min	11%	38%
	• *Nonventilated*			–14 mL/min	±103 mL/min	4%	32%
	• *nCPAP*			6.3 mL/min	±73 mL/min	2%	23%
	• *SIMV*			–29.6 mL/min	±98 mL/min	9%	31%
	• *HFOV*			–12.0 mL/min	±106 mL/min	4%	33%
Boet, 2016	79 preterms (31 ± 3.2 weeks); 451 paired measurements	EC vs. TTE (LVO)	NA	–0.21 L/min	±0.35 L/min (?) estimated (graph)	NA	NA

BR, Bioreactance method; CO, cardiac output; EC, electrical cardiometry; HFJV, high frequency jet ventilation; HFOV, high-frequency oscillatory ventilation; hsPDA, hemodynamically significant PDA; LBW, low birth weight; LOA, limits of agreement; LVO, left ventricular output; NA, not available; nCPAP, nasal continuous positive airway pressure; PDA, patent ductus arteriosus; PNA, postnatal age; SIMV, synchronized intermittent mandatory ventilation; TTE, transthoracic echocardiography; VLBW, very low birth weight. See references 71 to 77.

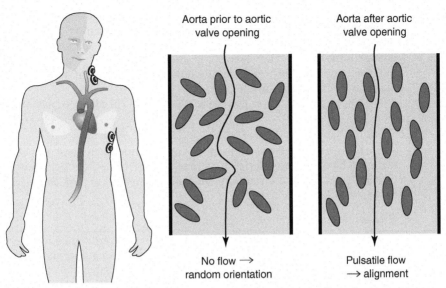

Fig. 14.5 Electrode arrangement and proposed orientation of red blood cells in the aorta prior to and shortly after aortic valve opening are shown.

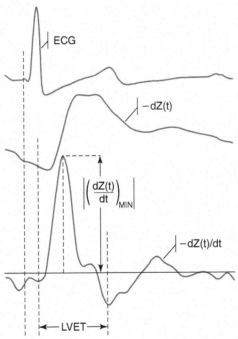

Fig. 14.6 Temporal course of surface electrocardiogram (ECG), the cardiac-related change of bioimpedance [−dZ(t)], and the rate of change of bioimpedance |−dZ(t)/dt|. The rate of change of bioimpedance is a calculated (i.e., artificial) signal waveform and used for waveform analysis (such as determination of minima and maxima). *LVET*, Left ventricular ejection time.

Very shortly after aortic valve opening, the pulsatile blood flow forces the red blood cells to align in parallel with the blood flow (mechanical properties of the disc-shaped red blood cells). The electrical current applied (f = 50 kHz) passes through the red blood cells more easily, which results in a lower voltage measurement and thus in a higher conductivity.

Fig. 14.6 illustrates the course of the surface ECG (waveform on top); −dZ(t) (second waveform from top); the calculated, artificial −dZ(t)/dt signal (third waveform from top); and the pulse plethysmogram (obtained by pulse oximetry; bottom waveform). The change from random orientation to alignment of red blood cells upon opening of the aortic valves generates a characteristic steep, beat-to-beat increase of conductivity (corresponding to a steep decrease of impedance). The red arrows point to the two states shown in the change-of-conductivity signal. The steeper the slope of the $-dZ(t)$ signal, or the higher the peak amplitude of $-dZ(t)/dt$, the quicker the alignment process and thus the higher the contractility of the heart.

The general formula to determine SV by means of bioimpedance (SV_{TEB}) is

$$SV_{TEB} = C_P \cdot \bar{v}_{FT} \cdot FT \tag{14.30}$$

where C_P is a patient constant, primarily derived from body mass and height, $\bar{v}_{FT}$ is the mean blood velocity during flow time, and FT is the flow time (left ventricular ejection time). $\bar{v}_{FT}$ is derived from the ohmic equivalent to peak aortic acceleration, $[-dZ(t)/dt]/Z0$.[69]

Bioreactance Method

The bioreactance (BR) method obtains its impedance cardiogram by solely looking at the phase of impedance—that is, the continuously changing shift of the voltage compared to the applied current ($f = 75$ kHz). The understanding is that a higher SV corresponds to a higher change of phase shift.

The general formula to determine SV by means of bioreactance (SV_X) is

$$SV_X = C_{PX} \cdot \Delta\theta \cdot FT \tag{14.31}$$

where C_{PX} is a patient constant, $\Delta\theta$ is the change of phase shift, and FT is the flow time (left ventricular ejection time).[70]

Compared with methods relying on the magnitude of bioimpedance, it is claimed that the BR is less prone to artifacts caused by motion, sensor placement, and excess thoracic fluids. In fact, the measurement of bioreactance or phase of bioimpedance does not reveal any information about quasi-static fluids.

Arterial Pulse Contour Analysis

Arterial pulse contour analysis (APCA) is based on the real-time estimation of SV derived from the arterial pressure wave form. This concept was first postulated by Frank in 1899, who suggested that the total peripheral resistance could be calculated from the time constant of diastolic aortic pressure decay and arterial compliance estimated by measuring aortic pulse wave velocity.[78] Cardiac output could subsequently be calculated by dividing blood pressure by the total peripheral resistance. The calculation of SV by calculating the area under the systolic part of the arterial pressure wave was described by Kouchoukos et al.[79] Wesseling et al. introduced the technique to calculate SV from the change in arterial blood pressure during systole and the aortic impedance,[80,81]

$$SV = \frac{\int dP/dt}{Z} \tag{14.32}$$

where SV = stroke volume, P = arterial pressure, t = time from end-diastole to end-systole, and Z = aortic impedance.

It should be noted that the configuration of the arterial pressure wave form can vary under different physiologic and pathologic circumstances. The arterial pressure wave form is the result of an initial pressure wave that is proportional to the SV and the pressure wave reflected back from the peripheral vasculature. The site of pressure registration will also influence the pressure wave configuration. Indeed, for the more distal vasculature, a higher systolic peak pressure, decreased diastolic pressure, higher pulse pressure, and nearly unchanged mean blood pressure are characteristic. Unfortunately there is no linear relationship between blood pressure and blood flow. This is primarily due to aortic impedance, which is influenced by aortic compliance, (vascular) resistance, and inductance (inertia of blood). The complexity of APCA is related to the dependency of the aortic impedance on both cardiac output and

Table 14.8 VALIDATION STUDIES OF ARTERIAL PULSE CONTOUR ANALYSIS IN "NEWBORNS"

Reference	Subjects	Comparison	CO, Mean	Mean Bias (Absolute)	LOA (Absolute)	Bias%	Error%
Calamandrei, 2008	48 Patients (2–45 kg); PICU; 48 paired measurements	PRAM vs. TTE	2.7 L/min	0.12 L/min	±0.66 L/min	4	24
Garisto, 2014	20 Patients (4.1–7.8 kg): cardiac surgery; 80 paired measurements	PRAM vs. BR	NA	5.7 mL/m²	±18.5 mL/m²	NA	92

BR, Bioreactance; *CO*, cardiac output; *LOA*, limits of agreement; *NA*, not available; *PICU*, pediatric intensive care unit; *PRAM*, pressure recording analytical method; *TTE*, transthoracic echocardiography.

aortic compliance. However, APCA could be very useful in monitoring the trend in SV or cardiac output, especially when it is calibrated by another (invasive) technology, such as TPTD (PiCCO) or lithium dilution (PulseCO). The ability to track fast changes in cardiac output by pulse contour analysis is limited, so a rather high frequency of calibration procedure might be needed.[34] PiCCO and PulseCO have been validated in children, but not in neonates.[82–84]

There are also systems available (PRAM, Mostcare, Vygon and Vigileo/FloTrac system, Edwards Life Sciences) that claim not to need prior calibration because of advanced algorithms used to translate the arterial pressure waveform to SV. The pressure recording analytical method (PRAM) has been validated in two studies in children, but the number of small infants was rather limited in these studies (Table 14.8).

Conclusion

Despite the availability of a number of technologies, cardiac output monitoring remains challenging in newborn infants. Unfortunately, none of the monitoring devices fulfill the characteristics of an ideal system (i.e., being accurate, precise, noninvasive, continuous, operator-independent, and inexpensive). Clinicians who use any method of cardiac output monitoring are obliged to thoroughly understand the basic principles of the applied technology and its respective advantages and limitations in order to prevent erroneous hemodynamic management. Newly designed systems of cardiac output monitoring must be carefully validated and evaluated for safety. The best candidates for cardiac output monitoring systems for clinical use in neonatal intensive care are TPID, TTE, TCD, TEB, and APCA.

In the selection of an appropriate cardiac output monitoring device, one should pay close attention to the accuracy and precision of the device, as well as to its feasibility and the safety risk it might pose to newborn infants. One needs to also consider whether measurement of precise intermittent absolute values or a reliable trend monitoring system would be the most appropriate in the given situation. In most currently available monitoring systems, noninvasiveness is unfortunately inversely related to accuracy; hence there will always be a compromise between these characteristics, as shown in Fig. 14.7.[87] Unfortunately, at present there is still no clinical gold standard for neonatal cardiac output monitoring that can be used to guide hemodynamic management.

It is also important to understand that an accurately measured cardiac output in the normal or even high reference range does not automatically imply adequate perfusion in all tissues. Cardiac output assessment will only provide information about global blood flow and oxygen delivery (see Chapter 1). The hemodynamic status of a newborn can only be adequately assessed with comprehensive hemodynamic monitoring, including cardiac output measurement (see Chapter 21).

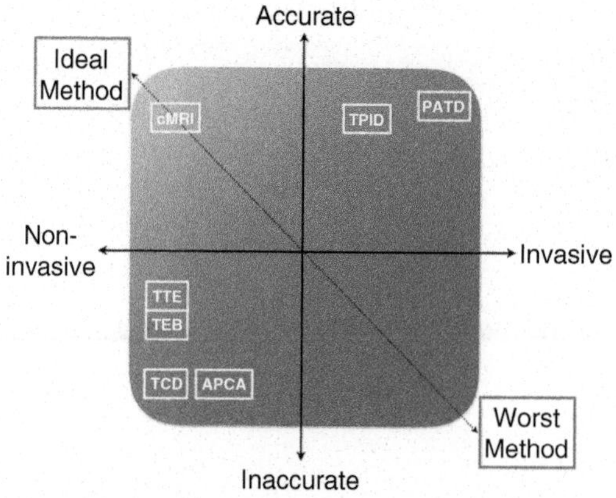

Fig. 14.7 Relation between invasiveness and accuracy. The level of invasiveness is shown on the *x*-axis with the degree of accuracy on the *y*-axis. Different methods of cardiac output monitoring are placed in this diagram. Of note, this classification is based on the subjective estimation of the authors and not on solid evidence. cMRI is almost an ideal method, but only regarding accuracy and noninvasiveness. On the contrary, its feasibility in daily clinical practice is extremely limited. *APCA*, Arterial pulse contour analysis; *cMRI*, cardiac magnetic resonance imaging; *PATD*, pulmonary artery thermodilution; *TCD*, transcutaneous Doppler; *TEB*, thoracic electrical bioimpedance; *TPID*, transpulmonary indicator dilution; *TTE*, transthoracic echocardiography. (Modified from Vincent JL, Pelosi P, Pearse R, et al: Perioperative cardiovascular monitoring of high-risk patients: a consensus of 12. *Crit Care* 19(1):224, 2015.)

Finally, it needs to be emphasized that without developing an accurate, noninvasive, continuous, easy-to-use, and appropriately validated technique to monitor cardiac output in the neonate, further advances in our understanding of transitional cardiovascular physiology and neonatal cardiovascular compromise and its treatment are unlikely to be achieved.

REFERENCES

1. Tibby SM, Hatherill M, Marsh MJ, et al.: Clinicians' abilities to estimate cardiac index in ventilated children and infants, *Arch Dis Child* 77(6):516–518, 1997.
2. Egan JR, Festa M, Cole AD, et al.: Clinical assessment of cardiac performance in infants and children following cardiac surgery, *Intensive Care Med* 31(4):568–573, 2005.
3. de Boode WP: Clinical monitoring of systemic hemodynamics in critically ill newborns, *Early Hum Dev* 86(3):137–141, 2010.
4. Lundell A, Bergqvist D, Mattsson E, et al.: Volume blood flow measurements with a transit time flowmeter: an in vivo and in vitro variability and validation study, *Clin Physiol* 13(5):547–157, 1993.
5. Hartman JC, Olszanski DA, Hullinger TG, et al.: In vivo validation of a transit-time ultrasonic volume flow meter, *J Pharmacol Toxicol Methods* 31(3):153–160, 1994.
6. Dean DA, Jia CX, Cabreriza SE, et al.: Validation study of a new transit time ultrasonic flow probe for continuous great vessel measurements, *ASAIO J* 42(5):M671–M676, 1996.
7. Gratama JW, Meuzelaar JJ, Dalinghaus M, et al.: Myocardial blood flow and VO2 in lambs with an aortopulmonary shunt during strenuous exercise, *Am J Physiol* 264(3 Pt 2):H938–H945, 1993.
8. Tibby SM, Hatherill M, Marsh MJ, et al.: Clinical validation of cardiac output measurements using femoral artery thermodilution with direct Fick in ventilated children and infants, *Intensive Care Med* 23(9):987–991, 1997.
9. Lemson J, de Boode WP, Hopman JCW, et al.: Validation of transpulmonary thermodilution cardiac output measurement in a pediatric animal model, *Pediatr Crit Care Med* 9(3):313–319, 2008.
10. Tibby S: Transpulmonary thermodilution: finally, a gold standard for pediatric cardiac output measurement, *Pediatr Crit Care Med* 9(3):341–342, 2008.
11. Bland JM, Altman DG: Statistical methods for assessing agreement between two methods of clinical measurement, *Lancet* 1(8476):307–310, 1986.
12. Critchley LA, Critchley JA: A meta-analysis of studies using bias and precision statistics to compare cardiac output measurement techniques, *J Clin Monit Comput* 15(2):85–91, 1999.
13. Cecconi M, Rhodes A, Poloniecki J, et al.: Bench-to-bedside review: the importance of the precision of the reference technique in method comparison studies–with specific reference to the measurement of cardiac output, *Crit Care* 13(1):201, 2009.
14. Critchley LA, Yang XX, Lee A: Assessment of trending ability of cardiac output monitors by polar plot methodology, *J Cardiothorac Vasc Anesth* 25(3):536–546, 2011.
15. Fick A: On the measurement of the blood quantity in the ventricles of the heart [Uber die Messung des Blutquantums in den Herzventrikeln]. In *Wurzburg Physikalische Medizinische Gesellschaft*, 1870.
16. de Boode WP: *Neonatal hemodynamic monitoring. validation in an experimental animal model [Thesis]*, Nijmegen, The Netherlands, 2010, Radboud University.

14

17. Stothers JK, Warner RM: Effect of feeding on neonatal oxygen consumption, *Arch Dis Child* 54(6):415–420, 1979.
18. Bauer J, Hentschel R, Linderkamp O: Effect of sepsis syndrome on neonatal oxygen consumption and energy expenditure, *Pediatrics* 110(6):e69, 2002.
19. Shiao SY: Oxygen consumption monitoring by oxygen saturation measurements in mechanically ventilated premature neonates, *J Perinat Neonatal Nurs* 20(2):178–189, 2006.
20. LaFarge CG, Miettinen OS: The estimation of oxygen consumption, *Cardiovasc Res* 4(1):23–30, 1970.
21. Krovetz LJ, Goldbloom S: Normal standards for cardiovascular data. I. examination of the validity of cardiac index, *Johns Hopkins Med J* 130(3):174–186, 1972.
22. Douglas AR, Jones NL, Reed JW: Calculation of whole blood CO_2 content, *J Appl Physiol* 1988;65(1):473–477, 1985.
23. De Boode WP, Hopman JCW, Daniels O, et al.: Cardiac output measurement using a modified carbon dioxide fick method: a validation study in ventilated lambs, *Pediatr Res* 61(3):279–283, 2007.
24. de Boode WP, Hopman JCW, Wijnen M, et al.: Cardiac output measurement in ventilated lambs with a significant left-to-right shunt using the modified carbon dioxide fick method, *Neonatology* 97(2):124–131, 2010.
25. Jaffe MB: Partial CO_2 rebreathing cardiac output–operating principles of the NICO system, *J Clin Monit Comput* 15(6):387–401, 1999.
26. Thome UH, Carroll W, Wu TJ, et al.: Outcome of extremely preterm infants randomized at birth to different $PaCO_2$ targets during the first seven days of life, *Biol Neonate* 90(4):218–225, 2006.
27. Fabres J, Carlo WA, Phillips V, et al.: Both extremes of arterial carbon dioxide pressure and the magnitude of fluctuations in arterial carbon dioxide pressure are associated with severe intraventricular hemorrhage in preterm infants, *Pediatrics* 119(2):299–305, 2007.
28. McKee LA, Fabres J, Howard G, et al.: $PaCO_2$ and neurodevelopment in extremely low birth weight infants, *J Pediatr* 155(2):217–221e1, 2009.
29. Jhanji S, Dawson J, Pearse RM: Cardiac output monitoring: basic science and clinical application, *Anaesthesia* 63(2):172–181, 2008.
30. Stewart GN: Researches on the circulation time and on the influences which affect it, *J Physiol* 22(3):159–183, 1897.
31. Stewart GN: The measurement of output of the heart, *Science* 5:137, 1897.
32. Hamilton WF: Simultaneous determination of the greater and lesser circulation time, of the mean velocity of blood flow through the heart and lungs and an approximation of the amount of blood actively circulating in the heart and lungs, *Am J Physiol* 85:337–378, 1928.
33. Hamilton WF, Moore JW, Kinsman JM, et al.: Studies on the circulation IV. Further analysis of the injection method, and changes in hemodynamics under physiological and pathological conditions, *Am J Physiol* 99:534–542, 1932.
34. Proulx F, Lemson J, Choker G, et al.: Hemodynamic monitoring by transpulmonary thermodilution and pulse contour analysis in critically ill children, *Pediatr Crit Care Med* 12(4):459–466, 2011.
35. McLuckie A, Murdoch IA, Marsh MJ, et al.: A comparison of pulmonary and femoral artery thermodilution cardiac indices in paediatric intensive care patients, *Acta Paediatr* 85(3):336–338, 1996.
36. Pauli C, Fakler U, Genz T, et al.: Cardiac output determination in children: equivalence of the transpulmonary thermodilution method to the direct fick principle, *Intensive Care Med* 28(7):947–952, 2002.
37. Lemson J, Eijk RJ, van der Hoeven JG: The "cross-talk phenomenon" in transpulmonary thermodilution is flow dependent, *Intensive Care Med* 32(7):1092, 2006.
38. Szekely A, Breuer T, Sapi E, et al.: Transpulmonary thermodilution in neonates undergoing arterial switch surgery, *Pediatr Cardiol* 32(2):125–130, 2011.
39. Linton RA, Band DM, Haire KM: A new method of measuring cardiac output in man using lithium dilution, *Br J Anaesth* 71(2):262–266, 1993.
40. Band DM, Linton RA, O'Brien TK, et al.: The shape of indicator dilution curves used for cardiac output measurement in man, *J Physiol* 498(Pt 1):225–229, 1997.
41. Kurita T, Morita K, Kawasaki H, et al.: Lithium dilution cardiac output measurement in oleic acid-induced pulmonary edema, *J Cardiothorac Vasc Anesth* 16(3):334–337, 2002.
42. Linton RA, Jonas MM, Tibby SM, et al.: Cardiac output measured by lithium dilution and transpulmonary thermodilution in patients in a paediatric intensive care unit, *Intensive Care Med* 26(10):1507–1511, 2000.
43. Krivitski NM, Kislukhin VV, Thuramalla NV: Theory and in vitro validation of a new extracorporeal arteriovenous loop approach for hemodynamic assessment in pediatric and neonatal intensive care unit patients, *Pediatr Crit Care Med* 9(4):423–428, 2008.
44. de Boode WP, van Heijst AFJ, Hopman JCW, et al.: Cardiac output measurement using an ultrasound dilution method: a validation study in ventilated piglets, *Pediatr Crit Care Med* 11(1):103–108, 2010.
45. Vrancken SL, de Boode WP, Hopman JC, et al.: Influence of lung injury on cardiac output measurement using transpulmonary ultrasound dilution: a validation study in neonatal lambs, *Br J Anaesth* 109(6):870–878, 2012.
46. Vrancken SL, de Boode WP, Hopman JC, et al.: Cardiac output measurement with transpulmonary ultrasound dilution is feasible in the presence of a left-to-right shunt: a validation study in lambs, *Br J Anaesth* 108(3):409–416, 2012.
47. Vrancken SL, van Heijst AF, Hopman JC, et al.: Hemodynamic volumetry using transpulmonary ultrasound dilution (TPUD) technology in a neonatal animal model, *J Clin Monit Comput* 29(5):643–652, 2015.
48. Vrancken SL, van Heijst AF, Hopman JC, et al.: Detection and quantification of left-to-right shunting using transpulmonary ultrasound dilution (TPUD): a validation study in neonatal lambs, *J Perinat Med*, 2016.

49. de Boode WP, van Heijst AFJ, Hopman JCW, et al.: Application of ultrasound dilution technology for cardiac output measurement: cerebral and systemic hemodynamic consequences in a juvenile animal model, *Pediatr Crit Care Med* 11(5):616–623, 2010.

50. Nusmeier A, de Boode WP, Hopman JCW, et al.: Cardiac output can be measured with the transpulmonary thermodilution method in a paediatric animal model with a left-to-right shunt, *Br J Anaesth* 107(3):336–343, 2011.

51. Lindberg L, Johansson S, Perez-de-Sa V: Validation of an ultrasound dilution technology for cardiac output measurement and shunt detection in infants and children, *Pediatr Crit Care Med* 15(2):139–147, 2014.

52. Crittendon I, III, Dreyer WJ, Decker JA, et al.: Ultrasound dilution: an accurate means of determining cardiac output in children, *Pediatr Crit Care Med* 13(1):42–46, 2012.

53. Floh AA, La Rotta G, Wermelt JZ, et al.: Validation of a new method based on ultrasound velocity dilution to measure cardiac output in paediatric patients, *Intensive Care Med* 39(5):926–933, 2013.

54. Taguchi N, Nakagawa S, Miyasaka K, et al.: Cardiac output measurement by pulse dye densitometry using three wavelengths, *Pediatr Crit Care Med* 5(4):343–350, 2004.

55. Milnor W: *Methods of Measurement*, Baltimore, 1982, Williams & Wilkins.

56. Greenfield JC Jr, Patel DJ: Relation between pressure and diameter in the ascending aorta of man, *Circ Res* 10:778–781, 1962.

57. Mark JB, Steinbrook RA, Gugino LD, et al.: Continuous noninvasive monitoring of cardiac output with esophageal Doppler ultrasound during cardiac surgery, *Anesth Analg* 65(10):1013–1020, 1986.

58. Chew MS, Poelaert J: Accuracy and repeatability of pediatric cardiac output measurement using Doppler: 20-year review of the literature, *Intensive Care Med* 29(11):1889–1894, 2003.

59. Kawahito S, Kitahata H, Tanaka K, et al.: Intraoperative transoesophageal echocardiography in a low birth weight neonate with atrioventricular septal defect, *Paediatr Anaesth* 13(8):735–738, 2003.

60. Mart CR, Fehr DM, Myers JL, et al.: Intraoperative transesophageal echocardiography in a 1.4-kg infant with complex congenital heart disease, *Pediatr Cardiol* 24(1):84–85, 2003.

61. Tibby SM, Hatherill M, Murdoch IA: Use of transesophageal Doppler ultrasonography in ventilated pediatric patients: derivation of cardiac output, *Crit Care Med* 28(6):2045–2050, 2000.

62. Tibby SM, Hatherill M, Durward A, et al.: Are transoesophageal Doppler parameters a reliable guide to paediatric haemodynamic status and fluid management? *Intensive Care Med* 27(1):201–205, 2001.

63. Raux O, Spencer A, Fesseau R, et al.: Intraoperative use of transoesophageal Doppler to predict response to volume expansion in infants and neonates, *Br J Anaesth* 108(1):100–107, 2012.

64. Cattermole GN, Leung PY, Mak PS, et al.: The normal ranges of cardiovascular parameters in children measured using the ultrasonic cardiac output monitor, *Crit Care Med* 38(9):1875–1881, 2010.

65. Patel N, Dodsworth M, Mills JF: Cardiac output measurement in newborn infants using the ultrasonic cardiac output monitor: an assessment of agreement with conventional echocardiography, repeatability and new user experience, *Arch Dis Child Fetal Neonatal Ed* 96(3):F206–F211, 2011.

66. Kanmaz HG, Sarikabadayi YU, Canpolat E, et al.: Effects of red cell transfusion on cardiac output and perfusion index in preterm infants, *Early Hum Dev* 89(9):683–686, 2013.

67. Phillips RA, Paradisis M, Evans NJ, et al.: Cardiac output measurement in preterm neonates: validation of USCOM against echocardiography [abstract], *Critical Care* 10(Suppl 1):144, 2006.

68. Kubicek WG, Karnegis JN, Patterson RP, et al.: Development and evaluation of an impedance cardiac output system, *Aerosp Med* 37(12):1208–1212, 1966.

69. Bernstein DP, Osypka MJ: *Apparatus and method for determining an approximation of the stroke volume and the cardiac output of the heart*, U.S. Patent No. 6,511,438, 2003.

70. Keren H, Simon AB: *System, method and apparatus for measuring blood flow and blood volume*, U.S. Patent No. 8,388,545, 2013.

71. Noori S, Drabu B, Soleymani S, et al.: Continuous non-invasive cardiac output measurements in the neonate by electrical velocimetry: a comparison with echocardiography, *Arch Dis Child Fetal Neonatal Ed* 97(5):F340–F343, 2012.

72. Weisz DE, Jain A, McNamara PJ, et al.: Non-invasive cardiac output monitoring in neonates using bioreactance: a comparison with echocardiography, *Neonatology* 102(1):61–67, 2012.

73. Grollmuss O, Gonzalez P: Non-invasive cardiac output measurement in low and very low birth weight infants: a method comparison, *Front Pediatr* 2:16, 2014.

74. Song R, Rich W, Kim JH, et al.: The use of electrical cardiometry for continuous cardiac output monitoring in preterm neonates: a validation study, *Am J Perinatol* 31(12):1105–1110, 2014.

75. Weisz DE, Jain A, Ting J, et al.: Non-invasive cardiac output monitoring in preterm infants undergoing patent ductus arteriosus ligation: a comparison with echocardiography, *Neonatology* 106(4):330–336, 2014.

76. Torigoe T, Sato S, Nagayama Y, et al.: Influence of patent ductus arteriosus and ventilators on electrical velocimetry for measuring cardiac output in very-low/low birth weight infants, *J Perinatol* 35(7):485–489, 2015.

77. Boet A, Jourdain G, Demontoux S, et al.: Stroke volume and cardiac output evaluation by electrical cardiometry: accuracy and reference nomograms in hemodynamically stable preterm neonates, *J Perinatol*, 2016.

78. Frank O: Die Grundform des arteriellen Pulses. Erste Abhandlung. Mathematische Analyze, *Z Biol* 37:483–526, 1899.

79. Kouchoukos NT, Sheppard LC, McDonald DA: Estimation of stroke volume in the dog by a pulse contour method, *Circ Res* 26(5):611–623, 1970.

80. Wesseling KH, de Witt B, Weber AP, et al.: A simple device for the continuous measurement of cardiac output. Its model basis and experimental verification, *Adv Cardiovasc Physiol* 5:1–52, 1983.

81. Jansen JR, Wesseling KH, Settels JJ, et al.: Continuous cardiac output monitoring by pulse contour during cardiac surgery, *Eur Heart J* 11(Suppl I):26–32, 1990.
82. Mahajan A, Shabanie A, Turner J, et al.: Pulse contour analysis for cardiac output monitoring in cardiac surgery for congenital heart disease, *Anesth Analg* 97(5):1283–1288, 2003.
83. Kim JJ, Dreyer WJ, Chang AC, et al.: Arterial pulse wave analysis: an accurate means of determining cardiac output in children, *Pediatr Crit Care Med* 7(6):532–535, 2006.
84. Fakler U, Pauli C, Balling G, et al.: Cardiac index monitoring by pulse contour analysis and thermo-dilution after pediatric cardiac surgery, *J Thorac Cardiovasc Surg* 133(1):224–228, 2007.
85. Calamandrei M, Mirabile L, Muschetta S, et al.: Assessment of cardiac output in children: a comparison between the pressure recording analytical method and Doppler echocardiography, *Pediatr Crit Care Med* 9(3):310–312, 2008.
86. Garisto C, Favia I, Ricci Z, et al.: Pressure recording analytical method and bioreactance for stroke volume index monitoring during pediatric cardiac surgery, *Paediatr Anaesth* 25(2):143–149, 2015.
87. Vincent JL, Pelosi P, Pearse R, et al.: Perioperative cardiovascular monitoring of high-risk patients: a consensus of 12, *Crit Care* 19(1):224, 2015.

14

CHAPTER 15

Cardiac Magnetic Resonance Imaging in the Assessment of Systemic and Organ Blood Flow and the Function of the Developing Heart

Anthony N. Price, David J. Cox, and Alan M. Groves

- Cardiac magnetic resonance (CMR) imaging techniques provide non-invasive assessments of the newborn circulation with high accuracy and repeatability.
- Cine CMR produces three-dimensional assessments of chamber volumes and myocardial mass.
- Phase contrast CMR can quantify blood flow in any major vessel.
- CMR techniques have provided normative ranges for neonatal left and right ventricular development, quantification of patent ductus arteriosus (PDA) shunt volume, and guided optimization of ultrasound techniques.

This chapter describes the emerging role of cardiovascular magnetic resonance (CMR) in the assessment of neonatal hemodynamics. While at the time of publication this approach remains in its infancy, the technique has begun to demonstrate its value in providing highly detailed insight into the pathophysiology of the neonatal circulation. CMR is also increasingly utilized for the assessment of structural congenital heart disease in infancy, but the reader is directed to other excellent reviews for discussions of this topic.[1,2]

CMR in adults is now acknowledged as the gold standard clinical assessment of ventricular function, cardiomyopathy, myocarditis, and complex congenital heart disease. The use of magnetic resonance imaging (MRI) in the brain is similarly the standard of care for assessment in newborns with encephalopathy, pathology of the premature brain, and developmental and genetic abnormalities.

CMR assessments of neonatal hemodynamic function are neither simple nor inexpensive, but they can be highly accurate and noninvasive. This chapter summarizes areas of neonatal hemodynamics where there is significant residual uncertainty over pathophysiology and management; provides a background to application of CMR in adult and newborns; discusses the current and emerging CMR techniques; and describes areas where CMR has already advanced understanding of developmental cardiovascular physiology, and where in the future it may contribute to changes in the care of critically ill preterm and term neonates with cardiovascular compromise.

Our hope is that as co-location of MRI technology with neonatal intensive care units (NICUs) becomes more common, CMR will fulfill its significant promise to advance clinical research and support improvements in mortality and morbidity in the vulnerable newborn through enhanced hemodynamic monitoring and support.

Current Understanding of Neonatal Hemodynamics

As discussed in a number of chapters in this book, the most prematurely born infants remain at high risk of death and disability.[3] While in the past respiratory disease was the primary cause of death, high quality research has improved preterm respiratory care, such that an increasing proportion of deaths occur due to episodes of sepsis or necrotizing enterocolitis,[4] where impaired myocardial function[5] and failing peripheral vascular control often make circulatory failure the final mechanism of death.

Circulatory failure is also central to the pathophysiology of the key morbidities of premature birth. The long-term sequelae of preterm birth carry an estimated annual socioeconomic burden of greater than £3 billion in the UK[6] and greater than $26 billion in the United States.[7] Failing cardiac function causes cerebral hypoperfusion,[8] and episodes of low cerebral blood flow are central to the pathophysiology of preterm brain injury, which causes long-term disability (see Chapters 7 and 26).[9] Limitations in clinicians' ability to adequately assess circulatory function[10] impair both the ability to tailor care in individual infants and the conduct of adequate trials of the impact of potential therapies. Improving circulatory management is therefore a research priority in preterm infants.[11]

Circulatory Physiology and Assessment

All circulatory function relies on the interplay of preload, contractility, and afterload (see Chapter 1). The preterm transitional circulation is further complicated by the persistence of fetal shunt pathways (foramen ovale and ductus arteriosus), which may significantly alter circulatory dynamics. A robust assessment of the newborn circulation therefore needs to quantify preload, contractility, afterload, and systemic and organ perfusion.

Unfortunately, the current methods fall short of this ideal; in particular, routine clinical monitoring of circulatory status in the neonatal unit still relies heavily on arterial blood pressure.[12,13] However, systemic arterial blood pressure is the product of systemic blood flow and systemic vascular resistance and cannot itself distinguish between the two. While clinicians presumably feel that monitoring systemic blood pressure is a screening tool for low systemic perfusion, in fact blood pressure in itself is at best weakly predictive of volume of blood flow,[14] and some studies have suggested no[15] or even an inverse[16] relationship between blood pressure and flow in newborn preterm infants. Other clinical assessments, such as capillary refill time or volume of urine output, also have limited value in indicating circulatory health.[14]

A range of technologies are now entering "prime time" for hemodynamic assessment in the neonatal unit. Point of care cardiac ultrasound (see Chapters 10 to 13) leads the way and has produced important advances in the understanding of circulatory physiology, with an increasing role in the assessment of circulatory status at the bedside. Established techniques are being improved upon,[17,18] and newer modalities are emerging and undergoing optimization.[19,20] Cardiac ultrasound currently provides only snapshots of hemodynamic status, so continuous monitoring techniques such as impedance monitoring[21] (see Chapter 14) and near-infrared spectroscopy[22] (see Chapters 17 and 18) are also reaching the point of clinical utility. Finally, the evolving systems capable of real-time, comprehensive, and mostly noninvasive, continuous cardiorespiratory and neurocritical care monitoring and data acquisition at the bedside provide an approach, with the potential of addressing many of the presently unanswered questions and unresolved controversies (see Chapter 21). CMR will again play a key role in helping improve our understanding of the interplay among important hemodynamic factors during transition and in pathologic conditions, in addition to assessing the response to various treatment approaches in neonates with hemodynamic compromise.

A key step for all new modalities is robust validation in the population of interest. In the current absence of a gold standard assessment of cardiac function in the premature infant, CMR has a role as a validation tool—its accuracy and repeatability in newborns[23-26] are consistently outperforming that of cardiac ultrasound,[27] near-infrared spectroscopy,[28] and impedance monitoring.[29] Outside the early newborn period (where transfer of a sick newborn to an MRI scanner, even one located on the NICU, is challenging), the accuracy of CMR in quantifying volume of blood flow and myocardial mass is providing valuable insights into circulatory physiology and cardiac development.

Cardiac Magnetic Resonance in Adults and Newborns

A comprehensive discussion of magnetic resonance (MR) physics is beyond the scope of this textbook, but a few basic principles may be pertinent. The underlying principle of MR relies upon the fact that certain atomic nuclei possess an intrinsic magnetic moment, if they contain an odd number of protons or neutrons. This is also identified as nuclei having the property of nonzero spin. When placed in a strong magnetic field, these nuclei align either with, or against, the field; a small proportion align with the field, leading to a net magnetization. The effect is proportional to the field strength and ultimately leads to the level of signal available in MRI—hence the drive for increasing the field strength of magnets in clinical imaging. The resulting net magnetization rotates or "precesses" around the axis of the magnetic field at a set rate depending on the field strength and the gyromagnetic ratio of the nuclei. This rate of precession (or resonance) is known as the *Larmor* frequency.

The aligned equilibrium magnetization can be manipulated by radiofrequency (RF) pulses applied at the resonant frequency; subsequently, the perturbed magnetization will then emit its own RF signal as it rotates in the magnetic field. This is measured using closely coupled receiver coils. Images are produced by localizing the abundance of spins by the use of magnetic field gradients. Hydrogen atoms consisting of a single proton, provide the strongest signal of all relevant atoms and are also the most abundant in the body. Image contrast may be based on the concentrations of protons or how they interact with their magnetic environment, which is detected by changes in their relaxation rate. In-flow effects can provide additional contrast; this is particularly useful to CMR, where blood flow provides "fresh" magnetization compared with saturated signals of more static tissue. Alternatively, in phase contrast (PC) MR, spins are "labeled" according to their velocity by applying additional encoding magnetic field gradients, producing a signal dependent on their velocity through the direction of the applied field, analogous to that achieved with Doppler ultrasound.

CMR In Adults

Cardiac MR techniques have significantly advanced our understanding of cardiovascular physiology and pathophysiology in adults and are now considered the gold standard functional assessment tool.[30] These noninvasive assessments of cardiac health are now being gained faster, in more detail, and with greater sophistication than ever before. The range of techniques available have been summarized in a number of recent reviews.[31,32] The key benefits of CMR in the adult population are the ability to quantify the component factors of circulatory function and the improved repeatability over echocardiography for the assessment of quantitative measures. Critically, improved repeatability also translates into a reduction in the patient numbers required to prove a hypothesis in research studies.[33]

CMR In Newborns

It is clear that functional CMR will not become a routine clinical assessment tool for the sick newborn infant in the foreseeable future; imaging acutely ill children and infants remains challenging. It is more feasible, especially for more stable newborns, when an MR scanner is located within the neonatal unit. A growing number of centers are installing either dedicated neonatal[34] or full-size adult scanners,[35] bringing "point of care MRI" closer to reality. Our group's patient care system for very low birth weight infants undergoing MRI has been described,[35] demonstrating that MR scans can safely be performed in the newborn population while maintaining respiratory, circulatory, and thermal stability. We have now performed cardiac MR examinations in more than 350 newborn preterm and term infants without any adverse events. Functional CMR images have been successfully obtained in infants weighing less than 600 g and at 25 weeks' corrected gestation. For the research data presented that follows, all infants were studied purely for research purposes, with signed parental consent and ethics committee or institutional review board approval. Scans were

15

carried out using dedicated neonatal scanners installed within the Neonatal Intensive Care Units at Hammersmith and St. Thomas's Hospitals (Philips 3.0 Tesla Achieva systems [Best, Netherlands]).

In all cases, cardiac MR images are obtained after infants have been allowed to fall into a natural sleep after a feeding, with careful swaddling. Neither sedative medication nor anesthesia is used. Infants are scanned with oxygen saturation, heart rate, and continuous temperature monitoring; a pediatrician/neonatologist or trained neonatal nurse should be in attendance throughout each scan. Protection from acoustic noise is achieved by applying moldable dental putty to the ears and covering them with neonatal ear muffs (Natus Minimuffs, Natus Medical Inc., San Carlos, California).[35] The application of an acoustic hood can further reduce disturbance from scanner noise.[36] Scans can be performed free-breathing or with the provision of mechanical ventilation, nasal continuous positive airway pressure, or high flow or low flow oxygen therapy, as clinically indicated. In older subjects, respiratory motion causes significant image degradation requiring breath-holds, the use of image navigators to coordinate acquisition with diaphragmatic movement, or advanced postprocessing to account for respiratory motion. However, in neonates, high quality cardiac images are obtainable without the need for sedation/anesthesia or respiratory navigation, presumably due to the relatively small degrees of diaphragmatic excursion. Performing scans free-breathing both improves the acceptability of the technique and limits scan acquisition times. The gating of scan acquisitions to the infant's cardiac cycle remains vital for adequate imaging. This is best achieved using a four-lead vector cardiogram (VCG), as a standard electrocardiogram (ECG) can be significantly degraded by the magnetic fields in the MRI environment. VCG gating can be carried out prospectively or retrospectively. In general, retrospective gating is preferred, as this technique allows imaging throughout the entire cardiac cycle and gives additional flexibility to adapt to the variable heart rate seen in the newborn.

Adult CMR studies are increasingly performed at higher (3.0 Tesla) field strengths. Discussion on the specific challenges faced when imaging at higher field strengths is outside the scope of this chapter.[37] However, in brief, the main drive to higher field systems comes from the increased signal offered as field strength increases, which may confer a substantial benefit for imaging small neonates. The major challenges faced in performing CMR in neonates arise from the need to significantly increase image resolution, both spatially, due to the size of the heart, and temporally, due to the rapid heart rates. These requirements place significant increased demands on the scanner hardware. In addition, the standard imaging protocols applied to adults may not be directly transferable, and thus require modification to be used for scanning small neonates. The initial process of image optimization that we have undergone to improve image quality has previously been described.[23,26]

Current and Emerging Cardiovascular Magnetic Resonance Techniques

Cine CMR

Cine CMR plays a central role in any CMR assessment by producing time-resolved images of the heart that can be used to analyze cardiac function. Typically, in adults, an MR acquisition method known as steady-state free procession (SSFP) is used because it provides images with excellent contrast between blood and muscle while also having very high signal-to-noise efficiency. The technique applies rapid repetitive RF pulses and subsequently acquires data, referenced relative to the VCG trace to allow retrospective reordering, that can produce dynamic images of the beating heart. However, applying this technique at higher fields (3.0 T and above) is challenging and in particular requires the maintenance of a very uniform background magnetic field through careful shimming of field inhomogeneities. Cine images acquired in the newborn infant typically have a temporal resolution of around 10 to 20 milliseconds, a spatial (in-plane) resolution of 1 mm, a slice thickness of 4 to 5 mm, and can be acquired in around 30 seconds per slice, with multiple averages. Scans can be acquired in any imaging plane, with example four-chamber and short-axis views shown (Fig. 15.1).[26,38]

However, the key utility of cine CMR comes from acquiring a stack of contiguous short axis images to encompass the entire volume of the left and right ventricles. Endocardial and epicardial borders can be traced at end-diastole and end-systole at each level of the stack of images to reconstruct three-dimensional (3-D) models of ventricular function using freely available software packages (e.g., Segment, http://medviso.com/products/segment/; Fig. 15.2). These models are constructed directly from imaging of the whole heart without the assumptions on ventricular geometry, which weaken the equivalent two-dimensional echocardiographic estimations.

Cine CMR techniques can therefore provide data on cardiac preload (end-diastolic volume), cardiac contractility (ejection fraction), cardiac output (stroke volume), and myocardial volume from these 3-D models. In addition to enabling assessments of cardiac preload and ejection fraction, which have not previously been readily assessed by echocardiography, our data demonstrate that these quantitative CMR measures have significantly improved repeatability compared with traditional echocardiographic methods[23] (discussed later).

PC CMR

PC CMR techniques require additional flow encoding gradients alongside a reference acquisition collected in quick succession. Any static tissue will have the same phase between acquisitions. Moving objects experience a different magnetic field between the flow encoded and reference acquisition, and therefore accumulate a phase directly (and quantifiably) proportional to the velocity of tissue or (more often) blood. Utilizing

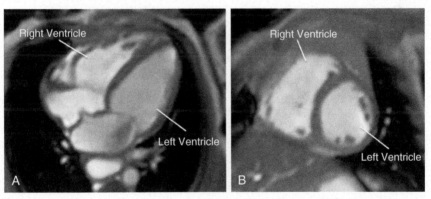

Fig. 15.1   Four chamber (A) and short axis (B) views obtained with steady state free procession sequences in a preterm infant.

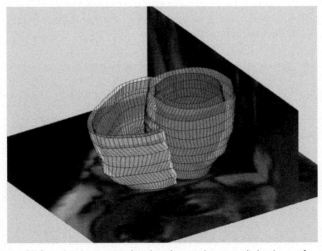

Fig. 15.2   Quantification of left and right ventricular chamber and myocardial volumes from a stack of cine images using Segment software.

this technique with VCG-synchronized cine (time-resolved) acquisition means that the flow of blood can be directly measured throughout the cardiac cycle. PC slices can be again placed in any orientation, allowing the quantification of volume of flow in any large blood vessel. PC images acquired in the newborn infant have a temporal resolution of 10 to 20 milliseconds, and with sequence optimization and dedicated receiver coil technology, images can now be acquired with a spatial (in-plane) resolution of 0.4 to 0.6 mm and a slice thickness of 4 mm in around 90 seconds.[24]

The particular value of PC imaging in the neonate lies in quantification of flow at multiple points in the circulation. The persistence of fetal shunt pathways in the preterm neonate means that neither left nor right ventricular output represents true systemic or pulmonary perfusion. Cardiac MR allows quantification of flow in the superior vena cava (SVC) and descending aorta (DAo), both of which are considered to be markers of true systemic perfusion in the preterm neonate.[39,40] In addition, flow can be assessed in the internal carotid and basilar arteries,[25,41] the sum of which equates to total brain blood flow.

PC MRI is a highly validated technique in the adult. Our data also demonstrate that quantification of SVC and DAo flow with PC CMR has significantly improved repeatability[23,24] compared with prior echocardiographic cohorts[39,40] (discussed later). This may be because echocardiographic techniques measure diameter, which then has to be squared to estimate the area and multiplied by the measured velocity time integral of blood flow, producing a potential multiplication of errors.[18,42] In contrast, PC MRI techniques measure velocity in each voxel across the vessel area, and total flow is estimated by averaging the signal over each of these voxels, so potentially smoothing out errors. The sum of SVC and DAo flow volumes correlates closely with left ventricular (LV) output when the ductus is closed,[24] providing further validation of the techniques and supporting the notion that both SVC flow and DAo flow are reasonable surrogates for systemic perfusion.

Three-Dimensional PC CMR

While two-dimensional (2-D) PC techniques allow quantification of flow within a single blood vessel, 3-D techniques allow for the visualization of flow in entire regions of the body. Specialist postprocessing software is commercially available, which allows the user to trace the path of a notional bolus of blood from within any vessel, throughout the cardiac cycle. We have applied these techniques in newborn infants and utilized MRI flow software (GTFlow, GyroTools LLC, Zurich, Switzerland) to visualize flow in the aortic arch and pulmonary arteries (Fig. 15.3).

The technique has also allowed for the visualization of flow through a patent ductus arteriosus in neonates[43] and demonstrated neonatal disruption of the adult physiologic intracardiac flow patterns which theoretically maintain the kinetic energy of blood flow within the cardiac chambers.[44] 3-D PC techniques may have the greatest value in the visualization of flow in infants with structural congenital heart disease (discussed later).

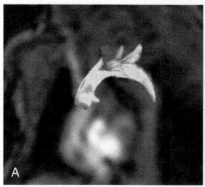 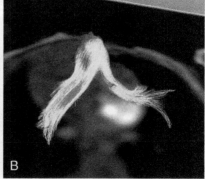

Fig. 15.3   Three-dimensional phase contrast imaging in a term newborn infant showing aortic arch (A) visualized from subject's left side, and pulmonary bifurcation (B) visualized from the subject's back.

Assessment of Myocardial Motion

A number of MR techniques give the potential for noninvasive quantification of myocardial motion. Myocardial tagging techniques use "magnetization preparation" pulses to transiently saturate myocardial tissue along set lines or grids, producing low signal areas. These "tags" are then distorted by the motion of the cardiac musculature. A number of techniques are in use in adults, although these require adaptation for use in the preterm neonate. Further candidates for development in the newborn are complementary spatial modulation of magnetization,[45] which has been shown to have improved tag persistence and temporal resolution in adults, automated analysis packages such as harmonic phase,[46] and automated feature tracking applications.[47] Once adapted for use in the newborn infant, motion assessment techniques may be able to provide quantitative measures of radial, longitudinal, and rotational motion of the heart, enhancing understanding of the development of intrinsic myocardial contractility.

"Atlasing" of Cine CMR Images

The definition of an imaging atlas is an alignment of data from different domains, which enables the querying of relations from multiple domains to create "the big picture." Atlases help overcome the significant intersubject variability in anatomy and function, which makes medical image interpretation challenging through the creation and use of common reference spaces that provide frameworks facilitating inter- and intrasubject comparison. The concept of an atlas can be applied to examine anatomical or functional differences within individuals in a population or to provide robust longitudinal assessment of a subject or cohort over time. Though significant image postprocessing is required, atlases provide statistically powerful representations of normal and abnormal cardiac anatomy, geometry, function, and development.[48] The application of atlasing technology in the adult has already provided unique insights into cardiac remodeling, occurring as a response to hypertension,[49] obesity,[50] and preterm birth[51] (discussed later).

Validation of CMR in the Newborn

As previously mentioned, robust validation is a key step in the development of all new imaging modalities. We have previously shown robust validation of neonatal PC MRI sequences against a gold standard ex-vivo flow phantom ($R^2 = 0.995$).[23] We have validated PC MRI against volumes of cardiac output generated from stacks of cine MR images (95% limits of agreement $\pm$ 16.6%)[26] and have internally validated PC sequences of systemic perfusion by comparing left ventricular output (LVO) with the sum of SVC and descending aortic flow in neonates without a ductus arteriosus (95% limits of agreement $\pm$ 13.2%).[24] Lastly, we have demonstrated that the scan-rescan repeatability of flow estimates from PC CMR is significantly better than flow estimates from echocardiography (95% limits of agreement for MRI $\pm$ 12%,[24] limits of agreement for echocardiography 30% to 50%).[18,27,40,42]

Role of Cardiovascular Magnetic Resonance in the Study of Neonatal Hemodynamics

As acknowledged previously, functional CMR will not become a routine clinical assessment tool for the sick newborn infant in the foreseeable future. However, as a research tool, the technique can contribute significantly to the study of neonatal hemodynamics in a number of areas.

Provision of Normative Data

Our group has constructed normal ranges for LV output, end-diastolic volume, end-systolic volume, and ejection fraction from cine MR images (Fig. 15.4).

These data were produced from a cohort of 75 infants with median (range) birth weight 1886 g (790 to 4140 g), birth gestation 33 weeks (25 to 42 weeks), postnatal age at scan 9 days (1 to 73 days), weight at scan 2192 g (790 to 4140 g), and gestation at scan 35 weeks (28 to 42 weeks). Forty-six infants had been admitted to

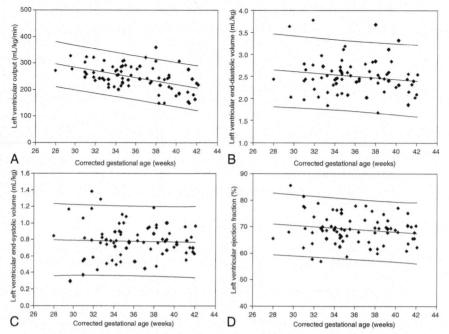

Fig. 15.4   Normal ranges by corrected gestational age at scan for steady state free precession assessment of left ventricular output (A), end-diastolic volume (B), end-systolic volume (C), and ejection fraction (D). (Reproduced with permission Groves AM, Chiesa G, Durighel G, et al: Functional cardiac MRI in preterm and term newborns, *Arch Dis Child Fetal Neonatal Ed* 96(2):F86–F91, 2011.)

the neonatal unit; 29 were term or near-term infants from the postnatal ward. The normal range for LV output decreased with increasing gestation, while chamber volumes and ejection fraction were stable across gestations. The lower limits of the population normal (2.5th percentile) were 1.8 mL/kg, 0.4 mL/kg, and 58%, for end-diastolic volume, end-systolic volume, and ejection fraction, respectively. We have similarly constructed a nomogram for left and right ventricular outputs and SVC and DAo flow volumes from a cohort of 28 newborns with confirmed ductal closure (Fig. 15.5). Once again, normal ranges for cardiac output and systemic blood flow volume decreased with increasing gestation at scan.

Quantification of PDA Shunt Volume

We have previously demonstrated that the sum of SVC and DAo flow volumes correlates closely with LV output when the ductus arteriosus is closed.[24] By extrapolation, when the ductus arteriosus is patent, the volume of shunt can be estimated as the difference between LV output and the sum of SVC and DAo flow (Fig. 15.6).[24]

Using this approach, we have been able to demonstrate that shunt through the PDA can account for up to 74% of the LV output in preterm infants. Despite this high shunt volume, at least outside the transitional period, LV output increases significantly, such that the volume of systemic blood flow approximates the normal range.[24] By examining the relationship between ductal shunt volume quantified by MRI and commonly used echocardiographic markers of PDA shunt volume, we have also demonstrated that the presence of diastolic flow reversal in the DAo is the most predictive marker of high volume ductal steal (Table 15.1).[24]

Guiding the Development of Emerging Cardiac Ultrasound Techniques

As discussed previously and in Chapters 10 to 13, point-of-care cardiac ultrasound has produced important advances in the understanding of circulatory physiology and plays a leading role in the assessment of circulatory status at the bedside. Traditional techniques are evolving, and newer modalities are emerging. A central aim of our

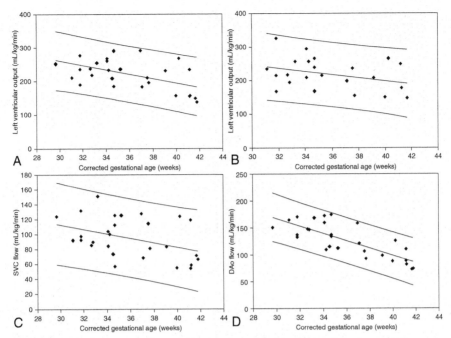

Fig. 15.5 Normal ranges by corrected gestational age at scan for phase contrast magnetic resonance imaging assessment of left ventricular output (A), right ventricular output (B), superior vena caval (SVC) flow (C), and descending aortic (DAo) flow (D). (Reproduced with permission from Groves AM, Chiesa G, Durighel G, et al: Functional cardiac MRI in preterm and term newborns, *Arch Dis Child Fetal Neonatal Ed* 96(2):F86–F91, 2011.)

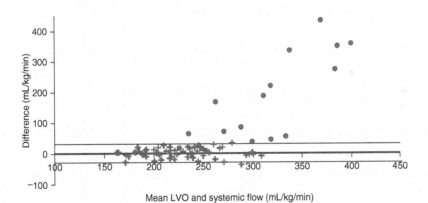

Fig. 15.6 Ductal shunt volume: Bland–Altman plot of LVO and total systemic blood flow (superior vena cava + descending aortic flow volume). Control infants (*crosses*) and PDA infants (*circles*). Ductal shunt ranged between 6.4% and 74.2% of LVO. (Reproduced with minor alterations Broadhouse KM, Price AN, Durighel G, et al: Assessment of PDA shunt and systemic blood flow in newborns using cardiac MRI, *NMR Biomed* 26:1135–1141, 2013.)

TABLE 15.1 R^2 AND *P* VALUES FOR THE LINEAR REGRESSION BETWEEN DUCTAL SHUNT VOLUME AS A PERCENTAGE OF LVO AND THE FOUR ECHO MEASURES

Echocardiography Measures	R^2	*P* Value
DAo regurgitant fraction	0.84	<.001
PDA diameter	0.63	<.001
LA:Ao ratio	0.59	.001
End-diastolic/max. ductal flow velocity	0.55	.004

Ao, Aorta; *DAo*, descending aorta; *LA*, left atrium; *PDA*, patent ductus arteriosus.

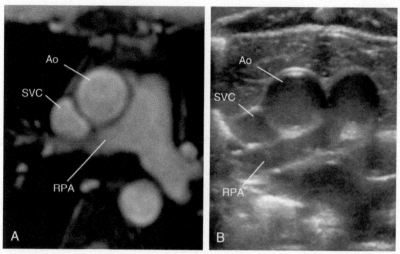

Fig. 15.7   Axial (cross-sectional) view of the superior vena cava (SVC) adjacent to the ascending aorta (Ao) at the level of the right pulmonary artery (RPA) visualized by magnetic resonance imaging (A) and echocardiography (B).

drive to develop cardiac MRI for the newborn was to use it to power improvements in cardiac ultrasound measurements, an approach also applied in older subjects.[52–57] As proof of concept, we performed paired MRI and ultrasound assessments of LV output and SVC flow volume in a cohort of newborns. While echocardiography and MRI showed good agreement for LVO ($R^2 = 0.83$), the agreement between measures of SVC flow was much weaker ($R^2 = 0.22$).[58] MRI also suggested that the cause for some of this variability may be the noncircular outline of the SVC (Fig. 15.7A).

We therefore propose that quantification of the SVC area directly from an axial rather than the traditional sagittal view might reduce measurement variability.[58] In a subsequent cohort of infants, we demonstrated that combining ultrasound quantification of SVC area from axially oriented imaging (see Fig. 15.7B), with quantification of SVC flow velocity from images acquired in a plane superior to the vessel (as previously suggested by Harabor et al.),[59] produces significant improvements in correlation with MRI ($R^2 = 0.77$ vs. 0.26).[18] This modified ultrasound approach also shows improved scan-rescan repeatability and improved repeatability of offline analysis.[18] While normative data using this modified approach are currently limited and validation in the hands of other operators has not yet been demonstrated, at least one expert in the field is suggesting that the modified approach, standardized against MRI measures, could be adopted as the new standard approach.[17]

In the future we hope that highly detailed CMR assessments of cardiac volumes and blood flows will be applied to power improvements in other cardiac ultrasound measures such as 3-D ultrasound, tissue Doppler imaging, and speckle tracking modalities.

Cardiac Remodeling Following Premature Birth

There are currently data emerging that suggest that the long-term pattern of heart growth and function may be altered by premature birth. Lewandowski et al. have assessed young adults with cardiac MRI and demonstrated significant increases in biventricular mass (Fig. 15.8) and decreases in biventricular contractility in those born prematurely.[51,60] They have also applied MR atlasing (as described previously) to demonstrate that the heart of young adults born prematurely also has characteristic alterations in shape and orientation (see Fig. 15.8).[51]

Our group has begun to study the phenomenon of early preterm ventricular remodeling through the creation of computational atlases of the preterm ventricles in the neonatal period. Our initial data suggest altered ventricular postnatal development associated with prematurity can be observed in the newborn period. By term-corrected age, infants born prematurely have an increase in their LV mass, which is proportional to their degree of prematurity (Fig. 15.9) and specific alterations in

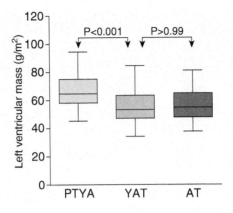

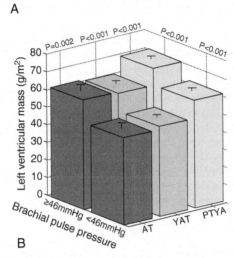

A

B

Fig. 15.8 Left ventricles of young adults born prematurely have increased myocardial mass compared with term-born controls (A). Increases in myocardial mass are independent of brachial pulse pressure (B). PTYA indicates preterm-born young adults (blue); YAT, term-born young adults (green) and AT, older term-born adults (red). (Reproduced from Lewandowski AJ, Augustine D, Lamata P, et al: Preterm heart in adult life: cardiovascular magnetic resonance reveals distinct differences in left ventricular mass, geometry and function, *Circulation* 127(2):197-2016, 2013.)

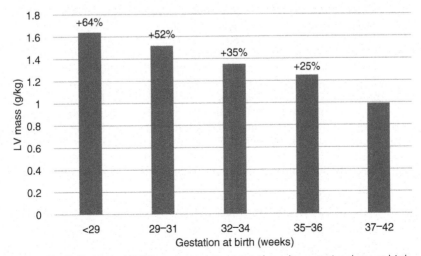

Fig. 15.9 Left ventricular (LV) mass at term corrected age by gestational age at birth.

15

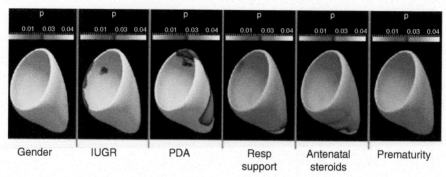

Fig. 15.10 Cardiac atlasing facilitates generalized linear modeling of associations with left ventricular (LV) remodeling in the newborn. Prematurity, antenatal steroid use, and duration of respiratory support are independently associated with statistically significant *(blue)* increases in LV wall thickness. Gender, intrauterine growth restriction (IUGR), and patency of the ductus arteriosus have less significant impact.

LV geometry identified by principal component analysis. The predominant alteration in geometry is increased sphericity of the left ventricle, a finding that has now been replicated by echocardiography in preterm infants with patent ductus arteiosus.[61] Prolonged patency of the ductus arteriosus also appears to be associated with increased LV mass as assessed by both MRI[38] and echocardiography.[61] However, LV mass may return to normal following spontaneous or forced closure of the PDA.[38,61] While further longitudinal studies are planned to examine the long-term clinical effects of these early changes, in adult populations the degree of increased LV mass and sphericity we observe in preterm neonates would be associated with substantially higher rates of heart failure and cardiac mortality.

Computational atlasing of preterm neonatal MR images also allows for multiple regression analysis of associations of altered ventricular wall thickness, with degree of prematurity, duration of respiratory support, and antenatal steroid administration showing the strongest independent associations with increased LV wall thickness (Fig. 15.10).

Cardiovascular Magnetic Resonance in the Fetus

Fetal MRI has been in use for a number of years, but until recently has generally been limited to imaging static structures in the fetal brain and body. However, CMR of the fetus is now being demonstrated, not only to depict cardiovascular anatomy[62] but also function.[63] There are obvious major challenges in imaging such a small rapidly moving structure within the constraints of the maternal torso: resolution (both spatial and temporal), motion (fetal breathing movements, bulk fetal movement, and maternal respiration), in addition to synchronizing data to the fetal heart rate. Specially adapted devices such as MR-compatible cardiotocography,[64] Doppler ultrasound,[65] and ECG[66] have been tested, but significant challenges remain during sporadic fetal movements. Novel developments in acquisition and reconstruction are now allowing for the fetal heartbeat to be directly detected from the data themselves using self-consistency terms in the reconstruction of data.[67] This has led to pioneering work to map the distribution of flow within the fetal circulation using PC-MRI.[68,69] Techniques in fetal CMR are still progressing; further approaches are utilizing highly accelerated real-time MRI with retrospective image-based cardiac synchronization, motion correction, and image registration in order to also address the problem of fetal and maternal motion.[70] Although fetal CMR is still in its infancy, it is likely that it may soon prove to be a reliable tool for the assessment of cardiac function in utero.

Advantages and Disadvantages of Functional Cardiovascular Magnetic Resonance Imaging

The multiple advantages of CMR imaging in terms of the complexity and repeatability of circulatory assessment have been described previously. It is important to also acknowledge the disadvantages of the technique, the most significant being access to the MR scanner. In addition, specialist cardiac radiographers are required for optimal image acquisition, and MR physicists have an important role to play in optimizing the methodology. The process of CMR imaging requires physical movement of the neonate from the NICU to the MR scanning suite. While this is an additional handling episode, we have been able to demonstrate that the process can occur without apparent adverse effects.[35] The potential for adverse effects from the imaging modality itself must be considered; however, MR imaging is considered safe, provided it is performed within internationally agreed on limits.[71] The risk of metallic objects either causing skin burns during the scan or becoming projectile as they approach the main magnetic field are both significant. A thorough metal checking process to prevent these complications is mandatory.[71]

Summary

Functional CMR imaging is feasible in the newborn infant and may contribute significantly to understanding circulatory function and development in this population. The detailed assessments provided, and the robust repeatability of the techniques, may allow conclusions to be drawn from interventional studies in relatively small numbers of infants.

Acknowledgments

We are grateful to Prof. David Edwards, Prof. Reza Razavi, Prof. Jo Hajnal, Miss Giuliana Durighel, Dr. Kathryn Broadhouse, Dr. Anna Finnemore, Dr. David Cox, and the staff of Queen Charlotte's and Chelsea Hospital and St. Thomas's Hospital Neonatal Units for their assistance with the project.

REFERENCES

1. Valsangiacomo Buechel ER, Grosse-Wortmann L, Fratz S, et al.: Indications for cardiovascular magnetic resonance in children with congenital and acquired heart disease: an expert consensus paper of the Imaging Working Group of the AEPC and the Cardiovascular Magnetic Resonance Section of the EACVI, *Eur Heart J Cardiovasc Imaging* 16(3):281–297, 2015.
2. Chan FP, Hanneman K: Computed tomography and magnetic resonance imaging in neonates with congenital cardiovascular disease, *Semin Ultrasound CT MR* 36(2):146–160, 2015.
3. Marlow N, Wolke D, Bracewell MA, et al.: Neurologic and developmental disability at six years of age after extremely preterm birth, *N Engl J Med* 352(1):9–19, 2005.
4. Doyle LW, Gultom E, Chuang SL, et al.: Changing mortality and causes of death in infants 23-27 weeks' gestational age, *J Paediatr Child Health* 35(3):255–259, 1999.
5. Ng PC, Li K, Wong RP, et al.: Proinflammatory and anti-inflammatory cytokine responses in preterm infants with systemic infections, *Arch Dis Child Fetal Neonatal Ed* 88(3):F209–F213, 2003.
6. Mangham LJ, Petrou S, Doyle LW, et al.: The cost of preterm birth throughout childhood in England and Wales, *Pediatrics* 123(2):e312–e327, 2009.
7. Behrman R, Stith Butler A: *Preterm Birth: Causes, Consequences, and Prevention/Committee on Understanding Premature Birth and Assuring Healthy Outcomes, Board on Health Sciences Policy*, Washington, 2007, The National Academies Press.
8. Kusaka T, Okubo K, Nagano K, et al.: Cerebral distribution of cardiac output in newborn infants, *Arch Dis Child Fetal Neonatal Ed* 90(1):F77–F78, 2005.
9. Volpe JJ: Neurobiology of periventricular leukomalacia in the premature infant, *Pediatr Res* 50(5):553–562, 2001.
10. Kluckow M: Low systemic blood flow and pathophysiology of the preterm transitional circulation, *Early Hum Dev* 81(5):429–437, 2005.
11. Jobe AH: The cardiopulmonary system: research and training opportunities, *J Perinatol* 26(Suppl 2):S5–S7, 2006.
12. Sehgal A, Osborn D, McNamara PJ: Cardiovascular support in preterm infants: a survey of practices in Australia and New Zealand, *J Paediatr Child Health* 48(4):317–323, 2012.
13. Stranak Z, Semberova J, Barrington K, et al.: International survey on diagnosis and management of hypotension in extremely preterm babies, *Eur J Pediatr* 173(6):793–798, 2014.
14. Osborn DA, Evans N, Kluckow M: Clinical detection of low upper body blood flow in very premature infants using blood pressure, capillary refill time, and central-peripheral temperature difference, *Arch Dis Child Fetal Neonatal Ed* 89(2):F168–F173, 2004.
15. Tyszczuk L, Meek J, Elwell C, et al.: Cerebral blood flow is independent of mean arterial blood pressure in preterm infants undergoing intensive care, *Pediatrics* 102(2 Pt 1):337–341, 1998.
16. Groves AM, Kuschel CA, Knight DB, et al.: The relationship between blood pressure and blood flow in newborn preterm infants, *Arch Dis Child Fetal Neonatal Ed* 93(1):F29–F32, 2008.
17. Evans N: Towards more accurate assessment of preterm systemic blood flow, *Arch Dis Child Fetal Neonatal Ed* 102(1):F2–F3, 2017.
18. Ficial B, Bonafiglia E, Padovani EM, et al.: A modified echocardiographic approach improves reliability of superior vena caval flow quantification, *Arch Dis Child Fetal Neonatal Ed* 102(1):F7–F11, 2017.

15

19. Levy PT, Dioneda B, Holland MR, et al.: Right ventricular function in preterm and term neonates: reference values for right ventricle areas and fractional area of change, *J Am Soc Echocardiogr* 28(5):559–569, 2015.

20. Levy PT, Machefsky A, Sanchez AA, et al.: Reference ranges of left ventricular strain measures by two-dimensional speckle-tracking echocardiography in children: a systematic review and meta-analysis, *J Am Soc Echocardiogr* 29(3):209–225, 2016.

21. Noori S, Drabu B, Soleymani S, et al.: Continuous non-invasive cardiac output measurements in the neonate by electrical velocimetry: a comparison with echocardiography, *Arch Dis Child Fetal Neonatal Ed* 97(5):F340–F343, 2012.

22. Hyttel-Sorensen S, Pellicer A, Alderliesten T, et al.: Cerebral near infrared spectroscopy oximetry in extremely preterm infants: phase II randomised clinical trial, *BMJ* 350:g7635, 2015.

23. Groves AM, Chiesa G, Durighel G, et al.: Functional cardiac MRI in preterm and term newborns, *Arch Dis Child Fetal Neonatal Ed* 96(2):F86–F91, 2011.

24. Broadhouse KM, Price AN, Durighel G, et al.: Assessment of PDA shunt and systemic blood flow in newborns using cardiac MRI, *NMR Biomed* 26:1135–1141, 2013.

25. Varela M, Groves AM, Arichi T, et al.: Mean cerebral blood flow measurements using phase contrast MRI in the first year of life, *NMR Biomed* 25(9):1063–1072, 2012.

26. Price AN, Malik SJ, Broadhouse KM, et al.: Neonatal cardiac MRI using prolonged balanced SSFP imaging at 3T with active frequency stabilization, *Magn Reson Med* 70(3):776–784, 2013.

27. Chew MS, Poelaert J: Accuracy and repeatability of pediatric cardiac output measurement using Doppler: 20-year review of the literature, *Intensive Care Med* 29(11):1889–1894, 2003.

28. Hessel TW, Hyttel-Sorensen S, Greisen G: Cerebral oxygenation after birth—a comparison of INVOS((R)) and FORE-SIGHT near-infrared spectroscopy oximeters, *Acta Paediatr* 103(5):488–493, 2014.

29. Taylor K, Manlhiot C, McCrindle B, et al.: Poor accuracy of noninvasive cardiac output monitoring using bioimpedance cardiography [PhysioFlow(R)] compared to magnetic resonance imaging in pediatric patients, *Anesth Analg* 114(4):771–775, 2012.

30. Finn JP, Nael K, Deshpande V, et al.: Cardiac MR imaging: state of the technology, *Radiology* 241(2):338–354, 2006.

31. Rajiah P, Tandon A, Greil GF, Abbara S: Update on the role of cardiac magnetic resonance imaging in congenital heart disease, *Curr Treat Options Cardiovasc Med* 19(1):2, 2017.

32. Greulich S, Arai AE, Sechtem U, Mahrholdt H: Recent advances in cardiac magnetic resonance, *F1000Res* 5:2253, 2016.

33. Grothues F, Smith GC, Moon JC, et al.: Comparison of interstudy reproducibility of cardiovascular magnetic resonance with two-dimensional echocardiography in normal subjects and in patients with heart failure or left ventricular hypertrophy, *Am J Cardiol* 90(1):29–34, 2002.

34. Tkach JA, Merhar SL, Kline-Fath BM, et al.: MRI in the neonatal ICU: initial experience using a small-footprint 1.5-T system, *AJR Am J Roentgenol* 202(1):W95–W105, 2014.

35. Merchant N, Groves A, Larkman DJ, et al.: A patient care system for early 3.0 Tesla magnetic resonance imaging of very low birth weight infants, *Early Hum Dev* 85(12):779–783, 2009.

36. Hughes EJ, Winchman T, Padormo F, et al.: A dedicated neonatal brain imaging system, *Magn Reson Med* 78:794–804, 2017.

37. Gutberlet M, Noeske R, Schwinge K, et al.: Comprehensive cardiac magnetic resonance imaging at 3.0 Tesla: feasibility and implications for clinical applications, *Invest Radiol* 41(2):154–167, 2006.

38. Broadhouse KM, Finnemore AE, Price AN, et al.: Cardiovascular magnetic resonance of cardiac function and myocardial mass in preterm infants: a preliminary study of the impact of patent ductus arteriosus, *J Cardiovasc Magn Reson* 16:54, 2014.

39. Groves AM, Kuschel CA, Knight DB, et al.: Echocardiographic assessment of blood flow volume in the SVC and descending aorta in the newborn infant, *Arch Dis Child Fetal Neonatal Ed* 93(1):F24–F28, 2008.

40. Kluckow M, Evans N: Superior vena cava flow in newborn infants: a novel marker of systemic blood flow, *Arch Dis Child Fetal Neonatal Ed* 82(3):F182–F187, 2000.

41. Benders MJ, Hendrikse J, De Vries LS, et al.: Phase-contrast magnetic resonance angiography measurements of global cerebral blood flow in the neonate, *Pediatr Res* 69(6):544–547, 2011.

42. Lee A, Liestol K, Nestaas E, et al.: Superior vena cava flow: feasibility and reliability of the off-line analyses, *Arch Dis Child Fetal Neonatal Ed* 95(2):F121–F125, 2010.

43. Broadhouse KM, Price AN, Finnemore AE, et al.: 4D phase contrast MRI in the preterm infant: visualisation of patent ductus arteriosus, *Arch Dis Child Fetal Neonatal Ed* 100(2):F164, 2015.

44. Groves AM, Durighel G, Finnemore A, et al.: Disruption of intracardiac flow patterns in the newborn infant, *Pediatr Res* 71(4 Pt 1):380–385, 2012.

45. Ibrahim el SH, Stuber M, Schar M, et al.: Improved myocardial tagging contrast in cine balanced SSFP images, *JMRI* 24(5):1159–1167, 2006.

46. Pan L, Prince JL, Lima JA, et al.: Fast tracking of cardiac motion using 3D-HARP, *IEEE Trans Biomed Eng* 52(8):1425–1435, 2005.

47. Claus P, Omar AM, Pedrizzetti G, et al.: Tissue tracking technology for assessing cardiac mechanics: principles, normal values, and clinical applications, *JACC Cardiovasc Iimaging* 8(12):1444–1460, 2015.

48. Young AA, Frangi AF: Computational cardiac atlases: from patient to population and back, *Exp Physiol* 94(5):578–596, 2009.

49. de Marvao A, Dawes TJ, Shi W, et al.: Precursors of hypertensive heart phenotype develop in healthy adults: a high-resolution 3D MRI study, *JACC Cardiovasc imaging* 8(11):1260–1269, 2015.

50. Corden B, de Marvao A, Dawes TJ, et al.: Relationship between body composition and left ventricular geometry using three dimensional cardiovascular magnetic resonance, *J Cardiovasc Magn Reson* 18(1):32, 2016.

51. Lewandowski AJ, Augustine D, Lamata P, et al.: Preterm heart in adult life: cardiovascular magnetic resonance reveals distinct differences in left ventricular mass, geometry, and function, *Circulation* 127(2):197–206, 2013.

52. Muraru D, Spadotto V, Cecchetto A, et al.: New speckle-tracking algorithm for right ventricular volume analysis from three-dimensional echocardiographic data sets: validation with cardiac magnetic resonance and comparison with the previous analysis tool, *Eur Heart J Cardiovasc Imaging* 17(11):1279–1289, 2016.

53. Choi J, Hong GR, Kim M, et al.: Automatic quantification of aortic regurgitation using 3D full volume color Doppler echocardiography: a validation study with cardiac magnetic resonance imaging, *Int J Cardiovasc Imaging* 31(7):1379–1389, 2015.

54. Laser KT, Houben BA, Korperich H, et al.: Calculation of pediatric left ventricular mass: validation and reference values using real-time three-dimensional echocardiography, *J Am Soc Echocardiogr* 28(3):275–283, 2015.

55. Ebtia M, Murphy D, Gin K, et al.: Best method for right atrial volume assessment by two-dimensional echocardiography: validation with magnetic resonance imaging, *Echocardiography* 32(5):734–739, 2015.

56. Zhang QB, Sun JP, Gao RF, et al.: Feasibility of single-beat full-volume capture real-time three-dimensional echocardiography for quantification of right ventricular volume: validation by cardiac magnetic resonance imaging, *Int J Cardiol* 168(4):3991–3995, 2013.

57. Borzage M, Heidari K, Chavez T, et al.: Phase-contrast MR imaging contradicts impedance cardiography stroke volume determination, *Am J Crit Care*, 2017. In Press.

58. Ficial B, Finnemore AE, Cox DJ, et al.: Validation study of the accuracy of echocardiographic measurements of systemic blood flow volume in newborn infants, *J Am Soc Echocardiogr* 26(12):1365–1371, 2013.

59. Harabor A, Fruitman D: Comparison between a suprasternal or high parasternal approach and an abdominal approach for measuring superior vena cava Doppler velocity in neonates, *J Ultrasound Med* 31(12):1901–1907, 2012.

60. Lewandowski AJ, Bradlow WM, Augustine D, et al.: Right ventricular systolic dysfunction in young adults born preterm, *Circulation* 128(7):713–720, 2013.

61. de Waal K, Phad N, Collins N, et al.: Cardiac remodeling in preterm infants with prolonged exposure to a patent ductus arteriosus, *Congenit Heart Dis* 12(3):364–372, 2017.

62. Lloyd DF, van Amerom JF, Pushparajah K, et al.: An exploration of the potential utility of fetal cardiovascular MRI as an adjunct to fetal echocardiography, *Prenat Diagn* 36(10):916–925, 2016.

63. Roy CW, Seed M, van Amerom JF, et al.: Dynamic imaging of the fetal heart using metric optimized gating, *Magn Reson Med Sci* 70(6):1598–1607, 2013.

64. Yamamura J, Kopp I, Frisch M, et al.: Cardiac MRI of the fetal heart using a novel triggering method: initial results in an animal model, *J Magn Reson Imaging* 35(5):1071–1076, 2012.

65. Kording F, Yamamura J, Lund G, et al.: Doppler ultrasound triggering for cardiovascular MRI at 3T in a healthy volunteer study, *Magn Reson Med Sci*, 2016.

66. Paley MN, Morris JE, Jarvis D, et al.: Fetal electrocardiogram (fECG) gated MRI, *Sensors (Basel)* 13(9):11271–11279, 2013.

67. Jansz MS, Seed M, van Amerom JF, et al.: Metric optimized gating for fetal cardiac MRI, *Magn Reson Med* 64(5):1304–1314, 2010.

68. Seed M, van Amerom JF, Yoo SJ, et al.: Feasibility of quantification of the distribution of blood flow in the normal human fetal circulation using CMR: a cross-sectional study, *J Cardiovasc Magn Reson* 14:79, 2012.

69. Prsa M, Sun L, van Amerom J, et al.: Reference ranges of blood flow in the major vessels of the normal human fetal circulation at term by phase-contrast magnetic resonance imaging, *Circulation Cardiovasc Imaging* 7(4):663–670, 2014.

70. van Amerom JF, Lloyd DF, Price AN, et al.: Fetal cardiac cine imaging using highly accelerated dynamic MRI with retrospective motion correction and outlier rejection, *Magn Reson Med*, 2017.

71. Shellock FG, Crues JV: MR procedures: biologic effects, safety, and patient care, *Radiology* 232(3):635–652, 2004.

15

Assessment of Organ and Peripheral Blood Flow

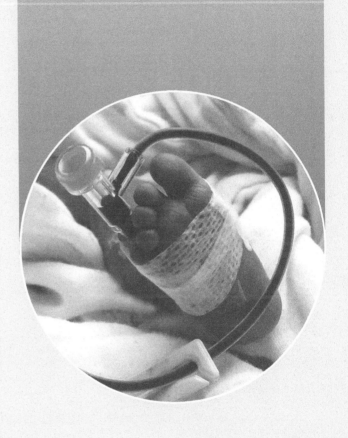

CHAPTER 16

Methods to Assess Organ Blood Flow in the Neonate

Gorm Greisen

- Almost all methods for measuring cerebral blood flow (CBF) have been applied to newborn infants.
- The normal global CBF in healthy newborn infants is likely to be only approximately 20 mL/100 g/min.
- Flow imaging with magnetic resonance imaging (and positron emission tomography) yields expected patterns with high flow to the brainstem, midbrain, cerebellum, and central gray matter and intermediate flows to cortex.
- Monitoring of cerebral oxygenation may serve as a surrogate for CBF, but its clinical value is still undetermined.

This chapter describes the methods available to assess organ blood flow in the neonate and discusses their strengths, weaknesses, and sources of errors. Most detail is given on Doppler ultrasound and diffuse optical methods with near-infrared (NIR) light because these are the most practical methods. The focus is on the measurement of blood flow to the brain (cerebral blood flow [CBF]) because this is where almost all the experience is. A brief section at the end addresses the experience with assessment of blood flow to other organs.

Organ blood flow is usually expressed in mL/min because this is the most descriptive unit when an organ is supplied from a single artery and/or drained via a single vein. Indeed, in animal experimentation the simplest method to measure blood flow to an organ is to drain the venous outflow into a calibrated container. The description of blood flow in mL/min has been used to judge the flow to an organ expressed as a fraction of cardiac output. Whether this fraction changes during development or under pathologic conditions, such as hypoxia, arterial hypotension, and/or low cardiac output states, is an important and clinically relevant question in the field of developmental physiology and pathophysiology. Finally, to allow comparisons among groups of infants of different gestational age and thus body weight, it is useful to normalize blood flow for body weight and express it as mL/min/kg.

However, organ blood flow can also be expressed in mL/100 g tissue/min. This measure may refer to an organ as a whole or to a specific region or compartment in a given organ, depending on the method of measurement. The simplest methods to assess organ blood flow use the Fick principle for inert tracers: "Flow equals the rate of change in tissue concentration of tracer divided by the arteriovenous concentration difference of the tracer." This measure is especially useful to assess the flow in relation to metabolism and organ function.

It is important to emphasize that blood flow is a complex and dynamic variable. Aside from physiologic fluctuations in organ blood flow governed by the changes in functional activity and thus the metabolic demand of a given organ, blood flow may significantly change within seconds under pathologic conditions, such as with abrupt changes in blood pressure or the onset of hypoxia. In addition, blood flow may vary from one part of an organ to the other, as during functional activation, or, during stress, the distribution may change markedly.

For several decades, authors studying the management of circulation during provision of intensive care to the neonate have been pointing out the need to consider blood flow, rather than only arterial blood pressure. Therefore thoughtful neonatal practice would include the use of indirect measures of blood flow, such as skin color, peripheral–core temperature difference, capillary refill time, urine output, and lactic acidosis. Unfortunately, these indirect signs of tissue perfusion either lack sensitivity and specificity (i.e., peripheral–core temperature difference, capillary refill time) or do not represent the changes in the hemodynamic status in a timely manner (i.e., urine output and lactic acidosis).

As for the methods available for the more direct assessment of organ blood flow in neonates, very few units routinely use these tools. Why is this so?

There are three main reasons why assessment of organ blood flow has not become routine in clinical practice. First, none of the many methods used for research has achieved broader application because none satisfies the requirements in terms of ease of use, precision, accuracy, noninvasiveness, and cost. In reality, therefore no method is truly available to clinicians who want to upgrade their clinical practice. Methods using "standard" equipment (e.g., ultrasound) require much skill and expensive equipment, whereas the ones, which in principle are "push-button" methods, require special instruments. Second, no method has truly sufficient enough precision. From this standpoint, for research purposes a method of measurement is appropriate if it is unbiased, even if it lacks high precision. Accordingly, although the findings in an individual infant may be imprecise (i.e., uncertain), it is still possible to achieve meaningful and statistically significant results by analysis of the findings from groups of infants. However, for clinical use, it is absolutely necessary that a single measurement is sufficiently precise. Third, research on organ blood flow in neonates has focused on physiology and pathophysiology and done little in the way of defining the clinical benefit of having measures of blood flow in ill infants. This means that there is minimal incentive for the clinician to overcome the difficulties presented earlier.

Doppler Ultrasound

Doppler ultrasound to assess changes in CBF was first used in neonates in 1979.[1] Because clinical and research interest focused on CBF during this time, several methods, including Doppler ultrasound, were introduced to assess blood flow to the brain of the neonate. The use of Doppler ultrasound for functional echocardiography in the neonate is described in Chapter 10 in detail.

Doppler Principle

According to the Doppler principle, the frequency shift of the reflected sound (the "echo") is proportional to the velocity of the reflector. Because erythrocytes in blood reflect ultrasound, blood flow velocity can be measured based on simple physics. The equation states that the frequency shift equals the flow velocity multiplied by the emitted frequency divided by the speed of sound in the tissue. However, there are several factors that need to be taken into consideration and corrected for with the use of the Doppler principle. First, the apparent velocity has to be corrected for the angle between the blood vessel and the ultrasound beam. Second, it should be kept in mind that multiple frequencies are detected when performing an ultrasound study of a vessel, because the flow velocity decreases from the center of the bloodstream toward the vessel wall. In addition, even the vessel wall itself contributes to the signal. Finally, the velocity is pulsating in nature because it is faster in systole than in diastole (Fig. 16.1).

First Instruments

The instruments of the 1970s and early 1980s were continuous wave (with no resolution of depth, with no image, and a crude mean frequency shift estimator). Finding an arterial signal was done blindly, using general anatomic knowledge and an audible

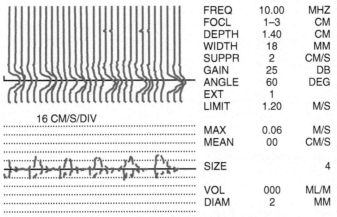

FREQ	10.00	MHZ
FOCL	1–3	CM
DEPTH	1.40	CM
WIDTH	18	MM
SUPPR	2	CM/S
GAIN	25	DB
ANGLE	60	DEG
EXT	1	
LIMIT	1.20	M/S
MAX	0.06	M/S
MEAN	00	CM/S
SIZE		4
VOL	000	ML/M
DIAM	2	MM

16 CM/S/DIV

Fig. 16.1 Output from a prototype Doppler instrument with multiple gates built in the late 1980s. The vertical lines represent the mean velocity detected in each of the 128 gates every 50 ms. Together, the 128 gates span 18 mm; that is, approximately 0.15 mm is covered by each gate. The probe was placed on the neck of a newborn infant to measure flow in the common carotid artery. The flow profile is parabolic, as expected, and steeper during systole. From the flow profile, the diameter can be estimated to be approximately 3 mm at 60-degree angle of insonation. This is the principle behind color-coded Doppler ultrasound. As a result of the speed of data processing, new instruments have the Doppler information as part of the two-dimensional ultrasound image. The vessel diameter is then read from the color image by the investigator using electronic calipers. Two principles can be used to estimate mean flow velocity for volumetric Doppler. The sample volume is set so that the entire vessel is covered. The machine can weigh the received mixture of frequency shifts (i.e., velocities) by their intensity (i.e., by the mass of erythrocytes flowing at each velocity). However, intensity is not a perfect measure of mass and not all ultrasound transducers produce homogeneous sonification of the entire vessel. Alternatively, the maximum velocity can be used and divided by a factor of 2. This corresponds to equality of the volume of a parabola with a cylinder of half the height. Maximum frequency is normally well measured, but the method will fail if the flow profile is not parabolic.

signal with the frequency shift in the 50 to 500 Hz range while searching for the loudest pulsating signal with the highest pitch. This left the angle and the true spatial average undetermined, and therefore the scale of measurement is uncertain. Indices of pulsatility (resistance index = [(peak systolic flow velocity − end diastolic flow velocity)/end diastolic flow velocity] and pulsatility index = [(peak systolic flow velocity − end diastolic flow velocity)/mean flow velocity]) are used since these indices are independent of the angle of insonation.

Indices of Pulsatility

Indices of pulsatility reflect downstream resistance to flow. The pulsatility in the umbilical artery has achieved great clinical importance in fetal monitoring.[2] However, in newborn infants the resistance index in the anterior cerebral artery was only weakly associated with CBF as measured by ^{133}Xe clearance.[3] In addition, more sophisticated modeling reveals that arterial blood pressure pulsatility and arterial wall compliance are just as important determinants of the indices of pulsatility as is the downstream resistance.[4] In summary, Doppler data on resistance indices may be biased. However, in a seminal clinical study the pulsatility index was shown to carry independent prognostic ability in term infants with neonatal hypoxic-ischemic encephalopathy.[5] With increased computational capacity, it has become possible to make full two-dimensional Doppler images at full spatial resolution and a sufficient time resolution to track the cardiac cycle—called fast Doppler. This allows measurement of indices of resistance in all vessels in the field and thereby will allow the study of functional activation and localized pathology.[6] Central hemodynamics will not bias local differences in pulsatility, but differences in local artery wall compliance may still be mistaken for local vasodilation or vasoconstriction.[4]

Blood Flow Velocity

Since the 1980s, duplex scanning combining imaging and Doppler, range-gating limiting flow detection to a small sample volume, and frequency analysis allowing proper estimation of maximum and mean frequency shift has been possible and all contributed to more reliable measurement of blood flow velocity. However, if arterial diameter is not measured, it is not straightforward to compare one infant with another, one organ with another, and even one state with another in the same infant because arterial diameter varies dynamically in the immature individual.[7,8]

Volumetric Measurements

Absolute organ blood flow in mL/min equals flow velocity (cm/s) multiplied by arterial cross-sectional area (cm^2). To measure left and right ventricular output, the diameters of the ascending aorta and the pulmonary trunk, respectively, need to be precisely determined. The diameter of these two major vessels is 6 to 10 mm, and an error of 0.5 mm on the first generation of duplex scanners translated to a reproducibility of 10% to 15%. Recently, for measurement of superior vena cava (SVC) flow at the vessel's entry into the right atrium with a diameter of 3 to 6 mm, a reproducibility of SVC flow of 14% was reported using a 7-MHz transducer.[9] With the advent of color-coded imaging and the use of higher ultrasound frequencies, volumetric measurement of distributary arteries has also become possible in the newborn. For instance, measurement of blood flow in the right common carotid artery with a diameter of 2 to 3 mm was reported to have a reproducibility of 10% to 15% using a 15-MHz transducer, and that in both internal carotid and both vertebral arteries with diameters of 1 to 2 mm was found to be 7% for the sum of the blood flows in the four arteries using a 10-MHz transducer[10,11] and the mean value 14 mL/100 g/min for infants born at 32 to 33 weeks' gestation and 19 mL/100 g/min for infants born at term.[12]

Diffuse Optical Methods Using Near-Infrared Light

NIR spectroscopy (NIRS) is also discussed in Chapters 17 and 18. The first clinical research use of this technology was carried out in newborns.[13] Quantitative spectroscopy (NIRS) was subsequently performed in 1986.[12] After 40 years, more than 300 published papers on diffuse optics with NIR in newborns have been published combining a variety of methodology with a range of physiologic and pathophysiologic questions. The great advantages are that it is noninvasive, usually inherently safe, and may potentially be bedside, continuous, and quantitative.

Geometry

The newborn infant's head is ideally suited for study with NIR. The overlying tissues are relatively thin, which ensures that the signal is dominated by brain tissue, including both the white and gray matter. NIR can be performed with the light applied to one side of the head and received on the other side (transmission mode) in the low birth weight infant with biparietal diameters from 6 to 8 cm. For every centimeter of source-detector (optode) separation, the intensity of the received light is reduced by a factor of 50 to 100. In transmission mode the results may be interpreted as "global." Larger babies can be investigated only with the emitting and receiving fibers in an angular arrangement (reflection mode), usually with both optodes on the same side of the head. In this situation a smaller volume of brain tissue between the optodes is investigated. This may be chosen on purpose, also in smaller babies, to obtain "regional" results. When the source-detector separation is less than 2 cm, the extracerebral tissues are more influential.

Algorithms and Wavelengths for Spectroscopy

The purpose of spectroscopy is to measure the concentrations of the various chromophores, light-absorbing molecules, particularly hemoglobin. The number of wavelengths used has varied from two to six. With the use of different wavelengths, the mathematical algorithms used to measure oxyhemoglobin (O_2Hb), deoxyhemoglobin (HHb), and the cytochrome aa3 oxidase difference signal[14] have differed.[15] This makes direct comparison of results difficult.

Pathlength

The pathlength of light traversing the tissue must be known to calculate concentrations (i.e., to measure quantitatively). The pathlength in tissue exceeds the geometric distance between the optodes by a factor of 3 to 6, and this factor is named the differential pathlength factor.

Measurement of Cerebral Blood Flow Using Oxyhemoglobin as Tracer

Measurement of blood flow in absolute terms is possible by NIRS and is based on the Fick principle and uses a rapid change in arterial O_2Hb as the intravascular tracer.[16] By using the change in the oxygenation index ($\Delta OI = (\Delta[O_2Hb] - \Delta[HHb])/2$) observed after a small sudden change in the arterial concentration of oxygen, CBF (in mL/100 g/min) can be calculated as $CBF = \Delta OI/(k \times \int SaO_2 \times dt)$, where ΔOI is measured in units of μmol/L, and k = Hgb × 1.05 × 100. Hgb is blood hemoglobin in mmol/L (tetraheme), SaO_2 is given in percent, and t is time in minutes (Fig. 16.2).

During the measurement of CBF, cerebral blood volume (CBV) and oxygen extraction must be constant and the period of measurement must be less than the cerebral transit time (approximately 10 seconds). This method of CBF measurement also has significant practical limitations. For instance, in infants with severe lung disease, arterial oxygen saturation (SaO_2) may be fixed at a low level despite administration of oxygen, whereas in infants with normal lungs, SaO_2 is near 100% in room air. Finally, manipulation of SaO_2 may not always be safe. CBF measured this way has a reported reproducibility of 17% to 24% and has been validated against ^{133}Xe clearance in sick newborns.[17,18] These comparisons constitute important direct external validation of NIRS in the brain of human neonates.

Indocyanine Green as an Alternative Tracer

In the past a dye, indocyanine green (ICG), given by intravenous injection, has been used in place of oxygen.[19–21] Because this requires measurement of the arterial ICG concentration during the injection, an alternative, a *blood flow index,* can

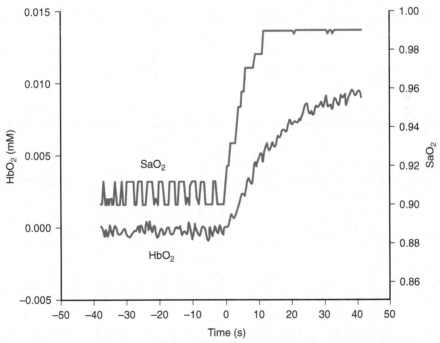

Fig. 16.2 Measurement of cerebral blood flow by near-infrared spectroscopy (NIRS) in a newborn infant. Arterial saturation (as monitored by a pulse oximeter; SaO_2) is stable at 90% to 91% until the concentration of oxygen in the inspired gas is increased at time 0. Within a few seconds the arterial saturation rises to 95% and greater. The rise in cerebral concentration of oxyhemoglobin (O_2Hb) is slower due to the time it takes for the more highly oxygenated arterial blood to fill the vascular bed of the brain. By restricting the analysis to the first 6 to 8 seconds because it is assumed that the venous saturation is still unchanged, a simplified version of the Fick principle can be used. NIRS using an intravascular tracer and measuring over a few seconds gives results of "global" cerebral blood flow similar to the result obtained with the use of ^{133}Xe clearance. Xenon is a diffusible tracer equilibrating between blood and tissue. Washout is much slower, and measurements are made over 8 to 15 minutes.

be calculated as the rise time in cerebral ICG concentration after a rapid intravenous injection.[22] This has a satisfactory coefficient of variability of 10% and has been used to study cerebral autoregulation directly during epinephrine injection.[23]

Calculating Cerebral Blood Flow from Cerebral Blood Volume

CBV may be estimated directly by NIRS from quantitation of the total hemoglobin concentration, and changes in CBV can be used as a surrogate measure of changes in CBF, using a conversion factor (the Grubb coefficient). The appropriateness of this has been substantiated in newborns by comparing the reactions to changes in arterial CO_2 tension[24] and during functional activation.[25]

Diffuse Correlation Spectroscopy

NIR equipment based on lasers can emit highly coherent light waves. When reflected from stationary reflectors in tissue, the coherence tends to decay slowly over 1 to 100 µs, whereas when the light is reflected from moving particles (in tissue this means red blood cells) the coherence decays more rapidly. The autocorrelation as a function of time therefore can be used as the *blood flow index*. The blood flow index has been correlated to Doppler ultrasound in preterm infants and to arterial spin labeling by magnetic resonance imaging (MRI) in neonates with congenital heart disease.[26-28]

Cerebral Oxygenation as a Surrogate for Blood Flow

The metabolic rate for oxygen varies little, except during seizures or due to heavy sedation/anesthesia, and arterial oxygenation is almost always known and, if needed, kept within rather narrow limits. In such circumstances, it is reasonable to see cerebral oxygenation primarily as an indicator of blood flow, or more appropriately, of oxygen delivery (i.e., the product of blood flow, arterial oxygen saturation, and blood hemoglobin concentration).

Cerebral oxygenation represents the mean oxygen saturation of the hemoglobin in all types of blood vessels in the tissue. In terms of interpretation, it is not known how much of the signal originates from blood in the arteries, capillaries, or veins. Data in piglets suggest that the arterial-to-venous ratio is approximately 1:2[29] but may vary and that the arterial fraction may increase during hypoxemia[30] and hypovolemic hypotension.[31]

Quantification

Three different principles are being used to measure hemoglobin-oxygen saturation in absolute terms. With spatially resolved spectroscopy (SRS), the detection of the transmitted light at two or more different distances from the light-emitting optode allows monitoring of the absolute concentration of oxyhemoglobin (O_2Hb) as a proportion of the total hemoglobin concentration (tHb), that is, the hemoglobin saturation.[32] This quantity is called (regional or cerebral) tissue oxygenation, (StO_2), or tissue oxygenation index (TOI). The measurement depends on the tissue being optically homogeneous, which is unlikely to be the case. Nevertheless, TOI values close to cerebrovenous values have been found, and appropriate changes in TOI have been documented with changes in arterial oxygen saturation and arterial partial pressure of carbon dioxide (Pco_2); SRS is simple and relatively cheap, and the devices are simple to handle and approved for clinical use. The other two principles are time-resolved spectroscopy, which detects the time of flight of very short light pulses, and phase shift spectroscopy, which detects the phase shift and phase modulation of a continuous frequency-modulated source of light.[33,34] These are more technically demanding, less commonly used, but able to determine the absorption and scattering of light separately and therefore likely to be more reliable.

Bias of Tissue Oxygen Saturation

Tissue oxygenation cannot be compared directly with any other measurement because it represents the findings in a mixture of blood in the arteries, capillaries, and veins. Interestingly, though, StO_2 has been validated on the head of young infants with heart disease during cardiac catheterization.[35] In this study, across an StO_2 range of 40%

to 80%, the mean value was almost identical to oxygen saturation in jugular venous blood as measured by co-oximetry. This suggests a significant negative bias as, in addition to venous blood, the StO_2 also represents arterial and capillary blood. This bias is likely to differ between different types of instruments.[36–38]

Precision of the Tissue Oxygen Saturation

Replacing the sensor of SRS instruments multiple times in newborns and young infants, the limits of agreement after optode replacement were found to be at least −15% to +16%.[39,40] For comparison, arterial hemoglobin oxygen saturation can be measured by pulse oximetry with limits of agreement of ±6% (two times absolute root mean [squared]).

Importance of the Low Precision of the Tissue Oxygen Saturation

Cerebrovenous saturation is tightly regulated, with the normal values between 60% and 70%. During hypoxemia, or cerebral ischemia, when CBF decreases without a change in cerebral oxygen consumption, cerebrovenous saturation falls. However, a 30% decrease in the CBF will lead to only a drop from 70% to 60% in the cerebrovenous oxygen saturation—and hence less in tissue oxygenation—which is well within the limits of the error of measurement.

Covariance of Cerebral Oxygenation and Arterial Blood Pressure as an Indication of Cerebral Autoregulation

During long-term cerebral monitoring of cerebral oxygenation as a surrogate for blood flow, the covariance with arterial blood pressure may be used as a measure of cerebral autoregulation. First, only changes lasting 10 seconds or more will reflect the "static" autoregulation (i.e., the full capacity of the cerebral vasculature to buffer changes in perfusion pressure) (see Chapter 2). Simple time-domain analysis may be better than more sophisticated frequency domain analysis,[41] although solving the problem of directionality of the covariance may help.[42] However, hours of data are typically required to obtain a reliable estimate, and it is difficult to avoid the bias that high variability in the blood pressure will give a better signal-to-noise ratio.

Magnetic Resonance Imaging

Although MRI is discussed in detail in Chapter 15, this chapter reviews the basics of the methodology for the measurement of blood flow. In the simplest way, global CBF may be estimated by imaging the four arteries in the neck and multiplying their cross-sectional area with the blood flow velocity, estimated by the loss of magnetization caused by fresh blood (water) flowing into the plane of imaging, also called *phase contrast imaging*.[43] It is thus quite similar to volumetric Doppler ultrasound (see earlier) and is possible in newborns, although more complex and not a bedside method. The results are in mL/s and can be related to body weight or to brain weight, as estimated from brain volume measured during the same procedure by MRI. An average global CBF of 15 mL/100 g/min in 10 healthy term infants with a test-retest variability of only 7% has been reported.[44]

Flow Imaging

Arterial spin labeling is performed by applying the radiofrequency pulse to a thick slice (slab) at the base of the skull. This labels the blood in segments of the large arteries supplying the brain. After allowing for the arterial transit time (a little less than a second) to pass, imaging of as many slices as technically possible commences. Regions with higher flow will contain more labeled blood (the bolus distribution principle) and hence a higher signal. Flow is quantified by measuring the relative difference in signal intensity divided by the duration of the labeling pulse. This method also requires correcting for the blood-brain water partition coefficient, any incomplete arterial labeling, and the imaging delay compared with the relaxation time in the blood.[45] This method was first used in 25 neonates with congenital heart disease during normal ventilation and during inhalation of added CO_2.[46] All babies were mechanically ventilated and sedated. Mean slice CBF was 19.7 ± 9.2 mL/100 g/min and 40.1 ± 20.3 mL/100 g/min before and during CO_2 inhalation, respectively, giving an overall CBF-CO_2 reactivity of 1 mL/Torr or 35% change per kPa. In nonsedated preterm infants near expected time of delivery and normal term infants, local CBF ranging from 39 mL/100 g/min in basal ganglia to 10 mL/100 g/min in white matter was found.[47] Improved computational capacity has allowed the development of multiple ("pseudocontinuous") arterial spin labeling, and this is also possible in newborns and appears to provide better signal-to-noise ratio and slightly higher values of CBF (25 mL/100 g/min).[48] However, the limits of agreement between the values of global CBF obtained by the two techniques was as much as ± 15 mL/100 g/min.

^{133}Xe Clearance

^{133}Xe is a radioactive isotope and chemically inert. Measurement of CBF by ^{133}Xe clearance is based on a modification of the Kety-Schmidt method, that is, $dC_t/dt = F \times (C_a - C_v)$. If instantaneous equilibration between brain and venous blood is assumed, the venous concentrations can be derived from tissue concentrations as measured by external detection of the gamma radiation emitted by the ^{133}Xe in the brain. Thus the need for jugular vein catheterization can be circumvented. When xenon is given intravenously dissolved in saline, the arterial concentration can be estimated by external detection over the chest, assuming equilibrium between alveolar air and arterial blood. In the small neonatal brain, ^{133}Xe clearance provides a measure of global CBF because the detector samples from a brain volume of approximately 200 mL has a reproducibility of 10% to 15%.[49,50] In a group of preterm infants without or with mild respiratory distress, the mean CBF was 20.5 mL/100 g/min, whereas in a group of preterm infants who were mechanically ventilated and sedated the mean CBF was 11.8 mL/100 g/min.[51]

Single-Photon Emission Computed Tomography

Tomographic images of radiotracer localization may be obtained by methods similar to computed x-ray tomography. Gamma-emitting decays (photons) across the brain are detected by a number of collimated detectors from a large number of angles around the head circumference. Slowly rotating gamma cameras may image the distribution of radioactively labeled substances, such as ^{131}I-iodoamphetamine or ^{99m}Tc-HMPAO (hexamethylpropylene amine oxime), that fix in tissue at first passage.[52-54] The advantage is that the tracer may be injected intravenously at any time, whereas the imaging may take place several hours later. Their disadvantage is that only the distribution of flow can be obtained without the ability to calculate absolute flows.

Stable Xenon-Enhanced Computed Tomography

This method is also a variant of the Kety-Schmidt method. Detection of the tracer (stable or nonradioactive xenon) in the brain is based on the high density of xenon to x-rays. By performing repeated x-ray computed tomography (CT) scans during inhalation of 35% xenon, brain saturation can be followed. In principle, the spatial resolution is as good as it is for conventional CT scanning. However, the low brain-blood partition coefficient of xenon in the newborn brain results in a low signal-to-noise ratio. Despite these limitations, very low levels of CBF have been documented in young, brain-dead infants.[55] With the advent of xenon-inhalation for neuroprotection, this technique may be used more frequently again.

Positron Emission Tomography

Positron emission tomography (PET) is similar to single-photon emission tomography in image reconstruction but differs in that PET uses the fact that positron annihilation results in two photons emitted always at an angle of 180 degrees. Therefore localization is achieved by accepting only the counts that occur simultaneously at

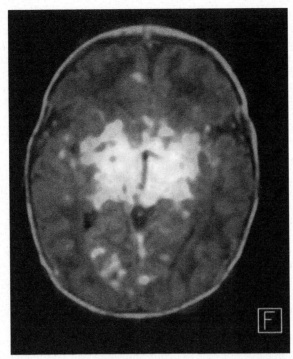

Fig. 16.3   Flow image in infant born after 40 weeks' gestation with a birth weight of 3260 g, on the second post-natal day during natural sleep, using a hybrid positron emission tomography/magnetic resonance scanner. Fourteen megabecquerel (MBq) ^{15}O-labeled water was used, resulting in a radiation dose of 0.3 mSv, which allows research for the purpose of "Increases in knowledge leading to health benefits."[67] The input function was taken from voxels in the left ventricle, imaged simultaneously. The global cerebral blood flow was 22.2 mL/100 g/min. (From Andersen JB, Lindberg U, Olesen OV, et al.: Hybrid PET/MRI imaging in healthy unsedated newborn infants with quantitative rCBF measurements using 15O-water PET. *Journal of Cerebral Blood Flow & Metabolism* 2018 Jan 1:0271678X17751835.)

two oppositely positioned detectors, collimation is not needed, and the sensitivity is better at high resolution. Biologically relevant positron-emitting isotopes exist (e.g., ^{11}C, ^{13}N, and ^{15}O), and many biochemical substances can be labeled. PET is ideally suited for receptor studies using specific ligands because imaging and quantification can be done with picomoles of tracer. Because the positron-emitting isotopes are very short-lived (2 minutes to 2 hours), PET requires a nearby cyclotron facility.

Finally, CBF, CBV, cerebral oxygen extraction fraction, and the cerebral metabolic rates of oxygen and glucose may all be measured by PET.[56–59] With the newest PET scanners, CBF imaging can be done with better spatial resolution and a lower dose of isotope at a level allowing nontherapeutic research in children (Fig. 16.3).[60]

Other Methods

The Kety-Schmidt method was developed specifically to measure blood flow to the brain and was applied to newborns.[61–63] Fifteen percent nitrous oxide, a freely diffusible inert gas, is administered by inhalation, and tracer concentration is measured in arterial and jugular venous blood and is therefore difficult to apply. Venous occlusion plethysmography is a standard method for measurement of limb blood flow and has been used to estimate jugular blood flow,[64] but low skull compliance yields falsely low values of cranial blood flow. The transcephalic electrical impedance is slightly pulsatile, and this correlates with CBF,[65] but, although it appears well suited for long-term monitoring, it has not been developed.

Flow to Other Organs

Doppler ultrasound has been used in newborns for measuring indices of resistance and/or flow velocity in the renal, celiac, superior mesenteric, carotid, and vertebral arteries. A few volumetric studies have been published: although recent studies have given plausible values, the earlier studies appear to have overestimated flow, most likely caused by overestimation of arterial cross-sectional area due to insufficient resolution at 5 MHz (see Chapter 11). Arterial spin labeling and phase-contrast imaging by magnetic resonance (MR) may also become possible for organs with a well-defined arterial supply, whereas this is not necessary for PET.

Flow to the forearm or lower leg can easily be measured by venous occlusion and NIRS (see Chapter 17). Recently, it was shown that the modulation (amplitude) of the plethysmographic signal of a pulse oximeter correlates well with flow.[53,66]

Conclusion

This chapter describes a number of methods. Nearly all were tried in newborns because they had worked in adults and because of the need to gather more information about normal brain function and blood supply, brain injury, and long-term neurodevelopmental sequelae of prematurity, perinatal insult, or critical neonatal illness. None of these methods has really been established as a reference, but the "consensus" is that the normal global CBF in healthy term newborn infants is approximately 20 mL/100 g/min, and it is somewhat lower in preterm infants.

Quoting the late Niels Lassen, my mentor in the measurement of CBF, "A method [measuring CBF] must have acceptable precision with a reproducibility of about 10%, and be able to demonstrate a plausible CBF-CO_2 reactivity and a reasonable CBF-MABP (mean arterial blood pressure) autoregulation in patients with a normal brain." To be used for acute clinical care in newborns, it must furthermore be feasible and safe in the intensive care unit and it must be possible to relate the values to a clinically relevant ischemic threshold and continuously monitor the changes. Unfortunately, no method so far has lived up to these requirements.

REFERENCES

1. Bada HS, Hajjar W, Chua C, et al.: Noninvasive diagnosis of neonatal asphyxia and intraventricular hemorrhage by Doppler ultrasound, *J Pediatr* 95:775–779, 1979.
2. Neilson JP, Alfirevic Z: Doppler ultrasound for fetal assessment in high risk pregnancies, *Cochrane Database Syst Rev* 2, 2006.
3. Greisen G, Johansen K, Ellison PH, et al.: Cerebral blood flow in the newborn infant: comparison of Doppler ultrasound and 133-Xenon clearance, *J Pediatr* 104:411–418, 1984.
4. Greisen G: Analysis of cerebroarterial Doppler flow velocity waveforms in newborn infants: towards an index of cerebrovascular resistance, *J Perinat Med* 4:181–187, 1986.
5. Levene MI, Sands C, Grindulis H, et al.: Comparison of two methods of predicting outcome in perinatal asphyxia, *Lancet* 67–69, 1985.
6. Demené C, Pernot M, Biran V, et al.: Ultrafast Doppler reveals the mapping of cerebral vascular resistivity in neonates, *J Cereb Blood Flow Metab* 34(6):1009–1017, 2014.
7. Drayton MR, Skidmore R: Vasoactivity of the major intracranial arteries in newborn infants, *Arch Dis Child* 62:236–240, 1987.
8. Malcus P, Kjellmer I, Lingman G, et al.: Diameters of the common carotid artery and aorta change in different directions during acute asphyxia in the fetal lamb, *J Perinat Med* 19:259–267, 1991.
9. Kluckow M, Evans N: Superior vena cava flow in newborn infants: a novel marker of systemic blood flow, *Arch Dis Child* 82:F182–F187, 2000.
10. Sinha AK, Cane C, Kempley ST: Blood flow in the common carotid artery in term and preterm infants: reproducibility and relation to cardiac output, *Arch Dis Child* 91:31–35, 2006.
11. Ehehalt S, Kehrer M, Goelz R, et al.: Cerebral blood flow volume measurement with ultrasound: interobserver reproducibility in preterm and term neonates, *Ultrasound Med Biol* 31:191–196, 2005.
12. Kehrer M, Krägeloh-Mann-I Goeltz M, et al.: The development of cerebral perfusion in healthy preterm and term neonates, *Neuropediatrics* 34:281–286, 2003.
13. Brazy JE, Lewis DV, Mitnisk MH, et al.: Noninvasive monitoring of cerebral oxygenation in preterm infants: preliminary observation, *Pediatrics* 75:217–225, 1985.
14. Wyatt JS, Cope M, Delpy DT, et al.: Quantification of cerebral oxygenation and haemodynamics in sick newborn infants by near infrared spectrophotometry, *Lancet* 2:1063–1066, 1986.
15. Matcher SJ, Elwell CE, Cooper CE, et al.: Performance of several published tissue near infrared spectroscopy algorithms, *Anal Biochem* 227:54–68, 1995.
16. Edwards AD, Wyatt JS, Richardson CE, et al.: Cotside measurement of cerebral blood flow in ill newborn infants by near-infrared spectroscopy, *Lancet* 2:770–771, 1988.
17. Skov L, Pryds O, Greisen G: Estimation cerebral blood flow in newborn infants: comparison of near infrared spectroscopy and ^{133}Xe clearance, *Pediatr Res* 30:570–573, 1991.
18. Bucher HU, Edwards AD, Lipp AE, et al.: Comparison between near infrared spectroscopy and 133Xenon clearance for estimation of cerebral blood flow in critically ill preterm infants, *Pediatr Res* 33:56–60, 1993.

19. Patel J, Marks K, Roberts I, et al.: Measurement of cerebral blood flow in newborn infants using near infrared spectroscopy with indocyanine green, *Pediatr Res* 643:34–39, 1998.
20. Brown DW, Picot PA, Naeini JG, et al.: Quantitative near infrared spectroscopy measurement of cerebral hemodynamics in newborn piglets, *Pediatr Res* 51:564–570, 2002.
21. Kusaka T, Okubo K, Nagano K, et al.: Cerebral distribution of cardiac output in newborn infants, *Arch Dis Child Fetal Neonatal Ed* 90:F77–F78, 2005.
22. Wagner BP, Gertsch S, Ammann RA, et al.: Reproducibility of the blood flow index as noninvasive, bedside estimation of cerebral blood flow, *Intensive Care Med* 29(2):196–200, 2003.
23. Wagner BP, Ammann RA, Bachmann DC, et al.: Rapid assessment of cerebral autoregulation by near-infrared spectroscopy and a single dose of phenylephrine, *Pediatr Res* 69:436–441, 2011.
24. Pryds O, Greisen G, Skov L, et al.: The effect of PaCO2 induced increase in cerebral blood volume and cerebral blood flow in mechanically ventilated, preterm infants. Comparison of near infra-red spectrophotometry and 133Xenon clearance, *Pediatr Res* 27:445–449, 1990.
25. Roche-Labarbe N, Fenoglio A, Radhakrishnan H, et al.: Somatosensory evoked changes in cerebral oxygen consumption measured non-invasively in premature neonates, *Neuroimage* 85(Pt 1):279–286, 2014.
26. Buckley EM, Cook NM, Durduran T, et al.: Cerebral hemodynamics in preterm infants during positional intervention measured with diffuse correlation spectroscopy and transcranial Doppler ultrasound, *Opt Express* 17:12571–12581, 2009.
27. Durduran T, Zhou C, Buckley EM, et al.: Optical measurement of cerebral hemodynamics and oxygen metabolism in neonates with congenital heart defects, *J Biomed Opt* 15:037004, 2010.
28. Jain V, Buckley EM, Licht DJ, et al.: Cerebral oxygen metabolism in neonates with congenital heart disease quantified by MRI and optics, *J Cereb Blood Flow Metab* 34(3):380–388, 2014.
29. Brun NC, Moen A, Borch K, et al.: Near-infrared monitoring of cerebral tissue oxygen saturation and blood volume in newborn piglets, *Am J Physiol* 273:H682–H686, 1997.
30. Wong FY, Alexiou T, Samarasinghe T, et al.: Cerebral arterial and venous contributions to tissue oxygenation index measured using spatially resolved spectroscopy in newborn lambs, *Anesthesiology* 113(6):1385–1391, 2010.
31. Rasmussen MB, Eriksen VR, Andresen B, et al.: Quantifying cerebral hypoxia by near-infrared spectroscopy tissue oximetry: the role of arterial-to-venous blood volume ratio, *J Biomed Opt* 22(2):25001, 2017.
32. Suzuki S, Takasaki S, Ozaki T, et al.: A tissue oxygenation monitor using NIR spatially resolved spectroscopy, *SPIE* 3597:582–592, 1999.
33. Ijichi S, Kusaka T, Isobe K, et al.: Quantification of cerebral hemoglobin as a function of oxygenation using near-infrared time-resolved spectroscopy in a piglet model of hypoxia, *J Biomed Opt* 10:024–026, 2005.
34. Zhao J, Ding HS, Hou XL, et al.: In vivo determination of the optical properties of infant brain using frequency-domain near-infrared spectroscopy, *J Biomed Opt* 10:024–028, 2005.
35. Nagdyman N, Fleck T, Schubert S, et al.: Comparison between cerebral tissue oxygenation index measured by near-infrared spectroscopy and venous jugular bulb saturation in children, *Intensive Care Med* 31:846–850, 2005.
36. Hessel TW, Hyttel-Sorensen S, Greisen G: Cerebral oxygenation after birth—a comparison of INVOS(®) and FORE-SIGHT™ near-infrared spectroscopy oximeters, *Acta Paediatr* 103(5):488–493, 2014.
37. Hyttel-Sorensen S, Kleiser S, Wolf M, et al.: Calibration of a prototype NIRS oximeter against two commercial devices on a blood-lipid phantom, *Biomed Opt Express* 4(9):1662–1672, 2013.
38. Kleiser S, Nasseri N, Andresen B, et al.: Comparison of tissue oximeters on a liquid phantom with adjustable optical properties, *Biomed Opt Express* 7(8):2973–2992, 2016.
39. Dullenkopf A, Kolarova A, Schulz G, et al.: Reproducibility of cerebral oxygenation measurement in neonates and infants in the clinical setting using the NIRO 300 oximeter, *Pediatr Crit Care Med* 6:344–347, 2005.
40. Sorensen LC, Greisen G: Precision of measurement of cerebral tissue oxygenation index using near infrared spectroscopy in term and preterm infants, *J Biomed Op* 11:05400, 2006.
41. Eriksen VR, Hahn GH, Greisen G: Cerebral autoregulation in the preterm newborn using near-infrared spectroscopy: a comparison of time-domain and frequency-domain analyses, *J Biomed Opt* 20(3):037009, 2015.
42. Riera J, Cabañas F, Serrano, et al.: New developments in cerebral blood flow autoregulation analysis in preterm infants: a mechanistic approach, *Pediatr Res* 79(3):460–465, 2016.
43. Benders MJ, Hendrikse J, de Vries LS, et al.: Phase contrast magnetic resonance angiography measurements of global cerebral blood flow in the neonate, *Pediatr Res* 69(6):544–547, 2011.
44. Liu P, Huang H, Rollins N, et al.: Quantitative assessment of global cerebral metabolic rate of oxygen (CMRO2) in neonates using MRI, *NMR Biomed* 27:332–340, 2014.
45. Wang J, Licht DJ, Jahng GH, et al.: Pediatric perfusion imaging using arterial spin labelling, *J Magn Res Imag* 18:404–413, 2003.
46. Licht DJ, Wang J, Silvestre DW, et al.: Preoperative cerebral blood flow is diminished in neonates with severe congenital heart defects, *J Thorac Cardiovasc Surg* 128:841–849, 2004.
47. Miranda MJ, Olofsson K, Sidaros K: Noninvasive measurements of regional cerebral perfusion in preterm and term neonates by magnetic resonance arterial spin labeling, *Pediatr Res* 60:359–363, 2006.
48. Boudes E, Gilbert G, Leppert IR, et al.: Measurement of brain perfusion in newborns: pulsed arterial spin labeling (PASL) versus pseudo-continuous arterial spin labeling (pCASL), *Neuroimage Clin* 6:126–133, 2014.

16

49. Greisen G, Pryds O: Intravenous ^{133}Xe clearance in preterm neonates with respiratory distress. Internal validation of CBF-infinity as a measure of global cerebral blood flow, *Scand J Clin Lab Invest* 48:673–678, 1988.
50. Greisen G, Trojaborg W: Cerebral blood flow, PaCO2 changes, and visual evoked potentials in mechanically ventilated, preterm infants, *Acta Paediatr Scand* 76:394–400, 1987.
51. Greisen G: Cerebral blood flow in preterm infants during the first week of life, *Ata Pædiatr Scand* 75:43–51, 1986.
52. Rubinstein M, Denays R, Ham HR, et al.: Functional imaging of brain maturation in humans using iodine ^{123}I-iodoamphetamine and SPECT, *J Nucl Med* 30:1982–1985, 1989.
53. Denays R, Ham H, Tondear M, et al.: Detection of bilateral and symmetrical anomalies in technecium-99 HMPAO brain SPECT studies, *J Nucl Med* 33:485–490, 1992.
54. Chiron C, Raynaud C, Maziere B, et al.: Changes in regional cerebral blood flow during brain maturation in children and adolescents, *J Nucl Med* 33:696–703, 1992.
55. Ashwal S, Schneider S, Thompson J: Xenon computed tomography measuring blood flow in the determination of brain death in children, *Ann Neurol* 25:539–546, 1989.
56. Volpe JJ, Herscovitch P, Perlman JM, et al.: Positron emission tomography in the newborn. extensive impairment of regional cerebral blood flow with intraventricular hemorrhage and hemorrhagic cerebral involvement, *Pediatrics* 72:589–601, 1983.
57. Powers WJ, Raichle ME: Positron emission tomography and its application to the study of cerebrovascular disease in man, *Stroke* 16:361–376, 1985.
58. Chugani HT, Phelps ME, Mazziotta JC: Positron emission tomography study of human brain functional development, *Ann Neurol* 22:487–497, 1987.
59. Altman DI, Perlman JM, Volpe JJ, et al.: Cerebral oxygen metabolism in newborns, *Pediatrics* 92:99–104, 1993.
60. Andersen JB, Henning WS, Lindberg U, et al.: Positron emission tomography/magnetic resonance hybrid scanner imaging of cerebral blood flow using (15)O-water positron emission tomography and arterial spin labeling magnetic resonance imaging in newborn piglets, *J Cereb Blood Flow Metab* 35(11):1703–1710, 2015.
61. Garfunkel JM, Baird HW, Siegler J: The relationship of oxygen consumption to cerebral functional activity, *J Pediatr* 44:64–72, 1954.
62. Sharples PM, Stuart AG, Aynsley-Green A, et al.: A practical method of serial bedside measurement of cerebral blood flow and metabolism during neurointensive care, *Arch Dis Child* 66:1326–1332, 1991.
63. Frewen TC, Kissoon N, Kronick J, et al.: Cerebral blood flow, cross-brain oxygen extraction, and fontanelle pressure after hypoxic-ischemic injury in newborn infants, *J Pediatr* 118:265–271, 1991.
64. Cross KW, Dear PRF, Hathorn MKS, et al.: An estimation of intracranial blood flow in the newborn infant, *J Physiol* 289:329–345, 1979.
65. Colditz P, Greisen G, Pryds O: Comparison of electrical impedance and ^{133}Xe clearance for the assessment of cerebral blood flow in the newborn infant, *Pediatr Res* 24:461–464, 1988.
66. Zaramella P, Freato F, Quaresima V, et al.: Foot pulse oximeter perfusion index correlates with calf muscle perfusion measured by near-infrared spectroscopy in healthy neonates, *J Perinatol* 25:417–422, 2005.
67. *European Commission.* https://ec.europa.eu/energy/sites/ener/files/documents/099_en.pdf, 1998.

CHAPTER 17

Near-Infrared Spectroscopy and Its Use for the Assessment of Tissue Perfusion in the Neonate

Suresh Victor, Petra Lemmers, and Michael Weindling

17

- **Continuous quantitative measurements desirable for clinical practice were not possible using original continuous wave instruments for several years.**
- **Spatially resolved spectroscopy is a development of NIRS which allowed continuous measurements.**
- **Large interindividual and intraindividual differences between absolute values from different monitors have been reported requiring further technological developments in the field.**

Light-based approaches to the assessment of a tissue's oxygen status are attractive to the clinician because they provide the possibility of continuous noninvasive measurements. For example, pulse oximetry, which relies on emission and absorption of light in red and infrared frequencies (660 and 940 nm, respectively), has become widely used in clinical practice. However, this technology measures only hemoglobin oxygen saturation, which is variably related to the partial pressure of oxygen in arterial blood and not oxygen delivery. The arterial oxygen saturation is estimated by measuring the transmission of light through the pulsatile tissue bed; the microprocessor analyzes the changes in light absorption due to pulsatile arterial flow and ignores the component of the signal that is nonpulsatile that results from blood in the veins and tissues. Near-infrared (NIR) spectroscopy technology takes this further and uses light in the NIR range (700 to 1000 nm).

Using one NIR spectroscopy technique (the continuous wave method with partial venous occlusion, described in more detail later), venous oxygen saturation (Svo_2) can be determined, and, from this, oxygen delivery and consumption can be measured. Blood flow can also be measured by continuous wave NIR spectroscopy and the Fick approach, either with a bolus of oxygen or with dye.[1,2] However, these methods allow only for intermittent measurements, and, more recently, another NIR spectroscopy technique (the time-of-flight method, also described in more detail later) has been used to measure an index of tissue oxygenation continuously.[3] Cytochrome activity can also be assessed, but this has not been used in any regular clinical or even research application.[4,5]

NIR spectroscopy instrumentation consists of fiber optic bundles or optodes placed either on opposite sides of the tissue being interrogated (usually a limb or the head of a baby) to measure transmitted light or close together to measure reflected light. Light enters through one optode, and a fraction of the photons are captured by a second optode and conveyed to a measuring device. Multiple light emitters and detectors can also be placed in a headband to provide tomographic imaging of the brain.

This chapter reviews the principles of NIR spectroscopy, quantifies physiologic variables, and reports clinically relevant observations that have been made using this technology. Clinical aspects of the use of NIR spectroscopy in neonatology are discussed in Chapter 18.

Principles of Near-Infrared Spectroscopy

NIR spectrophotometers are applied in the food industry, geologic surveys, and in laboratory analysis. Jöbsis et al. first introduced its use for human tissue in 1977.[6] Since 1985 NIR spectrophotometers have been used in newborn infants.

NIR spectroscopy relies on three important phenomena:
- Human tissue is relatively transparent to light in the NIR region of the spectrum.
- Pigmented compounds known as *chromophores* absorb light as it passes through biologic tissue.
- In tissue, there are compounds whose absorption differs depending on their oxygenation status.

Human tissues contain a variety of substances whose absorption spectra at NIR wavelengths are well defined. They are present in sufficient quantities to contribute significant attenuation to measurements of transmitted light. The concentration of some absorbers, such as water, melanin, and bilirubin, remains virtually constant with time. However, the concentrations of some absorbing compounds, such as oxygenated hemoglobin (HbO_2), deoxyhemoglobin (HbR), and oxidized cytochrome oxidase (Cyt aa3), vary with tissue oxygenation and metabolism. Therefore changes in light absorption can be related to changes in the concentrations of these compounds.

Dominant absorption by water at longer wavelengths limits spectroscopic studies to less than approximately 1000 nm. The lower limit of wavelength is dictated by the overwhelming absorption of HbR less than 650 nm. However, between 650 and 1000 nm, it is possible with sensitive instrumentation to detect light that has traversed 8 cm of tissue.[7]

The absorption properties of hemoglobin alter when it changes from its oxygenated to its deoxygenated form. In the NIR region of the spectrum, the absorption of the hemoglobin chromophores (HbR and HbO_2) decreases significantly compared with that observed in the visible region. However, the absorption spectra remain significantly different in this region. This allows spectroscopic separation of the compounds using only a few sample wavelengths. HbO_2 has its greatest absorbency at 850 nm. Absorption by HbR is maximum at 775 nm, so measurement at this wavelength enables any shift in hemoglobin oxygenation to be monitored. The isosbestic points (the wavelength at which light absorbance of a substance is constant during a chemical reaction) for HbR and HbO_2 are at 590 and 805 nm, respectively. These points may be used as reference points where light absorption is independent of the degree of saturation.

The major part of the NIR spectroscopy signal is derived from hemoglobin, but other hemoglobin compounds, such as carboxyhemoglobin, also absorb light in the NIR region.[8] However, the combined error due to ignoring these compounds in the measurement of the total hemoglobin (HbT) signal is probably less than 1% in normal blood. Nevertheless, when monitoring skeletal muscle using NIR spectroscopy, myoglobin and oxymyoglobin must also be considered because their NIR absorbance characteristics are similar to hemoglobin.

Near-Infrared Spectrophotometers

Three different methods of using NIR light for monitoring tissue oxygenation are currently used:
- Continuous wave method[9–11]
- Time-of-flight method (also known as time-domain or time-resolved)[12]
- Frequency domain method[11]

The *continuous wave method* has a very fast response but registers relative change only, and it is therefore not possible to make absolute measurements using this technique. Nevertheless, these instruments have been widely used for research studies.[1,2,5,13–25] The *time-of-flight method* needs extensive data processing but provides more accurate measurements. It enables one to explore different information provided by the measured signals and has the potential to become a valuable tool in research and clinical environments. The third approach, which uses *frequency domain or phase modulation technology*, has a lower resolution than that of the time-of-flight method but has the potential to provide estimates of oxygen delivery sufficiently quickly for clinical purposes. Thus frequency domain or phase modulation

Table 17.1 EXTINCTION COEFFICIENTS OF OXYGENATED HEMOGLOBIN
AND HEMOGLOBIN AND DIFFERENT WAVELENGTHS

Wavelength (nm)	HbO$_2$	Hb
772	0.71	1.36
824	0.983	0.779
844	1.07	0.778
907	1.2520	0.892

Hb, Hemoglobin; *HbO$_2$*, oxygenated hemoglobin.

technology is potentially the best candidate in the neonatal intensive care setting and for bedside use. The principles used in the three methods are described later.

Continuous Wave Instruments

In continuous wave spectroscopy, changes in tissue chromophore concentrations from the baseline value can be obtained from the modified Beer-Lambert law.[9] The original Beer-Lambert law describes the absorption of light in a nonscattering medium and states that, for an absorbing compound dissolved in a nonabsorbing medium, the attenuation is proportional to the concentration of the compound in the solution and the optical pathlength. Therefore $A = E \times C \times P$, where A = absorbance (no units), E = extinction coefficient or molar absorptivity (measured in L/mol/cm), P = pathlength of the sample (measured in cm), and C = concentration of the compound (measured in mol/L). Wray and colleagues characterized the extinction coefficient of hemoglobin and HbO$_2$ between the wavelengths of 650 and 1000 nm.[26] The extinction coefficients determined by them at four specific wavelengths are as shown in Table 17.1. Mendelson and colleagues showed that the absorption coefficients of fetal and adult hemoglobin are virtually identical.[27]

However, the application of the Beer-Lambert law in its original form has limitations. Its linearity is limited by:

- Deviation in the absorption coefficient at high concentrations (>0.01 M) due to electrostatic interaction between molecules in close proximity; fortunately, such concentrations are not met in biologic media;
- Scattering of light due to particulate matter in the sample; and
- Ambient light.

When light passes through tissue, it is scattered because of differences in the refractive indices of various tissue components. The effect of scattering is to increase the pathlength traveled by photons and the absorption of light within the tissue. Cell membranes are the most important source of scattering. In neonates, skin and bone tissue become important when the optodes are placed less than 2.5 cm apart.[28]

Thus for light passing through a highly scattering medium, the Beer-Lambert law has been modified to include an additive term, K, due to scattering losses, and a multiplier to account for the increased optical pathlength due to scattering.

Where the true optical distance is known as the differential pathlength (DP), P is the pathlength of the sample, and the scaling factor is the DP factor (L): thus DP = $P \times L$. The modified Beer-Lambert law, which incorporates these two additions, is then expressed as $A = P \times L \times E \times C + K$, where A is absorbance, P is the pathlength, E is the extinction coefficient, C is the concentration of the compound, and K is a constant. Unfortunately, K is unknown and is dependent on the measurement geometry and the scattering coefficient of the tissue investigated. Hence this equation cannot be solved to provide a measure of the absolute concentration of the chromophore in the medium. However, if K is constant during the measurement period, it is possible to determine a change in concentration (ΔC) of the chromophore from a measured change in attenuation (ΔA). Therefore $\Delta A = P \times L \times E \times \Delta C$, or

$$\Delta C = \Delta A / P \times L \times E$$

The DP factor describes the actual distance traveled by light. Because it is dependent on the amount of scattering in the medium, its measurement is not straightforward. The DP factor has been calculated on human subjects of different ages and in various tissues. Van der Zee and colleagues and Duncan and colleagues conducted optical pathlength measurements on human tissue and their results are as shown in Table 17.2.[28,29]

Table 17.2   DIFFERENTIAL PATHLENGTH FACTORS

	Van der Zee et al.[28]	Duncan et al.[29]
Preterm head	3.8 ± 0.57	—
Term head	—	4.99 ± 0.45
Adult forearm	3.59 ± 0.78	4.16 ± 0.78

Table 17.3   INVERSE MATRIX COEFFICIENTS FOR HEMOGLOBIN, OXYGENATED HEMOGLOBIN, AND CYTOCHROME aa3 AT DIFFERENT WAVELENGTHS

	774 nm	825 nm	843 nm	908 nm
Hb	1.363	−0.9298	−0.7538	0.6747
HbO_2	−0.7501	−0.5183	−0.0002	1.8881
Cyt aa3	−0.1136	0.7975	0.4691	−1.0945

Cyt aa3, Cytochrome oxidase; Hb, hemoglobin; HbO_2, oxygenated hemoglobin.

There is a small change in optical pathlength with gestation, but this is negligible and a constant relationship is assumed.[30] Despite gross changes in oxygenation and perfusion before and after death in experimental animals, the optical pathlength at NIR wavelengths was found to be nearly constant (maximum difference <9%).[31]

In a medium containing several chromophores (C_1, C_2, and C_3) the overall absorbance is simply the sum of the contributions of each chromophore. Therefore:

$$A = (E_1C_1 + E_2C_2 + E_3C_3) P \times L$$

For a medium containing several chromophores C_1, C_2, C_3:

$$\Delta C_1 = Q_1 \Delta A_1 + R_1 \Delta A_2 + S_1 \Delta A_3 + T_1 \Delta A_4$$

$$\Delta C_2 = Q_2 \Delta A_1 + R_2 \Delta A_2 + S_2 \Delta A_3 + T_2 \Delta A_4$$

$$\Delta C_3 = Q_3 \Delta A_1 + R_3 \Delta A_2 + S_3 \Delta A_3 + T_3 \Delta A_4$$

where ΔA_1, ΔA_2, ΔA_3, and ΔA_4 represent changes in absorption at wavelengths such as 774, 825, 843, and 908 nm. ΔC_1, ΔC_2, and ΔC_3 represent changes in the concentrations of C_1, C_2, and C_3 (such as HbR, HbO_2, and Cyt aa3). The 12 values of Q, R, S, and T are functions of the absorption coefficients of HbR, HbO_2, and Cyt aa3. They are termed *NIR coefficients*. Because the pathlength is wavelength dependent, a modification of these inverse matrix coefficients is listed in Table 17.3.[32]

Examples of instruments using continuous wave technology are the NIRO 500 and NIRO 100 (Hamamatsu Photonic, Hamamatsu City, Japan).

Spatially Resolved Spectroscopy

The continuous wave method, which measures only the intensity of light, is very reliable, but allows only relative or trend measurements due to the lack of information available about pathlength.[9] To address this problem using current continuous wave instruments, multiple optodes operating simultaneously are placed around the head. This allows for a pathlength correction, but only when the tissue being interrogated is assumed to be homogeneous. This modification is called spatially resolved spectroscopy. It has a reasonable signal-to-noise ratio, and the depth of brain tissue, which can be measured from the surface, varies typically between 1 and 3 cm.

Spatially resolved spectroscopy measures hemoglobin oxygen saturation. The NIRO 300 (Hamamatsu Photonics) and the INVOS 5100 (Somanetics, Troy, Michigan) both measure cerebral hemoglobin oxygen saturation and return a single numerator but use different terminology: tissue oxygenation index (TOI) from the NIRO 300 and regional oxygen saturation (rSO_2) from the INVOS 5100. In contrast to standard continuous wave NIR spectroscopy, this technique gives absolute values. A light detector measures TOI with three sensors at different distances from the light source. Scatter and absorption attenuate light passing into tissue. If the distance between the light source and the sensor is large enough (>3 cm), the isotropy of scatter distribution becomes so homogeneous that the loss due to scatter is the same at the three sensors. TOI is calculated according to the diffusion equation as follows:

$$\text{TOI}\,(\%) = \frac{K_{HbO_2}}{K_{HbO_2} + K_{HbR}}$$

where K is the constant scattering contribution. A similar concept is used in calculating regional oxygen saturation (rSO_2).

Dullenkopf and associates examined the reproducibility of cerebral TOI.[33] There was good agreement for sensor-exchange experiments (removing the sensor and reapplying another sensor at the same position), and simultaneous left-to-right forehead measurements revealed only small differences (<5%) and no significant differences between corresponding values.[33] The same group also showed that much of the variability of cerebral TOI was due to cerebral Svo_2.[34] A point about methodology for assessing the reliability of such tests was made by Sorensen and Greisen, who showed that optodes needed to be reapplied and measured at least five times before the precision of the mean value could be assumed to be comparable with pulse oximetry.[35] There was a mean difference of 8.5% (95% CI, 5.4% to 11.6%) when two probes were placed on the same patient's head at different positions.[36]

Quaresima and colleagues concluded that TOI reflected mainly the saturation of the intracranial venous compartment of circulation.[37] Variation in the results of studies aimed at correlating TOI with jugular venous bulb oximetry is likely due to assumptions made about the distribution of cerebral blood between arterial and venous compartments. Several studies used a fixed ratio of 25:75,[38–40] but Watzman and colleagues described an arterial-to-venous ratio of 16:84 in normoxia, hypoxia, and hypocapnia and also observed considerable biologic individual variability.[38–41]

Time-of-Flight Instruments

This time-resolved technique consists of emitting a very short laser pulse into an absorbing tissue and recording the temporal response (time-of-flight) of the photons at some distance from the laser source.[12] This method uses a mathematical approximation that is based on diffusion theory to allow for the separation of effects due to light absorbance from those due to light scattering. Thus the time-of-flight method permits differentiation of one tissue from another. In addition, the scattering component provides further useful information, which may be used for imaging. Functional imaging is an exciting application of the time-of-flight method because, in conjunction with hemoglobin status, scattering changes, which can be mapped optically, may provide information about the electrical and vascular interaction, which determines the functional status of the brain. Disadvantages of this technique, which still need to be addressed, are the large amount of data, which means that data are collected and analyzed relatively slowly (minutes), and information obtained at the bedside is not displayed instantaneously but rather a few minutes later.

There have been only a few reports on the use of time-of-flight instruments in neonates.[3] Measurements in neonates at the bedside have not been possible because of the size and the cost of typical laboratory equipment needed for these measurements. However, a new portable time-resolved spectroscopy (TRS) device (TRS-10, Hamamatsu Photonics K.K.), which has a high data acquisition rate, was recently used clinically. This TRS system can be used (1) for continuous absolute quantification of hemodynamic variables and (2) for better estimation of light-scattering properties by measurement of DP factors.

Frequency Domain Instruments

The frequency domain method is based on the modulation of a laser light at given frequencies.[11] Frequency domain instruments determine the absorption coefficient and reduce scattering coefficient of the tissue by measuring alternating current (AC), direct current (DC), and phase change as functions of distance through the tissue.

This method allows for correction of the detected signal for the different scattering effects of the fluid and tissue components of the brain using data-processing algorithms. Moreover, the phase and amplitude shifts can be used for localization of the signal. Because pathlength is measured directly, the hemoglobin saturation can be measured to ±5% in in vitro models and ±10% in piglets. Problems include noise and leakage associated with the high-frequency signal, but the devices are very compact and appropriate for bedside/incubator use.

Frequency domain NIR spectroscopy allows the absolute quantification of cerebral hemoglobin oxygen saturation and cerebral blood volume.[42]

Diffuse correlation spectroscopy was developed for in vivo applications to measure microvascular cerebral blood flow index (CBFi) noninvasively in deep biologic tissue without the injection of external contrasts. Using concurrent frequency domain measures of cerebral hemoglobin oxygen saturation and diffuse correlation spectroscopy measures of CBFi, cerebral oxygen consumption (Vo_2) can be calculated.[43,44]

Examples of instruments using this frequency domain technology are manufactured by ISS, Inc., Champaign, Illinois.

Measurements of Physiologic Variables

As previously stated, continuous wave NIR spectroscopy does not give absolute quantitative measurements. To derive quantitative values for physiologic variables, it is necessary to produce changes in the concentrations of the measured chromophore. This has been done by changing the volume of the cerebral venous compartment, either by tilting the subject head-down or, as we have done, by partial venous occlusion, or by using changes in cerebral blood volume induced by ventilation.[20,45,46] By observing the ratio of the changes in chromophores or the change in chromophore concentration in comparison to another measured variable, it is possible to calculate different physiologic variables.

Some assumptions are made. It is assumed that the receiving and transmitting fiber optodes do not move in position and that the distance between the optodes and the scattering characteristics of the tissue remain constant during a measurement. In addition, for cerebral measurements, it is assumed that there is no contribution to the NIR spectroscopy signal from extracerebral hemoglobin.[47]

Continuous wave NIR spectroscopy has been used in a number of ways to make measurements relevant to neonatal cerebral and peripheral hemodynamics. The technique has been used to measure peripheral and cerebral Svo_2 and cerebral and peripheral blood flow.

Venous Oxygen Saturation

Intermittent measurements of both cerebral and peripheral Svo_2 have been made using this technology.[16,20,45,46,48] The assumption is that in a steady state, arterial and venous blood flows are equal. The approach for measuring both cerebral and peripheral Svo_2 is similar, namely to induce a brief increase in the venous compartment (and hence in the concentration of venous hemoglobin) and then to measure that change.

Cerebral Venous Oxygen Saturation

Three techniques have been described for the measurement of cerebral Svo_2 using NIR spectroscopy.[20,45,46] Each involves the calculation of cerebral Svo_2 from the relative changes in HbO_2 and HbT (the sum of oxygenated and deoxygenated hemoglobin) that occur when there is an increase in the venous blood volume of the brain. As mentioned earlier, this is achieved by gravity using a tilt technique, or by partial jugular venous occlusion, or by using changes in cerebral blood volume induced by ventilation.[20,45,46]

The partial jugular venous occlusion technique for the measurement of cerebral Svo_2 was developed by our group in Liverpool, United Kingdom, and validated by Yoxall and colleagues.[20] To establish a baseline, the NIR spectroscopic data were monitored for a short period when no changes were made. Then a brief jugular venous occlusion was made using gentle pressure on the side of the neck over the jugular vein. The compression lasted for approximately 5 to 10 seconds, after which the pressure was released. The brief partial compression of the jugular vein led to an increase in the blood volume in the head. Because there was no arterial occlusion and the occlusion was brief, all the increase in hemoglobin concentration monitored using NIR spectroscopy may be assumed to be due to venous blood within the head. The relative changes in HbO_2 concentration and HbT concentration monitored could then be used to calculate the saturation of venous blood within the tissue studied.

The venous saturation every 0.5 second for 5 seconds following the occlusion was calculated from the change in the concentration of HbO_2 (ΔHbO_2) as a proportion of the change in HbT concentration (ΔHbT). Therefore

$$\text{Cerebral } S_V O_2 = \frac{\Delta HbO_2}{\Delta HbT}$$

This partial jugular venous occlusion technique was validated by comparison with Svo_2 measured by co-oximetry from blood obtained from the jugular bulb during cardiac catheterization.[20] Fifteen children were studied, aged 3 months to 14 years (median, 2 years).[20] Cerebral Svo_2 by co-oximetry ranged from 36% to 80% (median, 60%).[20] The mean difference (co-oximeter–NIR spectroscopy) was 1.5%.[20] Limits of agreement were −12.8% to 15.9%.[20]

Peripheral Venous Oxygen Saturation

Peripheral Svo_2 can be measured by two methods using NIR spectroscopy.[16,49] One approach, which is described in more detail later, involves measuring changes following venous occlusion. It is similar to that used for cerebral Svo_2 and was developed by Wardle and colleagues for preterm infants by adapting a method described and validated by De Blasi and colleagues in adult patients.[16,50] Another approach is a method involving the use of oxygen as an intravascular tracer, and it can be used in the same way that measurements of cerebral blood flow (CBF) are made (see later).[49]

In the venous occlusion method, the optodes were positioned on the upper arm. A brief venous occlusion with a blood pressure cuff around the upper arm was achieved by manually inflating the cuff to 30 mm Hg for approximately 5 to 10 seconds. This compression of the arm resulted in a rise in the blood volume within the forearm. Because the venous occlusion was brief and there was no arterial occlusion, all the measured increase in hemoglobin within the tissues monitored was assumed to be due to an increase in the venous blood. During the initial part of a venous occlusion, hemoglobin accumulated in the tissues, owing to cessation of venous flow, and the rate of hemoglobin flow was equal to the rate of tissue hemoglobin accumulation during the initial part of the occlusion.

Changes in HbR and HbO_2 concentration were used to calculate the saturation of venous blood within the forearm tissues. Data were recorded and analyzed as for NIR spectroscopic measurements of cerebral Svo_2 using partial jugular venous occlusion:

$$\text{Peripheral } S_V O_2 = \frac{\Delta HbO_2}{\Delta HbT}$$

The Svo_2 measurements using the venous occlusion technique made both from the forearms of adults and babies have been compared with co-oximetry measurements. The agreement between the methods was close.[21,22] In 19 adult volunteers, there was a significant correlation between forearm Svo_2 measured by NIR spectroscopy and Svo_2 of superficial venous blood measured by co-oximetry ($r = .7$, $P < .0001$).[22] When the study was repeated in 16 newborn infants, there was again a significant correlation between the two measurements ($r = .85$, $P < .0001$).[21] The mean difference between the two techniques was 6%, and the limits of agreement were between −5.1% and +17.1%.[21]

After venous saturation (using partial venous occlusion and continuous wave NIR spectroscopy) and arterial saturation (using pulse oximetry) are known, fractional oxygen extraction (FOE) can be measured (see later).

Blood Flow

NIR spectroscopy has also been used as a research tool for measuring cerebral and peripheral blood flow. The methods are described later.

From the measurements made using partial venous occlusion, hemoglobin flow (Hb flow) can also be calculated from the slope of a line through the ΔHbT values during the first 2 seconds of an occlusion, using a least squares method (i.e., the rate of increase of HbT within the forearm is used to calculate Hb flow):

$$\text{Hb flow} = \int \Delta \text{HbT } dt$$

and

$$\text{Blood flow} = \frac{\text{Hb flow}}{[\text{Hb}]}$$

where [Hb] is hemoglobin concentration.

Blood flow (mL/100 mL/min) is calculated by dividing Hb flow (μmol/100 mL/min) by venous [Hb] in μmol/mL. Because the molecular weight of hemoglobin is 64,500 g/mol, blood flow is:

$$\frac{\text{Hb flow} \times 6.45}{[\text{Hb}]}$$

where blood flow is in mL/100 mL/min, Hb flow is in μmol/100 mL/min, and [Hb] is in g/dL.

An alternative approach to measure flow by NIR spectroscopy is to use a bolus of oxidized hemoglobin as a nondiffusible intravascular tracer.[1,2,25] In this technique the monitoring optodes were positioned on the infant's head in the temporal or frontal region of the same side. The measurement is based on the Fick principle, which states that the amount of a nondiffusible intravascular tracer accumulated in a tissue over a time t is equal to the amount delivered in the arterial blood minus the amount removed in the venous blood. If the blood transit time for the brain (t) is less than 6 seconds, then the amount removed by venous flow will be zero and so increase in tissue tracer content is equal to the amount of tracer delivered by arterial blood flow. Hence the amount of HbO_2 delivered by arterial flow is arterial Hb flow $\times \int_0^t \Delta Sao_2$, where $\int_0^t \Delta Sao_2$ is the rate of increase in arterial oxygen saturation (Sao_2) and is measured by pulse oximetry. The equation can be rearranged as:

$$\text{Hb flow} = \frac{\Delta \text{HbO}_2}{\int_0^t \Delta Sao_2 \ dt}$$

HbT content [HbT] must remain constant through the measurement. The rise in HbO_2 must therefore be accompanied by an equal fall in HbR. To increase the signal-to-noise ratio ΔHbO_2 is substituted by $\Delta HbD/2$ where $HbD = HbO_2 - HbR$. The equation now reads:

$$\text{Hemoglobin flow} = \frac{\Delta \text{HbD}}{\int_0^t \Delta Sao_2 \ dt}$$

where the hemoglobin flow is in μmol/L/min. The Sao_2 is increased by approximately 5% over less than 6 seconds. Because Sao_2 is measured peripherally and the HbD is measured on the forehead, there may be an interval of not more than 2 seconds between the rises of each.

Because the molecular weight of hemoglobin is 64,500 g/mol and the tissue density of the brain is 1.05, CBF (mL/100 g/min) is:

$$\frac{\text{Hb} \times 6.14}{[\text{Hb}]}$$

where Hb flow is in μmol/L/min and [Hb] is in g/dL.

The oxygen tracer technique has a major drawback in that it self-selects infants within a range of oxygen requirement. Infants who are saturating close to 100% in room air or in small amounts of oxygen cannot increase their oxygen saturations

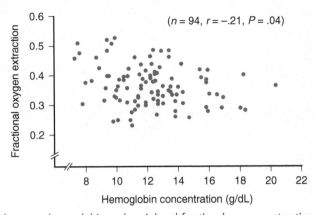

Fig. 17.1   Correlation between hemoglobin and peripheral fractional oxygen extraction. (Reproduced with permission from Wardle SP, Yoxall CW, Crawley E, Weindling AM: Peripheral oxygenation and anemia in preterm babies, *Pediatr Res* 44:125, 1998.)

any further with an oxygen bolus. In addition, infants who are on or close to 100% oxygen cannot be given an oxygen bolus.

Physiologic Observations Using Near-Infrared Spectroscopy

Oxygen Delivery

Oxygen delivery (Do_2) is the total amount of oxygen delivered to the tissue per minute.[51] Cerebral oxygen delivery is usually measured as milliliters of oxygen per 100 g of brain tissue per minute (mL/100 g/min).[23]

As dissolved oxygen is negligible, oxygen delivery can be calculated from the following formula[23]:

$$Do_2 = \text{cardiac output} \times ([Hb] \times Sao_2 \times 1.39)$$

where 1.39 is the oxygen-carrying capacity of hemoglobin. Although this formula gives the oxygen delivery to the entire body, oxygen delivery to the brain = CBF × ([Hb] × Sao_2 × 1.39). Similarly, oxygen delivery to the peripheral tissue = peripheral blood flow × ([Hb] × Sao_2 × 1.39).

Factors Determining Oxygen Delivery

From the equation Do_2 = cardiac output × ([Hb] × Sao_2 × 1.39), it can be seen that the factors affecting oxygen delivery to the brain are blood flow, hemoglobin concentration, and arterial oxygen saturation. Any one of these measurements alone does not adequately describe oxygen delivery. For example, Do_2 to an organ may be inadequate due to decreased CBF despite the presence of normal oxygen saturation and hemoglobin levels.

Effect of Anemia

Despite the importance of hemoglobin in oxygen transport, HbT concentration is a relatively poor indicator of the adequacy of the provision of oxygen to the tissues and may not accurately reflect tissue oxygen availability.[48] This has been demonstrated in various studies using NIR spectroscopy and is summarized later.

Only a weak but statistically significant negative correlation was demonstrated between blood hemoglobin concentration and cerebral FOE in 91 preterm infants and between blood hemoglobin concentration and peripheral FOE ($n = 94$, $r = -.21$, $P = .04$; Fig. 17.1).[16,18] The authors also compared the cerebral FOE of anemic and nonanemic preterm infants, with a relatively small difference in blood hemoglobin concentration between the two groups. There was no significant difference between the cerebral FOE of anemic compared with nonanemic preterm infants.[18] However, cerebral FOE decreased immediately after blood transfusion, suggesting that acute changes may produce an effect.[18]

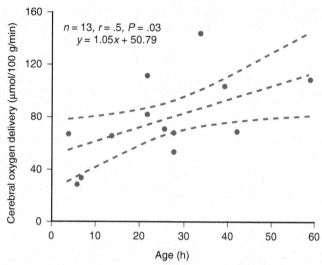

Fig. 17.2 Plot of cerebral oxygen delivery against time from birth in hours. There is a significant increase in cerebral oxygen delivery during the measurement, demonstrated by using weighted Pearson correlation coefficient. (Reproduced with permission from Kissack CM, Garr R, Wardle SP, Weindling AM: Cerebral fractional oxygen extraction is inversely correlated with oxygen delivery in the sick, newborn, preterm infant, *J Cereb Blood Flow Metab* 25:545, 2005.)

Peripheral D_{O_2} increased while peripheral V_{O_2} remained constant after blood transfusion in asymptomatic but not in symptomatic anemic infants.[45] In contrast, observations from animals and adult humans have shown little change in cerebral S_{VO_2} during anemic hypoxia.[52,53]

Cerebral Oxygen Delivery

Cerebral D_{O_2} has been calculated using the measurements of CBF in preterm infants.[23] The median cerebral D_{O_2} in infants between 24 and 41 weeks' gestation was 83.2 μmol/100 g/min (range, 33.2 to 172.3).[23] Cerebral D_{O_2} overall increases with gestational age ($n = 20$, $\rho = .56$, $P < .012$) and particularly during the first 3 days after birth (Fig. 17.2).[23,54]

Cerebral Blood Flow

Mean global CBF is extremely low in preterm infants and increases with postnatal and gestational age.[50] Using NIR spectroscopy, the median of CBF in preterm infants was 9.3 mL/100 g/min (range, 4.5 to 28.3).[23] Similar ranges have been reported by others using the same technique.[1,25,55] The finding of extremely low CBF in preterm infants using NIR spectroscopy is consistent with measurements of CBF using the xenon clearance technique and using positron emission tomography.[56,57] CBF values of less than 5.0 mL/100 g/min in the normal or near normal brain of the preterm infant are considerably less than the value of 10 mL/100 g/min that is considered to be the threshold for viability in the adult human brain.[58] The very low values of blood flow in the cerebral white matter in the human preterm infant also suggest that there is a small margin of safety between normal and critical cerebral ischemia.[58]

Using the oxygen tracer technique and NIR spectroscopy, CBF was found to increase over the first 3 days after birth in infants between 24 and 31 weeks' gestation.[1] In infants between 24 and 34 weeks' gestation, CBF was independent of mean arterial blood pressure and decreased with a decrease in transcutaneous carbon dioxide levels.[25]

NIR spectroscopy was used to investigate the effects of intravenously administered indomethacin (0.1 to 0.2 mg/kg) on cerebral hemodynamics and D_{O_2} in 13 very preterm infants treated for patent ductus arteriosus.[54] Seven infants received indomethacin by rapid injection (30 seconds) and six by slow infusion (20 to 30 minutes).[59] In all infants, CBF, D_{O_2}, blood volume, and the reactivity of blood volume to changes in arterial carbon dioxide tension fell sharply after indomethacin.[54] There were no differences in the effects of rapid versus slow infusion.[59]

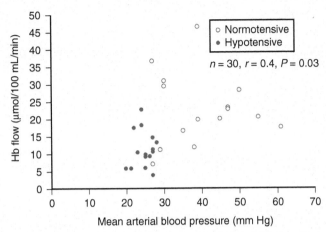

Fig. 17.3   Relationship between mean blood pressure and peripheral hemoglobin flow. (Reproduced with permission from Wardle SP, Yoxall CW, Weindling AM: Peripheral oxygenation in hypotensive preterm babies, *Pediatr Res* 45:343, 1999.)

Peripheral Blood Flow

As described earlier, NIR spectroscopy measures forearm blood flow from the data acquired by the venous occlusion technique.[17,49,50] Using this technique, De Blasi and colleagues found that the forearm blood flow in adults at rest was 1.9 ± 0.8 mL/100 mL/min, increasing after exercise to 8.2 ± 2.9 mL/100 mL/min.[50] These values correlated well with those made using forearm plethysmography.[50]

The partial venous occlusion technique was used to study peripheral oxygen delivery in hypotensive preterm infants between 26 and 29 weeks' gestation.[16] In preterm infants a significant correlation was determined between mean blood pressure and peripheral blood flow (Fig. 17.3).[16,60] Preterm infants with low mean arterial blood pressure of 25 mm Hg had median peripheral blood flow of 4.6 mL/100 mL/min. This was significantly lower than the median peripheral blood flow of 8.3 mL/100 mL/min in infants with higher mean arterial blood pressure of 39 mm Hg.[16] After treatment of hypotension, the median (interquartile range) forearm oxygen delivery increased significantly from 37 μmol/100 mL/min to 64 μmol/100 mL/min (Fig. 17.4).[16] The median (interquartile range) forearm V_{O_2} increased significantly from 11.0 μmol/100 mL/min to 21.7 μmol/100 mL/min (see Fig. 17.4).[16]

In a study investigating peripheral oxygen delivery and anemia, forearm blood flow did not correlate with the fetal hemoglobin fraction or the red cell volume[48] or change after transfusion of both symptomatic and asymptomatic anemic preterm infants.[48] However, the same study showed a significant positive correlation between forearm blood flow and postnatal age.[48]

Oxygen Consumption

V_{O_2} is defined as the total amount of oxygen consumed by the tissue per minute.[51] The amount of oxygen required by a tissue depends on the functional state of the component cells. Some tissues such as the brain, liver, and renal cortex have persistently high oxygen demands, whereas other tissues such as the spleen have low oxygen demands. Other tissues such as skeletal muscle have variable oxygen demands.

The units for cerebral V_{O_2} are milliliters of oxygen per 100 g of brain tissue per minute.[23] V_{O_2} can be calculated from the following formula[23]:

$$VO_2 = \text{cardiac output} \times [Hb] \times (SaO_2 - SvO_2) \times 1.39$$

and cerebral or peripheral V_{O_2} = cerebral or peripheral blood flow × [Hb] × (Sa_{O_2} – Sv_{O_2}) × 1.39, where 1.39 is the oxygen-carrying capacity of hemoglobin.

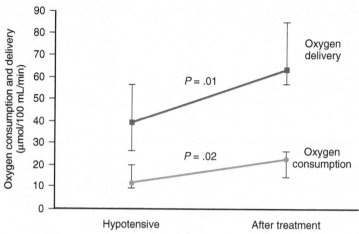

Fig. 17.4 Changes in forearm oxygen delivery and oxygen consumption after treatment for hypotension. (Reproduced with permission from Wardle SP, Yoxall CW, Weindling AM: Peripheral oxygenation in hypotensive preterm babies, *Pediatr Res* 45:343, 1999.)

Cerebral Venous Oxygen Saturation and Consumption

By combining measurement of CBF using ^{133}Xe clearance and estimation of cerebral Svo_2 using NIR spectroscopy and head tilt, cerebral Vo_2 was calculated as 1.0 mL/100 g/min in nine preterm infants and 1.4 mL/100 g/min in 10 asphyxiated term infants.[45]

We used NIR spectroscopy with partial jugular venous occlusion to determine cerebral Svo_2 and an oxygen bolus to measure CBF in 20 infants (median gestation, 27 weeks; range, 24 to 41 weeks).[23] The median cerebral Vo_2 was 0.52 mL/100 g/min (range, 0.19 to 1.76), and it increased with maturity in line with cerebral Do_2 (see later) and, presumably, increasing cerebral metabolism.[23]

Peripheral Venous Oxygen Saturation and Consumption

NIR spectroscopy has been used to study Svo_2 and Vo_2 in the forearm of preterm infants. Peripheral Svo_2 when measured by co-oximetry was generally slightly higher than that measured by NIR spectroscopy, and this difference was more pronounced at higher levels of SvO_2.[21] This relationship was significant ($r = .528$, $P < .05$, $n = 16$).

In a study comparing forearm Vo_2 in anemic preterm infants before and after blood transfusion, no differences were found.[48] This was regardless of whether infants were symptomatic or asymptomatic prior to transfusion.[48]

Peripheral Vo_2 increased significantly after treatment of hypotensive preterm infants.[16] In that study the treatment of hypotension consisted mainly of treatment with dopamine, which is known to stimulate metabolic activity particularly within muscle tissue.[16]

The relationship between the use of dopamine and Vo_2 has also been studied using NIR spectroscopy. In a study examining peripheral oxygenation in hypotensive preterm babies, treatment of hypotension using volume and/or dopamine increased forearm Do_2 and Vo_2 but did not affect FOE.[16] Low-dose dopamine infusion in young rabbits did not alter cerebral hemodynamics and oxygenation.[61]

Fractional Oxygen Extraction

FOE is the amount of oxygen consumed as a fraction of oxygen delivery.[52] It has also been called *oxygen extraction ratio, oxygen extraction,* and *oxygen extraction fraction*[51,55,62] and is the ratio of Vo_2 to oxygen delivery (Do_2). Vo_2/Do_2 is calculated as follows.[18,51]

Because Vo_2 = cardiac output × [(Hb × 1.39) × (Sao_2 − Svo_2)] and Do_2 = cardiac output × (Hb × 1.39) × Sao_2, then by simplifying the equation:

$$VO_2/DO_2 = (SaO_2 - SvO_2)/SaO_2.$$

Therefore FOE can be calculated if the Sao_2 and Svo_2 are known. Svo_2 is measured using the methods described earlier, and peripheral Sao_2 is measured by

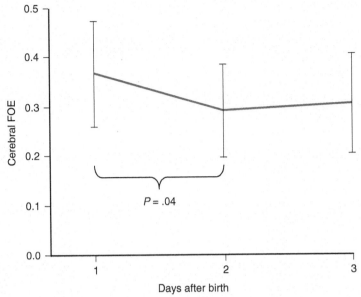

Fig. 17.5 Changes in cerebral fractional oxygen extraction (FOE) during the first 3 days after birth in sick, extremely preterm infants. Data are plotted as means with standard deviations. There is a significant decrease in cerebral fractional oxygen extraction between days 1 and 2. (Reproduced with permission from Kissack CM, Garr R, Wardle SP, Weindling AM: Cerebral fractional oxygen extraction is inversely correlated with oxygen delivery in the sick, newborn, preterm infant, *J Cereb Blood Flow Metab* 25:545, 2005.)

pulse oximetry (cerebral Sao_2 is assumed to be equal to peripheral Sao_2 as measured by pulse oximetry). The amount of oxygen dissolved in blood is considered to be negligible.

FOE varies from organ to organ and with levels of activity.[15] Measurements of FOE for the whole body produce a range of approximately 0.15 to 0.33.[15] That is, the body consumes 15% to 33% of the oxygen transported. The heart and brain are likely to have consistently high values of FOE during active states.[15] Mean cerebral FOE was 0.292 (SD = 0.06) when measured using NIR spectroscopy and partial jugular venous occlusion in 41 preterm infants (median gestation, 29 weeks; range, 27 to 31 weeks).[18] In that study, there appeared to be no relationship between cerebral FOE and gestational age or postnatal age (median, 9 days; range, 6 to 19 days).[18] However, when cerebral FOE was measured over the first 3 days after birth, there was a significant decrease in cerebral FOE between days 1 and 2, suggesting an increase in CBF and cerebral oxygen delivery (Fig. 17.5).[14,54,60]

Conclusions

This chapter reviewed the principles of NIR spectroscopy and its use in the quantification of oxygen delivery, FOE, and Vo_2. Continuous quantitative measurements desirable for clinical practice were not possible using the original continuous wave instruments, and this limited NIR spectroscopy for several years to clinical research studies because significant offline processing of data was required. Spatially resolved spectroscopy is a development of NIR spectroscopy that allowed continuous measurements. There is confusion with the terminology used between different manufacturers: the NIRO 200NX (Hamamatsu Photonics K.K.) defines TOI; the INVOS 5100c (Somanetics/Covidien, Mansfield, Massachusetts) describes rSO_2. More importantly, large interindividual and intraindividual differences between absolute values from different monitors have been reported, requiring further technological developments in the field.

REFERENCES

1. Meek JH, Tyszczuk L, Elwell CE, et al.: Cerebral blood flow increases over the first three days of life in extremely preterm neonates, *Arch Dis Child Fetal Neonatal Ed* 78:F33–F37, 1998.
2. Meek JH, Tyszczuk L, Elwell CE, et al.: Low cerebral blood flow is a risk factor for severe intraventricular haemorrhage, *Arch Dis Child Fetal Neonatal Ed* 81:F15–F18, 1999.
3. Ijichi S, Kusaka T, Isobe K, et al.: Developmental changes of optical properties in neonates determined by near-infrared time resolved spectroscopy, *Pediatr Res* 58:568–573, 2005.
4. Dani C, Bertini G, Reali MF, et al.: Brain hemodynamic changes in preterm infants after maintenance dose caffeine and aminophylline treatment, *Biol Neonate* 78:27–32, 2000.
5. Urlesberger B, Pichler G, Gradnitzer E, et al.: Changes in cerebral blood volume and cerebral oxygenation during periodic breathing in term infants, *Neuropediatrics* 31:75–81, 2000.
6. Jöbsis FF, Keizer JH, LaManna JC, et al.: Reflectance spectrophotometry of cytochrome aa3 in vivo, *J Appl Physiol* 43:858–872, 1977.
7. Irwin MS, Thorniley MS, Dore CJ, et al.: Near infra-red spectroscopy: a non-invasive monitor of perfusion and oxygenation within the microcirculation of limbs and flaps, *Br J Plast Surg* 48:14–22, 1995.
8. Mancini DM, Bolinger L, Li H, et al.: Validation of near-infrared spectroscopy in humans, *J Appl Physiol* 77:2740–2747, 1994.
9. Stankovic MR, Maulik D, Rosenfeld W, et al.: Role of frequency domain optical spectroscopy in the detection of neonatal brain hemorrhage—a newborn piglet study, *J Matern Fetal Med* 9:142–149, 2000.
10. Tsuji M, duPlessis A, Taylor G, et al.: Near infrared spectroscopy detects cerebral ischemia during hypotension in piglets, *Pediatr Res* 44:591–595, 1998.
11. Fantini S, Hueber D, Franceschini MA, et al.: Non-invasive optical monitoring of the newborn piglet brain using continuous-wave and frequency-domain spectroscopy, *Phys Med Biol* 44:1543–1563, 1999.
12. Alfano RR, Demos SG, Galland P, et al.: Time-resolved and nonlinear optical imaging for medical applications, *Ann N Y Acad Sci* 838:14–28, 1998.
13. Kissack CM, Garr M, Wardle SP, et al.: Postnatal changes in cerebral oxygen extraction in the preterm infant are associated with intraventricular haemorrhage and haemorrhagic parenchymal infarction but not periventricular leukomalacia, *Pediatr Res* 56:111–116, 2004.
14. Kissack CM, Garr R, Wardle SP, et al.: Cerebral fractional oxygen extraction in very low birth weight infants is high when there is low left ventricular output and hypocarbia but is unaffected by hypotension, *Pediatr Res* 55:400–405, 2004.
15. Wardle SP, Yoxall CW, Weindling AM: Cerebral oxygenation during cardiopulmonary bypass, *Arch Dis Child* 78:26–32, 1998.
16. Wardle SP, Yoxall CW, Weindling AM: Peripheral oxygenation in hypotensive preterm babies, *Pediatr Res* 45:343–349, 1999.
17. Wardle SP, Weindling AM: Peripheral oxygenation in preterm infants, *Clin Perinatol* 26:947–966, 1999.
18. Wardle SP, Yoxall CW, Weindling AM: Determinants of cerebral fractional oxygen extraction using near infrared spectroscopy in preterm neonates, *J Cereb Blood Flow Metab* 20:272–279, 2000.
19. Wardle SP, Weindling AM: Peripheral fractional oxygen extraction and other measures of tissue oxygenation to guide blood transfusions in preterm infants, *Semin Perinatol* 25:60–64, 2001.
20. Yoxall CW, Weindling AM, Dawani NH, et al.: Measurement of cerebral venous oxyhemoglobin saturation in children by near-infrared spectroscopy and partial jugular venous occlusion, *Pediatr Res* 38:319–323, 1995.
21. Yoxall CW, Weindling AM: The measurement of peripheral venous oxyhemoglobin saturation in newborn infants by near infrared spectroscopy with venous occlusion, *Pediatr Res* 39:1103–1106, 1996.
22. Yoxall CW, Weindling AM: Measurement of venous oxyhaemoglobin saturation in the adult human forearm by near infrared spectroscopy with venous occlusion, *Med Biol Eng Comput* 35:331–336, 1997.
23. Yoxall CW, Weindling AM: Measurement of cerebral oxygen consumption in the human neonate using near infrared spectroscopy: cerebral oxygen consumption increases with advancing gestational age, *Pediatr Res* 44:283–290, 1998.
24. Meek JH, Elwell CE, McCormick DC, et al.: Abnormal cerebral haemodynamics in perinatally asphyxiated neonates related to outcome, *Arch Dis Child Fetal Neonatal Ed* 81:F110–F115, 1999.
25. Tyszczuk L, Meek J, Elwell C, et al.: Cerebral blood flow is independent of mean arterial blood pressure in preterm infants undergoing intensive care, *Pediatrics* 102(2 Pt 1):337–341, 1998.
26. Wray S, Cope M, Delpy DT, et al.: Characterization of the near infrared absorption spectra of cytochrome aa3 and haemoglobin for the non-invasive monitoring of cerebral oxygenation, *Bioch Biophys Acta* 933:184–192, 1988.
27. Mendelson Y, Kent JC, Mendelson Y, et al.: Variations in optical absorption spectra of adult and fetal hemoglobins and its effect on pulse oximetry, *IEEE Trans Biomed Eng* 36:844–848, 1989.
28. van der Zee P, Cope M, Arridge SR, et al.: Experimentally measured optical pathlengths for the adult head, calf and forearm and the head of the newborn infant as a function of inter optode spacing, *Adv Exp Med Biol* 316:143–153, 1992.
29. Duncan A, Meek JH, Clemence M, et al.: Optical pathlength measurements on adult head, calf and forearm and the head of the newborn infant using phase resolved optical spectroscopy, *Phys Med Biol* 40:295–304, 1995.

30. Duncan A, Meek JH, Clemence M, et al.: Measurement of cranial optical pathlength as a function of age using phase resolved near infrared spectroscopy, *Pediatr Res* 39:889–894, 1996.

31. Delpy DT, Arridge SR, Cope M, et al.: Quantitation of pathlength in optical spectroscopy, *Adv Exp Med Biol* 248:41–46, 1989.

32. Essenpreis M, Cope M, Elwell CE, et al.: Wavelength dependence of the differential pathlength factor and the log slope in time-resolved tissue spectroscopy, *Adv Exp Med Biol* 333:9–20, 1993.

33. Dullenkopf A, Kolarova A, Schulz G, et al.: Reproducibility of cerebral oxygenation measurement in neonates and infants in the clinical setting using the NIRO 300 oximeter, *Pediatr Crit Care Med* 6:378–379, 2005.

34. Weiss M, Dullenkopf A, Kolarova A, et al.: Near-infrared spectroscopic cerebral oxygenation reading in neonates and infants is associated with central venous oxygen saturation, *Paediatr Anaesth* 15:102–109, 2005.

35. Sorensen LC, Greisen G: Precision of measurement of cerebral tissue oxygenation index using near-infrared spectroscopy in preterm neonates, *J Biomed Opt* 11:054005, 2006.

36. Sorensen LC, Leung TS, Greisen G: Comparison of cerebral oxygen saturation in premature infants by near-infrared spatially resolved spectroscopy: observations on probe-dependent bias, *J Biomed Opt* 13:064013, 2008.

37. Quaresima V, Sacco S, Totaro R, et al.: Noninvasive measurement of cerebral hemoglobin oxygen saturation using two near infrared spectroscopy approaches, *J Biomed Opt* 5:201–205, 2000.

38. Henson LC, Calalang C, Temp JA, et al.: Accuracy of a cerebral oximeter in healthy volunteers under conditions of isocapnic hypoxia, *Anesthesiology* 88:58–65, 1998.

39. Kurth CD, Levy WJ, McCann J: Near-infrared spectroscopy cerebral oxygen saturation thresholds for hypoxia-ischemia in piglets, *J Cereb Blood Flow Metab* 22:335–341, 2002.

40. Pollard V, Prough DS, DeMelo AE, et al.: Validation in volunteers of a near-infrared spectroscope for monitoring brain oxygenation in vivo, *Anesth Analg* 82:269–277, 1996.

41. Watzman HM, Kurth CD, Montenegro LM, et al.: Arterial and venous contributions to near-infrared cerebral oximetry, *Anesthesiology* 93:947–953, 2000.

42. Franceschini MA, Thaker S, Themelis G, et al.: Assessment of infant brain development with frequency-domain near-infrared spectroscopy, *Pediatr Res* 61(5 Pt 1):546–551, 2007.

43. Roche-Labarbe N, Carp SA, Surova A, et al.: Noninvasive optical measures of CBV, StO(2), CBF index, and rCMRO(2) in human premature neonates' brains in the first six weeks of life, *Hum Brain Mapp* 31:341–352, 2010.

44. Dehaes M, Aggarwal A, Lin PY, et al.: Cerebral oxygen metabolism in neonatal hypoxic ischemic encephalopathy during and after therapeutic hypothermia, *J Cereb Blood Flow Metab* 34(1):87–94, 2014.

45. Skov L, Pryds O, Greisen G, et al.: Estimation of cerebral venous saturation in newborn infants by near infrared spectroscopy, *Pediatr Res* 33:52–55, 1993.

46. Wolf M, Duc G, Keel M, et al.: Continuous noninvasive measurement of cerebral arterial and venous oxygen saturation at the bedside in mechanically ventilated neonates, *Crit Care Med* 25:1579–1582, 1997.

47. Owen-Reece H, Smith M, Elwell CE, et al.: Near infrared spectroscopy, *Br J Anaesth* 82:418–426, 1999.

48. Wardle SP, Yoxall CW, Crawley E, et al.: Peripheral oxygenation and anemia in preterm babies, *Pediatr Res* 44:125–131, 1998.

49. Edwards AD, Richardson C, van der ZP, et al.: Measurement of hemoglobin flow and blood flow by near-infrared spectroscopy, *J Appl Physiol* 75:1884–1889, 1993.

50. De Blasi RA, Ferrari M, Natali A, et al.: Noninvasive measurement of forearm blood flow and oxygen consumption by near-infrared spectroscopy, *J Appl Physiol* 76:1388–1393, 1994.

51. Leach RM, Treacher DF: The pulmonary physician in critical care 2: oxygen delivery and consumption in the critically ill, *Thorax* 57:170–177, 2002.

52. Borgstrom L, Johannsson H, Siesjo BK: The influence of acute normovolemic anemia on cerebral blood flow and oxygen consumption of anesthetized rats, *Acta Physiol Scand* 93:505–514, 1975.

53. Paulson OB, Parving HH, Olesen J, et al.: Influence of carbon monoxide and of hemodilution on cerebral blood flow and blood gases in man, *J Appl Physiol* 35:111–116, 1973.

54. Kissack CM, Garr R, Wardle SP, et al.: Cerebral fractional oxygen extraction is inversely correlated with oxygen delivery in the sick, newborn, preterm infant, *J Cereb Blood Flow Metab* 25:545–553, 2005.

55. Greisen G: Cerebral blood flow and energy metabolism in the newborn, *Clin Perinatol* 24:531–546, 1997.

56. Pryds O, Greisen G, Skov LL, et al.: Carbon dioxide-related changes in cerebral blood volume and cerebral blood flow in mechanically ventilated preterm neonates: comparison of near infrared spectrophotometry and [133]xenon clearance, *Pediatr Res* 27:445–449, 1990.

57. Altman DI, Powers WJ, Perlman JM, et al.: Cerebral blood flow requirement for brain viability in newborn infants is lower than in adults, *Ann Neurol* 24:218–226, 1988.

58. Volpe JJ: Neurobiology of periventricular leukomalacia in the premature infant, *Pediatr Res* 50:553–562, 2001.

59. Edwards AD, Wyatt JS, Richardson C, et al.: Effects of indomethacin on cerebral haemodynamics in very preterm infants, *Lancet* 335:1491–1495, 1990.

60. Victor S, Weindling AM, Appleton RE, et al.: Relationship between blood pressure, electroencephalograms, cerebral fractional oxygen extraction and peripheral blood flow in very low birth weight newborn infants, *Pediatr Res* 59:314–319, 2006.

17

61. Koyama K, Mito T, Takashima S, et al.: Effects of phenylephrine and dopamine on cerebral blood flow, blood volume, and oxygenation in young rabbits, *Pediatr Neurol* 6:87–90, 1990.
62. Hayashi T, Watabe H, Kudomi N, et al.: A theoretical model of oxygen delivery and metabolism for physiologic interpretation of quantitative cerebral blood flow and metabolic rate of oxygen, *J Cereb Blood Flow Metab* 23:1314–1323, 2003.

C

CHAPTER 18

Clinical Applications of Near-Infrared Spectroscopy in Neonates

Petra Lemmers, Laura Dix, Gunnar Naulaers, and Frank van Bel

- The status of cerebral oxygenation is not always represented appropriately by systemic arterial oxygenation. Oxygenation monitoring of the brain by near-infrared spectroscopy (NIRS) is therefore an important additive measure in neonatal intensive care.

- Monitoring cerebral oxygenation by NIRS—in addition to arterial saturation monitoring by pulse oximetry, blood pressure, and brain function by amplitude-integrated electroencephalography—can help to prevent brain damage as well as unnecessary treatment of the neonate.

- Cerebral oxygenation can be stabilized in the neonate by using a dedicated treatment guideline in combination with cerebral oxygenation monitoring by NIRS.

Survival of the extremely preterm infant has greatly improved over the past decades. However, perinatal brain damage with adverse neurodevelopmental outcome continues to affect a considerable number of these infants.[1-7] Although the etiology of brain damage is multifactorial and partly unknown (see Chapters 7 and 8), hypoxia, hyperoxia, specific and nonspecific inflammation, and hemodynamic instability during the first days of postnatal life play an important role.[8-14] It is clear that further advances in survival and improvements in neurodevelopmental outcome can be achieved only if we learn more about the underlying pathophysiology so that more effective treatment modalities can be established. The first step in this direction is to develop the ability to continuously monitor clinically relevant hemodynamic variables and, if possible, treat the underlying condition at an early stage. Continuous monitoring of physiologic parameters such as heart rate, blood pressure, arterial oxygen saturation (SaO_2), temperature, and, with increasing frequency, electrical activity of the brain using amplitude-integrated electroencephalography (aEEG) have been integrated into the monitoring practices of neonatal intensive care units (NICUs). aEEG has recently been introduced into neonatal intensive care as a novel monitoring technique to continuously assess cerebral function. Both the aEEG background patterns and analysis of the raw EEG signal have been used for the evaluation of neurologic function. The fewer number of channels compared with the classic full EEG improves its applicability, and the use of aEEG seems to have increased in neonatal intensive care.[15,16] Other novel techniques used to continuously monitor additional hemodynamic parameters, such as cardiac output, are discussed in detail in Chapters 14 and 21.

Discontinuous techniques to assess cerebral condition—such as cranial ultrasound, Doppler flow-velocity measurements, and (advanced) magnetic resonance imaging (MRI)—have also been increasingly integrated into the care of the sick neonate (see Chapters 10, 15, and 16). However, these techniques do not provide continuous information on the perfusion and oxygenation of the neonatal brain, and MRI is not a bedside technique, at least at present.

Thus we need a reliable and practical clinical tool that monitors oxygenation of the neonatal brain noninvasively and continuously so that conditions potentially leading to brain injury can be recognized in a timely manner. A promising method is monitoring cerebral oxygenation by NIRS.[17–21]

As discussed in Chapter 17 in detail, the use of NIRS to monitor cerebral perfusion and oxygenation was first described by Jobsis in 1977.[22] Since then, a great number of studies have been performed measuring cerebral oxygenation and assessing cerebral blood flow, cerebral blood volume, and fractional oxygen extraction (CFOE) in neonates using instruments based mainly on the Beer-Lambert law, which relates the attenuation of light to the properties of a material through which light is traveling. The early instruments were designed for research work; accordingly they remained difficult to use in the clinical setting due to movement artifacts and because absolute values were not provided.[17] The introduction of spatially resolved spectroscopy made it possible to use a new approach to monitor cerebral oxygenation in the clinical setting. Spatially resolved spectroscopy measures the absorption of the emitted light by two or more detectors. By using the diffusion equation, absolute values can be calculated assuming that the scattering for the different distances is constant.[23,24] Another method is to subtract the measurement of the closest detector from the measurement of the farthest detector so as to minimize the influence of the superficial tissue layers. For instruments using this algorithm, further calibration in vitro and in vivo is still in progress. As also discussed in Chapter 17, the different NIRS instruments used at present have different principles of measurement and different wavelengths, optode distances, and types (laser or LED) and numbers of light emitters. However, they all measure the status of cerebral oxygenation by using either the tissue oxygenation index (TOI) or regional cerebral oxygen saturation (rScO$_2$). Despite the different approaches, the measures of cerebral oxygenation reflect mixed tissue oxygen saturation by assuming that the contribution to the perfusion of the tissue interrogated is 25%, 5%, and 70% by the arteries, capillaries, and veins, respectively. The value is provided as an absolute number that can be measured continuously and over prolonged periods of time.[25]

For most of the instruments, a good correlation with jugular venous oxygen saturation has been documented.[26,27] The values are not identical, however, primarily because TOI and rScO$_2$ reflect the changes in oxygenation in the arterial, capillary, *and* venous compartments. A comparison in adults between the different monitoring techniques during changes in oxygenation and changes in the partial pressure of arterial carbon dioxide (PaCO$_2$) has also yielded a good correlation between the TOI and rScO$_2$.[28,29] In addition, in comparing the left and right sides of the brain, the Bland-Altman limits of agreement for rScO$_2$ were −8.5 to +9.5%, with even smaller limits during stable SaO$_2$ values between 85% and 97%.[30] However, due to the limitations of the technology (see Chapters 17 and 21), it is obvious that these measurements are better used for trend measurements rather than precise tissue oxygenation values.

Clinical monitoring of cerebral oxygenation by NIRS has already become routine in pediatric and adult intensive care and during cardiac surgical procedures in all age groups.[28,31–33] However, although information concerning brain tissue oxygenation may be important in considering the type and timing of an intervention and in assessing its impact on outcome, the use of NIRS has not yet been universally implemented in the daily care of neonates in the NICU. Although the accumulating evidence supporting the use of NIRS in clinical practice is encouraging, the information available is still not overwhelmingly convincing.

In addition to TOI or CrSO$_2$, cerebral fractional tissue oxygen extraction (cFTOE) is another important NIRS parameter. Cerebral fractional tissue oxygen extraction is derived from rScO$_2$ and SaO$_2$ based on the formula: SaO$_2$ − rScO$_2$ / SaO$_2$. Thus cFTOE is a surrogate indicator of the actual CFOE, which can be measured with the validated jugular venous occlusion technique (see Chapter 17).[27,34] Naulaers et al. reported a positive correlation between NIRS-calculated cFTOE and actual fractional oxygen extraction of the brain in a newborn piglet model.[35] Because cFTOE is a ratio of two variables, an increase might indicate either reduced oxygen delivery to the brain with constant oxygen consumption or increased cerebral oxygen consumption not satisfied by oxygen delivery. The opposite is true in the case of a decrease in the cFTOE, reflecting either a decrease in oxygen extraction because of decreased oxygen utilization or an increase in oxygen delivery to the brain while cerebral oxygen consumption has remained unchanged. Obviously both parameters might change at the same time, although relatively rapid changes in cerebral oxygen utilization are less common. Although NIRS-derived cFTOE is a less accurate parameter compared with fractional oxygen extraction determined by the jugular occlusion technique, the clear advantage of cFTOE is that we can now continuously assess cerebral oxygen extraction.[36,37]

Feasibility of Near-Infrared Spectroscopy–Monitored Regional Cerebral Oxygen Saturation and Cerebral Fractional Tissue Oxygen Extraction in Clinical Practice in the Neonatal Intensive Care Unit

In order to assess the utility of NIRS-monitored $rScO_2$ in clinical practice, it is essential to also obtain data on the signal-to-noise ratio and the inter- and intrapatient variability. As compared with pulse oximetry-measured SaO_2, a reliable and accepted trend monitor for systemic arterial oxygenation, the signal-to-noise ratio is larger for NIRS-measured $rScO_2$.[19] However, when the signal is averaged over a longer period (e.g., over 30 to 60 seconds), a reliable NIRS signal can be obtained with an acceptable signal-to-noise ratio.[19] With respect to intrapatient variability, differences of up to 7% or more have been reported when subsequent measurements are performed with repeated placement of the NIRS sensor. The limits of agreement after sensor replacement are in the range of −17% to +17%.[19,21,38] These values are more than double the limits of agreement for SaO_2.[34] On the other hand, Menke et al. described a good reproducibility of NIRS-measured $rScO_2$ with an intermeasurement variance only slightly higher than the physiologic baseline variation.[39] In comparing values during simultaneous monitoring of the left and right frontoparietal regions of the brain, limits of agreement of 7% to 9% have been reported.[30] Moreover, it appears that the experience of the investigator also plays an important role in the quality of the information obtained.

Reference values of $rScO_2$ or TOI during normal arterial oxygen saturations have been reported in several studies including preterm neonates. Of note is that not all studies incorporated postnatal age or the clinical status of the infant in reporting their findings. Mean values (±SD) of $rScO_2$ or TOI ranged between 61% and 75% (from ±7% to ±12%), or values comparable with those obtained in adults (Table 18.1).[21,29,38,40–48]

Over the past decade or so, more and more NIRS devices with special neonatal or pediatric sensors and algorithms have become available. Before interpreting the absolute values, however, attention must be paid to the differences between the old and new sensors. Indeed, studies have shown that in neonates, the newer, smaller sensors may measure up to 15% higher values compared with the previously used adult sensors.[49] Therefore reference values for the neonatal or pediatric sensors in preterm and term neonates are needed before their implementation in clinical practice. Indeed, a large study by Alderliesten et al. of 999 preterm infants has recently provided reference values for $rScO_2$ and cFTOE for different types of sensors.[48] Graphs of reference value curves allow for bedside interpretation of NIRS-monitored cerebral oxygenation (Fig. 18.1). These reference values can then be used for comparison with values obtained during conditions that may affect cerebral oxygenation (discussed later).

Importantly, an association between $rScO_2$ values in neonates and functional or histologic compromise of the brain has been documented. Several animal studies in newborn piglets and one human study in neonates with hypoplastic left heart syndrome who underwent open heart surgery have reported that $rScO_2$ or TOI values lower than 35% to 45% for more than 30 to 90 minutes are associated with functional (mitochondrial dysfunction or energy failure) and/or histologic damage,

Table 18.1   REFERENCE VALUES [MEAN (±SD)] OF REGIONAL CEREBRAL OXYGEN SATURATION/TISSUE OXYGEN INDEX (%) IN ADULTS AND IN TERM AND PRETERM NEONATES

Adults		67% (±8)	$n = 94$ (40)
		66% (±8)	$n = 19$ (rScO$_2$/TOI) (29)
		68%–76%	$n = 9$ (rScO$_2$) (47)
		61.5 (±6.1)	$n = 14$ (rScO$_2$) (45)
Term neonates/infants	Day 12 [0–365]	61% (±12)	$n = 155$ (TOI) (41)
	Day 4.5 [0–190]	63% (±12)	$n = 20$ (TOI) (38)
	8 min after birth	68% (IQR 55–80)	$n = 20$ (46)
Preterm neonates (GA <32 weeks)	Day 1	57% (54–66)	$n = 15$ (TOI) (21)
	Day 2	66% (62–82)	
	Day 3	76% (68–80)	
	NA	75% (±10.2)	$n = 253$ (TOI) (42)
	>Day 7	66% (±8.8)	$n = 40$ (rScO$_2$) (43)
	Day 1	70% (±7.4)	$n = 38$ (rScO$_2$) (44)
	Day 2	71% (±8.8)	
	Day 3	70% (±7.8)	
	Day 1–3	62%–71% (±7)	$n = 999$ (rScO$_2$) (48)

The interpatient variance of TOI/rScO$_2$ in these studies was larger than for pulse oximetry-measured oxygen saturation. Reference values for preterm infants are within the same range as the reference values of adults, infants, and term neonates.

GA, Gestational age; rScO$_2$, regional cerebral oxygen saturation; TOI, tissue oxygen index.

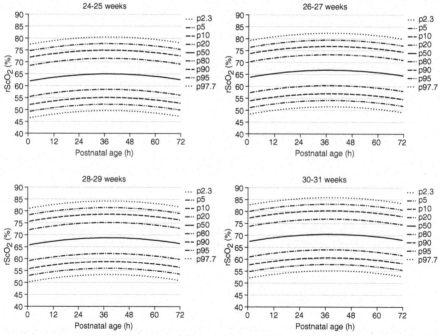

Fig. 18.1   Regional cerebral oxygen saturation (rScO$_2$) reference value curves for neonates of (A) 24 to 25 weeks' gestation, (B) 26 to 27 weeks' gestation, (C) 28 to 29 weeks' gestation, and (D) 30 to 31 weeks' gestation. The line patterns depict different percentiles: *dotted lines* indicate p2.3 and p97.7; *dash-dot-dot-dash lines* indicate p5 and p95; *dashed lines* indicate p10; and p90; *dash-dot-dash* lines indicate p20 and p80, and *solid lines* indicate p50. (As published by Alderliesten T, Dix L, Baerts W, et al.: Reference values of regional cerebral oxygen saturation during the first 3 days of life in preterm neonates. *Pediatr Res* 79(1-1):55–64, 2016.)

especially in the hippocampus (a brain region very vulnerable to hypoxia in the perinatal period).[50–52] Moreover, a number of studies, mostly performed in adult cardiac intensive care units, have reported that a 20% decrease from the baseline or an absolute rScO$_2$ value of less than 50% before intervention is associated with hypoxic-ischemic brain lesions.[53,54] Thus these findings suggest that rScO$_2$ values below 45% to 50% for a prolonged period of time should be avoided if possible. A large international randomized controlled clinical trial has investigated whether it is possible

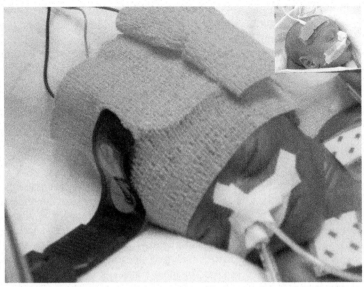

Fig. 18.2 Application of the near infrared sensor to the head of a preterm infant in the frontoparietal position using an elastic bandage. The inset shows the application of the sensor with an adhesive tape. (Published with parental permission.)

to detect and prevent cerebral oxygenation outside the assumed normal limits of 55% to 85% with NIRS monitoring to prevent neurologic injury and improve neurodevelopmental outcome.[55] The SafeBoosc II trial (Safeguarding the Brains of Our Smallest Children) randomized infants to either visible or shielded NIRS registration of cerebral oxygenation and compared the burden of hypoxia and hyperoxia between the two groups.[56] Infants with visible NIRS tracings spent a significantly shorter time outside the normal range mainly due to a reduction in the hypoxic burden because of clinical interventions. These findings indicate that unfavorable cerebral oxygen saturations can be detected by NIRS and prevented by timely interventions.[56]

Similar to the bedside detection and prevention of prolonged cerebral *hypoxia*, continuous monitoring of $rScO_2$ can also contribute to the prevention of prolonged cerebral *hyperoxia*, especially in the extremely preterm infant who is particularly prone to oxygen toxicity. The importance of avoiding hyperoxia has been increasingly recognized, as an association between normal oxygen saturations and improved long-term neurodevelopmental outcome in extremely preterm infants has been documented.[14,57,58] With these considerations and the presented data in mind, NIRS-monitored $rScO_2$ or TOI and NIRS-derived cFTOE are likely to play an important role in monitoring and improving cerebral oxygenation in sick neonates into the future.

Clinical Applications

Application of the Sensor and Its Pitfalls

The most important issue regarding the clinical application of noninvasive monitoring of cerebral oxygenation by NIRS is the ability to perform reliable, long-term monitoring in the most immature and unstable neonate without disturbing the infant. A critical part of initiating the process is the application of the sensor to the head. With appropriate placement, the sensor will allow reliable monitoring of the $rScO_2$ or TOI for a number of days without damaging the vulnerable skin, particularly of the very preterm infant. In addition, the sensor in place should not limit access to performing ultrasound studies of the brain, placement of electrodes for aEEG monitoring, and attachment of CPAP devices. In our experience, application of the NIRS sensor with a soft dark elastic bandage to the frontoparietal region of the head provides protection from ambient light and does not irritate or damage the skin of even the smallest infants while allowing reliable monitoring of $rScO_2$ for extended periods of time. Fig. 18.2 shows an example of the application of the NIRS sensor used in all of our clinical studies.[17] Alternatively, application of sensors using the original adhesive tape on the skin is possible, and this method is advocated by the manufacturers for most commercially available sensors (see Fig. 18.2).

Introduction of the system with structured theoretical courses and practical training for nurses and medical staff is a very important prerequisite for the successful use of this monitoring method in clinical practice. In addition, staff education about the potential benefits and risks of using NIRS is of great importance. In gaining experience, nursing staff in the authors' institutions have been able to recognize inappropriate transducer placement, improper transducer fixation, or insufficient transducer shielding. In our experience, this resulted in extended periods of uninterrupted and reliable $rScO_2$ monitoring even in the smallest infants (<600 g) comparable with pulse oximetry-monitored SaO_2. In monitoring and interpreting the values in daily clinical practice, one must be aware of several pitfalls. We have already discussed the importance of proper sensor application to prevent movement artifacts and the effect of ambient light. Yet despite these precautionary measures, phototherapy light will sometimes cause disturbances in $rScO_2$ monitoring. Accordingly, covering the sensor with an additional dark sheet during periods of phototherapy is recommended to ensure more reliable signal acquisition. Other factors such as dislocation of the NIRS sensor or the presence of hair, hematoma, edema, and/or other materials such as the plasters of the aEEG electrodes on the head can also cause disturbances of the NIRS signal. Interestingly, the influence of the curvature of the skull and head circumference seems negligible.[48]

Relation to Other Monitoring Devices

NIRS-monitored changes in brain oxygenation, represented by $rScO_2$ (or TOI) and cFTOE, generate important information in addition to that obtained from other monitoring devices such as pulse oximetry-monitored SaO_2, indwelling blood pressure monitoring, and heart rate/ electrical brain activity monitors. Monitoring SaO_2 is necessary to calculate cFTOE, as described earlier. The relationship between blood pressure and $rScO_2$ may provide information about the presence or lack of cerebral blood flow autoregulation (see Chapters 2 and 21).[59–62] As for the use of aEEG in combination with NIRS, our group has reported that persistent and unusually high $rScO_2$ values in term infants with severe perinatal asphyxia—probably due to profound vasodilation with or without vasoparalysis of the cerebral vascular bed and a decreased utilization of oxygen—were strongly associated with an abnormal aEEG pattern after the first postnatal day and adverse neurodevelopmental outcome at 2 years of age.[63] These findings indicate that the monitoring of cerebral oxygenation and oxygen extraction with NIRS along with other parameters reveals conditions at an early stage that might be associated with poor long-term outcomes.[56] The combination of the different parameters monitored can also be used in pharmacodynamic research. Medications given to neonates often have effects on both cerebral metabolism and hemodynamics; thus using the combination of NIRS, aEEG, and hemodynamic parameters such as blood pressure and heart rate will provide additional valuable information. An example is the use of propofol, which has direct effects on both blood pressure and cerebral metabolism.[64] Further research in neurovascular coupling in preterm infants is ongoing.[65] Finally, efforts to develop a comprehensive, real-time cardiorespiratory and neurocritical care monitoring system are described in Chapter 21.

Clinical Conditions Associated With Low Regional Cerebral Oxygen Saturation

Perlman et al. reported first that ductal steal has an impact on cerebral perfusion and is a risk factor for cerebral damage in the preterm infant.[66] Thus a hemodynamically significant patent ductus arteriosus (PDA) is a condition potentially associated with decreased oxygen delivery to the brain due to the impact of the diastolic runoff in the cerebral vessels and the associated changes in perfusion pressure on cerebral oxygen delivery throughout the entire cardiac cycle. Several recent reports using NIRS-monitored $rScO_2$ found a substantial decrease in cerebral oxygenation to sometimes critically low values in the presence of a hemodynamically significant PDA but with recovery to normal values after successful ductal closure.[67–69] The ductal diameter is the echocardiographic ductal characteristic that is best related to $rScO_2$, with the largest diameter resulting in the lowest $rScO_2$ values.[69] It appears that infants with a hemodynamically significant PDA unresponsive to pharmacologic closure with cyclooxygenase (COX) inhibitors are especially at risk before and during surgical ligation. Indeed, in a study of 20 infants, we found extremely low $rScO_2$ and high cFTOE values before and during ligation.[70] Infants undergoing surgical ligation of the ductus are often exposed to low $rScO_2$ values for a prolonged period of time, which may adversely affect brain development.[71] It was shown that the $rScO_2$ values before ductal closure are significantly associated with cerebellar growth as measured by MRI, with potential negative implications for neurodevelopment.[72] Moreover, early ductal screening and treatment seems to reduce in-hospital mortality.[73]

The monitoring of cerebral oxygenation has provided us with early information on the impact of left-to-right shunting across the duct on cerebral oxygenation as well as on the effectiveness of the treatment initiated to close the PDA. Fig. 18.3A provides a representative example of the impact of a hemodynamically significant PDA on cerebral oxygenation and the effect of successful pharmacologic closure of the duct with indomethacin. It should be noted that, unlike ibuprofen, indomethacin decreases and stabilizes cerebral blood flow via mechanisms independent of the drug's effect on the COX enzyme.

Another frequently encountered condition often related to low $rScO_2$ values is systemic hypotension. Hypotension can arise from various conditions including but not restricted to hypovolemia, myocardial dysfunction, the presence of a hemodynamically significant PDA, and specific (e.g., sepsis) or nonspecific inflammation or immaturity associated inability of the vascular bed to maintain an appropriate peripheral vascular resistance (see Chapters 1, 26, and 27). Although blood pressure is one of the most frequently measured hemodynamic variables in neonatal intensive care, the lower limits of the gestational and postnatal age–dependent normal blood pressure ranges are not known (see Chapter 3). These limits depend on a number of additional factors such as the underlying pathology, the ability of the individual patient to compensate with increasing blood flow to the vital organs, and maintenance of a proper autoregulatory capacity of the cerebrovascular bed (see Chapters 1, 2, and 19). Accordingly, evidence is emerging that a simple cutoff value based on gestational age is insufficient in establishing the diagnosis of hypotension (decreased perfusion pressure and blood flow in the vital organs along with decreased oxygen delivery) in an individual patient. The term *permissive hypotension* has been increasingly used to describe low blood pressure values without signs of impaired perfusion (see Chapter 3).[74–76] Accordingly, the ability to assess cerebral oxygenation is an important tool to evaluate the status of end-organ perfusion. If cerebral oxygenation and extraction are within the normal range in an otherwise hemodynamically stable infant, the presence of low blood pressure might call for further observation instead of the initiation of treatment (see Chapters 1 and 26). However, more information is needed before we can safely identify which neonates with low blood pressure might benefit from which treatment, and large trials are currently being conducted to answer these questions (see Chapters 3, 26, and 29).

Prematurity is a risk factor for impaired or absent autoregulatory ability of the cerebral vascular bed, and critically ill infants seem to be even more affected (see Chapter 2).[77,78] Impaired autoregulation is a risk for adverse neurodevelopmental outcome (see Chapters 2 and 7) and might be one of the causes of insufficient oxygen delivery to the immature brain.[61,79] Cerebral autoregulation can be calculated with NIRS-monitored $rScO_2$ combined with simultaneously monitored mean arterial blood pressure.[14,60–62,80] This approach assumes that cerebral metabolic rate, hemoglobin (Hb) concentration, and the proportion of arterial and venous blood perfusing the brain remain constant and that SaO_2 does not change. Accordingly, when a change in blood pressure is not associated with changes in cerebral oxygenation as assessed by $rScO_2$, cerebral autoregulation is presumed to be present. However, when there is an impairment or total lack of cerebral autoregulation, changes in blood pressure will have an immediate effect on cerebral oxygenation and thus on

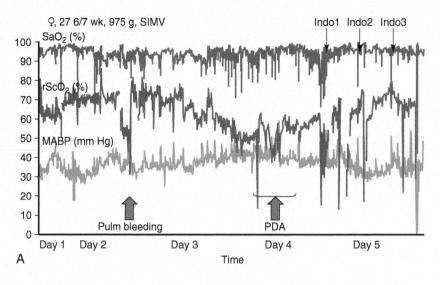

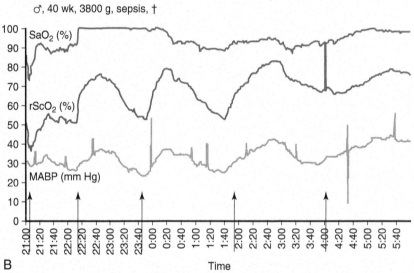

Fig. 18.3 (A) Representative patterns including artifacts of arterial oxygen saturation (SaO$_2$; *red line*), regional cerebral oxygen saturation (rScO$_2$; *black line*), and mean arterial blood pressure (MABP; *light red line*) in a male preterm neonate of 27 and 6/7 weeks' gestation with severe respiratory distress syndrome during the first 5 postnatal days. The infant received exogenous surfactant and was mechanically ventilated. The infant's course was complicated by pulmonary hemorrhage on day 2 *(arrow)*. Although the pulmonary hemorrhage could have been an early indication of pulmonary overcirculation due to a patent ductus arteriosus (PDA), the infant developed a hemodynamically significant PDA only on day 4 *(arrow)*; it was closed by indomethacin *(arrows)*. Note the decrease in rScO$_2$ (starting on day 3) to values below 50% at the time of diagnosis of the hemodynamically significant PDA and the recovery of rScO$_2$ after the ductus closed on day 5. See text for details. (B) Patterns of SaO$_2$ *(red line)*, rScO$_2$ *(black line)*, and MABP *(light red line)* over 8 hours in an infant with severe sepsis and systemic hypotension. The hypotension was treated with volume expansion and vasopressor-inotropes *(arrows)*. Changes in rScO$_2$ mirrored the changes in blood pressure, suggesting a pressure-passive cerebral circulation with lack of autoregulation of cerebral blood flow. *SIMV,* Synchronized mechanical ventilation.

rScO$_2$. Indeed, the findings of Tsuji et al. and Wong et al. suggest that infants lacking cerebral blood flow autoregulation assessed by NIRS compared with gestational age–matched infants with intact cerebral autoregulation have impaired short- and long-term central nervous system outcomes.[61,77] Several approaches are currently being tested for the continuous and real-time assessment of cerebral blood flow autoregulation.[62,80,81] Fig. 18.3B shows an example of the use of NIRS-monitored rScO$_2$ to assess the autoregulatory ability of the cerebral vascular bed. The main concern in using this approach is that the NIRS signal is also influenced by parameters other than blood pressure (see earlier) and that changes in PaCO$_2$ directly affect cerebral

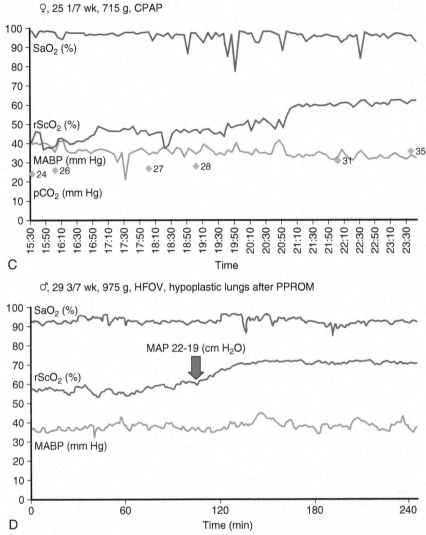

Fig. 18.3, cont'd (C) Patterns of SaO_2 *(red line)*, $rScO_2$ *(black line)*, and MABP *(light red line)* in an extremely preterm infant on continuous positive airway pressure (CPAP) on the first postnatal day. Despite normal blood pressure values and arterial saturations, $rScO_2$ was very low (<50%). Although this infant was breathing spontaneously, she hyperventilated on CPAP to very low $PaCO_2$ values *(grey rhomboids)*. Only when $PaCO_2$ increased to greater than 30 mm Hg did $rScO_2$ normalize, suggesting resolution of the cerebral hypoperfusion caused by hypocapnia-induced cerebral vasoconstriction. See text for details. (D) Patterns of SaO_2 *(red line)*, $rScO_2$ *(black line)*, and MABP *(light red line)* in an infant with hypoplastic lungs following prolonged premature rupture of the membranes. This infant was ventilated with high-frequency oscillatory ventilation (HFOV) with very high mean airway pressures (MAPs; 22 cm H_2O). Note the increase in $rScO_2$ after decreasing MAP from 22 to 19 cm H_2O, indicating that the earlier MAP was likely inappropriately high and affected preload and thus cardiac output negatively.

perfusion. Therefore, in addition to understanding the complexity of assessing the changes in cerebral perfusion by NIRS, appropriate monitoring and correction are necessary.

Of note is that recent findings suggest that the use of NIRS to monitor $rScO_2$ during the first 12 postnatal hours may identify very preterm neonates at higher risk for the development of periventricular or intraventricular hemorrhage during the second and third postnatal days (see Chapter 6).[82]

As alluded to earlier, $PaCO_2$ is another important parameter and the most powerful one that influences brain perfusion. Indeed, changes in $PaCO_2$ cause more robust changes in cerebral blood flow than changes in blood pressure outside the autoregulatory range (see Chapter 2). Hypocapnia directly decreases cerebral blood flow by inducing vasoconstriction, and thus reducing $rScO_2$ and increasing

♀, 27 wk, 1075 g, CPAP

E

1 = ♂ 40 5/7 wk; 4290 g; Apgar 0/1/5
2 = ♂ 40 2/7 wk; 3050 g; Apgar 1/1/2

F

Fig. 18.3, cont'd   (E) Patterns of SaO_2 (red line), $rScO_2$ (black line), and MABP (light red line) in an infant on CPAP with severe apnea treated with stimulation and supplemental oxygen administration. The $rScO_2$ increased to very high values and decreased to baseline only after the infant had been weaned off of supplemental oxygen. See text for details. (F) Patterns of $rScO_2$ (black and red lines) and central temperature (red line) in two term infants with hypoxic ischemic encephalopathy after severe perinatal asphyxia treated with moderate total-body cooling (33.5°C) during the first 72 postnatal hours. The first infant had a normal magnetic resonance imaging (MRI) scan after having been rewarmed on day 5 and subsequently was found to have a favorable neurodevelopmental outcome. The second infant had an adverse outcome with severe abnormalities on MRI on day 5. The first infant showed normal $rScO_2$ values during hypothermia (time points: admission [adm] until rewarming [rew]) and also during and after rewarming (time points t + 2 [2 hours after starting the process of rewarming] until t108 [108 postnatal hours]). The second infant had normal $rScO_2$ values on admission, which increased to high $rScO_2$ values at 24 hours of age (t24) and beyond. Persistently high $rScO_2$ values after 24 hours of age have been shown to be independently associated with adverse neurodevelopmental outcomes in infants with hypoxic ischemic encephalopathy following severe perinatal asphyxia. This is thought to be due to decreased utilization of oxygen and the inappropriately high oxygen delivery secondary to vasodilation/vasoparalysis.

cFTOE, whereas hypercapnia induces vasodilatation, with increased $rScO_2$ and reduced cFTOE values. Accordingly, even small changes in $PaCO_2$ within the normal range may affect the neonatal brain.[83] Therefore monitoring $rScO_2$ and cFTOE together can be used as a noninvasive approach to identify changes in $PaCO_2$ provided that cerebral metabolic rate and the proportion of arterial and venous blood flow in the brain remain constant and Hb concentration and SaO_2 do not change during the period of interrogation.[84] Fig. 18.3C is an example of a preterm infant with low $PaCO_2$ and $rScO_2$ values. Only when $PaCO_2$ increased to greater than 30 mm Hg did $rScO_2$ recover.

Table 18.2   CONDITIONS WITH LOW OR HIGH REGIONAL CEREBRAL OXYGEN SATURATION

Low rScO$_2$	High rScO$_2$
PDA	Oxygen therapy
During PDA ligation	• PPHN
Hypotension	• Pneumothorax
Lack of cerebral autoregulation	• Apnea
Hypoxia	Perinatal asphyxia
Hypocapnia	Hypercapnia
Anemia	SGA
High mean airway pressure	

The most important clinical conditions associated with low rScO$_2$ (<-2 SD) and high rScO$_2$ values (>2 SD) in the preterm infant.
PDA, Patent ductus arteriosus; *PPHN*, persistent pulmonary hypertension of the neonate; *rScO$_2$*, regional cerebral oxygen saturation; *SGA*, small for gestational age.

18

Preterm infants with severe respiratory distress syndrome often require ventilator support, sometimes with high mean, inspiratory, and/or end-expiratory pressures on conventional ventilators or with high-frequency oscillatory ventilation. The associated increase in intrathoracic pressure might decrease preload and thus cardiac output, resulting in a negative impact on cerebral hemodynamics with impaired cerebral oxygenation.[85] Indeed, the monitoring of rScO$_2$ has revealed this association in real time; its use might contribute to early recognition and the introduction of corrective measures to prevent such complications (see Fig. 18.3D).[86]

Another potential cause of decreased brain oxygenation is severe anemia. Anemia may have an even more profound effect on cerebral oxygen delivery in neonates with hypotension receiving mechanical ventilation with high mean airway pressures. Studies have shown an improvement in cerebral oxygenation following red blood cell transfusion, with the strongest effect in infants with the lowest pretransfusion cerebral oxygen saturation.[87] Van Hoften et al. have documented normalization of rScO$_2$ following packed red blood cell transfusions in 33 preterm infants and concluded that cerebral oxygenation in these infants may be at risk at Hb concentrations of less than 6 mmol/L (9.7 g/dL).[88] As discussed earlier, increased cFTOE (>0.4) is indicative of an oxygen supply-and-demand imbalance, which may also improve with red blood cell transfusions.[89] This suggests a potential role for NIRS monitoring to identify infants with high cFTOE (and low rScO$_2$) who might benefit from red blood cell transfusions.[90,91]

Infants with congenital cyanotic heart disease are at particularly high risk of compromised cerebral circulation. Most of these infants have baseline rScO$_2$ values below 55% with SaO$_2$ values in the range of 70% to 85%. Noteworthy is the fact that an rScO$_2$ value of 55% is below the 2 SD of "normal" values defined by our data for preterm neonates. Thus neonates with congenital heart disease, even if it is a noncyanotic but duct-dependent lesion, are at risk for cerebral damage. This is especially the case in combination with the risk factors discussed earlier, including low systemic perfusion, hypotension, and/or abnormal PaCO$_2$ values.

Infants with cardiac and noncardiac anomalies may require surgery shortly after birth. Neonatal surgery is also related to adverse neurodevelopmental outcome, including both the procedure itself and the anesthesia.[92,93] Importantly, peri- and postoperative NIRS monitoring of rScO$_2$ is useful to detect deteriorations; it has the potential to improve the stability of cerebral oxygenation and is predictive of cerebral injury.[94,95] Indeed, by using cerebral NIRS monitoring, we can detect episodes of hypoxia in an even more reliable fashion than with SaO$_2$ monitoring by pulse oximetry during the surgical procedure.[96,97]

Table 18.2 summarizes the clinical conditions associated with low rScO$_2$ values.

Clinical Conditions Associated With High Regional Cerebral Oxygen Saturation Values

NIRS-monitored rScO$_2$ may also be helpful in detecting hyperoxemia. Hyperoxemia has been increasingly linked with adverse long-term outcomes, especially in the extremely preterm neonate.[10,13,14]

Oxygen supplementation is the major cause of periods of hyperoxemia. Spontaneously breathing preterm infants are often treated with additional oxygen supplementation to accelerate normalization of partial arterial oxygen pressure and SaO_2. Brief but repetitive episodes of hyperoxemia occur relatively frequently during recovery from apnea and bradycardia episodes in these infants as well as when additional oxygen is provided before routine care or endotracheal intubation (see Fig. 18.3E). In addition, hyperoxemia often occurs in preterm or term neonates receiving prolonged oxygen therapy for severe respiratory distress syndrome, persistent pulmonary hypertension of the newborn, pneumothorax, or severe bronchopulmonary dysplasia. Hyperoxia still occurs frequently despite the increased awareness that oxygen therapy for some of these conditions is obsolete and harmful and that uncontrolled oxygen administration in itself is harmful under any circumstances unless the SaO_2 is successfully maintained in a gestational and postnatal age-appropriate range. Furthermore, even if oxygen saturation is carefully monitored, oxygen supplementation during episodes of apnea of prematurity can still result in hyperoxemia. One of the reasons for our inability to curtail the occurrence of hyperoxemia is because pulse oximetry–measured SaO_2 is not sensitive enough when SaO_2 is above 95%. In such cases, concomitant monitoring of cerebral oxygenation may, at least in part, be helpful to minimize the occurrence of potentially harmful hyperoxic episodes.

Episodes of hypercapnia cause an increase in brain perfusion and thus can contribute to cerebral hyperoxemia, especially in infants ventilated with additional oxygen supplementation. Again, NIRS-monitored $rScO_2$ may be used as an adjunct monitoring technique to aid in appropriately adjusting the oxygen therapy or to initiate CO_2 evaluation.

Preterm infants who are born small for gestational age (SGA) show higher cerebral oxygenation after birth compared with their appropriately grown peers.[98] Intrauterine growth restriction prompts the redistribution of the fetus's blood to the vital organs, including the brain, resulting in a higher cerebral oxygen saturation that persists after birth. Clinicians should be aware of this in interpreting the NIRS-monitored cerebral oxygenation in SGA infants.[99]

In addition to its use as a diagnostic tool to assess cerebral oxygen delivery and extraction, NIRS-monitored $rScO_2$ has been shown to be useful in predicting the long-term prognosis of infants with hypoxic-ischemic encephalopathy following perinatal asphyxia. Our group has reported that abnormally high values of $rScO_2$ (>85% to 90%) in these infants during the first 24 postnatal hours are strongly and independently associated with an adverse neurodevelopmental outcome at 2 years of age.[95] The high $rScO_2$ values are thought to be caused by low oxygen extraction due to a decrease in the metabolic activity of the injured brain, the inappropriately high cerebral oxygen delivery due to cerebral vasodilatation, and vasoparalysis along with the potential loss of cerebral autoregulation. Even when neonates with hypoxic-ischemic encephalopathy are treated with therapeutic hypothermia to prevent secondary injury associated with the ischemia-reperfusion cycle, the pattern of $rScO_2$ changes keeps its prognostic value in relation to long-term neurodevelopmental outcome (see Fig. 18.3F).[100]

Conditions related to high $rScO_2$ values are also summarized in Table 18.2.

Conclusion

Recent data indicate that NIRS-monitored cerebral oxygen saturation and extraction as measured by $rScO_2$ (or TOI) and cFTOE are of great value and have been increasingly incorporated into the standard clinical monitoring regimen in neonatal intensive care. Its noninvasive and bedside nature and the possibility of monitoring the brain continuously and directly are among its attractive features. However, the inter- and intrapatient variability of the measurements and the fact that NIRS is a trend monitor rather than a technique capable of directly monitoring cerebral perfusion in absolute values remain obstacles to overcome. Substantial changes in the NIRS-monitored $rScO_2$ (i.e., in cerebral oxygenation) can alert the caregiver to the fact that potentially harmful changes in brain oxygenation are occurring, thus providing opportunities for intervention. NIRS monitoring has shown its usefulness in several clinical conditions, and reliable reference values are now available that increase its clinical applicability. Finally, the information provided by the use of this technology has improved our understanding of the limitations of our knowledge and led to the initiation of appropriately designed observational and interventional trials so that the interventions used in clinical practice can be critically tested.

REFERENCES

1. Younge N, Goldstein RF, Bann CM, et al.: Survival and neurodevelopmental outcomes among periviable infants, *N Engl J Med* 376(7):617–628, 2017.
2. Anderson PJ, Doyle LW: Cognitive and educational deficits in children born extremely preterm, *Semin Perinatol* 32(1):51–58, 2008.
3. Wood NS, Costeloe K, Gibson AT, et al.: The EPICure study: associations and antecedents of neurological and developmental disability at 30 months of age following extremely preterm birth, *Arch Dis Child Fetal Neonatal Ed* 90(2):F134–F140, 2005.
4. Wilson-Costello D, Friedman H, Minich N, et al.: Improved neurodevelopmental outcomes for extremely low birth weight infants in 2000-2002, *Pediatrics* 119(1):37–45, 2007.
5. Wilson-Costello D, Friedman H, Minich N, et al.: Improved survival rates with increased neurodevelopmental disability for extremely low birth weight infants in the 1990s, *Pediatrics* 115(4):997–1003, 2005.
6. Samara M, Marlow N, Wolke D, et al.: Pervasive behavior problems at 6 years of age in a total-population sample of children born at </= 25 weeks of gestation, *Pediatrics* 122(3):562–573, 2008.
7. Wolke D, Samara M, Bracewell M, et al.: Specific language difficulties and school achievement in children born at 25 weeks of gestation or less, *J Pediatr* 152(2):256–262, 2008.
8. Logitharajah P, Rutherford MA, Cowan FM: Hypoxic-ischemic encephalopathy in preterm infants: antecedent factors, brain imaging, and outcome, *Pediatr Res* 66(2):222–229, 2009.
9. Dammann O, Allred EN, Kuban KC, et al.: Systemic hypotension and white-matter damage in preterm infants, *Dev Med Child Neurol* 44(2):82–90, 2002.
10. Deulofeut R, Critz A, Adams-Chapman I, et al.: Avoiding hyperoxia in infants < or = 1250 g is associated with improved short- and long-term outcomes, *J Perinatol* 26(11):700–705, 2006.
11. Perlman JM, McMenamin JB, Volpe JJ: Fluctuating cerebral blood-flow velocity in respiratory-distress syndrome. Relation to the development of intraventricular hemorrhage, *N Engl J Med* 309(4):204–209, 1983.
12. Van Bel F, Van de Bor M, Stijnen T, et al.: Aetiological role of cerebral blood-flow alterations in development and extension of peri-intraventricular haemorrhage, *Dev Med Child Neurol* 29(5):601–614, 1987.
13. Klinger G, Beyene J, Shah P, et al.: Do hyperoxaemia and hypocapnia add to the risk of brain injury after intrapartum asphyxia? *Arch Dis Child Fetal Neonatal Ed* 90(1):F49–F52, 2005.
14. Gerstner B, DeSilva TM, Genz K, et al.: Hyperoxia causes maturation-dependent cell death in the developing white matter, *J Neurosci* 28(5):1236–1245, 2008.
15. Shah NA, Van Meurs KP, Davis AS: Amplitude-integrated electroencephalography: a survey of practices in the United States, *Am J Perinatol* 32(8):755–760, 2015.
16. Appendino JP, McNamara PJ, Keyzers M, et al.: The impact of amplitude-integrated electroencephalography on NICU practice, *Can J Neurol Sci* 39(3):355–360, 2012.
17. van Bel F, Lemmers P, Naulaers G: Monitoring neonatal regional cerebral oxygen saturation in clinical practice: value and pitfalls, *Neonatology* 94(4):237–244, 2008.
18. Dix LM, van Bel F, Lemmers PM: Monitoring cerebral oxygenation in neonates: an update, *Front Pediatr* 5:46, 2017.
19. Greisen G: Is near-infrared spectroscopy living up to its promises? *Semin Fetal Neonatal Med* 11(6):498–502, 2006.
20. Kissack CM, Garr R, Wardle SP, et al.: Cerebral fractional oxygen extraction in very low birth weight infants is high when there is low left ventricular output and hypocarbia but is unaffected by hypotension, *Pediatr Res* 55(3):400–405, 2004.
21. Naulaers G, Morren G, Van Huffel S, et al.: Cerebral tissue oxygenation index in very premature infants, *Arch Dis Child Fetal Neonatal Ed* 87(3):F189–F192, 2002.
22. Jobsis FF: Noninvasive, infrared monitoring of cerebral and myocardial oxygen sufficiency and circulatory parameters, *Science* 198(4323):1264–1267, 1977.
23. Matcher SJ, Cooper CE: Absolute quantification of deoxyhaemoglobin concentration in tissue near infrared spectroscopy, *Phys Med Biol* 39(8):1295–1312, 1994.
24. Suzuki STS, Ozaki T, Kobayashi Y: A tissue oxygenation monitor using NIR spatially resolved spectrsoscopy, *PROc SPIE* 3597:582–592, 1999.
25. Watzman HM, Kurth CD, Montenegro LM, et al.: Arterial and venous contributions to near-infrared cerebral oximetry, *Anesthesiology* 93(4):947–953, 2000.
26. Nagdyman N, Fleck T, Schubert S, et al.: Comparison between cerebral tissue oxygenation index measured by near-infrared spectroscopy and venous jugular bulb saturation in children, *Intensive Care Med* 31(6):846–850, 2005.
27. Yoxall CW, Weindling AM, Dawani NH, et al.: Measurement of cerebral venous oxyhemoglobin saturation in children by near-infrared spectroscopy and partial jugular venous occlusion, *Pediatr Res* 38(3):319–323, 1995.

18

28. Thavasothy M, Broadhead M, Elwell C, et al.: A comparison of cerebral oxygenation as measured by the NIRO 300 and the INVOS 5100 near-infrared spectrophotometers, *Anaesthesia* 57(10): 999–1006, 2002.

29. Yoshitani K, Kawaguchi M, Tatsumi K, et al.: A comparison of the INVOS 4100 and the NIRO 300 near-infrared spectrophotometers, *Anesth Analg* 94(3):586–590, 2002.

30. Lemmers PM, van Bel F: Left-to-right differences of regional cerebral oxygen saturation and oxygen extraction in preterm infants during the first days of life, *Pediatr Res* 65(2):226–230, 2009.

31. Murkin JM: NIRS: a standard of care for CPB vs. an evolving standard for selective cerebral perfusion? *J Extra Corpor Technol* 41(1):P11–P14, 2009.

32. Hoffman GM: Neurologic monitoring on cardiopulmonary bypass: what are we obligated to do? *Ann Thorac Surg* 81(6):S2373–S2380, 2006.

33. Williams GD, Ramamoorthy C: Brain monitoring and protection during pediatric cardiac surgery, *Semin Cardiothorac Vasc Anesth* 11(1):23–33, 2007.

34. Yoxall CW, Weindling AM: The measurement of peripheral venous oxyhemoglobin saturation in newborn infants by near infrared spectroscopy with venous occlusion, *Pediatr Res* 39(6): 1103–1106, 1996.

35. Naulaers G, Meyns B, Miserez M, et al.: Use of tissue oxygenation index and fractional tissue oxygen extraction as non-invasive parameters for cerebral oxygenation. A validation study in piglets, *Neonatology* 92(2):120–126, 2007.

36. Wardle SP, Yoxall CW, Weindling AM: Cerebral oxygenation during cardiopulmonary bypass, *Arch Dis Child* 78(1):26–32, 1998.

37. Wardle SP, Yoxall CW, Weindling AM: Determinants of cerebral fractional oxygen extraction using near infrared spectroscopy in preterm neonates, *J Cereb Blood Flow Metab* 20(2):272–279, 2000.

38. Dullenkopf A, Kolarova A, Schulz G, et al.: Reproducibility of cerebral oxygenation measurement in neonates and infants in the clinical setting using the NIRO 300 oximeter, *Pediatr Crit Care Med* 6(3):344–347, 2005.

39. Menke J, Voss U, Moller G, et al.: Reproducibility of cerebral near infrared spectroscopy in neonates, *Biol Neonate* 83(1):6–11, 2003.

40. Misra M, Stark J, Dujovny M, et al.: Transcranial cerebral oximetry in random normal subjects, *Neurol Res* 20(2):137–141, 1998.

41. Weiss M, Dullenkopf A, Kolarova A, et al.: Near-infrared spectroscopic cerebral oxygenation reading in neonates and infants is associated with central venous oxygen saturation, *Paediatr Anaesth* 15(2):102–109, 2005.

42. Sorensen LC, Greisen G: Precision of measurement of cerebral tissue oxygenation index using near-infrared spectroscopy in preterm neonates, *J Biomed Opt* (5)11:054005, 2006.

43. Petrova A, Mehta R: Near-infrared spectroscopy in the detection of regional tissue oxygenation during hypoxic events in preterm infants undergoing critical care, *Pediatr Crit Care Med* 7(5):449–454, 2006.

44. Lemmers PM, Toet M, van Schelven LJ, et al.: Cerebral oxygenation and cerebral oxygen extraction in the preterm infant: the impact of respiratory distress syndrome, *Exp Brain Res* 173(3):458–467, 2006.

45. Olopade CO, Mensah E, Gupta R, et al.: Noninvasive determination of brain tissue oxygenation during sleep in obstructive sleep apnea: a near-infrared spectroscopic approach, *Sleep* 30(12):1747–1755, 2007.

46. Fauchere JC, Schulz G, Haensse D, et al.: Near-infrared spectroscopy measurements of cerebral oxygenation in newborns during immediate postnatal adaptation, *J Pediatr* 156(3):372–376, 2010.

47. Macleod DIK, Vacchiano C: Simultaneous comparison of Fore-sight and INVOS cerebral oximeters to jugular bulb and arterial co-oximetry measurements in healthy volunteerd, *SCA Suppl* 108:101–104, 2009.

48. Alderliesten T, Dix L, Baerts W, et al.: Reference values of regional cerebral oxygen saturation during the first 3 days of life in preterm neonates, *Pediatr Res* 79(1-1):55–64, 2016.

49. Dix LM, van Bel F, Baerts W, et al.: Comparing near-infrared spectroscopy devices and their sensors for monitoring regional cerebral oxygen saturation in the neonate, *Pediatr Res* 74(5):557–563, 2013.

50. Hou X, Ding H, Teng Y, et al.: Research on the relationship between brain anoxia at different regional oxygen saturations and brain damage using near-infrared spectroscopy, *Physiol Meas* 28(10):1251–1265, 2007.

51. Kurth CD, McCann JC, Wu J, et al.: Cerebral oxygen saturation-time threshold for hypoxic-ischemic injury in piglets, *Anesth Analg* 108(4):1268–1277, 2009.

52. Dent CL, Spaeth JP, Jones BV, et al.: Brain magnetic resonance imaging abnormalities after the Norwood procedure using regional cerebral perfusion, *J Thorac Cardiovasc Surg* 131(1):190–197, 2006.

53. Sakamoto T, Hatsuoka S, Stock UA, et al.: Prediction of safe duration of hypothermic circulatory arrest by near-infrared spectroscopy, *J Thorac Cardiovasc Surg* 122(2):339–350, 2001.

54. Hoffman GMGN, Stuth EA, Berens RJ, et al.: NIRS-derived somatic and cerebral saturation difference provides non-invasive real time hemodynamic assessment of cardiogenic shoch and anaerobic metabolism, *Anesthesiology* 101:A1448, 2004.

55. Hyttel-Sorensen S, Austin T, van Bel F, et al.: Clinical use of cerebral oximetry in extremely preterm infants is feasible, *Dan Med J* 60(1):A4533, 2013.

56. Hyttel-Sorensen S, Pellicer A, Alderliesten T, et al.: Cerebral near infrared spectroscopy oximetry in extremely preterm infants: phase II randomised clinical trial, *BMJ* 350:g7635, 2015.

57. Tin W: Optimal oxygen saturation for preterm babies. Do we really know? *Biol Neonate* 85(4):319–325, 2004.

58. Chow LC, Wright KW, Sola A, Group COAS: Can changes in clinical practice decrease the incidence of severe retinopathy of prematurity in very low birth weight infants? *Pediatrics* 111(2):339–345, 2003.

59. De Smet D, Vanderhaegen J, Naulaers G, et al.: New measurements for assessment of impaired cerebral autoregulation using near-infrared spectroscopy, *Adv Exp Med Biol* 645:273–278, 2009.

60. Brady KM, Lee JK, Kibler KK, et al.: Continuous time-domain analysis of cerebrovascular autoregulation using near-infrared spectroscopy, *Stroke* 38(10):2818–2825, 2007.

61. Wong FY, Leung TS, Austin T, et al.: Impaired autoregulation in preterm infants identified by using spatially resolved spectroscopy, *Pediatrics* 121(3):e604–e611, 2008.

62. Brady KM, Mytar JO, Lee JK, et al.: Monitoring cerebral blood flow pressure autoregulation in pediatric patients during cardiac surgery, *Stroke* 41(9):1957–1962, 2010.

63. Toet MC, Lemmers PM, van Schelven LJ, et al.: Cerebral oxygenation and electrical activity after birth asphyxia: their relation to outcome, *Pediatrics* 117(2):333–339, 2006.

64. Smits A, Thewissen L, Caicedo A, et al.: Propofol dose-finding to reach optimal effect for (semi-) elective intubation in neonates, *J Pediatr* 179:54.e9–60.e9, 2016.

65. Kozberg MG, Ma Y, Shaik MA, et al.: Rapid postnatal expansion of neural networks occurs in an environment of altered neurovascular and neurometabolic coupling, *J Neurosci* 36(25):6704–6717, 2016.

66. Perlman JM, Hill A, Volpe JJ: The effect of patent ductus arteriosus on flow velocity in the anterior cerebral arteries: ductal steal in the premature newborn infant, *J Pediatr* 99(5):767–771, 1981.

67. Lemmers PM, Toet MC, van Bel F: Impact of patent ductus arteriosus and subsequent therapy with indomethacin on cerebral oxygenation in preterm infants, *Pediatrics* 121(1):142–147, 2008.

68. Underwood MA, Milstein JM, Sherman MP: Near-infrared spectroscopy as a screening tool for patent ductus arteriosus in extremely low birth weight infants, *Neonatology* 91(2):134–139, 2007.

69. Dix L, Molenschot M, Breur J, et al.: Cerebral oxygenation and echocardiographic parameters in preterm neonates with a patent ductus arteriosus: an observational study, *Arch Dis Child Fetal Neonatal Ed*, 2016.

70. Lemmers PM, Molenschot MC, Evens J, et al.: Is cerebral oxygen supply compromised in preterm infants undergoing surgical closure for patent ductus arteriosus? *Arch Dis Child Fetal Neonatal Ed* 95(6):F429–F434, 2010.

71. Weisz DE, More K, McNamara PJ, et al.: PDA ligation and health outcomes: a meta-analysis, *Pediatrics* 133(4):e1024–e1046, 2014.

72. Lemmers PM, Benders MJ, D'Ascenzo R, et al.: Patent ductus arteriosus and brain volume, *Pediatrics* (4)137, 2016.

73. Roze JC, Cambonie G, Marchand-Martin L, et al.: Association between early screening for patent ductus arteriosus and in-hospital mortality among extremely preterm infants, *JAMA* 313(24):2441–2448, 2015.

74. Dempsey EM, Barrington KJ: Evaluation and treatment of hypotension in the preterm infant, *Clin Perinatol* 36(1):75–85, 2009.

75. Noori S, Seri I: Evidence-based versus pathophysiology-based approach to diagnosis and treatment of neonatal cardiovascular compromise, *Semin Fetal Neonatal Med* 20(4):238–245, 2015.

76. Alderliesten T, Lemmers PM, van Haastert IC, et al.: Hypotension in preterm neonates: low blood pressure alone does not affect neurodevelopmental outcome, *J Pediatr* 164(5):986–991, 2014.

77. Tsuji M, Saul JP, du Plessis A, et al.: Cerebral intravascular oxygenation correlates with mean arterial pressure in critically ill premature infants, *Pediatrics* 106(4):625–632, 2000.

78. Wong FY, Silas R, Hew S, et al.: Cerebral oxygenation is highly sensitive to blood pressure variability in sick preterm infants, *PLoS One* 7(8):e43165, 2012.

79. Soul JS, Hammer PE, Tsuji M, et al.: Fluctuating pressure-passivity is common in the cerebral circulation of sick premature infants, *Pediatr Res* 61(4):467–473, 2007.

80. Caicedo A, De Smet D, Naulaers G, et al.: Cerebral tissue oxygenation and regional oxygen saturation can be used to study cerebral autoregulation in prematurely born infants, *Pediatr Res* 69(6):548–553, 2011.

81. Caicedo A, Alderliesten T, Naulaers G, et al.: A new framework for the assessment of cerebral hemodynamics regulation in neonates using NIRS, *Adv Exp Med Biol* 876:501–509, 2016.

82. Noori S, McCoy M, Anderson MP, et al.: Changes in cardiac function and cerebral blood flow in relation to peri/intraventricular hemorrhage in extremely preterm infants, *J Pediatr* 164:264–270, 2014.

83. Dix LWL, de Vries L, Groenendaal F, et al.: Carbon dioxide fluctuations are associated with changes in cerebral oxygenation and electrical activity in preterm infants, *J Pediatr* S0022-3476(17):30590–30595, 2017.

84. Vanderhaegen J, Naulaers G, Vanhole C, et al.: The effect of changes in tPCO2 on the fractional tissue oxygen extraction—as measured by near-infrared spectroscopy—in neonates during the first days of life, *Eur J Paediatr Neurol* 13(2):128–134, 2009.

85. Milan A, Freato F, Vanzo V, et al.: Influence of ventilation mode on neonatal cerebral blood flow and volume, *Early Hum Dev* 85(7):415–419, 2009.

86. Hellstrom-Westas L, Rosen I, Svenningsen NW: Cerebral function monitoring during the first week of life in extremely small low birthweight (ESLBW) infants, *Neuropediatrics* 22(1):27–32, 1991.

87. Seidel D, Blaser A, Gebauer C, et al.: Changes in regional tissue oxygenation saturation and desaturations after red blood cell transfusion in preterm infants, *J Perinatol* 33(4):282–287, 2013.

18

88. van Hoften JC, Verhagen EA, Keating P, et al.: Cerebral tissue oxygen saturation and extraction in preterm infants before and after blood transfusion, *Arch Dis Child Fetal Neonatal Ed* 95(5): F352–F358, 2010.

89. Andersen CC, Karayil SM, Hodyl NA, et al.: Early red cell transfusion favourably alters cerebral oxygen extraction in very preterm newborns, *Arch Dis Child Fetal Neonatal Ed* 100(5):F433–F435, 2015.

90. Banerjee J, Aladangady N: Biomarkers to decide red blood cell transfusion in newborn infants, *Transfusion* 54(10):2574–2582, 2014.

91. Mintzer JP, Parvez B, Chelala M, et al.: Monitoring regional tissue oxygen extraction in neonates <1250 g helps identify transfusion thresholds independent of hematocrit, *J Neonatal Perinatal Med* 7(2):89–100, 2014.

92. Morriss Jr FH, Saha S, Bell EF, et al.: Surgery and neurodevelopmental outcome of very low-birth-weight infants, *JAMA Pediatr* 168(8):746–754, 2014.

93. Stolwijk LJ, Lemmers PM, Harmsen M, et al.: Neurodevelopmental outcomes after neonatal surgery for major noncardiac anomalies, *Pediatrics* 137(2):e20151728, 2016.

94. Durandy Y, Rubatti M, Couturier R: Near infrared spectroscopy during pediatric cardiac surgery: errors and pitfalls, *Perfusion* 26(5):441–446, 2011.

95. Toet MC, Flinterman A, Laar I, et al.: Cerebral oxygen saturation and electrical brain activity before, during, and up to 36 hours after arterial switch procedure in neonates without pre-existing brain damage: its relationship to neurodevelopmental outcome, *Exp Brain Res* 165(3):343–350, 2005.

96. Cruz SM, Akinkuotu AC, Rusin CG, et al.: A novel multimodal computational system using near-infrared spectroscopy to monitor cerebral oxygenation during assisted ventilation in CDH patients, *J Pediatr Surg* 51(1):38–43, 2016.

97. Koch HW, Hansen TG: Perioperative use of cerebral and renal near-infrared spectroscopy in neonates: a 24-h observational study, *Paediatr Anaesth* 26(2):190–198, 2016.

98. Cohen E, Baerts W, Alderliesten T, et al.: Growth restriction and gender influence cerebral oxygenation in preterm neonates, *Arch Dis Child Fetal Neonatal Ed* 101(2):F156–F161, 2016.

99. Cohen E, Baerts W, van Bel F: Brain-sparing in intrauterine growth restriction: considerations for the neonatologist, *Neonatology* 108(4):269–276, 2015.

100. Lemmers PM, Zwanenburg RJ, Benders MJ, et al.: Cerebral oxygenation and brain activity after perinatal asphyxia: does hypothermia change their prognostic value? *Pediatr Res* 74(2):180–185, 2013.

CHAPTER 19

Assessment of the Microcirculation in the Neonate

Ian M.R. Wright, M.J. Stark, and R.M. Dyson

Key Points

- The microvasculature is the largest single component of the cardiovascular system.
- There are tools to assess microvascular function that can be used in the smallest infants.
- Differences in microvascular function are seen in relation to gestational age, postnatal age, and sex of the infant.
- Changes in microvascular flow relate to neonatal illness severity and clinical risk factors.
- Underlying differences in the physiologic mediators of microvascular dilation have been demonstrated in the most-at-risk infants.
- Microvascular changes may represent the first cardiovascular changes of long-term health programming.

Why Assess the Microcirculation?

The cardiorespiratory system is crucial in the perinatal adaptation of the human neonate to extrauterine life. Most infants who die do so in the first few days after delivery and exhibit evidence of cardiovascular compromise. The cardiovascular system, as detailed in other chapters of this book, has a number of crucial components that affect the overall performance of the system, including the pump, circulating volume, and peripheral vasculature (see Chapters 1, 2, 3, and 21). It is being increasingly recognized that a key component of the peripheral vasculature, the microvasculature, exerts a significant influence on the overall function of the peripheral vasculature. Specifically, the microvasculature, as opposed to the macrovascular conductance vessels, is crucially important in the delivery of oxygen and nutrients to the tissues of the entire body. In addition, the flow within the microvasculature reflects the combined action of the central, macrohemodynamic components of the circulation and thus the end point of total cardiovascular efficiency. Despite this, the dynamic physiologic changes that occur in the microvasculature of the preterm neonate in the immediate transitional period are not completely characterized.

So what comprises the microvascular system? Current accepted definitions of microvascular components include, from proximal to distal, arterioles, capillaries, arteriolar-venular shunts, and venules.[1] In practice, these components represent all vascular tissue less than 100 μm in diameter. Lymphatic function, which is not discussed here, can also significantly influence overall microvascular function, but studies in the neonatal population remain limited.[2] The microvasculature has regional and organ-specific specialization but also has global function and responses. It therefore represents one of the largest virtual "organs" in the body. As nearly all tissue needs to be in close approximation to a blood supply for oxygen and nutrient delivery and removal of waste products, the microvasculature is all-pervasive.[3] It has been estimated that the capillary component of the microvasculature alone covers greater than a 6000 m² cross-sectional area in the adult. Further more, at least 5% of circulating blood volume is in the capillaries at any time, with the capillary system having the ability to increase this capacity by more than fourfold. Similar estimations have not been undertaken in the newborn. However, since the newborn is rapidly growing and has a less organized capillary network,[4] its capillary system may possess even greater proportional capacity.

Those involved with newborn care are mostly aware of microvascular growth in the context of the retina, with retinopathy of prematurity (ROP) remaining a significant cause of blindness in the preterm population. ROP studies have also allowed us to understand more about growth and development of the microvasculature during extrauterine adaptation. This includes the role of oxygenation levels in vascular growth, the importance of angiogenic and vascular "pruning" factors in the growing tree (e.g., vascular endothelial growth factor and the prorenin/angiotensin system).[5–7] The same process of angiogenesis, vasculogenesis, and remodeling are similarly going on throughout the developing preterm infant. Thus understanding the biology and physiology in the microvasculature contributes to understanding cardiovascular compromise at different gestational and postnatal ages and the role the microvasculature plays in certain long-term consequences of prematurity.

The drive to study and understand microcirculatory status has led to the development and use of a number of methods for the assessment of the microcirculation in preterm or sick term newborns. This chapter reviews the sites and techniques that have been used, outlines current understanding, and addresses the relationship of these microvascular findings to the macrocirculation in the preterm and sick term neonate.

Where to Study the Microcirculation in the Human Newborn?

As the microcirculation is ubiquitous throughout the body, the possibilities for observation and measurement are widespread. In animal models a number of techniques have been used to assess microcirculation in a selection of vascular beds, including laser Doppler flowmetry (LDF) in the skin, muscle, brain, liver, gastrointestinal tract, and kidneys; videomicroscopy in the brain, skin, and gut; as well as Xenon clearance blood flow measurement techniques.[8–18] Techniques employing the use of microspheres or perfusate casts, limited to animal work, are reviewed elsewhere.[19] The noninvasive requirements for human investigation in the preterm neonate have led to peripheral sites being targeted. Methods employed include heat conductance, skin temperature changes, laser Doppler, videomicroscopy (sublingual, retinal, and scleral), Xenon clearance, saturation oximetry, transcutaneous carbon dioxide measurement, thermography, near infrared spectroscopy (skin, muscle, and cerebral), and direct videomicroscopic observation of red cell flux in the nail fold capillaries.[20–37] These techniques have all demonstrated changes during the transitional period in the few days after birth.

The skin is the most easily accessible site in neonates and has received the most attention. As the skin has some very specialized microvascular functions, such as thermoregulation, it has been questioned as to how representative it is of the microcirculation in general. However, despite skin blood flow demonstrating a variety of adaptive responses, it is part of the wider microcirculation.[38] Many of the signals that govern microvascular response are systemic and affect all vascular beds to some degree. This may be particularly the case in the first few days of postnatal life in the preterm infant, where locally adaptive responses in the dermal circulation are impaired.[39] Moreover, even in adults, significant and generalizable systemic microvascular changes have been documented in highly specialized peripheral sites (e.g., the nail folds).[40]

Many of the techniques used previously are now considered too invasive or difficult in the nonsedated neonate,[41] with other indirect measures of questionable reliability.[42] With emerging techniques such as NIRS discussed elsewhere (see Chapters 16, 17, and 18), LDF and videomicroscopy will be the main techniques discussed in this chapter. While the focus is principally on skin microvascular flow, studies of the retinal circulation are also included in the context of vascular programming.

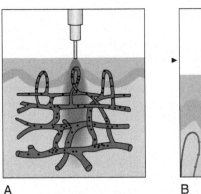 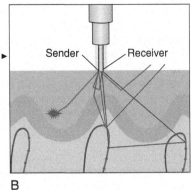

Fig. 19.1   Principle of laser Doppler flowmetry method. (A) Laser extends to subcapillary plexus. (B) Principle of back scatter and Doppler shift. (Perimed AB: Laser Doppler monitoring 2017. http://www.perimed-instruments.com/laser-doppler-monitoring.)

Laser Doppler Imaging

There are currently two systems using laser Doppler or related techniques. Although this chapter focuses on LDF, laser Doppler imaging (LDI) can also be used and may prove of increasing value in the neonatal field.[43] LDI uses a scanning laser beam over the area of interest and maps the cutaneous blood flow of a larger area than LDF. This leads to increased reproducibility for LDI compared with LDF.[44] LDI is also noncontact in nature and thus could be used in clinical situations where skin contact is not possible or desirable.[45] LDI is, however, more superficial and has limited ability to study the dynamics of dilator or constrictor responses. Despite the introduction of laser speckle contrast instruments, which can assess skin microvascular reactivity with excellent reproducibility,[46] the ability of LDF to provide a constant measure of perfusion and perform dynamic measures at relatively low cost means LDF remains the most widely used technique.

Laser Doppler Flowmetry

Microvascular laser Doppler has been used extensively in the newborn infant.[9,47–56] LDF uses the Doppler shift of a low-energy laser beam with a wavelength of 780 nm to quantify microvascular perfusion. The light is delivered to the tissue by a fiberoptic cable, where it is scattered by both stationary structures and moving blood cells. When scattered by moving cells, the light frequency is Doppler shifted in proportion to cell flux (defined as the product of mean velocity and cell number) in the few cubic millimeters of measured volume. The output is detected by fiberoptic receiving fibers of the same probe (Fig. 19.1), processed, and stored using proprietary software, which varies among the device brands. Although directly proportional to tissue perfusion, laser Doppler measurements provide a semiquantitative measure of blood flow, expressed as arbitrary perfusion units (PU) dependent on the output voltage (1 PU = 10 mV), but standardized by international agreement among manufacturers.[44,57–59] When the recording site is standardized, the reproducibility of LDF is high, with poorer reproducibility seen when the recording site is varied.[60–62]

In adults, arteries penetrating the subcutaneous tissue branch into several precapillary arterioles (30 to 80 μm). These pass into venous plexuses organized parallel to the skin surface, after forming 8 to 10 capillary loops orientated perpendicular to the skin surface.[63] In term neonates this network is much less organized, and the arteriolar-venular anastomoses and the capillary loops are poorly developed, not forming a more adult-type network until approximately 4 months of age.[64] The preterm skin microcirculation is even less developed. LDF measures flow to the depth of the subpapillary plexus in children and adults, but in the newborn it measures well into the subcutaneous microcirculation and therefore should be less affected by thermoregulatory shunts and other adaptive capillary loop mechanisms. In healthy term neonates, baseline skin blood flow has been shown to decrease during the first few postnatal days.[65–68]

Active stimulations of the microvasculature during LDF assessment may provide more detailed information of microvascular function by allowing for the interrogation of both endothelial and other pathways. These stimuli include postocclusive hyperemia, thermal hyperemia, and the microvascular response to iontophoresis of vasoactive medication.

Postocclusive Reactive Hyperemia

Postocclusive reactive hyperemia (PORH) has been used in conditions such as diabetes and variations have been linked to cardiovascular risk factors.[69–71] In neonates the test is performed by placing a sphygmomanometer cuff proximal to a limb-sited LDF probe. The cuff is then inflated to suprasystolic levels, holding for a designated length of time and then releasing the pressure as quickly as possible.[59] PORH is characterized by a transient increase in skin blood flow above baseline levels that is mediated by endothelium-dependent pathways. There has been some debate about the length of the occlusion time required, balancing the need to obtain the best response with patient comfort and safety. While 3 minutes of occlusion time has been proposed for adults, in the newborn a 1-minute occlusion period produces an adequate response.[72]

PORH may be expressed as an absolute value, an increase above baseline, a percentage increase above baseline, or a percentage relative to baseline, with the maximum increase in hyperemia-perfusion ($PORH_{max}$) being the most commonly reported variable. In addition, the time to reach peak hyperemia-perfusion (T_p) has been said to relate to the stiffness of the microvascular system.[59] This variable is not currently widely used in the acute assessment of the neonate but may be relevant to the assessment of long-term programming effects in the follow-up of premature infants.[73]

Local Thermal Hyperemia

Local thermal hyperemia is elicited by warming of the skin, causing direct vasodilatation of a given area. Heating can be applied to the whole environment, but in neonates is usually applied to the area of the LDF probe.[59] Several different thermostatically regulated probes are available which ensure a constant temperature at the site of the probe to both reduce study variability and enable elicitation of thermal stimuli responses.[59,62] In adults, applying a temperature change over a 20-minute period is the most common practice, but this is less suitable in the unstable preterm neonate, and thus shorter protocols have evolved. The most frequently employed protocol resembles those of Roustit and colleagues, with an initial rapid temperature increase to 40°C and then a sequential further increase to 44°C over a period of 5 minutes.[62] Maximum vasodilatation is measured at the end of the first minute at 44°C.

Two different mechanisms have been implicated in the response to thermal stimulation within the skin microvasculature. The initial response is mediated through nociceptive nerve pathways and via neurogenic reflexes and locally released vasoactive substances, including calcitonin gene-related peptide and nitric oxide.[74] The subsequent increase in microvascular blood flow over a longer period of time and/or at higher temperatures is thought to be mediated through the more classic endothelium-dependent nitric oxide pathways.[75]

Iontophoresis

Iontophoresis enables the transfer of soluble ions, including vasoactive molecules and hormonal moderators of vascular control, into body tissues using a small direct electrical current, clinically best known for using pilocarpine for cystic fibrosis sweat testing. A variety of vasoactive molecules and hormonal moderators of vascular control may be driven into the skin.[76,77] Acetylcholine (ACh), the classical paradigm-test for endothelium-dependent vasodilation, is the standard transdermal drug used in microvascular assessment, with relaxation occurring via nonnitric oxide, nonprostanoid endothelium-dependent hyperpolarization.[78,79] Iontophoresis in conjunction with LDF allows real-time interrogation of physiologic responses (Fig. 19.2). It can also been used with LDI systems, where a whole skin patch can be tested.

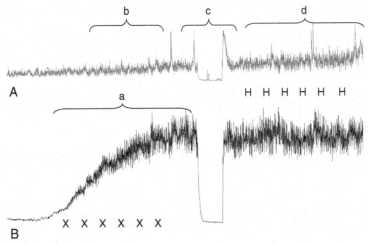

Fig. 19.2 An example of laser Doppler flowmetry (LDF) trace. LDF trace acquired using the periflux 5000 system, periont iontophoresis system, and perisoft software (Perimed AB, Järfälla, Sweden). Trace A is from a standard heated small angled probe; trace B is a simultaneous tracing from a larger heated iontophoresis probe. *Section a* demonstrates acetylcholine iontophoresis response (*X* represents iontophoretic dose applied); *Section b*, baseline trace; *Section c*, occlusion and reperfusion; *Section d*, thermal response (poor in this subject). (*H* represents 1°C surface temperature increments at skin surface; max 44°C.)

Videomicroscopy

Videomicroscopy, orthogonal polarized spectral (OPS) imaging, and later generation sidestream dark field (SDF) techniques all allow for the investigation of both microvasculature function and structure. Videomicroscopy has been widely used in adult populations, specifically in the intensive care setting, where persistent microcirculatory alterations in the sublingual area have been identified as predictors of adverse outcome.[80] Sublingual videomicroscopy in the newborn infant may be inconsistent due to small patient size and limited cooperation during assessment. However, the skin is thin enough in neonates to permit transcutaneous microcirculatory imaging, allowing studies during transition in both preterm and term neonates,[81] in babies experiencing respiratory distress or septic changes,[82] during transfusion,[23] or during whole-body cooling,[83,84] providing further insight into the (dys)function of newborn microvasculature. An extensive review of this technique was written by Kuiper et al.[85]

SDF imaging uses a green illumination light (wavelength 548 nm) that is maximally absorbed by oxy- and deoxy-hemoglobin. Surrounding tissue reflects this light, creating contrast, thereby allowing the visualization of red blood cells moving through the microvasculature. Second-generation SDF imaging is the most widely used videomicroscopy imaging system employed currently in pediatric studies. Third-generation systems, employing incident dark field (IDF) imaging, boast several technical improvements, potentially giving improved imaging resolution, but the neonatal literature on the use of these systems remains limited. A complete review of the technical aspects of OPS, SDF, and IDF, including comparisons between the technologies, can be found in the papers by van Elteren et al.[86] and Milstein et al.[87] The full range of videomicroscopy values using SDF in the immediate postnatal days and by sex are summarized for term infants by Wright et al.[88]

Microvasculature of the Neonate Studied by Laser Doppler Flowmetry and Videomicroscopy

Peripheral microvascular blood flow is subject to considerable changes during the first days of postnatal life, a period of marked circulatory vulnerability, especially in preterm infants. Myogenic and neural control of skin blood flow must be rapidly established during this period to allow appropriate thermoregulation to take place.[89]

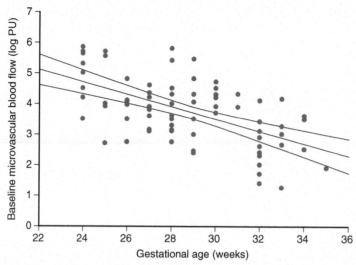

Fig. 19.3   Relationship between gestational age and baseline microvascular blood flow at 24 hours of postnatal age for all infants 24 to 36 weeks' gestation ($r = .624$, $P < .001$, Spearman r). *PU*, Laser Doppler perfusion units. (Stark MJ, Clifton VL, Wright IM: Sex-specific differences in peripheral microvascular blood flow in preterm infants. *Pediatr Res.* 63(4):415–419, 2008.)

LDF and OPS/SDF imaging have allowed detailed characterization of the relationship between peripheral microvascular blood flow and measures of neonatal physiologic and cardiovascular stability in infants during the immediate posttransitional period.

Neonatal Peripheral Microvascular Blood Flow and Gestational Age at Birth

Previously published findings on the influence of gestational age on baseline peripheral cutaneous blood flow are conflicting.[30,50,90–95] Some authors found no influence of gestational age on blood flow.[90] Other investigators reported an inverse relationship between baseline blood flow and increasing gestational age, whereas a few reported a higher baseline flow with increasing gestational age.[30,91–93] The apparent lack of consensus most likely reflects methodologic differences, with different patient groups, timing, and methods used.

Our data from two large cohorts of premature infants revealed a significant inverse relationship between LDF-measured baseline microvascular blood flow at 24 and 72 hours of age and gestational age (Fig. 19.3).[9,48] This relationship was complicated by the demonstration of a close interaction of gestational age and sex of the infant (discussed later), although some parameters appeared to be related to gestational age alone. Interestingly, the effect of thermal stimulation was most marked in the more immature infants.[48] Previous studies have reported no difference in skin vasodilatation to local thermal stimulation between preterm and term infants.[68,96] However, they focused on infants born after 30 weeks' gestation or studied the subjects at the end of the first postnatal week when variability in the response to thermal stimulation appears to resolve.[96,97] Further more, more recent studies using non-LDF methods to investigate microvascular blood flow support our observation of a thermal response being present even in the most preterm neonate.[98]

Neonatal Peripheral Microvascular Blood Flow, Postnatal Age, and Clinical Status

While alterations in microvascular function have been described in association with common clinical problems such as sepsis and polycythemia in the immediate postnatal period, it is the role of the microvasculature in the process of cardiovascular adaptation following preterm birth that is perhaps of the greatest interest.[99,100] With most extremely preterm infants that are going to die demonstrating clinical deterioration

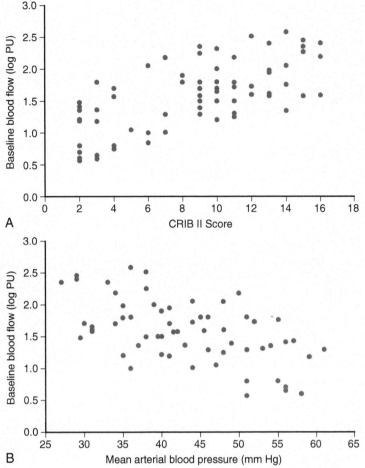

Fig. 19.4 (A) Relationship between baseline microvascular blood flow (log PU) at 24 hours of age and clinical illness severity determined by the Clinical Risk Index for Babies (CRIB) II score in infants of ≤32 weeks' gestation (n = 74). r^2 = .442, P < .001, multiple linear regression controlling for gestational age. (B) Relationship between baseline microvascular blood flow (log PU) at 24 hours of age and mean arterial blood pressure (mm Hg). r^2 = −.563, P < .001, multiple linear regression controlling for gestational age. *PU*, Perfusion units. (Stark MJ, Clifton VL, Wright IM: Microvascular flow, clinical illness severity and cardiovascular function in the preterm infant. *Arch Dis Child Fetal Neonatal Ed.* 93(4):F271–F274, 2008.)

in the first 72 hours following delivery, it is the influence of the relatively short-term postnatal preterm adaptation in microvascular blood flow that is potentially of the most importance and clinical relevance.[101]

Despite evidence from the animal literature and observational data in human neonates, the relationship between peripheral microvascular blood flow and measures of neonatal physiologic and cardiovascular stability in the immediate postnatal period had not been characterized until recently.[102] There is emerging evidence that the changes in early microvascular flow are of clinical significance. LDF measurements of peripheral microvascular blood flow have been shown to exhibit significant relationships with both clinical illness severity (Fig. 19.4A) and concomitant measures of cardiovascular function—in particular blood pressure (see Fig. 19.4B) in preterm infants during the first days of postnatal life.[103]

The underlying processes that explain these associations between peripheral microvascular blood flow and physiologic instability remain incompletely characterized. One explanation for the apparent discrepancy between early low central flow measures and high microvascular flow at 24 hours could be temporal change, with a period of low systemic perfusion followed by reperfusion.[104] Our recent human and animal data suggest though that this is not a significant effect.[9] Further more, we have preliminary evidence that structural maturation could underlie the changes

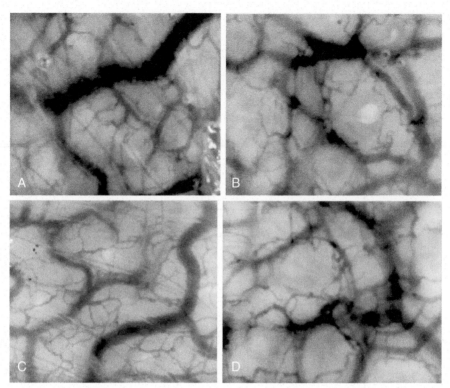

Fig. 19.5   Stills taken from microvascular videos on infants showing developmental changes with increasing gestation. (A) Male less than 28 weeks' gestation. (B) Male at term. (C) Female less than 28 weeks' gestation. (D) Female at term. Note change from three-dimensional network to more planar structured plexus with maturity. All images acquired at 24 hours of postnatal age using Microscan (Amsterdam, The Netherlands) sidestream darkfield videomicroscope.

in microvasculature function and apparent maldistribution of blood flow (Fig. 19.5), but definitive studies are still to be completed. Finally, another distributive scenario may contribute to this paradox. It is possible that a significant component to the observed peripheral increased microvascular flow may actually be on the venular side. This would lead to an apparent increase in flow by LDF assessment, but with an accompanying significant increase in capacitance. Such an effect would decrease preload with associated decreased cardiac output.[105] Further videomicroscopic studies, in combination with direct cardiac output and blood pressure measurements (see Chapters 3, 14, and 16), may contribute to clarification of this possibility.

Among the major forms of cardiovascular shock (see Chapters 1, 26 to 30), assessment of peripheral blood flow by techniques such as LDF may identify the presence of maldistributive shock.[106] This state is characterized by high blood flow recorded in shunting vessels but low blood flow in the nutritive components of the microvasculature. This clinical scenario characteristically demonstrates high LDF blood flow but anaerobic metabolism and lactic acid accumulation. Studies in babies with increased neonatal inflammatory markers, but without proven infection, have demonstrated increased flow using SDF videomicroscopy, but blood flow distribution was not documented.[107] To date, studies investigating the relationship between measured baseline microvascular flow and lactate have not shown any clear pattern of association.[108]

Neonatal Peripheral Microvascular Blood Flow and Sex

Sex-related differences in respiratory and circulatory parameters have been observed following preterm birth, with male sex associated with higher morbidity and both early and later mortality.[98,109–112] The need for cardiovascular support and the incidence of vasopressor-resistant hypotension are significantly higher in extremely preterm male infants during the first postnatal day.[110] Abnormal regulation of peripheral microvascular blood flow resulting in vasodilation and decreased peripheral vascular resistance may contribute to the development of circulatory compromise following preterm birth (see Chapters 1 and 26).

Recent studies have investigated sex-specific differences in basal peripheral microvascular blood flow and the functional ability of the microvasculature to respond to vasoactive stimuli in preterm infants in the immediate postnatal period. These show a significantly higher baseline flow in male versus female infants, with the effect increasing with decreasing gestation.[9,49] This sex-dependent dimorphic response is lost by 72 hours postnatal age. Vasodilation to ACh iontophoresis at 24 hours of age in the most immature infants (24 to 28 weeks' gestation) is significantly increased in males, above their already increased baseline flow. The underlying mechanisms resulting in this sex-specific dimorphic pattern of microvascular function have not been fully elucidated, but there are significant sex-related differences in the function of the gasotransmitters, nitrogen oxide, carbon monoxide (CO), and hydrogen sulfide (H_2S), and the interactions among them.[4,51,113,114] Clinically these sex-specific differences in microvascular function occur at a time of circulatory transition to the extrauterine environment, and thus could influence the transitional circulation and contribute to the higher rates of hypotension and low systemic blood flow in the first postnatal day observed in males.

Sex-dependent dimorphic differences in peripheral microvascular blood flow and function are also observed in term infants born following pregnancies complicated by mild-to-moderate late-gestation preeclampsia.[50] Female infants at 6 hours of age exhibit LDF-derived baseline microvascular blood flow that is similar to females of normotensive mothers, followed by significantly increased flow at 24 and 72 hours. Conversely, male infants do not demonstrate a temporal change in blood flow in the presence of preeclampsia but are significantly more vasodilated than males of nonpreeclamptic mothers at 6 hours of age. The transient nature of these findings supports the notion that differences in production and/or response to vasoactive mediators and/or neural control, and not structural differences, are responsible. Interestingly, these findings might lend support to the evolutionary theory for the persistence of preeclampsia to sustain brain growth in the presence of placental restriction, as male and female fetuses have different strategies to preserve growth and development.[115,116]

Intriguingly, there is evidence that the presence of a male or female fetus also exerts different effects on the maternal circulation in preeclamptic pregnancies.[117] Mothers pregnant with a male fetus demonstrate increased microvascular constriction and a lack of response to the vasodilator corticotropin-releasing hormone when compared with preeclamptic women pregnant with a female fetus. This has been proposed to be an attempt by the male fetus to improve uteroplacental nutritional supply, ensuring the maintenance of growth in the face of placental insufficiency.

Developmental changes in peripheral microvascular blood flow thus show relationships with gestation, sex, clinical illness, severity, and disease state. Variations in microcirculatory function might therefore contribute to observed cardiovascular maladaptation in early neonatal life. Cardiovascular maladaptation and the resultant hypotension and low systemic and organ blood flow are common problems in preterm infants, yet there is little outcome-based clinical evidence showing improvement in short- or long-term morbidity and mortality in response to commonly used treatments (see Chapters 1 and 26 to 30). Understanding the potential mechanisms of the response of the microvasculature to cardiovascular adaptation after preterm birth and in response to treatment therefore remains of significant clinical and research relevance.

Retinography and Cardiovascular Programming

In this chapter, we have focused on microvascular flow and its interaction with hemodynamic measures and clinically relevant risk factors in the premature infant during the first few postnatal days. In most studies, microvascular differences between risk groups are no longer evident by 1 week of age. However, there are concerns that the effects of the fetal and neonatal periods may have much longer lasting cardiovascular repercussions. The developmental origin of health and disease model has demonstrated that early influences not only produce local, short-term effects but also long-term programming conditions. Recent data suggest that some of these outcomes may be associated with changes in the microvasculature. The Atherosclerosis Risk in Communities (ARIC) study demonstrated that retinal microvascular changes were more common in individuals who went on to develop metabolic disease and appeared significantly earlier than changes in blood pressure or metabolic changes.[118] Further studies have shown microvascular changes as early as 6 to 9 years of age that may represent early markers, or even causal components, in the development of obesity, hypertension, and diabetes.[119,120] Those who are most at risk of future hypertensive disease, including indigenous populations, have been shown to have retinal microvascular differences from as early as the neonatal period.[36,121,122] With preterm neonates at greater risk of hypertension in later life, a risk highest for females,[123] it is possible that those factors that protect female neonates from the adverse effects of microvascular dilatation in the first few days of postnatal life increase the later risk for cardiovascular dysfunction. Further long-term cohort studies of preterm infants using videomicroscopy and retinography may help clarify this speculation.

Future Applications in Neonatal Medicine

Apart from the potential to predict future metabolic and cardiovascular trajectory, what other future developments are likely to be seen in the area of microvascular physiology in the neonate? The establishment and clarification of novel mechanisms, such as the role and mechanism of action of newer gasotransmitters, has the potential for new treatments to influence these pathways. Further studies need to be undertaken to determine if assessment of the microvasculature can aid in the decision to employ particular treatment strategies and to understand the specific microvascular effects of common neonatal therapies. Finally, the development and understanding of easy, reliable measures of the status and function of the microvasculature, at both the clinical and research levels, are likely to occur.

Summary and Conclusions

In this chapter we have discussed some of the tools and techniques used to understand more about the newborn microvasculature—most specifically in the preterm infant. Microvascular flow is increased in the first day of postnatal life in premature infants with poorer outcome; specifically in those of male sex, earlier gestational age, and higher clinical severity score. This appears to be a systemic effect, associated with known vasomediators, including less well-known gasotransmitters, such as CO and H_2S. It is clear that more work needs to be done to understand both neonatal microvascular function and control and the long-term consequences of microvascular dysfunction in the neonatal period. Importantly, current and future studies of the whole cardiovascular system of the newborn should include a detailed review of microvascular behavior to understand the system in its entirety.

REFERENCES

1. Hall JE: The microcirculation and the lymphatic system: capillary fluid exchange, interstitial fluid, and lymph flow. In Hall JE, editor: *Guyton and Hall Textbook of Medical Physiology*, ed 13, Philadelphia, 2016, Saunders/Elsevier, pp 189–201.
2. von der Weid PY, Rahman M, Imtiaz MS, et al.: Spontaneous transient depolarizations in lymphatic vessels of the guinea pig mesentery: pharmacology and implication for spontaneous contractility, *Am J Physiol Heart Circ Physiol* 295(5):H1989–H2000, 2008.
3. Skapinker R, Rothberg AD: Postnatal regression of the tunica vasculosa lentis, *J Perinatol* 7(4): 279–281, 1987.
4. Wright IMR, Dyson RM: Microcirculation of the newborn. In Lenasi H, editor: *Microcirculation revisited—from molecules to clinical practice: intech*, 2016.
5. McGregor ML, Bremer DL, Cole C, et al.: Retinopathy of prematurity outcome in infants with prethreshold retinopathy of prematurity and oxygen saturation >94% in room air: the high oxygen percentage in retinopathy of prematurity study, *Pediatrics* 110(3):540–544, 2002.

6. Rajappa M, Saxena P, Kaur J: Ocular angiogenesis: mechanisms and recent advances in therapy, *Adv Clin Chem* 50:103–121, 2010.
7. Wilkinson-Berka JL, Miller AG, Binger KJ: Prorenin and the (pro)renin receptor: recent advances and implications for retinal development and disease, *Curr Opin Nephrol Hypertens* 20(1):69–76, 2011.
8. Dyson RM, Palliser HK, Kelleher MA, et al.: The guinea pig as an animal model for studying perinatal changes in microvascular function, *Pediatr Res* 71(1):20–24, 2012.
9. Dyson RM, Palliser HK, Lakkundi A, et al.: Early microvascular changes in the preterm neonate: a comparative study of the human and guinea pig, *Physiol Rep* 2(9), 2014.
10. Newman JM, Dwyer RM, St-Pierre P, et al.: Decreased microvascular vasomotion and myogenic response in rat skeletal muscle in association with acute insulin resistance, *J Physiol* 587(Pt 11):2579–2588, 2009.
11. Wauschkuhn CA, Witte K, Gorbey S, et al.: Circadian periodicity of cerebral blood flow revealed by laser-Doppler flowmetry in awake rats: relation to blood pressure and activity, *Am J Physiol Heart Circ Physiol* 289(4):H1662–H1668, 2005.
12. Abu-Amara M, Yang SY, Quaglia A, et al.: Effect of remote ischemic preconditioning on liver ischemia/reperfusion injury using a new mouse model, *Liver Transpl* 17(1):70–82, 2011.
13. Krouzecky A, Matejovic M, Radej J, et al.: Perfusion pressure manipulation in porcine sepsis: effects on intestinal hemodynamics, *Physiol Res* 55(5):527–533, 2006.
14. Hammad FT, Davis G, Zhang XY, et al.: Intra- and post-operative assessment of renal cortical perfusion by laser Doppler flowmetry in renal transplantation in the rat, *Eur Surg Res* 32(5):284–288, 2000.
15. Taccone FS, Su F, Pierrakos C, et al.: Cerebral microcirculation is impaired during sepsis: an experimental study, *Crit Care* 14(4):R140, 2010.
16. Treu CM, Lupi O, Bottino DA, et al.: Sidestream dark field imaging: the evolution of real-time visualization of cutaneous microcirculation and its potential application in dermatology, *Arch Dermatol Res* 303(2):69–78, 2011.
17. Daudel F, Freise H, Westphal M, et al.: Continuous thoracic epidural anesthesia improves gut mucosal microcirculation in rats with sepsis, *Shock* 28(5):610–614, 2007.
18. Hughes S, Brain S, Williams G, et al.: Assessment of blood flow changes at multiple sites in rabbit skin using a 133Xenon clearance technique, *J Pharmacol Toxicol Methods* 32(1):41–47, 1994.
19. Glenny RW, Bernard S, Brinkley M: Validation of fluorescent-labeled microspheres for measurement of regional organ perfusion, *J Appl Physiol (1985)* 74(5):2585–2597, 1993.
20. de Boode WP: Clinical monitoring of systemic hemodynamics in critically ill newborns, *Early Hum Dev* 86(3):137–141, 2010.
21. Oh W, Lind J: Body temperature of the newborn infant in relation to placental transfusion, *Acta Paediatr Scand* (Suppl 172):35+, 1967.
22. Stromberg B, Oberg PA, Sedin G: Transepidermal water loss in newborn infants. X. Effects of central cold-stimulation on evaporation rate and skin blood flow, *Acta Paediatr Scand* 72(5):735–739, 1983.
23. Genzel-Boroviczeny O, Christ F, Glas V: Blood transfusion increases functional capillary density in the skin of anemic preterm infants, *Pediatr Res* 56(5):751–755, 2004.
24. Wellhoner P, Rolle D, Lonnroth P, et al.: Laser-Doppler flowmetry reveals rapid perfusion changes in adipose tissue of lean and obese females, *Am J Physiol Endocrinol Metab* 291(5):E1025–E1030, 2006.
25. Benaron DA, Parachikov IH, Friedland S, et al.: Continuous, noninvasive, and localized microvascular tissue oximetry using visible light spectroscopy, *Anesthesiology* 100(6):1469–1475, 2004.
26. Vallee F, Mateo J, Dubreuil G, et al.: Cutaneous ear lobe Pco(2) at 37 degrees C to evaluate microperfusion in patients with septic shock, *Chest* 138(5):1062–1070, 2010.
27. Merla A, Di Romualdo S, Di Donato L, et al.: Combined thermal and laser Doppler imaging in the assessment of cutaneous tissue perfusion, *Conf Proc IEEE Eng Med Biol Soc* 2007:2630–2633, 2007.
28. De Felice C, Latini G, Vacca P, et al.: The pulse oximeter perfusion index as a predictor for high illness severity in neonates, *Eur J Pediatr* 161(10):561–562, 2002.
29. Pellicer A, Bravo Mdel C: Near-infrared spectroscopy: a methodology-focused review, *Semin Fetal Neonatal Med* 16(1):42–49, 2011.
30. Wu PY, Wong WH, Guerra G, et al.: Peripheral blood flow in the neonate; 1. Changes in total, skin, and muscle blood flow with gestational and postnatal age, *Pediatr Res* 14(12):1374–1378, 1980.
31. Top AP, Ince C, Schouwenberg PH, et al.: Inhaled nitric oxide improves systemic microcirculation in infants with hypoxemic respiratory failure, *Pediatr Crit Care Med* 12(6):e271–e274, 2011.
32. Norman M, Herin P, Fagrell B, et al.: Capillary blood cell velocity in full-term infants as determined in skin by videophotometric microscopy, *Pediatr Res* 23(6):585–588, 1988.
33. Bucher HU, Edwards AD, Lipp AE, et al.: Comparison between near infrared spectroscopy and 133Xenon clearance for estimation of cerebral blood flow in critically ill preterm infants, *Pediatr Res* 33(1):56–60, 1993.
34. Baenziger O, Jaggi JL, Mueller AC, et al.: Cerebral blood flow in preterm infants affected by sex, mechanical ventilation, and intrauterine growth, *Pediatr Neurol* 11(4):319–324, 1994.
35. Ahmad S, Wallace DK, Freedman SF, et al.: Computer-assisted assessment of plus disease in retinopathy of prematurity using video indirect ophthalmoscopy images, *Retina* 28(10):1458–1462, 2008.
36. Kandasamy Y, Smith R, Wright IM: Retinal microvasculature measurements in full-term newborn infants, *Microvasc Res* 82(3):381–384, 2011.

37. Ormerod LD, Fariza E, Webb RH: Dynamics of external ocular blood flow studied by scanning angiographic microscopy, *Eye (Lond)* 9(Pt 5):605–614, 1995.

38. Johnson JM, Kellogg Jr DL: Local thermal control of the human cutaneous circulation, *J Appl Physiol (1985)* 109(4):1229–1238, 2010.

39. Fluhr JW, Darlenski R, Taieb A, et al.: Functional skin adaptation in infancy—almost complete but not fully competent, *Exp Dermatol* 19(6):483–492, 2010.

40. Cutolo M, Sulli A, Smith V: Assessing microvascular changes in systemic sclerosis diagnosis and management, *Nat Rev Rheumatol* 6(10):578–587, 2010.

41. Kunzek S, Quinn MW, Shore AC: Does change in skin perfusion provide a good index to monitor the sympathetic response to a noxious stimulus in preterm newborns? *Early Hum Dev* 49(2):81–89, 1997.

42. Osborn DA, Evans N, Kluckow M: Clinical detection of low upper body blood flow in very premature infants using blood pressure, capillary refill time, and central-peripheral temperature difference, *Arch Dis Child Fetal Neonatal Ed* 89(2):F168–F173, 2004.

43. Millet C, Roustit M, Blaise S, et al.: Comparison between laser speckle contrast imaging and laser Doppler imaging to assess skin blood flow in humans, *Microvasc Res* 82(2):147–151, 2011.

44. Rajan V, Varghese B, van Leeuwen TG, et al.: Review of methodological developments in laser Doppler flowmetry, *Lasers Med Sci* 24(2):269–283, 2009.

45. Turner J, Belch JJ, Khan F: Current concepts in assessment of microvascular endothelial function using laser Doppler imaging and iontophoresis, *Trends Cardiovasc Med* 18(4):109–116, 2008.

46. Roustit M, Millet C, Blaise S, et al.: Excellent reproducibility of laser speckle contrast imaging to assess skin microvascular reactivity, *Microvasc Res* 80(3):505–511, 2010.

47. Weindling M, Paize F: Peripheral haemodynamics in newborns: best practice guidelines, *Early Hum Dev* 86(3):159–165, 2010.

48. Stark MJ, Clifton VL, Wright IM: Microvascular flow, clinical illness severity and cardiovascular function in the preterm infant, *Arch Dis Child Fetal Neonatal Ed* 93(4):F271–F274, 2008.

49. Stark MJ, Clifton VL, Wright IM: Sex-specific differences in peripheral microvascular blood flow in preterm infants, *Pediatr Res* 63(4):415–419, 2008.

50. Stark MJ, Clifton VL, Wright IM: Neonates born to mothers with preeclampsia exhibit sex-specific alterations in microvascular function, *Pediatr Res* 65(3):292–295, 2009.

51. Stark MJ, Clifton VL, Wright IM: Carbon monoxide is a significant mediator of cardiovascular status following preterm birth, *Pediatrics* 124(1):277–284, 2009.

52. Stark MJ, Hodyl NA, Wright IM, et al.: The influence of sex and antenatal betamethasone exposure on vasoconstrictors and the preterm microvasculature, *J Matern Fetal Neonatal Med* 24(10):1215–1220, 2011.

53. Ishiguro A, Sekine T, Kakiuchi S, et al.: Skin and subcutaneous blood flows of very low birth weight infants during the first 3 postnatal days, *J Matern Fetal Neonatal Med* 23(6):522–528, 2010.

54. Ishiguro A, Sekine T, Suzuki K, et al.: Changes in skin and subcutaneous perfusion in very-low-birth-weight infants during the transitional period, *Neonatology* 100(2):162–168, 2011.

55. Ishiguro A, Suzuki K, Sekine T, et al.: Skin blood flow as a predictor of intraventricular hemorrhage in very-low-birth-weight infants, *Pediatr Res* 75(2):322–327, 2014.

56. Ishiguro A, Sakazaki S, Itakura R, et al.: Peripheral blood flow monitoring in an infant with septic shock, *Pediatr Int* 56(5):787–789, 2014.

57. Perimed AB. Laser Doppler monitoring 2017. http://www.perimed-instruments.com/laser-doppler-monitoring.

58. Kubli S, Waeber B, Dalle-Ave A, et al.: Reproducibility of laser Doppler imaging of skin blood flow as a tool to assess endothelial function, *J Cardiovasc Pharmacol* 36(5):640–648, 2000.

59. Smits GJ, Roman RJ, Lombard JH: Evaluation of laser-Doppler flowmetry as a measure of tissue blood flow, *J Appl Physiol* 61(2):666–672, 1986.

60. Cracowski JL, Minson CT, Salvat-Melis M, et al.: Methodological issues in the assessment of skin microvascular endothelial function in humans, *Trends Pharmacol Sci* 27(9):503–508, 2006.

61. Agarwal SC, Allen J, Murray A, et al.: Comparative reproducibility of dermal microvascular blood flow changes in response to acetylcholine iontophoresis, hyperthermia and reactive hyperaemia, *Physiol Meas* 31(1):1–11, 2010.

62. Yvonne-Tee GB, Rasool AH, Halim AS, et al.: Reproducibility of different laser Doppler fluximetry parameters of postocclusive reactive hyperemia in human forearm skin, *J Pharmacol Toxicol Methods* 52(2):286–292, 2005.

63. Kolarsick PAJ, Kolarsick MA, Goodwin C: Anatomy and physiology of the skin, *J Dermatol Nurs* 3(4):203–213, 2011.

64. Fagrell B: Peripheral vascular diseases. In Shepard AP, Oberg PA, editors: *Laser Doppler Blood Flowmetry*, Norwell, MA, 1990, Kluwer Academic.

65. Celander O, Marild K: Reactive hyperaemia in the foot and calf of the newborn infant, *Acta Paediatr* 51:544–552, 1962.

66. Ahlsten G, Ewald U, Tuvemo T: Impaired vascular reactivity in newborn infants of smoking mothers, *Acta Paediatr Scand* 76(2):248–253, 1987.

67. Suichies HE, Brouwer C, Aarnoudse JG, et al.: Skin blood flow changes, measured by laser Doppler flowmetry, in the first week after birth, *Early Hum Dev* 23(1):1–8, 1990.

68. Stromberg B, Riesenfeld T, Sedin G: Laser Doppler measurement of skin blood flow in newborn infants, *Pediatr Res* 19(10):1128–28, 1985.

69. Perera P, Kurban AK, Ryan TJ: The development of the cutaneous microvascular system in the newborn, *Br J Dermatol* 82:86–91, 1970.

70. Yamamoto-Suganuma R, Aso Y: Relationship between post-occlusive forearm skin reactive hyperaemia and vascular disease in patients with type 2 diabetes—a novel index for detecting micro- and macrovascular dysfunction using laser Doppler flowmetry, *Diabet Med* 26(1):83–88, 2009.
71. Wilson SB, Jennings PE, Belch JJ: Detection of microvascular impairment in type 1 diabetics by laser Doppler flowmetry, *Clin Physiol* 12(2):195–208, 1992.
72. Strain WD, Chaturvedi N, Hughes A, et al.: Associations between cardiac target organ damage and microvascular dysfunction: the role of blood pressure, *J Hypertens* 28(5):952–958, 2010.
73. Tee GB, Rasool AH, Halim AS, et al.: Dependence of human forearm skin postocclusive reactive hyperemia on occlusion time, *J Pharmacol Toxicol Methods* 50(1):73–78, 2004.
74. Norman M: Preterm birth—an emerging risk factor for adult hypertension? *Semin Perinatol* 34(3):183–187, 2010.
75. Magerl W, Treede RD: Heat-evoked vasodilatation in human hairy skin: axon reflexes due to low-level activity of nociceptive afferents, *J Physiol* 497(Pt 3):837–848, 1996.
76. Minson CT, Berry LT, Joyner MJ: Nitric oxide and neurally mediated regulation of skin blood flow during local heating, *J Appl Physiol (1985)* 91(4):1619–1626, 2001.
77. Sekkat N, Kalia YN, Guy RH: Porcine ear skin as a model for the assessment of transdermal drug delivery to premature neonates, *Pharm Res* 21(8):1390–1397, 2004.
78. Clifton VL, Crompton R, Read MA, et al.: Microvascular effects of corticotropin-releasing hormone in human skin vary in relation to estrogen concentration during the menstrual cycle, *J Endocrinol* 186(1):69–76, 2005.
79. Morris SJ, Shore AC: Skin blood flow responses to the iontophoresis of acetylcholine and sodium nitroprusside in man: possible mechanisms, *J Physiol* 496(Pt 2):531–542, 1996.
80. Wiessner R, Gierer P, Schaser K, et al.: Microcirculatory failure of sublingual perfusion in septic-shock patients. Examination by OPS imaging and PiCCO monitoring, *Zentralbl Chir* 134(3):231–236, 2009.
81. Schwepcke A, Weber FD, Mormanova Z, et al.: Microcirculatory mechanisms in postnatal hypotension affecting premature infants, *Pediatr Res* 74(2):186–190, 2013.
82. Alba-Alejandre I, Hiedl S, Genzel-Boroviczeny O: Microcirculatory changes in term newborns with suspected infection: an observational prospective study, *Int J Pediatr* 2013:768784, 2013.
83. Fredly S, Fugelseth D, Nygaard CS, et al.: Noninvasive assessments of oxygen delivery from the microcirculation to skin in hypothermia-treated asphyxiated newborn infants, *Pediatr Res* 79(6):902–906, 2016.
84. Fredly S, Nygaard CS, Skranes JH, et al.: Cooling effect on skin microcirculation in asphyxiated newborn infants with increased C-reactive protein, *Neonatology* 110(4):270–276, 2016.
85. Kuiper JW, Tibboel D, Ince C: The vulnerable microcirculation in the critically ill pediatric patient, *Crit Care* 20(1):352, 2016.
86. van Elteren HA, Ince C, Tibboel D, et al.: Cutaneous microcirculation in preterm neonates: comparison between sidestream dark field (SDF) and incident dark field (IDF) imaging, *J Clin Monit Comput* 29(5):543–548, 2015.
87. Milstein DMJ, Bezemer R, Ince C: Sidestream dark-field (SDF) video microscopy for clinical imaging of the microcirculation. In Leahy MJ, editor: *Microcirculation Imaging*, ed 1, Wiley-VCH Verlag GmbH, 2012.
88. Wright IM, Latter JL, Dyson RM, et al.: Videomicroscopy as a tool for investigation of the microcirculation in the newborn, *Physiol Rep* 4(19), 2016.
89. Buus NH, Simonsen U, Pilegaard HK, et al.: Nitric oxide, prostanoid and non-NO, non-prostanoid involvement in acetylcholine relaxation of isolated human small arteries, *Br J Pharmacol* 129(1):184–192, 2000.
90. Rutter N: The dermis, *Semin Neonatol* 5(4):297–302, 2000.
91. Beaufort-Krol GC, Suichies HE, Aarnoudse JG, et al.: Postocclusive reactive hyperaemia of cutaneous blood flow in premature newborn infants, *Acta Paediatr Scand Suppl* 360:20–25, 1989.
92. Berg K, Celander O: Circulatory adaptation in the thermoregulation of fullterm and premature newborn infants, *Acta Paediatr Scand* 60(3):278–284, 1971.
93. Riley ID: Hand and forearm blood flow in full term and premature infants; a plethysmographic study, *Clin Sci* 13(3):317–320, 1954.
94. Jahnukainen T, van Ravenswaaij-Arts C, Jalonen J, et al.: Dynamics of vasomotor thermoregulation of the skin in term and preterm neonates, *Early Hum Dev* 33(2):133–143, 1993.
95. Celander O, Marild K: Regional circulation and capillary filtration in relation to capillary exchange in the foot and calf of the newborn infant, *Acta Paediatr* 51:385–400, 1962.
96. Beinder E, Trojan A, Bucher HU, et al.: Control of skin blood flow in pre- and full-term infants, *Biol Neonate* 65(1):7–15, 1994.
97. Jahnukainen T, Lindqvist A, Jalonen J, et al.: Reactivity of skin blood flow and heart rate to thermal stimulation in infants during the first postnatal days and after a two-month follow-up, *Acta Paediatr* 85(6):733–738, 1996.
98. Genzel-Boroviczeny O, Seidl T, Rieger-Fackeldey E, et al.: Impaired microvascular perfusion improves with increased incubator temperature in preterm infants, *Pediatr Res* 61(2):239–242, 2007.
99. Martin H, Norman M: Skin microcirculation before and after local warming in infants delivered vaginally or by caesarean section, *Acta Paediatr* 86(3):261–267, 1997.
100. Poschl JM, Weiss T, Fallahi F, et al.: Reactive hyperemia of skin microcirculation in septic neonates, *Acta Paediatr* 83(8):808–811, 1994.

101. Norman M, Fagrell B, Herin P: Skin microcirculation in neonatal polycythaemia and effects of haemodilution. Interaction between haematocrit, vasomotor activity and perfusion, *Acta Paediatr* 82(8):672–677, 1993.

102. Kent AL, Wright IM, Abdel-Latif ME, et al.: Mortality and adverse neurologic outcomes are greater in preterm male infants, *Pediatrics* 129(1):124–131, 2012.

103. Molnar J, Nijland MJ, Howe DC, et al.: Evidence for microvascular dysfunction after prenatal dexamethasone at 0.7, 0.75, and 0.8 gestation in sheep, *Am J Physiol Regul Integr Comp Physiol* 283(3):R561–R567, 2002.

104. Kluckow M, Evans N: Superior vena cava flow in newborn infants: a novel marker of systemic blood flow, *Arch Dis Child Fetal Neonatal Ed* 82(3):F182–F187, 2000.

105. Eiby YA, Lumbers ER, Headrick JP, et al.: Left ventricular output and aortic blood flow in response to changes in preload and afterload in the preterm piglet heart, *Am J Physiol Regul Integr Comp Physiol* 303(7):R769–R777, 2012.

106. den Uil CA, Klijn E, Lagrand WK, et al.: The microcirculation in health and critical disease, *Prog Cardiovasc Dis* 51(2):161–170, 2008.

107. Weidlich K, Kroth J, Nussbaum C, et al.: Changes in microcirculation as early markers for infection in preterm infants–an observational prospective study, *Pediatr Res* 66(4):461–465, 2009.

108. Hussain F, Gilshenan K, Gray PH: Does lactate level in the first 12 hours of life predict mortality in extremely premature infants? *J Paediatr Child Health* 45(5):263–267, 2009.

109. Khoury MJ, Marks JS, McCarthy BJ, et al.: Factors affecting the sex differential in neonatal mortality: the role of respiratory distress syndrome, *Am J Obstet Gynecol* 151(6):777–782, 1985.

110. Elsmen E, Hansen Pupp I, Hellstrom-Westas L: Preterm male infants need more initial respiratory and circulatory support than female infants, *Acta Paediatr* 93(4):529–533, 2004.

111. Henderson-Smart DJ, Hutchinson JL, Donoghue DA, et al.: Prenatal predictors of chronic lung disease in very preterm infants, *Arch Dis Child Fetal Neonatal Ed* 91(1):F40–F45, 2006.

112. Stevenson DK, Verter J, Fanaroff AA, et al.: Sex differences in outcomes of very low birthweight infants: the newborn male disadvantage, *Arch Dis Child Fetal Neonatal Ed* 83(3):F182–F185, 2000.

113. Dyson RM, Palliser HK, Latter JL, et al.: A role for H2S in the microcirculation of newborns: the major metabolite of H2S (thiosulphate) is increased in preterm infants, *PLoS One* 9(8):e105085, 2014.

114. Dyson RM, Palliser HK, Latter JL, et al.: Interactions of the gasotransmitters contribute to microvascular tone (dys)regulation in the preterm neonate, *PLoS One* 10(3):e0121621, 2015.

115. Chaline J: Increased cranial capacity in hominid evolution and preeclampsia, *J Reprod Immunol* 59(2):137–152, 2003.

116. Clifton VL: Review: sex and the human placenta: mediating differential strategies of fetal growth and survival, *Placenta* 31(Suppl):S33–S39, 2010.

117. Stark MJ, Dierkx L, Clifton VL, et al.: Alterations in the maternal peripheral microvascular response in pregnancies complicated by preeclampsia and the impact of fetal sex, *J Soc Gynecol Investig* 13(8):573–578, 2006.

118. Sharrett AR, Hubbard LD, Cooper LS, et al.: Retinal arteriolar diameters and elevated blood pressure: the Atherosclerosis Risk in Communities Study, *Am J Epidemiol* 150(3):263–270, 1999.

119. Li LJ, Cheung CY, Chia A, et al.: The relationship of body fatness indices and retinal vascular caliber in children, *Int J Pediatr Obes* 6(3–4):267–274, 2011.

120. de Jongh RT, Serne EH, RG IJ, et al.: Microvascular function: a potential link between salt sensitivity, insulin resistance and hypertension, *J Hypertens* 25(9):1887–1893, 2007.

121. Kandasamy Y, Smith R, Wright IM: Retinal microvascular changes in low-birth-weight babies have a link to future health, *J Perinat Med* 40(3):209–214, 2012.

122. Kandasamy Y, Smith R, Wright IM, et al.: Relationship between birth weight and retinal microvasculature in newborn infants, *J Perinatol* 32(6):443–447, 2012, https://doi.org/10.1038/jp.2011.118.

123. Kistner A, Jacobson L, Jacobson SH, et al.: Low gestational age associated with abnormal retinal vascularization and increased blood pressure in adult women, *Pediatr Res* 51(6):675–680, 2002.

Comprehensive and Predictive Monitoring

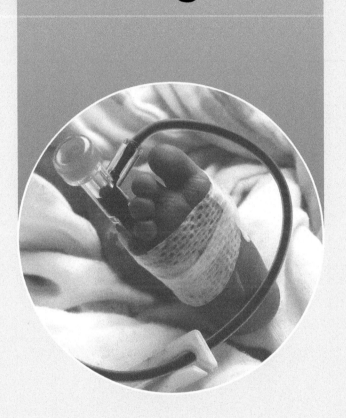

CHAPTER 20

Heart Rate and Cardiorespiratory Analysis for Sepsis and Necrotizing Enterocolitis Prediction

Brynne A. Sullivan and Karen D. Fairchild

- Sepsis and necrotizing enterocolitis (NEC) are major causes of mortality and morbidity for preterm infants in the neonatal intensive care unit (NICU), and earlier detection and treatment are likely to improve outcomes.
- Abnormal heart rate characteristics (HRC) of decreased variability and transient decelerations occur in some infants with sepsis and NEC. These abnormal patterns often begin hours or even days before more obvious clinical signs become apparent, and they cannot be discerned through conventional heart rate monitoring.
- An HRC monitor (HeRO monitor) was developed as an early warning system for sepsis in NICU patients. The HRC index incorporates three measures (heart rate variability, sample asymmetry, and sample entropy) and is the fold-increased risk an infant will experience a clinical deterioration consistent with sepsis in the next 24 hours.
- Display of the HRC index to clinicians was shown to reduce all-cause mortality by 22% and sepsis-associated mortality by 40% in a randomized trial of 3003 very low birthweight preterm infants.
- Adding analysis of respiratory characteristics to HRC may improve predictive monitoring algorithms. For example, cross-correlation of heart rate and oxygen saturation can detect deceleration-desaturation episodes that may accompany sepsis-associated apnea.
- Predictive monitoring is a screening tool that supplements but does not replace clinical judgment.
- Adding targeted biomarker screening to continuous physiomarker monitoring (HRC or combined cardiorespiratory metrics) may assist in decisions about testing and therapy.

Predictable Systemic Inflammatory Crises in the Neonatal Intensive Care Unit

Preterm infants are susceptible to late-onset sepsis and necrotizing enterocolitis (NEC), which, despite preventative efforts, continue to be major causes of mortality and morbidity in this population. Recent epidemiologic surveys indicate that the incidence of septicemia has decreased amongst very low birth weight infants (VLBW <1500 g) from about 25%[1,2] to about 15%,[3] due in part to improved hand and central line hygiene[4] and increased breast-milk feeding.[5] Unfortunately the incidence of NEC has not fallen in the same time period, remaining at about 5% to 10%.[6,7] Mortality related to septicemia and NEC is reported in the range of 15% to 20%,[1,8,9] and survivors have a higher risk of long-term neurodevelopmental impairment compared with age-matched preterm infants without these complications.[10,11]

Adverse outcomes may be attributed in part to brain damage from circulating inflammatory mediators[12–14] and also to cardiovascular compromise, leading to ischemic or hypoxic tissue damage.[15,16] Early prediction or detection of sepsis and NEC, prior to overt clinical deterioration, should lead to improved short- and long-term outcomes.

In this chapter we will briefly discuss the value of prenatal or early postnatal risk-based scores that incorporate cardiovascular data for prediction of adverse events or conditions diagnosed days or weeks later. We will then focus on early warning scores that reflect a systemic inflammatory response and predict *imminent* clinical deterioration from sepsis or NEC. We will primarily describe heart rate characteristics (HRC) monitoring, since this is the area that has the largest body of research and development. We will also discuss changes in breathing patterns and in cardiorespiratory interactions that may occur in the early phases of these potentially catastrophic illnesses. We will address important questions and controversies and present challenges and future directions for research in this field.

Of note, the terminology throughout the chapter will include heart rate variability (HRV) and HRC. HRC include HRV together with other measurements that reflect potentially pathologic heart rate (HR) patterns in preterm infants, such as repetitive brief decelerations.

Risk Prediction Incorporating Prenatal Heart Rate Data

Predicting the risk of future adverse events can be useful for clinical and research purposes and can include both fetal and early postnatal assessment of cardiovascular compromise. Abnormal fetal HRC of decreased variability and superimposed decelerations are commonly used as an indication of fetal distress and are associated with adverse perinatal outcomes.[17–19] These abnormal fetal HRC can be an indicator of acidemia, uteroplacental insufficiency, or a systemic inflammatory response and may predict the risk for postnatal ischemic or inflammatory conditions. A study in growth-restricted human fetuses drew a link between low HRV and increased middle cerebral artery perfusion, a measure of impaired tissue oxygen delivery that could predict ischemic complications postnatally.[20] In fetal sheep, the intrauterine administration of an inflammatory stimulus led to depressed fetal HRV and was associated postnatally with intestinal inflammation and altered mucosal integrity,[21] which could increase the risk of NEC and intestinal perforation if this finding translates to human fetuses.

The problem with current methods of assessing fetal HR is that they are primarily qualitative and prone to interobserver variation, which limits the predictive value for future adverse events.[22–24] Moorman and colleagues, who developed the neonatal HRC index monitor described later in this chapter, also developed quantitative methods for analyzing abnormal fetal HRC (low variability and superimposed decelerations) and showed good correlation between this quantitative assessment and obstetricians' impressions of "nonreassuring fetal HR."[25] More work is needed to determine whether quantitative measures of fetal HRC provide information that could impact perinatal and postnatal management in a way that improves neonatal outcomes.

Early Postnatal Predictors of Late Events or Outcomes

Assessment of HR, oxygenation, and perfusion in the first minutes, hours, and days after birth can provide important information about the well-being of newborn infants that might be useful for prediction of adverse events or outcomes diagnosed much later. Well-known examples of scores used to assess newborns in the first minutes to hours after birth are the Apgar, Score for Neonatal Acute Physiology (SNAP), Score for Neonatal Acute Physiology (SNAP) Perinatal Extension-II (SNAPPE-II), and Clinical Risk Indicator for Babies (CRIB-II) scores. The Apgar score includes assessment of HR, breathing, oxygenation, and other variables in the first minutes after birth and has some association with mortality and adverse neurologic outcomes.[26] The SNAPPE-II[27] and CRIB-II[28] were developed to measure the severity of illness and mortality risk in NICU patients using clinical and laboratory indices in the first 12 hours after birth. Metabolic acidosis (reflecting cardiovascular compromise) is incorporated into both of these scores, and lowest blood pressure is included in SNAPPE-II. The advantage of these scores is that they do not require specialized monitoring equipment, but the disadvantage is that they require some effort to retrieve the data and perform the calculations. While these scores were designed to predict mortality, they have been found to predict other adverse outcomes,[29,30] but serial assessment beyond the day of birth does not appear to accurately predict mortality or morbidities such as septicemia or NEC.[31,32]

A number of groups have sought to identify new physiologic metrics in the first hours or days after birth to predict later adverse events in preterm infants. One study found low HRV in the high-frequency spectrum in the first week after birth in preterm infants who developed NEC.[33] Another study reported that a "PhysiScore" that included low HRV in the first 3 hours after birth predicted morbidities including sepsis in a small cohort of preterm infants.[34] Early assessment of the HRC index was also studied for its ability to predict later events or outcomes. A high average HRC index in the first week after birth (reflecting low HRV and decelerations) was associated with late-onset septicemia but did not predict NEC after adjusting for gestational age (GA).[29]

Further research is needed to determine whether the analysis of fetal or early postnatal HR patterns can identify infants at high risk for various pathologies. Validated risk scores identifying the highest risk infants among the inherently high-risk preterm population could lead to targeted strategies to prevent or mitigate the damage from sepsis and NEC. Illness severity or risk scores may also be used as an objective measure of patient acuity for stratification in clinical trials, for comparing outcomes between units, or for resource allocation.[35]

Risk Prediction for Imminent Clinical Deterioration

Early warning systems, in contrast to the risk scores described previously, are designed to detect subtle pathologic signs predicting imminent deterioration before clinicians would recognize that a patient is ill. Often there are changes in vital sign patterns such as HRV and respiratory rate variability that would not be detected by even the most vigilant and experienced clinicians through inspection of conventional intensive care unit (ICU) monitors.[36,37] In preterm infants this is especially true, since signs of sepsis or NEC such as apnea with associated HR deceleration and oxygen desaturation are nonspecific and occur in healthy preterm infants. A continuously displayed risk score might detect a worsening in the cardiorespiratory pattern over an infant's prior baseline.

Fig. 20.1 depicts the potential value of early warning systems for detection of sepsis before there are obvious clinical signs. A key point with any such system is that clinician judgment is not replaced but supplemented, as reflected in the figure by the clinician carefully evaluating an infant with a rising risk score and considering the appropriate course of action. The decision about whether to obtain cultures and start antibiotics would incorporate an assessment of the infant's risk factors, clinical signs, vital sign trends, and laboratory data. Another key point is that for early warning systems to improve patient outcomes, there needs to be a significant time interval between the risk score rising and the time when clinicians using conventional systems would have recognized illness and initiated interventions. How much lead time is required to improve outcomes is debatable, but likely to be more than a few hours. With the HRC index monitor described later in this chapter, some infants have "spikes" in their score several days prior to clinical deterioration, which might reflect a sepsis prodrome and the opportunity for earlier intervention.[38]

Heart Rate Regulation by the Autonomic Nervous System

In order to optimally utilize the data presented by the HRC monitor, it is important to have a basic understanding of regulation of HR in health and disease. Beat-to-beat

20

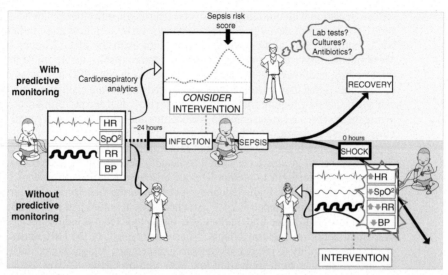

Fig. 20.1 Cardiorespiratory predictive monitoring for sepsis. The bottom scenario depicts a conventional neonatal intensive care unit practice with standard vital sign display. Once overt clinical or vital sign abnormalities associated with sepsis are recognized, the infant may be in an advanced stage of illness and is more likely to progress to shock and adverse outcomes. The top scenario depicts the potential impact of predictive monitoring. Validated cardiorespiratory algorithms are run and a sepsis risk score is displayed, which alerts clinicians that the infant might be getting sick. The clinician then considers the score in the context of clinical signs and decides whether to wait and watch closely, to perform laboratory or biomarker tests, or to send cultures and start antibiotics. With earlier intervention, the infant has a greater chance of recovery without end-organ damage. *BP*, Blood pressure; *HR*, heart rate; *RR*, respiratory rate; *SpO₂*, oxygen saturation.

HRV is regulated by the autonomic nervous system (ANS). Sympathetic activation leads to the release of norepinephrine, which acts on beta adrenergic receptors in the sinoatrial node to trigger acceleration in the HR. Parasympathetic activation leads to the release of acetylcholine, which binds to muscarinic cholinergic receptors leading to transient slowing of the HR.[39] In the healthy state, the two branches of the ANS are balanced, with sympathetic activity associated with low-frequency HRV (0.04 to 0.15 Hz) and parasympathetic activity associated with high-frequency HRV (0.15 to 0.4 Hz in adults). In conditions of stress, adrenal glucocorticoid release leads to sympathetic nervous system activation (the so-called fight-or-flight response), which increases the HR. The parasympathetic nervous system, in contrast, generally regulates organ functions that occur when the body is not acutely stressed (so-called rest-and-digest responses) but is also important in regulating the systemic inflammatory response.

Blood pressure and breathing impact HR and HRV through feedback systems. In the arterial baroreflex, an acute increase in blood pressure leads to decreased sympathetic and increased parasympathetic tone, with an associated decline in HR. Baroreflex sensitivity may be depressed in pathologic conditions such as congestive heart failure, leading to low HRV.[40] Respiratory sinus arrhythmia (RSA) is a normal reflex whereby HR increases during inhalation and decreases during exhalation. The basis of RSA is thought to be increased intrathoracic pressure as the lungs fill, causing decreased venous return to the heart. The decline in pressure in the right atrium leads to increased sympathetic and decreased parasympathetic output and a rise in HR, keeping cardiac output stable. On exhalation the process is reversed, leading to HR deceleration. Sepsis can impact respiratory rate and blood pressure, thereby indirectly altering HRV, but pathogens and inflammatory mediators also exert direct effects on adrenergic and cholinergic responses.[41,42]

The ANS not only regulates HR but also plays a critical role in host defense.[43] In the cholinergic anti-inflammatory response, vagus nerve activation leads to suppression of inflammatory cytokine release following binding of acetylcholine to nicotinic cholinergic receptors on leukocytes. The transient decelerations in HR seen in the course of sepsis and NEC may thus, at least in part, represent a protective parasympathetic nervous system response to pathogens or tissue damage.

Measurement of Heart Rate Variability Using Linear (Time and Frequency Domain) and Nonlinear Mathematical Methods

Research in complex physiologic systems has grown exponentially over the past several decades, leading to a more complete understanding of methods to analyze HRV.[44] Basic time series analysis involves measuring the standard deviation of interheartbeat (RR) intervals. After removing or replacing an artifact (e.g., noisy signal due to motion or loose leads), detection of R wave peaks in the QRS complex is performed. Ectopic or blocked beats are then discounted so that only normal RR intervals are analyzed. A frequently used measurement is therefore called SDNN, or standard deviation of normal-to-normal beats. Two other commonly used time domain measures are the root mean square of successive differences (RMSSD) and the proportion of intervals, which differ by more than 50 milliseconds from the prior interval (pNN50)[45] and can be an indicator of parasympathetic activity. Since neonates have a faster HR and shorter RR intervals than adults, pNN20 may be more appropriate than pNN50. HRV can also be assessed in terms of mathematical moments of probability,[46] including mean (first moment), variance (second moment), skewness (third moment), and kurtosis (fourth moment). Skewness and kurtosis both describe the shape of a probability distribution, where skewness measures the asymmetry and direction of the tails and kurtosis measures its sharpness or flatness. When considering a histogram of all HRs for an infant for a specific period of time, skewness and kurtosis can be used to assess the relative number and depth of decelerations compared with accelerations.

Frequency domain measurement of HRV may also be performed to quantify low- and high-frequency fluctuations, with the former related to sympathetic nervous system activity and the latter thought to primarily reflect parasympathetic (vagal) activity. Power spectrum analysis identifies dominant periodic variation in HR over time, thereby separating frequency components. Sympathetic HR activation occurs more slowly, in the range of about 0.04 to 0.15 Hz, or one cycle of increasing and decreasing HR every 7 to 25 seconds. Parasympathetic responses occur much faster, resulting in high-frequency HRV in the range of 0.15 to 0.4 Hz in adults, or one cycle of rise and fall in HR every 2.5 to 7 seconds. This corresponds to the frequency of respirations in adults and represents RSA, as described previously. While the presence of RSA reflected as high-frequency HRV is commonly used in adults to assess parasympathetic nervous system functioning, the evidence linking RSA to HRV in neonates is limited.[47–50] The rapid and irregular respiratory rate of neonates makes RSA analysis more complicated, with some studies using a frequency of 0.4 to 1 Hz (respiratory rate 24 to 60) for power spectrum analysis. If the respiratory rate is more than half the HR (e.g., RR 70 and HR 120), a phenomenon termed *cardiac aliasing* may occur, which leads to the inaccurate estimation of the magnitude of RSA contribution to HRV.[51,52]

In addition to the linear mathematical methods for time and frequency HRV analysis, nonlinear equations may also be used, which account for the nonstationarity of interbeat intervals.[44,53,54] One commonly used measure is detrended fluctuation analysis (DFA), which quantifies the magnitude of self-similarity or fractal-like correlation of interbeat intervals within a time series. This analysis calculates short- and long-term α values from RR-interval time series that represent a fractal scaling exponent.[55] DFA of HR or blood pressure time series data have been used to predict intraventricular hemorrhage (IVH) in preterm infants.[56,57] Various entropy measurements can also be used to assess HRV.[44] Sample entropy is a measurement related to approximate entropy that removes bias in short time series and was incorporated into the HRC index algorithm to account for both decreased variability and transient decelerations prior to neonatal sepsis.[58]

Developmental and Pathologic Factors Impacting Heart Rate Variability and Heart Rate Characteristics

Over the course of postnatal development, HR declines from about 150 beats per minute in preterm infants in the first week after birth to 135 beats per minute by 30 to

40 weeks of postmenstrual age (PMA),[59] and with this decline in baseline HR there may be increased beat-to-beat variability. In addition, an increase in HRV with postnatal development occurs due to a lag in maturation of the parasympathetic nervous system, with relatively higher sympathetic tone in the initial weeks after birth.[60] All components of the HRC index described later in this chapter (HRV, sample entropy, and sample asymmetry) have been found to change with increasing gestational and PMA,[29,61] likely reflecting both physiologic maturation and stabilization of the cardiorespiratory and other systems.[62]

Decreased HRV occurs in a number of acute or chronic disease processes across the age spectrum. In adults, low HRV has been associated with heart disease, renal failure, diabetes, smoking, brain injury, and sepsis.[40] HRV depression can have prognostic significance and has been linked to mortality and other adverse outcomes after myocardial infarction[63,64] in patients with chronic heart failure[65,66] and in patients with renal failure on hemodialysis.[67] In fetuses, good beat-to-beat variability is seen as reassuring, whereas low HRV is a sign of distress and may be associated with poor perfusion, acidosis, or a fetal systemic inflammatory response triggered by intrauterine infection. In preterm infants in the NICU, infection is an important cause of decreased HRV and abnormal HRC.

Tachycardia may occur in some neonates with sepsis due to sympathetic activation or hypovolemia but is not an ideal component of early warning systems, since it is usually a late sign associated with advanced illness. In the HRC monitor randomized controlled trial (RCT), HR was not higher within 24 hours of diagnosis of 488 cases of septicemia in 1489 VLBW infants, as compared with HR at other times during the NICU stay (159 vs. 160 beats per minute).[68] Another study of 1065 VLBW infants with 186 cases of septicemia or NEC also did not find higher HR in the 24-hour period before diagnosis compared with time periods without those illnesses (161 vs. 158 beats per minute).[69] More subtle changes in HR patterns must therefore be used in early warning algorithms.

Two elements of abnormal HRC in sepsis in preterm infants are decreased HRV and repetitive, transient decelerations. The decline in HRV is caused in part by elevated circulating levels of inflammatory cytokines. This was shown in a mouse model in which the administration of *Escherichia coli* lipopolysaccharide or a single cytokine, tumor necrosis factor alpha, led to reduced HRV.[41] Interleukin-6 elevation has also been linked to low HRV in both animal and human sepsis-like illnesses.[70,71] In both animal and human studies, administration of glucocorticoids has been shown to reduce cytokine levels and increase HRV.[43]

Transient HR decelerations in sepsis may be associated with apnea, or they may occur during regular breathing or on mechanical ventilation. Vagus nerve firing appears to be a major mechanism, and thus these transient decelerations may reflect activation of the cholinergic anti-inflammatory response.[43] In a mouse model, intraperitoneal injection of various bacterial or fungal pathogens very quickly led to repetitive, brief drops in HR during regular breathing.[42] These decelerations were terminated by atropine and associated with activation of vagal nuclei in the brainstem, demonstrating both afferent and efferent signaling in response to pathogens. In this mouse model, the repetitive decelerations did not recur on repeat injections of the same pathogen a few hours or even days after the initial injection, indicating that there was desensitization to the vagal stimulus.

Development of the Heart Rate Characteristics Index Monitor

Based on the observation of abnormal HRC in neonates with sepsis, a team of clinicians, mathematicians, and engineers at the University of Virginia, in partnership with a company, Medical Predictive Science Corporation, developed an HRC monitor (HeRO or *He*art *R*ate *O*bservation monitor) as an early warning system for neonatal sepsis. The idea was to detect subtle changes in HRC that occur in the hours or even days before an infant develops more obvious clinical signs of illness, prompting initiation of therapy. Earlier therapy could then, at least theoretically, avert worsening of the systemic inflammatory response and improve outcomes.

The challenge in developing the HRC index was to derive an algorithm that reflects more than decreased variability, since the transient decelerations observed in preterm infants with sepsis would inflate the HRV measurement toward a "healthy" level. Extensive work went into analysis of electrocardiogram data to develop a statistical model for prediction of sepsis incorporating measurements of HRV and transient decelerations.[72] Electrocardiography (ECG) data from day 7 after birth until NICU discharge were analyzed in 316 preterm infants, with 155 episodes of culture-positive sepsis or sepsis-like illness (culture-negative but treated with a full course of antibiotics due to a high clinical suspicion of sepsis). The ECG signal was analyzed in blocks of 4096 heartbeats (about 25 to 30 minutes of data) and then divided into 6-hour epochs for further analysis with summary statistics and clinical correlation. The 6-hour epoch including the sepsis event was not analyzed, since this period was considered likely to contain obvious clinical signs of illness. The 14-day period after diagnosis was also "blacked out," since this was considered a recovery period. The 6-hour epoch preceding the one with the sepsis or sepsis-like event was hypothesized to contain abnormal HRC, a preclinical signature of sepsis, and all other times during the NICU stay were considered "well." Multiple models were tested for the ability to distinguish sick from well ECG patterns, and the best predictive algorithm included weighted measurements of three HRC components:

1. Standard deviation of RR intervals
2. Sample asymmetry, which quantifies decelerations relative to accelerations[73]
3. Sample entropy, which describes the regularity of fluctuations[58]

The HRC index is the output of a logistic regression model using these measures and represents the fold-increased risk of sepsis being diagnosed in the subsequent 24 hours compared with the risk of sepsis at all times. The algorithm was externally validated on a similar number of infants at a second center and in both groups was highly associated with imminent diagnosis of sepsis.[72]

The HRC index monitor is connected to the standard bedside monitor and does not require extra connections to the infant. It captures the ECG signal and runs the HRC algorithm, and then averages the data from the previous 12 hours and displays an updated score every hour. The averaging step smoothes the score to minimize false-positive spikes related to transient, short-lived events that impact HR patterns. Fig. 20.2 shows three screenshots of the HRC index monitor showing normal HRC and two abnormal patterns with acute and chronic low variability and decelerations, resulting in a high HRC index.

It is important to note that although the HRC index (HeRO score) was designed for early *detection* of sepsis, it identifies HR patterns that *predict* imminent clinical deterioration. If, for example, the baseline risk for being diagnosed with sepsis for a preterm infant on any given day in the NICU is 2%, then a score of 3 indicates there is a 6% chance the infant will be diagnosed with suspected or proven sepsis at some point in the next 24 hours. Essentially, a rise in the score indicates that there is a physiologic change in the infant, and clinicians should consider whether that change might indicate an acute systemic inflammatory response due to infection, other illness, or nonspecific stimulus.

An important question in evaluating any new risk predictor such as the HRC index is whether it adds information beyond standard tools. In the case of neonatal sepsis, standard diagnosis involves evaluating clinical signs and laboratory tests. The HRC index was analyzed in comparison and in addition to abnormal laboratory tests (hyperglycemia, metabolic acidosis, a high or low leukocyte count, and elevated ratio of immature to total neutrophils) in 678 infants with 149 episodes of blood culture–proven sepsis.[74] From 6 to 24 hours prior to the positive blood culture, an HRC index above the 90th percentile had a higher odds ratio for septicemia than laboratory values, and logistic regression models showed that there was a significant additive value for sepsis prediction when the HRC index was added to laboratory values. Another study sought to determine whether HRC monitoring adds information to the conventional diagnosis of sepsis, using a combination of

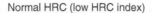

Normal HRC (low HRC index)

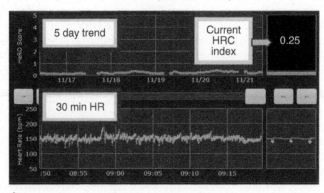

A

Acute HRC index spike

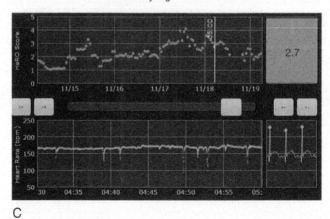

B

Chronically high HRC index

C

Fig. 20.2 **Heart rate characteristics (HRC) index monitor screenshots.** The individual patient display shows the 5-day trend in the HRC index, the last 30 minutes of heart rate (HR), and the current HRC index. There is also an option to scroll back in time to see earlier trends. (A) Normal HRC, with good variability and normal ratio of decelerations to accelerations, and a corresponding low HRC index. (B) Acute increase or "spike" in the HRC index. At the time indicated by the yellow arrow, the HRC index had increased from 1 to more than 3, and the corresponding 30 minutes HR tracing shows decreased variability with skewing of the HR to more and deeper decelerations and few accelerations. (C) Chronically high HRC index. In the previous 5 days the HRC index waxed and waned, increasing above 3 several times, with the corresponding HR tracing showing transient decelerations on a background of low variability. In addition to individual patient views, the HRC monitor has a "whole unit view" and a "pod view" that allows clinicians to see scores and trends for multiple patients at once.

clinical and laboratory signs.[75] A clinical score was developed, with points given for feeding intolerance, increased apnea, increased respiratory support, lethargy or hypotonia, temperature instability, hyperglycemia, low or high leukocyte count, or immature:total neutrophil ratio of greater than 0.2. Both the clinical score and the HRC index rose prior to sepsis diagnosis, and combining the two gave better predictive value than either value alone.

Does Heart Rate Characteristics Monitoring Improve Outcomes of Infants in the Neonatal Intensive Care Unit?

This question was addressed in a large, multicenter, randomized clinical trial in which 3003 VLBW infants at nine centers had their HRC index monitored.[76] After obtaining parental consent, the infants were randomized either to have their score displayed or not displayed to clinicians. Clinicians were educated about how the score was developed and instructed to evaluate infants whose scores were rising, but there was no mandated intervention for testing or treatment of infection. The primary outcome of days alive and not on mechanical ventilation in the 120 days after randomization was not significantly different in the display versus control infants. However, all-cause mortality, which was a secondary end point, was significantly reduced to 8.1% from 10.2% ($P = .04$). This 22% relative reduction in mortality translated to one extra survivor for 48 VLBW infants or 23 extremely low birth weight infants monitored. Slightly more blood cultures were obtained (1.8 per month vs. 1.6, $P = .05$) but there was no significant difference in total antibiotic days (15.7 days vs. 15.0, $P = .31$) in HRC display compared with control infants.

In a subanalysis of the 3003 VLBW infants in the RCT, there were 974 episodes of septicemia in 700 infants, and the incidence of septicemia was 23% in both the display and control groups.[38] Among the infants with septicemia, who were of significantly lower GA than those without, the number of total antibiotic days throughout the NICU stay was statistically significantly higher in the display versus control infants (32 vs. 29 days, $P = .047$). Mortality within 30 days of septicemia was 40% lower when the HRC index was displayed to clinicians (11.8% in the display group and 19.6% in the control group). An important question is whether the mortality reduction was due to earlier treatment, and this cannot be answered with certainty since the exact time that an infant becomes septicemic is unknown. To explore this question, an analysis of HRC index spikes was performed. Focusing on acute, large increases in the HRC index of 3 above the prior 5-day baseline, 34% of control infants had a spike in the week prior to diagnosis of septicemia, whereas only 22% of HRC index display infants had a prediagnosis spike ($P < .01$). This led to the hypothesis that some infants have a sepsis prodrome with abnormal HRC prior to overt deterioration, and treating in this phase of illness may lead to improved outcomes.

Can Other Adverse Events Be Predicted by the Heart Rate Characteristics Index?

A high HRC index during the NICU stay was shown to be associated with an increased risk of death within 7 days in a study of VLBW infants.[77] Another study found that the average HRC index in the first day after birth predicted the risk for death prior to NICU discharge and performed similarly for mortality prediction, compared with established illness severity scores SNAPPE-II and CRIB-II.[29] In this study, the average HRC index over the first week was also associated with risk of bronchopulmonary dysplasia (BPD) and late onset septicemia but was not predictive of NEC. The first-day HRC index was also significantly higher in infants with severe IVH, but whether this reflected IVH that had already occurred or identified a pattern associated with later development of IVH could not be determined. Several other studies have found that a high HRC index is associated with adverse neurologic outcomes. In 65 VLBW infants, a high cumulative HRC index throughout the NICU stay was associated with an increased risk of cerebral palsy and lower scores on the Bayley Scale of Infant Development-II at 12 to 18 months.[78] Another study focusing on extremely low birth weight infants found that the average HRC index in the first 28 days after birth was higher in infants with head ultrasound findings of grade III to IV IVH or cystic periventricular leukomalacia than in those with grade I to II IVH or normal head ultrasound.[79] Higher average HRC index also correlated with white matter injury in those infants with brain magnetic resonance imaging (MRI) and with death or Bayley motor or mental developmental index less than 70 in those with neurodevelopmental testing at 1 year of age.

Since depressed HRV reflects ANS dysfunction, the HRC index could be useful for estimating the severity of brain injury following an asphyxial event. In term infants undergoing hypothermia therapy for hypoxic ischemic encephalopathy, low HRV and a high HRC index in the first 24 hours after birth were associated with moderate to severe findings on electroencephalogram (EEG) and MRI.[61] HRV was also about 50% lower in infants who died compared with those who survived.

Another potential application of the HRC index is the prediction of respiratory failure in preterm infants in the NICU. In a study of 96 urgent, unplanned intubations in 51 infants, multiple physiologic parameters were tested and the HRC index was the best-performing individual predictor of intubation within the next 24 hours, with a receiver operating curve (ROC) area of 0.81.[50]

Limitations of the Heart Rate Characteristics Index

As illustrated in the previous section, the HRC index is not specific for sepsis. In a study of large spikes in the HRC index (3 above a 5-day baseline) with the score not displayed to clinicians, about half were associated with suspected or proven sepsis, urinary tract infection, or NEC. A third of these large spikes on a low baseline were associated with respiratory deterioration without suspected infection, and 14% had no apparent clinical correlate.[80] Of note, many infants with chronic illnesses have a chronically elevated or frequently spiking score, including infants with significant lung disease or severe IVH, and this is a significant confounding variable for use of the HRC index.

Since the HRC index was designed as a continuous risk indicator and was evaluated with predictiveness curves, diagnostic measures such as sensitivity and positive predictive accuracy of particular thresholds have not been formally studied.[76,81] In a randomized clinical trial of 3003 infants, 79% of the 974 cases of septicemia were associated with an HRC index greater than 2 in the 24 hours prior, but the positive predictive value of a score of 2 is very low, since it indicates the fold-increased risk in infants whose baseline risk on any given day is low. The low positive predictive value of the HRC index was demonstrated in a retrospective analysis at a single center over a 3-year period, in which 5% of infants with a score 2 or higher and 9% with a score 5 or higher had a bloodstream infection.[82] This highlights that clinician acumen is of paramount importance to assess the score in the context of other clinical risks, signs, and laboratory tests to avoid overuse of antibiotics.

Would Adding Clinical, Laboratory, or Biomarker Data Improve Predictive Algorithms?

The major risk predictor for sepsis and NEC is GA, and timing of these illnesses can be predicted by chronologic or PMA, with late-onset septicemia generally occurring at several weeks' chronologic age[38] and the timing of the occurrence of NEC being inversely related to GA at birth.[83] A predictive model including demographics (birth weight, GA, and postnatal age) and the HRC index for more than 600 infants at two centers had a higher ROC area for sepsis risk compared with either model alone.[72] Another study of 1065 VLBW infants reported that adding PMA to cardiorespiratory analysis substantially increased the ROC area for detection of septicemia or NEC.[69] Other demographic risk factors such as gender, race, and ethnicity appear to have only a small impact on risk for sepsis and NEC.[84] Clinical risk factors that increase the risk for septicemia and NEC and might be incorporated into predictive algorithms include the presence of an intravascular catheter, mechanical ventilation, and formula feeding.

Adding laboratory or biomarker tests may also improve the diagnostic utility of continuous physiomarker screening. Conventional laboratory tests including leukocyte count and immature:total neutrophil ratio were shown to have additive value when combined with the HRC index.[74] Multiple sepsis biomarkers have been tested, and C-reactive protein, which is readily available in most hospitals with short turnaround time, might serve as a good adjunct sepsis screen.[85] For example, when there is an acute worsening of the HRC index or other vital sign pattern but clinical data do not necessarily support testing and treating for infection, a serum C-reactive protein level might serve as a "tie-breaker" to assist in management decisions. However, serum cytokine testing has been shown to have better diagnostic value than CRP for detecting culture-positive sepsis.[86] In a study of 226 blood cultures obtained at the time of suspected sepsis in NICU patients with HRC index monitoring (including 33 positive cultures), a low interleukin 6 (IL-6) level had a strong association with a negative blood culture.[87] Cytokines may be useful biomarkers for NEC as well,[88] but cytokine testing is not currently available in most hospitals. Other sepsis and NEC biomarkers are under investigation and may assist in either prediction or detection of illness in ICU patients.[89-91] An important consideration in both physiomarker screening and biomarker testing is to balance sensitivity and specificity to avoid unnecessary testing or extra antibiotic therapy, which can have detrimental consequences.

The addition of demographic, clinical, or laboratory data into predictive algorithms makes the process more complicated, requiring either manual data entry or creation of a system for automated data transfer. An alternative is to present a vital sign-based score and allow clinicians to factor this in with other known risks and clinical and laboratory data to make decisions about further testing and therapies.

Would Adding Respiratory Analysis Improve Predictive Algorithms?

Preterm infants commonly have changes in respiratory rate during inflammatory illnesses such as sepsis and NEC. Tachypnea is a component of the systemic inflammatory response syndrome and is incorporated into a number of adult early warning scores for sepsis, including the quick Sepsis Organ Failure Assessment.[92] Preterm infants may also become tachypneic when septic, but even more common is an increase in central apnea, mediated at least in part by the release of prostaglandins[93] and inflammatory cytokines.[94] Since tachypnea and apnea are also common among healthy preterm infants, measuring a change in respiratory rate compared with an individual infant's prior baseline will be more useful than absolute values in predicting imminent clinical deterioration. There are a number of confounding variables for the analysis of respiratory rate in NICU patients. Impedance signals are used to detect breaths and contain significant artifact from motion, lead misplacement, and cardiac activity. Since healthy infants have irregular respirations and monitors capture very high and very low respiratory rates, frequent sampling and averaging would be necessary to detect true tachypnea. Also, many preterm infants have baseline tachypnea due to chronic lung disease, and an increase in respiratory rate may reflect an exacerbation of lung disease rather than sepsis. For these reasons, analysis of apnea is more likely to be a useful adjunct measurement in predictive algorithms.

Research in apnea of prematurity requires the analysis of large amounts of vital sign data over long periods of time. Recent developments in "big data science" have enabled research teams to collect, store, and analyze terabytes of continuously sampled bedside monitor waveform and vital sign data. The group at the University of Virginia that developed the HRC index monitor also developed an automated algorithm for analyzing the chest impedance and electrocardiogram waveforms and pulse oximeter data for episodes of very low amplitude signal accompanied by a drop in HR and oxygen saturation (apnea, bradycardia, desaturation [ABD] events).[95] One finding from this system, through the analysis of more than 1000 preterm infants during their entire NICU stay, is that about a third of preterm infants had a significant increase in ABD events in the day prior to diagnosis of septicemia (signs of sepsis and positive blood culture), compared with 2 days prior.[96] Periodic breathing, a normal breathing pattern in both preterm and term infants characterized by repetitive cycles of brief apneic pauses and fast breaths, also increased in the day prior to septicemia diagnosis in some infants.[97] Both apnea and periodic breathing also increased the day prior to NEC diagnosis. These findings suggest that combined cardiorespiratory algorithms may be superior to HR algorithms in early warning systems, and that these algorithms may perform better for infants not on mechanical ventilation.

Cardiorespiratory Interactions

Pauses in breathing of more than 10 seconds in duration often entrain a decline in HR and/or oxygen saturation. In periodic breathing, even shorter pauses in breathing may also entrain small decelerations and desaturations. These HR and arterial oxygen saturation (SpO_2) declines in periodic breathing are usually not deep enough to trigger bedside monitor alarms for bradycardia and desaturation, and even with longer central apnea events, HR and SpO_2 may not fall below alarm thresholds. New analyses would therefore be needed to identify subtle changes in cardiorespiratory patterns in the preclinical phase of sepsis. Another important consideration is how to distinguish physiologic from pathologic (sepsis-associated) apnea and periodic breathing. Research thus far indicates the difference has to do more with quantity rather than quality of the immature breathing patterns. Preterm infants can have very long central apnea events (>60 seconds with slow onset of bradycardia) in the absence of an acute illness,[98] whereas an acute increase in the *number* of ABD events or percentage of time spent in periodic breathing over an infant's prior baseline may occur in the early phases of sepsis or NEC.[96,97]

Since apnea analysis is complicated, the University of Virginia research group sought surrogate metrics to use in predictive algorithms. In a two-center study of 1065 VLBW infants, three vital signs (HR, RR, SpO_2) were analyzed for the entire NICU stay (131 infant-years' data), including in the 24 hours prior to the diagnosis of 186 cases of septicemia or NEC.[69] The mean and standard deviation of each vital sign and cross-correlation of all pairs of vital signs were analyzed. The mean HR was only slightly higher in the day prior to diagnosis, compared with all times (161 vs. 158 beats per minute), and there was no significant difference in mean respiratory rate (50 vs. 51 breaths per minute). The best single vital sign metric for distinguishing "sick" from "well" was a cross-correlation of HR-SpO_2. This is an indicator of co-trending of HR and SpO_2, allowing a lag time of up to 30 seconds, and can be measured using the XCorr function in MatLab (Mathworks, Natick, Massachusetts). The value for XCorr can be positive (signals moving in the same direction; e.g., deceleration-desaturation that may occur with apnea or periodic breathing) or negative (signals moving in opposite directions; e.g., tachycardia-desaturation that may occur during periods of agitation). A high (positive) XCorr-HR-SpO_2 was commonly associated with deceleration-desaturation, with a lag time of about 8 to 15 seconds, and was found to be associated with central apnea. To a lesser extent, high XCorr was associated with a high percentage of time spent in periodic breathing with dual entrainment of HR and SpO_2. Interestingly, some infants on ventilators had increased XCorr HR-SpO_2 in the hours leading up to the diagnosis of sepsis or NEC, indicating that this metric does not always correspond to central apnea and periodic breathing. Deceleration-desaturation episodes on mechanical ventilation may represent airway obstruction or vagus nerve activation, which can impact both HR and respiratory function and thus the contribution of the ventilated infant to pulmonary gas exchange.

Two other types of cardiorespiratory interactions that are more difficult to quantify in preterm infants are cardiorespiratory coupling (heartbeats synchronized to breaths) and cardioventilatory coupling (breaths synchronized to heartbeats). Cardiorespiratory coupling, also termed RSA, refers to an increase in HR during inhalation and decrease during exhalation, mediated by changes in sympathetic and parasympathetic balance (as discussed earlier). Although this has been demonstrated in both term and preterm infants, particularly during quiet sleep,[99,100] it is difficult to measure, due to the factors discussed in the section on HRV analysis. Cardioventilatory coupling is also difficult to quantify but appears to be present in preterm and term infants and to be dependent on sleep state and position.[101] Most studies on cardiorespiratory coupling and cardioventilatory coupling include a relatively small number of infants. However, in a study of 1202 NICU infants with chest impedance and ECG analyzed over the entire NICU stay, a breath-by-breath measure that analyzed the respiratory phase at which each heartbeat fell found evidence of cardiorespiratory interaction 18% of the time, which corresponded to some degree with cardioventilatory coupling but not with RSA.[102] Cardiorespiratory interactions increased over the course of postnatal development in the NICU but did not vary based on GA.

Pulse Oximetry-Based Algorithms: Are "Small Data" as Good as "Big Data"?

Pulse oximetry data on pulse rate and SpO_2 are generally measured every 1 to 2 seconds (0.5 to 1 Hz), compared with chest impedance and electrocardiogram waveform data recorded from multiple leads, which cumulatively amount to greater than 500 Hz. Since most centers do not have adequate computer storage or processing capacity for this degree of continuous "big data" analysis, efforts are under way to develop pulse oximetry-based algorithms for sepsis detection. These algorithms would be able to incorporate not only abnormal HRC (decreased variability and decelerations) but also cardiorespiratory interactions and SpO_2, which may provide clues to either risk for or presence of sepsis or NEC.[33,103] In the two-center study of vital signs of 1065 preterm infants referred to earlier in this chapter, in addition to the finding of rising cross-correlation of HR-SpO_2 prior to sepsis and NEC, mean SpO_2 was also significantly different in the "sick" versus "well" periods (91% vs. 94%).[69] The pulse oximetry signal also contains information that might correlate with perfusion, such as pulsatility index (PI) and plethysmography variability index (PVI). Limited evidence suggests that low or declining PI might indicate poor perfusion in preterm infants[104] and animal models,[105] but normative data are lacking, and there are insufficient data to support the use of PI to guide clinical care. PVI appears to be of some value in adults for determining volume status[106] but has not been shown to be of value in neonates.[107]

Other Systems for Predictive Monitoring in Infant and Adult Intensive Care Unit Patients

Several other systems are under development for the detection of sepsis in preterm infants in the NICU. A platform called Artemis, which analyzes multiple streams of NICU data using IBM InfoSphere Streams software, is undergoing testing in Canada.[108] Another software platform called RALIS (Integralis-Global, Israel) allows clinicians to input clinical and vital sign data every 2 hours, including body weight, temperature, HR, respiratory rate, and episodes of bradycardia and oxygen desaturation. From these variables a score is calculated from 0 to 10, with 5 considered a threshold for a possible diagnosis of sepsis.[109] Further testing on these and other early warning systems is needed to determine their impact on outcomes.

In adult ICU populations, vital sign pattern analysis is also being tested for its ability to predict sepsis and other adverse clinical events. One example is Continuous Individual Multiorgan Variability Analysis software, which can report on low HRV and respiratory rate variability associated with sepsis[110] and multiorgan dysfunction syndrome.[23] Another group developed TREWS (Targeted Real-time Early Warning Score) for septic shock in adult ICU patients.[111] Mining data from more than 16,000 patients in the MIMIC II Clinical Database, they used supervised machine learning on more than 50 vital sign and clinical parameters and developed an algorithm to predict septic shock, which occurred in 2200 patients. The TREWS algorithm had better sensitivity than an existing early warning system (MEWS, Modified Early Warning Score) and identified patients a median of 28 hours before the onset of shock.

Process of Developing Early Warning Systems

A great deal of work is involved in developing and testing early warning systems to improve patient outcomes. Generally the steps are as follows:

1. **Identify a clinical problem** for which early intervention might lead to improved outcomes. Sepsis and NEC are good examples in the NICU, since earlier administration of antibiotics, discontinuation of enteral feeding, closer monitoring of hemodynamic and respiratory status, and administration of intravenous fluids or medications to support blood pressure might lead to lower risk of mortality, organ dysfunction, and short- and long-term morbidities. Prediction of imminent respiratory failure requiring intubation or IVH are two other events for which predictive algorithms have been developed.[50,56] For these adverse events, it is less clear whether preventative interventions exist beyond the current standard of care for all preterm infants, or whether prediction will improve outcomes.

2. **Collect physiologic and clinical data** on a very large number of at-risk patients and annotate the date and time of the clinical event of interest. A large number of events are required for effective modeling, to account for individual variation in vital signs and illness presentation, and to avoid statistical problems such as overfitting. As a general rule, there should be at least 10 events for every variable included in the model.[112] Since sepsis and NEC occur in only about 15%[3] and 5% to 10%[6,7] of very low birthweight infants, respectively, having data on at least several hundred (ideally >1000) infants is required to develop robust predictive algorithms. Another important consideration is settling on a definition of the event. For the HRC index previously described, the algorithm was modeled on both clinical and culture-proven sepsis, whereas other studies have used blood culture-positive sepsis as the event of interest.[69] Another issue is determining which data periods to use as ill versus well for modeling; it is likely that detection at least 12 hours prior to overt clinical deterioration would be required to improve outcomes. Censoring out time periods in which potentially confounding medical interventions are present is another consideration for predictive modeling.[111] For example, preterm infants frequently have nonspecific clinical signs prompting "sepsis rule-outs" (several days of antibiotics with negative cultures), and including these periods in the "well" category for modeling may lead to lower diagnostic utility measures. Finally, removing artifact from the vital sign data is a critical step, and the methodology for this continues to evolve.[113]

3. **Have experienced clinicians inspect vital signs** in the hours and days leading up to the event to determine whether there are expected or unexpected cardiorespiratory patterns in individual infants or in groups of infants. Known sepsis-associated changes should be sought, such as tachycardia, tachypnea, and apnea with bradycardia and desaturation. Unexpected patterns may also be found in individual patients and then should be evaluated in healthy and sick time periods in the larger group. For example there might be a persistent decline in HR or SpO_2 compared with prior baseline, a change in respiratory rate variability, or in mechanically ventilated patients with ventilator data available, a decrease in patient-triggered breaths representing decreased respiratory drive that often accompanies bacterial or viral infection in preterm infants.[114]

4. **Have experienced data scientists** (computer scientists, engineers, mathematicians, and/or statisticians) **analyze vital sign data** using various approaches. Standard approaches include time series analyses and multivariate logistic regression. One disadvantage of logistic regression is that it will pick up monotonic relationships only, whereas some vital signs or laboratory changes are not one-directional. For example, respiratory rate, temperature, or white blood cell count may be high or low in sepsis. Newer statistical approaches include supervised or unsupervised machine learning methods. Often, both approaches yield similar results, but it is possible that machine learning methodologies will uncover novel pathologic patterns or combinations of data that lead to useful algorithms.

5. **Test models** of single and combined vital sign metrics for their ability to predict/detect illness in the hours and days prior to diagnosis. This involves deciding on

the time of onset of illness. For sepsis, the time of a positive blood culture might be used as "time zero," and for NEC, the time of an abdominal x-ray that led to diagnosis and initiation of therapy. Signs of illness may have been recognized hours before these events, but annotation of the time of first clinical suspicion is often not available in the medical record. For the HRC index, ECG data from the 6-hour period around the time of diagnosis was not included in algorithm development, on the assumption that clinicians might have already recognized signs of illness in those hours.

6. **Determine whether addition of demographic or laboratory data** improve on vital sign algorithms. Often, change in area under the ROC curve is used. The contribution of each variable to a model may be assessed by a Wald chi square statistic or likelihood ratio test.

7. **Internally and externally validate the algorithm** on patients from different centers. This is a key step since differences in patient populations or in clinical care practices between institutions may impact the diagnostic utility of a predictive algorithm. For example, target range for SpO_2, modes of respiratory support, and dosing of caffeine can impact SpO_2 and apnea, and algorithms that include these variables may have different performance in different NICUs.

8. **Compare performance of the new algorithm with existing scores or algorithms.** This can be done by determining the difference in ROC area or by calculating a Net Reclassification Improvement Index,[115] which is the fraction of cases correctly reclassified as having or not having the condition using the new test compared with an established test.

9. **Develop a method for real-time display** of the new prediction score. There is evidence that visual representation extending beyond conventional waveform display is more likely to have a positive impact on patient outcomes.[116] Web-based data streaming and analysis methodology, including use of virtual machines, has evolved and is likely to be part of future prediction systems rather than algorithms run on a local server.[117,118]

10. **Test the impact** of displaying the new score on important clinical outcomes in large multicenter randomized trials.

Challenges and Future Directions for Predictive Monitoring Research

Electronic Medical Record Alerts and Alarms

Most hospitals in the United States have implemented electronic medical records, which contain a wealth of patient data entered in near-real time. Sepsis alerts may be built into these systems, whereby clinicians are notified about abnormal vital signs such as high respiratory rate or low blood pressure, or laboratory values such as high serum lactate that may indicate sepsis. The goal of these systems is to direct clinicians to the right patient at the right time, on the assumption that earlier interventions for sepsis or other life-threatening conditions will improve outcomes. Based on prior research, an optimal early warning system for NICU patients is likely to include not simply vital sign thresholds but also more complex calculations of cardiorespiratory patterns, perhaps with the addition in real-time of laboratory values or biomarker test results.

A critical component in developing early warning systems is how best to alert clinicians to abnormal results for individual patients. Alarms are a double-edged sword in the ICU, since some may be life-saving but most are not, and caregivers are distracted and desensitized by noncritical alarms. The HRC index monitor that is Food and Drug Administration cleared for use in the United States does not have an alarm, whereas the same monitor European Conformity marked for use in Europe was required to include an alarm. A visual alarm was designed that activates when the HRC index rises above 2 and disappears when a caregiver clicks on it to acknowledge the score. Determining a threshold for an alarm is complicated from both a clinical and a regulatory perspective. On the clinical side, since vital sign changes in neonatal sepsis are nonspecific, selecting a threshold with high sensitivity will lead to a high false-positive rate. An alternative to setting an alarm is to consider the output of the algorithm as a continuous risk indicator, and to use a very high or rising score as an alert that clinicians should carefully evaluate a patient and determine whether a new action is required based on the whole clinical picture.

The Importance of Data Sharing

Research in predictive monitoring will progress much quicker if centers endeavor to share deidentified vital sign and clinical data so that other researchers can formulate or test hypotheses that might lead to better algorithms. Systems are already in place for some degree of data sharing through PhysioNet and the associated PhysioBank and PhysioToolkit.[119] These were developed under the auspices of the National Center for Research Resources, part of the National Institutes of Health. PhysioBank contains archived digital recordings of physiologic signals and clinical information collected by multiple research groups from both healthy individuals and chronically or acutely ill patients with a variety of conditions. PhysioNet (http://www.physionet.org) is an online forum for dissemination of the data to biomedical researchers, with PhysioToolkit providing open source analytic software and online tutorials available for registered users. Within PhysioNet, researchers can gain access to the MIMIC databases. MIMIC-II, first released in 2010 and named "Multiparameter Intelligent Monitoring in Intensive Care," was updated in 2016 to MIMIC-III and was renamed "Medical Information Mart for Intensive Care," to reflect a broadening of the scope of data available.[120] It contains vital sign, laboratory, and clinical data from more than 53,000 adults admitted to critical care units at Beth Israel Deaconess Hospital in Boston from 2001 to 2012, and also includes some data on 7870 neonates admitted from 2001 to 2008. These data are available for research or education through a data use agreement. Expanding the shared vital sign and clinical data from NICU patients, through PhysioNet or other means, is likely to enhance predictive algorithm development and validation.

Conclusion

The HRC index was designed as a tool to assist clinicians in identifying infants at high risk for imminent deterioration from sepsis. A key question is whether adding respiratory analysis to HR analysis will lead to algorithms with improved diagnostic utility. Another important question is whether vital sign patterns in the first few days after birth can predict which infants, among the inherently high-risk preterm population, are most likely to develop sepsis or NEC, so that these infants might receive targeted preventative therapies or heightened surveillance that may not be beneficial or practicable for the whole population. Finally, determining the best way to display and alert clinicians to a high or rising risk score in individual patients is essential to developing a system that might improve short- and long-term outcomes.

REFERENCES

1. Stoll BJ, Hansen N, Fanaroff AA, et al.: Late-onset sepsis in very low birth weight neonates: the experience of the NICHD Neonatal Research Network, *Pediatrics* 110(2):285–291, 2002.
2. Vergnano S, Menson E, Kennea N, et al.: Neonatal infections in England: the NeonIN surveillance network, *Arch Dis Child Fetal Neonatal Ed* 96(1):F9–F14, 2011.
3. Ting JY, Synnes A, Roberts A, et al.: Association between antibiotic use and neonatal mortality and morbidities in very low-birth-weight infants without culture-proven sepsis or necrotizing enterocolitis, *JAMA Pediatr* 117(6):1979–1987, 2016.
4. Schulman J, Stricof R, Stevens TP, et al.: Statewide NICU central-line-associated bloodstream infection rates decline after bundles and checklists, *Pediatrics* 127(3):436–444, 2011.
5. Patel AL, Johnson TJ, Engstrom JL, et al.: Impact of early human milk on sepsis and health-care costs in very low birth weight infants, *J Perinatol* 33(7):514–519, 2013.
6. Yee WH, Soraisham AS, Shah VS, et al.: Incidence and timing of presentation of necrotizing enterocolitis in preterm infants, *Pediatrics* 129(2):e298–e304, 2012.
7. Stoll BJ, Hansen NI, Bell EF, et al.: Neonatal outcomes of extremely preterm infants from the NICHD Neonatal Research Network, *Pediatrics* 126(3):443–456, 2010.
8. Ra W, Holman RC, Stoll BJ, et al.: The epidemiology of necrotizing enterocolitis infant mortality in the United States, *Am J Public Health* 87(12):2026–2031, 1997.

9. Hornik CP, Fort P, Clark RH, et al.: Early and late onset sepsis in very-low-birth-weight infants from a large group of neonatal intensive care units, *Early Hum Dev* 88(2):S69–S74, 2012.

10. Stoll B, Hansen N, Adams-Chapman I: Neurodevelopmental and growth impairment among extremely low-birth-weight infants with neonatal infection, *JAMA* 292:2357–2365, 2004.

11. Wheater M, Rennie JM: Perinatal infection is an important risk factor for cerebral palsy in very-low-birthweight infants, *Dev Med Child Neurol* 42(6):364–367, 2000.

12. Deguchi K, Mizuguchi M, Takashima S: Immunohistochemical expression of tumor necrosis factor alpha in neonatal leukomalacia, *Pediatr Neurol* 14(1):13–16, 1996.

13. Volpe JJ: Neurobiology of periventricular leukomalacia in the premature infant, *Pediatr Res* 50(5):553–562, 2001.

14. Duncan J, Cock M, Scheerlinck J, et al.: White matter injury after repeated endotoxin exposure in the preterm ovine fetus, *Pediatr Res* 52(6):941–949, 2002.

15. Inder T, Volpe J: Mechanisms of perinatal brain injury, *Semin Neonatol* 5(1):3–16, 2000.

16. O'Shea J, Ma A, Lipsky P: Cytokines and autoimmunity, *Nat Rev Immunol* 2(1):37–45, 2002.

17. Burrus DR, O'Shea Jr TM, Veille JC, et al.: The predictive value of intrapartum fetal heart rate abnormalities in the extremely premature infant, *Am J Obs Gynecol* 171(4):1128–1132, 1994.

18. Williams KP, Galerneau F: Intrapartum fetal heart rate patterns in the prediction of neonatal acidemia, *Am J Obs Gynecol* 188(3):820–823, 2003.

19. Parer JT, King T, Flanders S, et al.: Fetal acidemia and electronic fetal heart rate patterns: is there evidence of an association? *J Matern Neonatal Med* 19(5):289–294, 2006.

20. Stampalija T, Casati D, Monasta L, et al.: Brain sparing effect in growth-restricted fetuses is associated with decreased cardiac acceleration and deceleration capacities: a case-control study, *Br J Obstet Gynocol* 123(12):1947–1954, 2016.

21. Liu HL, Garzoni L, Herry C, et al.: Can monitoring fetal intestinal inflammation using heart rate variability analysis signal incipient necrotizing enterocolitis of the neonate? *Pediatr Crit Care Med* 17(4):e165–e176, 2016.

22. Chauhan SP, Klauser CK, Woodring TC, Sanderson M, Magann EF, Morrison JC: Intrapartum non-reassuring fetal heart rate tracing and prediction of adverse outcomes: interobserver variability, *Am J Obstet Gynecol* 199(6):623.e1–623.e5, 2008.

23. Frasch M, Xu Y, Stampalija T, et al.: Correlating multidimensional fetal heart rate variability analysis with acid-base balance at birth, *Physiol Meas* 35(12):L1–L12, 2014.

24. Behar J, Zhu T, Oster J, et al.: Evaluation of the fetal QT interval using non-invasive fetal ECG technology, *Physiol Meas* 37(9):1392, 2016.

25. Cao H, Lake DE, Ferguson JE, et al.: Toward quantitative fetal heart rate monitoring, *IEEE Trans Biomed Eng* 53(1):111–118, 2006.

26. Thorngren-Jerneck K, Herbst A: Low 5-minute Apgar score: a population-based register study of 1 million term births, *Obstet Gynecol* 98(1):65–70, 2001.

27. Richardson DK, Corcoran JD, Escobar GJ, et al.: SNAP-II and SNAPPE-II: simplified newborn illness severity and mortality risk scores, *J Pediatr* 138(1):92–100, 2001.

28. Parry G, Tucker J, Tarnow-Mordi W: CRIB II: an update of the clinical risk index for babies score, *Lancet* 361(9371):1789–1791, 2003.

29. Sullivan BA, McClure C, Hicks J, et al.: Early heart rate characteristics predict death and morbidities in preterm infants, *J Pediatr* 174:57–62, 2016.

30. Dorling JS, Field DJ, Manktelow B: Neonatal disease severity scoring systems, *Arch Dis Child Fetal Neonatal Ed* 90(1):F11–F16, 2005.

31. Lim L, Rozycki HJ: Postnatal SNAP-II scores in neonatal intensive care unit patients: relationship to sepsis, necrotizing enterocolitis, and death, *J Matern Neonatal Med* 21(6):415–419, 2008.

32. Meadow W, Frain L, Ren Y, et al.: Serial assessment of mortality in the neonatal intensive care unit by algorithm and intuition: certainty, uncertainty, and informed consent, *Pediatrics* 109(5):878–886, 2002.

33. Doheny KK, Palmer C, Browning KN, et al.: Diminished vagal tone is a predictive biomarker of necrotizing enterocolitis-risk in preterm infants, *Neurogastroenterol Motil* 26(6):832–840, 2014.

34. Saria S, Rajani AK, Gould J, et al.: Integration of early physiological responses predicts later illness severity in preterm infants, *Sci Transl Med* 2(48):48ra65, 2010.

35. Gagliardi L, Cavazza A, Brunelli A, et al.: Assessing mortality risk in very low birthweight infants: a comparison of CRIB, CRIB-II, and SNAPPE-II, *Arch Dis Child Fetal Neonatal Ed* 89(5):F419–F422, 2004.

36. Buchan CA, Bravi A, Seely AJE: Variability analysis and the diagnosis, management, and treatment of sepsis, *Curr Infect Dis Rep* 14(5):512–521, 2012.

37. Sullivan BA, Fairchild KD: Predictive monitoring for sepsis and necrotizing enterocolitis to prevent shock, *Semin Fetal Neonatal Med* 20:255–261, 2015.

38. Fairchild K, Shelonka R, Kaufman D, et al.: Septicemia mortality reduction in neonates in a heart rate characteristics monitoring trial, *Pediatr Res* 74(5):570–575, 2013.

39. Fairchild KD, O'Shea TM: Heart rate characteristics: physiomarkers for detection of late-onset neonatal sepsis, *Clin Perinatol* 37(3):581–598, 2010.

40. Rajendra AU, Paul Joseph K, Kannathal N, et al.: Heart rate variability: a review, *Med Biol Eng Comput* 44(12):1031–1051, 2006.

41. Fairchild KD, Saucerman JJ, Raynor LL, et al.: Endotoxin depresses heart rate variability in mice: cytokine and steroid effects, *Am J Physiol Regul Integr Comp Physiol* 297(4):R1019–R1027, 2009.

42. Fairchild KD, Srinivasan V, Moorman JR: Gaykema RP a, Goehler LE. Pathogen-induced heart rate changes associated with cholinergic nervous system activation, *Am J Physiol Regul Integr Comp Physiol* 300(2):R330–R339, 2011.

43. Huston J, Tracey K: The pulse of inflammation- heart rate variability the cholinergic anti inflammatory pathway and immplications for therapy 2011, *J Intern Med* 269(1):45–53, 2011.

44. Bravi A, Longtin A, Seely AJ: Review and classification of variability analysis techniques with clinical applications, *Biomed Eng Online* 10(1):90, 2011.

45. Camm A, Malik M, Bigger J, et al.: Heart rate variability: Standards of measurement, physiological interpretation, and clinical use, *Eur Heart J* 17(5):354–381, 1996.

46. Griffin MP, Moorman JR: Toward the early diagnosis of neonatal sepsis and sepsis-like illness using novel heart rate analysis, *Pediatrics* 107(1):97–104, 2001.

47. Thompson CR, Brown JS, Gee H, Taylor EW: Heart rate variability in healthy term newborns: the contribution of respiratory sinus arrhythmia, *Early Hum Dev* 31(3):217–228, 1993.

48. Dykes FD, Ahmann PA, Baldzer K, et al.: Breath amplitude modulation of heart rate variability in normal full term neonates, *Pediatr Res* 20(4):301–308, 1986.

49. Divon MY, Winkler H, Yeh SY, et al.: Diminished respiratory sinus arrhythmia in asphyxiated term infants, *Am J Obstet Gynecol* 155(6):1263–1266, 1986.

50. Clark MT, Vergales BD, Paget-Brown AO, et al.: Predictive monitoring for respiratory decompensation leading to urgent unplanned intubation in the neonatal intensive care unit, *Pediatr Res* 73(1):104–110, 2013.

51. Chang KL, Monahan KJ, Griffin MP, et al.: Comparison and clinical application of frequency domain methods in analysis of neonatal heart rate time series, *Ann Biomed Eng* 29(9):764–774, 2001.

52. Rother M, Witte H, Zwiener U, et al.: Cardiac aliasing—a possible cause for the misinterpretation of cardiorespirographic data in neonates, *Early Hum Dev* 20(1):1–12, 1989.

53. Voss A, Schroeder R, Vallverdu M, et al.: Linear and nonlinear heart rate variability risk stratification in heart failure patients, *2008 Comput Cardiol* 557–560, 2008.

54. Lin C-W, Wang J-S, Chung P-C: Mining physiological conditions from heart rate variability analysis, *IEEE Comput Intell Mag* 5:50–58, 2010.

55. Peña MA, Echeverría JC, García MT, et al.: Applying fractal analysis to short sets of heart rate variability data, *Med Biol Eng Comput* 47(7):709–717, 2009.

56. Tuzcu V, Nas S, Ulusar U, et al.: Altered heart rhythm dynamics in very low birth weight infants with impending intraventricular hemorrhage, *Pediatrics* 123(3):810–815, 2009.

57. Zhang Y, Chan GSH, Tracy MB, et al.: Detrended fluctuation analysis of blood pressure in preterm infants with intraventricular hemorrhage, *Med Biol Eng Comput* 51:1051–1057, 2013.

58. Lake DE, Richman JS, Griffin MP, et al.: Sample entropy analysis of neonatal heart rate variability, *Am J Physio Regul Integr Comp Physiol* 283(3):789–797, 2002.

59. Chatow U, Davidson S, Reichman BL, et al.: Development and maturation of the autonomic nervous system in premature and full-term infants using spectral analysis of heart rate fluctuations, *Pediatr Res* 37(3):294–302, 1995.

60. Mazursky J, Birkett C, Bedell K, et al.: Development of baroreflex influences on heart rate variabilty in preterm infants, *Early Hum Dev* 53(1):37–52, 1998.

61. Vergales BD, Zanelli S, Matsumoto J, et al.: Depressed heart rate variability is associated with abnormal EEG, MRI, and death in neonates with hypoxic ischemic encephalopathy, *Am J Perinatol* 31(10):855–862, 2013.

62. Griffin MP, O'Shea TM, Bissonette EA, et al.: Abnormal heart rate characteristics are associated with neonatal mortality, *Pediatr Res* 55(5):782–788, 2004.

63. Kleiger RE, Miller JP, Bigger Jr JT, et al.: Decreased heart rate variability and its association with increased mortality after acute myocardial infarction, *Am J Cardiol* 59(4):256–262, 1987.

64. Tsuji H, Larson MG, Venditti Jr FJ, et al.: Impact of reduced heart rate variability on risk for cardiac events. The Framingham Heart Study, *Circulation* 94(11):2850–2855, 1996.

65. La Rovere MT, Bigger Jr JT, Marcus FI, et al.: Baroreflex sensitivity and heart-rate variabiltiy in prediction of total cardiac mortality after myocardial infarction, *Lancet* 351(9101):478–484, 1998.

66. Sandercock GRH, Brodie DA: The role of heart rate variability in prognosis for different modes of death in chronic heart failure, *Pacing Clin Electrophysiol* 29(8):892–904, 2006.

67. Oikawa K, Ishihara R, Maeda T, et al.: Prognostic value of heart rate variability in patients with renal failure on hemodialysis, *Int J Cardiol* 32(6):516–520, 2008.

68. Lake DE, Fairchild KD: Reply: heart rate predicts sepsis, *J Pediatr* 161(4):770–771, 2012.

69. Fairchild K, Lake D, Kattwinkel J, et al.: Vital signs and their cross-correlation in sepsis and NEC: a study of 1065 very low birth weight infants in two NICUs, *Pediatr Res*, 2016.

70. Durosier LD, Herry CL, Cortes M, et al.: Does heart rate variability reflect the systemic inflammatory response in a fetal sheep model of lipopolysaccharide-induced sepsis? *Physiol Meas* 36(10):2089–2102, 2015.

71. Kuwaki T, Moriguchi T, Hirasawa H: Depress heart rate variability is associated with high IL-6 blood level and decline in the blood pressure in septic patients, *Crit Care* 28(5):549–553, 2007.

72. Griffin MP, O'Shea TM, Bissonette EA, et al.: Abnormal heart rate characteristics preceding neonatal sepsis and sepsis-like illness, *Pediatr Res* 53(6):920–926, 2003.

73. Kovatchev BP, Farhy LS, Cao H, et al.: Sample asymmetry analysis of heart rate characteristics with application to neonatal sepsis and systemic inflammatory response syndrome, *Pediatr Res* 54(6):892–898, 2003.

74. Griffin M, Lake D, Moorman J: Heart rate characteristics and laboratory tests in neonatal sepsis, *Pediatrics* 115(4):937–941, 2005.

75. Griffin MP, Lake DE, O'Shea TM, et al.: Heart rate characteristics and clinical signs in neonatal sepsis, *Pediatr Res* 61:222–227, 2007.

76. Moorman JR, Carlo WA, Kattwinkel J, et al.: Mortality reduction by heart rate characteristic monitoring in very low birth weight neonates: a randomized trial, *J Pediatr* 159(6):900.e1–906.e1, 2011.

77. Griffin MP, Lake DE, Bissonette EA, et al.: Heart rate characteristics: novel physiomarkers to predict neonatal infection and death, *Pediatrics* 116(5):1070–1074, 2005.

78. Addison K, Griffin MP, Moorman JR, et al.: Heart rate characteristics and neurodevelopmental outcome in very low birth weight infants, *J Perinatol* 29(11):750–756, 2009.

79. Fairchild KD, Sinkin RA, Davalian F, et al.: Abnormal heart rate characteristics are associated with abnormal neuroimaging and outcomes in extremely low birth weight infants, *J Perinatol* 34(5): 375–379, 2014.

80. Sullivan BA, Grice SM, Lake DE, et al.: Infection and other clinical correlates of abnormal heart rate characteristics in preterm infants, *J Pediatr* 164(4):775–780, 2014.

81. Pepe MS, Feng Z, Huang Y, et al.: Integrating the predictiveness of a marker with its performance as a classifier, *Am J Epidemiol* 167(3):362–368, 2008.

82. Coggins SA, Weitkamp J-H, Grunwald L, et al.: Heart rate characteristic index monitoring for bloodstream infection in an NICU: a 3-year experience, *Arch Dis Child Fetal Neonatal Ed* 101(4):F329–F332, 2016.

83. Stone ML, Tatum PM, Weitkamp J-H, et al.: Abnormal heart rate characteristics before clinical diagnosis of necrotizing enterocolitis, *J Perinatol* 33(11):847–850, 2013.

84. Seeman SM, Mehal JM, Haberling DL, et al.: Infant and maternal risk factors related to necrotising enterocolitis-associated infant death in the United States, *Acta Paediatr Int J Paediatr* 105(6):e240–e246, 2016.

85. Weitkamp J-H, Aschner JL: Diagnostic Use of C-reactive protein (CRP) in assessment of neonatal sepsis, *Neoreviews* 6(11):e508–e515, 2005.

86. Zhou M, Cheng S, Yu J, Lu Q: Interleukin-8 for diagnosis of neonatal sepsis: a meta-analysis, *PLoS One* 10(5), 2015.

87. Raynor LL, Saucerman JJ, Akinola MO, et al.: Cytokine screening identifies NICU patients with Gram-negative bacteremia, *Pediatr Res* 71(3):261–266, 2012.

88. Maheshwari A, Schelonka R, Dimmitt R: Cytokines associated with necrotizing enterocolitis in extremely-low-birth-weight infants, *Pediatr Res* 76(1):100–108, 2014.

89. Ng PC, Lam HS: Diagnostic markers for neonatal sepsis, *Curr Opin Pediatr* 18(2):125–131, 2006.

90. Skibsted S, Jones AE, Puskarich MA, et al.: Biomarkers of endothelial cell activation in early sepsis, *Shock* 39(5):427–432, 2013.

91. Berkhout DJC, Niemarkt HJ, Buijck M, et al.: Detection of sepsis in preterm infants by fecal volatile organic compounds analysis: a proof of principle study, *J Pediatr Gastroenterol Nutr*, 2016.

92. Seymour CW, Liu VX, Iwashyna TJ, et al.: Assessment of clinical criteria for sepsis: for the Third International Consensus Definitions for Sepsis and Septic Shock (Sepsis-3), *J Am Med Assoc* 315(8):762–774, 2016.

93. Siljehav V, Olsson Hofstetter A, Jakobsson P-J, et al.: mPGES-1 and prostaglandin E2: vital role in inflammation, hypoxic response, and survival, *Pediatr Res* 72(5):460–467, 2012.

94. Jafri A, Belkadi A, Zaidi SIA, et al.: Lung inflammation induces IL-1 expression in hypoglossal neurons in rat brainstem, *Respir Physiol Neurobiol* 188(1):21–28, 2013.

95. Lee H, Rusin CG, Lake DE, et al.: A new algorithm for detecting central apnea in neonates, *Physiol Meas* 33(1):1–17, 2012.

96. Fairchild K, Mohr M, Paget-Brown A, et al.: Clinical associations of immature breathing in preterm infants: part 1—central apnea, *Pediatr Res* 80(1):21–27, 2016.

97. Patel M, Mohr M, Lake D, et al.: Clinical associations with immature breathing in preterm infants. part 2: periodic breathing, *Pediatr Res*, 2016.

98. Mohr M, Vergales B, Lee H, et al.: Very long apnea events in preterm infants, *J Appl Physiol* 118(5):558–568, 2015.

99. Hathorn MK: The rate and depth of breathing in new-born infants in different sleep states, *J Physiol* 243(1):101–113, 1974.

100. Hathorn MKS: Respiratory modulation of heart rate in newborn infants, *Early Hum Dev* 20(2):81–99, 1989.

101. Elder DE, Larsen PD, Galletly DC, et al.: Cardioventilatory coupling in preterm and term infants: effect of position and sleep state, *Respir Physiol Neurobiol* 174(1–2):128–134, 2010.

102. Clark MT, Rusin CG, Hudson JL, et al.: Breath-by-breath analysis of cardiorespiratory interaction for quantifying developmental maturity in premature infants, *J Appl Physiol* 112(5):859–867, 2012.

103. Askie LM, Brocklehurst P, Darlow BA, et al.: NeOProM: Neonatal Oxygenation Prospective Meta-analysis Collaboration study protocol, *BMC Pediatr* 11(1):6, 2011.

104. De Felice C, Goldstein MR, Parrini S, et al.: Early dynamic changes in pulse oximetry signals in preterm newborns with histologic chorioamnionitis, *Pediatr Crit Care Med* 7(2):138–142, 2006.

105. Hummler HD, Engelmann A, Pohlandt F, et al.: Decreased accuracy of pulse oximetry measurements during low perfusion caused by sepsis: is the perfusion index of any value? *Intensive Care Med* 32(9):1428–1431, 2006.

20

106. Forget P, Lois F, De Kock M: Goal-directed fluid management based on the pulse oximeter-derived pleth variability index reduces lactate levels and improves fluid management, *Anesth Analg* 111(4):910–914, 2010.
107. Sahni R: Noninvasive monitoring by photoplethysmography, *Clin Perinatol* 39(3):573–583, 2012.
108. McGregor C, Catley C, James A, et al.: Next generation neonatal health informatics with artemis. In *Studies in Health Technology and Informatics*, 2011, pp 115–119, vol. 169.
109. Gur I, Riskin A, Markel G, et al.: Pilot study of a new mathematical algorithm for early detection of late-onset sepsis in very low-birth-weight infants, *Am J Perinatol* 32(4):321–330, 2015.
110. Bravi A, Green G, Longtin AA, et al.: Monitoring and identification of sepsis development through a composite measure of heart rate variability, *PLoS One* 7(9):e45666, 2012.
111. Henry KE, Hager DN, Pronovost PJ, et al.: A targeted real-time early warning score (TREWScore) for septic shock, *Sci Transl Med* 7(299):299ra122, 2015.
112. Peduzzi P, Concato J, Feinstein AR, et al.: Importance of events per independent variable in proportional hazards regression analysis II. Accuracy and precision of regression estimates, *J Clin Epidemiol* 48(12):1503–1510, 1995.
113. Hravnak M, Chen L, Dubrawski A, et al.: Real alerts and artifact classification in archived multi-signal vital sign monitoring data: implications for mining big data, *J Clin Monit Comput* 30(6):875–888, 2016.
114. Firestone KS, Beck J, Stein H: Neurally adjusted ventilatory assist for noninvasive support in neonates, *Clin Perinatol* 43(4):707–724, 2016.
115. Pencina M, D'Agostino R, Steyerberg E: Extensions of net reclassification improvement calculations to measure usefulness of new biomarkers, *Stat Med* 30(1):11–21, 2011.
116. Kamaleswaran R, McGregor C: A review of visual representations of physiologic data, *JMIR Med informatics* 4(4):e31, 2016.
117. Dieterich JM, Hartke B: Error-safe, portable, and efficient evolutionary algorithms implementation with high scalability, *J Chem Theory Comput* 12(10):5226–5233, 2016.
118. Xiao M, Jiang G, Cao J, Zheng W: *Local Bifurcation analysis of a delayed fractional-order dynamic mdel of dual congestion control algorithms*, IEEE, 2016.
119. Goldberger AL, Amaral LA, Glass L, et al.: PhysioBank, PhysioToolkit, and PhysioNet: components of a new research resource for complex physiologic signals, *Circulation* 101(23):E215–E220, 2000.
120. Johnson AEW, Pollard TJ, Shen L, et al.: MIMIC-III, a freely accessible critical care database, *Sci Data* 3:160035, 2016.

CHAPTER 21

Comprehensive, Real-Time Hemodynamic Monitoring and Data Acquisition: An Essential Component of the Development of Individualized Neonatal Intensive Care

Timur Azhibekov, Sadaf Soleymani, Willem-Pieter de Boode, Shahab Noori, and Istvan Seri

21

- Accurate assessment of the hemodynamic status in critically ill neonates requires blood pressure measurements to be interpreted in the context of indirect (clinical signs) and direct (measurements and assessments) indicators of systemic circulation (cardiac output) and regional organ blood flow.

- Further validation of emerging technological approaches to evaluate systemic circulation and regional blood flow in a continuous and noninvasive manner is necessary.

- Comprehensive monitoring systems allow continuous and simultaneous collection of physiologic data on multiple hemodynamic parameters in real time. Inclusion of a motion-activated video-recording device enables analyzing objectively collected information in the context of the various clinical events taking place at the bedside.

- Addition of the modules to assess functional status of a given organ allows correlation of the hemodynamic changes with functional activity of the interrogated organ (with a primary focus on the brain).

- In a neonate, complex physiologic interactions such as baroreceptor reflex sensitivity, an indicator of the autonomic control of the circulation (heart and peripheral vascular resistance), and cerebral autoregulation can be reliably evaluated only using comprehensive monitoring systems.

- Computational modeling using large amounts of the physiometric data obtained is the next step in identifying physiologic trends that predict the development of cardiovascular compromise. The development of algorithms then enables timely application of pathophysiology- and evidence-based interventions.

- Relevant genetic information obtained via genome sequencing coupled with physiometric data may allow further stratification of patient subpopulations based on their individual risk of developing cardiovascular compromise and subsequent complications, such as periventricular/intraventricular hemorrhage, and allows prediction of the potential response to particular interventions. This approach will serve as the foundation of the development of individualized medicine in neonatology.

Recent advances in biomedical research and technology have allowed clinicians to obtain significantly more clinically relevant physiologic, biochemical, and genetic information that could be useful in the diagnosis and management of various conditions. It is fair to state that neonatology has become one of the rapidly evolving subspecialties at the frontier of this progress. However, the field of neonatal hemo-dynamics, although being extensively investigated in basic and animal laboratory and clinical research settings, remains inadequately understood. Accordingly, we continue to have difficulties in establishing reliable criteria for the diagnosis of the most common deviations from physiology, such as neonatal hypotension, especially during the period of immediate postnatal transition. This, in turn, leads to a paucity of established, evidence-based guidelines on when and how to intervene in a neonate presenting with these conditions.[1] Thus we must recognize the significant limitations of our current understanding of a number of clinically relevant aspects of neonatal cardiovascular physiology and pathophysiology and acknowledge the existing vast differences in opinions on diagnostic criteria and treatment approaches in neonatal intensive care in general and neonatal cardiovascular pathophysiology in particular.

The next logical step in identifying individual patients with early signs of hemo-dynamic compromise is to develop and implement comprehensive hemodynamic monitoring systems that enable continuous and real-time monitoring and acquisi-tion of multiple hemodynamic parameters of systemic and regional blood flow and oxygen demand-delivery coupling. The information obtained can then be used to design and execute clinical trials in subpopulations of neonates exhibiting common hemodynamic features and targeted by a given intervention. Only this approach will enable timely identification of the individual patient in the future in whom a trial-tested, individualized management plan can be used and the response to the patho-physiology- and evidence-based interventions monitored.

Limitations of Conventional Monitoring

Multiple studies have shown an association between severe cardiovascular compro-mise and increased morbidity and mortality in affected patients.[2-6] Although there is some evidence for improved outcome in hypotensive preterm infants responding to vasopressor-inotropes with increases in blood pressure and cerebral blood flow,[7,8] essentially none of the suggested interventions or medications used (dopamine, epi-nephrine, dobutamine, milrinone, or vasopressin) has been properly studied to deter-mine the actual impact of the treatment on clinically relevant medium- and long-term outcomes.[9-13]

The failure to identify effective interventions for the treatment of neonatal hemo-dynamic compromise stems from several unresolved challenges. The cardiovascular system of the newborn undergoes rapid changes during transition to extrauterine life, and these changes are greatly affected by multiple intrinsic and extrinsic factors. Such factors include, but are not limited to, individual variations in the degree of immaturity based on gestational and postnatal age, coexisting comorbidities includ-ing the need for positive pressure ventilation, the complex interactions between sys-temic and regional blood flow, and underlying genetic heterogeneity.

Another fundamental challenge is the lack of a pathophysiology- and evidence-based definition of neonatal hypotension (see Chapters 1 and 3). Measurements of blood pressure with or without the use of indirect clinical indicators of perfusion remain the major criterion in the assessment of the hemodynamic status and the need for interventions.[13-15] Normative blood pressure values in preterm and term infants have been reported in population-based studies, and mean arterial blood pressure increases with increasing gestational and postnatal age (see Chapter 3).[16,17] However, blood pressure within the normal range for a given gestational and postna-tal age does not necessarily reflect normal organ blood flow. And, similarly, abnor-mally low blood pressure values do not automatically translate into compromised organ blood flow (see Chapters 1 and 3). So, for patients of the same gestational age and degree of maturity, the same blood pressure values can be associated with either adequate or compromised systemic and organ perfusion. More so, even for the same patient under different conditions and points in time, the same blood pres-sure values may represent adequate or compromised systemic and/or organ perfu-sion. The reason for such significant limitations of using the blood pressure alone as an indicator of hemodynamic compromise lies in the fact that blood pressure is determined by the interaction between systemic blood flow represented by effective cardiac output (CO) and systemic vascular resistance. Thus the same values of blood pressure, the dependent variable, can result from different combinations of the other two, independent, variables. In the early, compensated phase of shock, blood pressure remains within the normal range, whereas nonvital organ perfusion has, by definition, decreased. Because many pathophysiologic mechanisms may lead to inadequate organ blood flow, whether they affect effective CO, systemic vascular resistance, or both, failure to recognize these changes leads to delay in initiation of treatment, exhaustion of limited compensatory mechanisms, and a resultant progression to the uncompensated phase of shock with obvious signs of decreased organ perfusion and oxygen delivery. On the other hand, unnecessary treatment might also be started if the condition is thought to have reached the treatment threshold when, in reality, systemic and/or regional blood flow is maintained. In addition, identification of the primary pathophysiologic mechanism that could prompt appropriately targeted intervention becomes significantly more challenging when reliable information on the status of the macrocirculation and/or tissue oxygen delivery is not readily available.

Other conventional hemodynamic parameters (heart rate and SpO_2), even if continuously monitored along with blood pressure, as well as capillary refill time, urine output, and serum lactate levels, have significant limitations for timely and accurate assessment of both the cardiovascular status and the response to interventions aimed to treat the hemodynamic compromise. Therefore inclusion of targeted assessment of systemic blood flow and regional organ perfusion becomes paramount to overcome these limitations and identify at-risk patients in a timely manner and intervene appropriately.

Assessment of Systemic and Regional Blood Flow

Systemic Blood Flow

The essential component in bedside assessment of systemic perfusion is measurement of CO. Several diagnostic modalities are available for such measurements, with functional cardiac magnetic resonance imaging (*fc*MRI) being now considered a "gold standard." However, several factors, such as the need for expensive equipment, highly trained personnel, sedation, and transportation of the patient to MRI suite, as well as its noncontinuous nature, limit the use of *fc*MRI for routine bedside assessment.[18] Accordingly, *fc*MRI remains mostly used in research settings (see Chapter 15).

Bedside functional echocardiography (*f*ECHO) offers noninvasive, real-time, yet noncontinuous, assessment of CO in addition to other important parameters such as myocardial contractility, estimates of preload and afterload, etc. (see Chapters 10, 11, 12, and 13). Precision of *f*ECHO is within the acceptable range for technology used for clinical applications and is approximately 30%.[19] It has increasingly become an integral part of routine bedside neonatal assessment[20-22]; however, to ensure accurate and reliable measurements, it requires appropriate training and sufficient practice.[23,24] More so, a number of important limitations of *f*ECHO need to be accounted for when assessment of systemic circulation is performed at the bedside. Unlike in older children and adults when left ventricular output (LVO) can be used as a surrogate of systemic blood flow with confidence, transitional changes of the cardiovascular system in a neonate may significantly affect LVO because it will no longer represent only systemic blood flow. For example, in the presence of a hemodynamically significant patent ductus arteriosus (*hs*PDA) when substantial left-to-right shunting takes place, the resultant increase in LVO represents both systemic and ductal (pulmonary) blood flow. Relying on LVO in such cases will lead to significant overestimation of systemic blood flow that can, in reality, be either within the normal range or decreased. Right ventricular output (RVO) has also been suggested for assessment of systemic perfusion. However, with significant left atrial overload from pulmonary overcirculation in the presence of a *hs*PDA, left-to-right atrial shunting via the patent foramen ovale (PFO) will result in an increased RVO.[25,26]

Thus RVO in such cases reflects both systemic venous return and transatrial left-to-right flow through the PFO. Alternatively, superior vena cava (SVC) flow, which is not affected by the presence of either interatrial or transductal shunts, has been studied and proposed as a surrogate of systemic perfusion.[27] Although not without its own limitations, decreased SVC flow has been associated with adverse short- and long-term outcomes.[2,4] Finally and of utmost importance, in any situation when congenital heart disease is suspected clinically or has been prenatally diagnosed, a formal echocardiographic evaluation must be performed and interpreted by a pediatric cardiologist.

Impedance electrical cardiometry (IEC) enables continuous and noninvasive assessment of CO using the changes in thoracic bioimpedance during the cardiac cycle (see Chapter 14). Beat-to-beat measurements of stroke volume (SV) and CO have been validated in term neonates without cardiovascular compromise,[28] as well as in preterm neonates, including those requiring low-dose inotropic support and/or mechanical ventilation.[29-31] The reported precision of the method was similar to that of fECHO (approximately 30%). Preliminary normative data for CO measured by IEC in both preterm and term neonates,[31,32] and the effects of PDA ligation on systemic perfusion,[33] have also been published. However, in all three studies,[31-33] CO data collection was noncontinuous.

Another, similar noninvasive technique of continuous monitoring of CO in preterm and term neonates has been studied recently.[34,35] To measure CO, this technique uses the changes in bioreactance (i.e., electrical capacitive and inductive properties of the thorax) as reflected by the relative phase shift of an injected current.[36] However, based on the consistent underestimation of LVO,[34,35] the wide limits of agreement, and the increasing bias over time with continuous use,[35] this technique seems to be inferior to fECHO in its current form.

Organ Blood Flow

Near-infrared spectroscopy (NIRS) uses the principle of the different absorbency patterns of near-infrared light by oxyhemoglobin and deoxyhemoglobin to measure tissue oxygenation index or regional tissue oxygen saturation (rSO_2) (see Chapters 17 and 18). Thus NIRS also provides information on tissue oxygen extraction in vital and nonvital organs. Therefore it allows the *indirect* assessment of organ blood flow noninvasively and in a continuous manner. Indeed, with caution, it can be used as a surrogate of organ blood flow[37,38] provided that SpO_2, the metabolic rate for oxygen, the ratio of arterial-to-venous blood flow in the target organ, and hemoglobin concentration during the assessment period remain stable.

A growing body of evidence supports the clinical use of NIRS in neonates, particularly for assessment of cerebral tissue oxygen saturation ($CrSO_2$). A number of studies have reported on the changes in $CrSO_2$ in preterm and term neonates during transition[39-41] and investigated the association between changes in $CrSO_2$ and adverse short- and long-term outcomes.[42-45] Of note is that the earlier studies have significant limitations due to the noncontinuous assessment of $CrSO_2$. This methodologic problem has, for instance, resulted in contradicting reports on the association between changes in $CrSO_2$ and the development of periventricular/intraventricular hemorrhage (P/IVH) in preterm neonates (see Chapters 6 and 7). Both increased mean $CrSO_2$ along with decreased mean fractional tissue oxygen extraction (FTOE)[42] and, conversely, decreased $CrSO_2$ along with increased FTOE values[44] have been reported in preterm neonates that developed P/IVH during the first few postnatal days compared with controls. When the systemic and cerebral hemodynamic changes were investigated in extremely preterm neonates, using intermittent assessment of cardiac function by fECHO and mean velocity in the middle cerebral artery (MCA) by Doppler ultrasound *along with continuous* $CrSO_2$ monitoring, the identified early pattern of hemodynamic changes in preterm neonates later inflicted by P/IVH suggested a plausible pathophysiologic explanation for such discrepancies in the reported findings (see Chapter 7).[43] Affected neonates demonstrated initial systemic and cerebral hypoperfusion followed by improvement in both systemic and cerebral blood flow as indicated by the increase in CO, MCA mean velocity, and

CrSO$_2$ during the subsequent 20 to 44 hours and preceding detection of P/IVH. Of note is that partial pressure of arterial carbon dioxide (PaCO$_2$) also increased prior to detection of P/IVH. These observations support the hypoperfusion-reperfusion hypothesis as the major hemodynamic pathophysiologic factor in the development of P/IVH and underscore the advantages of continuous regional tissue oxygen saturation (rSO$_2$) monitoring in neonates using NIRS technology. Furthermore, findings of a number of studies investigating the changes in CrSO$_2$ in conjunction with other hemodynamic parameters and brain functional activity have enabled the assessment of cerebral autoregulation dynamics and its potential clinical implications in preterm and term neonates under different conditions (see later).

Peripheral Perfusion and Microcirculation

The observations on the gender-specific differences in vascular tone regulation and peripheral perfusion in preterm and term neonates and the findings that, in patients with sepsis or anemia, changes in microcirculation precede the changes in other hemodynamic parameters or laboratory values indicate the importance of the assessment of microcirculation in the overall evaluation of the neonate.

Perfusion index (PI), defined as the ratio of the pulsatile and nonpulsatile components of the photoelectric plethysmographic signal of pulse oximetry, has been used as a marker of peripheral perfusion.[46-50] However, likely due to the high coefficient of variation of the measurements, the PI is not considered informative during early transition in both preterm and term neonates.[51-53] In addition, whether the PI can be used reliably in the clinical setting for monitoring of perfusion in patients with *hs*PDA remains uncertain. Although, compared with neonates with a non-*hs*PDA or no PDA, some studies reported a significant difference in preductal and postductal PI values in patients with a *hs*PDA during the first days after delivery,[54] others reported no effect of ductal flow and/or its persistence on PI.[55] Moreover, the presence of the reported preductal and postductal gradient in both preterm[56] and term neonates during the first several postnatal day seems to resolve by postnatal day 5.[57]

Several other methods are currently available to assess peripheral perfusion and the microcirculation (see also Chapter 19). They include, but are not limited to, orthogonal polarization spectral (OPS) imaging, side-stream dark-field (SDF) imaging,[58-63] laser Doppler flowmetry,[64-67] and visible light technology.[68,69] Videomicroscopy techniques (OPS and SDF) allow direct visualization of the microcirculation. However, their bedside use in neonates has been limited to intermittent assessments of peripheral perfusion rather than continuous monitoring. Although continuous recording of the images can be done, real-time assessment and interpretation remain challenging at this point, with motion and pressure artifacts posing a significant problem. A newer technique, incident dark-field imaging appears to be superior to SDF in image quality and accuracy of assessment of the microcirculation in preterm neonates but also bears the limitation of noncontinuous evaluation.[70] On the other hand, laser Doppler flowmetry offers the capability of continuous monitoring and has been also used in the neonatal population. The main limitations of the technology include inability to evaluate absolute flow properties and thus allowing only assessment of the relative changes in flow over time, low temporal resolution requiring measurement times of approximately 1 minute and technical challenges (motion artifacts) to maintain proper probe position on the patient for an extended period of time. A newer laser-based technology, laser speckle contrast imaging (LSCI)[71-74] addresses the issue of temporal resolution with significantly faster measurement times. However, similar to laser Doppler flowmetry, it provides only relative measurements of flux. In addition, LSCI has not been studied in the neonate yet. Assessment of the microcirculation using visible light technology has been reported.[75] However, little is known about its utility in the neonatal population.[76]

Table 21.1 summarizes the tools available for bedside monitoring of the various physiologic parameters discussed in this section.

Comprehensive Monitoring Systems

A growing body of evidence underscores the importance of, and the need for incorporating, multiple physiologic parameters when evaluating the hemodynamic status of

21

Table 21.1 SYSTEMIC AND REGIONAL HEMODYNAMIC PARAMETERS FREQUENTLY MONITORED IN NEONATES

	Parameter	Technology/Method	Purpose and Acquisition [C, I or C/I]
Systemic perfusion (BP and CO)	Heart rate	ECG (electrodes)	In conjunction with stroke volume gives flow status [C]
	BP	Arterial line/cuff (oscillometry; Doppler-US)	Perfusion pressure [C/I]
	Stroke volume/CO	ECG	Systemic, pulmonary (CO) and organ blood flow, cardiac function [I]
		IEC	Systemic blood flow (CO) and SV [C]
Systemic oxygenation	SpO_2	Pulse oximetry	Oxygenation on the arterial side [C]
CO_2 status	TCOM	CO_2 diffusion through skin	Potential effect on cerebral vasculature (changes in CBF) [C]
Regional perfusion	Regional O_2 saturation	NIRS	Tissue oxygenation and (indirectly) organ perfusion [C]
Peripheral perfusion	Microcirculation (oxygenation; blood flow velocity; capillary recruitment)	Visible light technology Laser Doppler flowmetry OPS, SDF, and IDF	Peripheral perfusion [C] Peripheral perfusion [C] Peripheral perfusion [I]
Indirect assessment of perfusion	Capillary Refill Time	Visual	Systemic perfusion (indirectly) [I]
	Delta T (C-P)	Temperature	Systemic perfusion (indirectly) [I]
	Color	Visual	Peripheral perfusion [I]
Organ function	Brain electrical activity	aEEG	Assessment of brain activity [C]
	Urine Output	Urinary catheter	Assessment of renal function [I]

Physiologic parameters of systemic blood flow (BP and CO) and oxygenation, carbon dioxide production and elimination, regional (organ) and peripheral (microcirculation) blood flow, and organ (brain) function (aEEG) with corresponding assessment tools are listed that can be monitored at the bedside, along with the indirect methods used in clinical practice to evaluate perfusion and organ function. Data acquisition can be continuous [C], intermittent [I], or both [C/I]. *aEEG*, Amplitude-integrated electroencephalography; *BP*, blood pressure; *CBF*, cerebral blood flow; *CO*, cardiac output; *Delta T (C-P)*, difference core and peripheral temperature; *ECG*, echocardiography; *IDF*, incident dark-field (imaging); *IEC*, impedance electrical cardiometry; *OPS*, orthogonal polarization spectral (imaging); *SDF*, side-stream dark-field (imaging); *SV*, stroke volume; *TCOM*, transcutaneous CO_2 monitoring; *US*, ultrasonography. Modified from Azhibekov T, Noori S, Soleymani S, Seri I: Transitional cardiovascular physiology and comprehensive hemodynamic monitoring in the neonate: relevance to research and clinical care. *Semin Fetal Neonatal Med* 19:45–53, 2014.

neonates. Increasingly, investigators have combined data from different monitoring tools to improve their diagnostic and prognostic value. Such an approach frequently provides valuable insights into the underlying physiologic processes, as well as the pathophysiology, of the cardiovascular compromise that would not be possible with monitoring tools used in isolation.[77-80] As an example, cerebral autoregulation (i.e., the ability of the brain to maintain cerebral blood flow during fluctuations of blood pressure within a certain blood pressure range [see Chapter 2]),[81] has been studied using the interaction between the two aforementioned parameters (blood pressure and cerebral blood flow). Significant advances have been made in both studying cerebral autoregulation[82] and improving our prognostic capability in preterm neonates,[83] especially in those at risk for the development of P/IVH, and in term neonates with hypoxic-ischemic encephalopathy undergoing therapeutic hypothermia.[84,85] Inclusion of continuous monitoring of $PaCO_2$, the most important and powerful regulator of cerebral blood flow,[86-88] has the potential to provide additional information about the complex interactions between $PaCO_2$, cerebral blood flow, and other hemodynamic parameters. This is of importance because significant alterations in $PaCO_2$ (both hypocapnia and hypercapnia) have been associated with adverse short- and long-term outcomes.[43,89,90]

Currently, clinical and conventional physiologic data are collected and documented manually in the patient's chart or recorded automatically from the bedside monitors to the patient's electronic medical records. However, this information is typically documented on an hourly or bi-hourly basis only, intervals that are unacceptable for appropriate monitoring of the rapid and dynamic changes characteristic of the cardiovascular system. To be able to accurately assess the overall hemodynamic status, identify relevant changes in a timely manner, and understand the intricate interplay among the different hemodynamic parameters, these data need to be collected at much higher frequencies (sampling rates) and be time-stamped to other relevant clinical events. The development of comprehensive hemodynamic monitoring systems enables real-time, simultaneous, and continuous collection of physiologic data in a reliable and comprehensive manner for subsequent analysis and assessment of the complex interactions among multiple hemodynamic parameters that may change significantly in a matter of seconds or minutes. Such systems include various monitoring tools enabling concomitant evaluation of both systemic and regional perfusion and oxygen delivery and other physiologic parameters that play a role in cardiovascular regulation and adaptation along with monitoring the functional status of specific organs (Fig. 21.1). Advances in biomedical technology and computer science have improved the capabilities of comprehensive monitoring systems to collect and store increasing sets of complex physiometric data. However, the caveats regarding their accuracy, feasibility, reliability, and need for validation across various subpopulations have to be emphasized.[91,92] Finally and as previously discussed, the utility of the monitoring systems is determined by the comprehensiveness of the monitored hemodynamic parameters.

A previously described hemodynamic monitoring "tower" developed by the authors[91,92] was the first step in the process to enable practical, continuous, and simultaneous monitoring and acquisition of neonatal hemodynamic data at high sampling rates in real time, initially designed for research applications. It integrates conventionally used technologies to continuously monitor heart rate, blood pressure, SpO_2, transcutaneous CO_2 tension, and respiratory rate with other technologies such as IEC for beat-to-beat measurements of SV and CO, and NIRS for continuous monitoring of rSO_2 changes in vital (brain) and nonvital (kidney, intestine, and/or muscle) organs. The "tower" incorporates these various parameters onto a comprehensive patient monitor using conventional or VueLink modules (Phillips, Palo Alto, California). The continuous stream of measurements is then acquired through the analog output of the monitor via the use of an analog-to-digital converter and data-acquisition system onto a laptop computer. A motion-activated camera with the same time stamp is used to capture the bedside events that could affect the accuracy and interpretation of the collected data. This functionality aids in differentiating between true fluctuations of physiologic data versus equipment malfunction (lead disconnection, electrode/optode displacement) or other potential artifacts related to provision of routine clinical care and procedures. Another unique advantage of the "tower" is its ability to operate as a mobile, stand-alone unit that could be used at any bedside, space permitting.

Collection of all the data with a single monitoring device enables automatic data synchronization and avoids the need to match different time stamps so that simultaneous minute-to-minute changes and interactions between various parameters can be reliably analyzed. Relevant clinical events such as fluid bolus administration, titration of vasoactive medications or treatment of a PDA, transfusion of blood products, intubation/extubation, and change in respiratory support are manually documented by the bedside nurse on a dedicated flowsheet. Fig. 21.2 demonstrates an example of an approximately 1-hour and 10-minute period of processed patient data that was acquired using the hemodynamic monitoring "tower" when the clinicians' assumption of the patient's hemodynamic status was not fully supported by the data obtained by comprehensive hemodynamic monitoring. Fig. 21.3 demonstrates the hemodynamic changes that were observed during various events related to routine patient care and extubation. Retrospective review of the video data captured by the motion-activated camera during the study period enabled identification and accurate time-stamping of these events. Without the concomitant

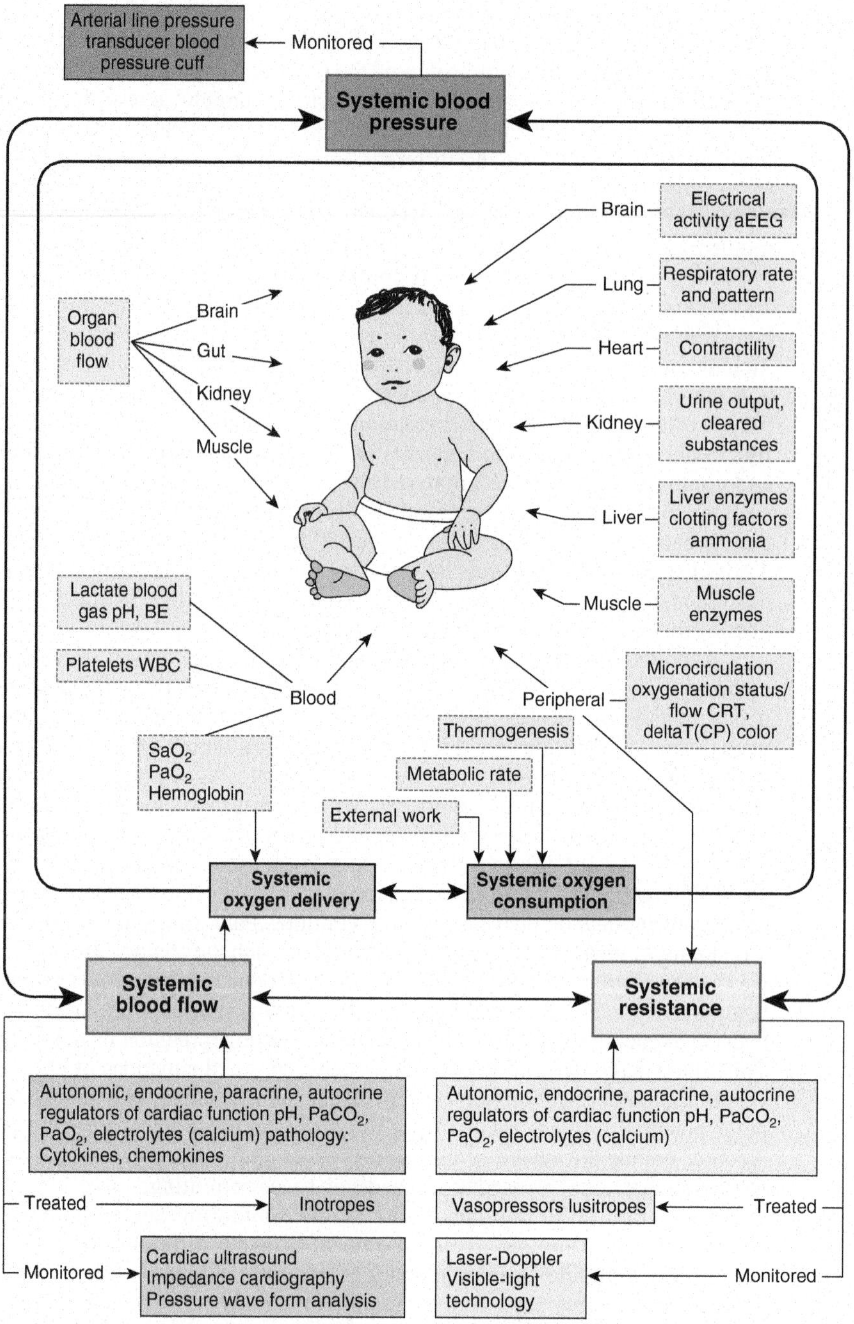

Fig. 21.1 **Comprehensive neonatal hemodynamic monitoring.** Physiologic parameters and tools available to provide a global (outside the square) and regional (inside the square) assessment of developmental hemodynamics. Global monitoring of the relationship among systemic flow, blood pressure and resistance, and arterial/venous oxygen content provides information on systemic oxygen delivery and consumption. Regionally monitored parameters provide direct or indirect information on specific organ blood flow and function and vital versus nonvital blood flow regulatory assignment. aEEG, Amplitude-integrated electroencephalography; BE, base excess; CRT, capillary refill time; $PaCO_2$, arterial partial pressure of carbon dioxide; PaO_2, arterial partial pressure of oxygen; SaO_2, arterial oxygen saturation; WBC, white blood cell. (Modified from Azhibekov T, Noori S, Soleymani S, Seri I: Transitional cardiovascular physiology and comprehensive hemodynamic monitoring in the neonate: relevance to research and clinical care. Semin Fetal Neonatal Med 19:45–53, 2014.)

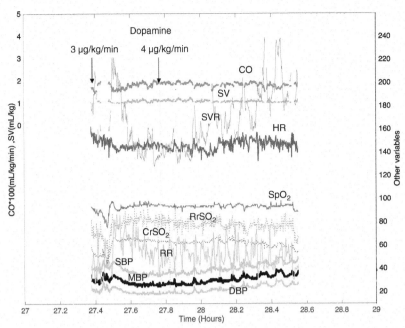

Fig. 21.2 An approximately one-hour and 10-imute tracing selected from the comprehensive hemodynamic monitoring recording of a 1-day old 27 weeks' gestation (BW 1020 g) preterm infant with respiratory failure on volume-guarantee ventilation. Patient received low doses of dopamine as she was considered to be hypotensive. Yet, renal rSO$_2$ was consistently higher than cerebral rSO$_2$; a pattern frequently seen in normotensive neonates suggesting that the patient's mean blood pressure in the high 20 mm Hg-range with a cardiac output of ~200 mL/kg/min was most likely appropriate to ensure normal oxygen deliver to the organs. Accordingly, based on the data obtained by the comprehensive monitoring system, this patient did not meet the criteria of systemic hypotension. During the recording shown, cardiac output remained unchanged while blood pressure and thus calculated systemic vascular resistance (SVR) increased. The increase in blood pressure from ~25 mm hg to ~40 mm Hg was associated with a small but apparent decrease in cerebral and renal rSO$_2$ from ~65% and ~82% to ~60% and ~77%, respectively while SpO$_2$ remained unchanged. At the time of these changes dopamine was being administered at 3 and 4 μg/kg/min at 27.4 and 27.8 hours, respectively. The findings might be explained by the development of slight vasoconstriction in response to low-dose dopamine or it might be due to spontaneous changes in SVR due to autonomic nervous system immaturity/dysregulation and/or physiologic fluctuations in vascular resistance. CO, Cardiac output (x100 mL/kg/min); CrSO$_2$, cerebral regional tissue oxygen saturation (%); DBP, diastolic blood pressure (mm Hg); HR, heart rate (beat/min); MBP, mean blood pressure (mm Hg); RR, respiratory rate (breath/min); RrSO$_2$, renal regional tissue oxygen saturation (%); SBP, systolic blood pressure (mm Hg); SpO$_2$, peripheral oxygen saturation (%); SV, stroke volume (mL/kg); SVR, calculated systemic vascular resistance (mmHg × min × mL^{-1}).

video component, proper interpretation of the physiologic data would have been challenging if not impossible.

On a larger scale, hospital-wide systems are now also available from third-party vendors (e.g., Bernoulli Enterprize [Cardiopulmonary Corporation, Connecticut] or BedMaster [Excel Medical Electronics, Florida]). Using hospital data networks, these systems acquire output data from bedside monitors and other devices (e.g., ventilators, infusion pumps) from multiple patients and route it to central servers for storage and subsequent data processing and analysis. The collected physiologic data can then be retrieved in real-time or retrospectively as a data spreadsheet or as waveforms when applicable. Various software packages are available to process these data so that the parameters of interest can be viewed, scored, transformed, and/ or analyzed. Flexibility of the output format allows analyzing various combinations of parameters, such as blood pressure and CrSO$_2$ to evaluate cerebral autoregulation, or rSO$_2$ and SpO$_2$ to calculate FTOE.

We have previously described a recently developed hospital-wide system ("Bernoulli" system) for comprehensive collection of physiometric data that is currently in place in the authors' institution at Children's Hospital Los Angeles.[93] Although the crucial task of obtaining feasible, reliable, and accurate documentation

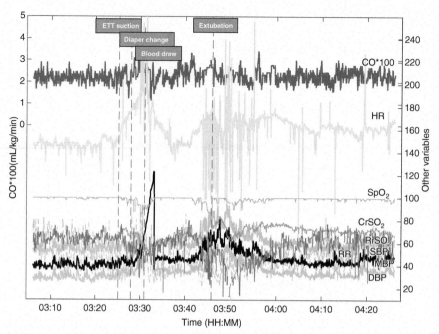

Fig. 21.3 A 90-min segment of prospectively collected continuous recording of nine hemodynamic parameters in a 3-day-old preterm neonate born at 28 weeks' gestation (birth weight, 920 g). Retrospective review of the data from the motion-activated camera allowed time-stamping of the clinical events on the fig. The video recording revealed that the increase in heart rate along with changes in blood pressure at approximately the 03:25 mark corresponded to the time of endotracheal tube (ETT) suctioning, followed by a diaper change and then a blood draw (also represented by the artificial increase in blood pressure). Increased heart rate and blood pressure variability 10 min later corresponds to the time of extubation. *CO,* Cardiac output; *CrSO₂,* Cerebral regional tissue oxygen concentration (rSO_2); *DBP,* diastolic blood pressure; *HR,* heart rate; *MBP,* mean blood pressure; *RR,* respiratory rate; *RrSO₂,* renal rSO_2; *SBP,* systolic blood pressure; *SpO₂,* arterial oxygen saturation.

of therapeutic interventions remains largely unresolved, and these interventions are still documented manually, we are now capable of retrieving information from a wider range of bedside equipment, including infusion pumps that now transmit data on medication administration and dosage changes to a central data server. However, the data stream from the infusion pumps and the bedside monitors are not yet synchronized and therefore still require manual time stamp confirmation during data processing and analysis. Nevertheless, it is an important step forward to improve accuracy and reliability of data collection. Fig. 21.4 illustrates the hemodynamic changes seen during titration of dopamine infusion administered for low blood pressure in a patient who had been monitored using the Bernoulli system.

Automated collection of physiologic datasets has a number of inherent challenges. These include, but are not limited to, intermittent data fall-out (patient movements or maneuvers by the care team, sensor dislodgement, or erroneous measurements during sensor calibration) and the presence of noise and artifacts. Thorough and systematic cleaning of the data is a time-consuming and challenging task, but it is crucial to address these issues prior to data analysis. Furthermore, information about data variability such as the coefficient of variation should also be available for all variables studied. Without this information, one would not be able to interpret changes in the trend of a given hemodynamic parameter, because we need to know what level of changes can be considered *normal variability* and which are *pathologic.*

The next step in the process is performing the analysis of the processed data that can potentially advance our understanding of the physiologic characteristics of a parameter and/or a relationship between two or more parameters. As an example, heart rate and blood pressure characteristics can be used to assess autonomic nervous system function; indeed, heart rate variability (HRV) and baroreflex sensitivity can indirectly quantify autonomic activity.

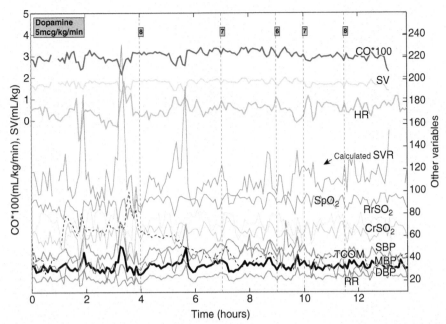

Fig. 21.4 Real-time continuous recording of 11 hemodynamic parameters prospectively collected over a 12-h period in a 10-day-old preterm neonate born at 25 weeks' gestation (birth weight, 825 g) with multiple morbidities related to prematurity. Treatment of hypotension was initiated with dopamine infusion at 5 μg/kg/min (start of infusion not shown) and increased to 8 μg/kg/min (at the 4-h mark), with gradual increase in arterial blood pressure. This increase was most likely mediated by an increase in SVR via *alpha*-receptor activation because no apparent increase in CO was observed. $RrSO_2$ increased along with the increase in blood pressure, whereas $CrSO_2$ remained essentially unchanged. The observed blood pressure fluctuations up to 20 mm Hg in magnitude did not coincide with the timing of changes in the dose of dopamine and likely represent spontaneous fluctuations in peripheral vascular resistance. Interestingly, the fluctuations were not accompanied by similar abrupt increases in $CrSO_2$. $CrSO_2$, as expected, followed the changes in SpO_2 instead, suggesting that autoregulation of cerebral blood flow was likely intact in this 10-day-old patient. Hemodynamic data were collected at the sampling rate of 0.2 Hz. For visual assessment of the trends, a smoothing function using the median value of 24 consecutive samples, which is equivalent to a 2-min interval, was applied. The exact time of the adjustments of the dose of dopamine was entered manually after data collection was complete based on the nursing documentation. *CO*, Cardiac output; $CrSO_2$, cerebral tissue oxygen saturation; *DBP*, diastolic blood pressure; *HR*, heart rate; *MBP*, mean blood pressure; *RR*, respiratory rate; $RrSO_2$, renal tissue oxygen saturation; *SBP*, systolic blood pressure; SpO_2, arterial oxygen saturation; *SV*, stroke volume; *SVR*, systemic vascular resistance; *TCOM*, transcutaneous pCO₂ measurements. (Modified from Azhibekov T, Soleymani S, Lee BH, Noori S, Seri I: Hemodynamic monitoring of the critically ill neonate: an eye on the future. *Semin Fetal Neonatal Med* 20:246–254, 2015.)

HRV is a well-established noninvasive measure of autonomic control of the heart. It provides a powerful means of monitoring the interplay between the sympathetic and parasympathetic nervous systems.[94,95] Both parasympathetic and sympathetic activities modulate the R-R interval at the low-frequency (LF) range, whereas parasympathetic activity modulates it in the higher-frequency (HF) range. Fast Fourier transformation for power spectral density analysis can be used to measure R-R interval variability distribution as a function of the frequency.[94] LF and HF components are calculated based on the frequency bands identified for infants as 0.03 to 0.2 Hz and 0.3 to 2 Hz, respectively.[96,97]

The baroreceptor reflex buffers changes in systemic blood pressure by adjusting HR and peripheral vascular resistance (Fig. 21.5). Evaluation of baroreceptor sensitivity can provide insights into the ability of a neonate to redistribute blood flow via changes in peripheral vascular resistance. HR changes are mediated by both the parasympathetic and sympathetic nervous system, whereas a change in vascular resistance is mediated through the sympathetic system.[98,99] Baroreceptor function is measured as the slope of the sigmoid-shaped blood pressure and R-R interval relationship at the operating physiologic point, referred to as baroreceptor reflex sensitivity (Fig. 21.6).[100] It is typically measured during a change (increase or decrease) in the blood pressure that is pharmacologically induced. Because it is rarely practical or ethical

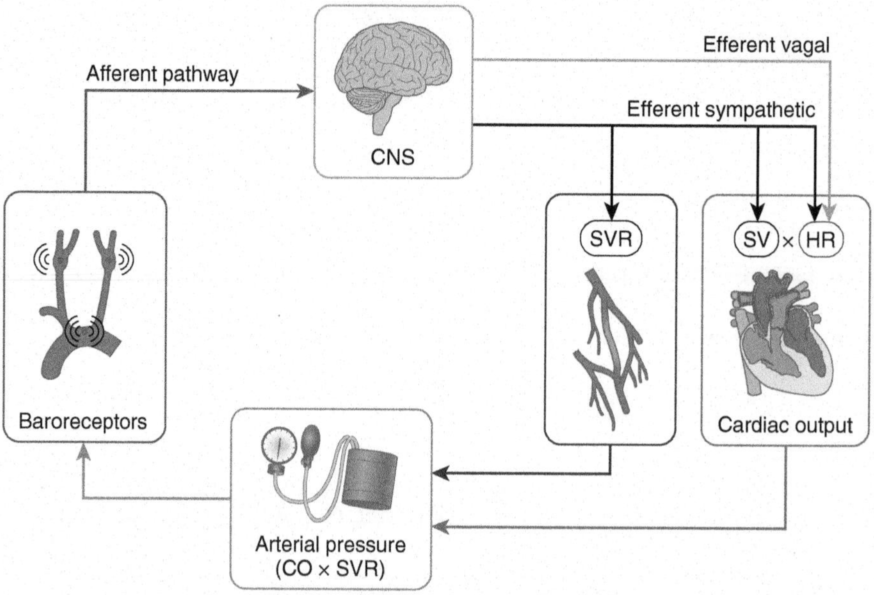

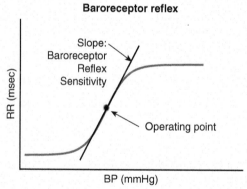

Fig. 21.5 Interactions between cardiovascular nervous system *(CNS)* and autonomic nervous system. Changes in blood pressure are sensed by baroreceptors in the aorta or carotid sinus. The information is sent, via afferent nerves, to the cardiac regulatory center in the brain, which in turn initiates changes in vagal and sympathetic tone. In response to a sudden increase in blood pressure a decrease in sympathetic tone and an increase in parasympathetic tone ensues. Decrease in sympathetic signal causes vasodilation in the vessels (↓ systemic vascular resistance *[SVR]*), decrease in contractility (↓ stroke volume *[SV]*), and slower firing rate of the sinoatrial (SA) node (↓ heart rate *[HR]*); all of which result in lowering the blood pressure. The elevated parasympathetic tone decreases the SA node firing rate and also contributes to lowering of the blood pressure by decreasing the HR. *CO,* Cardiac output.

Fig. 21.6 Baroreceptor function is measured as the slope of the sigmoid shaped blood pressure *(BP)* and *R-R* interval relationship at the operating physiologic point, referred to as baroreceptor reflex sensitivity. (From Andriessen P, Oetomo SB, Peters C, Vermeulen B, Wijn PF, Blanco CE. Baroreceptor reflex sensitivity in human neonates: the effect of postmenstrual age. *J Physiol.* 2005;568:333–341.)

to pharmacologically modify the blood pressure in neonates for diagnostic purposes, researchers have used spontaneous fluctuation in blood pressure and the R-R interval. Using transfer function analysis, baroreceptor reflex sensitivity is then calculated as a transfer gain using the ratio of the amplitude of the output signal (R-R interval) to that of the input signal (systolic blood pressure) at LF range.[100] Table 21.2 summarizes the available information on baroreceptor reflex sensitivity in neonates.[100,101]

Another example includes cerebral autoregulation. Newer analytic approaches have laid the ground for further improvements in our understanding of cerebral hemodynamics and its autoregulation (see Chapter 2).[102,103] In addition, a number of other approaches to study cerebral autoregulation have been reported in the literature, including correlation analysis using statistical principles,[104] spectral analysis techniques of coherence function or the transfer function analysis,[79,105-108] and, more recently, wavelet coherence analysis.[109]

Table 21.2 BARORECEPTOR REFLEX SENSITIVITY IN NEONATES

Method	Sequence Method (Drouin et al., 1997[101])		Spectral Method (Andriessen et al., 2005[100])		
GA	GA: 26–39 $N = 14$	GA: 40–41 $N = 5$	PMA 28–32 ($n = 16$)	PMA 32–37 ($n = 10$)	PMA 37–42 ($n = 6$)
Baroreceptor reflex sensitivity value (ms/mm Hg) Mean (SD) or Median (range)	4.07 (2.19)	10.23 (2.92)	4.6 (3.1–5.4)	7.5 (5.2–10.1)	15.0 (11.8–19.7)

Comparison of baroreceptor reflex sensitivity (BRS) value using the sequence and spectral methods in neonates. In the sequence method, BRS is calculated using the mean slope of the linear regression of the R-R intervals vs. systolic blood pressure (SBP). In the spectral method, BRS is calculated using the low frequency (0.04–0.15 Hz) transfer function gain between SBP and the R-R interval. *GA*, Gestational age; *PMA*, postmenstrual age (weeks).

From Research to Individualized Neonatal Intensive Care

Due to a number of limitations, comprehensive hemodynamic monitoring systems are still being used mostly for research purposes. Overall, the implementation and maintenance of such a system is a challenging and time-consuming process that, in addition to the financial cost, requires very close collaboration between the vendor, the institution's biomedical engineering and information technology departments, hospital administration, and the members of the multidisciplinary team of healthcare providers (physicians, respiratory therapists, and nurses). The enormous amount of continuously growing data requires additional infrastructure to store and organize the data, as well as the involvement of computer scientists and experts in bioinformatics to assist with large data handling and analysis. In addition, because the collected data represent protected health information, protection of patients' rights and confidentiality is mandatory, and all related processes to access the data for research and quality improvement purposes must comply with federal, state, and hospital-wide regulations, policies, and procedures. However, once established, accurately collected and appropriately stored data from such multimodular monitoring systems will serve as an invaluable resource for multiple research ideas and quality improvement activities that extend far beyond cardiovascular physiology alone.

For clinical application, with close collaboration among researchers in basic science and translational and clinical research, biostatisticians, computer and bioinformatics scientists, biomedical engineers, and scientists in other specialties, analysis of the information obtained via comprehensive hemodynamic monitoring can potentially reveal pathognomonic trends and patterns that may precede changes in systemic and organ perfusion. Therefore such a system with the required infrastructural support enables the development of algorithms to predict impending hemodynamic compromise and the responsiveness of a given patient to a particular intervention. As an example of such an effort, analysis of HRV allowed developing a heart rate characteristics monitoring system to identify neonates at risk for developing sepsis, and it has subsequently been shown to decrease mortality from late onset neonatal sepsis.[110,111] In the pediatric and adult critical care literature, similar findings of continuous monitoring of dynamic changes in cardiovascular parameters in response to various factors have also been reported.[112] Clinical applications of functional hemodynamic monitoring data include the ability to detect shock in the compensated phase prior to decompensation[113,114] and the prediction of the patient's responsiveness to fluid administration.[115-118]

Computational modeling is one of the approaches that enables such transition from research findings to advances in intensive care where decision-making needs to take place quickly in the setting of large amounts of patient data that have to be included and analyzed. Computational models serve as a mathematical representation of human physiology and/or pathophysiology and assist in improving our understanding of the interrelationship among various parameters or estimating the unknown ones, thus aiding in the diagnosis and management of certain conditions. They also allow experimenting with potential interventions and procedures in the model before trialing them in patient care.[119] Hemodynamic data obtained via comprehensive monitoring can be used to validate mathematical models aiming at predicting cardiovascular responses to distinct stimuli. As an example of such mathematical models, PNEUMA, a comprehensive and physiologically realistic computer model, has been developed and described in the adult literature.[120] It incorporates cardiovascular, respiratory, and autonomous nervous systems and was originally designed to study cardiorespiratory mechanisms of breathing in adults with sleep disorders. The model has been adapted by the authors to neonatal physiology to study the effects of PDA on systemic, pulmonary, and organ blood flow, as well as the ability to *predict* hemodynamic and autonomic nervous system changes in response to surgical closure of the PDA. Hemodynamic and/or respiratory changes associated with PDA ligations have been studied in both animal models[121] and premature infants.[33,122] Despite differences in the study designs, measurement techniques, and time intervals, all studies reported similar changes, with decreases in SV and CO and increases in SVR immediately following ductal closure. These changes, when monitored for up to 24 hours, gradually improved over time. Fig. 21.7 demonstrates the acute hemodynamic and autonomic changes following PDA ligation as predicted by a modified PNEUMA model[123] that align with the published literature (Fig. 21.8). Preliminary data from the authors' institution provide an example of the hemodynamic changes observed in a preterm neonate when PDA ligation was captured using the Bernoulli system (Fig. 21.9). Of note is that validation of the predictive capabilities of the model in neonates still requires further work.

Another important factor being increasingly recognized is genetic variability and its impact on individual susceptibility to certain external adverse factors, characteristics of the disease process, and response to particular interventions. Advances in molecular genetics and genetic epidemiology and the increasingly simplified access to data provided by whole genome sequencing will open another era of hemodynamic research and aid in the appreciation and better understanding of the multilayered nature of cardiovascular physiology and pathophysiology. Theoretically the advantages of studying the neonatal population,[93] and exploring the associations between genetic variability and phenotypic presentations will likely lead to identification of genetic variants associated with particular cardiovascular disease processes in discrete subpopulations of neonates or to understanding therapeutic efficacy or inefficacy of the pharmacologic agents used in the treatment of neonatal cardiovascular compromise.

To support this hypothesis, an increasing number of genome-wide association studies report identified genetic polymorphisms that are associated with certain hemodynamic parameters such as blood pressure,[124] resting heart rate,[125,126] HRV,[127] and cardiac function.[128] These findings provide new insights into underlying biologic mechanisms of the interindividual variability of the hemodynamic parameters and their interaction with potentially important diagnostic and therapeutic applications. For example, single nucleotide polymorphisms (SNPs) have been identified that are associated with the response pattern to different classes of antihypertensive medications, such as diuretics and angiotensin II receptor blockers.[129,130] Moreover, SNPs associated with genetic predisposition to presenting with a PDA in preterm neonates have also been reported.[131,132]

Lastly, inclusion of the tools that assess functional status of target organs, such as amplitude-integrated electroencephalography, into comprehensive hemodynamic monitoring systems will allow the development of predictive models for short-term neonatal outcomes such as P/IVH and long-term outcomes such as neurodevelopmental scores. With the incorporation of solitary data such as neuroimages, biomarkers, and SNPs, these multimodular monitoring systems will contribute to the creation of a new generation of real-time clinical decision support tools to refine individualized medical care plans and improve survival and quality of life for critically ill neonates.

To change from a *population-focused medicine* using evidence from large clinical trials enrolling patients with little to no consideration for individual patient characteristics to *individualized medicine*, we need to make radical changes in our

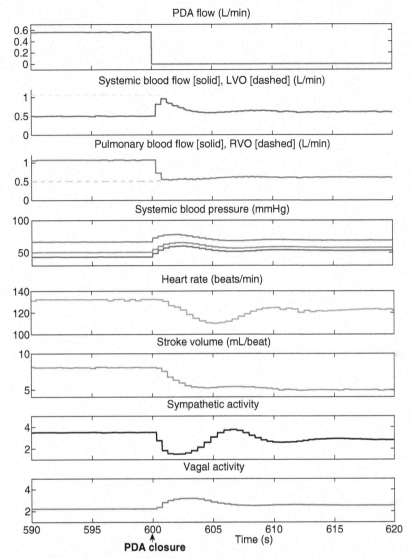

Fig. 21.7　Computer simulation of the acute hemodynamic and autonomic changes of the sudden closure of a moderate PDA. Systolic, mean, and diastolic blood pressure is represented in the systemic blood pressure panel. See text for details. *LVO*, Left ventricular output; *PDA*, patent ductus arteriosus; *RVO*, right ventricular output. (Modified from Soleymani S, Khoo MCK, Noori S, Seri I: Modeling of neonatal hemodynamics during PDA closure. *Conf Proc Annu Int Conf IEEE Eng Med Biol Soc IEEE Eng Med Biol Soc Annu Conf* 2015:1886–1889, 2015 and Azhibekov T, Soleymani S, Lee BH, Noori S, Seri I: Hemodynamic monitoring of the critically ill neonate: an eye on the future. *Semin Fetal Neonatal Med* 20:246–254, 2015.)

approach, first perhaps for patients requiring intensive or complex clinical care. Indeed, the recent recognition of the need to develop and use comprehensive monitoring and data acquisition systems, harness mathematical analysis to develop predictive algorithms, and incorporate machine learning and artificial intelligence allows us to advance our ability to predict the future and are the first steps in this direction.[38,133]

Conclusion

In summary, despite multiple attempts to define neonatal hypotension, develop criteria for initiating interventions, and/or identify the most appropriate, pathophysiology-targeted treatment to normalize blood pressure and organ perfusion, these and other related hemodynamic questions remain mostly unanswered. The challenges to define

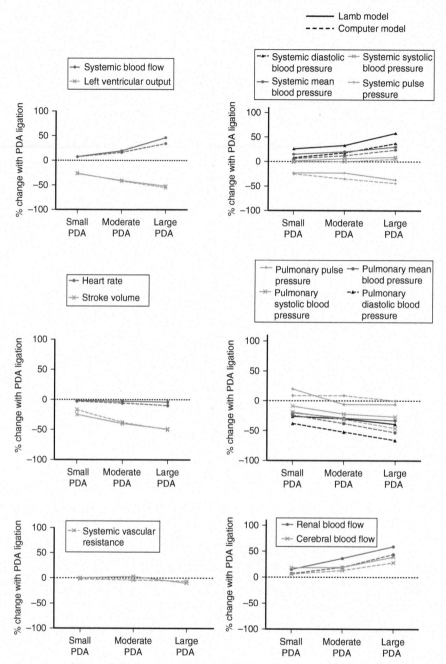

Fig. 21.8 Changes in various cardiovascular and respiratory parameters in response to patent ductus arteriosus *(PDA)* ligation as determined in a lamb model[121] *(solid lines)* and predicted by PNEUMA computer model *(dashed lines)*. The data are presented as percent change from baseline occurring once the PDA is closed. Stratification is based on the size of the duct: small, moderate, and large PDA.

hypotension include variations in blood pressure values based on gestational and postnatal age and existing comorbidities (lung disease, infection, etc.), and the fact that, in patients of the same gestational and postnatal age and degree of maturity, the same blood pressure value can be associated with either adequate or compromised systemic and organ perfusion. Even in the same patient under different conditions and at different points in time, the same blood pressure value can represent adequate or compromised systemic and/or organ perfusion. Without comprehensive evaluation using additional data that accurately represent both blood pressure and systemic and organ blood flow and oxygen delivery in neonates at risk, timely diagnosis of

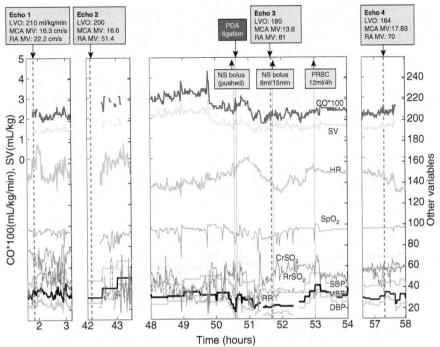

Fig. 21.9 Real-time recording of 10 hemodynamic parameters prospectively collected in an 11-day-old preterm neonate born at 25 weeks' gestation (birth weight, 810 g) undergoing patent ductus arteriosus *(PDA)* ligation. This mechanically ventilated neonate had received two courses of indomethacin without success. PDA ligation is marked in *red* at approximately the 50.5-h mark. The four functional echocardiographic/Doppler ultrasound assessments of left ventricular output *(LVO)*, middle cerebral artery, and renal artery mean velocity *(MCA MV* and *RA MV*, respectively) are displayed in *light red* boxes. Administration of normal saline *(NS* bolus) and packed red blood cells *(PRBCs)* are displayed in *grey* boxes. Immediately prior to ligation, the significant decrease in blood pressure (BP) was likely precipitated by the anesthesia and mediated via a decrease in the systemic vascular resistance. Administration of a normal saline bolus (possibly through an increase in preload) and ligation of PDA (by the sudden removal of the shunt) resulted in a BP increase primarily via an increase in the effective CO (both SV and HR increased). The subsequent decrease in HR to the "preligation range" accompanied by a more prominent decrease in SV (below the preligation values) within 1 hour resulted in a significant decrease in the CO and thus in BP. $CrSO_2$ did not show significant changes in absolute values. However, the fluctuations in $CrSO_2$ following the ligation appear to be less related to changes in SpO_2 and BP, suggesting an improvement in cerebral autoregulation. $RrSO_2$, instead, increased significantly following PDA ligation and fluid administration, concomitantly with an increase in RA MV as estimated by Doppler ultrasound. These changes likely represent improved nonvital organ blood flow after removal of the left-to-right PDA shunt. Hemodynamic parameters: Left Y axis depicts SV (mL) and CO (100 mL/min) and the right Y axis shows the values for SpO_2, $CrSO_2$ and $RrSO_2$ (%), HR and RR (1/min), SBP, MBP, and DBP (mm Hg). *CO,* Cardiac output; $CrSO_2$, cerebral regional tissue oxygen saturation; *DBP,* diastolic blood pressure; *HR,* heart rate; *MBP,* mean blood pressure; *RR,* respiratory rate; $RrSO_2$, renal regional tissue oxygen saturation; *SBP,* systolic blood pressure; SpO_2, arterial oxygen saturation; *SV,* stroke volume.

impending cardiovascular compromise and an appropriate, pathophysiology-targeted decision to intervene with the most appropriate medication in the given individual remain challenging, if not impossible.

At present, comprehensive hemodynamic monitoring systems are being used primarily for research applications. The use of these novel systems capable of continuous data monitoring and acquisition, sophisticated data handling, and analysis of large physiologic data sets with validation of the findings followed by the development of management algorithms requires a truly multidisciplinary approach with close collaboration among clinicians and researchers of different specialties, biomedical engineers, statisticians, and computer scientists. The ultimate goal is to be able to *predict the future with reasonable certainty*. This goal can be accomplished by identifying discrete neonatal subpopulations that have a significantly higher risk for the development of severe hemodynamic instability or its complications, based on genetic susceptibility, perinatal factors, and/or the presence of early signs of impending compromise, and applying pathophysiology-targeted interventions that are the most beneficial and the least harmful in the given patient. As a result, the novel information obtained will contribute to clinically relevant improvements in neonatal care in the future, including a decrease in morbidity and mortality associated with cardiovascular instability in the neonatal period and improvement in relevant long-term outcomes. Comprehensive hemodynamic monitoring will not improve outcome by itself. This can be accomplished only when early detection of circulatory failure is followed by optimized and *individualized* hemodynamic management. Gaining insight into the underlying pathophysiology and monitoring the effects of therapeutic interventions will further contribute to the benefits gained from the use of comprehensive hemodynamic monitoring and data acquisition. Finally, these systems and the inherent need for the use of a multidisciplinary approach will serve as the foundation to use mathematical analysis to develop predictive algorithms and use machine learning and artificial intelligence to predict the future instead of continuing to only react to advancing pathophysiologic events.

REFERENCES

1. Seri I, Evans J: Controversies in the diagnosis and management of hypotension in the newborn infant, *Curr Opin Pediatr* 13:116–123, 2001.
2. Kluckow M: Low superior vena cava flow and intraventricular haemorrhage in preterm infants, *Arch Dis Child - Fetal Neonatal Ed* 82:F188–F194, 2000.
3. Osborn DA, Evans N, Kluckow M: Hemodynamic and antecedent risk factors of early and late periventricular/intraventricular hemorrhage in premature infants, *Pediatrics* 112:33–39, 2003.
4. Hunt RW, Evans N, Rieger I, Kluckow M: Low superior vena cava flow and neurodevelopment at 3 years in very preterm infants, *J Pediatr* 145:588–592, 2004.
5. Fanaroff JM, Wilson-Costello DE, Newman NS, et al.: Treated hypotension is associated with neonatal morbidity and hearing loss in extremely low birth weight infants, *Pediatrics* 117:1131–1135, 2006.
6. Pellicer A, et al.: Early systemic hypotension and vasopressor support in low birth weight infants: impact on neurodevelopment, *Pediatrics* 123:1369–1376, 2009.
7. Pellicer A, et al.: Cardiovascular support for low birth weight infants and cerebral hemodynamics: a randomized, blinded, clinical trial, *Pediatrics* 115:1501–1512, 2005.
8. Vesoulis ZA, et al.: Response to dopamine in prematurity: a biomarker for brain injury? *J Perinatol Off J Calif Perinat Assoc* 36:410, 2016.
9. Roze JC, Tohier C, Maingueneau C, et al.: Response to dobutamine and dopamine in the hypotensive very preterm infant, *Arch Dis Child* 69:59–63, 1993.
10. Osborn D, Evans N, Kluckow M: Randomized trial of dobutamine versus dopamine in preterm infants with low systemic blood flow, *J Pediatr* 140:183–191, 2002.
11. Paradisis M, Evans N, Kluckow M, Osborn D: Randomized trial of milrinone versus placebo for prevention of low systemic blood flow in very preterm infants, *J Pediatr* 154:189–195, 2009.
12. Bidegain M, et al.: Vasopressin for refractory hypotension in extremely low birth weight infants, *J Pediatr* 157:502–504, 2010.
13. Batton B, et al.: Use of antihypotensive therapies in extremely preterm infants, *Pediatrics* 131:e1865–e1873, 2013.
14. Dempsey EM, Barrington KJ: Diagnostic criteria and therapeutic interventions for the hypotensive very low birth weight infant, *J Perinatol Off J Calif Perinat Assoc* 26:677–681, 2006.
15. Stranak Z, et al.: International survey on diagnosis and management of hypotension in extremely preterm babies, *Eur J Pediatr* 173:793–798, 2014.
16. Batton B, Batton D, Riggs T: Blood pressure during the first 7 days in premature infants born at postmenstrual age 23 to 25 weeks, *Am J Perinatol* 24:107–115, 2007.
17. Lee J, Rajadurai VS, Tan KW: Blood pressure standards for very low birthweight infants during the first day of life, *Arch Dis Child Fetal Neonatal Ed* 81:F168–F170, 1999.
18. Groves AM, et al.: Functional cardiac MRI in preterm and term newborns, *Arch Dis Child - Fetal Neonatal Ed* 96:F86–F91, 2011.
19. Chew MS, Poelaert J: Accuracy and repeatability of pediatric cardiac output measurement using Doppler: 20-year review of the literature, *Intensive Care Med* 29:1889–1894, 2003.
20. Kluckow M, Seri I, Evans N: Functional echocardiography: an emerging clinical tool for the neonatologist, *J Pediatr* 150:125–130, 2007.
21. Kluckow M: Functional echocardiography in assessment of the cardiovascular system in asphyxiated neonates, *J Pediatr* 158:e13–e18, 2011.
22. De Waal K, Kluckow M: Functional echocardiography; from physiology to treatment, *Early Hum Dev* 86:149–154, 2010.
23. Mertens L, et al.: Targeted neonatal echocardiography in the neonatal intensive care unit: practice guidelines and recommendations for training: Eur. J. Echocardiogr. J. Work. Group Echocardiogr, *Eur Soc Cardiol* 12:715–736, 2011.
24. De Boode WP, et al.: Recommendations for neonatologist performed echocardiography in Europe: consensus statement endorsed by European Society for Paediatric Research (ESPR) and European Society for Neonatology (ESN), *Pediatr Res* 80:465–471, 2016.

21

25. Evans N, Iyer P: Assessment of ductus arteriosus shunt in preterm infants supported by mechanical ventilation: effect of interatrial shunting, *J Pediatr* 125:778–785, 1994.
26. Evans N, Iyer P: Incompetence of the foramen ovale in preterm infants supported by mechanical ventilation, *J Pediatr* 125:786–792, 1994.
27. Kluckow M: Superior vena cava flow in newborn infants: a novel marker of systemic blood flow, *Arch Dis Child - Fetal Neonatal Ed* 82:F182–F187, 2000.
28. Noori S, Drabu B, Soleymani S, Seri I: Continuous non-invasive cardiac output measurements in the neonate by electrical velocimetry: a comparison with echocardiography, *Arch Dis Child - Fetal Neonatal Ed* 97:F340–F343, 2012.
29. Song R, Rich W, Kim JH, et al.: The use of electrical cardiometry for continuous cardiac output monitoring in preterm neonates: a validation study, *Am J Perinatol* 31:1105–1110, 2014.
30. Grollmuss O, Gonzalez P: Non-invasive cardiac output measurement in low and very low birth weight infants: a method comparison, *Front Pediatr* 2:16, 2014.
31. Boet A, Jourdain G, Demontoux S, De Luca D: Stroke volume and cardiac output evaluation by electrical cardiometry: accuracy and reference nomograms in hemodynamically stable preterm neonates, *J Perinatol Off J Calif Perinat Assoc* 36:748–752, 2016.
32. Hsu K-H, et al.: Hemodynamic reference for neonates of different age and weight: a pilot study with electrical cardiometry, *J Perinatol Off J Calif Perinat Assoc* 36:481–485, 2016.
33. Lien R, Hsu K-H, Chu J-J, et al.: Hemodynamic alterations recorded by electrical cardiometry during ligation of ductus arteriosus in preterm infants, *Eur J Pediatr*, 2014. https://doi.org/10.1007/s00431-014-2437-9.
34. Weisz DE, Jain A, McNamara PJ, EL-Khuffash A: Non-invasive cardiac output monitoring in neonates using bioreactance: a comparison with echocardiography, *Neonatology* 102:61–67, 2012.
35. Weisz DE, Jain A, Ting J, et al.: Non-invasive cardiac output monitoring in preterm infants undergoing patent ductus arteriosus ligation: a comparison with echocardiography, *Neonatology* 106:330–336, 2014.
36. Keren H, Burkhoff D, Squara P: Evaluation of a noninvasive continuous cardiac output monitoring system based on thoracic bioreactance, *Am J Physiol Heart Circ Physiol* 293:H583–589, 2007.
37. Van Bel F, Lemmers P, Naulaers G: Monitoring neonatal regional cerebral oxygen saturation in clinical practice: value and pitfalls, *Neonatology* 94:237–244, 2008.
38. Azhibekov T, Noori S, Soleymani S, Seri I: Transitional cardiovascular physiology and comprehensive hemodynamic monitoring in the neonate: relevance to research and clinical care, *Semin Fetal Neonatal Med* 19:45–53, 2014.
39. Binder C, et al.: Cerebral and peripheral regional oxygen saturation during postnatal transition in preterm neonates, *J Pediatr* 163:394–399, 2013.
40. Mukai M, et al.: Tissue oxygen saturation levels from fetus to neonate, *J Obstet Gynaecol Res*, 2017. https://doi.org/10.1111/jog.13295.
41. Tamussino A, et al.: Low cerebral activity and cerebral oxygenation during immediate transition in term neonates– a prospective observational study, *Resuscitation* 103:49–53, 2016.
42. Alderliesten T, et al.: Cerebral oxygenation, extraction, and autoregulation in very preterm infants who develop peri-intraventricular hemorrhage, *J Pediatr* 162:698–704, 2013.e2.
43. Noori S, McCoy M, Anderson MP, et al.: Changes in cardiac function and cerebral blood flow in relation to peri/intraventricular hemorrhage in extremely preterm infants, *J Pediatr* 164:264–270, 2014.e1–e3.
44. Verhagen EA, et al.: Cerebral oxygenation in preterm infants with germinal matrix-intraventricular hemorrhages, *Stroke J Cereb Circ* 41:2901–2907, 2010.
45. Verhagen EA, et al.: Cerebral oxygenation is associated with neurodevelopmental outcome of preterm children at age 2 to 3 years, *Dev Med Child Neurol* 57:449–455, 2015.
46. Lima AP, Beelen P, Bakker J: Use of a peripheral perfusion index derived from the pulse oximetry signal as a noninvasive indicator of perfusion, *Crit Care Med* 30:1210–1213, 2002.
47. De Felice C, Latini G, Vacca P, Kopotic RJ: The pulse oximeter perfusion index as a predictor for high illness severity in neonates, *Eur J Pediatr* 161:561–562, 2002.
48. De Felice C, et al.: Early postnatal changes in the perfusion index in term newborns with subclinical chorioamnionitis, *Arch Dis Child Fetal Neonatal Ed* 90:F411–F414, 2005.
49. Takahashi S, et al.: The perfusion index derived from a pulse oximeter for predicting low superior vena cava flow in very low birth weight infants, *J Perinatol* 30:265–269, 2010.
50. Bagci S, et al.: A pilot study of the pleth variability index as an indicator of volume-responsive hypotension in newborn infants during surgery, *J Anesth* 27:192–198, 2013.
51. Unal S, et al.: Perfusion index assessment during transition period of newborns: an observational study, *BMC Pediatr* 16:164, 2016.
52. Kroese JK, et al.: The perfusion index of healthy term infants during transition at birth, *Eur J Pediatr* 175:475–479, 2016.
53. Hawkes GA, O'Toole JM, Kenosi M, et al.: Perfusion index in the preterm infant immediately after birth, *Early Hum Dev* 91:463–465, 2015.
54. Khositseth A, Muangyod N, Nuntnarumit P: Perfusion index as a diagnostic tool for patent ductus arteriosus in preterm infants, *Neonatology* 104:250–254, 2013.
55. Vidal M, et al.: Perfusion index and its dynamic changes in preterm neonates with patent ductus arteriosus, *Acta Paediatr Oslo Nor. 1992* 102:373–378, 2013.

56. Kinoshita M, Hawkes CP, Ryan CA, Dempsey EM: Perfusion index in the very preterm infant, *Acta Paediatr Oslo Nor.1992* 102:e398–e401, 2013.
57. Hakan N, Dilli D, Zenciroglu A, et al.: Reference values of perfusion indices in hemodynamically stable newborns during the early neonatal period, *Eur J Pediatr* 173:597–602, 2014.
58. Groner W, et al.: Orthogonal polarization spectral imaging: a new method for study of the microcirculation, *Nat Med* 5:1209–1212, 1999.
59. Genzel-Boroviczény O, Strötgen J, Harris AG, et al.: Orthogonal polarization spectral imaging (OPS): a novel method to measure the microcirculation in term and preterm infants transcutaneously, *Pediatr Res* 51:386–391, 2002.
60. Genzel-Boroviczény O, Seidl T, Rieger-Fackeldey E, et al.: Impaired microvascular perfusion improves with increased incubator temperature in preterm infants, *Pediatr Res* 61:239–242, 2007.
61. Genzel-Boroviczény O, Christ F, Glas V: Blood transfusion increases functional capillary density in the skin of anemic preterm infants, *Pediatr Res* 56:751–755, 2004.
62. Weidlich K, et al.: Changes in microcirculation as early markers for infection in preterm infants—an observational prospective study, *Pediatr Res* 66:461–465, 2009.
63. Van den Berg VJ, et al.: Reproducibility of microvascular vessel density analysis in sidestream dark-field-derived images of healthy term newborns, *Microcirc N. Y. N 1994* 22:37–43, 2015.
64. Kubli S, Feihl F, Waeber B: Beta-blockade with nebivolol enhances the acetylcholine-induced cutaneous vasodilation, *Clin Pharmacol Ther* 69:238–244, 2001.
65. Yvonne-Tee GB, Rasool AHG, Halim AS, Rahman ARA: Reproducibility of different laser Doppler fluximetry parameters of postocclusive reactive hyperemia in human forearm skin, *J Pharmacol Toxicol Methods* 52:286–292, 2005.
66. Stark MJ, Clifton VL, Wright IMR: Neonates born to mothers with preeclampsia exhibit sex-specific alterations in microvascular function, *Pediatr Res* 65:292–295, 2009.
67. Stark MJ, Clifton VL, Wright IMR: Sex-specific differences in peripheral microvascular blood flow in preterm infants, *Pediatr Res* 63:415–419, 2008.
68. Benaron DA, et al.: Continuous, noninvasive, and localized microvascular tissue oximetry using visible light spectroscopy, *Anesthesiology* 100:1469–1475, 2004.
69. Liu FWH, et al.: Design of a visible-light spectroscopy clinical tissue oximeter, *J Biomed Opt* 10:2005. 044005–044005–9.
70. Van Elteren HA, Ince C, Tibboel D, et al.: Cutaneous microcirculation in preterm neonates: comparison between sidestream dark field (SDF) and incident dark field (IDF) imaging, *J Clin Monit Comput* 29:543–548, 2015.
71. Briers D, et al.: Laser speckle contrast imaging: theoretical and practical limitations, *J Biomed Opt* 18:066018, 2013.
72. Sun S, et al.: Comparison of laser Doppler and laser speckle contrast imaging using a concurrent processing system, *Opt Lasers Eng* 83:1–9, 2016.
73. Ansari MZ, Humeau-Heurtier A, Offenhauser N, et al.: Visualization of perfusion changes with laser speckle contrast imaging using the method of motion history image, *Microvasc Res* 107:106–109, 2016.
74. Ansari MZ, Kang E-J, Manole MD, et al.: Monitoring microvascular perfusion variations with laser speckle contrast imaging using a view-based temporal template method, *Microvasc Res* 111:49–59, 2017.
75. Amir G, et al.: Visual light spectroscopy reflects flow-related changes in brain oxygenation during regional low-flow perfusion and deep hypothermic circulatory arrest, *J Thorac Cardiovasc Surg* 132:1307–1313, 2006.
76. Noori S, Drabu B, McCoy M, Sekar K: Non-invasive measurement of local tissue perfusion and its correlation with hemodynamic indices during the early postnatal period in term neonates, *J Perinatol* 31:785–788, 2011.
77. Verhagen EA, Hummel LA, Bos AF, Kooi EMW: Near-infrared spectroscopy to detect absence of cerebrovascular autoregulation in preterm infants, *Clin. Neurophysiol* 125:47–52, 2014.
78. Tsuji M, et al.: Cerebral intravascular oxygenation correlates with mean arterial pressure in critically ill premature infants, *Pediatrics* 106:625–632, 2000.
79. Soul JS, et al.: Fluctuating pressure-passivity is common in the cerebral circulation of sick premature infants, *Pediatr Res* 61:467–473, 2007.
80. Ter Horst HJ, Verhagen EA, Keating P, Bos AF: The relationship between electrocerebral activity and cerebral fractional tissue oxygen extraction in preterm infants, *Pediatr Res* 70:384–388, 2011.
81. Greisen G: Autoregulation of cerebral blood flow in newborn babies, *Early Hum Dev* 81:423–428, 2005.
82. Caicedo A, et al.: Cerebral tissue oxygenation and regional oxygen saturation can be used to study cerebral autoregulation in prematurely born infants, *Pediatr Res* 69:548–553, 2011.
83. Alderliesten T, et al.: Hypotension in preterm neonates: low blood pressure alone does not affect neurodevelopmental outcome, *J Pediatr* 164:986–991, 2014.
84. Ancora G, et al.: Early predictors of short term neurodevelopmental outcome in asphyxiated cooled infants. A combined brain amplitude integrated electroencephalography and near infrared spectroscopy study, *Brain Dev* 35:26–31, 2013.
85. Gucuyener K, et al.: Use of amplitude-integrated electroencephalography (aEEG) and near infrared spectroscopy findings in neonates with asphyxia during selective head cooling, *Brain Dev* 34:280–286, 2012.
86. Wolf ME: Functional TCD: regulation of cerebral hemodynamics–cerebral autoregulation, vasomotor reactivity, and neurovascular coupling, *Front Neurol Neurosci* 36:40–56, 2015.

87. Kaiser JR, Gauss CH, Williams DK: The effects of hypercapnia on cerebral autoregulation in ventilated very low birth weight infants, *Pediatr Res* 58:931–935, 2005.

88. Noori S, Anderson M, Soleymani S, Seri I: Effect of carbon dioxide on cerebral blood flow velocity in preterm infants during postnatal transition, *Acta Paediatr* 103:e334–e339, 2014.

89. Kaiser JR, Gauss CH, Pont MM, Williams DK: Hypercapnia during the first 3 days of life is associated with severe intraventricular hemorrhage in very low birth weight infants, *J Perinatol* 26:279–285, 2006.

90. McKee LA, et al.: PaCO$_2$ and neurodevelopment in extremely low birth weight infants, *J Pediatr* 155:217–221, 2009.e1.

91. Soleymani S, Borzage M, Seri I: Hemodynamic monitoring in neonates: advances and challenges, *J Perinatol* 30:S38–S45, 2010.

92. Soleymani S, Borzage M, Noori S, Seri I: Neonatal hemodynamics: monitoring, data acquisition and analysis, *Expert Rev Med Devices* 9:501–511, 2012.

93. Azhibekov T, Soleymani S, Lee BH, et al.: Hemodynamic monitoring of the critically ill neonate: an eye on the future, *Semin Fetal Neonatal Med* 20:246–254, 2015.

94. Malik M, et al.: Heart rate variability. Standards of measurement, physiological interpretation, and clinical use. Task force of the European Society of Cardiology and the North American Society of Pacing and Electrophysiology, *Eur Heart J* 17:354–381, 1996.

95. Rajendra Acharya U, Paul Joseph K, Kannathal N, et al.: Heart rate variability: a review, *Med Biol Eng Comput* 44:1031–1051, 2006.

96. Schechtman VL, Harper RM, Kluge KA, et al.: Correlations between cardiorespiratory measures in normal infants and victims of sudden infant death syndrome, *Sleep* 13:304–317, 1990.

97. Regalado MG, Schechtman VL, Khoo MC, Bean XD: Spectral analysis of heart rate variability and respiration during sleep in cocaine-exposed neonates, *Clin Physiol Oxf Engl* 21:428–436, 2001.

98. Ursino M: Interaction between carotid baroregulation and the pulsating heart: a mathematical model, *Am J Physiol* 275:H1733–H1747, 1998.

99. Dat M, Jennekens W, Bovendeerd P, van Riel D: *Modeling cardiovascular autoregulation of the preterm infant*, Wiley-Blackwell, 2010.

100. Andriessen P, et al.: Baroreceptor reflex sensitivity in human neonates: the effect of postmenstrual age, *J Physiol* 568:333–341, 2005.

101. Drouin E, Gournay V, Calamel J, et al.: Assessment of spontaneous baroreflex sensitivity in neonates, *Arch Dis Child Fetal Neonatal Ed* 76:F108–F112, 1997.

102. Caicedo A, et al.: A new framework for the assessment of cerebral hemodynamics regulation in neonates using NIRS, *Adv Exp Med Biol* 876:501–509, 2016.

103. Kleiser S, et al.: Characterizing fluctuations of arterial and cerebral tissue oxygenation in preterm neonates by means of data analysis techniques for nonlinear dynamical systems, *Adv Exp Med Biol* 876:511–519, 2016.

104. Lemmers PMA, Toet M, van Schelven LJ, van Bel F: Cerebral oxygenation and cerebral oxygen extraction in the preterm infant: the impact of respiratory distress syndrome, *Exp Brain Res* 173:458–467, 2006.

105. De Smet D, et al.: The partial coherence method for assessment of impaired cerebral autoregulation using near-infrared spectroscopy: potential and limitations, *Adv Exp Med Biol* 662:219–224, 2010.

106. Kuo TB, Chern CM, Sheng WY, et al.: Frequency domain analysis of cerebral blood flow velocity and its correlation with arterial blood pressure, *J Cereb Blood Flow Metab* 18:311–318, 1998.

107. Wong FY, et al.: Impaired autoregulation in preterm infants identified by using spatially resolved spectroscopy, *Pediatrics* 121:e604–e611, 2008.

108. Zhang R, Zuckerman JH, Giller CA, et al.: Transfer function analysis of dynamic cerebral autoregulation in humans, *Am J Physiol* 274:H233–H241, 1998.

109. Tian F, Tarumi T, Liu H, et al.: Wavelet coherence analysis of dynamic cerebral autoregulation in neonatal hypoxic-ischemic encephalopathy, *Neuroimage Clin* 11:124–132, 2016.

110. Fairchild KD, O'Shea TM: Heart rate characteristics: physiomarkers for detection of late-onset neonatal sepsis, *Clin Perinatol* 37:581–598, 2010.

111. Fairchild KD, et al.: Septicemia mortality reduction in neonates in a heart rate characteristics monitoring trial, *Pediatr Res* 74:570–575, 2013.

112. Pinsky MR: Functional haemodynamic monitoring, *Curr Opin Crit Care* 20:288–293, 2014.

113. Creteur J, et al.: The prognostic value of muscle StO$_2$ in septic patients, *Intensive Care Med* 33:1549–1556, 2007.

114. Mesquida J, et al.: Prognostic implications of tissue oxygen saturation in human septic shock, *Intensive Care Med* 38:592–597, 2012.

115. Michard F, et al.: Relation between respiratory changes in arterial pulse pressure and fluid responsiveness in septic patients with acute circulatory failure, *Am J Respir Crit Care Med* 162:134–138, 2000.

116. Berkenstadt H, et al.: Stroke volume variation as a predictor of fluid responsiveness in patients undergoing brain surgery, *Anesth Analg* 92:984–989, 2001.

117. Lanspa MJ, Grissom CK, Hirshberg EL, et al.: Applying dynamic parameters to predict hemodynamic response to volume expansion in spontaneously breathing patients with septic shock, *Shock Augusta Ga* 39:155–160, 2013.

118. García MIM, Cano AG, Romero MG: Dynamic arterial elastance to predict arterial pressure response to volume loading in preload-dependent patients, *Crit Care* 15:R15, 2011.

119. Neal M: Patient-specific modeling for critical care. In Kerckhoffs R, editor: *Patient-specific modeling of the cardiovascular system*, 2010, Springer, pp 81–94.

120. Ivanova O, K Khoo M: Simulation of spontaneous cardiovascular variability using PNEUMA, *Conf Proc Annu Int Conf IEEE Eng Med Biol Soc IEEE Eng Med Biol Soc Annu Conf* 6:3901–3904, 2004.

121. Clyman RI, Mauray F, Heymann MA, Roman C: Cardiovascular effects of patent ductus arteriosus in preterm lambs with respiratory distress, *J Pediatr* 111:579–587, 1987.

122. Weisz DE, Jain A, Ting J, et al.: Non-invasive cardiac output monitoring in preterm infants undergoing patent ductus arteriosus ligation: a comparison with echocardiography, *Neonatology* 106: 330–336, 2014.

123. Soleymani S, Khoo MCK, Noori S, Seri I: Modeling of neonatal hemodynamics during PDA closure, *Conf Proc Annu Int Conf IEEE Eng Med Biol Soc IEEE Eng Med Biol Soc Annu Conf* 2015:1886–1889, 2015.

124. International Consortium for Blood Pressure Genome-Wide Association Studies, et al.: Genetic variants in novel pathways influence blood pressure and cardiovascular disease risk, *Nature* 478:103–109, 2011.

125. Eijgelsheim M, et al.: Genome-wide association analysis identifies multiple loci related to resting heart rate, *Hum Mol Genet* 19:3885–3894, 2010.

126. Mezzavilla M, et al.: Insight into genetic determinants of resting heart rate, *Gene* 545:170–174, 2014.

127. Newton-Cheh C, et al.: Genome-wide association study of electrocardiographic and heart rate variability traits: the Framingham heart study, *BMC Med Genet* 8(Suppl 1):S7, 2007.

128. Vasan RS, et al.: Genetic variants associated with cardiac structure and function: a meta-analysis and replication of genome-wide association data, *JAMA* 302:168–178, 2009.

129. Turner ST, et al.: Genomic association analysis identifies multiple loci influencing antihypertensive response to an angiotensin II receptor blocker, *Hypertension* 59:1204–1211, 2012.

130. Turner ST, et al.: Genomic association analysis of common variants influencing antihypertensive response to hydrochlorothiazide, *Hypertension* 62:391–397, 2013.

131. Angiotensin II type 1 receptor A1166C polymorphism and prophylactic indomethacin treatment induced ductus arteriosus closure in very low birth weig. - PubMed - NCBI. Available at: https://www.ncbi.nlm.nih.gov/pubmed/12904590.

132. Dagle JM, et al.: Determination of genetic predisposition to patent ductus arteriosus in preterm infants, *Pediatrics* 123:1116–1123, 2009.

133. Obermeyer Z, Emanuel EJ: Predicting the future - big data, machine learning, and clinical medicine, *N Engl J Med* 375:1216–1219, 2016.

Patent Ductus Arteriosus

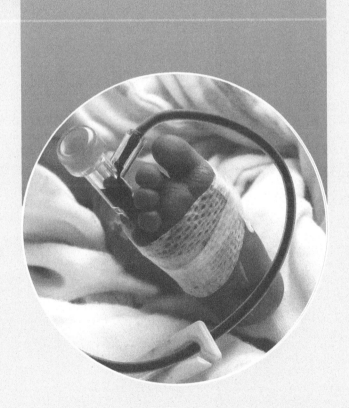

CHAPTER 22

Diagnosis, Evaluation, and Monitoring of Patent Ductus Arteriosus in the Very Preterm Infant

Afif Faisal El-Khuffash, Patrick Joseph McNamara, and Shahab Noori

- Although presence of a patent ductus arteriosus (PDA) can easily be confirmed with ultrasound, diagnosis of a hemodynamically significant PDA is more challenging and not standardized.

- Evaluation of a PDA for hemodynamic and clinical significance should include assessment of the magnitude of ductal shunt volume, the ability of the heart to accommodate and compensate for the shunt, and the impact of the shunt on the pulmonary and systemic circulations.

- Clinical characteristics such as gestational and chronologic age, extent of cardiopulmonary support, and presence of other variables that may either enhance or mitigate the potential detrimental effects of a PDA can be useful in the evaluation of the hemodynamic and clinical significance of a PDA.

- Scoring systems based on clinical characteristics, ultrasound measurements and other technologies such as near-infrared spectroscopy may be useful in evaluation and monitoring of a PDA in the future.

The diagnosis and management of a patent ductus arteriosus (PDA) with cardiorespiratory and thus clinical relevance in preterm neonates poses a major challenge in neonatal medicine. It is the most common cardiovascular abnormality in premature infants. The majority (~70%) of infants born at a gestational age of less than 29 weeks will have a persistent PDA by the end of the first week of age.[1] PDA is associated with several morbidities and mortality; however, a cause-and-effect relationship between the presence of a PDA and important short- and long-term clinical outcomes has never been definitively established. In addition, due to limitations in study design of randomized control trials and the retrospective nature of cohort studies reporting clinical outcomes, the impact of various approaches to treatment (conservative, medical, and surgical) on outcomes is unclear. As a result, treatment strategies (particularly modality and timing) vary between centers.[2]

Developmental Role of the Ductus Arteriosus

The ductus arteriosus (DA) connects the main pulmonary artery to the descending aorta and is necessary for fetal survival. In the fetus the left ventricle receives oxygenated blood, returning from the placenta via the inferior vena cava and through the foramen ovale, and delivers it mainly to the upper part of the body. The right ventricle receives the majority of blood draining from the superior vena cava (SVC) and a proportionately lower amount of oxygenated blood from the umbilical venous system. Due to high pulmonary vascular resistance (PVR), the majority (80% to 90% depending on the gestational age of the fetus) of right ventricular output flows from the pulmonary artery to the descending aorta across the DA; hence the DA modulates flow to the lower part of the body. Similarly, the patent foramen ovale (PFO) is the route which modulates the delivery of oxygenated blood to the head and neck. Following birth, there is a sudden rise in left ventricular afterload, resulting from the loss of the low resistance placental circulation. This is accompanied by the aeration of the lungs, resulting in a fall in PVR and an increase in pulmonary blood flow. This results in a change in the organ of gas exchange from the placenta to the lungs. The DA eventually closes (first functionally and then anatomically) over the subsequent days in term infants. However, in preterm infants the DA can remain patent for a prolonged period of time for a variety of reasons.

Regulation of Ductal Tone and Constriction

In term infants, closure of the PDA occurs within the first 48 hours after birth. Closure of the DA occurs in two phases. The first phase, "functional closure," involves narrowing of the lumen within the first hours after birth by smooth muscle constriction and the second phase, "anatomic remodeling," consists of occlusion of the residual lumen by extensive neointimal thickening and loss of muscle media smooth muscle over the next few days.

The rate and degree of initial "functional" closure are determined by the balance between factors (mediators, second messengers and channels, among others) that favor constriction (oxygen, endothelin, calcium channels, catecholamines, and Rho kinase) and those that oppose it (intraluminal pressure, prostaglandins [PGs], nitric oxide [NO], carbon monoxide, potassium channels, cyclic adenosine monophosphate [AMP], and cyclic guanosine monophosphate). PGs play a key role in the regulation of ductal tone, especially during the first few postnatal weeks. PGE_2 is the most important factor in the regulation of DA tone during fetal development and acts on G protein–coupled E-prostanoid receptors to maintain ductal patency. It is generated from arachidonic acid by cyclooxygenase-1 (COX-1) and COX-2, the COX component of $PG-H_2$ synthase, followed by peroxidation by the same enzyme complex and, finally, by the action of PGE synthase (see Chapter 23). COX-2 plays a major role in maintaining ductal patency during fetal life.[3] The current approach to medical therapy exploits this mechanism by the use of nonselective COX inhibitors such as indomethacin and ibuprofen and also by the use of acetaminophen, a peroxidase inhibitor, to close the DA postnatally.

Low oxygen tension in the fetus is another important factor for maintaining ductal patency.[4] Following birth, the rise in oxygen tension promotes an oxygen-mediated constriction which is facilitated by the inhibition of the potassium voltage channels (Kv channels) present on the ductal smooth muscle cells and function to keep the cells in a hyperpolarized state.[5] The presence of oxygen leads to depolarization, which in turn activates L-type calcium channels, allowing an influx of calcium into the smooth muscle cells causing constriction. A countermechanism via the mitochondrial electron transport chain serves as the intrinsic oxygen-sensing mechanism which regulates this constrictive effect via formation of reactive oxygen radicals which inhibit Kv channels.[6] Interestingly, in vitro studies using rings of human DA tissue incubated in relatively low oxygen tension conditions (to mimic conditions of prematurity) for several days selectively fail to constrict in response to oxygen. This may explain, at least in part, failure of the DA to close in preterm infants.

The fall in PG levels following birth (due to the loss of placental PG production and increase in its removal by the lungs), accompanied by the rise in oxygen tension promotes the functional closure of the DA over the first 24 to 48 postnatal hours. After functional DA closure is achieved, the smooth muscle cells migrate from the media to the subendothelial layer, leading to neointimal formation.[7] Expansion of the neointima (by hyaluron, migrating smooth muscle cells, and proliferating endothelia) forms protrusions, or mounds, that permanently occlude the already constricted lumen.[8,9] This process results in an interruption of the blood supply to the innermost cellular layer, resulting in hypoxia and cell death.[10] The presence of intramural vasa vasorum is essential to ensure adequate provision of oxygen and nutrition to the thicker wall of the DA at term. During postnatal constriction, the intramural tissue pressure obliterates vasa vasorum flow in the muscle media. The ensuing ischemic and hypoxic insult inhibits local PGE_2 and NO production, induces local production of hypoxia-inducible factors (HIF) like HIF-1α and vascular endothelial growth factor (VEGF) (which play critical roles in smooth muscle migration into the neo-intima), and produces smooth muscle apoptosis in the muscle media. In addition, monocytes/macrophages adhere to the ductus wall and appear to be necessary for ductus remodeling.[11]

Resistance to Ductal Closure in Premature Infants

In contrast, in preterm infants the DA frequently fails to constrict or undergo anatomic remodeling after birth. The incidence of persistent PDA is inversely related to gestational age.[12] This is due to several mechanisms. The intrinsic tone of the extremely immature ductus (<70% of gestation) is decreased compared with the ductus at term.[13] This may be due to the presence of immature smooth muscle myosin isoforms, with a weaker contractile capacity,[14-17] and to decreased Rho kinase expression and activity.[18-20] Calcium entry through L-type calcium channels also appears to be impaired in the immature ductus.[19-21] In addition, the potassium channels, which inhibit ductus contraction, change during gestation from K_{Ca} channels not regulated by oxygen tension to K_V channels, which can be inhibited by increased oxygen concentrations.[22-24] The reduced expression and function of the putative oxygen-sensing K_V channels in the immature ductus appear to contribute to ductus patency in several animal species.[20,22,24]

In most mammalian species the major factor that prevents the preterm ductus from constricting after birth is its increased sensitivity to the vasodilating effects of PGE_2 and NO.[25] The increased sensitivity of the preterm ductus to PGE_2 is due to increased cyclic AMP signaling. There is both increased cyclic AMP production, due to enhanced PG receptor coupling with adenylyl cyclase, and decreased cyclic AMP degradation by phosphodiesterase in the preterm ductus.[26,27] As a result, inhibitors of PG production (e.g., indomethacin, ibuprofen, mefenamic acid, paracetamol) are usually effective agents in promoting ductus closure in the premature infant. Premature infants also have elevated circulating concentrations of PGE_2 due to the decreased ability of the premature lung to clear circulating PGE_2.[28] In the preterm newborn, circulating concentrations of PGE_2 can reach the pharmacologic range during episodes of bacteremia and necrotizing enterocolitis and are often associated with reopening of a previously constricted DA.[29]

Little is known about the factors responsible for the changes that occur with advancing gestation. A recent study showed advancing gestation alters gene expression in pathways involved with oxygen-induced constriction, contractile protein maturation, tissue remodeling, and PG and NO signaling.[30] Prenatal administration of glucocorticoids significantly reduces the incidence of PDA in premature humans and animals.[31-36] Although postnatal glucocorticoid or corticosteroid administration also reduces the incidence of PDA, glucocorticoid (dexamethasone) or corticosteroid (hydrocortisone) treatment, especially if it is given in the immediate postnatal period or combined with administration of COX inhibitors, respectively, has been associated with increased incidence of several other neonatal morbidities.[37,38] The patient's genetic background also seems to play a significant role in determining persistent ductus patency. Several single nucleotide polymorphisms in candidate genes have been identified that are associated with PDA in preterm infants: angiotensin receptor (ATR) type 1,[39] interferon γ (IFN-γ),[40] estrogen receptor-alpha PvuII,[41] transcription factor AP-2B (TFAP2B), PGI synthase, and TRAF1.[42] Studies suggest that an interaction between preterm birth and TFAP2B may be responsible for the PDAs that occur in some preterm infants: TFAP2B is uniquely expressed in ductus smooth muscle and regulates other genes that are important in ductus smooth muscle development.[43] Mutations in TFAP2B result in patency of the DA in mice and humans[44] and TFAP2B polymorphisms are associated with the PDA in preterm infants (especially those that are unresponsive to indomethacin).[42] Expression of SLCO2A1 and NOS3 genes (involved with PG reuptake/metabolism and NO production, respectively) is decreased in the DA from non-Caucasians.[30] This may lead to an increase in PG and decrease in NO concentrations, thereby making ductal patency more PG dependent and possibly explaining the clinical finding of a better response to indomethacin in non-Caucasians.[30,45,46]

Neointimal mounds are less well developed and often fail to occlude the lumen in preterm infants (especially those born before 28 weeks' gestation). The preterm ductus is a much thinner vessel than the full-term ductus; therefore there is no need for vasa vasorum because the vessel wall is nourished with oxygen via diffusion through luminal blood flow (vasa vasorum first appear in the outer ductus wall after 28 weeks' gestation when the vessel wall thickness increases beyond 400 μm). As a result, unless the ductus lumen is completely obliterated, the preterm ductus is less likely to develop profound hypoxia as it constricts after birth. Without a strong hypoxic signal, neointimal expansion is markedly diminished, resulting in mounds that fail to occlude the residual lumen.[8,11,47,48]

Pathophysiologic Continuum of the Ductal Shunt in Preterm Infants

During fetal life, low systemic vascular resistance (SVR) due to the low resistance placenta, combined with elevated PVR result in pulmonary artery–to-aorta ("right-to-left") flow across the DA. During normal neonatal transition, increased SVR associated with umbilical cord clamping occurs in parallel to a longitudinal decrease in PVR precipitated by ventilation and increase in pulmonary blood flow. The degree of right-to-left ductal shunt decreases to equally bidirectional within 5 minutes of birth, becomes mostly left to right by 10 to 20 minutes, and entirely left to right by 24 hours of age.[49,50]

In preterm neonates the size and direction of the ductal shunt will have a variable impact on pulmonary and systemic hemodynamics. The shunt may be conceptualized within a physiologic continuum between life-sustaining conduit, neutral bystander, and pathologic entity. In infants with critical congenital heart disease, patency of the DA may be necessary to support pulmonary (e.g., tricuspid atresia) or systemic (e.g., critical aortic stenosis) blood flow. In severe persistent pulmonary hypertension of the newborn (PPHN), the postnatal failure of pulmonary arterioles to relax (e.g., due to asphyxia, respiratory distress syndrome) results in high PVR and persistence of a right-to-left ductal shunt. The latter shunt may reduce right ventricular afterload and support postductal systemic blood flow, albeit with deoxygenated blood. A bidirectional shunt in milder cases of PPHN may play a neutral role, merely permitting the noninvasive estimation of the systemic-pulmonary pressure gradient.

If the DA remains patent after birth, preterm infants who experience the expected fall in PVR may be susceptible to the effects of a large systemic-to-pulmonary (left-to-right) shunt. Blood flows across the PDA continuously in systole and diastole, resulting in volume overload of the pulmonary artery, pulmonary veins, and left heart. Shunt volume *(Q)* is directly proportional to the fourth power of the ductal radius *(r)* and the aortopulmonary pressure gradient (ΔP) and is inversely proportional to the ductal length *(L)* and blood viscosity (η). It is important to consider the relative contributions of each component to shunt volume

$$Q = \frac{\Delta P \Pi r^4}{8\,L\eta}$$

Increased pulmonary blood flow (termed pulmonary overcirculation) may lead to alveolar edema, reduced pulmonary compliance, and increased need for respiratory support. Increased blood flow to the left heart results in dilatation and increased end-diastolic pressures in the left ventricle and atrium. In the setting of immature diastolic function present in preterm infants, the increase in end-diastolic pressure can significantly contribute to the evolution of pulmonary venous hypertension and pulmonary hemorrhage (see later discussion). The increase in pulmonary blood flow occurs at the expense of systemic blood flow. Left-to-right shunting across the PDA (referred to as ductal steal) will lead to systemic hypoperfusion that may result in organ dysfunction. In addition, ductal steal from the descending aorta associated with a PDA, shorter diastolic (and coronary perfusion) times due to tachycardia, and increased myocardial oxygen demand may result in subendocardial ischemia. This pathophysiologic cascade is thought to explain, at least in part, the relation between a PDA and adverse outcomes.

Myocardial Adaptation in Preterm Infants to Patent Ductus Arteriosus

Cardiac output is the result of the interactions between preload, afterload, intrinsic myocardial contractility, and heart rate. Under normal conditions and in the absence of a PDA, the left cardiac output of a neonate is in the range of 150 to 300 mL/kg/min. The presence of a PDA results in increased pulmonary blood flow and left atrial (LA) volume and a resultant increase in left ventricular preload. Studies have consistently shown a higher left ventricle end-diastolic volume (preload) when the DA is open with a predominantly left-to-right shunting pattern. According to the Starling curve, the increase in myocardial muscle fiber stretch from higher preload augments stroke volume. Indeed, most studies have demonstrated a significantly increased left ventricular output (LVO) in the presence of a PDA with predominantly left-to-right shunting.[51-60] In the presence of a PDA, the low-resistance pulmonary vascular bed is in parallel with the systemic vascular bed. This results in a reduction of left ventricle afterload, which, in combination with the increased preload, enhances the myocardium's ability to increase its stroke volume. However, in the clinical setting the presence of a PFO alters the effects of a PDA on left ventricular stroke volume by decompressing the left atrium.[61]

There are significant differences in both the structure and function of the myocardium between preterm and term neonates, and older children and adults. These differences place the immature myocardium at a disadvantage as far as contractility is concerned.[62] Furthermore, because coronary blood flow takes place primarily during diastole, myocardial performance might be adversely affected if diastolic blood pressure is low in the presence of a PDA. Some early studies suggested that myocardial ischemia may occur in the presence of a hemodynamically significant PDA (hsPDA).[63] More recently, studies have demonstrated compromised coronary artery perfusion and the presence of high cardiac-specific troponin levels (indicative of myocardial damage) in the presence of a PDA, suggesting a detrimental effect on myocardial perfusion and potential ischemia.[64,65]

Some authors have suggested that because higher preload is associated with a greater stretch of myocardial fibers, myocardial contractility should increase in the presence of a PDA, along with the increased LVO. They speculate that a lack of change in myocardial contractility, in the presence of a PDA, indicates deterioration of myocardial function. However, using a relatively load-independent measure of myocardial contractility, Barlow et al. showed that hsPDA had no effect on contractility.[66] More recent studies, using more advanced functional parameters such as strain, have also failed to demonstrate worsening function in the presence of the PDA.[67-69] Preservation of left ventricular function occurs despite significant changes in left ventricle morphology over the first 4 postnatal weeks. This includes an increase in LA volume, left ventricle end-diastolic volume, left ventricle sphericity index (indicating a more globular heart), and left ventricle filling pressure.[70]

The potential impact that a PDA has on right ventricular function remains poorly understood. Changes seen in the left ventricle are a consequence of pulmonary overcirculation described previously. Conversely, systemic hypoperfusion may result in a reduction in the right ventricle preload (even in the presence of a left-to-right PFO shunt). In addition, prolonged exposure to increased pulmonary blood flow may promote an increase in PVR and a resultant increase in right ventricular afterload. Recent studies have demonstrated reduced right ventricular function evident as early as day 7 in infants with a large PDA.[71] The clinical relevance of these changes to left or right ventricle function and morphology and their potential impact on the evolution of PDA-associated morbidities is currently unknown.

22

Effects of Patent Ductus Arteriosus on Blood Pressure

Blood pressure is the product of the interaction between cardiac output and peripheral vascular resistance (see Chapter 3). In general, systolic blood pressure is primarily affected by changes in stroke volume, whereas diastolic blood pressure is mainly reflective of changes in peripheral vascular resistance. Traditionally, low diastolic blood pressure has been considered the hallmark of an hsPDA and many studies have supported this notion.[58,66] Studies that specifically looked at the relationship between blood pressure and PDA have shown similar decreases in both systolic and diastolic blood pressure (and therefore no change in the pulse pressure), at least during the first postnatal week.[72,73] Infants born at weights between 1000 and 1500 g with a PDA have slight, but nonsignificant, decreases in systolic, diastolic, and mean blood pressures. In contrast, infants born at less than 1000 g and with a PDA have significantly lower systolic, diastolic, and mean blood pressures but no change in pulse pressure.[73] Because stroke volume increases and vascular resistance decreases in the presence of a PDA, one might expect that systolic blood pressure be maintained despite the decrease in diastolic pressure. Unfortunately, cardiac output, ductal shunt volume, and peripheral resistance were not measured in any of these studies, making it difficult to determine the cause for the lack of a wide pulse pressure. In immature animals a decrease in the diastolic and mean blood pressure occurs even when the shunt is small, whereas a significant decrease in systolic blood pressure occurs only when the PDA shunt is moderate or large.[53] In a more recent cohort of 141 preterm infants less than 29 weeks' gestation, systolic blood pressure in infants with a PDA by the first postnatal week was only slightly lower than those without a PDA. However, diastolic and mean blood pressure were lower by the end of the first postnatal week, which translates into a higher pulse pressure (Fig. 22.1).[1] In this group, LVO was higher and diastolic flow in systemic vessels was lower, possibly explaining those findings (Fig. 22.2). PDA may also contribute to development of hypotension, even during the transitional period, a time period when high-volume ductal shunts are thought to be uncommon. A study found evidence for a possible role of a moderate-large PDA in vasopressor-dependent hypotension.[74] Similarly, PDA is reported to be an independent risk factor for refractory hypotension.[75]

Effects of a Hemodynamically Significant Patent Ductus Arteriosus on Organ Perfusion

Despite the ability of the left ventricle to increase its output in the face of a left-to-right ductus shunt, organ blood flow distribution is significantly altered. Interestingly, redistribution of systemic blood flow occurs even with small shunts.[53] Blood flow to the skin, bone, and skeletal muscle is most likely to be affected first by the left-to-right ductal shunt. The organs affected thereafter are the gastrointestinal tract and kidneys, due to a combination of decreased perfusion pressure (ductal steal) and localized vasoconstriction (compensatory measure). Indeed, mesenteric blood flow is decreased in both fasting and fed states in the presence of a PDA.[76] Significant decreases in blood flow to these organs may occur before there are signs of left ventricular compromise.[57,58] In addition, treatment strategies used to facilitate closure of the PDA, such as indomethacin, may have an effect on organ blood flow independent of the hemodynamic changes associated with the presence of an hsPDA.

Although cerebral blood flow (CBF) has also been assessed by near-infrared spectroscopy (NIRS) and magnetic resonance imaging (MRI) (see later and Chapter 16), blood flow velocity, measured by the Doppler technique, has been the most frequently used technique to assess changes in organ blood flow in the human neonate. In animal models, organ blood flow has also been measured by the microsphere technique or direct flow measurements. As discussed in Chapter 16 in detail, each of these techniques has significant limitations. Unfortunately, it is not currently feasible to continuously measure absolute blood flow to different organs in human neonates.

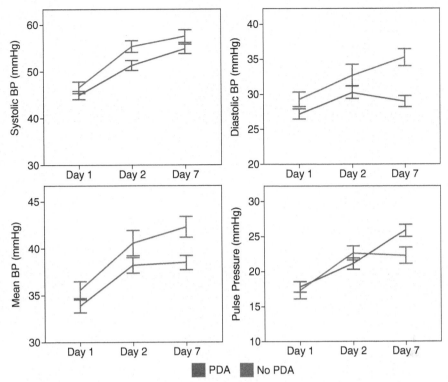

Fig. 22.1 Changes in systolic, diastolic, mean and pulse pressure in patent ductus arteriosus (PDA) and non-PDA infants over the first week of age. PDA infants represent those with a PDA greater than 1.5 mm on day 7 of age. Data represent means and standard error. *BP*, Blood pressure. (Data modified from El-Khuffash A, James AT, Corcoran JD, et al: A patent ductus arteriosus severity score predicts chronic lung disease or death before discharge. *J Pediatr* 167[6]:1354–1361, 2015.)

Using the Doppler technique with ultrasonography, the amount of blood flowing through a vessel is a function of the vessel diameter (cross-sectional area) and mean blood flow velocity. Because of the small size of the neonatal vessels (e.g., anterior cerebral artery [ACA] or middle cerebral artery [MCA]), accurate measurement of vessel diameter is not possible. In addition, the Doppler technique assumes that the diameter of the vessel remains constant during the cardiac cycle, a notion that has been repeatedly challenged. Despite these limitations, Doppler velocity measurements and velocity-derived indices have been shown to have acceptable correlations with more invasive measures of organ blood flow.[77-79] The most commonly used Doppler indicators of organ blood flow are systolic, diastolic, and mean blood flow velocities, velocity time integral, pulsatility index (PI), and resistive index (RI). Because the PI and RI are inversely related to flow, and directly related to vascular resistance, an increase in the PI or RI indicates a reduction in organ blood flow and/or an increase in the vascular resistance of the organ.

Cerebral Blood Flow

Although some studies suggest that CBF is maintained in the presence of an hsPDA,[52,58] most studies have shown a decrease in flow and a disturbance in cerebral hemodynamics.[53] Furthermore, indomethacin, one of the drugs used for pharmacologic closure of the PDA, has a direct, albeit, transient vasoconstrictive effect on the cerebral circulation, which is likely independent of the drug's effect on the COX enzyme.[80,81]

Using the Doppler technique, Perlman et al. demonstrated a decrease in diastolic blood flow velocity in the ACA of preterm infants in the presence of hsPDA.[82] Similarly, Lemmers et al. reported that an hsPDA had a negative impact on cerebral oxygenation that resolved after treatment with indomethacin.[83] Investigators have also observed retrograde diastolic flow and increased PI in the ACA in the presence of a PDA.[84] In contrast, Shortland et al. found no difference in ACA CBF velocity

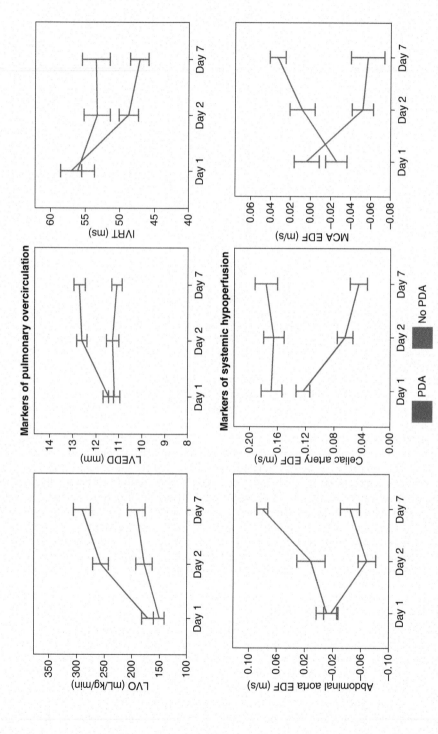

Fig. 22.2 Patterns of echocardiography markers in infants with and without a patent ductus arteriosus (PDA) over the first week of age. Divergence in echocardiography parameters becomes apparent within the first 48 hours following birth. "PDA infants" represents those with a PDA of greater than 1.5 mm on day 7 of age. Data represent means and standard error. *EDF,* End-diastolic frames; *IVRT,* isovolumic relaxation time; *LVO,* left ventricular output; *MCA,* middle cerebral artery; *LVEDD,* left ventricle end-diastolic dimension. (Data modified from El-Khuffash A, James AT, Corcoran JD, et al: A patent ductus arteriosus severity score predicts chronic lung disease or death before discharge. *J Pediatr* 167[6]:1354–1361, 2015.)

between infants with or without a PDA[85]; however, they did report that there was a higher incidence of periventricular leukomalacia (PVL) in the subgroup of infants with retrograde blood flow in the ACA.[85] A study showed progressive reduction in MCA end-diastolic flow velocity during the first postnatal week in extremely preterm infants.[86] These changes sharply contrasted to those without a PDA in whom the velocity progressively increased. Correlations between a hsPDA (assessed by the left atrial-to-aortic (LA:AO) ratio) and both end-diastolic velocity and RI in the ACA have also been made in very low birth weight (VLBW) infants.[87] These data suggest that CBF progressively decreases as left-to-right shunts across the PDA become larger. In preterm lambs[52] and humans,[58] CBF is maintained at a constant level in the presence of a PDA, as long as LVO is increased. It appears that the increase in cardiac output, at least to a certain point, ensures adequate cerebral perfusion (albeit with an altered pattern) in patients with a PDA. Indeed, Baylen et al. reported a decrease in CBF when cardiac output was compromised in preterm lambs with a PDA.[59]

Furthermore, a significant PDA is an independent predictor of low SVC flow (a surrogate for systemic blood flow and perhaps CBF) in preterm infants.[88] The effect of a PDA on SVC flow appears isolated to the first 12 hours after birth (when the myocardium has not yet adjusted to the postnatal increase in afterload). Even in the term neonate during the first few minutes after birth, the rapid change in ductal shunting to a left-to-right pattern may affect CBF, as suggested by the strong inverse relationship between net left-to-right ductal shunting and MCA mean velocity.[49] This finding supports the notion that absence of a compensatory increase in cardiac output may be, at least in part, responsible for the low CBF associated with a PDA in preterm neonates.

Superior Mesenteric and Celiac Artery Blood Flow

Intestinal hypoperfusion is a known risk factor for necrotizing enterocolitis (NEC). Studies evaluating blood flow to the abdominal organs in general, and to the superior mesenteric artery (SMA) in particular, have uniformly demonstrated a decrease in blood flow in the presence of a hsPDA. Diastolic flow reversal in the descending aorta has been reported as early as 4 hours after birth; flow reversal can be seen in 34% and 46% of very preterm infants with a large PDA, at 12 and 24 hours after birth, respectively.[89] In addition, administration of indomethacin appears to directly reduce not only CBF but also intestinal blood flow.

Studies using preterm lambs, during the first 10 hours after delivery,[53] demonstrate that even small ductal shunts (those <40% of the LVO) cause significant reductions in blood flow to the abdominal organs. The decrease in organ blood flow occurs despite significant increases in cardiac output and is due to the combined effects of decreased perfusion pressure and localized vasoconstriction. Similar findings were also reported by other investigators.[59] In premature primates, mesenteric blood flow is decreased in both fasting and fed states in the presence of a PDA.[76] Despite the changes in blood flow, oxygen consumption in the terminal ileum appears to be unaffected by the presence of a PDA in preterm lambs.[57]

Similar findings have been reported in premature human infants. Martin et al. reported retrograde diastolic flow in the descending aorta of preterm infants with a large PDA, which resolved after closure of the DA.[84] Similarly, Deeg et al.[90] and Coombs et al.[91] demonstrated a decrease in both the systolic and diastolic blood flow velocities in the SMA and celiac artery in preterm infants with a PDA. The diastolic blood flow abnormalities appeared to be greater in the SMA.[91] Using ultrasound, Shimada et al. assessed left cardiac output and abdominal aortic blood flow in VLBW infants before and after ductal closure and compared the findings with those obtained in patients without a PDA (Fig. 22.3).[58] Despite a higher left ventricular cardiac output in the PDA group, blood flow in the abdominal aorta was lower in the PDA group than in the controls. Abdominal aortic blood flow increased significantly after ductus closure. These changes in intestinal perfusion have led to concerns when feeding infants with a PDA.

As mentioned earlier, indomethacin treatment of a PDA also affects mesenteric blood flow[91,92] and compromises the premature intestine's ability to

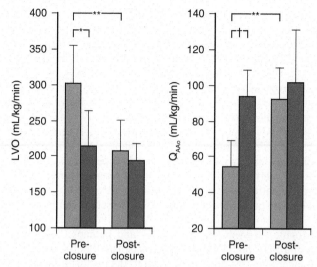

Fig. 22.3   Left ventricular output (LVO) and blood flow volume of the abdominal aorta (Q_{AAo}) before and after closure of ductus arteriosus by mefenamic acid. *Light red bars* represent the values for hemodynamically significant patent ductus arteriosus (hsPDA) group; *dark red bars* represent the values for group without hsPDA. Values are expressed as mean ± SD. *$P < .002$; **$P < .001$; †$P < .0001$. (From Shimada S, Kasai T, Konishi M, Fujiwara T: Effects of patent ductus arteriosus on left ventricular output and organ blood flows in preterm infants with respiratory distress syndrome treated with surfactant. *J Pediatr* 125:270–277, 1994.)

autoregulate its oxygen consumption.[57] On the other hand, ibuprofen, another nonselective COX inhibitor, mediates PDA closure without affecting mesenteric blood flow.[93] A recent meta-analysis comparing ibuprofen treatment of a PDA with indomethacin treatment suggests that ibuprofen may be associated with a lower incidence of NEC while being equally effective in producing PDA closure.[94]

Pulmonary Blood Flow

The decreased ability of the preterm infant to maintain active pulmonary vasoconstriction[95] may be responsible, at least in part, for the pulmonary presentation of a "large" left-to-right PDA shunt in preterm infants relatively early after delivery.[96,97] Therapeutic maneuvers, such as surfactant replacement, or prenatal conditions, such as intrauterine growth retardation, that lead to or are associated with an accelerated postnatal decrease in PVR can exacerbate the amount of left-to-right shunt and might result in an increased incidence of pulmonary hemorrhage.[98-100]

In premature animals a wide-open PDA increases the hydraulic pressures in the pulmonary vasculature, which in turn increases the rate of fluid transudation into the pulmonary interstitium.[101] Any increase in pulmonary microvascular perfusion pressure in premature infants with respiratory distress syndrome may also increase interstitial and alveolar lung fluid because of their low plasma oncotic pressures and increased capillary permeability. Leakage of plasma proteins into the developing lungs inhibits surfactant function and increases surface tension in the immature air sacs,[102] which are already compromised by surfactant deficiency. The increased fraction of inspired oxygen (FiO_2) and mean airway pressures required to overcome these early changes in compliance may contribute to the development of chronic lung disease.[103-105] Depending on the gestational age and the species examined, changes in pulmonary mechanics may occur as early as 1 day after birth or not before several days of exposure to the left-to-right PDA shunt.[106,107]

Although it is true that preterm animals with a PDA have increased fluid and protein clearance into the lung interstitium, due to an increase in pulmonary microvascular filtration pressure, a simultaneous increase in lung lymph flow appears to eliminate the excess fluid and protein from the lungs.[101] This compensatory increase in lung lymph flow acts as an "edema safety factor," inhibiting fluid accumulation in the lungs. As a result, there is no net increase in water or protein accumulation in the lungs and there is no change in pulmonary mechanics.[105,107-110] This delicate balance between the PDA-induced fluid filtration and lymphatic reabsorption is consistent with the observation, made in human infants, that closure of the DA within the first 24 hours after birth has no effect on the course of hyaline membrane disease. However, if lung lymphatic drainage is impaired, alveolar epithelial permeability is altered, and the likelihood of pulmonary and alveolar edema increases dramatically. After several days of mechanical ventilation, the residual functioning lymphatics are more easily overwhelmed by the same size ductus shunt that is well accommodated on the first day after delivery. As a result, it is not uncommon for infants with a persistent PDA to develop pulmonary edema and alterations in pulmonary mechanics at 7 to 10 days after birth. In these infants, improvement in lung compliance occurs following closure of the PDA.[105,111-115]

Not all of the changes associated with a PDA are necessarily detrimental to the immature infant with respiratory distress. The recirculation of oxygenated arterial blood through lungs that are not fully expanded can lead to improved levels of arterial partial pressure of oxygen (PaO_2).[53,116] Conversely, decreases in systemic arterial O_2 content have been observed following PDA closure, despite the absence of any alterations in pulmonary mechanics.

Clinical and Radiologic Diagnosis of Patent Ductus Arteriosus

The emergence of detectable clinical signs of PDA occurs when PVR declines and left heart volume loading and systemic arterial diastolic "steal" ensue. Cardiomegaly and tachycardia result in an active precordium, and diastolic hypotension leads to a wide pulse pressure and bounding central pulses and easily palpable peripheral pulses (e.g., palmar pulses).[117] A holosystolic murmur of irregular intensity is typically audible at the upper left sternal border. Pulmonary overcirculation manifests as radiographic engorgement, increased need for supplemental oxygen, and increased work of breathing. The clinical signs of PDA are generally apparent beyond the first postnatal week but lag behind the echocardiographic diagnosis of an hsPDA by nearly 2 days.[118]

A large left-to-right ductal shunt results in pulmonary overcirculation and left heart enlargement, which projects as LA and ventricular dilatation and increased pulmonary vascular markings on chest radiographs (Fig. 22.4). The electrocardiogram may demonstrate sinus tachycardia, LA enlargement, and left ventricular hypertrophy. Smaller ductal shunts may be associated with a normal radiograph and electrocardiogram. Of note, the electrocardiogram is not a reliable screening tool to identify an hsPDA.[119]

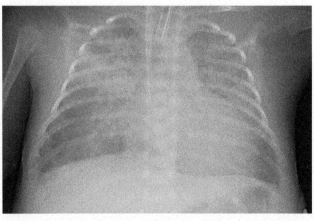

Fig. 22.4   Chest radiograph in a ventilated preterm infant with a large patent ductus arteriosus. Note the large heart shadow and the increased lung markings representing pulmonary overcirculation.

Echocardiographic Diagnosis and Assessment of a Patent Ductus Arteriosus

Ultrasound is the most reliable method of evaluating a PDA and has become the mainstay for diagnosis, disease staging, and treatment response monitoring. Evaluation and staging of DA shunt severity requires assessment of ductal size, transductal Doppler flow pattern, indices of pulmonary overcirculation and left heart volume loading, and surrogate markers of systemic hypoperfusion. Traditional assessments of the hemodynamic significance of a PDA have relied substantially on ductal diameter alone. Although ductal diameter is one of the most important determinants of ductal shunt volume (owing to the exponential relationship between ductal radius and flow), the use of ductal diameter, in isolation, to determine the hemodynamic significance of the ductal shunt should be avoided due to the potential for measurement error and the poor outcome-predictive ability of diameter alone. A comprehensive echocardiographic evaluation provides a more holistic picture with redundancies to mitigate measurement error within the individual echo parameters (Tables 22.1 and 22.2).

Ductus Arteriosus Size and Transductal Doppler Flow Pattern

Ductal diameter on two-dimensional echocardiography ≥1.5 mm on the first day after birth predicts the development of a clinically symptomatic PDA.[120] An hsPDA is characterized by an unrestrictive or arterial left-to-right flow pattern, with a very low diastolic velocity. Peak systolic velocity (PSV) of less than 1.5 m/s has been traditionally described as "unrestrictive." On the other hand, clinicians should recall that PSV may be elevated (>2.0 m/s) either in the setting of a restrictive ductal shunt or due to a very high-volume shunt promoted by low PVR. Peak PDA systolic

Table 22.1   ULTRASOUND PARAMETERS OF DUCTAL HEMODYNAMIC SIGNIFICANCE IN EXTREMELY PRETERM INFANTS (<29 WEEKS' GESTATION) AFTER THE FIRST POSTNATAL DAY

Parameter[a]	Hemodynamic Significance		
	Mild	Moderate	Severe
PDA Diameter			
2D diameter (mm)	<1.5	1.5–3	>3
PDA to LPA ratio	<0.5	0.5–1	>1
PDA Doppler			
Vmax (m/s)	>2.5	1.5–2.5	<1.5
Systolic to diastolic velocity ratio	<2	2–4	>4
LV chamber dilatation (Z score)	<+2.0	+2.0–+3.0	>+3.0
Pulmonary Overcirculation			
LA to Ao ratio	<1.5	1.5–2.0	>2.0
Mitral valve E to A ratio	<1	<1	>1
IVRT (milliseconds)	>40	30–40	<30
LPA Vmax diastole (m/s)	<0.3	0.3–0.5	>0.5
LVO (mL/kg/min)	<200	200–300	>300
PV D wave (m/s)	<0.35	0.35–0.45	>0.45
Systemic Hypoperfusion			
Abdominal Ao diastolic flow	Forward	Absent	Reversed
Celiac artery diastolic flow	Forward	Absent	Reversed
MCA diastolic flow	Forward	Forward	Absent/Reversed

[a]Applies beyond the first 48 hours.
2D, Two-dimensional; *Ao*, aorta; *IVRT*, isovolumic relaxation time; *LA*, left atrium; *LPA*, left pulmonary artery; *LV*, left ventricle; *LVO*, left ventricular output; *MCA*, middle cerebral artery; *PDA*, patent ductus arteriosus; *PV*, pulmonary vein; *Vmax*, maximum velocity.

Table 22.2 INTEROBSERVER VARIABILITY FOR ECHOCARDIOGRAPHY PARAMETERS

Parameter	Correlation Coefficient
Ductal diameter	0.85 (0.68–0.94)[a]
Left pulmonary artery diameter	0.62 (0.34–0.80)[a]
E to A ratio	0.90 (0.77–0.95)[a]
IVRT	0.84 (0.63–0.93)[a]
Aortic diameter	0.99 (0.80–0.95)[a]
Aortic velocity time index	0.79 (0.63–0.90)[a]
Left ventricular output	0.97 (0.94–0.99)[a]
LV end diastolic diameter	0.93 (0.86–0.97)[a]
LA to Ao ratio	0.65 (0.44–0.82)[a]
Descending aorta diastolic flow	0.75 (0.43–1.00)[b]
Celiac diastolic flow	0.88 (0.65–1.00)[b]

[a]Lin's concordance Correlation Coefficient.
[b]Kappa Coefficient.
Ao, Aorta; IVRT, isovolumic relaxation time; LA, left atrium; LV, left ventricle.

velocity should be interpreted in tandem with the "pulsatility" of the PDA Doppler pattern, which can be quantified using the ratio of the PDA PSV to minimum diastolic velocity (MDV).[121] The Doppler profile of a *restrictive PDA* is characterized by a high-velocity shunt throughout systole and diastole and a low PSV to MDV ratio (Fig. 22.5). In addition, transductal velocity ratio (PSV ratio of the pulmonary end over the aortic end of the ductus) has been shown to correlate with other indices of hemodynamic significance of PDA and has been proposed as a measure of the degree of ductal constriction.[122]

Pulmonary Overcirculation and Left Heart Loading

Pulmonary artery Doppler patterns and left heart inflow, dilatation, and output are surrogate markers of the pulmonary–to–systemic blood flow ratio (Qp to Qs). Left pulmonary artery antegrade diastolic velocity greater than 0.3 m/s correlates with a moderate PDA.[123] LVO of greater than 300 mL/kg/min on the first day after delivery predicts a later symptomatic PDA.[120] Subsequently, infants with a symptomatic PDA have significantly higher LVO (419 [305 to 562] mL/kg/min) than infants without PDA (221 ± 56 mL/kg/min), and LVO returns to normal after surgical ligation (246 [191 to 292] mL/kg/min).[124,125]

Left ventricle end-diastolic dimension (LVEDD), a surrogate for LV end-diastolic volume, is increased in infants with PDA and has been correlated with the need for medical and surgical treatment.[124] LVEDD increases with patient weight and may be compared with normative data from extremely preterm infants, although LVEDD greater than 15 mm/kg approximates the upper limit of normal.[126] In infants with a left-to-right shunt across the PDA, LA dilatation occurs due to volume loading from excessive pulmonary venous return. The LA to aortic root ratio (LA to Ao) is a commonly used echocardiographic index of LA dilatation. An LA:AO ratio greater than 1.5 has high sensitivity for a symptomatic PDA but is poorly predictive on the first postnatal day and may be unreliable in the presence of a large transatrial shunt that may unload the left heart (Fig. 22.6).[127] The early phase of filling (E wave) in preterm infants has a lower velocity than the late phase (A wave), resulting in an E to A wave ratio of less than 1. This relates to developmental immaturity of the preterm myocardium and impaired diastolic performance therein limiting early diastolic flow. LA pressure loading occurs due to progressive LV diastolic dysfunction associated with very large volume ductal shunts and drives early passive diastolic LV filling, resulting in a mitral E to A wave ratio greater than 1.[128] In addition, earlier mitral valve opening results in a shortened isovolumic relaxation time (<40 ms) (Fig. 22.7).[129]

Systemic Arterial Diastolic Flow Reversal

Ultrasound can be used to provide an estimate of systemic hypoperfusion by assessing Doppler flow patterns in certain blood vessels that are affected by ductal

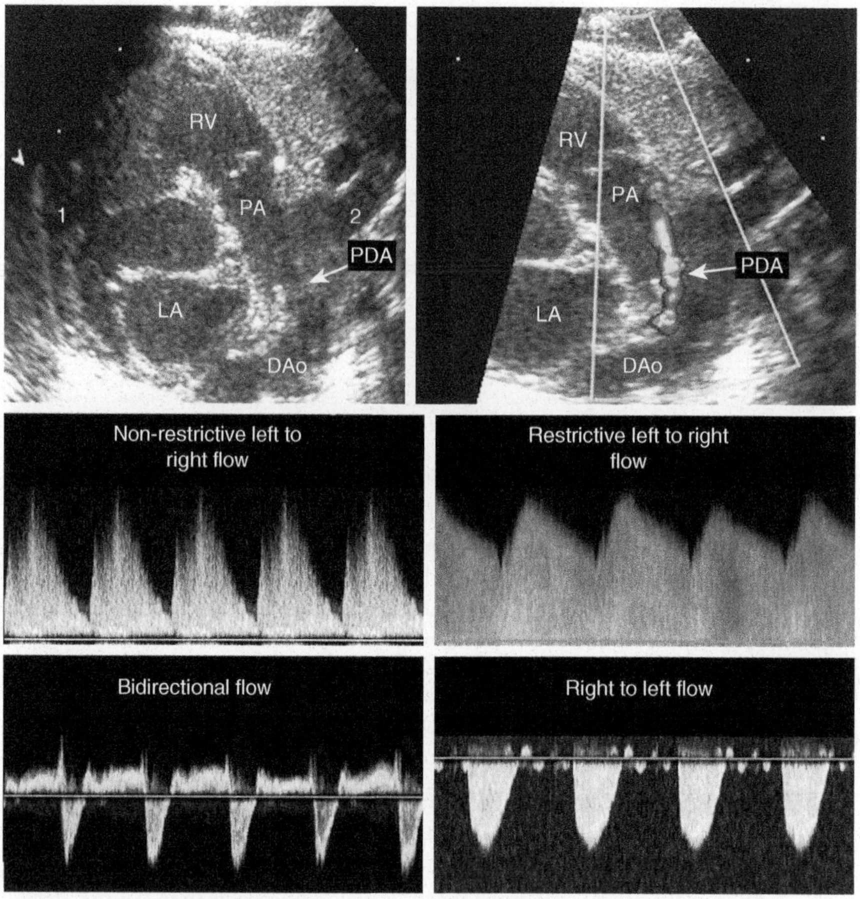

Fig. 22.5 Patent ductus arteriosus (PDA) two-dimensional (2D), color Doppler image, and Doppler flow patterns. The top panel demonstrates the PDA in 2D and color Doppler. *Pulsatile or nonrestrictive pattern*: characterized by a left-to-right shunt with an arterial waveform and high peak systolic velocity to end-diastolic velocity ratio. *Restrictive pattern*: characterized by high systolic and diastolic velocity and low peak systolic velocity to end-diastolic velocity ratio. *Bidirectional pattern*: elevated pulmonary pressures equal to or near systemic pressures; *Right-to-left flow pattern*: suprasystemic pulmonary pressures. *DAo*, Descending aorta; *LA*, left atrium; *RV*, right ventricle; *PA*, pulmonary artery.

steal: the abdominal aorta, the celiac trunk, and the MCA. Diastolic flow reversal in the abdominal aorta is the measurement that best correlates with cardiac MRI estimates of ductal shunt volume.[89] Reduced celiac artery flow (CAF), quantified as a CAF to LVO ratio of less than 0.1, correlates well with conventional echocardiographic indices of the hemodynamic significance of the PDA.[130] Aberrant diastolic flow in the SMA and MCA have been associated with a ductal shunt and improve after PDA ligation. However, their relevance to neonatal and neurodevelopmental outcomes is presently unknown.[131]

The Use of Biomarkers in Patent Ductus Arteriosus Assessment: Brain Natriuretic Peptide and N-Terminal Pro–Brain Natriuretic Peptide

In response to volume and pressure loading, myocytes in the left and right ventricles cleave pro–brain natriuretic peptide (BNP) into the biologically active BNP and the inactive amino-terminal pro-BNP (NTpBNP). BNP promotes natriuresis and diuresis to counteract the effects of LV volume loading secondary to a significant PDA. Studies have evaluated the reliability of BNP and NTpBNP measurements in various potential roles in clinical care, including the replacement of echocardiography for the diagnosis

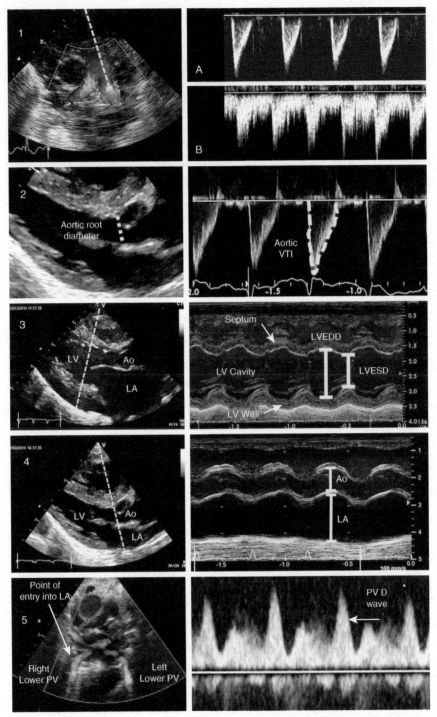

Fig. 22.6   Assessment of pulmonary overcirculation. (1) Measurement of diastolic flow in the left pulmonary artery. Panel (B) illustrates forward diastolic flow in the presence of significant left-to-right ductal flow. (2) Measurement of left ventricular output (LVO): increased LVO in the setting of a PDA indicates increased pulmonary venous return. (3) Measurement of LV diameter in diastole: increased LV diameter is another surrogate marker for increased LV end-diastolic volume. (4) LA to Ao ratio: atrial enlargement can be indexed to a relatively fixed aortic root diameter to further estimate the degree of increased LA volume. Ao, Aorta; LA, left atrium; LV, left ventricle; LVEDD, left ventricle end-diastolic dimension; LVESD, left ventricle end-systolic dimension; PDA, patent ductus arteriosus; PV, pulmonary vein; VTI, velocity time integral.

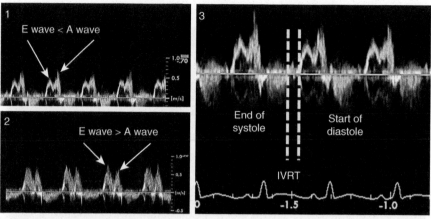

Fig. 22.7 Pulsed wave Doppler of left ventricular inflow across the mitral valve, demonstrating the early ("E") and late ("A," during atrial contraction) ventricular filling velocities. Transmitral valve left ventricle (LV) filling in normal term infants is characterized by a predominance of early diastolic ("E") filling, with limited late LV filling occurring during atrial contraction ("A"), resulting in an E to A ratio greater than 1.0. (1) Healthy preterm infants without a patent ductus arteriosus (PDA) have intrinsically decreased LV diastolic function, relying more on late atrial filling, and E to A ratio less than 1.0. (2 and 3) Preterm infants with a large PDA have increased left atrial pressure, which results in earlier mitral valve opening and drives early passive filling, leading to shortened isovolumetric relaxation time (<40 ms) and a "pseudonormalized" E to A ratio greater than 1.0. *IVRT*, Isovolumic relaxation time.

of PDA, the assessment of treatment response, the triage of patients for early targeted PDA screening, or as an add-on to echocardiography. The interpretation and integration of BNP and NTpBNP measurements into clinical care is hampered by the availability of multiple testing kits, each with a discrete reference range and published results in observational studies correlating these biomarkers with the development of a PDA.

Brain Natriuretic Peptide/N-Terminal Pro–Brain Natriuretic Peptide and the Diagnosis of Presymptomatic Patent Ductus Arteriosus

The early identification of asymptomatic ductal shunting would be clinically useful in centers seeking to administer targeted indomethacin prophylaxis but who have limited access to echocardiography. Umbilical cord concentrations of BNP are positively correlated with the subsequent postnatal development of symptomatic PDA.[132] In addition, NTpBNP concentrations on day 1 are inversely proportional to decreasing gestational age but are nonspecific for the diagnosis of PDA.[133] These findings suggest that factors other than PDA contribute to in utero and early postnatal changes in BNP/NTpBNP (such as elevated pulmonary pressures) because PDA shunting in this period is physiologic and rarely results in pathologic left heart volume overloading.

Both BNP and NTpBNP are predictive of an hsPDA after the second postnatal day and may be used to triage patients for echocardiographic evaluation or empiric therapy. Several cutoffs exist in the literature for both BNP and NTpBNP for the identification of a PDA. However, translation to clinical use is hampered by heterogeneity of the studies, the variety of cutoffs used based on the analytic method or exact timing of sampling, and the increasing availability of echocardiography in many neonatal intensive care units (NICUs).[134-136] In addition, infants with a PDA who respond to indomethacin treatment have greater absolute and relative decreases in BNP and NTpBNP than do nonresponders. However, there is significant overlap in the serum concentrations of these biomarkers among responders and nonresponders, meaning that echocardiography follow-up cannot be reliably replaced.

Near-Infrared Spectroscopy and Patent Ductus Arteriosus Assessment

NIRS offers the ability to noninvasively assess target organ blood flow, in particular, the brain and splanchnic circulation.[137] The ability to assess cerebral and mesenteric perfusion in real time may offer the ability to better appraise the hemodynamic impact a PDA has on these organs. This may also provide an insight into the pathologic basis for the associations between the PDA and important morbidities, aid in triaging PDAs into pathologic versus innocent bystanders, and help to determine which patients warrant treatment. NIRS may also enable the treating physician to monitor treatment response.

However, the studies using NIRS in infants with a PDA have yielded mixed results. Early evidence of the application of NIRS in PDA assessment in a pilot study of 29 infants suggested that PDAs receiving treatment were associated with lower pretreatment renal and skeletal muscle regional saturations. Following treatment, regional saturations "increased toward the range seen in patients who did not require treatment of a PDA."[138] Consistent with this finding, another study found lower cerebral oxygen saturation and higher extraction in the presence of PDA, with normalization of these values 24 hours after starting indomethacin.[83] A recent study of 380 infants less than 32 weeks' gestation demonstrated that regional cerebral oxygen saturations were inversely related to PDA diameter, suggesting that a larger ductal diameter may be associated with lower CBF.[139] A smaller study of 38 infants demonstrated that those with a large PDA had lower mesenteric tissue oxygenation and higher oxygen extraction. However, the study failed to demonstrate a relationship between PDA size (or presence) and cerebral or renal regional oxygenation when assessed before pharmacologic treatment within the first 28 days after birth.[140] In a similar study, van der Laan et al. also failed to demonstrate an association between renal or cerebral regional oxygenation and a significant PDA.[141] On the other hand, a small study found low renal but not cerebral regional oxygen saturation to be associated with a hemodynamically significant DA.[142] The differing results between these studies likely stem from the heterogeneity of the study participants, the timing of assessments (in relation to various confounders including the timing of feeds), the PDA characteristics, comorbidities, and the positioning of the sensors. Studies to date have not investigated the relationship between shunt volume and changes in regional tissue oxygenation, nor have they investigated the relationship between disturbed regional tissue oxygenation and important PDA-related morbidities.

A Comprehensive Appraisal of the Hemodynamic Significance of the Patent Ductus Arteriosus

A cause-and-effect relationship between a PDA and adverse short- and long-term outcomes has been difficult to elucidate. This may either stem from the possibility that no actual relationship exists or, a more likely scenario, a failure to date to accurately appraise and identify high-risk PDAs. This appraisal must be multifactorial, integrating surrogate measures of the magnitude of shunt volume, the ability of the heart to accommodate and compensate for the shunt, the impact of the shunt on the pulmonary and systemic circulations, and important clinical characteristics that may either enhance or mitigate the potential detrimental effects of a PDA (Fig. 22.8). The ability to accurately risk-stratify PDAs into those that are innocent bystanders and those likely to be pathologic is greatly enhanced if ultrasound measurements of ductal characteristics, markers of pulmonary overcirculation, and markers of systemic hypoperfusion are integrated with the clinical status to provide a comprehensive picture of the infants' well-being. The surrogate measures of shunt volume, degree of cardiac adaptation to the shunt, pulmonary overcirculation, and systemic hypoperfusion can be assessed by ultrasound shortly after birth. In the presence of an open ductus, as PVR falls and shunt volume increases during the first few postnatal days, these echocardiographic markers become increasingly more useful in determining the hemodynamic significance of the PDA (Fig. 22.9). However, delaying assessment could lead to a prolonged exposure to the potential detrimental effects of a PDA and mitigate the presumed benefits of early treatment.

Gestational age plays an independent role in the evolution of morbidities, and therefore it should be considered as an important factor in determining PDA significance. Infants at the lower gestational age brackets (≤26 weeks) are more likely to

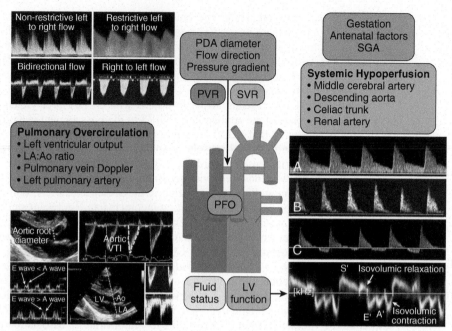

Fig. 22.8 Determinants of hemodynamic significance of a patent ductus arteriosus (PDA). Volume of the shunt, left ventricular function, and clinical parameters are all important in determining treatment. *Ao*, Aorta; *LA*, left atrium; *LV*, left ventricle; *PFO*, patent foramen ovale; *PVR*, pulmonary vascular resistance; *SGA*, small for gestational age; *SVR*, systemic vascular resistance; *VTI*, velocity time integral.

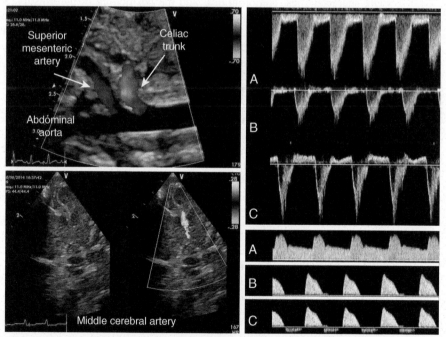

Fig. 22.9 Assessment of systemic hypoperfusion. Measurement of pulsed wave Doppler pattern in the celiac trunk, the abdominal aorta, and the middle cerebral artery can highlight the effect of left-to-right shunting across the patent ductus arteriosus. In the top Doppler panel, three abdominal aortic Doppler wave forms are illustrated demonstrating normal forward diastolic flow (A), absent diastolic flow (B), and reversed diastolic flow (C). A similar pattern can be seen in the lower Doppler panel, which is representative of celiac and middle cerebral arteries.

be predisposed to the effects of the pathophysiologic consequences of the PDA. In addition, important antenatal events (such as the administration of steroids, growth restriction, uteroplacental insufficiency), and maternal illness (such as preeclampsia and diabetes) can also set the scene for adverse events in the setting of a PDA. The role of left heart function, in particular diastolic function, is often also forgotten. As discussed, shunting into the pulmonary circulation in association with a PDA leads to increased pulmonary venous return and increased LV preload. Left heart diastolic function plays a key role in handling this increased blood volume returning to the heart. Compromised diastolic function secondary to the stiff immature myocardium may contribute to increased pulmonary venous pressure because it cannot accommodate the increased blood return to the left atrium, therefore worsening the effect of increased pulmonary blood flow. Impaired diastolic function in the setting of increased pulmonary venous return will lead to increased LA pressure and eventual pulmonary venous congestion. Therefore assessment of systolic and diastolic function of LV can provide valuable information on the significance of a PDA. In addition to ultrasound, biomarkers and NIRS may also be used in the future to provide a comprehensive approach to the management of PDA.

There have been recent attempts to devise a comprehensive PDA appraisal approach by relating early PDA characteristics and integrating them with important clinical features to facilitate the prediction of the evolution of PDA-associated morbidities, particularly respiratory morbidities such as bronchopulmonary dysplasia (BPD). Recent observational studies have demonstrated that a comprehensive echocardiographic assessment which incorporates several parameters discussed earlier applied at 24 to 48 hours of age and different scoring systems identify infants with a PDA that went on to develop severe periventricular/intraventricular hemorrhage, BPD, or death.[1,143-145] In addition, these markers may be able to predict poor neurodevelopmental outcome associated with a PDA.[146] It is plausible that applying a staging system for ductal disease severity at an earlier time point may facilitate better targeted treatment. In a recent multicenter prospective observational study of 141 infants with a gestational age of 26 ± 1.4 weeks, a comprehensive echocardiogram between 36 and 48 hours after delivery was performed.[147] The aim of the study was to assess whether a PDA severity score (PDAsc) incorporating markers of pulmonary overcirculation and LV diastolic function, in addition to the infant's gestation can predict BPD or death before discharge (BPD/death). In multiple logistic regression, five parameters were independently associated with BPD/death: gestation at birth, PDA diameter and flow velocity, LVO, and left ventricle left diastolic wave (LV A'wave). The PDAsc ranged from 0 (low risk) to 13 (high risk). Infants who developed BPD/death had a higher score than those who did not. A cutoff PDAsc of 5.0 had an area under the curve of 0.92 for the ability to predict BPD/death. A PDAsc cutoff of 5.0 has a sensitivity and specificity of 92% and 87%, respectively, and positive and negative predictive values of 92% and 82%, respectively. Other scoring systems are currently being investigated.[148]

Summary

PDA is a common problem in VLBW infants. The shunt across the PDA is primarily left to right in the immediate hours after birth. If the DA remains open, it results in a progressive increase in pulmonary overcirculation and left-sided cardiac volume overload, with accompanying systemic hypoperfusion. Despite the immaturity of the myocardium, the heart is capable of augmenting cardiac output even in VLBW neonates. The increase in cardiac output is a result of an increase in stroke volume without a significant change in heart rate. Because of the diversion of blood from the aorta to the pulmonary artery, the decrease in systolic, diastolic, and mean blood pressures, and the vasoconstriction that occurs in selected vascular beds, the increase in LVO does not lead to an increase or even maintenance of *effective* systemic blood flow. Both animal and human studies show compromised organ blood flow patterns, especially to organs supplied by the aorta distal to the PDA. Further research should focus on a comprehensive approach to the assessment recommended by the authors, the use of newer modalities, and the selection of infants who would most likely benefit from targeted treatment.

REFERENCES

1. El-Khuffash A, James AT, Corcoran JD, et al.: A patent ductus arteriosus severity score predicts chronic lung disease or death before discharge, *J Pediatr* 167(6):1354–1361.e2, 2015.
2. El-Khuffash A, Weisz DE, McNamara PJ: Reflections of the changes in patent ductus arteriosus management during the last 10 years, *Arch Dis Child Fetal Neonatal Ed*, 2016.
3. Guerguerian AM, Hardy P, Bhattacharya M, et al.: Expression of cyclooxygenases in ductus arteriosus of fetal and newborn pigs, *Am J Obstet Gynecol* 179(6 Pt 1):1618–1626, 1998.
4. Hermes-DeSantis ER, Clyman RI: Patent ductus arteriosus: pathophysiology and management, *J Perinatol* 26(Suppl 1):S14–S18, 2006.
5. Weir EK, Lopez-Barneo J, Buckler KJ, et al.: Acute oxygen-sensing mechanisms, *N Engl J Med* 353(19):2042–2055, 2005.
6. Michelakis ED, Rebeyka I, Wu X, et al.: O2 sensing in the human ductus arteriosus: regulation of voltage-gated K+ channels in smooth muscle cells by a mitochondrial redox sensor, *Circ Res* 91(6):478–486, 2002.
7. Francalanci P, Camassei FD, Orzalesi M, et al.: CD44-v6 expression in smooth muscle cells in the postnatal remodeling process of ductus arteriosus, *Am J Cardiol* 97(7):1056–1059, 2006.
8. Clyman RI: Mechanisms regulating the ductus arteriosus, *Biol Neonate* 89(4):330–335, 2006.
9. Silver MM, Freedom RM, Silver MD, et al.: The morphology of the human newborn ductus arteriosus: a reappraisal of its structure and closure with special reference to prostaglandin E1 therapy, *Hum Pathol* 12(12):1123–1136, 1981.
10. Clyman RI, Chan CY, Mauray F, et al.: Permanent anatomic closure of the ductus arteriosus in newborn baboons: the roles of postnatal constriction, hypoxia, and gestation, *Pediatr Res* 45(1):19–29, 1999.
11. Waleh N, Seidner S, McCurnin D, et al.: The role of monocyte-derived cells and inflammation in baboon ductus arteriosus remodeling, *Pediatr Res* 57(2):254–262, 2005.
12. Reller MD, Rice MJ, McDonald RW: Review of studies evaluating ductal patency in the premature infant, *J Pediatr* 122(6):S59–S62, 1993.
13. Kajino H, Chen YQ, Seidner SR, et al.: Factors that increase the contractile tone of the Ductus Arteriosus also regulate its anatomic remodeling, *Am J Physiol Regul Integr Comp Physiol* 281:R291–R301, 2001.
14. Brown S, Liu X-T, Ramaekers F, Rosenfeld C: Differential maturation in ductus arteriosus and umbilical artery smooth muscle during ovine development, *Pediatr Res* 51:34A, 2002.
15. Sakurai H, Matsuoka R, Furutani Y, et al.: Expression of four myosin heavy chain genes in developing blood vessels and other smooth muscle organs in rabbits, *Eur J Cell Biol* 69(2):166–172, 1996.
16. Colbert MC, Kirby ML, Robbins J: Endogenous retinoic acid signaling colocalizes with advanced expression of the adult smooth muscle myosin heavy chain isoform during development of the ductus arteriosus, *Circ Res* 78(5):790–798, 1996.
17. Reeve H, Tolarova S, Cornfield D, et al.: Developmental changes in K+ channel expression may determine the O2 response of the ductus arteriosus, *FASEB J* 11:420A, 1997.
18. Kajimoto H, Hashimoto K, Bonnet SN, et al.: Oxygen activates the Rho/Rho-Kinase pathway and induces RhoB and ROCK-1 expression in human and rabbit ductus arteriosus by increasing mitochondria-derived reactive oxygen species. A newly recognized mechanism for sustaining ductal constriction, *Circulation* 115:1777–1788, 2007.
19. Clyman RI, Waleh NS, Kajino H, et al.: Calcium-dependent and calcium-sensitizing pathways in the mature and immature ductus arteriosus, *Am J Physiol Regul Integr Comp Physiol* 293(4):R1650–R1656, 2007.
20. Cogolludo AL, Moral-Sanz J, Van der Sterren S, et al.: Maturation of O2 sensing and signalling in the chicken ductus arteriosus, *Am J Physiol Lung Cell Mol Physiol*, 2009.
21. Thebaud B, Wu XC, Kajimoto H, et al.: Developmental absence of the O2 sensitivity of L-type calcium channels in preterm ductus arteriosus smooth muscle cells impairs O2 constriction contributing to patent ductus arteriosus, *Pediatr Res* 63(2):176–181, 2008.
22. Waleh N, Reese J, Kajino H, et al.: Oxygen-induced tension in the sheep ductus arteriosus: effects of gestation on potassium and calcium channel regulation, *Pediatr Res* 65(3):285–290, 2009.
23. Wu C, Hayama E, Imamura S, et al.: Developmental changes in the expression of voltage-gated potassium channels in the ductus arteriosus of the fetal rat, *Heart Vessels* 22(1):34–40, 2007.
24. Thebaud B, Michelakis ED, Wu XC, et al.: Oxygen-sensitive Kv channel gene transfer confers oxygen responsiveness to preterm rabbit and remodeled human ductus arteriosus: implications for infants with patent ductus arteriosus, *Circulation* 110(11):1372–1379, 2004.
25. Clyman RI, Waleh N, Black SM, et al.: Regulation of ductus arteriosus patency by nitric oxide in fetal lambs. The role of gestation, oxygen tension and vasa vasorum, *Pediatr Res* 43:633–644, 1998.
26. Waleh N, Kajino H, Marrache AM, et al.: Prostaglandin E2–mediated relaxation of the ductus arteriosus: effects of gestational age on g protein-coupled receptor expression, signaling, and vasomotor control, *Circulation* 110(16):2326–2332, 2004.
27. Liu H, Manganiello VC, Clyman RI: Expression, activity and function of cAMP and cGMP phosphodiesterases in the mature and immature ductus arteriosus, *Pediatr Res* 64:477–481, 2008.
28. Clyman RI, Mauray F, Heymann MA, et al.: Effect of gestational age on pulmonary metabolism of prostaglandin E1 & E2, *Prostaglandins* 21(3):505–513, 1981.
29. Gonzalez A, Sosenko IR, Chandar J, et al.: Influence of infection on patent ductus arteriosus and chronic lung disease in premature infants weighing 1000 grams or less, *J Pediatr* 128(4):470–478, 1996.

30. Waleh N, Barrette AM, Dagle JM, et al.: Effects of advancing gestation and non-caucasian race on ductus arteriosus gene expression, *J Pediatr* 167(5):1033–1041.e2, 2015.
31. Collaborative Group on Antenatal Steroid Therapy: *Prevention of respiratory distress syndrome: effect of antenatal dexamethasone administration*, Publication No 85-2695: National Institutes of Health, 1985, p 44.
32. Clyman RI, Ballard PL, Sniderman S, et al.: Prenatal administration of betamethasone for prevention of patent ductus arteriosus, *J Pediatr* 98:123–126, 1981.
33. Clyman RI, Mauray F, Roman C, et al.: Effects of antenatal glucocorticoid administration on the ductus arteriosus of preterm lambs, *Am J Physiol* 241:H415–H420, 1981.
34. Momma K, Mishihara S, Ota Y: Constriction of the fetal ductus arteriosus by glucocorticoid hormones, *Pediatr Res* 15:19–21, 1981.
35. Thibeault DW, Emmanouilides GC, Dodge ME: Pulmonary and circulatory function in preterm lambs treated with hydrocortisone in utero, *Biol Neonate* 34:238–247, 1978.
36. Waffarn F, Siassi B, Cabal L, et al.: Effect of antenatal glucocorticoids on clinical closure of the ductus arteriosus, *Am J Dis Child* 137:336–338, 1983.
37. Watterberg KL, Gerdes JS, Cole CH, et al.: Prophylaxis of early adrenal insufficiency to prevent bronchopulmonary dysplasia: a multicenter trial, *Pediatrics* 114(6):1649–1657, 2004.
38. Group VONSS: Early postnatal dexamethasone therapy for the prevention of chronic lung disease, *Pediatrics* 108(3):741–748, 2001.
39. Treszl A, Szabo M, Dunai G, et al.: Angiotensin II type 1 receptor A1166C polymorphism and prophylactic indomethacin treatment induced ductus arteriosus closure in very low birth weight neonates, *Pediatr Res* 54(5):753–755, 2003.
40. Bokodi G, Derzbach L, Banyasz I, et al.: Association of interferon gamma T+874A and interleukin 12 p40 promoter CTCTAA/GC polymorphism with the need for respiratory support and perinatal complications in low birthweight neonates, *Arch Dis Child Fetal Neonatal Ed* 92(1):F25–F29, 2007.
41. Derzbach L, Treszl A, Balogh A, et al.: Gender dependent association between perinatal morbidity and estrogen receptor-alpha Pvull polymorphism, *J Perinat Med* 33(5):461–462, 2005.
42. Dagle JM, Lepp NT, Cooper ME, et al.: Determination of genetic predisposition to patent ductus arteriosus in preterm infants, *Pediatrics* 123(4):1116–1123, 2009.
43. Ivey KN, Sutcliffe D, Richardson J, et al.: Transcriptional regulation during development of the ductus arteriosus, *Circ Res* 103(4):388–395, 2008.
44. Zhao F, Weismann CG, Satoda M, et al.: Novel TFAP2B mutations that cause Char syndrome provide a genotype-phenotype correlation, *Am J Hum Genet* 69(4):695–703, 2001.
45. Cotton RB, Haywood JL, FitzGerald GA: Symptomatic patent ductus arteriosus following prophylactic indomethacin. A clinical and biochemical appraisal, *Biol Neonate* 60(5):273–282, 1991.
46. Chorne N, Jegatheesan P, Lin E, et al.: Risk factors for persistent ductus arteriosus patency during indomethacin treatment, *J Pediatr* 151(6):629–634, 2007.
47. Clyman RI, Seidner SR, Kajino H, et al.: VEGF regulates remodeling during permanent anatomic closure of the ductus arteriosus, *Am J Physiol* 282(1):R199–R206, 2002.
48. Kajino H, Goldbarg S, Roman C, et al.: Vasa vasorum hypoperfusion is responsible for medial hypoxia and anatomic remodeling in the newborn lamb ductus arteriosus, *Pediatr Res* 51(2):228–235, 2002.
49. Noori S, Wlodaver A, Gottipati V, et al.: Transitional changes in cardiac and cerebral hemodynamics in term neonates at birth, *J Pediatr* 160(6):943–948, 2012.
50. van Vonderen JJ, te Pas AB, Kolster-Bijdevaate C, et al.: Non-invasive measurements of ductus arteriosus flow directly after birth, *Arch Dis Child Fetal Neonatal Ed* 99(5):F408–F412, 2014.
51. Alverson DC, Eldridge MW, Johnson JD, et al.: Effect of patent ductus arteriosus on left ventricular output in premature infants, *J Pediatr* 102:754–757, 1983.
52. Baylen BG, Ogata H, Oguchi K, et al.: The contractility and performance of the preterm left ventricle before and after early patent ductus arteriosus occlusion in surfactant-treated lambs, *Pediatr Res* 19(10):1053–1058, 1985.
53. Clyman RI, Mauray F, Heymann MA, et al.: Cardiovascular effects of a patent ductus arteriosus in preterm lambs with respiratory distress, *J Pediatr* 111:579–587, 1987.
54. Clyman RI, Roman C, Heymann MA, et al.: How a patent ductus arteriosus effects the premature lamb's ability to handle additional volume loads, *Pediatr Res* 22:531–535, 1987.
55. Walther FJ, Kim DH, Ebrahimi M, et al.: Pulsed Doppler measurement of left ventricular output as early predictor of symptomatic patent ductus arteriosus in very preterm infants, *Biol Neonate* 56(3):121–128, 1989.
56. Lindner W, Seidel M, Versmold HJ, et al.: Stroke volume and left ventricular output in preterm infants with patent ductus arteriosus, *Pediatr Res* 27:278–281, 1990.
57. Meyers RL, Alpan G, Lin E, et al.: Patent ductus arteriosus, indomethacin, and intestinal distension: effects on intestinal blood flow and oxygen consumption, *Pediatr Res* 29:569–574, 1991.
58. Shimada S, Kasai T, Konishi M, et al.: Effects of patent ductus arteriosus on left ventricular output and organ blood flows in preterm infants with respiratory distress syndrome treated with surfactant, *J Pediatr* 125(2):270–277, 1994.
59. Baylen BG, Ogata H, Ikegami M, et al.: Left ventricular performance and regional blood flows before and after ductus arteriosus occlusion in premature lambs treated with surfactant, *Circulation* 67(4):837–843, 1983.
60. Tamura M, Harada K, Takahashi Y, et al.: Changes in left ventricular diastolic filling patterns before and after the closure of the ductus arteriosus in very-low-birth weight infants, *Tohoku J Exp Med* 182(4):337–346, 1997.

22

61. Evans N, Iyer P: Assessment of ductus arteriosus shunt in preterm infants supported by mechanical ventilation: effect of interatrial shunting, *J Pediatr* 125(5 Pt 1):778–785, 1994.
62. Noori S, Seri I: Pathophysiology of newborn hypotension outside the transitional period, *Early Hum Dev* 81(5):399–404, 2005.
63. Way GL, Pierce JR, Wolf RR, et al.: ST depression suggesting subendocardial ischemia in neonates with respiratory distress syndrome and patent ductus arteriosus, *J Pediatr* 95:609–611, 1979.
64. Arvind Sehgal PJM: Coronary artery hypo-perfusion is associated with impaired diastolic dysfunction in preterm infants after patent ductus arteriosus (PDA) ligation, *PAS*, 2007.
65. El-Khuffash AF, Molloy EJ: Influence of a patent ductus arteriosus on cardiac troponin T levels in preterm infants, *J Pediatr*, 2008.
66. Barlow AJ, Ward C, Webber SA, et al.: Myocardial contractility in premature neonates with and without patent ductus arteriosus, *Pediatr Cardiol* 25(2):102–107, 2004.
67. James AT, Corcoran JD, Breatnach CR, et al.: Longitudinal assessment of left and right myocardial function in preterm infants using strain and strain rate imaging, *Neonatology* 109(1):69–75, 2016.
68. Czernik C, Rhode S, Helfer S, et al.: Development of left ventricular longitudinal speckle tracking echocardiography in very low birth weight infants with and without bronchopulmonary dysplasia during the neonatal period, *PLoS One* 9(9):e106504, 2014.
69. Helfer S, Schmitz L, Buhrer C, et al.: Tissue doppler-derived strain and strain rate during the first 28 days of life in very low birth weight infants, *Echocardiography* 31(6):765–772, 2013.
70. de Waal K, Phad N, Lakkundi A, et al.: Cardiac function after the immediate transitional period in very preterm infants using speckle tracking analysis, *Pediatr Cardiol* 37(2):295–303, 2016.
71. James AT, Corcoran JD, Franklin O, et al.: Clinical utility of right ventricular fractional area change in preterm infants, *Early Hum Dev* 92:19–23, 2016.
72. Ratner I, Perelmuter B, Toews W, et al.: Association of low systolic and diastolic blood pressure with significant patent ductus arteriosus in the very low birth weight infant, *Crit Care Med* 13(6):497–500, 1985.
73. Evans N, Moorcraft J: Effect of patency of the ductus arteriosus on blood pressure in very preterm infants, *Arch Dis Child* 67(10 Spec No):1169–1173, 1992.
74. Liebowitz M, Koo J, Wickremasinghe A, et al.: Effects of prophylactic indomethacin on vasopressor-dependent hypotension in extremely preterm infants, *J Pediatr*, 2016.
75. Sarkar S, Dechert R, Schumacher RE, et al.: Is refractory hypotension in preterm infants a manifestation of early ductal shunting? *J Perinatol*, 2007.
76. McCurnin D, Clyman RI: Effects of a patent ductus arteriosus on postprandial mesenteric perfusion in premature baboons, *Pediatrics* 122(6):e1262–e1267, 2008.
77. Raju TN: Cerebral Doppler studies in the fetus and newborn infant, *J Pediatr* 119(2):165–174, 1991.
78. Greisen G, Johansen K, Ellison PH, et al.: Cerebral blood flow in the newborn infant: comparison of Doppler ultrasound and 133xenon clearance, *J Pediatr* 104(3):411–418, 1984.
79. Hansen NB, Stonestreet BS, Rosenkrantz TS, et al.: Validity of Doppler measurements of anterior cerebral artery blood flow velocity: correlation with brain blood flow in piglets, *Pediatrics* 72(4):526–531, 1983.
80. Chemtob S, Beharry K, Rex J, et al.: Prostanoids determine the range of cerebral blood flow autoregulation of newborn piglets, *Stroke* 21(5):777–784, 1990.
81. Laudignon N, Chemtob S, Bard H, et al.: Effect of indomethacin on cerebral blood flow velocity of premature newborns, *Biol Neonate* 54(5):254–262, 1988.
82. Perlman JM, Hill A, Volpe JJ: The effect of patent ductus arteriosus on flow velocity in the anterior cerebral arteries: ductal steal in the premature newborn infant, *J Pediatr* 99:767–771, 1981.
83. Lemmers PM, Toet MC, van Bel F: Impact of patent ductus arteriosus and subsequent therapy with indomethacin on cerebral oxygenation in preterm infants, *Pediatrics* 121(1):142–147, 2008.
84. Martin CG, Snider AR, Katz SM, et al.: Abnormal cerebral blood flow patterns in preterm infants with a large patent ductus arteriosus, *J Pediatr* 101:587–593, 1982.
85. Shortland DB, Gibson NA, Levene MI, et al.: Patent ductus arteriosus and cerebral circulation in preterm infants, *Dev Med Child Neurol* 32(5):386–393, 1990.
86. Breatnach CR, Franklin O, McCallion N, et al.: The effect of a significant patent ductus arteriosus on doppler flow patterns of preductal vessels: an assessment of the brachiocephalic artery, *J Pediatr* 180:279–281.e1, 2017.
87. Jim WT, Chiu NC, Chen MR, et al.: Cerebral hemodynamic change and intraventricular hemorrhage in very low birth weight infants with patent ductus arteriosus, *Ultrasound Med Biol* 31(2):197–202, 2005.
88. Kluckow M, Evans N: Low superior vena cava flow and intraventricular haemorrhage in preterm infants, *Arch Dis Child Fetal Neonatal Ed* 82(3):F188–F194, 2000.
89. Groves AM, Kuschel CA, Knight DB, et al.: Does retrograde diastolic flow in the descending aorta signify impaired systemic perfusion in preterm infants?, *Pediatr Res* 63(1):89–94, 2008.
90. Deeg KH, Gerstner R, Brandl U, et al.: Doppler sonographic flow parameter of the anterior cerebral artery in patent ductus arteriosus of the newborn infant compared to a healthy control sample, *Klin Padiatr* 198(6):463–470, 1986.
91. Coombs RC, Morgan MEI, Durin GM, et al.: Gut blood flow velocities in the newborn: effects of patent ductus arteriosus and parenteral indomethacin, *Arch Dis Child* 65:1067–1071, 1990.
92. Yanowitz TD, Yao AC, Werner JC, et al.: Effects of prophylactic low-dose indomethacin on hemodynamics in very low birth weight infants, *J Pediatr* 132(1):28–34, 1998.
93. Pezzati M, Vangi V, Biagiotti R, et al.: Effects of indomethacin and ibuprofen on mesenteric and renal blood flow in preterm infants with patent ductus arteriosus, *J Pediatr* 135(6):733–738, 1999.

94. Ohlsson A, Walia R, Shah S: Ibuprofen for the treatment of patent ductus arteriosus in preterm and/or low birth weight infants, *Cochrane Database Syst Rev* (4): CD003481, 2010.

95. Lewis AB, Heymann MA, Rudolph AM: Gestational changes in pulmonary vascular responses in fetal lambs in utero, *Circ Res* 39:536–541, 1976.

96. Jacob J, Gluck G, DiSessa T, et al.: The contribution of PDA in the neonate with severe RDS, *J Pediatr* 96(1):79–87, 1980.

97. Gersony WM, Peckham GJ, Ellison RC, et al.: Effects of indomethacin in premature infants with patent ductus arteriosus: results of a national collaborative study, *J Pediatr* 102:895–906, 1983.

98. Raju TNK, Langenberg P: Pulmonary hemorrhage and exogenous surfactant therapy—a metaanalysis, *J Pediatr* 123(4):603–610, 1993.

99. Alpan G, Clyman RI: Cardiovascular effects of surfactant replacement with special reference to the patent ductus arteriosus. In Robertson B, Taeusch HW, editors: *Surfactant Therapy for Lung Disease: Lung Biology in Health and Disease,* 84, New York, 1995, Marcel Dekker, Inc, pp 531–545.

100. Rakza T, Magnenant E, Klosowski S, et al.: Early hemodynamic consequences of patent ductus arteriosus in preterm infants with intrauterine growth restriction, *J Pediatr* 151(6):624–628, 2007.

101. Alpan G, Scheerer R, Bland RD, et al.: Patent ductus arteriosus increases lung fluid filtration in preterm lambs, *Pediatr Res* 30:616–621, 1991.

102. Ikegami M, Jacobs H, Jobe A: Surfactant function in respiratory distress syndrome, *J Pediatr* 102:443–447, 1983.

103. Brown E: Increased risk of bronchopulmonary dysplasia in infants with patent ductus arteriosus, *J Pediatr* 95:865–866, 1979.

104. Cotton RB, Stahlman MT, Berder HW, et al.: Randomized trial of early closure of symptomatic patent ductus arteriosus in small preterm infants, *J Pediatr* 93:647–651, 1978.

105. Clyman RI: Commentary: Recommendations for the postnatal use of indomethacin. An analysis of four separate treatment strategies, *J Pediatr* 128:601–607, 1996.

106. McCurnin D, Seidner S, Chang LY, et al.: Ibuprofen-induced patent ductus arteriosus closure: physiologic, histologic, and biochemical effects on the premature lung, *Pediatrics* 121(5):945–956, 2008.

107. Perez Fontan JJ, Clyman RI, Mauray F, et al.: Respiratory effects of a patent ductus arteriosus in premature newborn lambs, *J Appl Physiol* 63(6):2315–2324, 1987.

108. Shimada S, Raju TNK, Bhat R, et al.: Treatment of patent ductus arteriosus after exogenous surfactant in baboons with hyaline membrane disease, *Pediatr Res* 26:565–569, 1989.

109. Krauss AN, Fatica N, Lewis BS, et al.: Pulmonary function in preterm infants following treatment with intravenous indomethacin, *Am J Dis Child* 143:78–81, 1989.

110. Alpan G, Mauray F, Clyman RI: Effect of patent ductus arteriosus on water accumulation and protein permeability in the premature lungs of mechanically ventilated premature lambs, *Pediatr Res* 26:570–575, 1989.

111. Gerhardt T, Bancalari E: Lung compliance in newborns with patent ductus arteriosus before and after surgical ligation, *Biol Neonate* 38:96–105, 1980.

112. Naulty CM, Horn S, Conry J, et al.: Improved lung compliance after ligation of patent ductus arteriosus in hyaline membrane disease, *J Pediatr* 93:682–684, 1978.

113. Stefano JL, Abbasi S, Pearlman SA, et al.: Closure of the ductus arteriosus with indomethacin in ventilated neonates with respiratory distress syndrome. Effects of pulmonary compliance and ventilation, *Am Rev Respir Dis* 143(2):236–239, 1991.

114. Yeh TF, Thalji A, Luken L, et al.: Improved lung compliance following indomethacin therapy in premature infants with persistent ductus arteriosus, *Chest* 80(6):698–700, 1981.

115. Szymankiewicz M, Hodgman JE, Siassi B, et al.: Mechanics of breathing after surgical ligation of patent ductus arteriosus in newborns with respiratory distress syndrome, *Biol Neonate* 85(1):32–36, 2004.

116. Dawes GS, Mott JC, Widdicombe JG: The patency of the ductus arteriosus in newborn lambs and its physiological consequences, *J Physiol* 128:361–383, 1955.

117. Stuckey D: Palmar pulsation: a physical sign of patent ductus arteriosus in infancy, *Med J Aust* 44(19):681–682, 1957.

118. Skelton R, Evans N, Smythe J: A blinded comparison of clinical and echocardiographic evaluation of the preterm infant for patent ductus arteriosus, *J Paediatr Child Health* 30(5):406–411, 1994.

119. Shipton SE, van der Merwe PL, Nel ED: Diagnosis of haemodynamically significant patent ductus arteriosus in neonates– is the ECG of diagnostic help? *Cardiovasc J S Afr* 12(5):264–267, 2001.

120. Kluckow M, Evans N: Early echocardiographic prediction of symptomatic patent ductus arteriosus in preterm infants undergoing mechanical ventilation, *J Pediatr* 127(5):774–779, 1995.

121. Smith A, Maguire M, Livingstone V, et al.: Peak systolic to end diastolic flow velocity ratio is associated with ductal patency in infants below 32 weeks of gestation, *Arch Dis Child Fetal Neonatal Ed* 100(2):F132–F136, 2015.

122. Davies MW, Betheras FR, Swaminathan M: A preliminary study of the application of the transductal velocity ratio for assessing persistent ductus arteriosus, *Arch Dis Child Fetal Neonatal Ed* 82(3):F195–F199, 2000.

123. Hiraishi S, Horiguchi Y, Misawa H, et al.: Noninvasive Doppler echocardiographic evaluation of shunt flow dynamics of the ductus arteriosus, *Circulation* 75(6):1146–1153, 1987.

124. Lindner W, Seidel M, Versmold HT, et al.: Stroke volume and left ventricular output in preterm infants with patent ductus arteriosus, *Pediatr Res* 27(3):278–281, 1990.

125. Alverson DC, Eldridge MW, Johnson JD, et al.: Effect of patent ductus arteriosus on left ventricular output in premature infants, *J Pediatr* 102(5):754–757, 1983.

22

126. Zecca E, Romagnoli C, Vento G, et al.: Left ventricle dimensions in preterm infants during the first month of life, *Eur J Pediatr* 160(4):227–230, 2001.
127. Harling S, Hansen-Pupp I, Baigi A, et al.: Echocardiographic prediction of patent ductus arteriosus in need of therapeutic intervention, *Acta Paediatr* 100(2):231–235, 2011.
128. Sehgal A, McNamara PJ: Does echocardiography facilitate determination of hemodynamic significance attributable to the ductus arteriosus?, *Eur J Pediatr* 168(8):907–914, 2009.
129. Schmitz L, Stiller B, Koch H, et al.: Diastolic left ventricular function in preterm infants with a patent ductus arteriosus: A serial Doppler echocardiography study, *Early Human Development* 76(2): 91–100, 2004.
130. El-Khuffash A, Higgins M, Walsh K, et al.: Quantitative assessment of the degree of ductal steal using celiac artery blood flow to left ventricular output ratio in preterm infants, *Neonatology* 93(3): 206–212, 2008.
131. Hoodbhoy SA, Cutting HA, Seddon JA, et al.: Cerebral and splanchnic hemodynamics after duct ligation in very low birth weight infants, *J Pediatr* 154(2):196–200, 2009.
132. Mannarino S, Garofoli F, Cerbo RM, et al.: Cord blood, perinatal BNP values in term and preterm newborns, *Arch Dis Child Fetal Neonatal Ed* 95(1):F74, 2010.
133. Farombi-Oghuvbu I, Matthews T, Mayne PD, et al.: N-terminal pro-B-type natriuretic peptide: a measure of significant patent ductus arteriosus, *Arch Dis Child Fetal Neonatal Ed* 93(4):F257–F260, 2008.
134. Chen S, Tacy T, Clyman R: How useful are B-type natriuretic peptide measurements for monitoring changes in patent ductus arteriosus shunt magnitude?, *J Perinatol* 30(12):780–785, 2010.
135. El-Khuffash A, Molloy EJ: Are B-type natriuretic peptide (BNP) and N-terminal-pro-BNP useful in neonates?, *Arch Dis Child Fetal Neonatal Ed* 92(4):F320–F324, 2007.
136. Martinovici D, Vanden Eijnden S, Unger P, et al.: Early NT-proBNP is able to predict spontaneous closure of patent ductus arteriosus in preterm neonates, but not the need of its treatment, *Pediatr Cardiol* 32(7):953–957, 2011.
137. Murkin JM, Arango M: Near-infrared spectroscopy as an index of brain and tissue oxygenation, *Br J Anaesth* 103(Suppl 1):i3–i13, 2009.
138. Underwood MA, Milstein JM, Sherman MP: Near-infrared spectroscopy as a screening tool for patent ductus arteriosus in extremely low birth weight infants, *Neonatology* 91(2):134–139, 2007.
139. Dix L, Molenschot M, Breur J, et al.: Cerebral oxygenation and echocardiographic parameters in preterm neonates with a patent ductus arteriosus: an observational study, *Arch Dis Child Fetal Neonatal Ed*, 2016.
140. Petrova A, Bhatt M, Mehta R: Regional tissue oxygenation in preterm born infants in association with echocardiographically significant patent ductus arteriosus, *J Perinatol* 31(7):460–464, 2011.
141. van der Laan ME, Roofthooft MT, Fries MW, et al.: A hemodynamically significant patent ductus arteriosus does not affect cerebral or renal tissue oxygenation in preterm infants, *Neonatology* 110(2):141–147, 2016.
142. Chock VY, Rose LA, Mante JV, et al.: Near-infrared spectroscopy for detection of a significant patent ductus arteriosus, *Pediatr Res* 80(5):675–680, 2016.
143. El-Khuffash A, Barry D, Walsh K, et al.: Biochemical markers may identify preterm infants with a patent ductus arteriosus at high risk of death or severe intraventricular haemorrhage, *Arch Dis Child Fetal Neonatal Ed* 93(6):F407–F412, 2008.
144. Schena F, Francescato G, Cappelleri A, et al.: Association between hemodynamically significant patent ductus arteriosus and bronchopulmonary dysplasia, *J Pediatr*, 2015.
145. Gursoy T, Hayran M, Derin H, et al.: A clinical scoring system to predict the development of bronchopulmonary dysplasia, *Am J Perinatol* 32(7):659–666, 2015.
146. El-Khuffash AF, Slevin M, McNamara PJ, et al.: N-terminal pro natriuretic peptide and a patent ductus arteriosus scoring system predict death before discharge or neurodevelopmental outcome at 2 years in preterm infants, *Arch Dis Child Fetal Neonatal Ed* 96(2):F133–F137, 2011.
147. El-Khuffash A, James AT, Corcoran JD, et al.: A patent ductus arteriosus severity score predicts chronic lung disease or death before discharge, *J Pediatr* 167(6):1354–1361.e2, 2015.
148. Fink D, El-Khuffash A, McNamara PJ, et al.: Tale of two patent ductus arteriosus severity scores: similarities and differences, *Am J Perinatol*, 2017. https://doi.org/10.1055/s-0037-1605576.

CHAPTER 23

Pharmacologic Management of Patent Ductus Arteriosus in the Very Preterm Neonate

Prakesh S. Shah

- The clinical management of patent ductus arteriosus (PDA) in the very preterm neonate remains a controversial topic because the risks and benefits of medical or surgical interventions remain unclear.
- Nonsteroidal antiinflammatory drugs (NSAIDs) (indomethacin and ibuprofen) and acetaminophen are the most common and effective pharmacologic agents used for PDA closure.
- No major differences in the efficacy between the three agents have been reported in comparative effectiveness trials as far as closure of the PDA is concerned. However, there are differences among the drugs in their ability to directly affect cerebral perfusion and their side-effect profiles vary as well.
- Wide variations in the timing, dosage, and type of pharmacologic agent have been reported internationally.
- Conservative and pharmacologic management have become increasingly popular, resulting in less use of surgical ligation.

This chapter reviews the epidemiology and current state of pharmacologic management (prophylactic and therapeutic) of the patent ductus arteriosus (PDA) in the very preterm neonate. Until now, the optimal management of PDA has been controversial in the scientific community, with no clear consensus or generally accepted guidelines for management. Most of the dispute stems from several sources: the natural history of PDA, the hemodynamic significance of PDA (especially concerning its impact on cerebral oxygenation and its potential long-term consequences on neurodevelopment), variable efficacy of the available treatments, unpredictable side effects of pharmacologic and surgical therapy, and the lack of information on long-term outcomes associated with treatment. The wide variations in PDA management reported worldwide reflect our poor understanding of these uncertainties. Although efforts are underway to expand our current understanding of the condition, clinicians should continue to consider the risks and benefits of different treatment options when deciding the correct clinical course of action.

Apart from pharmacologic therapy, conservative management and surgical ligation of PDA are also used. Conservative management through watchful waiting may involve fluid restriction and supportive therapy. In contrast, pharmaceutical agents used for PDA either specifically reduce hemodynamically significant shunt effects or stimulate complete ductal closure. Pharmacologic agents stimulate PDA closure via inhibition of prostaglandin production, which plays a significant role in maintaining ductal patency in utero and during the first one to two postnatal weeks. These agents are specifically designed to target either cyclooxygenase (COX) or peroxidase (POX), the second and third enzymes, respectively, in the process of prostaglandin synthesis. These agents include the COX inhibitors indomethacin and ibuprofen and the POX inhibitor acetaminophen (paracetamol) (Fig. 23.1). Adding to the

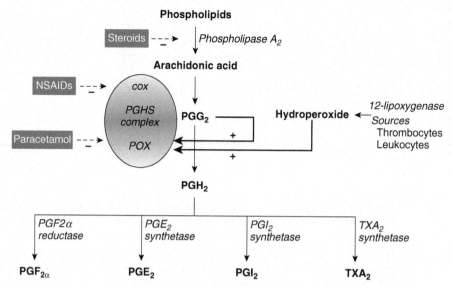

Fig. 23.1   The figure depicts arachidonic acid metabolism along with the inhibitory effects of medications and the stimulatory actions of endogenous substances on the enzymes of the pathway. See text for details. *COX*, Cyclooxygenase; *NSAID*, nonsteroidal antiinflammatory drugs; *PG*, prostaglandin (PG subtypes G_2, H_2, $F_{2\alpha}$, and I_2); *PGHS*, prostaglandin H_2 synthetase; *POX*, peroxidase; *TX*, thromboxane (TX subtype A_2). (Allegaert K, Anderson B, Simons S, van Overmeire B: Paracetamol to induce ductus arteriosus closure: is it valid? *Arch Dis Child* 98:462–466, 2013. Copyright: BMJ Publishing Group Ltd & Royal College of Paediatrics and Child Health.)

complexity of pharmacologic management is the question of when to treat, which may include prophylactic (treat all without assessing), early asymptomatic (detect and treat early before PDA becomes significant during first week after birth), and symptomatic (treat when PDA becomes clinically and hemodynamically significant) treatment.

Epidemiology of Patent Ductus Arteriosus Treatment

Variations in the management of PDA in very preterm and very low birth weight infants have been well reported in North America, Europe, Australia, and Asia. These differences have been described for all aspects of treatment, including if, when, and how to treat PDA. Surveys conducted over the past 20 years regarding the practitioner's approach to treatment of PDA have yielded consistently variable results. In North America a survey of 100 Canadian neonatologists in 1998 revealed a wide variation in practices regarding management of PDA both within and between centers.[1] Fluid restriction and indomethacin were used for treatment by 89% of neonatologists surveyed, whereas surgery was reserved for patients unresponsive to pharmacologic agents or who had contraindications. Use of echocardiography for diagnosis of PDA also varied among clinicians. Almost a decade later, 56 fellowship program directors in the United States were surveyed regarding the management of PDA.[2] A quarter of respondents were using prophylactic indomethacin for prevention of interventricular hemorrhage (IVH) and 9% used indomethacin to treat asymptomatic PDA. In cases of persistent PDA, three-quarters of respondents indicated use of more than one course of indomethacin, with nearly half reporting usage of two courses and half reporting three courses, if needed. Most respondents were keen on administering indomethacin for patients younger than 2 weeks and used echocardiographic criteria to determine PDA treatment.

Hoellering and Cooke also surveyed Australian and New Zealand neonatologists in 2007 for management of PDA in neonates of 28 weeks' gestation or less or birth weights less than 1000 g.[3] Expectant (or conservative) management of PDA was favored by 35% of clinicians, whereas 32% used echocardiographic-targeted prophylaxis, 16% used presymptomatic treatment, and 17% used a prophylactic approach; however, nearly half of participating units reported using more than one approach, often depending upon the preference of the individual practitioner. Interestingly, 86% of physicians used long courses of indomethacin and nearly one-quarter of respondents indicated that their approach was not influenced by published literature. This raises important questions regarding the level of effect that individual units or practitioners have on the outcomes of neonates with PDA.

In a survey of 24 European Societies of Neonatology and Perinatology, Guimaraes and colleagues reported data on 45 responses from 19 countries.[4] The majority of neonatal units used intravenous indomethacin (71%), followed by intravenous ibuprofen (36%) and oral ibuprofen (29%); some units reported use of multiple agents. Approximately half of the centers used a second course and a quarter used a third course of pharmacotherapy in the event of persistent patency of the ductus. Nearly all (96%) units treated hsPDA, but a quarter would also treat non-hsPDA. Only one neonatal unit preferred surgical ligation as the first line therapy. In France, nearly three-quarters of the 49 neonatal units surveyed between 2007 and 2008 reported the use of both clinical and echocardiographic criteria to decide on treatment for PDA, whereas the remaining relied on echocardiographic criteria alone.[5] Most units also used echocardiography to diagnose PDA, but the criteria used to describe hsPDA differed. All units used ibuprofen to treat PDA, with the majority of units using a standard course (see section "Ibuprofen" later). Between one-half to two-thirds of centers indicated a tendency to use a second course when either the first course failed or if the duct reopened after successful closure. In the event of contraindications to medical treatment or ductal malformation, 39% of units considered surgery as the primary treatment.

Irmesi et al.[6] recently collated information from published randomized trials of PDA management around the world. They identified that treatment with indomethacin and ibuprofen was more prevalent in the United States and Canada, whereas ibuprofen was the most often used agent in Europe. Worldwide variations in treatment were further validated in an international survey[7] of investigators from 317 neonatal units in 11 high-income countries. Japan, Finland, and the Tuscany region of Italy all routinely perform echocardiographic screening for PDA. Treatment rates of PDA based on routine echocardiography results alone, regardless of a patient's clinical status, ranged between 11% and 87% (11% of units in Canada; 13% in Illinois; 20% in Israel; 33% in Sweden; 41% in Spain; 50% in Switzerland; 58% in Australia and New Zealand; 75% in Finland; 75% in Tuscany, Italy; and 87% in Japan) among those who conduct echocardiography screening. Acetaminophen was used as the primary treatment for PDA in nine units (one unit each in Australia/New Zealand and Canada; two units in Illinois; and five units in Israel).

Apart from the survey data described previously, reports of actual practices in the management of PDA have been published. For instance, data on outborn extremely low birth weight neonates in a Pediatric Health Information System showed a steady decline in indomethacin use and increase in ibuprofen use (from 12.8% to 38.9%) between 2007 and 2010.[8] In another study, Hagadorn and colleagues examined trends in the management of PDA in 19 U.S. Children's hospitals between 2005 and 2014 and linked the data to neonatal outcomes.[9] Approximately three-quarters of infants with PDA were treated with pharmacologic management or surgery, with wide variation noted among hospitals. There was a steady decline in the number of neonates treated over the years, with the odds of treatment decreasing by 11% in each year of the study period. The trend of reducing treatment was temporally associated with a decline in mortality; however, the incidences of bronchopulmonary dysplasia (BPD), periventricular leukomalacia, retinopathy of prematurity (ROP,) and acute renal failure increased over that time. In a population-based cohort study, Edstedt Bonamy et al. evaluated regional variations and its relationship with outcomes in PDA management across 19 regions in 11 European countries between 2011 and 2012.[10] The proportion of neonates ≤31 weeks' gestation who received PDA treatment varied from 10% to 39% between units, and it was independent of perinatal characteristics of patients. Variations in PDA treatment rate did not correlate with neonatal outcomes.

In Canada, conservative management of PDA in neonates between 23 and 32 weeks' gestation increased from 14% to 38% between 2006 and 2012, whereas using pharmacotherapy alone and surgical treatment alone decreased from 58% to 49% and 7.1% to 2.5%, respectively, and both pharmacotherapy and surgical ligation dropped from 21% to 10% (all $P < .01$) during the same time period.[11] With an increase in conservative management, there was a reduction in the composite outcome of mortality or major morbidity between 2009 and 2012 compared with 2006 and 2008; however, there remains the possibility of confounding bias. Slaughter et al. attempted to adjust for residual confounding by incorporating clinician preference-based variation in practice as an instrument in their analyses.[12] They reported that although an infant's chance of receiving pharmacotherapy increased by 0.84% for each 1% increase in the hospital's annual pharmacotherapy rate for treatment of PDA, there was no association between pharmacotherapy and mortality and mortality or BPD in neonates of ≤28 weeks' gestation. This finding suggests that conservative management of PDA may be a rational approach for the population examined. However, we still do not know how to approach the individual patient (Chapter 21).

In a prospective cohort from France, Rozé et al. evaluated the role of early screening (before day 3 of postnatal life) in neonates <29 weeks' gestation.[13] The authors determined that screened infants were more likely to be treated for PDA than unexposed infants (55% vs. 43%; odds ratio [OR] 1.62, 95% confidence interval [CI] 1.32 to 2.00). Screened neonates were at lower odds of mortality (OR 0.73, 95% CI 0.54 to 0.98) and pulmonary hemorrhage (OR 0.60, 95% CI 0.38 to 0.95). However, when instrumental variable analyses using unit preference for early screening was conducted, there was no association between early screening and mortality (OR 0.62, 95% CI 0.37 to 1.04), suggesting that questions about screening, prophylaxis, and treatment could only best be answered in well-designed randomized trials. The variations reported above in both survey designs and in studies comparing the evolution of approaches and their relationship with outcomes indicate that the management of PDA is widely variable within neonatal units and at regional, national, and international levels.

Pharmacologic Interventions

Pharmacologic interventions for PDA can be divided into two groups: agents used for symptomatic treatment (i.e., management of heart failure) and agents that induce PDA closure. Based on symptoms associated with heart failure, diuretics such as furosemide have been used to reduce overall fluid overload and pulmonary edema formation. Thus far, three randomized controlled trials (RCTs) of furosemide for symptomatic PDA have been conducted, but none of them demonstrated any benefit.[14] On the contrary, increased prostaglandin synthesis following administration of furosemide[15] may contribute to ductal patency. Diuretics, particularly furosemide, are also associated with various side effects,[16] including electrolyte imbalance, nephrocalcinosis, and hearing impairment. The symptoms of heart failure associated with PDA in preterm neonates are usually managed by restricting fluid intake. Alternatively, digoxin is occasionally used for the management of heart failure;[17] however, justification of its use has been theoretical due to limited clinical evidence available.

As previously mentioned, the three main pharmacologic agents used to stimulate PDA closure include indomethacin, ibuprofen, and acetaminophen (paracetamol), each of which is described next. The complexity of management of PDA is summarized in Fig. 23.2, where strategies that have been tested in randomized trials are delineated.

Indomethacin

Mechanism of Action

Indomethacin is a potent and nonselective inhibitor of the COX enzyme and promotes PDA closure by inhibiting the synthesis of prostaglandins, including prostaglandin E2 (see Fig. 23.1).[18] The half-life of indomethacin is 4 to 5 hours longer

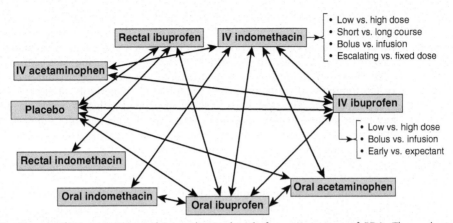

Fig. 23.2 Pharmacologic agents tested in randomized trials for management of PDA. Three pharmacologic agents have been tested against one another via different route of administration and even within each intervention different approaches are compared.

on average in preterm neonates less than 32 weeks' gestation compared with those greater than 32 weeks' gestation (17.2 ± 0.8 vs. 12.5 ± 0.5 hours) and thus, prolonged accumulation can occur in very preterm neonates.[19]

Route, Dose and Frequency

Although the most common route of administration of indomethacin is intravenous, it has been used orally, rectally, and intraarterially. Six studies of oral use (ranging between 9 and 74 neonates) have reported PDA closure rates of 66%–67%. Intraarterial use in 26 neonates was successful in 76% of cases, whereas a 66% closure rate was observed in a small group of neonates treated either orally ($n = 1$) or rectally ($n = 5$).[18] Both of these routes have not been widely used due to concerns of damage to mucosal layers from local direct effects of indomethacin, as well as the effects on prostaglandin synthesis inhibition affecting mucosal integrity of the gastrointestinal track, especially the ileum.

Intravenous indomethacin has been used in various dosing regimens.[18] Although the majority of studies use three standard doses of 0.1 to 0.2 mg/kg/dose 12 to 24 hours apart, many modifications of this strategy have been carried out. In one study, dose escalation of indomethacin starting from 0.2 mg/kg and increasing to 1 mg/kg in nonresponders resulted in a 98.5% PDA closure rate.[20] It should be noted that higher doses are typically associated with increased risk of side effects, which were not addressed in the study quoted.[20] In another study a high-dose (0.2 to 0.5 mg/kg/dose) and low-dose (0.1 mg/kg/dose) regimen of indomethacin were compared in cases of persistent PDA following conventional treatment with the three conventional doses described previously. Although the authors reported no difference in PDA closure rates (55% vs. 48%, respectively),[21] the infants exposed to the higher dosage displayed increased rates of renal compromise and moderate to severe retinopathy.

The usual duration for one course of indomethacin treatment is 48 to 72 hours. For some neonates, ductal closure can be a lengthy remodeling process and may need prolonged treatment. Five randomized trials compared PDA closure rates in neonates treated with a prolonged course of indomethacin versus routine treatment using a three-dose course and reported no difference in PDA closure rates but identified that an increased risk of necrotizing enterocolitis (NEC) was associated with longer indomethacin exposure (relative risk [RR] 1.87, 95% CI 1.07 to 3.27).[22] Some practitioners advocate for an echocardiogram to be performed after the last dose (third dose of a routine course) and to continue treatment until the duct closes. However, based on concerns of adverse side effects, a prolonged course is not recommended by most.

Typically, indomethacin is administered as a slow infusion to avoid rapidly rising concentrations characteristic of bolus infusions. The potential impact of indomethacin concentration on cerebral, renal, and splanchnic blood flow has led to recommendations for infusion to be carried out over a 20- to 30-minute time period. Studies have reported reduced blood flow,[23] and similar[24] or higher closure rates (81% vs. 43%, $P = .03$),[25] with bolus infusion compared with continuous infusion. However, as suggested by a previous systematic review, the evidence may be too limited to draw a conclusion regarding the superiority of either approach.[26] Pharmacokinetic data from a small series of neonates suggest that in neonates who had lower plasma levels, faster clearance, and shorter half-life, the drug was less effective. In addition, there was a 20-fold variation in the plasma levels 24 hours after indomethacin administration among neonates.[27]

Efficacy

Indomethacin is a potent medication for PDA closure, with historically proven rates of ductal closure. Closure rates following an initial course vary from 48% to 98.5% depending upon dose, duration, and method of administration.[18,28,29] Many times a repeat course is provided when either a PDA fails to close following the first course or reopens after initial closure. The success rates with a second course are approximately 40%–50%.[29] Very rarely is a third course of indomethacin attempted, because exposure to more than two courses has been associated with periventricular leukomalacia. It is unclear what pathologic mechanisms play a role in this association,[30] but the indomethacin-induced prolonged decrease in cerebral blood flow might contribute to this phenomenon. The efficacy of indomethacin declines with decreasing gestational age and increasing postnatal age.[31] Data regarding efficacy of indomethacin beyond 2 months of age suggest its ineffectiveness at this age.[18] Similarly, it is unclear whether indomethacin is as useful in the treatment of periviable neonates of 22 and 23 weeks' gestation because the efficacy decreases with decreasing gestational age. Of note is that most efficacy studies had very few infants in this gestational age range.

Timing of Administration

Indomethacin administration has been defined as prophylactic, early asymptomatic, and symptomatic treatment. Prophylactic use is employed in the first 12 hours after birth irrespective of the presence of a PDA. Because approximately half of preterm neonates with a gestational age of ≤28 weeks close their ductus arteriosus spontaneously, this strategy predisposes many neonates to overtreatment. The underlying basis of prophylactic administration is to reduce the impact of a PDA on hemodynamic instability before it becomes of sufficient size and to reduce the incidence and/or severity of peri/intraventricular hemorrhage (P/IVH). A systematic review and meta-analysis of 19 studies identified a significant reduction in the incidence of symptomatic PDA (RR 0.44, 95% CI 0.38 to 0.50) and need for surgical ligation of a PDA (RR 0.51, 95% CI 0.37 to 0.71) with prophylactic use compared with placebo.[32] Indomethacin use was also associated with reduced rates of any P/IVH (RR 0.88, 95% CI 0.80 to 0.98) and severe P/IVH (RR 0.66, 95% CI 0.53 to 0.82). However, there was no improvement in neurodevelopmental outcomes during early childhood despite a reduction in the severity of P/IVH.[33] This has created diverse opinions and practices regarding the use of prophylactic indomethacin in routine clinical settings. Certain subgroups, such as males and neonates less than 27 weeks' gestation, have been identified as potential candidates for prophylactic indomethacin. In addition, units with a higher underlying rate of P/IVH might use this approach because in this situation the benefits likely outweigh the risks of prophylactic indomethacin administration.

Using indomethacin during the "early asymptomatic phase" significantly lowers the number of patients exposed to the drug compared with prophylactic measures described previously, yet several patients who would have had a spontaneous closure will still be exposed. A systematic review of three RCTs reported a reduction in symptomatic PDA (RR 0.36, 95% CI 0.19 to 0.68) and duration of oxygen therapy following indomethacin use in the early asymptomatic phase; however, there was no difference in any other neonatal complications and no assessment of long-term neurodevelopmental outcomes.[34] An RCT compared treatment with indomethacin and a placebo within the first 12 hours after delivery in infants who positively screened for a "large" PDA, irrespective of their effects on hemodynamic status. The trial was stopped prematurely due to unavailability of indomethacin. There was a significant reduction in pulmonary hemorrhage (2% vs. 21%), early P/IVH (4.5% vs. 12.5%) and need for later medical treatment of PDA (20% vs. 40%) with early asymptomatic treatment. However, there was no difference in the primary outcome of death or abnormal head ultrasound findings.[35]

Another approach is to treat PDA when it becomes symptomatic or hemodynamically significant. This method prevents unnecessary exposure to indomethacin as far as the PDA is concerned. Early treatment is used to describe the administration of the medication within the first 5 postnatal days, whereas late treatment is considered to occur in the second week after birth. A meta-analysis of four trials conducted between 1980 and 1990 revealed a significant reduction in BPD (OR 0.39, 95% CI 0.21 to 0.76) and duration of mechanical ventilation in infants receiving early versus late symptomatic treatment.[36] Furthermore, in a randomized clinical trial, higher PDA closure rates were noted when treatment was begun on day 6 (73% vs. 44%, P < .001) and day 9 (91% vs. 78%, P < .05) versus later treatment.[37] However, there was no difference in the rate of surgical duct ligation. Infants treated early were more susceptible to side effects, such as lower urine output and higher creatinine levels, and experienced more severe adverse events. Two other studies, one RCT and one before-after study,[38,39] evaluated early versus late symptomatic treatment and concluded that delays in treatment are feasible and may reduce exposure to pharmacologic agents; yet, an increase in the combined outcome of death or BPD may result.[38]

Side Effects

Indomethacin produces alterations in cerebral, renal, and splanchnic blood flow in a concentration-dependent manner and thus can lead to side effects, including cerebral ischemia, renal dysfunction, and gut ischemia, and it also impairs platelet aggregation. Reduction of blood flow in the renal arteries occurs within the first 30 minutes of indomethacin administration and continues for 2 hours.[40] This can lead to elevations in urea and creatinine levels and even renal failure. Mucosal injury associated with indomethacin is secondary to effects on prostaglandin synthesis. Indomethacin is associated with spontaneous intestinal perforation, especially when given concomitantly with corticosteroids.[41] However, the association of indomethacin with NEC is a subject of debate because the occurrence of NEC could be due to the disturbance of blood flow in the presence of a hsPDA rather than indomethacin alone. Still, indomethacin is also known to reduce splanchnic blood flow during its administration, and therefore this cause-and-effect relationship remains unclear.[23] Because of concerns regarding intestinal blood flow, feeding is either discontinued, held, or sustained depending upon the attending medical team's preference; however, similar outcomes have been reported with each approach.[42]

Take-Home Message

Of all pharmacologic agents used to manage PDA, indomethacin is the most studied and used and is effective in treating PDA, with successful closure rates of approximately 70% with the first course and 50% with a repeat course. Recommended use includes a routine course of three doses after excluding contraindications, followed by repeat use for persistent PDA, if clinically indicated. Varying side effects, concerns over the impact of oral use on immature gastric mucosa, and the availability of other alternatives have led to a decrease in indomethacin use for treatment of PDA. Finally, the decrease in the rate of P/IVH with the use of prophylactic indomethacin might serve as an indication of its use in patients with higher risk of P/IVH (see Chapter 6).

Ibuprofen

Mechanism of Action

Ibuprofen is a nonselective COX inhibitor (see Fig. 23.1) that does not alter cerebral perfusion and has a significantly reduced effect on renal and gut perfusion. Ibuprofen inhibits COX-1 and COX-2 in a rapid and reversible manner. It is metabolized in the liver and excreted in urine, and thus physiologic impairment of hepatic or renal function may lead to adverse reactions.

Route, Dose, and Frequency

Ibuprofen can be given orally or intravenously. Although the peak levels are reached earlier with intravenous delivery, the elimination is slower after enteral administration and thus no adjustment in dose has been suggested for route of administration. The usual dose is 10 mg/kg on day 1, followed by two doses of 5 mg/kg 24 hours apart. However, suggestions for variable dosing based on advancing postnatal age (14-7-7 mg/kg for postnatal ages of 4 to 7 days and 20-10-10 mg/kg for postnatal ages >7 days)[43] due to increased clearance of ibuprofen after birth have been made. A reduced rate of failure to close the ductus arteriosus has been observed with high doses of ibuprofen compared with low doses (RR 0.27; 95% CI 0.11 to 0.64).[44] In a study of 60 preterm neonates with hsPDA, Pourarian et al.[45] reported a 70% ductal closure rate in infants treated with an oral high-dose ibuprofen regimen (20-10-10 mg/kg) compared with a 37% closure rate with standard dosing (10-5-5 mg/kg) with no difference in adverse renal or gastrointestinal side effects. Adaptive dosing in the form of continued doses of ibuprofen (up to six doses if PDA was not closed) was associated with an 88% closure rate (similar to indomethacin).[46] Doubling of the doses during the second course was associated with 60% closure rates compared with 10% in infants receiving the same dose when a consecutive treatment protocol was used, underscoring the need for further studies on ibuprofen dosing, pharmacokinetics, and pharmacodynamics.[47]

Several trials have also compared the efficacy of routes of administration. A systematic review of oral versus intravenous ibuprofen indicated a lower risk of failure to close a PDA with oral ibuprofen use (RR 0.41, 95% CI 0.27 to 0.64).[44] However, it should be noted that oral ibuprofen is associated with higher rates of gastrointestinal hemorrhage. Furthermore, higher rates of sustained closure have been observed after continuous infusion compared with bolus infusion (closure after one or two courses 86% in continuous infusion group versus 68% after one or two courses in the intermittent infusion group; $P = .02$).[48]

Ibuprofen is available in two preparations, ibuprofen lysine and ibuprofen-tris-hydroxymethyl-aminomethane (THAM). The association of ibuprofen use with pulmonary hypertension was initially thought to be specific to the ibuprofen-THAM preparation; however, in a cohort of 144 neonates who received ibuprofen treatment for PDA, 10 cases developed pulmonary arterial hypertension, of which 7 occurred in the intravenous ibuprofen-THAM group ($n = 100$), 2 in the oral ibuprofen group ($n = 40$), and 1 who received intravenous ibuprofen lysine preparation ($n = 4$). Risk factors for the development of pulmonary arterial hypertension were small for gestational age, maternal hypertension, and oligohydramnios.[49] In one retrospective study from Italy, it was identified that ibuprofen lysine was more effective than ibuprofen THAM in PDA ligation (73% vs. 51%, $P = .002$) when used prophylactically in neonates of ≤28 weeks' gestation.[50]

Efficacy

Similar to indomethacin, ibuprofen is also an effective agent for closure of the PDA. The response rate for the first and second course mimics that of indomethacin, with approximate closure rates of 70% and 50%, respectively. A detailed systematic review of studies evaluating the therapeutic use of ibuprofen revealed that oral ibuprofen reduces failure of PDA closure (RR 0.26, 95% CI 0.11 to 0.62) and intravenous ibuprofen reduces the need for rescue treatment (RR 0.71, 95% CI 0.51 to 0.99) in comparison with placebo treatment.[44] Ibuprofen has been compared with indomethacin in several RCTs. A systematic review[44] of these trials indicated that ibuprofen and indomethacin (both oral and intravenous) are similar in terms of their efficacy in ductal closure (RR 1.00, 95% CI 0.84 to 1.20), rates of PDA reopening after the first course (RR 1.28; 95% CI 0.48 to 3.38), need for surgical ligation (RR 1.07, 95% CI 0.76 to 1.50), or need for retreatment with either agent (RR 1.20, 95%

CI 0.76 to 1.90). In addition, ibuprofen was associated with a lower incidence of renal dysfunction (as indicated by its effect on urine output and serum creatinine), shorter duration of mechanical ventilation (−2.4 days; 95% CI −3.7 days to −1.0 day), and lower incidence of NEC (16 studies, 948 infants; RR 0.64, 95% CI 0.45 to 0.93). There were no differences in P/IVH, ROP, and survival or neurodevelopmental outcomes between the two agents.[44]

Timing of Administration

Similar to indomethacin, ibuprofen has also been used as a prophylactic agent, with an aim to reduce P/IVH. Use of oral or intravenous ibuprofen prophylactically reduces the incidence of PDA on postnatal day 3 (oral, RR 0.34, 95% CI 0.16 to 0.73; intravenous, RR 0.37, 95% CI 0.29 to 0.47) compared with placebo or no treatment but has no benefit on any other neonatal outcomes.[44]

Yoo et al. evaluated mortality and neonatal complications following the use of ibuprofen in two groups of neonates,[51] including 14 (15.4%) preterm infants of less than 28 weeks' gestation with clinical symptoms of hsPDA and 77 (84.6%) asymptomatic neonates with no evidence of hsPDA. Infants in the symptomatic group were of younger gestation (by 1 week) and lower birth weight (by 225 g) and had higher severity of illness scores. They also received more courses of ibuprofen. In a logistic regression analysis after adjustment for severity of illness, birth weight, birth year, and invasive ventilator care ≤2 postnatal days, there were no significant differences in mortality, frequency of secondary ligation, NEC, P/IVH, BPD, or death between the two groups. The authors concluded that treatment of asymptomatic or non-hsPDA may not be warranted.

In a randomized trial of infants of 23 to 32 weeks' gestation and weighing less than 1250 g, neonates with non-hsPDA were randomized to receive either early ibuprofen (*n* = 54) or treatment only when hsPDA was detected (*n* = 51).[39] The early ibuprofen group received treatment at a median age of 3 days, whereas the latter group received ibuprofen at a median of 11 days. Approximately half of the patients in the latter group never required ibuprofen. There was no difference in BPD, BPD or death, intestinal perforation, surgical NEC, grades 3 and 4 P/IVH, periventricular leukomalacia, sepsis, or ROP. Therefore this study suggests that infants with non-hsPDA do not benefit from early treatment. Although ibuprofen is an effective treatment for PDA in both forms (oral and intravenous), the impact of early treatment of PDA with ibuprofen on other neonatal conditions and neurodevelopmental outcomes is unknown.

Side Effects

Major side effects of ibuprofen include oliguria, high bilirubin levels, gastrointestinal hemorrhage, and pulmonary hypertension. The use of ibuprofen-THAM has been associated with higher rates of gastrointestinal complications,[52] as well as pulmonary hypertension.

Take-Home Message

Several studies have confirmed that ibuprofen has similar potency for PDA closure as indomethacin but carries a lower profile of side effects. Given that oral ibuprofen is as effective as intravenous ibuprofen and is likely to result in reduced side effects, it may be the preferred agent among practitioners for ductal closure.

Acetaminophen (Paracetamol)

Mechanism of Action

Acetaminophen acts on PDA closure through the inhibition of POX-mediated conversion of prostaglandin G_2 to prostaglandin H_2 (see Fig. 23.1). It has no peripheral vasoconstrictive effects, which may be considered as an advantage over the COX inhibitors.

Route, Dose, and Frequency

The compound's pharmacokinetics, including the route and dose of administration, have not been well studied compared with indomethacin and ibuprofen. Most case reports have evaluated acetaminophen after failure of PDA closure by routine measures. Several studies report the use of 15-mg/kg dose every 6 hours for 2 to 7 days.[53,54] However, effects on other neonatal and neurodevelopmental outcomes are poorly understood. The requirement for prolonged administration calls into question the efficacy of paracetamol because PDA closure may be related to time rather than drug administration. This is particularly relevant with paracetamol because there is a paucity of placebo-controlled RCTs. Most studies have used oral acetaminophen; however, some have reported on the use of its intravenous formulation, which is not readily available in North America.

Efficacy

A total of seven RCTs (Table 23.1)[55-61] and several case series and reports have examined the efficacy of acetaminophen. Overall, most of the randomized studies have assessed acetaminophen treatment as a primary medical therapy, whereas the majority of case series and reports have described the use of acetaminophen after failure with COX inhibitors.[62] The efficacy of acetaminophen in randomized studies has been similar to any other comparator treatment via any route. The most current Cochrane review analyzes only the first two published trials and highlights the need for more information on efficacy and long-term safety of the intervention.[63] PDA closure rates range from 70.5% to 100% with acetaminophen use. Because most studies have only described acetaminophen use for PDA in neonates greater than 28 weeks' gestational age, data for extremely preterm neonates is limited and the efficacy and side effects of acetaminophen in this population remain unanswered.[53]

Timing of Administration

Harkin and colleagues[59] provide the only available evidence to date regarding pro- phylactic use of acetaminophen irrespective of the PDA status, which suggests that nearly two-thirds of patients receiving a placebo have spontaneous closure of a PDA. This finding, along with similar results from indomethacin and ibuprofen studies, highlights concerns regarding prophylaxis. All remaining RCTs have compared the primary use of acetaminophen when the PDA was either clinically or hemodynami- cally significant, although the criteria for defining hsPDA have varied.

Side Effects

Side effects of acetaminophen generally include hepatotoxicity, as well as hemo- dynamic and thermodynamic effects. Therapeutic doses of acetaminophen used for analgesic purposes do not result in acute side effects. The oral preparation of acet- aminophen is often diluted significantly prior to administration due to concerns of the solution's high osmolality and the potentially associated risk for the subsequent devel- opment of NEC. Viberg and colleagues[64] showed that exposure to paracetamol during a critical period of brain development can induce long-lasting effects on cognitive function in mice and alter the adult response to paracetamol. Moreover, acute neonatal exposure in mice also led to altered locomotor activity and affected spatial learning in adulthood. Avella-Garcia et al.[65] followed children of 1 year and 5 years of age who were exposed to maternal intake of acetaminophen before 32 weeks' gestation. The authors found that prenatal exposure to acetaminophen may alter attention function at 5 years of age, while affecting males and females differently. However, this study suf- fers from issues of inexact delineation of the quantity, timing, and duration of mater- nal acetaminophen intake. Through analyzing data from a population-based cohort in Denmark, Liew et al.[66] reported that prenatal use of acetaminophen was associated with a higher risk of hyperkinetic disorder (hazard ratio 1.37, 95% CI 1.19 to 1.59), need for attention-deficit/hyperactivity disorder treatment (hazard ratio 1.29, 95% CI 1.15 to 1.44), and attention-deficit/hyperactivity disorder–like behaviors at 7 years of age (RR 1.13, 95% CI 1.01 to 1.27). There was also some evidence for a dose-response relationship. Finally, in an ecologic analysis, Bauer and Kriebel[67] reported that coun- try-level autism was correlated with rates of circumcision. Given that this procedure is often accompanied by the use of acetaminophen for pain management, the possibility of an associative link has been entertained. Further data on both the side effects and the impact of acetaminophen on neurodevelopmental outcomes are clearly needed.

Table 23.1   RANDOMIZED CONTROLLED TRIALS OF ACETAMINOPHEN

Author	Population	Acetaminophen	Control	Results
Dang et al. 2013[56]	≤34 weeks GA, age ≤14 days, echocardiographic diagnosis of hsPDA	Oral 15 mg/kg/q6h for 3 days (n = 80)	Oral ibuprofen 10 mg/kg followed by 5 mg/kg/q24h for two doses (n = 80)	Overall ductal closure 81% in acetaminophen group compared with 79% in ibuprofen group (P = .69)
Oncel et al. 2014[60]	≤30 weeks GA, ≤1250 g BW, and postnatal age 48–96 h who had echocardiographically confirmed significant PDA	Oral 15 mg/kg/q6h for 3 days (n = 40)	Oral ibuprofen 10 mg/kg followed by 5 mg/kg/q24h for two doses (n = 40)	Overall ductal closure rate 97.5% in acetaminophen group vs. 95% in ibuprofen group
Dash et al. 2015[57]	BW ≤1500 g and echocardiographically significant PDA within first 48 h of age	Oral 15 mg/kg/q6h for 7 days (n = 36)	Intravenous indomethacin 0.2 mg/kg/d for 3 days (n = 37)	Overall closure rate was 100% in acetaminophen group vs. 94.6% in intravenous indomethacin group (P = .13)
Harkin et al. 2016[59]	≤32 weeks GA irrespective of PDA status (prophylactic trial)	Intravenous 20 mg/kg within 24 h of birth, then 7.5 mg/kg/q6h for 4 days (n = 23)	0.45% saline as placebo (n = 25)	Ductal closure was 80% in acetaminophen group vs. 64% in placebo group. Four (17%) in acetaminophen group and 3 (12%) in placebo group required treatment of PDA
Yang et al. 2016[61]	<37 weeks GA, symptomatic PDA (clinical and echocardiographic)	Oral 15 mg/kg/q6h for 3 days (n = 44)	Oral ibuprofen 10 mg/kg followed by 5 mg/kg/q24h for two doses (n = 43)	Ductal closure rate 70.5% in acetaminophen group vs. 76.7% in ibuprofen group (P = .51)
Bagheri et al. 2016[55]	<37 weeks GA, ≤14 days of age with hsPDA	Oral 15 mg/kg/q6h for 3 days (n = 67)	Oral ibuprofen 20 mg/kg, followed by 10 mg/kg/q24h for two doses (n = 62)	Overall ductal closure rate 91% in acetaminophen group vs. 90.3% in ibuprofen group (P = .89)
El-Mashad et al. 2017[58]	<28 weeks GA or <1500 g BW in the first 2 weeks of life with hsPDA	Intravenous 15 mg/kg/q6h for 3 days (n = 100)	*Group 1:* Intravenous ibuprofen 10 mg/kg followed by 5 mg/kg/q24h for two doses (n = 100) *Group 2:* Intravenous indomethacin 0.2 mg/kg/q12h for three doses (n = 100)	Overall ductal closure 88% with acetaminophen, 83% with ibuprofen and 89% with indomethacin

BW, Birth weight; *GA,* gestational age; *hsPDA,* hemodynamically significant PDA; *PDA,* patent ductus arteriosus.

Take-Home Message

Studies evaluating the efficacy of acetaminophen as a primary agent for treatment of a PDA have emerged, along with studies using acetaminophen in patients not responding to a COX-inhibitor. Future efforts should address the optimal duration of therapy and its effectiveness in extremely preterm neonates, who are now the most likely candidates for treatment. In addition, potential long-term effects of neonatal acetaminophen administration on neurodevelopment need to be examined.

Comparison of the Three Pharmacologic Agents

All three agents have been tested against one another in various combinations (see Fig. 23.1), with no major differences observed in the rate of PDA closure, failure of PDA closure, or any other neonatal outcomes with the exemption of the effect of pro-phylactic indomethacin on decreasing the rate of P/IVH. These comparisons include seven RCTs testing oral indomethacin versus oral ibuprofen (RR 0.82, 95% CI 0.52 to 1.29),[68] 12 studies of intravenous indomethacin versus intravenous ibuprofen (RR 1.03, 95% CI 0.74 to 1.43),[68] three small studies of intravenous indomethacin versus oral ibuprofen (RR 0.94, 95% CI 0.56 to 1.60),[69] and two RCTs of oral paracetamol versus oral ibuprofen (RR 0.83, 95% CI 0.60 to 1.15[56]; RR 1.22, 95% CI 0.57 to 2.62[60]). Although these individual comparisons noted similar efficacies between pharmacologic agents, variations in side effects were observed. With more evidence emerging from recent trials (see Table 23.1), it is essential to update some of the existing systematic reviews with careful attention to the population(s) included and rates of open-label treatment in the study.

To date, only one randomized study has evaluated all three agents (paracetamol, ibuprofen, and indomethacin) relative to each other.[58] In this prospective study, pre-term neonates less than 28 weeks' gestation or with birth weights of less than 1500 g who were diagnosed with an hsPDA by echocardiography and clinical examination were randomized to one of the three intervention groups (100 in each arm). The first group received a dose of 15 mg/kg of intravenous paracetamol every 6 hours for 3 days; the second group received a dose of 10 mg/kg of intravenous ibuprofen on day 1, followed by 5 mg/kg once a day for 2 days; and the third group received three doses of 0.2 mg/kg of intravenous indomethacin 12 hours apart. Patients received a second course of the same treatment regimen if the PDA failed to close. Overall, there was no difference in the rate of ductal closure after the first (80% vs. 77% vs. 81%) or second course (88% vs. 83% vs. 87%) of paracetamol, ibuprofen, and indomethacin, respectively. There was also no difference in neonatal complications and side effects between all groups, with the exception of a higher occurrence of intestinal bleeding in the indomethacin- and ibuprofen-treated patients ($P < .05$).[58] A future network meta-analysis has been designed to comparatively evaluate all three agents for their relative superiority with respect to efficacy and safety, of which the results are eagerly awaited.[70]

Conclusions and Implications for Practice and Research

Diagnosis of PDA, especially significant PDA, remains a challenge. Although echo-cardiographic characteristics have been identified, they are not reliable enough to effectively identify cases of clinically significant PDA where treatment can lead to better long-term outcomes (these concepts are further discussed in Chapters 22 and 25). Even in cases in which perturbation of blood flow to splanchnic organs has been identified, the choice and timing of treatment remains uncertain. Worldwide trends in the management of PDA are constantly changing and remain unpredict-able. Increasingly more neonates are managed conservatively or via pharmacologic intervention. At the same time, the number of infants receiving surgical ligation is declining, which most often is offered as a last resort (Chapter 24). Indomethacin and ibuprofen remain the mainstays of medical management, whereas acetaminophen is emerging as a potentially less toxic option with similar efficacy to the COX inhibitors. The pharmacokinetic profile and appropriateness of dosing of these agents in infants treated later (after the first few days) and dosing in the more immature infant (<26 weeks) needs further study. The effects of such approaches on long-term neurodevelopmental and cardiovascular health are not known.

To better guide clinicians in the management of PDA, further understanding of the systemic changes caused by the condition is required. The identification of biochemical or imaging biomarkers that signal affected organ blood flow arising from the systematic diversion of blood to the lungs by a significant PDA may complement current diagnostic tools. Furthermore, the identification of mechanisms by which higher pulmonary vascular flow secondary to hsPDA affects the developing lungs and pulmonary blood flow regulation may help to guide the development of new therapies because not all neonates with higher flow develop pulmonary edema and hemorrhage.[71] Pharmacokinetics and pharmacodynamics of all three agents are very poorly studied, and future studies should build that component in to their design so that such questions can be answered simultaneously rather than as afterthoughts. Ideally, randomized controlled studies would be the preferred approach to evaluate the impact of diagnostic tests or therapeutic interventions. However, large cohorts could also be studied with careful selection of analytical techniques that incorporate as many residual confounding variables as possible (propensity score methods, instrumental variable analyses) and answer two critical biases associated with the assessment of long-term outcomes of PDA—confounding by indication or contraindication, and survival bias.[72] Future studies will need to try to account for these biases when assessing the impact of therapies on survival free of neurodevelopmental impairment. In the meantime, clinicians will continue debating the risks and benefits of various treatment options until enough evidence is available to establish generally accepted guidelines for the management of PDA in the preterm neonate. Finally, using comprehensive, real-time monitoring and data acquisition systems along with mathematical modeling and machine learning (Chapter 21), differences among individual patients affecting PDA rates, rates of spontaneous closure, and the patient's response to the different treatment approaches could also be recognized and modeled to the phenotypic profile of the given patient.

REFERENCES

1. Lai LS, McCrindle BW: Variation in the diagnosis and management of patent ductus arteriosus in premature infants, *Paediatr Child Health* 3:405–410, 1998.
2. Amin SB, Handley C, Carter-Pokras O: Indomethacin use for the management of patent ductus arteriosus in preterms: a web-based survey of practice attitudes among neonatal fellowship program directors in the United States, *Pediatr Cardiol* 28:193–200, 2007.
3. Hoellering AB, Cooke L: The management of patent ductus arteriosus in Australia and New Zealand, *J Paediatr Child Health* 45:204–209, 2009.
4. Guimaraes H, Rocha G, Tome T, et al.: Non-steroid anti-inflammatory drugs in the treatment of patent ductus arteriosus in European newborns, *J Matern Fetal Neonatal Med* 22(Suppl 3):77–80, 2009.
5. Brissaud O, Guichoux J: Patent ductus arteriosus in the preterm infant: a survey of clinical practices in French neonatal intensive care units, *Pediatr Cardiol* 32:607–614, 2011.
6. Irmesi R, Marcialis MA, Anker JV, et al.: Non-steroidal anti-inflammatory drugs (NSAIDs) in the management of patent ductus arteriosus (PDA) in preterm infants and variations in attitude in clinical practice: a flight around the world, *Curr Med Chem* 21:3132–3152, 2014.
7. Variations in management of patent ductus arteriosus and use of echocardiography in preterm neonates <29 weeks gestation: an international survey, *Pediatric Academic Societies Meeting*. May 6-9, 2017, 2017.
8. ElHassan NO, Bird TM, King AJ, et al.: Variation and comparative effectiveness of patent ductus arteriosus pharmacotherapy in extremely low birth weight infants, *J Neonatal Perinatal Med* 7:229–235, 2014.
9. Hagadorn JI, Brownell EA, Trzaski JM, et al.: Trends and variation in management and outcomes of very low-birth-weight infants with patent ductus arteriosus, *Pediatr Res* 80:785–792, 2016.
10. Edstedt Bonamy AK, Gudmundsdottir A, Maier RF, et al.: Patent ductus arteriosus treatment in very preterm infants: a European population-based cohort study (EPICE) on variation and outcomes, *Neonatology* 111:367–375, 2017.
11. Lokku A, Mirea L, Lee SK, et al.: Trends and outcomes of patent ductus arteriosus treatment in very preterm infants in canada, *Am J Perinatol*, 2016.

23

12. Slaughter JL, Reagan PB, Newman TB, et al.: Comparative effectiveness of nonsteroidal anti-inflammatory drug treatment vs no treatment for patent ductus arteriosus in preterm infants, *JAMA Pediatr* 164354, 2017.

13. Roze JC, Cambonie G, Marchand-Martin L, et al.: Association between early screening for patent ductus arteriosus and in-hospital mortality among extremely preterm infants, *JAMA* 313:2441–2448, 2015.

14. Brion LP, Campbell DE: Furosemide for symptomatic patent ductus arteriosus in indomethacin-treated infants, *Cochrane Database Syst Rev* CD001148, 2000.

15. Toyoshima K, Momma K, Nakanishi T: In vivo dilatation of the ductus arteriosus induced by furosemide in the rat, *Pediatr Res* 67:173–176, 2010.

16. Lee BS, Byun SY, Chung ML, et al.: Effect of furosemide on ductal closure and renal function in indomethacin-treated preterm infants during the early neonatal period, *Neonatology* 98:191–199, 2010.

17. Tripathi A, Black GB, Park YM, et al.: Prevalence and management of patent ductus arteriosus in a pediatric medicaid cohort, *Clin Cardiol* 36:502–506, 2013.

18. Pacifici GM: Clinical pharmacology of indomethacin in preterm infants: implications in patent ductus arteriosus closure, *Paediatr Drugs* 15:363–376, 2013.

19. Bhat R, Vidyasagar D, Fisher E, et al.: Pharmacokinetics of oral and intravenous indomethacin in preterm infants, *Dev Pharmacol Ther* 1:101–110, 1980.

20. Sperandio M, Beedgen B, Feneberg R, et al.: Effectiveness and side effects of an escalating, stepwise approach to indomethacin treatment for symptomatic patent ductus arteriosus in premature infants below 33 weeks of gestation, *Pediatrics* 116:1361–1366, 2005.

21. Jegatheesan P, Ianus V, Buchh B, et al.: Increased indomethacin dosing for persistent patent ductus arteriosus in preterm infants: a multicenter, randomized, controlled trial, *J Pediatr* 153:183–189, 2008.

22. Herrera C, Holberton J, Davis P: Prolonged versus short course of indomethacin for the treatment of patent ductus arteriosus in preterm infants, *Cochrane Database Syst Rev* CD003480, 2007.

23. Christmann V, Liem KD, Semmekrot BA, et al.: Changes in cerebral, renal and mesenteric blood flow velocity during continuous and bolus infusion of indomethacin, *Acta Paediatr* 91:440–446, 2002.

24. Hammerman C, Glaser J, Schimmel MS, et al.: Continuous versus multiple rapid infusions of indomethacin: effects on cerebral blood flow velocity, *Pediatrics* 95:244–248, 1995.

25. de Vries NK, Jagroep FK, Jaarsma AS, et al.: Continuous indomethacin infusion may be less effective than bolus infusions for ductal closure in very low birth weight infants, *Am J Perinatol* 22:71–75, 2005.

26. Gork AS, Ehrenkranz RA, Bracken MB: Continuous infusion versus intermittent bolus doses of indomethacin for patent ductus arteriosus closure in symptomatic preterm infants, *Cochrane Database Syst Rev* CD006071, 2008.

27. Brash AR, Hickey DE, Graham TP, et al.: Pharmacokinetics of indomethacin in the neonate. Relation of plasma indomethacin levels to response of the ductus arteriosus, *N Engl J Med* 305: 67–72, 1981.

28. Gersony WM, Peckham GJ, Ellison RC, et al.: Effects of indomethacin in premature infants with patent ductus arteriosus: results of a national collaborative study, *J Pediatr* 102:895–906, 1983.

29. Godambe S, Newby B, Shah V, et al.: Effect of indomethacin on closure of ductus arteriosus in very-low-birthweight neonates, *Acta Paediatr* 95:1389–1393, 2006.

30. Sangem M, Asthana S, Amin S: Multiple courses of indomethacin and neonatal outcomes in premature infants, *Pediatr Cardiol* 29:878–884, 2008.

31. Achanti B, Yeh TF, Pildes RS: Indomethacin therapy in infants with advanced postnatal age and patent ductus arteriosus, *Clin Invest Med* 9:250–253, 1986.

32. Fowlie PW, Davis PG, McGuire W: Prophylactic intravenous indomethacin for preventing mortality and morbidity in preterm infants, *Cochrane Database Syst Rev* CD000174, 2010.

33. Schmidt B, Roberts RS, Fanaroff A, et al.: Indomethacin prophylaxis, patent ductus arteriosus, and the risk of bronchopulmonary dysplasia: further analyses from the Trial of Indomethacin Prophylaxis in Preterms (TIPP), *J Pediatr* 148:730–734, 2006.

34. Cooke L, Steer P, Woodgate P: Indomethacin for asymptomatic patent ductus arteriosus in preterm infants, *Cochrane Database Syst Rev* CD003745, 2003.

35. Kluckow M, Jeffery M, Gill A, et al.: A randomised placebo-controlled trial of early treatment of the patent ductus arteriosus, *Arch Dis Child Fetal Neonatal Ed* 99:F99–F104, 2014.

36. Clyman RI: Recommendations for the postnatal use of indomethacin: an analysis of four separate treatment strategies, *J Pediatr* 128:601–607, 1996.

37. Van OB, Van de Broek H, Van LP, et al.: Early versus late indomethacin treatment for patent ductus arteriosus in premature infants with respiratory distress syndrome, *J Pediatr* 138:205–211, 2001.

38. Kaempf JW, Wu YX, Kaempf AJ, et al.: What happens when the patent ductus arteriosus is treated less aggressively in very low birth weight infants?, *J Perinatol* 32:344–348, 2012.

39. Sosenko IR, Fajardo MF, Claure N, et al.: Timing of patent ductus arteriosus treatment and respiratory outcome in premature infants: a double-blind randomized controlled trial, *J Pediatr* 160:929–935, 2012.

40. Pezzati M, Vangi V, Biagiotti R, et al.: Effects of indomethacin and ibuprofen on mesenteric and renal blood flow in preterm infants with patent ductus arteriosus, *J Pediatr* 135:733–738, 1999.

41. Attridge JT, Clark R, Walker MW, et al.: New insights into spontaneous intestinal perforation using a national data set: (1) SIP is associated with early indomethacin exposure, *J Perinatol* 26:93–99, 2006.

42. Louis D, Torgalkar R, Shah J, et al.: Enteral feeding during indomethacin treatment for patent ductus arteriosus: association with gastrointestinal outcomes, *J Perinatol* 36:544–548, 2016.

43. Hirt D, Van OB, Treluyer JM, et al.: An optimized ibuprofen dosing scheme for preterm neonates with patent ductus arteriosus, based on a population pharmacokinetic and pharmacodynamic study, *Br J Clin Pharmacol* 65:629–636, 2008.

44. Ohlsson A, Walia R, Shah SS: Ibuprofen for the treatment of patent ductus arteriosus in preterm or low birth weight (or both) infants, *Cochrane Database Syst Rev* CD003481, 2015.

45. Pourarian S, Takmil F, Cheriki S, et al.: The effect of oral high-dose ibuprofen on patent ductus arteriosus closure in preterm infants, *Am J Perinatol* 32:1158–1163, 2015.

46. Su BH, Lin HC, Chiu HY, et al.: Comparison of ibuprofen and indometacin for early-targeted treatment of patent ductus arteriosus in extremely premature infants: a randomised controlled trial, *Arch Dis Child Fetal Neonatal Ed* 93:F94–F99, 2008.

47. Decobert F, Kampf F, Durrmeyer X, et al.: Efficiency of a double-dosed second ibuprofen course for the closure of patent ductus arteriosus in extremely premature infants, *E-PAS* 5842.4, 2008.

48. Lago P, Salvadori S, Opocher F, et al.: Continuous infusion of ibuprofen for treatment of patent ductus arteriosus in very low birth weight infants, *Neonatology* 105:46–54, 2014.

49. Kim SY, Shin SH, Kim HS, et al.: Pulmonary arterial hypertension after ibuprofen treatment for patent ductus arteriosus in very low birth weight infants, *J Pediatr* 179:49–53, 2016.

50. De Carolis MP, Bersani I, De RG, et al.: Ibuprofen lysinate and sodium ibuprofen for prophylaxis of patent ductus arteriosus in preterm neonates, *Indian Pediatr* 49:47–49, 2012.

51. Yoo H, Lee JA, Oh S, et al.: Comparison of the mortality and in-hospital outcomes of preterm infants treated with ibuprofen for patent ductus arteriosus with or without clinical symptoms attributable to the patent ductus arteriosus at the time of ibuprofen treatment, *J Korean Med Sci* 32:115–123, 2017.

52. Gournay V, Roze JC, Kuster A, et al.: Prophylactic ibuprofen versus placebo in very premature infants: a randomised, double-blind, placebo-controlled trial, *Lancet* 364:1939–1944, 2004.

53. El-Khuffash A, Jain A, Corcoran D, et al.: Efficacy of paracetamol on patent ductus arteriosus closure may be dose dependent: evidence from human and murine studies, *Pediatr Res* 76:238–244, 2014.

54. Hammerman C, Bin-Nun A, Markovitch E, et al.: Ductal closure with paracetamol: a surprising new approach to patent ductus arteriosus treatment, *Pediatrics* 128:e1618–e1621, 2011.

55. Bagheri MM, Niknafs P, Sabsevari F, et al.: Comparison of oral acetaminophen versus ibuprofen in premature infants with patent ductus arteriosus, *Iran J Pediatr* 26:e3975, 2016.

56. Dang D, Wang D, Zhang C, et al.: Comparison of oral paracetamol versus ibuprofen in premature infants with patent ductus arteriosus: a randomized controlled trial, *PLoS One* 8:e77888, 2013.

57. Dash SK, Kabra NS, Avasthi BS, et al.: Enteral paracetamol or intravenous indomethacin for closure of patent ductus arteriosus in preterm neonates: a randomized controlled trial, *Indian Pediatr* 52:573–578, 2015.

58. El-Mashad AE, El-Mahdy H, El AD, et al.: Comparative study of the efficacy and safety of paracetamol, ibuprofen, and indomethacin in closure of patent ductus arteriosus in preterm neonates, *Eur J Pediatr* 176:233–240, 2017.

59. Harkin P, Harma A, Aikio O, et al.: Paracetamol accelerates closure of the ductus arteriosus after premature birth: a randomized trial, *J Pediatr* 177:72–77, 2016.

60. Oncel MY, Yurttutan S, Erdeve O, et al.: Oral paracetamol versus oral ibuprofen in the management of patent ductus arteriosus in preterm infants: a randomized controlled trial, *J Pediatr* 164:510–514, 2014.

61. Yang B, Gao X, Ren Y, et al.: Oral paracetamol vs. oral ibuprofen in the treatment of symptomatic patent ductus arteriosus in premature infants: a randomized controlled trial, *Exp Ther Med* 12:2531–2536, 2016.

62. Terrin G, Conte F, Oncel MY, et al.: Paracetamol for the treatment of patent ductus arteriosus in preterm neonates: a systematic review and meta-analysis, *Arch Dis Child Fetal Neonatal Ed* 101:F127–F136, 2016.

63. Ohlsson A, Shah PS: Paracetamol (acetaminophen) for prevention or treatment of pain in newborns, *Cochrane Database Syst Rev* 10:CD011219, 2016.

64. Viberg H, Eriksson P, Gordh T, et al.: Paracetamol (acetaminophen) administration during neonatal brain development affects cognitive function and alters its analgesic and anxiolytic response in adult male mice, *Toxicol Sci* 138:139–147, 2014.

65. Avella-Garcia CB, Julvez J, Fortuny J, et al.: Acetaminophen use in pregnancy and neurodevelopment: attention function and autism spectrum symptoms, *Int J Epidemiol*, 2016.

66. Liew Z, Ritz B, Rebordosa C, et al.: Acetaminophen use during pregnancy, behavioral problems, and hyperkinetic disorders, *JAMA Pediatr* 168:313–320, 2014.

67. Bauer AZ, Kriebel D: Prenatal and perinatal analgesic exposure and autism: an ecological link, *Environ Health* 12:41, 2013.

68. Ohlsson A, Walia R, Shah SS: Ibuprofen for the treatment of patent ductus arteriosus in preterm and/or low birth weight infants, *Cochrane Database Syst Rev* CD003481, 2013.

69. Neumann R, Schulzke SM, Buhrer C: Oral ibuprofen versus intravenous ibuprofen or intravenous indomethacin for the treatment of patent ductus arteriosus in preterm infants: a systematic review and meta-analysis, *Neonatology* 102:9–15, 2012.

70. Mitra S, Florez ID, Tamayo ME, et al.: Effectiveness and safety of treatments used for the management of patent ductus arteriosus (PDA) in preterm infants: a protocol for a systematic review and network meta-analysis, *BMJ Open* 6:e011271, 2016.

71. El-Khuffash A, Weisz DE, McNamara PJ: Reflections of the changes in patent ductus arteriosus management during the last 10 years, *Arch Dis Child Fetal Neonatal Ed* 101:F474–F478, 2016.

72. Weisz DE, More K, McNamara PJ, et al.: PDA ligation and health outcomes: a meta-analysis, *Pediatrics* 133:e1024–e1046, 2014.

23

Surgical Management of Patent Ductus Arteriosus in the Very Preterm Infant and Postligation Cardiac Compromise

Dany Weisz, Joseph Ting, and Patrick McNamara

24

- Surgical ligation is a therapeutic option for persistent large patent ductus arteriosus (PDA) after unsuccessful medical therapy, although additional research is needed to determine the clinical and echocardiography characteristics associated with improved outcomes compared with conservative management.

- Prophylactic surgical ligation in the first postnatal days is generally unnecessary due to the availability of pharmacologic therapy, the possibility of spontaneous ductal closure and the potential for coexistent pulmonary arterial hypertension.

- Epidemiologic associations between PDA ligation and increased neonatal morbidity and neurodevelopmental impairment may be due to residual bias from confounding by indication, rather than a true detrimental causal effect of PDA surgery.

- Transcatheter closure of PDA is an emerging therapeutic approach that requires further study as an alternate to open surgical ligation.

- Postligation cardiac syndrome, characterized by oxygenation and ventilation failure and systemic hypotension with onset 6 to 12 hours postoperatively, is common in preterm infants and likely related to increased left ventricular afterload.

- The early targeted administration of intravenous milrinone to preterm infants with low cardiac output in the immediate postoperative period may ameliorate the hemodynamic significance of postligation cardiac syndrome.

- The approach to the acutely unstable postoperative infant should include consideration of postligation cardiac syndrome, nonspecific inflammatory response, potential surgical complications, adrenal insufficiency, and the possibility of occult infection (specific inflammation).

Surgical ligation is an immediate and definitive method for closure of patent ductus arteriosus (PDA). However, the selection of preterm infants for surgical treatment remains one of the most enduring controversies in neonatal medicine. There is marked center-to-center variation in the incidence of ligation among extremely low birth weight (ELBW) infants. Overall rates of ligation reported by international neonatal networks are decreasing,[1,2] although the reasons behind this secular trend are likely multifactorial.

Observational studies have associated PDA surgery with adverse neonatal outcomes and neurodevelopmental impairment (NDI) in early childhood, although bias due to residual confounding threatens the validity of these studies. Infants treated with surgical ligation undergo major rapid changes in systemic hemodynamics which commonly lead to postoperative cardiorespiratory instability. In addition, given that dependence on mechanical ventilation is the *sine qua non* of referring an infant for PDA surgery, the increasing availability and use of advanced noninvasive methods of ventilation may permit earlier endotracheal extubation of extremely preterm infants. Consequently, clinician perceptions of the merits of surgical intervention may differ, prompting them to avoid PDA surgery with the hope of spontaneous ductal closure, yet this management strategy has not been rigorously evaluated.

As a result, contemporary practice is dominated by considerable uncertainty regarding the role of surgical ligation. In this chapter, we review the evidence regarding the benefits and risks of PDA surgery in very preterm neonates and provide a pathophysiology-based management paradigm to guide perioperative care in these high-risk infants.

Patent Ductus Arteriosus Ligation: Evidence of Benefit Versus Harm in Randomized Clinical Trials

A limited number of randomized clinical trials, all conducted more than 3 decades ago, have evaluated the impact of surgical ligation in preterm infants on neonatal outcomes (Table 24.1). Two trials were conducted prior to the routine use of indomethacin treatment to pharmacologically achieve earlier ductal closure. Cotton et al.[3] randomized 25 very low birth weight preterm infants (mean gestational age [GA] 28 weeks) with a clinical diagnosis of symptomatic PDA and requiring invasive mechanical ventilation at 1 week of postnatal life to surgical ligation versus ongoing medical management, which consisted of diuretic and digoxin therapy. Infants treated with surgical ligation had a significantly shorter time to successful extubation (median 6 vs. 22 days after enrollment, $P < .05$).[3] In contrast, Levitsky et al.[4] randomized 31 moderately preterm infants (mean GA 31 weeks) with respiratory distress syndrome and clinically diagnosed PDA to ligation or medical management.[4] There were no differences in neonatal outcomes, although nearly half of the medically treated group was ultimately treated with surgery.

Only one trial, involving 154 preterm infants (median GA 28 to 29 weeks) with symptomatic PDA despite conservative management, compared surgical ligation versus a first course of indomethacin therapy. Infants randomized to ligation had a higher incidence of severe retinopathy of prematurity (ROP), and there were no other differences in neonatal outcomes.[5] Cassady et al.[6] reported reduced rates of necrotizing enterocolitis (NEC; 30% vs. 8%, $P = .002$) in ELBW preterm infants undergoing prophylactic ligation on the first postnatal day,[6] although a recent post hoc secondary analysis reported an increased risk of moderate-severe bronchopulmonary dysplasia (BPD) in surgically treated infants.[7]

Taken together, the common salient feature of trials of PDA ligation is a lack of external validity to permit their interpretation within contemporary practice. Although dependence on mechanical ventilation has remained the most common indication for referring infants for surgical treatment, advances in respiratory care (e.g., exogenous surfactant therapy, inline flow sensors, and noninvasive positive pressure ventilation) have dramatically altered the trajectory of mechanical ventilation for respiratory distress syndrome, including earlier endotracheal extubation. The advent of prophylactic indomethacin and the concept of exposing all infants (potentially including some with pathologically elevated pulmonary vascular resistance) to the incipient risks of early surgical ductal closure render prophylactic ligation untenable in modern practice. In addition, echocardiography is currently the definitive and integral method of assessing the magnitude of the ductal shunt and guiding management. This modality was conspicuously absent in these older trials alongside a limited, and predominantly clinical, definition of hemodynamic significance. Finally, over the past decade, surgical treatment has become uncommon in infants

Table 24.1 RANDOMIZED CLINICAL TRIALS OF SURGICAL PATENT DUCTUS ARTERIOSUS LIGATION COMPARED WITH MEDICAL MANAGEMENT

Author (Year)	Size	Population	Intervention	Comparison	Outcome	Results		
						Ligation group	Comparator group	P-value
Levitsky et al.[4] (1976)	$n = 31$	• Mean BW 1383 g (range 550–2000); mean GA 31 weeks • All patients had RDS and clinical diagnosis of PDA and remained symptomatic after treatment with digoxin ± diuretics • Blood transfusions administered to maintain HCT > 40%	Ligation ($n = 8$)	No additional treatment, with ligation as backup ($n = 23$) Rescue ligation: 11/23 (48%)	Survival (in-hospital)	4 (50%)	16 (70%)	.32[a]
Cotton et al.[3] (1978)	$n = 25$	• Birthweight < 1500 g (mean GA 28–29 weeks) • All patients had clinical diagnosis of PDA who remained symptomatic and dependent on invasive ventilation at 1 week despite treatment with digoxin and strategies to reduce pulmonary edema (diuretics, fluid restriction, distending airway pressure) • Blood transfusions administered to maintain HCT > 40%	Ligation ($n = 10$)	No additional treatment with ligation as backup ($n = 15$) Rescue ligation: 2/15 (13%)	Survival (in-hospital) Duration of endotracheal intubation (median)	9 (90%) 6 days	12 (80%) 22 days	.50[a] <.05
Gersony et al.[5] (1983)	$n = 154$	• Mean GA 28–29 weeks • Clinical and echocardiography diagnosis (PDA signs, cardiorespiratory compromise, with patency and LA:Ao ≥ 1.15 on echocardiogram) • Remained symptomatic despite medical management with diuretics, fluid restriction or digoxin	Ligation ($n = 79$)	Indomethacin ($n = 75$) Rescue ligation: 25/75 (33%)	Survival (in-hospital) BPD ROP (III or IV) NEC ≥ 14 days invasive ventilation	67 (85%) 31 (39%) 12 (15%) 5 (6%) 22 (30%)	58 (77%) 23 (31%) 3 (4%) 5 (7%) 22 (32%)	.3 .3 .02 .9 .84[a]
Cassady et al.[6] (1989) and Clyman et al.[7] (2009) [post hoc analysis]	$n = 84$	• Birthweight < 1000 g • Required supplemental oxygen on first day of life	Prophylactic ligation within 24 h of birth ($n = 40$)	Standard treatment ($n = 44$) • Initial treatment with nCPAP for RDS or pulmonary edema • Rescue ligation [23/44 (52%), 7 occurring within 3 days of birth] if Qp:Qs > 3.0 or ventilator dependence with large left-to-right PDA shunt on echocardiography	Survival to 1 year NEC IVH III/IV[b] BPD[b] (Bancalari definition) Oxygen at 36 weeks[c] Mechanical ventilation at 36 weeks[c]	25 (63%) 3 (8%) 16/35 (46%) 14 (35%) 11(48%) 6 (26%)	26 (59%) 13 (30%) 23/41 (56%) 16 (36%) 4(21%) 0 (0%)	.75[a] .002 .37[a] .90[a] <.05 <.05

[a]Chi-square analysis performed using published data when comparison not presented in original publication.

[b]Incidence represents the number of infants with the condition out of the total number evaluated.

[c]Incidence shown represents survivors at 36 weeks' postmenstrual age (23 from prophylactic ligation arm and 19 from control arm).

BPD, Bronchopulmonary dysplasia; BW, birthweight; GA, gestational age; HCT, hematocrit; IVH, intraventricular hemorrhage; LA:Ao, left atrium to aortic root ratio; nCPAP, nasal continuous positive airway pressure; NEC, necrotizing enterocolitis; PDA, patent ductus arteriosus; Qp:Qs, pulmonary to systemic flow ratio; RDS, respiratory distress syndrome; ROP, retinopathy of prematurity.

born at GA ≥27 weeks and is typically only considered after pharmacotherapeutic closure has failed or was contraindicated, representing a population and therapeutic approach that has not been evaluated.

Patent Ductus Arteriosus Ligation and Outcomes: Associations from Observational Studies

Studies have reported increased neonatal morbidity and NDI in early childhood among infants treated with PDA ligation compared with medical management alone.[7-13] In these large retrospective cohort studies, infants were categorized by treatment assignment (conservative management, cyclooxygenase inhibitor [COXI] only, COXI followed by surgical ligation, or primary ligation) and outcomes compared between treatment groups.

In a large retrospective cohort study of preterm infants born less than 32 weeks' GA with a symptomatic PDA, Mirea et al. compared neonatal outcomes according to PDA treatment assignment.[8] After adjustment for antenatal and perinatal confounders, infants treated with surgical ligation had lower mortality but higher odds of BPD and ROP, compared with infants treated with medical management alone. Similarly, in a retrospective review of 426 ELBW infants, Kabra et al. detected higher BPD and ROP in 110 infants who underwent surgical ligation compared with 316 infants who received medical management only.[10] Higher rates of BPD among infants with PDA ligation was also detected by Madan et al. in a review of 2838 ELBW treated for symptomatic PDA.[11] Several studies also reported an association of PDA ligation with increased rates of NDI in early childhood.[10-13] A recent systematic review and metaanalysis of randomized trials and controlled observational studies demonstrated that compared with medically treated infants, ligated infants were more likely to develop BPD, severe ROP, and NDI, although with improved survival (Table 24.2).[14]

Retrospective epoch studies have reported a similar association between PDA ligation and NDI; specifically, an improvement in neurodevelopmental outcomes coincided with a reduced proportion of infants referred for surgical ligation. Wickremasinghe et al. evaluated 18- to 36-month neurodevelopmental outcomes after moving from an early, aggressive surgical approach (infants with echocardiographic evidence of PDA after medical therapy were immediately referred for surgery) to a delayed selection ligation approach (infants with a persistent PDA were referred for ligation if the PDA was clinically and echocardiographically significant). Infants in the selective ligation epoch were less likely to be treated with surgery (66% vs. 100%) and had less NDI (adjusted odds ratio [OR] 0.07, 95% confidence interval [CI] 0.00 to 0.96), potentially reflecting a benefit of avoiding ligation in infants with smaller ductal shunts.[15] These studies highlight the importance of the ascertainment of hemodynamic significance, particularly in appraising the merits of surgical intervention.

Aspects of PDA ligation that have been postulated to contribute to the risk of NDI include surgical and anesthesia effects and postoperative hemodynamic compromise. Vocal cord paresis is a common surgical complication and is associated with an increased risk of death, extubation failure and chronic lung disease, need for gastrostomy tube, and gastroesophageal reflux disease.[16-19] Recent studies have associated use of halothane gases for anesthesia in young children with NDI.[20-22] Preterm infants are at risk of postoperative hypotension and cardiogenic shock due to postligation cardiac syndrome (PLCS), which may result in cerebral hypoperfusion and injury.[23-28] Although it is important to acknowledge the clinical importance of these complications, causality is not implied.

In light of concerns regarding NDI and neonatal morbidities, the safety of PDA ligation has been questioned.[15,29-33] These concerns have been associated with a secular trend toward a reduction in infants being treated with surgical ligation in North American centers.[1,2] On the contrary, the reduction in ligation has been associated with increased BPD in one large American neonatal network, suggesting caution before imposing radical changes in practice (Fig. 24.1).[2]

Table 24.2 NEONATAL AND NEURODEVELOPMENTAL OUTCOMES REPORTED IN SELECT LARGE ADJUSTED OBSERVATIONAL STUDIES FOR INFANTS WITH A PATENT DUCTUS ARTERIOSUS TREATED WITH SURGICAL LIGATION COMPARED WITH MEDICAL MANAGEMENT ONLY

Study	Characteristics	Antenatal/Perinatal Confounders Adjusted	Postnatal Confounders Adjusted	Odds Ratio (95% Confidence Interval)[a]				
				Death or NDI	Death	NDI	Severe ROP	CLD
Kabra et al.[10] 2007	ELBW infants with symptomatic PDA. PDA ligation (n = 110). Medical only (n = 316)	GA, sex, ACS, multiples, mother's education, total dose indomethacin	None	1.55 (0.97, 2.50)	0.56 (0.29, 1.10)	1.98 (1.18, 3.30)	2.20 (1.19, 4.07)	1.81 (1.09, 3.03)
Madan et al.[11] 2009[b]	ELBW infants with PDA. Primary ligation (n = 135), Indo only (n = 1525), Indo and ligation (n = 775). No treatment (n = 403)	GA, BW, gender, ACS, center, prophylactic indomethacin, Apgar score, RDS, IUGR, antenatal infection, maternal marital status and age	Postnatal sepsis	1.03 (0.80, 1.33)	0.46 (0.35, 0.62)	1.53 (1.16, 2.03)	n/a	3.10 (2.26, 4.26)
Mirea et al.[8] 2012[c]	Infants with GA ≤ 32 weeks with PDA. Conservative (n = 577), Indo only (n = 2026), Indo + ligation (n = 626), Primary ligation (n = 327)	GA, ACS, multiples, gender, IUGR, SNAP II	None	n/a	0.41 (0.31, 0.54)	n/a	1.91 (1.51, 2.41)	2.30 (1.91, 2.77)
Bourgoin et al.[12] 2016[d]	Infants with GA ≤ 28 weeks with PDA. Conservative (n = 505), Ibuprofen only (n = 248), Ligation (n = 104)	gender, GA, BW Z-score, ACS, gestational hypertension, clinical chorioamnionitis, Apgar score, place of hospitalization, place of birth, year of birth, delivery characteristics	None	n/a	n/a	1.9 (1.1, 3.1)	n/a	n/a
Weisz et al.[47] 2017[e]	Infants with GA < 28 weeks with clinical and echo diagnosis of PDA. Ligation (n = 184). Medical treatment only (n = 570)	GA, IUGR, ACS, gender, multiples, SNAP II score ≥ 20, center	sepsis, severe IVH, inotropes, NEC >2, average daily mean airway pressure, No. days invasive ventilation, total dose of indomethacin, systemic corticosteroids	0.83 (0.52, 1.32)	0.09 (0.04, 0.21)	1.27 (0.78, 2.06)	1.61 (0.85, 3.06)	1.36 (0.78, 2.39)

ACS, Antenatal corticosteroids; BW, birthweight; CLD, chronic lung disease; ELBW, extremely low birthweight; GA, gestational age; Indo, indomethacin; IUGR, intrauterine growth restriction; IVH, intraventricular hemorrhage; NDI, neurodevelopmental impairment; NEC, necrotizing enterocolitis; PDA, patent ductus arteriosus; RDS, respiratory distress syndrome; ROP, retinopathy of prematurity; SNAP, score for neonatal acute physiology.
[a]Reference is medically treated infants
[b]Data shown for Indomethacin and Ligation vs. Indomethacin only. Sepsis was adjusted for in multivariable analysis; however, the timing of infection in relation to ductal closure was not specified.
[c]Data shown for any ligation vs. no ligation. This data was provided by the primary author and is unpublished.
[d]Compared ligation vs. conservative management.
[e]Postnatal confounders adjusted were those occurring prior to ductal closure during the period each infant was considered "at-risk" of surgical ligation

24

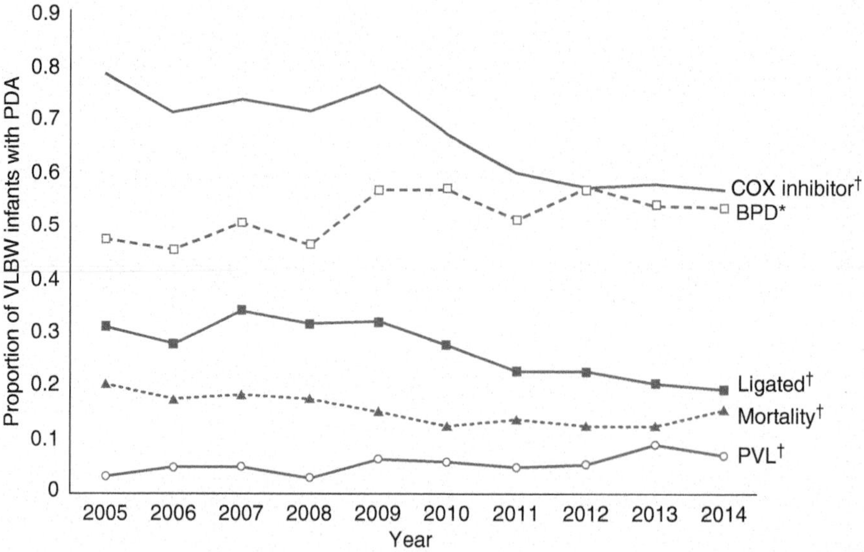

Fig. 24.1 Trends in treatment and outcomes among 5719 very low birth weight infants with patent ductus arteriosus at 19 US referral children's hospitals, 2005–2014. *$P < .01$; †$P < .001$. *BPD*, Bronchopulmonary dysplasia; *PDA*, patent ductus arteriosus; *PVL*, periventricular leukomalacia; *VLBW*, very low birth weight. (Reproduced from Hagadorn JI, Brownell EA, Traszki JM, et al.: Trends and variation in management and outcomes of very low birth weight infants with patent ductus arteriosus, *Pediatr Res* 80(6):785–792, 2016, with permission from Nature Publishing.)

Neonatal Morbidity, Neurodevelopmental Impairment, and Patent Ductus Arteriosus Ligation: Residual Bias in Observational Studies

Residual selection bias and bias due to confounding by indication threaten the validity of observational studies that have associated PDA ligation with increased neonatal morbidity and NDI but lower mortality compared with medical management alone. The divergence of these competing outcomes (lower mortality but increased BPD, ROP, and NDI) may be explained by several possible situations: "First, surgical ligation may improve the survival of infants with PDA but may be simultaneously neurologically detrimental, either directly through the surgery-associated inflammatory response or indirectly via worsening lung disease and ventilator dependency." Second, ligation may improve the survival of infants with PDA, but the infants referred for ligation are at higher preligation risk of NDI (confounding by indication and increased preligation illness severity). Finally, the decreased mortality may be a spurious finding influenced by survival bias (where moribund nonligated infants with a PDA die before becoming eligible for ligation), and the increase in NDI may be due to either a true detrimental effect of ligation, the effect of confounding by indication, or a combination of these two possibilities.

Studies to date have inadequately addressed confounding by indication—that infants referred for ligation may be more "ill" and/or have larger ductal shunts at the time of the decision to treat with surgery, compared with infants who are treated with medical management alone. Illness severity, characterized by postnatal morbidities such as periventricular/intraventricular hemorrhage (P/IVH), NEC, and sepsis, and parameters of physiologic instability such as hypotension, predict both neonatal morbidities and NDI (see Table 24.2).[9,34-37]

The intensity and duration of invasive mechanical ventilation is a particularly important confounder of the association between ligation and adverse outcomes. Prolonged ventilator dependence is a commonly used clinical criterion in the decision to treat with ligation (vs. medical management) and also strongly predicts neonatal morbidities such as BPD, ROP, and NDI.[38-41]

Survival bias may have influenced the reported lower mortality among ligated infants.[8,11,42,43] Ligation is generally undertaken later in life after failure of medical

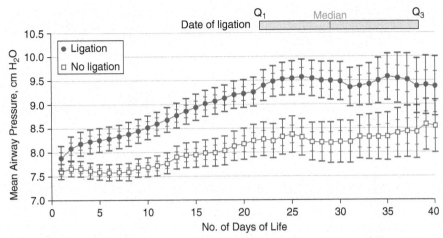

Fig. 24.2 Average daily mean airway pressure (cm H_2O) with 68% and 95% confidence intervals (CIs) over the first 40 days of postnatal life for medically treated *(black solid line)* vs. ligated infants *(red dashed line)*, respectively, prior to ductal closure. Infants no longer contributed data after the date of ductal closure, leading to the widening of CIs over time as the number of infants with persistent hemodynamically significant patent ductus arteriosus (PDA) diminished with time. The median date of ligation was day of life (DOL) #29 with interquartile range [DOL #22, DOL #38] *(solid pink box)*. The earliest date of ligation was on DOL #7. (Reproduced from Weisz DE, Mirea L, Rosenberg E, et al.: Patent ductus arteriosus ligation and death or neurodevelopmental impairment in extremely preterm infants, JAMA Pediatr 171(5):443–449, 2017, with permission.)

therapy, meaning that ligated infants are more likely to have already survived the critical period of high early neonatal mortality. This treatment paradigm implies that some of the sickest infants, treated initially with conservative management and/or COXIs, may have died prior to becoming "eligible" for ligation, resulting in selection bias in assembling the cohort of ligated infants. The possibility of survival bias is supported by studies which found no difference in mortality between medically and surgically treated groups of infants who both received treatments at a similar postnatal age.[5,8,9,11,44-46] Taken together, survival bias may be present and any beneficial effect of ligation on mortality requires additional study prior to clinicians being confident of a survival benefit of PDA surgery.

A recent large cohort study (*n* = 754) of extremely preterm infants with PDA compared neonatal and neurodevelopmental outcomes of infants treated with ligation versus medical treatment, while minimizing the effect of residual bias due to confounding by indication (see Table 24.2).[47] Multivariable logistic regression analysis was used to adjust for antenatal, perinatal, and postnatal, preductal closure confounders, including the duration and intensity of mechanical ventilation and morbidities such as NEC and sepsis. Infants treated with ligation had higher ventilation requirements than did infants who were not treated with ligation, a confounder not controlled for in studies to date (Fig. 24.2). As with previous observational studies, when adjusting only for antenatal and perinatal confounders, ligation was associated with increased BPD, ROP, and NDI. However, after further adjustment for postnatal, preductal closure confounders (e.g., burden of mechanical ventilation, sepsis), ligation was no longer associated with any adverse outcome.[47] This study suggests that the associations of ligation with adverse outcomes from earlier studies were likely due to confounding by indication rather than a true detrimental causal effect of ligation. These findings have direct clinical relevance; specifically, neonatologists and pediatric cardiac surgeons may now consider to no longer prioritize the risk of adverse neonatal and neurodevelopmental outcomes as a reason to avoid surgical PDA ligation.

Patent Ductus Arteriosus Ligation Decision: Timing, Patient Selection, and Staging

In contemporary practice the "PDA ligation decision" remains an enduring controversy for clinicians. There is currently a paucity of knowledge regarding the clinical and echocardiography characteristics of infants with persistent PDA who may benefit from ligation. The relative risks and benefits of rescue surgical ligation compared with conservative management are unknown. Although dependence on mechanical ventilation remains the primary criterion for surgical referral, the relative independent contribution of the PDA to ongoing respiratory insufficiency is, at present, difficult to quantify. Infants with similar echocardiography indices of PDA hemodynamic significance may have varying degrees of respiratory failure (severe to none) owing to differences in nascent lung disease of prematurity, pulmonary arterial pressure, and tolerance of the increased pulmonary blood flow from the ductal shunt.

Limited evidence from clinical trials and careful reflection on contemporary treatment practices provides some boundaries for surgical treatment, mostly by limiting the use of ligation in the first postnatal week. Although the trial by Cassady et al. reported reduced NEC with prophylactic ligation on the first postnatal day in ELBW infants, several factors render this practice now untenable.[6] First, prophylactic indomethacin has both relatively high efficacy for early closure and reduces all grades of P/IVH, providing a therapeutic alternative with additional benefit. Second, PDA ligation may result in increased right ventricular (RV) afterload, so early ligation may be harmful in preterm infants with increased pulmonary artery pressure, a common finding in severe respiratory distress syndrome. Finally, the natural history of ductal closure has been described, with many infants experiencing early spontaneous closure. Exposing all infants to the risk of prophylactic surgical ligation is therefore inappropriate.[48]

Epoch studies have reported that preterm infants treated with delayed selective ligation (surgical PDA closure after failure of medical therapy only if infants had concomitant respiratory failure, systemic hypotension, or signs of end-organ hypoperfusion) had improved rates of BPD and NDI compared with infants treated with early, routine ligation.[49] Ligation prior to the 10th postnatal day was independently associated with adverse outcomes.

Beyond the first 2 weeks after delivery, there is a paucity of data specifically addressing the impact of ligation versus conservative management in infants with persistent PDA after unsuccessful pharmacologic therapy. In most cases the persistent ductal shunt may be considered a chronic, consistent contributor to impaired pulmonary compliance. Infants with a persistent PDA may be considered for surgical ligation when the clinical and echocardiography evaluations identify a shunt of sufficient volume that may be actively contributing to respiratory insufficiency. Persistent dependence on invasive or noninvasive ventilation in combination with moderate-severe echocardiography indicators of hemodynamic significance suggests an impaired ability to compensate for the ductal shunt.

However, it is important to consider preterm infants who have clinical features of chronic end-organ hypoperfusion (systemic hypotension, renal failure, feeding intolerance) in the absence of an acute etiology (e.g., sepsis, NEC) accompanied by echocardiographic indices of a large ductal shunt. In these infants, echocardiographic indices are often in the "severe" range across all parameters, although there are little data regarding the direct clinical relevance of these deviations from normal (Table 24.3). Early surgical ligation after failure of medical therapy may be indicated for this subgroup of infants.

Preoperative and Intraoperative Management

Echocardiography should be performed at least within 48 hours of surgery to reevaluate PDA severity. Baseline hemoglobin, platelet count, and prothrombin time should be obtained. Adrenocorticotropin stimulation testing should be performed preoperatively to assess adrenal cortex responsiveness, which may be impaired in preterm infants with PDA.[50] Preoperative serum cortisol ≤750 nmol/L (≤27 µg/dL) after adrenocorticotropic hormone (ACTH) stimulation is associated with increased postoperative hypotension and respiratory failure.[51] On the other hand, routine preoperative stress-dose hydrocortisone was not associated with improved cardiovascular stability, regardless of GA.[52]

Table 24.3 ECHOCARDIOGRAPHY PARAMETERS OF DUCTAL HEMODYNAMIC SIGNIFICANCE

	Parameter	Hemodynamic Significance		
		Mild	Moderate	Severe
Ductus arteriosus size and flow pattern	PDA 2D diameter	<1.5 mm	1.5–2.5 mm	>2.5 mm
	PDA Doppler			
	Peak systolic velocity[a]	>2.5	1.5–2.5	<1.5
	Peak systolic velocity: minimum diastolic velocity	<2	2–4	>4
Pulmonary over-circulation/left heart loading	LV output (mL/kg/min)	<300	300–450	>450
	LV chamber size	Z-score < +1.5	+1.5 < Z < +2.5	+2.5 < Z-score
	LA hypertension			
	LA:Ao	<1.5	1.5–1.9	≥2.0
	Mitral valve E:A ratio[b]	<1		>1
	IVRT	>40 ms	30–40 ms	<30 ms
Systemic steal	Abdominal aorta	No diastolic reversal	Diastolic reversal	

[a]Very large left-to-right ductal shunts may have higher peak systolic velocities (>1.5 m/s), indicating high shunt volume (and low pulmonary vascular resistance) rather than flow restriction.

[b]Mitral valve E:A ratio >1 represents "pseudonormalization" and is suggestive of left atrial pressure loading.

Ao, Aorta; *IVRT*, isovolumic relaxation time; *LA*, left atrium; *LPA*, left pulmonary artery; *LV*, left ventricle; *Mitral Valve E:A*, Early-to-late (atrial contraction) inflow ratio.

Ligation is most commonly performed in an operating room or at the bedside in the neonatal intensive care unit (NICU), via a left lateral thoracotomy, and with application of a clip or ligature to the PDA. Previous studies have reported no significant differences in neonatal outcomes between an intrapleural or extrapleural approach.[53,54] The relative merits of the use of clip versus ligature in preterm infants have had mixed reports, with one study reporting reduced operation and anesthesia times and decreased bleeding[55] with clip application and other studies suggesting an increased risk of vocal cord paresis with clip use.[55-57]

Intraoperative anesthesia management may have a significant impact on an infant's perioperative outcome. A small randomized placebo-controlled trial found that the addition of higher-dose fentanyl to intraoperative anesthesia for preterm infants undergoing surgery resulted in lower hormonal stress responses to surgery and fewer postoperative metabolic and circulatory complications.[58] In a small retrospective cohort study of 33 preterm infants undergoing PDA ligation, a fentanyl dose of less than 10.5 µg/kg was associated with increased postoperative respiratory instability but not hypotension.[59] The use of higher fentanyl doses (25 to 30 µg/kg) in children undergoing cardiac surgery resulted in lower serum levels of glucose, epinephrine, ACTH, and cortisol. These findings suggest that higher-dose fentanyl (10 to 30 µg/kg) may provide effective anesthesia and contribute to less postoperative instability.

Care of the Preterm Infant After Patent Ductus Arteriosus Ligation

Physiologic Changes After Surgery

Reduction in left ventricle (LV) preload, surge in systemic vascular resistance (SVR), and reduced cardiac output

PDA ligation results in an instantaneous fall in LV preload (pulmonary venous return) and surge in LV afterload due to increased SVR,[60] culminating in an abrupt drop in LV output.[24] Using noninvasive electrical cardiometry to monitor hemodynamic changes intraoperatively, Lien et al. demonstrated that there was a significant decline in LV output and surge in SVR upon sudden termination of ductal shunting.[61] The deterioration in LV output was associated with a decrease in stroke volume rather than heart rate, and the magnitude of the reduction was particularly pronounced among ELBW infants.[61,62]

Myocardial dysfunction

PDA ligation in premature baboons resulted in impaired LV systolic performance and ventilation failure, coinciding with an increase in SVR.[63] LV fractional shortening (FS) deteriorates 6 to 12 hours after surgical ligation.[63] Similar findings have been confirmed with modern echocardiographic analysis in preterm infants, mostly in the past 10 years.[64,65] PDA ligation was found to be associated with a significant reduction in LV FS and mean velocity of circumferential fiber shortening, especially in the ELBW group.[66] The LV myocardial performance index, which incorporates the isovolumetric contraction and relaxation times and adjusts, at least in theory, for preload by accounting for the ejection time, deteriorated acutely after ligation, mimicking the changes in LV output.[60] LV efficiency, defined as the ratio of stroke volume to pressure-volume area, transiently deteriorates within 24 hours after ligation and then recovers to preoperative levels by 2 to 4 days after ligation.[67]

In a cohort of 19 very preterm infants evaluated with tissue Doppler imaging and myocardial deformation techniques after PDA ligation, systolic and diastolic LV tissue Doppler velocities and global LV longitudinal strain decreased immediately after ligation.[23] The former remained significantly lower than the preoperative levels at 18 hours, whereas the latter significantly improved 18 hours after the procedure.[23]

Notably, these longitudinal changes can be affected, to a certain extent, by the acute changes in loading conditions, rather than solely myocardial performance alone.[68] Noori postulated that there was a "resetting" of the set point of the Starling curve of the myocardium after a prolonged period of stretch so that the decrease in end-diastolic fiber length after ligation would result in a decrease in contractile force.[33] Saida et al. demonstrated that a larger preoperative LV internal dimension in diastole was predictive of a decrease in postoperative FS of the LV.[69]

Preterm infants have decreased sarcoplasmic reticulum and a poorly developed or absent T-tubule system in their myocytes; thus they have less mature excitation-contraction and relaxation mechanisms.[70,71] As a result the ability of the myocardium of premature neonates to respond to a sudden surge in SVR is limited compared with that of term neonates.[70] The risk of impaired LV systolic performance and associated clinical deterioration appears to be greater in more immature infants after PDA ligation.[66,72]

Hemodynamic changes in mesenteric and cerebral circulations

Doppler evaluation of systemic arteries, such as the celiac artery, superior mesenteric artery, renal artery, and cerebral arteries, demonstrates significant postoperative changes after ligation.[73] Hoodbhoy et al. reported a significant increase in average velocities in both the celiac and superior mesenteric arteries within 3 hours post-PDA ligation, but such a phenomenon was not found in the middle cerebral artery until 24 hours after surgery.[74] The normalization of Doppler estimates of diastolic flow after PDA ligation strongly implicates the PDA as the cause of abnormal preoperative diastolic flow in systemic arteries. However, the utility of these sonographic changes in managing postoperative care is unknown.

The reported association of PDA ligation and NDI has led to concerns regarding the effect of postoperative myocardial dysfunction and systemic hypotension on cerebral perfusion, especially in extremely preterm infants with reduced capacity for cerebrovascular autoregulation.[33] Leslie et al. evaluated cerebral electrical activity changes after ligation using amplitude-integrated electroencephalography and found a decrease in the lower trace margin and proportion of patients with trace continuity after surgery, independent of cardiac output status.[75] However, other studies that have used near-infrared spectroscopy to assess changes in regional cerebral oxygen saturation and cerebral blood flow have shown conflicting results.[33] The relationship of postoperative brain perfusion and later neurosensory impairment requires further evaluation.

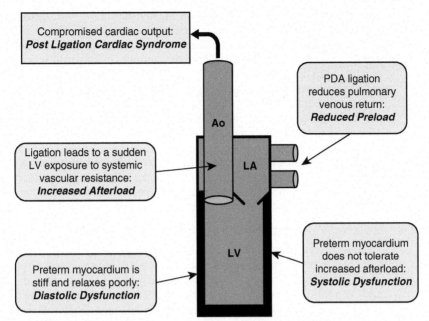

Fig. 24.3   Physiologic determinants of postligation cardiac syndrome. *Ao*, Aorta; *LA*, left atrium; *LV*, left ventricle; *PDA*, patent ductus arteriosus. (Reproduced from El-Khuffash A, Jain A, McNamara PJ: Ligation of the patent ductus arteriosus in preterm infants: understanding the physiology, *J Pediatr* 162(6):1100–1106, 2013, with permission from Elsevier.)

PLCS and Targeted Milrinone Prophylaxis

The postoperative course may be complicated by acute cardiorespiratory instability, termed PLCS, which occurs in up to half of infants and typically occurs between 6 and 12 hours after surgery.[26,60,68,76] The two components of PLCS are respiratory instability and systemic hypotension, manifesting as significant increases in fractional oxygen requirement, mean airway pressure, and the need for inotropic support.[26,60,77-79] Data suggest that increased LV afterload is a greater contributor to the pathophysiology of PLCS than reduced preload. Impairment in indices of LV systolic function and peak measures of LV afterload coincide with the clinical onset of PLCS at approximately 8 hours postoperatively.[66] In contrast, the effects of reduced LV preload, such as low LV output, are echocardiographically evident as early as 1 hour after surgery when the patient is clinically asymptomatic (Fig. 24.3).[80] Reduced preload may limit the immature myocardium's ability to maintain cardiac output under conditions of increased afterload and may be clinically important in select infants with coexisting severe acute inflammatory lesions (e.g., NEC) where capillary leak may reduce intravascular volume.

PDA ligation in preterm infants younger than 4 weeks old is associated with oxygenation failure, decreased systolic arterial pressure, and an increased need for cardiotropic support in the initial 24 postoperative hours.[77] Infants who had lower birth weight and GA, or higher ventilatory support had a higher risk of vasopressor-inotrope treatment after ligation.[68] Retrospective studies have failed to identify any relationship between surgical technique, anesthetic approach, or intraoperative fluid management and the development of hypotension.[79,81] Jain et al. reported that LV output of less than 200 mL/kg/min estimated by echocardiography 1 hour after PDA ligation was a sensitive predictor of systemic hypotension and the need for inotropes. Reduced tissue Doppler systolic indices (LV basal lateral peak systolic annular velocity (S′), basal septal S′ and basal RV S′) at 1 hour postoperatively correlate strongly with early low LV output, potentially providing an additional echocardiography indicator of infants at higher risk of PLCS.[80]

Milrinone, a selective phosphodiesterase III inhibitor, is a systemic vasodilator with lusitropic and positive inotropic effects which acts by inhibiting the hydrolysis of cyclic adenosine monophosphate in the myocardium.[76,82] Targeted early postoperative administration of an intravenous infusion of milrinone in infants with low cardiac output (<200 mL/kg/min) has been associated with a significant reduction in ventilation failure (48% to 15%), need for inotropes (56% to 19%), and the incidence of overall PLCS (44% to 11%).[26] Milrinone treatment was also associated with longitudinal improvement in tissue Doppler imaging and speckle-tracking echocardiography–derived indicators of systolic function within 18 hours, likely due to the effects of afterload reduction and improvement in myocardial systolic performance.[80] This practice is supported by a randomized placebo-controlled trial of universal prophylactic milrinone after open congenital heart disease surgery in a pediatric population, which demonstrated a 64% relative risk reduction in death or low cardiac output syndrome in the first 36 hours postoperatively in the milrinone group (26.7% vs. 9.6%, P = .007).[83] Postoperative milrinone treatment has not been evaluated in a randomized trial in preterm infants after PDA ligation.

Isolated Postoperative Respiratory Instability

Postoperatively, ligation of the PDA has been shown to improve pulmonary dynamic compliance, tidal volume, and minute ventilation.[84] However, not all patients exhibit immediate improvement; a subset develop early (4 to 12 hours after surgery) oxygenation or ventilation failure, requiring an escalation of respiratory support.[26,66]

In preterm baboons, PDA ligation was found to produce a significant increase in the expression of genes involved in pulmonary inflammation (COX-2, tumor necrosis factor (TNF)-α, and CD14) and a significant decrease in α-epithelial sodium channel (ENaC) expression, resulting in a decrease in the rate of alveolar fluid clearance.[85] This deleterious inflammatory response to the surgical procedure may, at least in part, mediate deterioration in lung function in preterm infants.[60]

Ting et al. reported that the incidence of oxygenation or ventilation failure remained high (51.2%) in preterm infants undergoing PDA ligation, despite the implementation of early targeted milrinone treatment, among infants with early echocardiographic evidence of low cardiac output.[79] Postoperative LV diastolic dysfunction, manifested by prolonged isovolumic relaxation time (IVRT) on early echocardiography, is associated with subsequent respiratory instability. This may be related to the inability of the premature LV, with a priori diastolic dysfunction, to adapt to the acute postligation increase in LV afterload, leading to further augmentation in LV filling pressures, secondary pulmonary venous hypertension, and oxygenation failure.[79] Infants with LV diastolic dysfunction may benefit from a higher dose of milrinone to exert its lusitropic effects, although an adequately powered prospective study is needed to address this hypothesis.[86]

Hypothalamic-Pituitary-Adrenal (HPA) Gland Axis and Postligation Cardiovascular Stability

The HPA axis is crucial in regulating organ maturational events, especially the increased concentration of β-adrenergic receptors in tissues, and effective cardiovascular responsiveness to endogenous and pharmacologic vasoactive agents.[87] Preterm infants are prone to life-threatening hypotension secondary to HPA axis immaturity, resulting from adrenocortical insufficiency.[88] Under stress, the premature adrenal gland may not respond appropriately to elevated ACTH, producing only a blunted cortisol response (see also Chapter 30).[89-91] Adrenal hypoperfusion secondary to chronic ductal "steal" has been postulated to be another contributory mechanism in infants with persistent PDA.[51] Clyman et al. found that infants with low cortisol concentrations after PDA ligation are more likely to develop postoperative catecholamine-resistant hypotension.[92]

Surgical Complications

There are little data regarding site-specific variability in the incidence of direct surgical complications. The frequency of these complications is likely to be influenced by surgical volumes and the expertise of the surgical operator.

Pneumothorax and Chylothorax

Prompt recognition and management of pneumothorax and chylothorax after ligation are essential to prevent cardiorespiratory compromise. Pneumothorax is typically the result of intrapleural accumulation of air either through the thoracotomy site or from alveolar rupture secondary to mechanical ventilation. There is a wide range of reported incidence rates, from 1.6% to 5.4%, depending on the inclusion criteria of the series.[16,93-95] Chylothorax is a rare but potentially devastating complication, which results from traumatic disruption of the thoracic duct or adjacent lymphatic channels.[94,96]

Phrenic Nerve Paralysis

Phrenic nerve injury resulting in transient or permanent diaphragmatic dysfunction after PDA ligation has been reported.[97,98] Neonates are especially vulnerable to the effects of diaphragmatic dysfunction due to supine positioning, dependence upon the diaphragm for optimal respiratory effort, the greater compliance of the chest wall, and the horizontal orientation of the rib cage.[99] In a case-control study of very low birth weight infants, Hsu et al. reported that infants with diaphragmatic paralysis had a longer duration of ventilator dependency (56 vs. 30 days) and a higher incidence of severe BPD (87% vs. 23%).[97] Predicting recovery continues to be difficult, and diaphragmatic plication may be needed in select patients.[97,98]

Injury or Ligation of Adjacent Structures

The anatomy of the premature infant is different from that of the older child and presents a risk for surgical inaccuracy.[100] The ductus arteriosus is commonly larger than the transverse aorta proximal to the left subclavian artery. The PDA may appear through the unopened pleura to be the aortic arch itself.[100] The aorta, left pulmonary artery, and left main stem bronchus have all been mistaken for the ductus arteriosus and ligated.[101-104] The aortic arch vessels must be carefully identified to avoid surgical misadventure, and echocardiography can be useful to understand postoperative hemodynamic changes as well as to ascertain ductal ligation.

Residual Ductal Shunting

Ductal division usually offers complete closure, whereas ligation has been reported to be associated with recurrences, due to either recanalization or incomplete closure.[105] Residual shunt after ductal interruption is almost always small or trivial and does not lead to hemodynamic compromise in neonates or children.[101] However, there is a lack of reports of incidence and complications associated with residual shunting in preterm infants.

Bleeding

The ductus tissue can be very fragile; major bleeding should be suspected when radiodense areas are found on a chest roentgenogram with unexplained hemodynamic compromise after surgery.[101]

Vocal Cord Paralysis

The left recurrent laryngeal nerve is a branch of the vagus nerve that loops around the aortic arch immediately adjacent to the ductus arteriosus, before traveling superiorly alongside the trachea to innervate the laryngeal muscles. This complex anatomic course places the left recurrent laryngeal nerve at risk of injury with surgical ligation of PDA, with possible iatrogenic left vocal fold paralysis (LVFP). There is a wide range of reported incidence rates (2.2% to 67%),* although the incidence is higher in ELBW infants (23% to 67%).[17,18,57] Risk factors for LVFP include lower birth weight and GA[18,19] and possibly surgical technique (vascular clip).[55-57]

LVFP may result in increased requirements for tube feeding, respiratory support, and length of hospital stay, as well as increased BPD.[17,18] Benjamin et al. reported persistent respiratory and feeding problems in the first 2 years of age after development of LVFP, with 86% (19/22) of affected infants developing reactive airway disease and 64% (14/22) requiring gastrostomy tube insertion for feeding.[17]

D

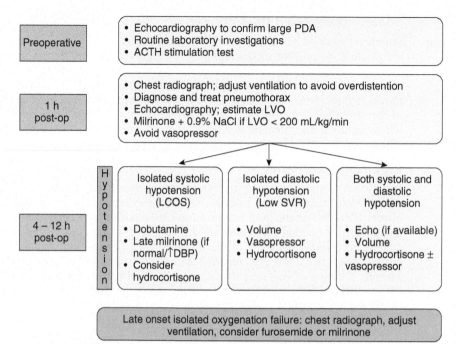

Fig. 24.4 Clinical algorithm for the immediate postoperative management of preterm infants undergoing patent ductus arteriosus *(PDA)* ligation. *ACTH*, Adrenocorticotropic hormone; *DBP*, diastolic blood pressure; *LCOS*, low cardiac output state; *LVO*, left ventricular output; *SVR*, systemic vascular resistance. (Modified from El-Khuffash A, Jain A, McNamara PJ: Ligation of the patent ductus arteriosus in preterm infants: understanding the physiology. *J Pediatr* 162(6):1100–1106, 2013, with permission from Elsevier.)

Resolution occurred in only 3% (2/66) of affected ELBW infants, with a median follow-up of 2 years, whereas respiratory symptoms, dysphagia, and dysphonia frequently persisted.[108] In a Norwegian follow-up study of young adults with a history of preterm birth and surgical closure of PDA, 7 of 13 subjects had LVFP, and they were noted to have lifelong symptoms in relation to vocal function as a result of the narrowed laryngeal entrance due to persistent paramedian position of the left vocal cord and anteromedial collapse of left supraglottic structures.[109] In summary, preterm infants (and especially ELBW infants) are at high risk of developing LVFP, which can result in increased in-hospital morbidity and persistent clinical symptoms in early childhood and even adulthood. Some laryngologists have proposed evaluating vocal fold mobility by laryngoscopy on all high-risk infants undergoing PDA ligation, regardless of the status of laryngeal symptoms.[107]

Early Postoperative Management

Immediate postoperative care should be directed at ruling out urgent surgical complications, such as pneumothorax and bleeding. A chest radiograph should be performed to confirm endotracheal tube placement and identify air leak or pulmonary overdistention. Preterm infants should remain invasively ventilated in the immediate postsurgical period and the mean airway pressure and tidal volume adjusted to optimize lung inflation and compliance. Infants may experience a rapid improvement in pulmonary compliance after ligation, owing to the rapid decrease in pulmonary capillary hydrostatic pressure. Failure to anticipate a need for reduction in positive end-expiratory pressure may lead to pulmonary overdistention with resultant impairment in systemic and pulmonary venous return and the potential for the development of a pneumothorax (Fig. 24.4).

Most preterm infants are hemodynamically stable in the immediate (<2 hours) postoperative period but demonstrate an abrupt increase in diastolic blood pressure due to the increased SVR associated with interruption of the ductal shunt. The presence of early (<4 hours) diastolic or combined (systolic and diastolic) hypotension is atypical and should prompt investigation for hemorrhage, obstruction to LV output (e.g., tension pneumothorax), severe pulmonary arterial hypertension, and causes of decreased SVR (e.g., adrenal insufficiency, sepsis). Intravascular volume expansion and intravenous stress-dose hydrocortisone can be considered. Vasoconstricting agents should be avoided in these infants in lieu of agents that improve LV systolic function and reduce afterload, such as dobutamine or milrinone. However, refractory diastolic hypotension without a clear etiology may be treated with judicious use of an intravenous infusion of dopamine or epinephrine, and hydrocortisone treatment should be considered early.

The immediate postoperative increase in diastolic blood pressure (and resultant rise in mean blood pressure) may mask a diminished postoperative systolic blood pressure indicative of acutely decreased LV systolic function. Systolic and diastolic blood pressures should therefore be distinctly measured, recorded, and evaluated in the postoperative period. The gradual development of isolated systolic hypotension, frequently due to declining LV systolic performance, may be managed with an intravenous infusion of dobutamine with isotonic volume expansion if preload is compromised.

Targeted neonatal echocardiography, if available, should be performed at 1 hour postoperatively to estimate LV output. Infants with LV output less than 200 mL/kg/min should be considered to receive an intravenous infusion of prophylactic milrinone at a starting dose of 0.33 μg/kg/min, administered with 10 mL/kg isotonic saline to augment preload and offset the decrease in SVR associated with milrinone. In centers without access to timely postoperative echocardiography, the administration of prophylactic intravenous milrinone to infants based on perioperative risk factors may be considered.[83] Care must be taken to ensure that milrinone is administered only to clinically stable infants demonstrating the expected postoperative hemodynamic effects, namely stable respiratory status and a rise in postoperative diastolic blood pressure and normal-to-increased systolic blood pressure. The pharmacokinetics of milrinone in this population have not been delineated; hence the administration of a bolus of milrinone is not currently recommended.

Transcatheter Closure of Patent Ductus Arteriosus

Percutaneous transcatheter closure of PDA has been well described in children and adults; however, this has not been widely applied in infants younger than 6 months, due to concerns regarding vascular access, overall patient fragility, contrast administration, and lack of a suitable device.[110] In recent years, transcatheter closure of a PDA has been successfully reported as an alternative to surgical ligation, with the potential benefits of being less invasive and shorter time of recovery of respiratory status, compared with surgical ligation.[111-115] Two primary methods are used for transcatheter PDA closure: coil and occluder devices (see also Chapter 32).[111] Zahn et al. reported that six premature infants ranging between 26 and 31 weeks GA underwent transcatheter PDA closure using the Amplatzer Vascular Plug II device at a median age of 21.5 days, with complete closure achieved and no procedure-related complications.[116] In their follow-up series of 24 extremely premature infants (mean procedural weight of 1249 g), they reported two complications, including two instances of device malposition and one instance of LPA stenosis, requiring an LPA stent.[110] Other complications described in case series or reports include femoral arterial thrombosis or coil/device malposition leading to embolization, aortic coarctation, or cardiac perforation.[112,113,117] Apart from the technical skills of the interventional cardiologist, the success and complication rates may be affected by the morphologic characterization of the PDA.[118]

Overall, transcatheter closure of PDA appears technically feasible in carefully selected symptomatic preterm infants in designated centers. A large prospective trial using appropriate devices designated for a preterm population is required to compare the effect of open surgical ligation versus transcatheter closure on acute postoperative cardiorespiratory instability and neonatal outcomes.

Summary: The Patent Ductus Arteriosus Ligation Decision and Postoperative Management—Present Uncertainty, Practice Variability, and An Urgent Need for Clarity

As neonatal intensive care has evolved over the past 4 decades, some clarity in the role of surgical PDA ligation has emerged. In contrast to older clinical trials of surgical ligation that enrolled moderately preterm infants, advances in care have relegated PDA ligation to being a treatment modality considered almost exclusively within the very preterm patient population (infants born ≤ 26 weeks' gestation). Although the PDA is associated (and potentially has a causal relationship) with severe early morbidity such as pulmonary hemorrhage and P/IVH, the efficacy of early pharmacotherapy has all but eliminated ligation from the treatment armamentarium within the first postnatal week. Surgical ligation is therefore now most often viewed as a therapeutic option for the "chronic" phase of a persistent symptomatic PDA, characterized by a variable (but difficult to quantify) effect on respiratory insufficiency. In contemporary practice, ligation typically occurs after the first 2 postnatal weeks.

The current paucity of research in determining the efficacy of surgical ligation versus conservative management after failure of medical therapy represents a major gap in clinical care. Previously reported associations of ligation with adverse neonatal and neurodevelopmental outcomes have rendered the "ligation decision" more challenging for clinicians, but these findings have likely been affected by bias from confounding by indication rather than representing a clear causal detrimental effect of PDA surgery. Accordingly, ligation may still be indicated for some infants, although there is a need for comprehensive methods of evaluation (e.g., echocardiography, pulmonary imaging, biomarkers) to reliably identify high-volume shunts whose surgical interruption may result in measurable short- and, at least, medium-term benefit. Predictors of infants who respond favorably (e.g., rapid endotracheal extubation) need to be established. Ultimately a randomized clinical trial of surgical ligation versus conservative management is necessary to assess the efficacy of this invasive intervention in an appropriately selected population. A transcatheter approach to ductal closure in the very immature infant is an exciting therapeutic alternative that is still in its infancy, but which has the potential to supersede open thoracotomy.

For infants who do undergo surgery, new insights over the past decade may help clinicians to maintain cardiorespiratory stability in the postoperative period. Increased LV afterload appears to be the main contributor to the development of PLCS while a decrease in the LV preload is likely also a contributory hemodynamic factor to the development of this presentation. Observational data in preterm infants and randomized placebo-controlled trials in the pediatric population support the targeted administration of intravenous milrinone. However, clinicians should maintain a thoughtful and pathophysiology-focused approach to the acutely unstable postoperative infant, considering the potential etiological role of surgical complications, adrenal insufficiency, and occult sepsis/NEC. Targeted neonatal echocardiography, if available, may provide valuable information to characterize the hemodynamic conditions and assist in the administration of targeted treatment.

REFERENCES

1. Lokku A, Mirea L, Lee SK, et al.: Trends and outcomes of patent ductus arteriosus treatment in very preterm infants in Canada, *Am J Perinatol* 2016.
2. Hagadorn JI, Brownell EA, Trzaski JM, et al.: Trends and variation in management and outcomes of very low birth weight infants with patent ductus arteriosus, *Pediatr Res* 80(6):785–792, 2016.
3. Cotton RB, Stahlman MT, Bender HW, et al.: Randomized trial of early closure of symptomatic patent ductus arteriosus in small preterm infants, *J Pediatr* 93(4):647–651, 1978.
4. Levitsky S, Fisher E, Vidyasagar D, et al.: Interruption of patent ductus arteriosus in premature infants with respiratory distress syndrome, *Ann Thorac Surg* 22(2):131–137, 1976.
5. Gersony WM, Peckham GJ, Ellison RC, et al.: Effects of indomethacin in premature infants with patent ductus arteriosus: results of a national collaborative study, *J Pediatr* 102(6):895–906, 1983.

6. Cassady G, Crouse DT, Kirklin JW, et al.: A randomized, controlled trial of very early prophylactic ligation of the ductus arteriosus in babies who weighed 1000 g or less at birth, *N Engl J Med* 320(23):1511–1516, 1989.

7. Clyman R, Cassady G, Kirklin JK, et al.: The role of patent ductus arteriosus ligation in bronchopulmonary dysplasia: reexamining a randomized controlled trial, *J Pediatr* 154(6):873–876, 2009.

8. Mirea L, Sankaran K, Seshia M, et al.: Treatment of patent ductus arteriosus and neonatal mortality/morbidities: adjustment for treatment selection bias, *J Pediatr* 161(4):689–694.e681, 2012.

9. Chorne N, Leonard C, Piecuch R, et al.: Patent ductus arteriosus and its treatment as risk factors for neonatal and neurodevelopmental morbidity, *Pediatrics* 119(6):1165–1174, 2007.

10. Kabra NS, Schmidt B, Roberts RS, et al.: Neurosensory impairment after surgical closure of patent ductus arteriosus in extremely low birth weight infants: results from the trial of indomethacin prophylaxis in preterms, *J Pediatr* 150(3):229–234, 234.e221, 2007.

11. Madan JC, Kendrick D, Hagadorn JI, et al.: Patent ductus arteriosus therapy: impact on neonatal and 18-month outcome, *Pediatrics* 123(2):674–681, 2009.

12. Bourgoin L, Cipierre C, Hauet Q, et al.: Neurodevelopmental outcome at 2 years of age according to patent ductus arteriosus management in very preterm infants, *Neonatology* 109(2):139–146, 2016.

13. Janz-Robinson EM, Badawi N, Walker K, et al.: Neurodevelopmental outcomes of premature infants treated for patent ductus arteriosus: a population-based cohort study, *J Pediatr* 167(5):1025–1032.e1023, 2015.

14. Weisz DE, More K, McNamara PJ, et al.: PDA ligation and health outcomes: a meta-analysis, *Pediatrics* 133(4):e1024–e1046, 2014.

15. Wickremasinghe AC, Rogers EE, Piecuch RE, et al.: Neurodevelopmental outcomes following two different treatment approaches (early ligation and selective ligation) for patent ductus arteriosus, *J Pediatr* 161(6):1065–1072, 2012.

16. Heuchan AM, Hunter L, Young D: Outcomes following the surgical ligation of the patent ductus arteriosus in premature infants in Scotland, *Arch Dis Child Fetal Neonatal Ed* 97(1):F39–F44, 2012.

17. Benjamin JR, Smith PB, Cotten CM, et al.: Long-term morbidities associated with vocal cord paralysis after surgical closure of a patent ductus arteriosus in extremely low birth weight infants, *J Perinatol* 30(6):408–413, 2010.

18. Clement WA, El-Hakim H, Phillipos EZ, et al.: Unilateral vocal cord paralysis following patent ductus arteriosus ligation in extremely low-birth-weight infants, *Arch Otolaryngol Head Neck Surg* 134(1):28–33, 2008.

19. Rukholm G, Farrokhyar F, Reid D: Vocal cord paralysis post patent ductus arteriosus ligation surgery: risks and co-morbidities, *Int J Pediatr Otorhinolaryngol* 76(11):1637–1641, 2012.

20. Flick RP, Katusic SK, Colligan RC, et al.: Cognitive and behavioral outcomes after early exposure to anesthesia and surgery, *Pediatrics* 128(5):e1053–e1061, 2011.

21. Ing C, DiMaggio C, Whitehouse A, et al.: Long-term differences in language and cognitive function after childhood exposure to anesthesia, *Pediatrics* 130(3):e476–e485, 2012.

22. Glatz P, Sandin RH, Pedersen NL, et al.: Association of anesthesia and surgery during childhood with long-term academic performance, *JAMA Pediatr* 171(1):e163470, 2017.

23. El-Khuffash AF, Jain A, Dragulescu A, et al.: Acute changes in myocardial systolic function in preterm infants undergoing patent ductus arteriosus ligation: a tissue Doppler and myocardial deformation study, *J Am Soc Echocardiogr* 25(10):1058–1067, 2012.

24. El-Khuffash AF, Jain A, McNamara PJ: Ligation of the patent ductus arteriosus in preterm infants: understanding the physiology, *J Pediatr* 162(6):1100–1106, 2013.

25. El-Khuffash AF, McNamara PJ: The patent ductus arteriosus ligation decision, *J Pediatr* 158(6):1037–1038, 2011.

26. Jain A, Sahni M, El-Khuffash A, et al.: Use of targeted neonatal echocardiography to prevent postoperative cardiorespiratory instability after patent ductus arteriosus ligation, *J Pediatr* 160(4):584–589, 2012.

27. Sehgal A, Francis JV, James A, et al.: Patent ductus arteriosus ligation and post-operative hemodynamic instability: case report and framework for enhanced neonatal care, *Indian J Pediatr* 77(8):905–907, 2010.

28. Sehgal A, McNamara PJ: Coronary artery perfusion and myocardial performance after patent ductus arteriosus ligation, *J Thorac Cardiovasc Surg* 143(6):1271–1278, 2012.

29. Clyman RI: Surgical ligation of the patent ductus arteriosus: treatment or morbidity? *J Pediatr* 161(4):583–584, 2012.

30. Clyman RI, Couto J, Murphy GM: Patent ductus arteriosus: are current neonatal treatment options better or worse than no treatment at all? *Semin Perinatol* 36(2):123–129, 2012.

31. Jhaveri N, Moon-Grady A, Clyman RI: Early surgical ligation versus a conservative approach for management of patent ductus arteriosus that fails to close after indomethacin treatment, *J Pediatr* 157(3):381–387, 2010.

32. Noori S: Patent ductus arteriosus in the preterm infant: to treat or not to treat? *J Perinatol* 30(Suppl):S31–S37, 2010.

33. Noori S: Pros and cons of patent ductus arteriosus ligation: hemodynamic changes and other morbidities after patent ductus arteriosus ligation, *Semin Perinatol* 36(2):139–145, 2012.

34. Chau V, Brant R, Poskitt KJ, et al.: Postnatal infection is associated with widespread abnormalities of brain development in premature newborns, *Pediatr Res* 71(3):274–279, 2012.

24

35. Schlapbach LJ, Aebischer M, Adams M, et al.: Impact of sepsis on neurodevelopmental outcome in a Swiss national cohort of extremely premature infants, *Pediatrics* 128(2):e348–e357, 2011.

36. Bonnard A, Zamakhshary M, Ein S, et al.: The use of the score for neonatal acute physiology-perinatal extension (SNAPPE II) in perforated necrotizing enterocolitis: could it guide therapy in newborns less than 1500 g? *J Pediatr Surg* 43(6):1170–1174, 2008.

37. Sonntag J, Grimmer I, Scholz T, et al.: Growth and neurodevelopmental outcome of very low birth-weight infants with necrotizing enterocolitis, *Acta Paediatr* 89(5):528–532, 2000.

38. Laughon M, O'Shea MT, Allred EN, et al.: Chronic lung disease and developmental delay at 2 years of age in children born before 28 weeks' gestation, *Pediatrics* 124(2):637–648, 2009.

39. Laughon MM, Langer JC, Bose CL, et al.: Prediction of bronchopulmonary dysplasia by postnatal age in extremely premature infants, *Am J Respir Crit Care Med* 183(12):1715–1722, 2011.

40. Onland W, Debray TP, Laughon MM, et al.: Clinical prediction models for bronchopulmonary dysplasia: a systematic review and external validation study, *BMC Pediatr* 13:207, 2013.

41. Van Marter LJ, Kuban KC, Allred E, et al.: Does bronchopulmonary dysplasia contribute to the occurrence of cerebral palsy among infants born before 28 weeks of gestation? *Arch Dis Child Fetal Neonatal Ed* 96(1):F20–F29, 2011.

42. Alexander F, Chiu L, Kroh M, et al.: Analysis of outcome in 298 extremely low-birth-weight infants with patent ductus arteriosus, *J Pediatr Surg* 44(1):112–117, 2009; discussion 117.

43. Moore GP, Lawrence SL, Maharajh G, et al.: Therapeutic strategies, including a high surgical ligation rate, for patent ductus arteriosus closure in extremely premature infants in a North American centre, *Paediatr Child Health* 17(4):e26–e31, 2012.

44. Merritt TA, DiSessa TG, Feldman BH: Closure of the patent ductus arteriosus with ligation and indomethacin: a consecutive experience, *J Pediatr* 93(4):639–646, 1978.

45. Cats BP, Van Ertbruggen I, Gerards LJ: Patent ductus arteriosus in premature infants [Dutch], *Tijdschr Kindergeneeskd* 48(4):107–111, 1980.

46. Zerella JT, Spies RJ, Deaver 3rd DC, et al.: Indomethacin versus immediate ligation in the treatment of 82 newborns with patent ductus arteriosus, *J Pediatr Surg* 18(6):835–841, 1983.

47. Weisz DE, Mirea L, Rosenberg E, et al.: Association of patent ductus arteriosus ligation with death or neurodevelopmental impairment among extremely preterm infants, *JAMA Pediatrics* 171(5):1–8, 2017.

48. Rolland A, Shankar-Aguilera S, Diomande D, et al.: Natural evolution of patent ductus arteriosus in the extremely preterm infant, *Arch Dis Child Fetal Neonatal Ed* 100(1):F55–F58, 2015.

49. Wickremasinghe AC, Rogers EE, Piecuch RE, et al.: Neurodevelopmental outcomes following two different treatment approaches (early ligation and selective ligation) for patent ductus arteriosus, *J Pediatr* 161(6):1065–1072, 2012.

50. Watterberg KL, Scott SM, Backstrom C, et al.: Links between early adrenal function and respiratory outcome in preterm infants: airway inflammation and patent ductus arteriosus, *Pediatrics* 105(2):320–324, 2000.

51. El-Khuffash AF, McNamara PJ, Lapointe A, et al.: Adrenal function in preterm infants undergoing patent ductus arteriosus ligation, *Neonatology* 104(1):28–33, 2013.

52. Satpute MD, Donohue PK, Vricella L, et al.: Cardiovascular instability after patent ductus arteriosus ligation in preterm infants: the role of hydrocortisone, *J Perinatol* 32(9):685–689, 2012.

53. Sersar SI, Mooty HA, Hafez MM, et al.: PDA ligation: trans or extrapleural approach, *Ann Thorac Surg* 80(5):1976, 2005; author reply 1976–1977.

54. Leon-Wyss J, Vida VL, Veras O, et al.: Modified extrapleural ligation of patent ductus arteriosus: a convenient surgical approach in a developing country, *Ann Thorac Surg* 79(2):632–635, 2005.

55. Mandhan PL, Samarakkody U, Brown S, et al.: Comparison of suture ligation and clip application for the treatment of patent ductus arteriosus in preterm neonates, *J Thorac Cardiovasc Surg* 132(3):672–674, 2006.

56. Spanos WC, Brookes JT, Smith MC, et al.: Unilateral vocal fold paralysis in premature infants after ligation of patent ductus arteriosus: vascular clip versus suture ligature, *Ann Otol Rhinol Laryngol* 118(10):750–753, 2009.

57. Zbar RI, Chen AH, Behrendt DM, et al.: Incidence of vocal fold paralysis in infants undergoing ligation of patent ductus arteriosus, *Ann Thorac Surg* 61(3):814–816, 1996.

58. Anand KJ, Sippell WG, Aynsley-Green A: Randomised trial of fentanyl anaesthesia in preterm babies undergoing surgery: effects on the stress response, *Lancet* 1(8527):243–248, 1987.

59. Janvier A, Martinez JL, Barrington K, et al.: Anesthetic technique and postoperative outcome in preterm infants undergoing PDA closure, *J Perinatol* 30(10):677–682, 2010.

60. Noori S, Friedlich P, Seri I, et al.: Changes in myocardial function and hemodynamics after ligation of the ductus arteriosus in preterm infants, *J Pediatr* 150(6):597–602, 2007.

61. Lien R, Hsu KH, Chu JJ, et al.: Hemodynamic alterations recorded by electrical cardiometry during ligation of ductus arteriosus in preterm infants, *Eur J Pediatr* 174(4):543–550, 2015.

62. Lindner W, Seidel M, Versmold HT, et al.: Stroke volume and left ventricular output in preterm infants with patent ductus arteriosus, *Pediatr Res* 27(3):278–281, 1990.

63. Taylor AF, Morrow WR, Lally KP, et al.: Left ventricular dysfunction following ligation of the ductus arteriosus in the preterm baboon, *J Surg Res* 48(6):590–596, 1990.

64. Nagata H, Yamamura K, Ihara K, et al.: Left ventricular efficiency after ligation of patent ductus arteriosus for premature infants, *Cardiol Young* 23:S110–S111, 2013.

65. El-Khuffash AF, Jain A, McNamara PJ: Ligation of the patent ductus arteriosus in preterm infants: Understanding the physiology, *J Pediatr* 162(6):1100–1106, 2013.

66. McNamara PJ, Stewart L, Shivananda SP, et al.: Patent ductus arteriosus ligation is associated with impaired left ventricular systolic performance in premature infants weighing less than 1000 g, *J Thorac Cardiovasc Surg* 140(1):150–157, 2010.
67. Nagata H, Ihara K, Yamamura K, et al.: Left ventricular efficiency after ligation of patent ductus arteriosus for premature infants, *J Thorac Cardiovasc Surg* 146(6):1353–1358, 2013.
68. Moin F, Kennedy KA, Moya FR: Risk factors predicting vasopressor use after patent ductus arteriosus ligation, *Am J Perinatol* 20(6):313–320, 2003.
69. Saida K, Nakamura T, Hiroma T, et al.: Preoperative left ventricular internal dimension in end-diastole as earlier identification of early patent ductus arteriosus operation and postoperative intensive care in very low birth weight infants, *Early Hum Dev* 89(10):821–823, 2013.
70. Fineman JR, Soifer SJ: The fetal and neonatal circulations. In Chang AC, Hanley FL, Wernovsky G, Wessel DL, editors: *Pediatric Cardiac Intensive Care*, Lippincott Williams & Wilkins, 1998.
71. Artman M, Mahony L, Teitel DF: *Chapter 3: Cardiovascular Physiology in Neonatal Cardiology*, ed 2, McGraw-Hill, 2011.
72. Rowland DG, Gutgesell HP: Noninvasive assessment of myocardial contractility, preload, and afterload in healthy newborn infants, *Am J Cardiol* 75(12):818–821, 1995.
73. Sehgal A, Coombs P, Tan K, et al.: Spectral Doppler waveforms in systemic arteries and physiological significance of a patent ductus arteriosus, *J Perinatol* 31(3):150–156, 2011.
74. Hoodbhoy SA, Cutting HA, Seddon JA, et al.: Cerebral and splanchnic hemodynamics after duct ligation in very low birth weight infants, *J Pediatr* 154(2):196–200, 2009.
75. Leslie AT, Jain A, El-Khuffash A, et al.: Evaluation of cerebral electrical activity and cardiac output after patent ductus arteriosus ligation in preterm infants, *J Perinatol* 33(11):861–866, 2013.
76. Kimball TR, Ralston MA, Khoury P, et al.: Effect of ligation of patent ductus arteriosus on left ventricular performance and its determinants in premature neonates, *J Am Coll Cardiol* 27(1):193–197, 1996.
77. Teixeira LS, Shivananda SP, Stephens D, et al.: Postoperative cardiorespiratory instability following ligation of the preterm ductus arteriosus is related to early need for intervention, *J Perinatol* 28(12):803–810, 2008.
78. Harting MT, Blakely ML, Cox Jr CS, et al.: Acute hemodynamic decompensation following patent ductus arteriosus ligation in premature infants, *J Invest Surg* 21(3):133–138, 2008.
79. Ting JY, Resende M, More K, et al.: Predictors of respiratory instability in neonates undergoing patient ductus arteriosus ligation after the introduction of targeted milrinone treatment, *J Thorac Cardiovasc Surg* 152(2):498–504, 2016.
80. El-Khuffash AF, Jain A, Weisz D, et al.: Assessment and treatment of post patent ductus arteriosus ligation syndrome, *J Pediatr* 165(1):46–52.e41, 2014.
81. Lemyre B, Liu L, Moore GP, et al.: Do intra-operative fluids influence the need for post-operative cardiotropic support after a PDA ligation? *Zhongguo Dang Dai Er Ke Za Zhi* 13(1):1–7, 2011.
82. Honerjager P: Pharmacology of bipyridine phosphodiesterase III inhibitors, *Am Heart J* 121(6 Pt 2):1939–1944, 1991.
83. Hoffman TM, Wernovsky G, Atz AM, et al.: Efficacy and safety of milrinone in preventing low cardiac output syndrome in infants and children after corrective surgery for congenital heart disease, *Circulation* 107(7):996–1002, 2003.
84. Szymankiewicz M, Hodgman JE, Siassi B, et al.: Mechanics of breathing after surgical ligation of patent ductus arteriosus in newborns with respiratory distress syndrome, *Biol Neonate* 85(1):32–36, 2004.
85. Waleh N, McCurnin DC, Yoder BA, et al.: Patent ductus arteriosus ligation alters pulmonary gene expression in preterm baboons, *Pediatr Res* 69(3):212–216, 2011.
86. Kalfa D, Krishnamurthy G, Cheung E: Patent ductus arteriosus surgical ligation: Still a lot to understand, *J Thorac Cardiovasc Surg* 152(2):505–506, 2016.
87. Liggins GC: The role of cortisol in preparing the fetus for birth, *Reprod Fertil Dev* 6(2):141–150, 1994.
88. Ng PC: Adrenocortical insufficiency and refractory hypotension in preterm infants, *Arch Dis Child Fetal Neonatal Ed*, 2016.
89. Hochwald O, Holsti L, Osiovich H: The use of an early ACTH test to identify hypoadrenalism-related hypotension in low birth weight infants, *J Perinatol* 32(6):412–417, 2012.
90. Ng PC, Lam CW, Fok TF, et al.: Refractory hypotension in preterm infants with adrenocortical insufficiency, *Arch Dis Child Fetal Neonatal Ed* 84(2):F122–F124, 2001.
91. Masumoto K, Kusuda S, Aoyagi H, et al.: Comparison of serum cortisol concentrations in preterm infants with or without late-onset circulatory collapse due to adrenal insufficiency of prematurity, *Pediatr Res* 63(6):686–690, 2008.
92. Clyman RI, Wickremasinghe A, Merritt TA, et al.: Hypotension following patent ductus arteriosus ligation: the role of adrenal hormones, *J Pediatr* 164(6):1449–1455.e1441, 2014.
93. Avsar MK, Demir T, Celiksular C, et al.: Bedside PDA ligation in premature infants less than 28 weeks and 1000 grams, *J Cardiothorac Surg* 11(1):146, 2016.
94. Kang SL, Samsudin S, Kuruvilla M, et al.: Outcome of patent ductus arteriosus ligation in premature infants in the East of England: a prospective cohort study, *Cardiol Young* 23(5):711–716, 2013.
95. Little DC, Pratt TC, Blalock SE, et al.: Patent ductus arteriosus in micropreemies and full-term infants: the relative merits of surgical ligation versus indomethacin treatment, *J Pediatr Surg* 38(3):492–496, 2003.

96. Newth CJL, Hammer J: Pulmonary Issues. In Chang AC, Hanley FL, Wernovsky G, Wessel DL, editors: *Pediatric Cardiac Intensive Care*, Lippincott Williams & Wilkins, 1998.
97. Hsu KH, Chiang MC, Lien R, et al.: Diaphragmatic paralysis among very low birth weight infants following ligation for patent ductus arteriosus, *Eur J Pediatr* 171(11):1639–1644, 2012.
98. de Leeuw M, Williams JM, Freedom RM, et al.: Impact of diaphragmatic paralysis after cardiothoracic surgery in children, *J Thorac Cardiovasc Surg* 118(3):510–517, 1999.
99. Smith BM, Ezeokoli NJ, Kipps AK, et al.: Course, predictors of diaphragm recovery after phrenic nerve injury during pediatric cardiac surgery, *Ann Thorac Surg* 96(3):938–942, 2013.
100. Fleming WH, Sarafian LB, Kugler JD, et al.: Ligation of patent ductus arteriosus in premature infants: importance of accurate anatomic definition, *Pediatrics* 71(3):373–375, 1983.
101. Chang AC, Wells W: Shunt lesions. In Chang AC, Hanley FL, Wernovsky G, Wessel DL, editors: *Pediatric Cardiac Intensive Care*, Lippincott Williams & Wilkins, 1998.
102. Jaffe RB, Orsmond GS, Veasy LG: Inadvertent ligation of the left pulmonary artery, *Radiology* 161(2):355–357, 1986.
103. Harris LL, Krishnamurthy R, Browne LP, et al.: Left main bronchus obstruction after patent ductus arteriosus ligation: an unusual complication, *Int J Pediatr Otorhinolaryngol* 76(12):1855–1856, 2012.
104. Kim D, Kim SW, Shin HJ, et al.: Unintended pulmonary artery ligation during PDA ligation, *Heart Surg Forum* 19(4):E187–E188, 2016.
105. Sorensen KE, Kristensen B, Hansen OK: Frequency of occurrence of residual ductal flow after surgical ligation by color-flow mapping, *Am J Cardiol* 67(7):653–654, 1991.
106. Pereira KD, Webb BD, Blakely ML, et al.: Sequelae of recurrent laryngeal nerve injury after patent ductus arteriosus ligation, *Int J Pediatr Otorhinolaryngol* 70(9):1609–1612, 2006.
107. Smith ME, King JD, Elsherif A, et al.: Should all newborns who undergo patent ductus arteriosus ligation be examined for vocal fold mobility? *Laryngoscope* 119(8):1606–1609, 2009.
108. Nichols BG, Jabbour J, Hehir DA, et al.: Recovery of vocal fold immobility following isolated patent ductus arteriosus ligation, *Int J Pediatr Otorhinolaryngol* 78(8):1316–1319, 2014.
109. Roksund OD, Clemm H, Heimdal JH, et al.: Left vocal cord paralysis after extreme preterm birth, a new clinical scenario in adults, *Pediatrics* 126(6):e1569–e1577, 2010.
110. Zahn EM, Peck D, Phillips A, et al.: Transcatheter closure of patent ductus arteriosus in extremely premature newborns: early results and midterm follow-up, *JACC Cardiovasc Interv* 9(23):2429–2437, 2016.
111. Perez KM, Laughon MM: What is new for patent ductus arteriosus management in premature infants in 2015? *Curr Opin Pediatr* 27(2):158–164, 2015.
112. Baspinar O, Sahin DA, Sulu A, et al.: Transcatheter closure of patent ductus arteriosus in under 6 kg and premature infants, *J Interv Cardiol* 28(2):180–189, 2015.
113. Roberts P, Adwani S, Archer N, et al.: Catheter closure of the arterial duct in preterm infants, *Arch Dis Child Fetal Neonatal Ed* 92(4):F248–F250, 2007.
114. Bentham J, Meur S, Hudsmith L, et al.: Echocardiographically guided catheter closure of arterial ducts in small preterm infants on the neonatal intensive care unit, *Catheter Cardiovasc Interv* 77(3):409–415, 2011.
115. Francis E, Singhi AK, Lakshmivenkateshaiah S, et al.: Transcatheter occlusion of patent ductus arteriosus in pre-term infants, *JACC Cardiovasc Interv* 3(5):550–555, 2010.
116. Zahn EM, Nevin P, Simmons C, et al.: A novel technique for transcatheter patent ductus arteriosus closure in extremely preterm infants using commercially available technology, *Catheter Cardiovasc Interv* 85(2):240–248, 2015.
117. Abu Hazeem AA, Gillespie MJ, Thun H, et al.: Percutaneous closure of patent ductus arteriosus in small infants with significant lung disease may offer faster recovery of respiratory function when compared to surgical ligation, *Catheter Cardiovasc Interv* 82(4):526–533, 2013.
118. Philip R, Waller 3rd BR, Agrawal V, et al.: Morphologic characterization of the patent ductus arteriosus in the premature infant and the choice of transcatheter occlusion device, *Catheter Cardiovasc Interv* 87(2):310–317, 2016.

CHAPTER 25

Pathophysiology Based Management of the Hemodynamically Significant Ductus Arteriosus in the Very Preterm Neonate

Chandra Rath and Martin Kluckow

- The simplistic "treat all or treat none" approach to management of a patent ductus arteriosus (PDA) has been increasingly challenged over the past few years as the variation in clinical and hemodynamic presentation has been realized.

- Spontaneous closure rates, poor efficacy of medical treatment, and high open-label treatment rates in clinical trials are among the major factors that have resulted in a lack of confidence in the usefulness of treating a PDA.

- The era of personalized medicine whereby the individual characteristics of the patient (genetics, physiology/pathophysiology, biochemistry, clinical variables) are taken into consideration when deciding on management is ideally suited for many of the neonatal hemodynamic treatment dilemmas, including PDA management.

- Understanding the clinical and hemodynamic variability of an individual patient's PDA may allow more specific decision-making around when to treat, what to treat, and with what treatment approach. In this regard, better evaluation tools and development of multiparameter scoring systems based on patient characteristics is likely to be increasingly important.

For many years now the default position of most neonatologists has been to treat the patent ductus arteriosus (PDA), particularly in the very low birth weight (VLBW) infant (<1500 g). More recently as our intensive care practices have evolved and the infants for whom we care do better, the need for medical treatment, particularly with the nonsteroidal antiinflammatory drugs (NSAIDs) has been increasingly questioned. The uncertainty has been driven by a number of factors, including our inability to identify infants who would most benefit from treatment, demonstrated high spontaneous closure rates, variable efficacy of the medications available, balancing the risks of side effects, and the failure of trials of treatment in nonspecific subgroups of infants to show clear short- or long-term benefits. However, it is not an all-or-none solution—there are likely to be a subset of newborns with a PDA which should be treated at an appropriate time to avoid possible deleterious effects from a significant left-to-right shunt. Identification of these infants has become a priority, to allow avoidance of side effects and unnecessary treatment. The key to selecting patients for treatment is likely to be understanding the individual pathophysiology (i.e., the effects that the PDA is having in a particular infant). The effects will be dependent on a number of underlying elements—the gestational age of the infant, the volume of any left-to-right shunt (related to the size of the PDA and the pressure difference across it), the effect of steal on the systemic circulation (blood pressure, blood flow to the brain, kidney, and gut), and the effect of pulmonary flooding on the

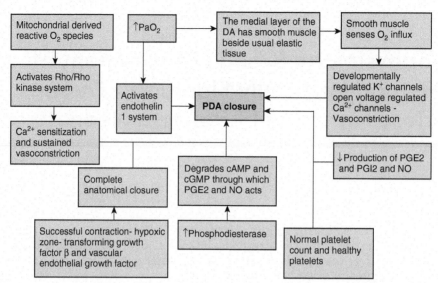

Fig. 25.1 A schematic diagram showing the relationship of all of the factors involved in closure of the patent ductus arteriosus *(PDA). cAMP*, Cyclic adenosine monophosphate; *cGMP*, cyclic guanosine monophosphate; *DA*, ductus arteriosus; *NO*, nitric oxide, *PaO₂*, partial pressure of oxygen; *PGI2*, prostacyclin, *PGE2*, prostaglandin E2.

pulmonary circulation (increased respiratory support needs and a subsequent relation to bronchopulmonary dysplasia [BPD] and risks of pulmonary hemorrhage). Clinician-performed ultrasound (CPU) of the heart in the neonatal intensive care unit (NICU), by the physician caring for the baby in a longitudinal setting is set to play an indispensable role in the selection of patients for treatment or no treatment and subsequently the overall management of PDA. Understanding how to assess the underlying elements of the pathophysiologic scenario potentially allows a more individualized decision to be made regarding the need for treatment.

Pathophysiology of Patent Ductus Arteriosus Closure

Understanding the pathophysiologic basis of natural ductus arteriosus (DA) closure is an important aspect of the logical approach to PDA management. Preterm PDA closure is different to term closure, and different clinical situations such as infections, pulmonary vascular resistance and its regulation, and the severity of the underlying lung disease may alter the usual ground rules of PDA closure. The underlying physiology of natural PDA closure is depicted in Fig. 25.1.

In most term babies, functional closure occurs by 24 hours of age.[1] Intimal ischemia and then necrosis result from the continued intense constriction of the muscular wall and the ductus eventually evolves into the ligamentum arteriosum and is permanently closed. The preterm DA does not follow the same course and is thus less likely to close spontaneously—the more immature the infant, the less the likelihood of early spontaneous closure.[2] The differences in the pathophysiology of closure between term and preterm PDA are outlined in Table 25.1.

Issues to be Considered When Deciding Whether to Treat the Patent Ductus Arteriosus

Spontaneous Closure Rates

Modern-day neonatology has come a long way with our vastly improved understanding of developmental cellular physiology, the advent of new technology, and introduction of better treatment modalities. Survival of neonates born greater than 30 weeks' gestation is almost 100%, and there has been a significant increase in the survival of extremely preterm infants. Due to reduced spontaneous ductal closure rates coupled with significant pulmonary-systemic pressure differences, extremely

Table 25.1 DIFFERENCES IN THE PATHOPHYSIOLOGY OF CLOSURE BETWEEN TERM AND PRETERM PATENT DUCTUS ARTERIOSUS

- Immature K^+ and Ca^{2+} channels lead to ineffective oxygen mediated closure in the preterm PDA
- Mitochondria-derived reactive O_2 species responsible for Rho/Rho-kinase signaling are decreased in the preterm PDA
- Failure to generate a true hypoxic zone by insufficient constriction prevents true anatomic closure which adds to risk of reopening in the preterm PDA
- Sensitivity to vasoconstrictor O_2 is reduced; however, sensitivity to vasodilator PGE2, PGI2, and NO is increased in the preterm PDA
- Duct-specific phosphodiesterase is reduced in the preterm PDA

PDA, Patent ductus arteriosus.

25

preterm infants (<28 weeks' gestation) are at higher risk of complications from the PDA both early on, where there are risks of acute left-to-right shunting with pulmonary flooding and relative reduction of blood flow on the systemic side, and later due to the prolonged effects of left-to-right shunting on the heart, brain, kidneys, intestines, and lungs. A PDA in a relatively mature preterm neonate is of less concern as the left-to-right shunt appears to be tolerated better and the cardiovascular system and cerebral autoregulation protective mechanisms are more developed. Despite this, the systematic meta-analyses regarding PDA treatment include many trials from greater than 20 years ago and trials that focused on larger, more mature infants of up to 33 to 34 weeks of gestation, where spontaneous closure in the first few days is almost inevitable.[3] Inclusion of both extremely preterm neonates and relatively mature neonates in the same study makes it difficult to understand the efficacy of treatment versus the effects of spontaneous closure. The protagonists of no treatment argue on the basis of these studies, despite them including a wide mix of gestational age groups, using poor diagnostic criteria for the PDA, with high rates of open-label treatment in the control group, small sample sizes, and/or often lacking objective criteria at randomization. Importantly, spontaneous closure in the placebo control arm of the randomized controlled trials, as well as high levels of open-label treatment in both trial arms (from 30% to 70%),[4] make the interpretation of outcomes in many of the PDA trials difficult at best. In fact, much of the "efficacy" of our current treatment drugs may be ascribed more to spontaneous closure rates, particularly in more mature infants, rather than the treatment itself. The real natural course of PDA in treatment-naïve extreme preterm neonates and the true efficacy of the medications used for treatment are therefore not well understood.

Recently, several groups have published data about the use of conservative treatment of the PDA. However, to date, these have been descriptive cohort studies only. In a study of the natural evolution of PDA in extremely low birth weight (ELBW) neonates,[5] the authors observed a 73% spontaneous DA closure rate in newborns born less than 28 weeks. However, deaths (both early and late), undiagnosed probable PDAs, and infants discharged home with persistent PDAs were excluded from the study. In the end, 41% of the neonates were excluded from the total sample size of 103, many of whom had morbidity and mortality that could be attributed to the PDA. For instance, causes of death of the excluded babies included pulmonary hemorrhage, severe periventricular/intraventricular hemorrhage (P/IVH), and hypoxic respiratory failure, all of which could be attributed to or at least made worse by a PDA, making the outcome of the study difficult to interpret. It should also be noted here that a high incidence of pulmonary hemorrhage (25% [23/91]) was observed in this study.[5] Similarly in another study,[6] the authors reported a 34% permanent closure rate of PDA in ELBW neonates. However, in this study the authors omitted 26% of the total sample size of preterm neonates because of death or comfort care. The use of x-ray and clinical presentation and not ultrasound to decide on treating the PDA also made these conclusions questionable.[6] However, this study made an important observation and estimated that, for each week of increase in gestational age greater than 23 weeks, the odds of spontaneous closure increase by a ratio of 1.5. There is a direct relationship between gestational age, birth weight, and persistence of the PDA.[6,7] Narayanan estimated the rate of spontaneous closure is approximately 31% in preterm neonates of 26 to 27 weeks' gestation during the first 3 to 4

450 Clinical Presentations and Treatment of Cardiovascular Compromise in the Neonate

postnatal days, whereas the spontaneous closure rate is approximately 21% at 24 and 25 weeks' gestation.[8] An Italian study also showed a 24% spontaneous closure rate in 23- to 27-week preterm neonates.[9] The majority of these studies were undertaken in a different era of neonatology than the current, where there is now increasing use of noninvasive ventilation and increasing survival of infants less than 25 weeks' gestational age. Therefore information about the natural history of PDA in the current day NICU is urgently needed. More recently, two larger observational studies of minimal/no treatment of the PDA have been published from the same group. The first study[10] compares three different PDA management approaches in 138 VLBW infants. Infants received either symptomatic, early targeted (during the first 48 hours), or conservative treatment. The authors found no short-term differences between the groups and a decreased rate of BPD in the conservative treatment group. The second, more contemporaneous study[11] is a retrospective cohort study in two European units which enrolled 297 VLBW infants—280 received conservative PDA management and 85% of PDA closed by hospital discharge with a median time to ductal closure of 71 days in infants of less than 26-weeks' gestation. Seventeen infants received treatment (13 medical, 4 surgical ligation—overall 10 closed before discharge). The 26 infants who died were not included in the primary analysis, although the authors comment that 16 of the 26 infants had a cause of death potentially related to a PDA. There was no increase in morbidity in the nontreated infants. A significant number of infants were discharged with an open PDA (50 overall or 17%), and by 1 year of age, 30 infants had closed the PDA. Thus the PDA remained open in 20 patients—this is a not insignificant impost on the healthcare system, requiring ongoing follow-up and possibly device-based closure in the future (see Chapter 32).

Beside gestation, other factors, which are probably responsible for patency of the DA include histologic chorioamnionitis, neonatal infectious diseases such as sepsis or necrotizing enterocolitis (NEC), neonatal respiratory distress syndrome (RDS) and mechanical ventilation, decreased platelet count within 24 hours after birth, hypoxia, low APGAR scores, and low birth weight.[12-15]

Consequences of a Patent Ductus Arteriosus

The argument that the PDA is an innocent bystander which may spontaneously close, rather than a condition causing pathology, is becoming more prevalent in neonatology.[16] Waiting for spontaneous closure implies acceptance of any long-term consequences of a PDA, and these consequences are in part related to the timing of intervention. The adverse effects of a PDA are probably related to the amount of time the infant is exposed to a left-to-right shunt.

Physiologically, a PDA can potentially harm a neonate by complications of pulmonary flooding and/or reduced systemic blood flow. Prolonged patency is associated with numerous adverse outcomes, including, prolongation of assisted ventilation and higher rates of BPD, pulmonary hemorrhage, P/IVH, periventricular leukomalacia (PVL), renal impairment, NEC, hypotension, and death.[7,17,32] The key issue is whether we can intervene at some point and prevent some or all of these complications, with minimal side effects of the treatment. Importantly, for *each individual infant*, there will be a different risk/benefit equation.

In most newborn babies, even in the first postnatal hours, the ductal shunt is pure left to right or bidirectional with a dominant left-to-right component, demonstrating that pulmonary pressures are usually subsystemic even shortly after birth. Using superior vena cava (SVC) flow as a surrogate measure of systemic blood flow, we showed a significant negative association between duct diameter and SVC flow at 5 hours of age, but this association was not significant on subsequent studies at 12, 24, and 48 hours. There was a significant association between early low systemic blood flow and development of P/IVH and later NEC, suggesting a possible mechanism by which PDA shunting might play an important role in the pathophysiology of these conditions.[18] There is also mounting evidence to suggest a PDA may cause pulmonary hemorrhage in preterm neonates because of the overload of the pulmonary circulation in the presence of a low pulmonary vasculature resistance and that early ductal treatment may prevent this.[19-21]

A PDA causes left-to-right shunting of blood, which may flood the lungs and cause pulmonary edema. Pulmonary edema reduces lung compliance, resulting in increased ventilator and oxygen requirements. All these factors together might contribute to the development of BPD. BPD is associated with the persistence of a hemodynamically significant PDA (hsPDA). Each week of a hemodynamically significant DA represented an added risk for BPD (Odds ratio, 1.7).[22] Similarly in another recent study but contrary to the study cited earlier by Letshwiti et al.,[10] extreme preterm newborns with PDA who were treated conservatively had a higher incidence of BPD compared with infants without PDA.[23] There is emerging but not unequivocal[10] evidence that a tolerant approach to PDA may be associated with a higher incidence of BPD, particularly if treatment is delayed till after the first postnatal week.[23-25] Use of multiparameter scoring systems may be predictive of future BPD and death—a high PDA severity score on day 2 was associated with these outcomes.[26]

A PDA may cause hemodynamic alterations, resulting in "steal" of blood from the systemic circulation, including the mesenteric arteries, with the consequences of decreased oxygen delivery to the gut and with the potential of tissue injury and NEC. Even a small PDA can reduce mesenteric artery flow and decrease the expected postprandial increase in blood flow.[27] Because reduced intestinal blood flow is a contributor to the development of NEC, PDA may be a causative factor for NEC.[28] In a study involving a relatively large number of neonates, PDA was an independent risk factor for the development of NEC in VLBW infants.[29]

There is ample evidence on the basis of Doppler and near-infrared spectroscopy (NIRS) studies to suggest that cerebral blood flow is reduced in the presence of a PDA.[27] In a based study using NIRS, cerebral tissue oxygen saturation was lowest in the group of newborns just prior to the surgical closure of PDA after a failed trial of medical treatment (indomethacin). The magnetic resonance imaging (MRI)-measured global and regional brain volume showed a trend toward lower volumes in the group that had met criteria for surgical ligation compared with the groups which were treated medically and did not have a PDA. The surgical group also had a statistically significant lower cerebellar volume compared with other groups. The authors attributed this observation to the prolonged exposure to left-to-right shunting because of the amount of time elapsed between the diagnosis of PDA and actual surgical closure.[30] PDA has an effect on cerebral hemodynamics, but whether it is causative for P/IVH in a small number of infants is a question which remains unanswered. Cerebral autoregulation is likely to play some role, particularly in immature infants, in protecting against P/IVH (see also Chapter 6). Intact autoregulation is variable in immature infants (see also Chapter 2),[31] and one of the risk factors for impaired autoregulation may be a PDA resulting in a period of reduced cerebral blood flow that might impair the autoregulatory mechanism. Early treatment with indomethacin may result in both closure of the PDA and protection against P/IVH, and this is one area where the evidence is strong. However, many clinicians are not convinced that early prophylactic treatment of the PDA is helpful, because of the lack of demonstration of improved neurodevelopmental outcomes in infants treated early with indomethacin,[42] PDA is also a risk factor for development of PVL.[32] Last but not the least, PDA is associated with a higher rate of mortality in preterm neonates.[7,17,32] In a retrospective study, after adjustment for perinatal factors, level of maturity, disease severity, and morbid pathologies, the hazard risk for death in neonates with a PDA was eightfold higher than in those with a closed ductus.[7] Exclusion of patients who died during the first 2 weeks or inclusion of those who underwent ductal ligation did not change the findings. In neonates born prior to 28 weeks of gestation, a PDA diameter ≥1.5 mm on postnatal day 3 was associated with greater odds of mortality.[33]

One of the aims of contemporary PDA management could be to identify and target a population which would be most likely to benefit from PDA treatment. To achieve this aim we need to address three key questions:
- When to treat a PDA?
- Which PDA to treat?
- How to treat a PDA?

When to Treat?

The time frame of treatment determines some of the likely outcomes. P/IVH and pulmonary hemorrhage are early complications of a PDA, usually developing during the first 3 to 7 days of postnatal life. There is reasonably good evidence that early treatment of the PDA (mainly with indomethacin) can prevent both P/IVH and pulmonary hemorrhage,[19,34] but to achieve this, treatment needs to have been given prior to entering the risk period (days 2 to 7) for these complications. Of note is that indomethacin, unlike ibuprofen, decreases cerebral blood flow and improves cerebral blood flow autoregulation at least in part independently of its inhibitory effect on prostaglandin synthesis.[35] Therefore the effect of prophylactic indomethacin on decreasing the rate of P/IVH[42] or white matter injury[36] is not only related to the drug-induced decrease/cessation of ductal shunting. Assessing whether PDA treatment can prevent later complications such as NEC or BPD, which have a multifactorial etiology and a longer development phase, is more difficult. There are some animal data to support prevention of BPD by early ductal closure. In a baboon model, surgical ligation on day 6 had no effect on lung histology; conversely, early indomethacin treatment improved pulmonary mechanics and minimized lung injury by limiting pulmonary blood flow.[37,38] Demonstrating this in the human infant is more difficult partly due to the multifactorial etiology but also because in most clinical trials there is no true placebo group. High open-label rates of treatment meant that many infants enrolled in PDA treatment trials still received NSAIDs—just at a later time point. Therefore the natural history of an untreated PDA in a clinical trial setting is relatively unknown.[25]

Clinical symptoms of an hsPDA such as a murmur, active precordium, high volume pulses, poor growth, and increased work of breathing are nonspecific and might develop later in the clinical course.[39,40] Signs of cardiac failure usually do not develop until the second or third postnatal week. Most PDA-related Randomized control trials (RCTs) were not designed to address the question of whether or not a symptomatic PDA should be treated during the neonatal period; they were designed instead to assess the relationship between timing of treatment and efficiency of PDA closure. By the time the DA declares itself, it may already be too late and it may have already contributed to the development of one of the complications of prematurity. Symptomatic treatment trials are scarce, and results did not show any major advantage in terms of prevention of adverse effects from the PDA.[41] Studies from the presurfactant and antenatal steroid era suggest early symptomatic treatment may reduce the duration of mechanical ventilation and BPD compared with late symptomatic treatment.[42]

The efficacy of NSAIDs commonly used for the treatment of PDA decreases with increasing postnatal age as the balance of vasodilators changes from a system regulated predominantly by prostaglandins to one regulated by other vasodilators.[43] Up to 85% of PDAs would close if the first dose of indomethacin was administered within 24 hours after birth, and the rate decreases to 48% if it were started 72 hours or more after birth.[44] So not only does early treatment potentially allow treatment in a period before significant complications appear, it will also increase the likelihood of successful closure. Another benefit of earlier treatment is fewer potential side effects—particularly gut-associated side effects such as spontaneous intestinal perforation (SIP) and NEC. In the early prophylactic treatment studies, there is no increased rate of gut-associated side effects.[19,45,46]

The value of early asymptomatic treatment is uncertain. A Cochrane analysis consisting of three small RCTs concluded that asymptomatic treatment might be associated with fewer subsequent PDAs, and there was a reduction in duration of supplemental oxygen. There were no reported long-term outcomes in the included trials. It should also be noted here that the population included in the trials were a mixed population and included neonates up to 1700 g.[47] Another trial subsequent to this Cochrane review using ibuprofen did not show any difference in terms of clinical outcome but showed a trend toward decreased PVL at 36 weeks' postmenstrual age.[48] One of the issues with asymptomatic treatment is that it exposes a lot of infants to the adverse effects of medical treatment, some of whom would probably not have required treatment and would have undergone spontaneous closure.

Prophylactic Treatment

It is clearly not known how long the DA can be left open without causing potential harmful effects. Prophylactic treatment, which is usually instituted within the first 24 hours after birth, is most widely studied and probably the most effective mode of PDA treatment. The Cochrane analysis that includes 19 trials comprising 2872 infants[34] concluded that prophylactic treatment with indomethacin has a number of immediate benefits, in particular a reduction in symptomatic PDA, the need for duct ligation, and decreased rate of P/IVH, particularly severe P/IVH. There was also a borderline decrease in PVL, ventriculomegaly, and other white matter abnormalities. The Cochrane analysis concluded that there is a statistically nonsignificant trend toward a decrease in pulmonary hemorrhage. It should be noted here that out of the four trials which were included for the analysis, three trials showed a significant decrease in the incidence. However, the large Trial of Indomethacin Prophylaxis in Preterm infants (TIPP)[45] did not show a statistically significant protection against pulmonary hemorrhage in the primary analysis, and with this trial added to the meta-analysis there was no benefit for pulmonary hemorrhage reduction overall.

It is noteworthy that on reanalysis of the TIPP trial, prophylactic indomethacin reduced the rate of *early* serious pulmonary hemorrhage, mainly through its action on PDA. There was an overall reduction of pulmonary hemorrhage by 35%, and a reduced risk for PDA explained 80% of the beneficial effect of prophylactic indomethacin on serious pulmonary bleeds.[49] Similarly in a relatively recent double-blinded RCT, early cardiac ultrasound-targeted treatment of a large PDA resulted in a significant reduction in *early* pulmonary hemorrhage.[19]

Although prophylactic indomethacin has been shown to decrease severe forms of P/IVH, the long-term effect on neurodevelopmental outcomes is equivocal and somewhat improved. The relevance of the long-term versus short-term outcomes debate regarding its value will continue. Neil Marlow in his scientific philosophy paper asked a very pertinent question—"Is the primary outcome (mortality and severe neuro disability) directly causally relevant to the intervention under study?" He argues death can be from a less prevalent factor, which is not adjusted for, and considers neurodevelopment and death as complex outcomes. We should not be afraid to regard 2-year outcomes as proof of safety rather than efficacy and therefore be reassured in using the treatment.[50] Certainly there is enough evidence to suggest that indomethacin does not adversely affect neurodevelopmental outcome.[51,52] Very few RCTs have compared neurodevelopmental outcome and death in the follow-up. Only one RCT, which has followed neonates up to school age, did not find any beneficial effect of indomethacin.[53] The TIPP trial's 18-month follow-up did not show any major difference between indomethacin and the control group in terms of severe neurodevelopmental outcome and death; however, controversy exists regarding the study design and the interpretation of these results. The argument pertains to inadequate sample size, later indomethacin exposure of the controls, and the low incidence of P/IVH, making it difficult to come to any meaningful conclusion about neurodevelopmental outcome despite this being by far the largest trial of this intervention. It has been suggested that the 18-month follow-up performed in TIPP, as in many other long-term follow-up studies, may have failed to detect subtle neurodevelopmental abnormalities that became evident later in childhood.[54] A recent population-based cohort study reported that treatment for PDA may be associated with a greater risk of adverse neurodevelopmental outcome at age 2 to 3 years.[55] However, in the analysis, the treatment group was more likely to have a lower birth weight, head circumference, gestational age, and APGAR scores. The treatment group was also more likely to undergo mechanical ventilation for a longer period with more comorbidity, including BPD, retinopathy of prematurity (ROP), and infection. This gives the impression that patients in the treatment group were generally sicker than those in the control group, highlighting one of the drawbacks of retrospective analysis of data. In addition, in the multivariate analysis for neurodevelopmental outcome, no adjustment was made for P/IVH and NEC.[55] It has been shown that there is a decrease in cerebral blood flow with increasing left-to-right shunt through a PDA, that indomethacin improves regional cerebral oxygenation in hsPDA, and that prolonged indomethacin exposure was the only variable independently associated with a lower risk of white matter injury or brain abnormality.[36,56,57] Males who received prophylactic indomethacin had significantly higher verbal scores when compared with control males.[58] Ment and colleagues described trends favoring the prophylactic indomethacin group in cognitive functioning, some of which became statistically significant with adjustment for certain baseline variables.[51] Therefore the question as to what effect prophylactic indomethacin has on neurodevelopment is still not answered.

There is little evidence to support or refute the role of a PDA in NEC. The only study showing a decreased incidence of NEC was an older, unique study in infants less than 1000 g after early prophylactic PDA ligation.[59] Studies have consistently shown a reduction in intestinal blood flow in the presence of a PDA, providing some plausibility for an association with gut injury and NEC. Mesenteric artery flow decreases despite an increase in left ventricular output (LVO). Superior mesenteric artery flow usually increases after feeding; however, this physiologic phenomenon is blunted in the presence of a PDA.[60-63] In another human study, higher rates of NEC and feeding intolerance were seen in infants with a large PDA.[64] Therefore we suspect PDA might play a role in the pathophysiology of NEC, and treatment may be able to reduce this complication. However, due to the decreasing incidence of NEC in many nurseries a very large trial would be required to prove causation.

From the previous discussion, it is clear that prophylactic treatment definitely gives short-term benefit against severe P/IVH and pulmonary hemorrhage. The treatment also reduces the incidence of symptomatic PDA and need for surgical ligation. Despite the clear short-term benefits, this has not translated into improved outcomes for surviving infants. Early prophylactic treatment may improve neurodevelopmental outcome, although available evidence has not conclusively supported this notion.[42]

Although a "prophylactic" treatment approach has several important benefits, it also results in overtreatment of a PDA that would have closed spontaneously. As per the previous discussion, it is probable that at least 30% of the PDAs in extremely premature newborns close spontaneously, and it is important to identify these patients to avoid unnecessary exposure to medications. If prophylactic treatment is desired, indomethacin is currently the drug of choice because ibuprofen has not as yet been shown to have similar short-term benefits. On the other side, there is little evidence to suggest that treating PDA when it becomes symptomatic is helpful in the long term,[65] rather we may lose an opportunity to prevent significant early complications.[19,45]

The Cochrane analysis that includes 19 trials comprising of 2872 infants showed a safe profile of prophylactic indomethacin. Increased serum creatinine, NEC, spontaneous perforation, thrombocytopenia, ROP, and excessive bleeding were not of concern. Oliguria and hyperbilirubinemia are short-term and reversible side effects.[34] Indomethacin treatment for PDA does not increase NEC risk and, in fact, may decrease the risk.[66] Indomethacin treatment is associated with an increased risk of intestinal perforation, especially when given after the first 24 hours or combined with systemic glucocorticoids.[67] Very early prophylactic treatment is feasible even in infants born at 23 to 24 weeks' gestation without any side effects of the drug.[68] However, these patients might be at risk for SIP if they are given systemic steroids during the first few days after indomethacin has been started.

If early prophylactic treatment could be targeted at only those with evidence of poor PDA constriction, then the benefits may be maximized and potential harms decreased. Identification and targeting of a particular subset of the population who are least likely to undergo closure of their PDA and are most vulnerable to complications are therefore priorities. Cardiac ultrasound is an obvious way to aid in identifying this subgroup of patients and it is in this area that the efforts of the author's group have been focused.

Different timings of interventions along with their advantages and disadvantages from a pathophysiologic viewpoint are shown in Fig. 25.2, with pros and cons listed in Table 25.2. A schematic representation of the relationship between various complications of prematurity, the postnatal age at which they commonly occur, and various treatment approaches is provided in Fig. 25.3.

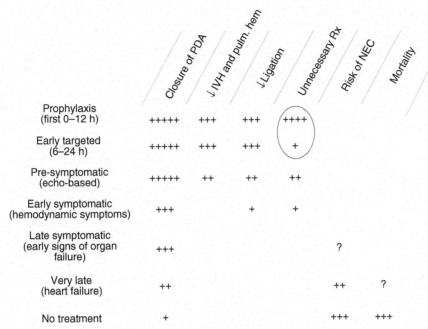

	Closure of PDA	↓ IVH and pulm. hem	↓ Ligation	Unnecessary Rx	Risk of NEC	Mortality
Prophylaxis (first 0–12 h)	+++++	+++	+++	++++		
Early targeted (6–24 h)	+++++	+++	+++	+		
Pre-symptomatic (echo-based)	+++++	++	++	++		
Early symptomatic (hemodynamic symptoms)	+++		+	+		
Late symptomatic (early signs of organ failure)	+++			?		
Very late (heart failure)	++			++	?	
No treatment	+				+++	+++

Fig. 25.2   The differing time points at which patent ductus arteriosus (PDA) treatment may be given are listed on the Y axis, and the consequences of treatment or nontreatment are listed along the top of the figure. Earlier treatment results in more short-term beneficial effects but at the cost of more infants receiving unnecessary treatment. Early targeted treatment using clinician-performed cardiac ultrasound to identify infants who fail to constrict the PDA results in earlier treatment, fewer side effects, and prevention from both intraventricular hemorrhage (IVH) and pulmonary hemorrhage while exposing fewer infants to unnecessary treatment. NEC, Necrotizing enterocolitis. Modified from Shahab Noori 2014, personal communication).

Table 25.2   SUMMARY OF THE PROS AND CONS OF DIFFERENT TREATMENT TIME POINTS

Treatment Type	Advantages	Disadvantages
Prophylactic (within 6–24 h of life, preferably within the first 12 h)	Most widely studied Some benefits (decreased IVH, pulmonary hemorrhage)	• Due to frequency of spontaneous closure, exposes a large number of infants to the side effects of NSAID treatment
Early asymptomatic (usually by day 3–7 on the basis of ultrasound/clinical signs)	Exposes fewer babies to the risks of treatment	• Few studies • By day 3 the damage may have already been done—particularly regarding IVH and pulmonary hemorrhage
Symptomatic (usually after postnatal day 3–4)	Exposes fewest babies to the risks of treatment	• Treatment is given later, which increases the chance of PDA-related morbidity and mortality • Closure rate is low • Few studies
Conservative (no medication or surgery)	No initial exposure to medication but risk of need for later treatment	• Unproven usefulness and safety profile • Nonstandardized approach

IVH, Intraventricular hemorrhage; NSAID, nonsteroidal antiinflammatory drugs; PDA, patent ductus arteriosus.

Which Patent Ductus Arteriosus to Treat?

From the available evidence, prophylactic treatment for a targeted population is probably the best approach we can offer as of now. We do not want to overexpose preterm neonates to the side effects of NSAIDs, and at the same time we do not want to delay treatment in order to avoid lower treatment success rates. The parameters to take in to consideration while making a decision to treat or not to treat the PDA include gestational age, postnatal age, level of respiratory support, existing

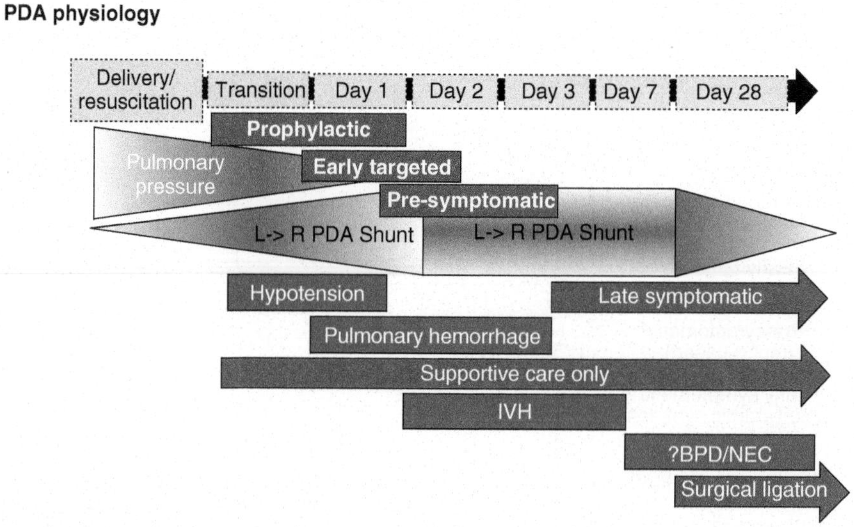

PDA physiology

Fig. 25.3 Diagram representing the different time points that ductal treatment may be considered versus the underlying pathophysiology. Treatment at earlier points means that there may be an opportunity to intervene in the developing pathophysiology. *BPD*, Bronchopulmonary dysplasia; *IVH*, intraventricular hemorrhage; *NEC*, necrotizing enterocolitis; *PDA*, patent ductus arteriosus.

comorbidities, ultrasound (US) features of PDA, including size and hemodynamic effect, and possibly cardiac biochemical markers. The definition of what constitutes an hsPDA varies between clinicians and centers, as well as between trials of PDA management. Investigators have used echocardiography alone, or in combination with physical examination findings and cardiac biochemical markers, in an attempt to more objectively define an hsPDA.

In the author's unit, we routinely consider early targeted prophylactic treatment for infants who are less than 28 weeks' gestation—more mature neonates need to have clinical symptoms as well as ultrasound evidence of a large volume left-to-right shunt before receiving treatment. Our real targets are infants who are born ≤26 weeks and who are most vulnerable to both short- and long-term adverse effects of PDA.

Bedside CPU plays an important role in the management of PDA in preterm neonates in our unit and many other units. Bedside CPU can diagnose the presence of a PDA more accurately than evaluation based on clinical signs, especially within the first 3 days after birth, and this reduces unnecessary treatment because of PDA misdiagnosis.[39] Bedside CPU allows for more timely and frequent assessment of PDA than does conventional echocardiography. By using PDA diameter measurement and flow pattern assessment, early CPU may identify large, nonconstricting PDAs which are unlikely to close spontaneously, thus reducing the duration of time spent in a hemodynamically compromised state with the associated risks of adverse outcomes.[69,70] In an RCT by the authors, early CPU-targeted PDA treatment reduced pulmonary hemorrhage and suggested a lower rate of P/IVH.[19] Continued PDA monitoring using serial CPU during indomethacin treatment can reduce the total dose and complications related to indomethacin treatment by facilitating earlier stopping of the treatment if the PDA is closed.[71,72] In countries where bedside CPU was more frequently used to diagnose PDA and where the clinicians had a proactive approach, the composite mortality/morbidity outcome and surgical ligation rate was lower compared to countries where bedside CPU was not so frequently used.[73] It is also a concern that infants with a delayed diagnosis of PDA may exceed the postnatal age for effective NSAID treatment. In a national population-based cohort of extremely preterm infants, screening echocardiography before postnatal day 3 was associated with lower in-hospital mortality and likelihood of pulmonary hemorrhage but not with differences in NEC, severe BPD, or severe cerebral lesions.[74]

The lack of a perceived long-term benefit of treatment strategies may relate to the marked variability in strategies in identifying an hsPDA. The definition of an

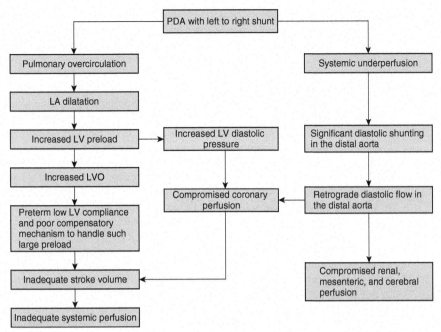

Fig. 25.4   Pathophysiology of patent ductus arteriosus *(PDA)* with a large left-to-right shunt and ultrasound targets. *LA,* Left atrium; *LV,* left ventricle; *LVO,* left ventricular output.

hsPDA remains controversial and thus varies significantly. Bedside CPU not only helps in diagnosing a PDA but also helps in deciding whether to treat and how and when to treat. A simplified version of PDA pathophysiology and CPU evaluation targets are depicted in Fig. 25.4.

Candidates for Patient Selection

Clinical

- Immaturity (<26 weeks' gestational age [GA])
- Low birthweight (<1000 g)
- Lack of antenatal steroids
- Male infant
- Maternal infection/chorioamnionitis
- Severe respiratory distress syndrome/mechanical ventilation
- Postnatal age less than 2 weeks

Ultrasound

- PDA diameter/flow pattern and peak left-to-right velocity
- Evidence of systemic steal—reverse flow in diastole in the descending aorta and/or cerebral arteries using Doppler
- Evidence of increased pulmonary blood flow—left pulmonary artery (LPA) diastolic velocity, increased pulmonary venous return velocity, increased left ventricular (LV) end-diastolic diameter
- Cardiac dilatation (increased left atrial to aortic root ratio), increased LVO
- Features of impaired myocardial performance—E wave to A wave ratio, LVO:SVC flow ratio, isovolumetric relaxation time, LV systolic time interval.

The details of techniques for measuring these parameters are discussed in Chapters 10 to 13. In this chapter, we shall discuss the clinical utility of these parameters in identifying hsPDA.

In the beginning, it should be remembered that the magnitude of ductal shunting is an interplay between systemic and pulmonary pressure/impedance, myocardial function, and size of the duct.

Ductal shunting cannot be simply estimated from a single ductal diameter measurement alone—this would be an oversimplification of a complex issue. The shunting of blood through the PDA is a complex interaction between the systemic and pulmonary pressure/impedance at both ends of the duct. There may be minimal shunting of blood in a large duct if the pulmonary systolic pressure is similar to or higher than the systemic systolic pressure. Beside this, the capability of the immature myocardium to handle the extra volume because of shunting through a PDA is also a consideration in the way that shunting will manifest. Various ultrasound parameters are determined in the assessment and evaluation of a PDA. In isolation, many of these parameters have a low sensitivity and specificity for determining the hemodynamic significance of a PDA. A ductal size of greater than 1.5 mm is generally considered to be large enough to cause significant hemodynamic disturbances.[75] However, this definition by itself has its drawbacks because it does not take into account the neonate's weight and the diameter measurement of a PDA itself has significant interuser variability. For example, a 2-mm PDA is expected to cause more hemodynamic disturbance in a 500-g weight baby than in a 1-kg weight baby. Sometimes the size of the PDA, if present, was defined as small, moderate, or large on the basis of the ratio of the smallest ductal diameter to the ostium of the left pulmonary artery (LPA) (PDA:LPA ratio). A ratio of ≥ 1 defined a large PDA, ≥ 0.5 but ≤ 1 a moderate PDA, and ≤ 0.5 a small PDA.[76] Ductal size may vary with oxygen saturation, surfactant treatment, or intravenous furosemide administration.[77] When a ductal size of 3 mm was considered, a significant correlation between ductal size and surrogate markers of pulmonary overcirculation was noted.[78] This diameter correlated significantly with ductal velocity, end-diastolic LPA flow, PDA diameter:LPA ratio, Left atrium:Aortic root (LA:Ao) ratio, and LVO:SVC ratio. In another study a ductal diameter of greater than 2 mm/kg measured from color Doppler at 72 hours of age was the most sensitive method for predicting a PDA in need of therapeutic intervention. The authors found ductus diameter to be the most important variable in determining the need for therapeutic intervention for PDA in preterm infants.[79] The PDA:LPA ratio could be used to identify and facilitate the treatment of a selected population destined to experience the development a symptomatic PDA. A ratio of 1 or more indicated a large PDA.[80] PDA size defined by PDA:LPA ratio at 3 days postnatal in combination with GA predicted spontaneous PDA closure.[81] Similarly the ductal diameter and body surface area ratio has been used to determine hsPDA, and a cutoff of greater than 14 is considered significant.[82]

The ideal way to measure a PDA shunt would be to quantify transductal flow or the total volume of shunt; however, a variable diameter across the course of the ductus and the nonlaminar nature of its flow makes this difficult. Different flow patterns have been defined in the literature, and these do give us some useful information about the hemodynamic significance of the duct.[83] A hsPDA will have a pulsatile flow pattern and a large unrestricted left-to-right flow.[79] The peak velocity at the end of diastole is usually zero or very low and implies an almost equal pulmonary and systolic pressure in diastole. Peak systolic flow velocity is usually less than 1.5 m/s, and if it increases above this there is usually constriction of the ductus. The ductal flow pattern is important not only from the hsPDA point of view but also from the perspective of relative pulmonary/systemic pressures. A pure or predominant right-to-left shunt through a PDA signifies pulmonary hypertension or significant systemic hypotension, often with offloading of the right ventricle such that closure of the duct may end up in a disastrous outcome with acute right ventricular cardiac failure. Many clinicians when faced with a bidirectional PDA flow would be reluctant to close the duct because of these concerns; however, closing of a clinically significant bidirectional duct, particularly if the right-to-left component is not more than 30% of the total cardiac cycle, is not absolutely contraindicated.[84] It should be noted here that myocardial function also plays an important role in direction of shunting through a patent duct, with impaired right ventricle (RV) function often resulting in less pulmonary blood flow and impaired LV function increasing the risk of right to left ductal shunting.

Pulmonary artery flow has a lamellar flow and is considered to be a surrogate of significant shunting. An LPA diastolic flow of greater than 0.2 m/s significantly correlates with the magnitude of the left-to-right shunt, but its impact on clinical outcome is unknown.[85] Pulsatility index (PI) refers to a variable reflecting the downstream resistance to blood flow in the vascular bed; therefore the PI of the LPA provides insight into right ventricular contractility, preload, and afterload.[86]

Left heart size and flow are useful surrogates of increased pulmonary blood flow and give useful insight into the magnitude of transductal flow. An increased LA:Ao ratio (usually >1.4), which is commonly used to ascertain ductal significance, lacks sensitivity and specificity. Measurement of a three-dimensional structure in two dimensions may be error prone. In addition, significant transatrial shunting may reduce the size of the LA by decompressing it, thereby giving a falsely low LA:Ao ratio even in the presence of significant pulmonary overload. The left atrium takes time to dilate and may not be a useful parameter to assess ductal significance in the first few postnatal days.[87] LVO also reflects a combination of increased pulmonary venous return and increased stroke volume to compensate for ductal runoff but has the same limitations as dilation of the left atrium. A large transatrial shunt, dehydration, and myocardial dysfunction may give rise to a relatively low LVO even in the setting of a large PDA. Here it should be noted that generally increased LVO implies adequate systemic blood flow. The LVO:SVC flow ratio may be a more reliable estimation of the ductal flow because it is unaffected by the transatrial flow, unlike other markers. The LVO reflects systemic plus ductal flow. The LVO:SVC flow ratio is potentially a more sensitive marker of ductal significance because LVO increases and SVC decreases with increases in ductal shunting. The LVO:SVC ratio correlates well with ductal size and is independent of the transatrial shunt.[78,86,88,89] Other features of increased blood flow, such as a mitral E wave to A wave ratio greater than 1, may suggest a hsPDA; however, this is not well validated.

An important sign of hemodynamic significance of the PDA is absence or reversal of aortic diastolic flow in the descending aorta and mesenteric arteries, also known as "ductal steal," which puts the infant at risk of hypoperfusion in the brain, splanchnic vessels, and renal vessels. Absent or retrograde diastolic flow in cerebral vessels is a constant feature of hsPDA but not in nonsignificant ducts, where cerebral vascular autoregulation plays an important role in maintaining cerebral perfusion.[90] In preterm infants less than 31 weeks' gestation with a ductal diameter of greater than 1.7 mm, descending aortic diastolic reversal was associated with a 35% decrease in descending aorta flow volume. However, the authors did not find any reduction in SVC flow and concluded that preterm infants with high-volume ductal shunt may have preserved upper body perfusion but reduced lower body perfusion.[91] Researchers have also tried to quantify the diastolic reversal and have suggested that a greater than 50% reversal is associated with hsPDA. The ratio of PI of the LPA to descending aorta has been proposed as another semiquantitative index that measures the downstream blood velocity in the pulmonary artery and descending aorta just distal to the PDA. Studies have shown stealing of blood in the superior mesenteric artery using this ratio.[63] Although all hsPDA's may have some component of reversal of flow which typically resolves after closure of the duct, its exact relationship to neonatal morbidity and mortality has not been well established.

In isolation, many of the discussed markers have low sensitivity and specificity and are prone to interobserver variability. Sehgal et al. have proposed a staging system and concluded that infants with a high composite score,[92] assigned according to the staging criteria at the time of treatment, were noted to have a higher incidence of subsequent chronic lung disease (CLD). The staging system is depicted in Table 25.3 as an example of a scoring system. A more complex PDA scoring system has been published using five factors that were independently associated with CLD/death (gestation at birth, PDA diameter, maximum flow velocity, LV output, and LV a′ wave). The PDA score had a range from 0 (low risk) to 13 (high risk). Infants who developed CLD/death had a higher score than those who did not.[26]

Assessment of an hsPDA does not stop with bedside CPU and gestation alone. The presence of respiratory distress syndrome and the use of mechanical ventilation may alter pulmonary vascular resistance and have a remarkable influence on left-to-right shunting through the open ductus. As neonatal care has improved there has been a dramatic move toward the use of noninvasive ventilation in even our smallest babies in the first days of life. However, in the same time frame we have become more conservative regarding treatment of the PDA. Invasive ventilation probably gives more protection against morbidities like pulmonary hemorrhage by keeping PDA shunting in check to some extent.

Table 25.3 ULTRASOUND PARAMETERS AND CLASSIFICATION INTO A SCORING SYSTEM
PERFORMED AT THE TIME OF PATENT DUCTUS ARTERIOSUS ASSESSMENT

Feature Quantified	Modality/Position of Sample Gate	Score 0	Score 1	Score 2	Score 3
Ductal features					
Transductal diameter (mm)	Two-dimensional, short axis view	0	<1.5	1.5–3	>3
Ductal velocity V_{max} (m/s)	PWD at pulmonary end of duct	0	>2	1.5–2	<1.5
Magnitude of ductal shunt					
PDA:LPA diameter			<0.5	≥0.5–1	≥1
Antegrade PA diastolic flow (cm/s)	PWD within main pulmonary artery	0	0–20	>20	
Antegrade LPA diastolic flow (cm/s)	PWD within left pulmonary artery	0	<30	30–50	>50
Left atrial to aortic ratio	M-mode, long axis view	1.13 ± 0.23[a]	<1.4:1	1.4–1.6:1	>1.6:1
Left ventricular to aortic ratio	M-mode, long axis view	1.86 ± 0.29[a]	–	2.15 ± 0.39[a]	≥2.5
Features of myocardial performance					
LVO/SVC flow ratio	PWD of flow in superior vena cava	2.4 ± 0.3[a]	–	–	≥4
E wave/A wave ratio	Transmitral Doppler	<1		1–1.5	>1.5
IVRT (ms)	Between mitral and aortic valves	>55	46–54	36–45	<35

[a]Mean ± SD.
Higher composite scores were correlated with increased risk of CLD (chronic lung disease).
CWD, Continuous wave Doppler; *IVRT*, isovolumic relaxation time; *LPA*, left pulmonary artery; *LVO*, left ventricular output; *PA*, pulmonary artery; *PDA*, patent ductus arteriosus; *PWD*, pulse wave Doppler; *SVC*, superior vena cava; V_{max}, maximum velocity.From Sehgal A, Paul E, Menahem S: Functional echocardiography in staging for ductal disease severity: role in predicting outcomes. *Eur J Pediatr.* 172(2):179–184, 2013.

After a CPU diagnosis of hsPDA is made, we take the infant's clinical condition in to consideration, in addition to the findings on ultrasound. If the PDA size is borderline on ultrasound and the infant has significant respiratory and oxygen support requirements, we would probably be more inclined to treat this infant than an infant who is in room air and on less support. Similarly, other factors such as GA, use of antenatal steroids, maternal chorioamnionitis, active pulmonary hemorrhage, P/IVH, renal function, metabolic acidosis, hyperdynamic precordium, hypotension, and other cardiac morbidities are also taken in to consideration and may make treatment more likely.

All infants who are born less than 28 weeks' gestational age undergo bedside ultrasound in the first 24 to 48 hours to ascertain the presence of and the hemodynamic significance of any PDA. It is important to use multiple markers such as PDA diameter, flow pattern, LPA diastolic flow, diastolic flow in descending aorta, transatrial flow, and LVO before deciding on hemodynamic significance. Some examples of PDA closure decision-making as practiced in our unit are discussed as follows to illustrate the variability in scenarios.

CASE STUDY 1

24 weeks GA on day 0
Antenatal steroid—No
Respiratory support—On ventilator (invasive) Peak inspiratory pressure
   (PIP)—22 cm H_2O, Peak end expiratory pressure (PEEP)—6 cm H_2O,
   Fraction of inspired oxygen (FiO$_2$)—50%
CPU—Duct size—3 mm, Flow—Growing pattern, LPA end diastole—0.4 m/s,
   reversal of diastolic flow in descending aorta, LVO—400 mL/kg/min

OUTCOME CASE STUDY 1

Medical closure of the PDA. Given indomethacin by 12 h of age

CASE STUDY 2

28 weeks GA on day 0
Antenatal steroid—Yes
Respiratory support—On continuous positive airway pressure (CPAP) 6 cm H_2O/FiO$_2$—30%
CPU—Duct size—2.5 mm, Flow—Pulsatile, LPA end diastole—0.3 m/s, some reversal of diastolic flow in descending aorta, LVO—300 mL/kg/min

OUTCOME CASE STUDY 2

Wait and watch

25

CASE STUDY 3

25 weeks GA on day 0
Antenatal steroid—Yes
Respiratory support—on CPAP 6 cm H_2O/FiO$_2$—21%
CPU—Duct size—4 mm, Flow—Growing pattern, LPA end diastole—0.4 m/s, reversal of diastolic flow in descending aorta, LVO—300 mL/kg/min

OUTCOME CASE STUDY 3

Medical closure even if the baby is not on much respiratory support. This is clearly a big PDA with other potential hemodynamic consequences.

CASE STUDY 4

27 weeks GA on day 0
Antenatal steroid—yes
Respiratory support—Ventilation (invasive) PIP—18 cm H_2O, PEEP—5 cm H_2O, FiO$_2$—70%
CPU—Duct size—3.5 mm, Flow—Pulmonary hypertension pattern, LPA end diastole—0.2 m/s, Antegrade diastolic flow in descending aorta, LVO—130 mL/kg/min

OUTCOME CASE STUDY 4

Wait even though the duct is big and baby is on significant respiratory support. This baby has a component of pulmonary hypertension.

CASE STUDY 5

24 weeks GA on day 0
Antenatal steroid—No
Respiratory support—Ventilation (invasive) PIP—18 cm H_2O, PEEP—5 cm H_2O, FiO$_2$—35%
CPU—Duct size—1.8 mm, Flow—Pulsatile, LPA end diastolic—0.3 m/s, Retrograde diastolic flow in the distal aorta, LVO—450 mL/kg/min

OUTCOME CASE STUDY 5

Medical closure of this duct. Even if the duct is not so big, the baby is at risk of complications and there is evidence of a significant left-to-right shunt.

CASE STUDY 6

26 weeks GA on day 8 with excessive weight gain
Antenatal steroid—Yes
Respiratory support—On CPAP 8 cm H_2O/FiO_2—50% (Gradual increase in respiratory support requirement)
CPU—Duct size—3.5 mm, Flow—Pulsatile, LPA end diastole—0.5 m/s, Retrograde diastolic flow in the distal aorta, LA:AO ratio—2.2, LVO—650 mL/kg/min

OUTCOME CASE STUDY 6

Attempt medical closure because there is evidence of a significant left-to-right shunt and some suggestion of early cardiac failure, albeit our success chance may be lower than on day 0.

CASE STUDY 7

27 weeks GA on day 9
Antenatal steroid—Yes
Respiratory support—On CPAP 6 cm H_2O/FiO_2—30% (steady respiratory support requirement)
CPU—Duct size—2.2 mm, Flow—Pulsatile, LPA end diastole—0.3 m/s, Some retrograde diastolic flow in the distal aorta, LA:AO ratio—1.7, LVO—250 mL/kg/min

OUTCOME CASE STUDY 7

Review in 3 to 4 days' time, monitoring the clinical condition and respiratory requirement.

CASE STUDY 8

27 weeks GA on day 0
Antenatal steroid—Yes
Respiratory support—On CPAP, 6 cm H_2O/FiO_2—25%
CPU—Duct size—3 mm, Flow—Growing pattern, LPA end diastole—0.3 m/s, Antegrade diastolic flow in the distal aorta, LVO—200 mL/kg/min

OUTCOME CASE STUDY 8

Review in 24 to 48 h. Although the duct is big, there is little evidence of left-to-right shunting.

CASE STUDY 9

25 weeks GA on day 21
Antenatal steroid—Yes
Respiratory support—On CPAP, 6 cm H_2O/FiO_2—30% Stable
CPU—Duct size—2.5 mm, Flow—Variable pattern, LPA end diastole—0.25 m/s, No diastolic flow in the distal aorta, LA:AO ratio—2.5, LVO—300 mL/kg/min

OUTCOME CASE STUDY 9

Review in 5 to 7 days. This infant is likely to have developed shunt tolerance.

Early prophylactic treatment undoubtedly exposes many infants to the side effects of treatment, and the early asymptomatic treatment option is not well explored. A definitive trial, comparing current standard treatment (pharmacologic treatment with supportive care) versus supportive care alone with no option for open-label treatment, is necessary to resolve doubts regarding the quality or conduct of prior studies. A recent Australian clinical trial (Selecting optimal Management of the ductus ARTeriosus Trial [SMART]), has been designed to address this particular issue and will hopefully give us an answer in the future. (ANZCTR—Trial No-ACTRN12616000195459).

Biochemical markers such as cardiac troponin T, N-terminal prohormone atrial natriuretic peptide, and B-type natriuretic peptide have been proposed individually or in conjunction with ultrasound to diagnose an hsPDA. The added benefit of biomarkers is unclear when ultrasound, the "gold standard" for diagnosis, is available. However, in places where ultrasound is unavailable, biochemical markers may be useful.

How to Treat?

We have three alternatives to treat a PDA: medical, surgical, and conservative. Among the three methods, medical intervention with NSAID is most widely used. Medical treatment is discussed in detail elsewhere in this book (Chapter 23).

There are concerns that the untested conservative treatment approach of fluid restriction, higher PEEP/CPAP, and diuretic therapy may do more harm than good. The Cochrane analysis of this approach showed a decreasing trend of PDA and NEC but at the expense of increased postnatal weight loss with a risk of dehydration.[93] Another prospective observational study of fluid restriction to 108 ± 10 mL/kg/day in neonates with gestational age 24.8 ± 1.1 weeks had no beneficial effects on pulmonary or systemic hemodynamics. Similarly, diuretic therapy is not useful, and a Cochrane analysis concluded that there is not enough evidence to support the administration of furosemide to premature infants treated with indomethacin for symptomatic PDA. Furosemide appears to be contraindicated in the presence of dehydration in these infants.[94] Use of furosemide in combination with indomethacin increased the incidence of acute renal failure but did not affect PDA closure rate in preterm infants.[95] Furosemide has also a theoretical risk of reopening the DA or keeping the DA patent because of its pro-prostaglandin properties. Contrary to all these studies, a retrospective observational time series has shown a significant decrease in BPD and ligation in the conservative group (restricted fluid and high PEEP) compared with the symptomatic and early treatment group. However, it should be noted here that the different groups were managed in different time periods and that it was a study in relatively bigger infants with birth weight less than 1500 g.[10] Adequate respiratory support has a definite role and is a part of the conservative management of PDA. Adequate lung recruitment by invasive or noninvasive ventilation minimizes left-to-right shunt through a PDA. Some form of conservative management at this stage is a definite adjunct to medical therapy, and ongoing trials incorporating these newer management approaches in a contemporary NICU population should provide more clarity about its role in the management of PDA into the future.

There is increasing concern about the utilization of surgical management of the PDA, and the issues around this are discussed in detail in Chapter 24. Immediate adverse effects are systemic hypotension, myocardial dysfunction, and possible respiratory deterioration. In the TIPP trial there was an increased incidence of ROP, BPD, neurosensory impairment, and cognitive delay after surgical intervention. However, the authors did not make any adjustment for the duration of exposure to a ductal shunt, which is thought to have contributed to these morbidities.[45] Most of the DA ligations were undertaken in the second or third postnatal week, so there is concern that the impact of prolonged cerebral and other organ blood flow disturbances from the PDA shunt itself might have been contributory to the adverse outcome seen after surgical ligation. In a prospective study, day 3 to 4 ductal diameter^2/birth weight index greater than 5 mm^2/kg, LA:Ao ratio greater than 1.5, and high volume of ductal shunting were statistically significant indicators of the need for surgical closure of the PDA in low birth weight preterm neonates.[96] There appears to be an international trend to a less aggressive approach to ductal ligation, reflecting concerns that ligation of a PDA may do more harm than good. This issue needs to be addressed by a randomized controlled trial, which most likely will never happen because of ethical concerns. In the authors' unit, the clinicians rarely opt for surgical closure, and there are several series describing very low ligation rates in the modern era. We consider surgical closure after two failed courses of medical treatment in the presence of ultrasound evidence of a large PDA with significant left-to-right shunt and ongoing/increasing oxygen and ventilatory needs.

Conclusion

Prophylactic indomethacin is the only approach in PDA management to date that has been convincingly studied and shown any effect on any outcome. However, there is reasonable evidence of lack of harm in all comparisons assessed (apart from transient oliguria/anuria) from medical treatment in the trials completed to date. On the other hand, we know almost nothing about the consequences of conservative treatment pathways. We have made some progress towards identifying ducts which are not likely to close. The next significant advances in management will be focused on demonstrating the safety of a purely conservative approach where no treatment is given to close the PDA. Development of evaluation tools that will be able to provide the clinician with more specific predictive data as to whether an infant is at risk of short- or medium-term complications of a significant left-to-right shunt will also be important. Part of this effort will be developing simpler ways to measure the volume of shunt in individual infants and incorporate these into standardized scoring systems. Until then it is important for clinicians to consider the individual circumstances of each patient, looking for signs of stability or decompensation, and directing treatment accordingly.

REFERENCES

1. Evans NJ, Archer LN: Postnatal circulatory adaptation in healthy term and preterm neonates, *Arch Dis Child* 65(1 Spec No):24–26, 1990.
2. Koch J, Hensley G, Roy L, et al.: Prevalence of spontaneous closure of the ductus arteriosus in neonates at a birth weight of 1000 grams or less, *Pediatrics* 117(4):1113–1121, 2006.
3. Zonnenberg I, de Waal K: The definition of a haemodynamic significant duct in randomized controlled trials: a systematic literature review, *Acta Paediatr* 101(3):247–251, 2012.
4. Evans N: Preterm patent ductus arteriosus: a continuing conundrum for the neonatologist? *Semin Fetal Neonatal Med* 20(4):272–277, 2015.
5. Rolland A, Shankar-Aguilera S, Diomande D, et al.: Natural evolution of patent ductus arteriosus in the extremely preterm infant, *Arch Dis Child Fetal Neonatal Ed* 100(1):F55–58, 2015.
6. Koch J, Hensley G, Roy L, et al.: Prevalence of spontaneous closure of the ductus arteriosus in neonates at a birth weight of 1000 grams or less, *Pediatrics* 117(4):1113–1121, 2006.
7. Noori S, McCoy M, Friedlich P, et al.: Failure of ductus arteriosus closure is associated with increased mortality in preterm infants, *Pediatrics* 123(1):e138–e144, 2009.
8. Narayanan M, Cooper B, Weiss H, Clyman RI: Prophylactic indomethacin: factors determining permanent ductus arteriosus closure, *J Pediatr* 136(3):330–337, 2000.
9. Dani C, Bertini G, Corsini I, et al.: The fate of ductus arteriosus in infants at 23-27 weeks of gestation: from spontaneous closure to ibuprofen resistance, *Acta Paediatr* 97(9):1176–1180, 2008.
10. Letshwiti JB, Semberova J, Pichova K, et al.: A conservative treatment of patent ductus arteriosus in very low birth weight infants, *Early Hum Dev* 104:45–49, 2017.
11. Semberova J, Sirc J, Miletin J, et al.: Spontaneous closure of patent ductus arteriosus in infants ≤1500 g, *Pediatrics* 2017.
12. Du JF, Liu TT, Wu H: [Risk factors for patent ductus arteriosus in early preterm infants: a case-control study], *Zhongguo Dang Dai Er Ke Za Zhi* 18(1):15–19, 2016.
13. Park HW, Choi YS, Kim KS, Kim SN: Chorioamnionitis and patent ductus arteriosus: a systematic review and meta-analysis, *PLoS One* 10(9):e0138114, 2015.
14. Qu XY, Zhou XF, Qu Y, et al.: [Risk factors for patent ductus arteriosus in neonates], *Zhongguo Dang Dai Er Ke Za Zhi* 13(5):388–391, 2011.
15. Pourarian S, Farahbakhsh N, Sharma D, et al.: Prevalence and risk factors associated with the patency of ductus arteriosus in premature neonates: a prospective observational study from Iran, *J Matern Fetal Neonatal Med* 1–5, 2016.
16. Benitz WE: Learning to live with patency of the ductus arteriosus in preterm infants, *J Perinatol* 31(Suppl 1):S42–S48, 2011.

17. Brooks JM, Travadi JN, Patole SK, et al.: Is surgical ligation of patent ductus arteriosus necessary? The Western Australian experience of conservative management, *Arch Dis Child Fetal Neonatal Ed* 90(3):F235–239, 2005.

18. Kluckow M, Evans N: Low superior vena cava flow and intraventricular haemorrhage in preterm infants, *Arch Dis Child Fetal Neonatal Ed* 82:188–194, 2000.

19. Kluckow M, Jeffery M, Gill A, Evans N: A randomised placebo-controlled trial of early treatment of the patent ductus arteriosus, *Arch Dis Child Fetal Neonatal Ed* 99(2):F99–F104, 2014.

20. Garland J, Buck R, Weinberg M: Pulmonary hemorrhage risk in infants with a clinically diagnosed patent ductus arteriosus: a retrospective cohort study, *Pediatrics* 94(5):719–723, 1994.

21. Lewis MJ, McKeever PK, Rutty GN: Patent ductus arteriosus as a natural cause of pulmonary hemorrhage in infants: a medicolegal dilemma, *Am J Forensic Med Pathol* 25(3):200–204, 2004.

22. Schena F, Francescato G, Cappelleri A, et al.: Association between hemodynamically significant patent ductus arteriosus and bronchopulmonary dysplasia, *J Pediatr* 166(6):1488–1492, 2015.

23. Chen HL, Yang RC, Lee WT, et al.: Lung function in very preterm infants with patent ductus arteriosus under conservative management: an observational study, *BMC Pediatr* 15:167, 2015.

24. Sadeck LS, Leone CR, Procianoy RS, et al.: Effects of therapeutic approach on the neonatal evolution of very low birth weight infants with patent ductus arteriosus, *J Pediatr (Rio J)* 90(6):616–623, 2014.

25. Clyman RI, Liebowitz M: Treatment and nontreatment of the patent ductus arteriosus: identifying their roles in neonatal morbidity, *J Pediatr* 2017.

26. El-Khuffash A, James AT, Corcoran JD, et al.: A patent ductus arteriosus severity score predicts chronic lung disease or death before discharge, *J Pediatr* 167(6):1354–1361.e1352, 2015.

27. Noori S: Patent ductus arteriosus in the preterm infant: to treat or not to treat? *J Perinatol* 30(Suppl): S31–S37, 2010.

28. Jhaveri N, Moon-Grady A, Clyman RI. Early surgical ligation versus a conservative approach for management of patent ductus arteriosus that fails to close after indomethacin treatment. *J Pediatr* 157(3):381–387.

29. Dollberg S, Lusky A, Reichman B, Network IN: Patent ductus arteriosus, indomethacin and necrotizing enterocolitis in very low birth weight infants: a population-based study, *J Pediatr Gastroenterol Nutr* 40(2):184–188, 2005.

30. Lemmers PM, Benders MJ, D'Ascenzo R, et al.: Patent ductus arteriosus and brain volume, *Pediatrics* 137(4), 2016.

31. Wong FY, Leung TS, Austin T, et al.: Impaired autoregulation in preterm infants identified by using spatially resolved spectroscopy, *Pediatrics* 121(3):e604–e611, 2008.

32. Chung MY, Fang PC, Chung CH, et al.: Risk factors for hemodynamically-unrelated cystic periventricular leukomalacia in very low birth weight premature infants, *J Formos Med Assoc* 104(8):571–577, 2005.

33. Sellmer A, Bjerre JV, Schmidt MR, et al.: Morbidity and mortality in preterm neonates with patent ductus arteriosus on day 3, *Archives of disease in childhood fetal and neonatal edition* 98(6):F505–510, 2013.

34. Fowlie PW, Davis PG, McGuire W: Prophylactic intravenous indomethacin for preventing mortality and morbidity in preterm infants, [Update of Cochrane Database Syst Rev. 2002;(3):CD000174; PMID: 12137607]. *Cochrane Database Syst Rev* (7):CD000174, 2010.

35. Chock VY, Ramamoorthy C, Van Meurs KP: Cerebral autoregulation in neonates with a hemodynamically significant patent ductus arteriosus, *J Pediatr* 160(6):936–942, 2012.

36. Miller SP, Mayer EE, Clyman RI, et al.: Prolonged indomethacin exposure is associated with decreased white matter injury detected with magnetic resonance imaging in premature newborns at 24 to 28 weeks' gestation at birth, *Pediatrics* 117(5):1626–1631, 2006.

37. McCurnin DC, Yoder BA, Coalson J, et al.: Effect of ductus ligation on cardiopulmonary function in premature baboons, *Am J Respir Crit Care Med* 172(12):1569–1574, 2005.

38. Chang LY, McCurnin D, Yoder B, et al.: Ductus arteriosus ligation and alveolar growth in preterm baboons with a patent ductus arteriosus, *Pediatr Res* 63(3):299–302, 2008.

39. Skelton R, Evans N, Smythe J: A blinded comparison of clinical and echocardiographic evaluation of the preterm infant for patent ductus arteriosus, *J Paediatr Child Health* 30:406–411, 1994.

40. Alagarsamy S, Chhabra M, Gudavalli M, et al.: Comparison of clinical criteria with echocardiographic findings in diagnosing PDA in preterm infants, *J Perinat Med* 33(2):161–164, 2005.

41. Gersony WM, Peckham GJ, Ellison RC, et al.: Effects of indomethacin in premature infants with patent ductus arteriosus: results of a national collaborative study, *J Pediatr* 102(6):895–906, 1983.

42. Clyman RI: Recommendations for the postnatal use of indomethacin: an analysis of four separate treatment strategies, *J Pediatr* 128(5 Pt 1):601–607, 1996.

43. Clyman RI, Couto J, Murphy GM: Patent ductus arteriosus: are current neonatal treatment options better or worse than no treatment at all? *Semin Perinatol* 36(2):123–129, 2012.

44. Yang CZ, Lee J: Factors affecting successful closure of hemodynamically significant patent ductus arteriosus with indomethacin in extremely low birth weight infants, *World J Pediatr* 4(2):91–96, 2008.

45. Schmidt B, Davis P, Moddemann D, et al.: Long-term effects of indomethacin prophylaxis in extremely-low-birth-weight infants, *N Engl J Med* 344(26):1966–1972, 2001.

46. Wadhawan R, Oh W, Vohr BR, et al.: Spontaneous intestinal perforation in extremely low birth weight infants: association with indometacin therapy and effects on neurodevelopmental outcomes at 18-22 months' corrected age, *Arch Dis Child Fetal Neonatal Ed* 98(2):F127–132, 2013.

47. Cooke L, Steer P, Woodgate P: Indomethacin for asymptomatic patent ductus arteriosus in preterm infants, *Cochrane Database Syst Rev* (2):CD003745, 2003.

25

48. Aranda JV, Clyman R, Cox B, et al.: A randomized, double-blind, placebo-controlled trial on intravenous ibuprofen L-lysine for the early closure of nonsymptomatic patent ductus arteriosus within 72 hours of birth in extremely low-birth-weight infants, *Am J Perinatol* 26(3):235–245, 2009.

49. Alfaleh K, Smyth JA, Roberts RS, et al.: Prevention and 18-month outcomes of serious pulmonary hemorrhage in extremely low birth weight infants: results from the trial of indomethacin prophylaxis in preterms, *Pediatrics* 121(2):e233–e238, 2008.

50. Marlow N: Is survival and neurodevelopmental impairment at 2 years of age the gold standard outcome for neonatal studies? *Arch Dis Child Fetal Neonatal Ed* 100(1):F82–84, 2015.

51. Ment LR, Vohr B, Allan W, et al.: Outcome of children in the indomethacin intraventricular hemorrhage prevention trial, *Pediatrics* 105(3 Pt 1):485–491, 2000.

52. Couser RJ, Hoekstra RE, Ferrara TB, et al.: Neurodevelopmental follow-up at 36 months' corrected age of preterm infants treated with prophylactic indomethacin, *Arch Pediatr Adolesc Med* 154(6):598–602, 2000.

53. Vohr BR, Allan WC, Westerveld M, et al.: School-age outcomes of very low birth weight infants in the indomethacin intraventricular hemorrhage prevention trial, *Pediatrics* 111(4 Pt 1):e340–e346, 2003.

54. Clyman RI, Saha S, Jobe A, Oh W: Indomethacin prophylaxis for preterm infants: the impact of 2 multicentered randomized controlled trials on clinical practice, *J Pediatr* 150(1):46–50.e42, 2007.

55. Janz-Robinson EM, Badawi N, Walker K, et al.: Network NICU. Neurodevelopmental outcomes of premature infants treated for patent ductus arteriosus: a population-based cohort study, *J Pediatr* 167(5):1025–1032.e1023, 2015.

56. Lemmers PM, Toet MC, van Bel F: Impact of patent ductus arteriosus and subsequent therapy with indomethacin on cerebral oxygenation in preterm infants, *Pediatrics* 121(1):142–147, 2008.

57. Noori S, Wlodaver A, Gottipati V, et al.: Transitional changes in cardiac and cerebral hemodynamics in term neonates at birth, *J Pediatr* 160(6):943–948, 2012.

58. Ment LR, Vohr BR, Makuch RW, et al.: Prevention of intraventricular hemorrhage by indomethacin in male preterm infants, *J Pediatr* 145(6):832–834, 2004.

59. Cassady G, Crouse DT, Kirklin JW, et al.: A randomized, controlled trial of very early prophylactic ligation of the ductus arteriosus in babies who weighed 1000 g or less at birth, *N Engl J med* 320(23):1511–1516, 1989.

60. McCurnin D, Clyman RI: Effects of a patent ductus arteriosus on postprandial mesenteric perfusion in premature baboons, *Pediatrics* 122(6):e1262–e1267, 2008.

61. Shimada S, Kasai T, Hoshi A, et al.: Cardiocirculatory effects of patent ductus arteriosus in extremely low-birth-weight infants with respiratory distress syndrome, *Pediatr Int* 45(3):255–262, 2003.

62. Coombs RC, Morgan ME, Durbin GM, et al.: Gut blood flow velocities in the newborn: effects of patent ductus arteriosus and parenteral indomethacin [see comments], *Arch Dis Child* 65:1067–1071, 1990.

63. Freeman-Ladd M, Cohen JB, Carver JD, Huhta JC: The hemodynamic effects of neonatal patent ductus arteriosus shunting on superior mesenteric artery blood flow, *J Perinatol* 25(7):459–462, 2005.

64. Havranek T, Rahimi M, Hall H, Armbrecht E: Feeding preterm neonates with patent ductus arteriosus (PDA): intestinal blood flow characteristics and clinical outcomes, *J Matern Fetal Neonatal Med* 28(5):526–530, 2015.

65. Benitz WE: Treatment of persistent patent ductus arteriosus in preterm infants: time to accept the null hypothesis? *J Perinatol* 30(4):241–252, 2010.

66. McPherson CGP, Smith M, Wilder W, et al.: Necrotizing enterocolitis in preterm infants with patent ductus arteriosus: does indomethacin increase the risk? *J Neonat-Perinat Med* 1(4):209–216, 2008.

67. Paquette L, Friedlich P, Ramanathan R, Seri I: Concurrent use of indomethacin and dexamethasone increases the risk of spontaneous intestinal perforation in very low birth weight neonates, *J Perinatol* 26(8):486–492, 2006.

68. Yoshimoto S, Sakai H, Ueda M, et al.: Prophylactic indomethacin in extremely premature infants between 23 and 24 weeks gestation, *Pediatr Int* 52(3):374–377, 2010.

69. Kluckow M, Seri I, Evans N: Functional echocardiography: an emerging clinical tool for the neonatologist, *J Pediatr* 150(2):125–130, 2007.

70. O'Rourke DJ, El-Khuffash A, Moody C, et al.: Patent ductus arteriosus evaluation by serial echocardiography in preterm infants, *Acta Paediatr* 97(5):574–578, 2008.

71. Su BH, Peng CT, Tsai CH: Echocardiographic flow pattern of patent ductus arteriosus: a guide to indomethacin treatment in premature infants, *Arch Dis Child Fetal Neonatal Ed* 81(3):F197–F200, 1999.

72. Carmo KB, Evans N, Paradisis M: Duration of indomethacin treatment of the preterm patent ductus arteriosus as directed by echocardiography, *J Pediatr* 155(6):819–822, 2009.

73. Isayama T, Mirea L, Mori R, et al.: Patent ductus arteriosus management and outcomes in Japan and Canada: comparison of proactive and selective approaches, *Am J Perinatol* 32(11):1087–1094, 2015.

74. Roze JC, Cambonie G, Marchand-Martin L, et al.: Association between early screening for patent ductus arteriosus and in-hospital mortality among extremely preterm infants, *JAMA* 313(24):2441–2448, 2015.

75. Evans N: Current controversies in the diagnosis and treatment of patent ductus arteriosus in preterm infants, *Adv Neonatal Care* 3(4):168–177, 2003.

76. Wald RM, Adatia I, Van Arsdell GS, Hornberger LK: Relation of limiting ductal patency to survival in neonatal Ebstein's anomaly, *Am J Cardiol* 96(6):851–856, 2005.

77. Sehgal A, McNamara PJ: The ductus arteriosus: a refined approach!, *Semin Perinatol* 36(2):105–113, 2012.

78. Sehgal A, Menahem S: Interparametric correlation between echocardiographic markers in preterm infants with patent ductus arteriosus, *Pediatr Cardiol* 34(5):1212–1217, 2013.
79. Harling S, Hansen-Pupp I, Baigi A, Pesonen E: Echocardiographic prediction of patent ductus arteriosus in need of therapeutic intervention, *Acta Paediatr* 100(2):231–235, 2011.
80. Ramos FG, Rosenfeld CR, Roy L, et al.: Echocardiographic predictors of symptomatic patent ductus arteriosus in extremely-low-birth-weight preterm neonates, *J Perinatol* 30(8):535–539, 2010.
81. Thankavel PP, Rosenfeld CR, Christie L, Ramaciotti C: Early echocardiographic prediction of ductal closure in neonates </= 30 weeks gestation, *J Perinatol* 33(1):45–51, 2013.
82. Tapia-Rombo CA, Gonzalez-Arenas M, Carpio-Hernandez JC, Santiago-Romo JE: [An index internal diameter ductus arteriosus/body surface area as a need for closure of duct in the preterm newborn], *Rev Invest Clin* 65(1):12–23, 2013.
83. Su BH, Watanabe T, Shimizu M, Yanagisawa M: Echocardiographic assessment of patent ductus arteriosus shunt flow pattern in premature infants, *Arch Dis Child Fetal Neonatal Ed* 77(1):F36–F40, 1997.
84. Ethington PN, Smith PB, Katakam L, et al.: Treatment of patent ductus arteriosus with bidirectional flow in neonates, *Early Hum Dev* 87(5):381–384, 2011.
85. Hirsimaki H, Kero P, Wanne O: Doppler ultrasound and clinical evaluation in detection and grading of patient ductus arteriosus in neonates, *Crit Care Med* 18:490–493, 1990.
86. Engur D, Deveci M, Turkmen MK: Early signs that predict later haemodynamically significant patent ductus arteriosus, *Cardiol Young* 26(3):439–445, 2016.
87. Iyer P, Evans N: Re-evaluation of the left atrial to aortic root ratio as a marker of patent ductus arteriosus, *Arch Dis Child* 70:F112–117, 1994.
88. El Hajjar M, Vaksmann G, Rakza T, et al.: Severity of the ductal shunt: a comparison of different markers, *Arch Dis Child Fetal Neonatal Ed* 90(5):F419–422, 2005.
89. Phillipos EZ, Robertson MA, Byrne PJ: Serial assessment of ductus arteriosus hemodynamics in hyaline membrane disease, *Pediatrics* 98(6 Pt 1):1149–1153, 1996.
90. Kupferschmid C, Lang D, Pohlandt F: Sensitivity, specificity and predictive value of clinical findings, m-mode echocardiography and continuous-wave doppler sonography in the diagnosis of symptomatic patent ductus arteriosus in preterm infants, *Eur J Pediatr* 147:279–282, 1988.
91. Groves AM, Kuschel CA, Knight DB, Skinner JR: Does retrograde diastolic flow in the descending aorta signify impaired systemic perfusion in preterm infants? *Pediatr Res* 63(1):89–94, 2008.
92. Sehgal A, Paul E, Menahem S: Functional echocardiography in staging for ductal disease severity: role in predicting outcomes, *Eur J Pediatr* 172(2):179–184, 2013.
93. Bell EF, Acarregui MJ: Restricted versus liberal water intake for preventing morbidity and mortality in preterm infants, *Cochrane Database Syst Rev* (12):CD000503, 2014.
94. Brion LP, Campbell DE: Furosemide for symptomatic patent ductus arteriosus in indomethacin-treated infants, *Cochrane Database Syst Rev* (3):CD001148, 2001.
95. Lee BS, Byun SY, Chung ML, et al.: Effect of furosemide on ductal closure and renal function in indomethacin-treated preterm infants during the early neonatal period, *Neonatology* 98(2):191–199, 2010.
96. Braulio R, Gelape CL, Araujo FD, et al.: Indicators of surgical treatment of patent ductus arteriosus in preterm neonates in the first week of life, *Rev Bras Cir Cardiovasc* 28(4):504–508, 2013.

25

Pathophysiology and Treatment of Neonatal Shock

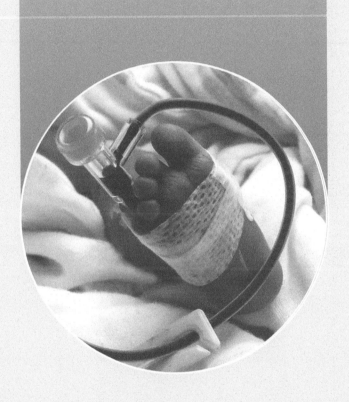

CHAPTER 26

Cardiovascular Compromise in the Preterm Infant During the First Postnatal Day

Martin Kluckow and Istvan Seri

- The very low birth weight infant is hemodynamically vulnerable due to a unique set of risk factors, which include an immature myocardium with poor response to afterload, immature autonomic vasoregulation, and thus ineffective cardiovascular compensatory mechanisms, propensity to develop specific or nonspecific inflammatory responses, the imposition of positive airway pressure, systemic to pulmonary shunts, and variability in the degree of placental restoration of blood volume according to cord clamp timing.

- The low cardiac output state that may then occur is associated with adverse outcomes, including neurological injury and potential long-term developmental impairment.

- Assessment of the degree of hemodynamic impairment is difficult, with reliance on standard hemodynamic assessment tools such as capillary refill time, acidosis, and blood pressure all having limitations, especially when used in isolation.

- Awareness of the risks of hemodynamic instability with appropriate treatment response may decrease the risk of some of the severe complications of prematurity.

- Point-of-care ultrasound by the clinician can assist in recognizing hemodynamic compromise and allow targeted management of the underlying problems.

The birth of a very low birth weight (VLBW) infant creates a unique set of circumstances that can adversely affect the cardiovascular system resulting in cardiovascular compromise. The cardiovascular system of the fetus is adapted to an in-utero environment that is constant and stable. The determinants of cardiac output, such as preload and afterload, are maintained in equilibrium without interference from the external factors that may affect a neonate born prematurely. Postnatal factors that can affect the cardiovascular function of the VLBW infant include perinatal asphyxia, sepsis, positive pressure respiratory support, unnecessary exposure to high oxygen concentration, and cord clamp time. During the immediate transitional period, these factors may alter preload and change afterload at the time of rapid transition from the fetal circulation, characterized by low systemic vascular resistance, to the postnatal neonatal circulation with higher peripheral vascular resistance. The predominantly systemic to pulmonary shunts at the atrial and ductal level through persisting fetal channels can further reduce potential systemic blood flow (Fig. 26.1).

The situation is made more complex by the difficulty in assessing the adequacy of the cardiovascular system in the VLBW infant. The small size of the infant and the frequent presence of shunting at both ductal and atrial level preclude the use of many of the routine cardiovascular assessment techniques used in children and adults to determine cardiac output. As a result, clinicians are forced to fall back on more

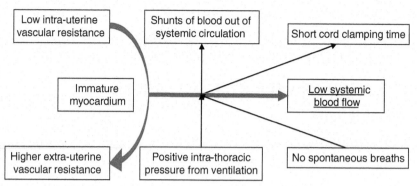

Fig. 26.1   Suggested model of how the various external and internal influences on the cardiovascular system of the very low birth weight infant can result in low systemic blood flow.

easily measured parameters such as the blood pressure. However, blood pressure is the dependent measure among the three determinants of systemic circulation, with cardiac output and systemic vascular resistance being the independent determinants. Accordingly, changes in the blood pressure do not necessarily reflect changes in the cardiac output and subsequent changes in organ blood flow and tissue oxygen delivery (see Chapters 1, 11, and 21).

Hypotension occurs in up to 30% of VLBW infants, with between 16% and 52% of these infants receiving treatment with volume expansion and up to 39% receiving vasopressors (see Chapter 3 for details).[1] More recent surveys of the management of extremely low birth weight (ELBW) infants have demonstrated treatment (fluid bolus or vasopressor administration) rates for hypotension up to 93% at 23 weeks' gestational age (GA) and up to 73% of infants at 27 weeks' GA.[2-4] Most treatment was commenced in the first 24 hours of postnatal life. Similarly, low systemic blood flow in the first 24 hours is seen in up to 35% of VLBW infants, but not all of these infants will have hypotension initially, though many will develop it.[5] Recent studies of the incidence of low superior vena cava (SVC) flow show a reduced incidence (18% to 21% of ELBW infants), possibly reflecting changes in obstetric and delivery room management, respiratory care, and perhaps fluid management of the neonate.[6,7] There is a wide variation in the assessment and management of cardiovascular compromise among both institutions and individual clinicians.[1,8] As with many other areas in medicine where there is variation in practice with multiple treatment options, the lack of good evidence for both when to treat cardiovascular compromise and whether treatment benefits the long-term outcome of infants underlies this uncertainty. This chapter explores the importance of the unique changes involved in the transitional circulation during the first postnatal day and how they impact the presentation, assessment, and management of neonatal cardiovascular compromise.

Definition of Hypotension and Its Relationship to Low Systemic Perfusion

The definition of normal blood pressure and hypotension is discussed in detail in Chapter 3. This chapter will focus on the relevance of these definitions to the VLBW infant. Hypotension can be defined as the blood pressure value where vital organ (brain) blood flow autoregulation is lost. If effective treatment is not initiated at this point, blood pressure may further decrease and reach a "functional threshold" when neuronal function is impaired, and then the "ischemic threshold" resulting in tissue ischemia with likely permanent organ damage.[9] Neither the blood pressure causing loss of autoregulation nor the critical blood pressure resulting in direct tissue damage has been clearly defined for the VLBW neonate in the immediate postnatal period.[10] The distinction between the three levels of hypotension is important, because although loss of autoregulation and cellular function *may* predispose to brain injury, reaching the ischemic threshold of hypotension by definition *is associated with direct tissue damage.* Finally, these thresholds may be affected by several factors, including gestational and postmenstrual age, the duration of hypotension, and the presence of acidosis and/or infection. Furthermore, these thresholds are thought to be specific to the individual patient and are affected by the neonate's ability to compensate in order to maintain adequate oxygen delivery to the organs (see Chapters 1 and 21).

Although the normal autoregulatory blood pressure range in the VLBW infant is not known, in clinical practice there are generally two definitions of early hypotension in widespread use:

- Mean blood pressure less than 30 mm Hg in any gestation infant in the first postnatal days. This definition is based on pathophysiologic associations between cerebral injury (white matter damage or intraventricular hemorrhage) and mean blood pressure less than 30 mm Hg,[11,12] and to a lesser degree on more recent data looking at the maintenance of cerebral blood flow (CBF) measured by near-infrared spectroscopy (NIRS)[13,14] and single-photon emission computed tomography (SPECT)[15] over a range of blood pressures, suggesting a reduction in CBF when a particular (28 to 30 mm Hg) mean blood pressure threshold is reached. It is important to note that although the 10th centile for infants of all GAs is at or above 30 mm Hg by the third postnatal day, in more immature infants, the 10th centile of mean blood pressure is lower than 30 mm Hg during the first 3 days.[16] Therefore it is too simplistic to use a single cutoff value for blood pressure across a range of gestational and postnatal ages.
- Mean blood pressure less than the GA in weeks during the first postnatal days, which roughly correlates with the 10th centile for age in tables of normative data.[11,17] This statistical definition has also been supported by professional body guidelines such as the Joint Working Group of the British Association of Perinatal Medicine.[18] Again this rule of thumb applies mainly in the first 24 to 48 hours of extrauterine life; after this time there is a gradual increase in the expected mean blood pressure such that most premature infants have a mean blood pressure greater than 30 mm Hg and thus above GA by postnatal day 3 (Chapter 3).[17]

The current definitions are not related to physiologic endpoints such as maintenance of organ blood flow or tissue oxygen delivery. However, most but not all studies using ^{133}Xe clearance, SPECT, or NIRS to assess changes in CBF found that the lower limit of the autoregulatory blood pressure range may be around 30 mm Hg, even in the 1-day-old ELBW neonate.[14,15,19-21] Indeed, preterm neonates with a mean blood pressure at or above 30 mm Hg appear to have intact static autoregulation of their CBF during the first postnatal day.[22] It is reasonable to assume that although the GA-equivalent blood pressure value is below the CBF autoregulatory range, this value is still higher than the suspected ischemic blood pressure threshold for the VLBW patient population.[21]

A confounding finding to the straightforward-appearing blood pressure-CBF relationship has been provided by a series of studies using SVC flow measurements to indirectly assess brain perfusion in the VLBW neonate with a focus on the ELBW infant in the immediate postnatal period.[5,23] The findings of these studies suggest that, in the ELBW neonate, blood pressure in the normal range may not always guarantee normal vital organ (brain) blood flow. Although caution is needed when interpreting these findings, as only approximately 30% of the blood in the SVC represents the blood coming back from the brain, in the preterm neonate (Chapter 2), animal and additional human data support this notion (see Chapter 6). In the compensated phase of shock, redistribution of blood flow from the nonvital organs (e.g., muscle, skin, kidneys, intestine, etc.) to the vital organs (brain, heart, adrenals), as well as neuroendocrine compensatory and local vascular mechanisms, ensure that blood pressure and organ blood flow to the vital organs are maintained within the normal range. With progression of the condition, shock enters its uncompensated phase, and blood pressure, vital organ perfusion and oxygen delivery also decrease. Since the immature myocardium of the ELBW neonate may not be able to compensate for the sudden increase in peripheral vascular resistance immediately following delivery, cardiac output may fall.[23,24] Yet despite the decrease in cardiac output, many ELBW neonates maintain their blood pressure in the normal range by redistributing blood flow to the organs that are vital at that particular developmental stage (see Chapter 6). As referred to earlier, data suggest that the rapidly developing cerebral cortex and white matter of the ELBW neonate have not yet reached vital organ assignments with appropriately developed vasodilatory responses when perfusion falls.[20,23,24] However, by the second to third postnatal days, forebrain vascular response matures and normal blood pressure is more likely to be associated with normal brain and systemic blood flow.[23,24]

26

The molecular mechanisms by which the vasculature of the cerebral cortex and white matter of the ELBW neonate mature rapidly and become "high-priority" vascular beds soon after delivery are unknown.[24,25]

The Transitional Circulation in the Very Low Birth Weight Infant

The traditional understanding of the changes occurring in the transitional circulation of the preterm infant suggests that atrial and ductal shunts in the first postnatal hours are of little significance and are bidirectional or primarily right to left in direction as a result of the higher pulmonary vascular resistance expected in the newborn premature infant.[26] In contrast to this understanding, longitudinal studies using bedside noninvasive ultrasound show significant variability in the time taken for the preterm infant to transition from the in-utero right ventricle (RV)-dominant, low resistance circulation to the biventricular, higher resistance postnatal circulation. Shortly after delivery, the severing of the umbilical vessels, the inflation of the lungs with air, and the associated changes in oxygenation lead to a sudden increase in resistance in the systemic circulation and a lowering of resistance in the pulmonary circulation. Cardiac output now passes in a parallel fashion through the pulmonary and the systemic circulation, except for the blood flow shunting through the closing fetal channels. The role of placental transfusion and the timing of cord clamp and how this affects transitional hemodynamics is discussed in Chapters 4 and 5.

In healthy term infants, the ductus arteriosus is functionally closed by the second postnatal day and the right ventricular pressure usually falls to adult levels by about 2 to 3 days after birth.[27,28] This constriction and functional closure of the ductus arteriosus is then followed by anatomical closure over the next 2 to 3 weeks. In contrast, in the VLBW infant there is frequently a failure of complete closure of both the foramen ovale and the ductus arteriosus in the expected time frame, probably due to structural immaturity and the immaturity of the mechanisms involved.[29,30] The persistence of the fetal channels in the setting of decreasing pulmonary pressures leads to blood flowing preferentially from the aorta to the pulmonary artery, resulting in a relative loss of blood from the systemic circulation and pulmonary circulatory overload. Contrary to traditional understanding, this systemic to pulmonary shunting can occur as early as the first postnatal hours, with recirculation of 50% or more of the normal cardiac output back into the lungs.[31] The myocardium subsequently attempts to compensate by increasing the total cardiac output. There can be up to a twofold increase in the left ventricular (LV) output by 1 hour of age, resulting primarily from an increased stroke volume, rather than increased heart rate.[32] A significant proportion of this increased blood flow is likely to be passing through the ductus arteriosus.[33] There is a wide range of early ductal constriction, with some infants able to effectively close or minimize the size of the ductus arteriosus within a few hours of birth, while others achieve an initial constriction followed by an increase in size of the ductus, and yet another group having a persistent large ductus arteriosus with no evidence of early constriction and subsequent limitation of shunt size.[34] Pulmonary blood flow can be more than twice the systemic blood flow as early as the first few postnatal hours, which may be enough to cause clinical effects, such as reduced systemic blood pressure and blood flow, increases in ventilatory requirements, or even pulmonary hemorrhagic edema.[34]

In utero, the fetal communications of the foramen ovale and ductus arteriosus result in a lack of separation between the left and right ventricular outputs, making it difficult to quantitate their individual contributions. In addition to heart rate, the ventricular systolic function is determined by the physiologic principles of preload (distension of the ventricle by blood prior to contraction), contractility (the intrinsic ability of the myocardial fibers to contract), and afterload (the combined resistance of the blood, the ventricular walls, and the vascular beds). The myocardium of the VLBW infant is less mature than that of a term infant with fewer mitochondria and less energy stores. This results in a limitation in the ability to respond to changes in the determinants of the cardiac output, in particular the afterload.[35,36] Consequently the myocardium of the VLBW infant, just like the fetal myocardium, is likely to be less able to respond to stresses that occur in the postnatal period, such as increased peripheral vascular resistance with the resultant increase in afterload. There is a significant

26

difference in the influence of determinants of cardiac output in the newborn premature infant with a dramatically increased afterload and changes in the preload caused by the inflation of the lungs. Furthermore, the effect of lung inflation on preload is different when lung inflation occurs by positive pressure ventilation rather than by the negative intrathoracic pressures generated by spontaneous breathing. The newborn ventricle is more sensitive to changes in the afterload, such that small changes can have large effects, especially if the preload and contractility are not optimized.[35]

Failure of the normal transitional changes to occur in a timely manner can result in impairment of cardiac function, leading to low cardiac output states and hypotension in the VLBW infant. As oxygen delivery is primarily related to the oxygen carrying capacity and the oxygen content of the blood and the volume of blood flow to the organ, delivery of oxygen to vital organs may be impaired where there is cardiovascular impairment.[37] Therefore the timely identification and appropriate management of early low cardiac output states and hypotension are of vital importance in the overall care of the VLBW infant.

Physiologic Determinants of the Blood Pressure in the Very Low Birth Weight Infant

The product of cardiac output and peripheral vascular resistance determines arterial blood pressure. The main influences on the cardiac output are the preload or blood volume and myocardial contractility. The peripheral vascular resistance is determined by the vascular tone, which in the presence of an unconstricted ductus arteriosus may not only be the systemic peripheral vascular resistance, but is also contributed to by the pulmonary vascular resistance. Myocardial contractility is difficult to assess in the newborn, as the accepted measures of contractility in the adult, such as the echocardiographic measure of fractional shortening, are adversely influenced by the asymmetry of the ventricles caused by the in utero right ventricular dominance. In this regard, the use of load-independent measures of cardiac contractility, such as mean velocity of fractional shortening or LV wall stress indices, may provide more useful information (Chapters 10 and 11; Fig. 26.2).[38] Some studies have found a

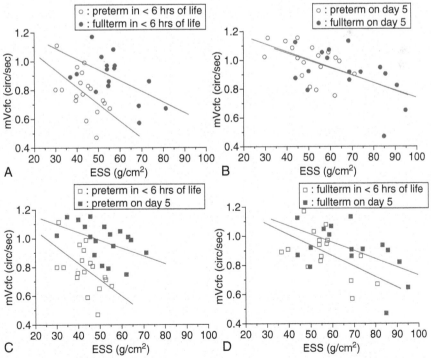

Fig. 26.2 Relationship between mean velocity of circumferential fiber shortening (mVcfs) and end-systolic wall stress (ESS) at <6 hours of age and on Day 5 in preterm and term infants demonstrating the different characteristics of this relationship with both postnatal age and maturity. (Reproduced with permission from Takahashi Y, Harada K, Kishkurno S, et al.: Postnatal left ventricular contractility in very low birth weight infants, *Pediatr Cardiol* 18(2):112–117, 1997.)

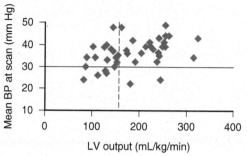

Fig. 26.3 The weak relationship between mean systemic blood pressure (BP) and simultaneously measured left ventricular (LV) output. Some infants with a mean BP greater than 30 mm Hg have critically low cardiac output (<150 mL/kg/min) and conversely some infants with normal LV output have low mean blood pressure. (Reproduced with permission from Kluckow M, Evans N: Relationship between blood pressure and cardiac output in preterm infants requiring mechanical ventilation. *J Pediatr* 129:506–512, 1996.)

relationship between myocardial dysfunction and hypotension in the preterm infant while others have not, even though a similar measurement method was used. Blood volume correlates poorly with blood pressure in hypotensive neonates.[39-42] Due to the unique characteristics of the newborn cardiovascular system discussed earlier, systemic blood pressure is closely related to changes in the systemic vascular resistance. As systemic vascular resistance cannot be measured directly, the measurement of cardiac output or systemic blood flow becomes an essential element in understanding the dynamic changes occurring in the cardiovascular system of the VLBW infant.

In the absence of simple techniques to measure cardiac output and systemic vascular resistance (Chapter 21), clinicians have tended to rely on blood pressure as the sole assessment of circulatory compromise. However, in the VLBW neonate with a closed ductus arteriosus during the first 24 to 48 hours, there is only a weak relationship between mean blood pressure and cardiac output (Fig. 26.3).[40] Relying on measurements of blood pressure alone can lead the clinician to make assumptions about the underlying physiology of the cardiovascular system that may be incorrect, especially during the period of early transition with the fetal channels open (Chapter 3). Indeed, many hypotensive preterm infants potentially have a normal or high LV output.[40,43,44] One of the reasons for this apparent paradox relates to the presence of a hemodynamically significant ductus arteriosus, which causes an increase in LV output while also causing a reduction in the overall systemic vascular resistance. In addition, variations in the peripheral vascular resistance may cause a change in the underlying cardiac output that does not affect the blood pressure. This phenomenon makes it possible for two infants with the same blood pressure to have markedly different cardiac outputs. Thus the physiologic determinants of blood pressure may affect the blood pressure in multiple ways—acting via an effect on cardiac performance and thus cardiac output, altering the vascular resistance, or sometimes altering both.

Clinical Determinants of Blood Pressure in the Very Low Birth Weight Infant

Gestational Age and Postnatal Age

Both GA and postnatal age are major determinants of the systemic blood pressure, as can be seen by examining nomograms and tables of normal blood pressure data (see Chapter 3). Generally, blood pressure is higher in more mature infants and progressively increases with advancing postnatal age. The reasons why blood pressure increases with postnatal age are unclear but are probably related to changes in the underlying vascular tone, mediated by various humoral regulators and possibly the upregulation of receptors involved in myocardial responses. Simultaneously, there are temporal physical changes in the transitional circulation, such as closure of the ductus arteriosus, which will affect both blood pressure and blood flow.

Use of Antenatal Glucocorticoid Therapy

There is evidence that sick VLBW infants have relative adrenal insufficiency and that this condition may be one of the underlying causes of cardiovascular dysfunction, with the propensity to inflammation in these patients contributing to the pathogenesis of clinical conditions such as bronchopulmonary dysplasia.[45-47] Low cortisol levels have been documented in hypotensive infants requiring cardiovascular support.[48] The use of antenatal glucocorticoids to assist in fetal lung maturation may therefore have an additional effect of improving neonatal blood pressure. Likely mechanisms for this effect include the acceleration of adrenergic receptor expression and maturation of myocardial structure and function. The enhanced adrenergic receptor expression also increases the sensitivity of the myocardium and peripheral vasculature to endogenous catecholamines.[49] Randomized controlled trials of the use of antenatal glucocorticoids have shown variable effects on the neonatal blood pressure. In some trials, there was an increase in the mean blood pressure of VLBW infants in the treated group, with a decreased need for cardiovascular support, while others have shown little difference between the mean blood pressures of infants whose mothers did or did not receive antenatal steroids.[50-53]

Blood Loss

Acute blood loss in the VLBW infant is unusual and can result from prenatal events such as fetomaternal hemorrhage; antepartum hemorrhage or twin-twin transfusion syndrome; or intrapartum events such as a tight nuchal cord, resulting in an imbalance between blood flow to and from the fetus or postnatally from a large subgaleal hematoma or hemorrhage into an organ such as the liver or brain. Acute blood loss can result in significant hypotension, but due to the immediate compensatory mechanisms of the cardiovascular system, this effect may be delayed. Similarly, a drop in the infant's hemoglobin level can also be delayed following significant acute hemorrhage.

Timing of Umbilical Cord Clamp

Both the volume of placental transfusion and the normal sequence of the transition can be affected by the timing of the clamping of the umbilical cord, with later clamping being associated with a smoother hemodynamic transition (at least in an animal model),[54] increased systemic blood pressure, and decreased need for cardiovascular support and blood transfusions.[55] An emerging concept of placental blood volume restoration is intriguing, whereby the perceived placental transfusion of "extra" blood is actually a rebalancing of the plasma volume lost due to the physiologically increased capillary permeability during labor, the blood volume lost into the placenta during labor and delivery, and the effect of immediate cord clamping on the "rebalancing" process itself. Indeed, immediate clamping of the cord deprives the preterm infant of the placental transfusion, and thus of the return to normal blood volume, and renders the infant hemodynamically vulnerable (see Chapter 4 for details).

Positive Pressure Ventilation

Many VLBW infants are exposed to positive pressure respiratory support in the first postnatal days. Positive end-expiratory pressure (PEEP) or nasal continuous positive airway pressure is often utilized to reduce the atelectasis resulting from the collapse of unstable alveoli when surfactant is lacking, particularly in more immature infants. Although surfactant deficiency is the main reason for the provision of positive pressure support in preterm neonates, other conditions such as sepsis, pneumonia, and immaturity of the lungs without surfactant deficiency also benefit from positive pressure support. The use of high ventilation pressures in the premature infant, especially with improving lung compliance, can result in secondary interference with cardiac function. Function can be impaired by a reduction in the preload from reduced systemic or pulmonary venous return, and/or direct compression of cardiac chambers, also resulting in a reduced stroke volume or an increase in afterload. This latter scenario is particularly concerning for the RV and may reduce cardiac output.[56] As the right and left sides of the heart are connected in series, a reduction in the RV output will in turn result in a reduction in the LV cardiac output.

Studies in VLBW infants have shown a fall-off in the systemic oxygen delivery if the PEEP was greater than 6 cm of water and a reduction in the cardiac output at a PEEP level of 9 cm water in mechanically ventilated infants.[57] However, as these findings were not normalized for lung compliance, their generalizability requires caution. A study of VLBW infants (mean GA 29 weeks) before and during treatment with mechanical ventilation for severe respiratory distress syndrome demonstrated a reduction in LV dimensions and filling rate, with a resultant decrease in the cardiac output by about 40% compared with control values. The addition of a packed cell blood transfusion prevented the decrease in ventricular size and reduction in cardiac output.[58] The blood pressure did not change significantly in the group where cardiac output dropped. In longitudinal clinical studies of blood pressure and blood flow, mean airway pressure has a consistently negative influence on both mean blood pressure and systemic blood flow.[23,40,59,60] Consequently, careful titration of the positive pressure to the underlying respiratory pathology is essential; however, more recent clinical studies have failed to demonstrate clinically relevant decreases in blood flow in the conventional range of pressure support.[61,62]

Patent Ductus Arteriosus (see Chapter 22)

A patent ductus arteriosus (PDA) may not be recognized clinically in the first days after delivery, as the flow through it is generally not turbulent and therefore no murmur is audible.[63] Despite this, the flow is almost always left-to-right or bidirectional, with a predominantly left-to-right pattern.[31] A PDA is usually thought to be associated with a low diastolic blood pressure, but some data suggest that it can be associated with both low diastolic and systolic blood pressure, making a PDA one of the possible causes of systemic hypotension.[64] As clinical detection of a PDA in the first postnatal days is difficult, cardiac ultrasound is required for early diagnosis.[63] The classic clinical signs of a murmur, bounding pulses, and a hyperdynamic precordium usually become evident only after the third postnatal day, making clinical detection much more accurate at that time.[63]

Calculated Systemic Vascular Resistance

There is a reciprocal relationship between the systemic vascular resistance and cardiac output in the healthy term, preterm, and sick ventilated infant.[65] This relationship is particularly important when considering the use of vasopressor-inotropes such as dopamine in preterm infants, where an increase in the peripheral vascular resistance can increase the blood pressure but have no impact on or even decrease the cardiac output.[66] The peripheral resistance varies markedly in the preterm infant and can be affected by numerous factors, including environmental temperature; carbon dioxide level; the maturity of the sympathoadrenal system; patency of the ductus arteriosus; presence of vasoactive substances such as catecholamines, prostacyclin, and nitric oxide; and sepsis.[34,65,67] It is important to note that in patients with a PDA the left ventricle is exposed to the combined pulmonary and systemic vascular resistance. The potential variability of the peripheral resistance in VLBW infants means that significant changes in cardiac output or blood flow cannot be identified by measurement of the systemic blood pressure alone.

Assessment of Cardiovascular Compromise in the Shocked Very Low Birth Weight Infant

Because of the wide variation in blood pressure levels at varying gestations and postnatal ages, some authors have cautioned against the simplicity of just treating low BP alone, but suggest that the clinician should look for some other evidence of hypoperfusion, such as decreased capillary return, oliguria, or metabolic acidosis.[68,69] The assessment of cardiovascular adequacy (i.e., tissue oxygen delivery in the VLBW infant) is more of a challenge than in infants and adults. Measures of cardiovascular function used in these groups, such as pulmonary wedge pressure, central venous pressure, and cardiac output measured via thermodilution, are impractical in the preterm infant due to their size and fragility and the frequent presence of cardiac shunting. Assessment usually consists of a mainly clinical appraisal of the perfusion via capillary refill time (CRT) and urine output, and the documentation of the pulse rate and blood pressure. The acid-base balance and evidence of lactic acidosis are further important adjuncts to this assessment, but unless serum lactate levels are serially monitored, changes in pH and base deficit may be misleading due to increased bicarbonate losses through the immature kidneys. Indeed, all of these parameters present specific limitations in the newborn' and particularly in the VLBW infant.

Capillary Refill Time

CRT is a widely used proxy of both cardiac output and peripheral resistance in neonates, and normal values have been documented for this group of infants.[70] A number of confounding factors lead to the CRT being potentially inaccurate, and these include the different techniques used (sites tested and pressing time), interobserver variability, ambient temperature, medications, and maturity of skin blood flow control mechanisms (see Chapter 19).[71] In addition, even in older children receiving intensive care, there is only a weak relationship between the CRT and other hemodynamic measures such as the stroke volume index.[72] A study investigating the relationship between a measure of systemic blood flow (SVC flow) and CRT in VLBW infants showed that a CRT of ≥3 seconds had only 55% sensitivity and 81% specificity for predicting low systemic blood flow. However, a markedly increased CRT of 4 seconds or more was more closely correlated with low blood flow states.[73]

Urine Output

Following urine output is useful in the assessment of cardiovascular well-being in the adult; however, the immature renal tubule in VLBW infants is inefficient at concentrating the urine and therefore has an impaired capacity to appropriately adjust urine osmolality and flow in the face of high serum osmolality.[74] As a result, even if the glomerular filtration rate is decreased markedly, there can be little change in urine output. In addition, the significant physiological decrease in urine output immediately after delivery further compromises our ability to appropriately assess the adequacy of urine output in the neonate. Finally, accurate measurement of urine output is not easy in VLBW infants, generally requiring collection via a urinary catheter or via a collection bag, both techniques being invasive with significant potential complications, and thus infrequently done in regular clinical practice.

Pulse Rate

A rising pulse rate is usually indicative of hypovolemia in the adult. The mechanism relies on a mature autonomic nervous system, with detection of reduced blood volume and then blood pressure via baroreceptors and subsequent increase in the heart rate in an attempt to sustain appropriate cardiac output. Neonates, especially preterm infants, have a faster baseline heart rate and an immature myocardium and autonomic nervous system, affecting the cardiovascular response to hypovolemia. There are many other influences on the heart rate in the immediate postnatal period, so it cannot be relied upon as an accurate assessment of cardiovascular status.

Metabolic Acidosis/Lactic Acidosis

After exhaustion of all compensatory mechanisms (Chapter 2), tissue hypoxia due to low arterial oxygen tension, inadequate systemic and organ blood flow, or a combination of these two factors, results in a switch to anaerobic metabolism at the cellular level. Reduced systemic blood flow may therefore result in an increase in the serum lactate. A combined lactate value of more than 4 mmol with prolonged CRT of more than 4 seconds predicts low SVC flow with 97% specificity.[75] Serum lactate levels have been correlated with illness severity and mortality in critically ill adults and in ventilated neonates with respiratory distress syndrome.[76-83] The normal lactate level in this group of infants is less than 2.5 mmol/L, and there is an association with mortality as the serum lactate level increases above this threshold.[81,82]

Blood Pressure (see Chapter 3)

Invasive measurement of the arterial blood pressure using a fluid-filled catheter and pressure transducer is usually performed either via an indwelling umbilical artery catheter in the descending aorta or a peripherally-placed arterial catheter. There is a strong correlation between blood pressure obtained via a peripheral artery catheter and that obtained via the umbilical artery.[84] The agreement between direct and indirect (noninvasive) measures of blood pressure is generally also good.[85-90] However, the noninvasive technique is more problematic in the VLBW infant, as it is more dependent on choice of the appropriate cuff size and is noncontinuous.[91] In the newborn, a cuff width-to-arm ratio between 0.45 and 0.55 increases the accuracy of indirect blood pressure measurements when compared with direct measures.[16] Accuracy of invasive blood pressure measurement is dependent on proper use of the equipment, including accurate placement of the transducer at the level of the heart, proper calibration of the system, and avoidance of blockages, air bubbles, or blood clots in the catheter line. With the increased use of noninvasive respiratory support, even in the smallest infants access to invasive blood pressure is becoming less common, resulting in the need for other ways to assess perfusion and cardiovascular adequacy.

Cardiac Output (see Chapter 14)

Invasive hemodynamic measures such as pulmonary artery thermodilution and mixed venous oxygen saturation monitoring are commonly used in adult intensive care to allow accurate and continuous assessment of the cardiovascular system. The size of both term and preterm infants with the associated difficulty of placing intracardiac catheters has precluded the use of such measures, especially in the group of infants less than 30 weeks' gestation. Another issue specific to premature infants is the potential inaccuracy of the dye dilution and thermodilution method in the presence of intracardiac shunts through the ductus arteriosus and the foramen ovale. Noninvasive methods of measuring cardiac output particularly Doppler ultrasound have become more popular, aided by improvements in image resolution and reductions in ultrasound transducer size. Doppler ultrasound was first used to noninvasively measure the cardiac output in neonates in 1982 and subsequently has been validated against more invasive techniques in children, neonates, and VLBW infants.[92,93] The expected coefficient of variation using Doppler compares favorably to that of indicator-dilution and thermodilution. Chapter 14 reviews other novel approaches such as impedance electrical cardiometry for the continuous beat-to-beat assessment of stroke volume and cardiac output in detail. Finally, another newer modality for measuring cardiac output is functional cardiac magnetic resonance imaging (MRI), which is envisaged to be predominantly a research tool at present (see Chapter 15).[94]

Monitoring of Peripheral and Mucosal Blood Flow

Laser Doppler and visible light technology (T-Stat) are techniques currently being assessed for usefulness in directly assessing systemic vascular resistance in neonates.[95,96] These techniques are further considered in Chapter 19.

Pulse Oximeter Derived Perfusion Index

The perfusion index is derived from the plethysmographic signal of a pulse oximeter, using a ratio of the pulsatile component (arterial) and the nonpulsatile components of the light reaching the detector. The perfusion index is measured noninvasively, displayed continuously, and subsequently has potential as a marker of low systemic blood flow. Several studies have validated the perfusion index against other measures of systemic blood flow, including SVC flow, and found it to be reasonably predictive of low flow states.[97] More recently, statistical analysis methods have been used to more carefully assess the quantitative features of the perfusion index signal in the first 24 postnatal hours and relate these to adverse outcomes.[98]

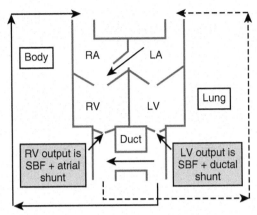

26

Fig. 26.4 Diagram demonstrating the points where right (RV) and left ventricular (LV) output are measured using Doppler ultrasound. The RV output will consist of the combined systemic venous return and any left-to-right shunting across the foramen ovale. The LV output will consist of the total pulmonary venous return and the blood destined to cross the ductus arteriosus. *LA*, Left atrium; *RA*, right atrium; *SBF*, systemic blood flow. (Reprinted with permission from Kluckow M, Evans N: Low systemic blood flow in the preterm infant. *Semin Neonatol* 6:75–84, 2001.)

Systemic Blood Flow

As discussed earlier, normal mean blood pressure does not guarantee normal LV output or CBF in preterm infants, even in the subgroup in whom the ductus arteriosus has closed (see Fig. 26.3).[24,40,44] Further problems arise in assessing systemic blood flow in the preterm infant, as a result of failure or delay of the normal circulatory transition and closure of the fetal channels. Indeed, the assumption that the LV and RV outputs are identical is often incorrect in the VLBW infant. Also, as discussed earlier, increased blood flowing through the PDA (ductal shunt) will be reflected in an increased LV output, and the blood flowing left-to-right through a patent foramen ovale (atrial shunt) will be reflected in an increased RV output (Fig. 26.4).[34]

Systemic blood flow falls dramatically in many extremely premature infants in the first hours after delivery, and this reduction in flow is usually associated with an increase in peripheral vascular resistance. A substantial proportion of these infants will initially have a "normal" blood pressure (i.e., they are in "compensated shock"; see Chapter 1). Of the VLBW infants who initially develop low systemic blood flow, about 80% will subsequently develop systemic hypotension. Accordingly, utilizing hypotension to direct cardiovascular interventions results in a considerable delay in identifying infants with low systemic blood flow and in some infants with low systemic blood flow not being recognized at all. Hypotension may also be associated with normal or even a high systemic blood flow, as frequently occurs in the preterm infant with persisting hypotension after the first postnatal days or those with "hyperdynamic" sepsis.[99] These infants generally have low systemic vascular resistance with peripheral vasodilation.

Short- and Long-Term Effects of Cardiovascular Compromise/Shock in the Very Low Birth Weight Infant

An important aim of intensive care management in VLBW infants is the maintenance of tissue oxygenation and the avoidance of impaired cerebral perfusion. CBF, which is an important determinant of cerebral oxygen delivery, is determined by the relationship of cerebral perfusion pressure, systemic blood flow, and the vascular resistance of the cerebral circulation. The process of cerebral autoregulation allows maintenance of a constant CBF in the face of variations in the blood pressure, systemic blood flow, and resistance within the autoregulatory range of mean blood pressure (see Chapter 2 for details). There is evidence that sick preterm infants may have impaired or lost CBF autoregulation, resulting in a pressure-passive cerebral circulation mirroring fluctuations in blood pressure.[100] Accordingly, CBF is low when there is systemic hypotension.[100] However, we do not know where the blood pressure lower elbow of the CBF autoregulatory curve is in preterm neonates (Chapter 2). It is also unclear at what level of hypotension ischemic tissue damage occurs. Interestingly, cerebral fractional oxygen extraction is not related to blood pressure until very low levels (<20 mm Hg) of mean blood pressure, suggesting that sufficient oxygen to meet cerebral demand can be delivered, even in the presence of hypotension (Chapters 2, 6 and 7).[24,37,101,102] This finding supports the concept that there is a difference between the autoregulatory and ischemic threshold of blood pressure, with the latter being reached only when increasing fractional cerebral oxygen extraction cannot compensate for the decreased oxygen delivery anymore. However, because of the differences among infants in their ability to compensate for the decreases in perfusion pressure and/or systemic blood flow, a single blood pressure value cannot be used to define the ischemic threshold for preterm infants, even with the same gestational and postnatal age (Chapters 2 and 21).

Several studies have suggested that autoregulation is intact in many preterm babies but appears to be compromised in a subgroup who seem to be at particularly high risk of peri/intraventricular hemorrhage (P/IVH).[103,104] High coherence between mean arterial blood pressure and measures of CBF/oxygenation indicates impaired cerebral autoregulation and is associated with subgroup of preterm infants at high risk of adverse outcome.[105] It has been suggested that infants suffering severe P/IVH are more likely to have blood-pressure-passive changes in CBF and oxygenation in the first postnatal days.[11-14,104]

Peri/Intraventricular Hemorrhage

A number of studies have described associations between low mean blood pressure and subsequent P/IVH, and neurological injury (see Chapters 3 and 6).[11,12,106-109] It was these observations of an association between systemic blood pressure and cerebral injury that led to current recommendations for the treatment of blood pressure. However, a large population-based study has not found systemic hypotension to be an independent risk factor for P/IVH in VLBW infants.[110] Importantly, there is no evidence from appropriately-designed, prospective, controlled clinical trials that the treatment of hypotension decreases the incidence of P/IVH and neurological injury. Further studies designed to establish or refute causation are ongoing, including the HIP (hypotension in prematurity) trial.

Periventricular Leukomalacia

The potential relationship between low CBF and white matter injury due to the specific vulnerability of the periventricular white matter in the preterm infant has led to concerns that hypotension may be a precursor of white matter injury. Observational data again have shown a relationship between hypotension (often mean arterial blood pressure below 30 mm Hg) and adverse cranial ultrasound findings.[12] However, as with P/IVH, larger population-based studies have failed to identify systemic hypotension as an independent risk factor for white matter injury.[111,112] It is conceivable that the pathogenesis of periventricular leukomalacia, just like that of P/IVH, is multifactorial, and in addition to changes in cerebral perfusion pressure, factors such as specific or nonspecific inflammation and oxidant injury play a significant role in its development. The relationship between hemodynamics and brain injury is further explored in Chapters 6 and 7.

Long-Term Neurodevelopmental Outcome

Hypotension in VLBW infants has been correlated with longer-term adverse neurodevelopmental outcome (see Chapter 3).[108,109,113,114] There are no prospective studies evaluating the effect of untreated hypotension on any important long-term outcomes; however, there is a prospective study showing that hypotensive preterm infants had a significant increase in adverse neurodevelopmental outcome at term.[115] Several retrospective studies have raised the possibility that preterm infants treated for hypotension may have a worse outcome than untreated infants—it is unclear whether the effect is due to the treatment or other factors associated with hypotension.[69,109,116] Of note is that assessing all hypotensive patients as one group, regardless of their initial underlying physiology or response to treatment, is a significant further limitation of the retrospective studies. Interestingly, the findings of the only prospective randomized clinical trial addressing this issue revealed that hypotensive preterm VLBW neonates had a higher rate of severe P/IVH compared with nonhypotensive controls.[116] However, the outcome of the hypotensive preterm neonates who responded to dopamine or epinephrine with an increase in blood pressure during the first postnatal day was the same as in the controls. Furthermore, there was no association between abnormal ultrasound findings and the use of vasopressors/inotropes. Finally, at 2- to 3-year follow-up, there was no difference in the rate of abnormal neurological outcome between survivors of the hypotensive and control groups. Although these findings provide some reassurance about the safety and potential benefits of vasopressors/inotropes for the treatment of early hypotension in VLBW neonates, the small sample size and the lack of an "untreated hypotensive group" limit the generalizability of the findings of this study.[116] In support of the latter findings, a recent retrospetive multicenter study (EPIPAGE 2) found that antihypotensive treatment was associated with higher survival without major morbidity and lower incidence of central nervous system abnormalities compared to untreated matched controls.[117]

A study of systemic blood flow in VLBW infants demonstrated an independent relationship between low systemic blood flow (particularly the duration of the insult) and adverse neurodevelopmental outcome at 3 years of age.[118]

Treatment Options in the Management of Cardiovascular Compromise/Shock in the Very Low Birth Weight Infant

The appropriate management of cardiovascular compromise/shock in the VLBW infant will vary according to the underlying physiology. The clinician must take into account a number of possible factors, including the infant's GA, postnatal age, measures of cardiovascular adequacy (such as cardiac output or systemic blood flow if available), and associated pathologic conditions. An early cardiac ultrasound can assist greatly in the diagnostic process by providing information about the presence, size, and direction of the ductus arteriosus shunt; presence of pulmonary hypertension; assessment of cardiac contractility; adequacy of venous filling; and measurement of cardiac output or systemic blood flow (Chapter 10).

Before instituting specific treatment for hypotension, potentially reversible causes such as a measurement error (transducer height in comparison to patient's right atrium, calibration of the transducer, air bubble, or blood clot in the measurement catheter), PDA, hypovolemia from blood or fluid loss, pneumothorax, use of excessive mean airway pressure, sepsis, and adrenal insufficiency should be considered and managed appropriately. Therapeutic options that have a cardiovascular physiologic basis for efficacy and have been subjected to clinical trial include volume loading (with crystalloid or colloid), vasopressor/inotropes and inotropic agents, hydrocortisone, and other glucocorticoids. Further details regarding the hemodynamically-based management of circulatory compromise and shock in the ELBW infant are reviewed in Chapter 29.

Conclusion

The appropriate assessment and treatment of the VLBW infant with cardiovascular impairment or shock requires the clinician to obtain adequate information about the etiology and underlying physiologic determinants of the condition. The clinician should be aware of the physiologic changes that occur in areas such as myocardial function and vital organ blood flow allocation in the first postnatal days. An understanding of the actions of the therapeutic options available and the specific effects of these treatments on the circulation of the VLBW infant is also important. The addition of a cardiac ultrasound to the assessment process provides information about the

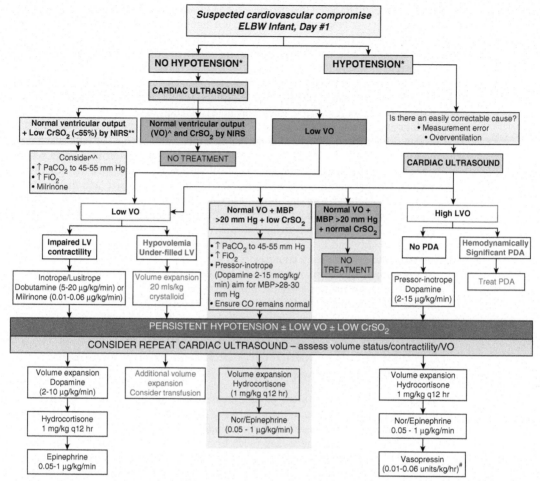

Fig. 26.5 Treatment of cardiovascular compromise based on assessment of blood pressure, cardiac ultrasound, and near-infrared spectroscopy (NIRS). *, Definition of hypotension per agreed upon criteria. **, Using NIRS with proposed cut-off value below which brain injury is more frequent.[119] ^, Use left VO in the absence of significant left-to-right PDA shunting; use right VO if significant left-to-right PDA shunting and insignificant foramen ovale shunting is present. ^^, Consideration based on recent data to be confirmed.[120,121] #, Vasopressin dose recommendation as per Rios and Kaiser.[122] *CO*, Cardiac output; *CrSO2*, cerebral tissue O_2 saturation; *ELBW*, extremely low birth weight; *FIO2*, fraction of inspired oxygen; *hr*, hour; *LV*, left ventricle; *LVO*, left ventricular output; *MBP*, mean blood pressure; *PaCO2*, arterial partial pressure of CO_2; *PDA*, patent ductus arteriosus; *VO*, ventricular output. (Structure originally adapted from Subhedar NV.[123])

size and shunt direction of the ductus arteriosus, the function of the myocardium and its filling, as well as the cardiac output and calculated peripheral vascular resistance. Fig. 26.5 summarizes the approach to management of hypotension in the ELBW infant using the additional information provided by ultrasound and NIRS.

REFERENCES

1. Al Aweel I, Pursley DM, Rubin LP, et al.: Variations in prevalence of hypotension, hypertension, and vasopressor use in NICUs, *J Perinatol* 21(5):272–278, 2001.
2. Laughon M, Bose C, Clark R: Treatment strategies to prevent or close a patent ductus arteriosus in preterm infants and outcomes, *J Perinatol* 27(3):164–170, 2007.
3. Rios DR, Moffett BS, Kaiser JR: Trends in pharmacotherapy for neonatal hypotension, *J Pediatr* 165(4):697–701.e1, 2014.
4. Stranak Z, Semberova J, Barrington K, et al.: International survey on diagnosis and management of hypotension in extremely preterm babies, *Eur J Pediatr* 173(6):793–798, 2014.
5. Kluckow M, Evans N: Superior vena cava flow in newborn infants: a novel marker of systemic blood flow, *Arch Dis Child Fetal Neonatal Ed* 82(3):F182–F187, 2000.
6. Miletin J, Dempsey EM, Miletin J, et al.: Low superior vena cava flow on day 1 and adverse outcome in the very low birthweight infant, *Arch Dis Child Fetal Neonatal Ed* 93(5):F368–F371, 2008.

7. Paradisis M, Evans N, Kluckow M, et al.: Randomized trial of milrinone versus placebo for prevention of low systemic blood flow in very preterm infants, *J Pediatr* 154(2):189–195, 2009.
8. Laughon M, Bose C, Allred E, et al.: Factors associated with treatment for hypotension in extremely low gestational age newborns during the first postnatal week, *Pediatrics* 119(2):273–280, 2007.
9. McLean CW, Noori S, Cayabyab R, et al.: Cerebral circulation and hypotension in the premature infant- diagnosis and treatment. In Perlman JM, editor: *Questions and controversies in neonatology - neurology*, ed 2, Philadelphia, 2011, Saunders/Elsevier, pp 3–27.
10. Seri I: Circulatory support of the sick preterm infant, *Semin Neonatol* 6(1):85–95, 2001.
11. Watkins AM, West CR, Cooke RW: Blood pressure and cerebral haemorrhage and ischaemia in very low birthweight infants, *Early Hum Dev* 19(2):103–110, 1989.
12. Miall-Allen VM, de Vries LS, Whitelaw AG: Mean arterial blood pressure and neonatal cerebral lesions, *Arch Dis Child* 62(10):1068–1069, 1987.
13. Tsuji M, Saul JP, du PA, et al.: Cerebral intravascular oxygenation correlates with mean arterial pressure in critically ill premature infants, *Pediatrics* 106(4):625–632, 2000.
14. Munro MJ, Walker AM, Barfield CP: Hypotensive extremely low birth weight infants have reduced cerebral blood flow, *Pediatrics* 114(6):1591–1596, 2004.
15. Borch K, Lou HC, Greisen G: Cerebral white matter blood flow and arterial blood pressure in preterm infants, *Acta Paediatr* 99(10):1489–1492, 2010.
16. Nuntnarumit P, Yang W, Bada-Ellzey HS: Blood pressure measurements in the newborn, *Clin Perinatol* 26(4):981–996, 1999.
17. Hegyi T, Carbone MT, Anwar M, et al.: Blood pressure ranges in premature infants. i. the first hours of life, *J Pediatr* 124(4):627–633, 1994.
18. Development of audit measures and guidelines for good practice in the management of neonatal respiratory distress syndrome: report of a joint working group of the British Association of Perinatal Medicine and the research unit of the Royal College of Physicians, *Arch Dis Child* 67(10): 1221–1227, 1992.
19. Greisen G, Borch K: White matter injury in the preterm neonate: the role of perfusion, *Dev Neurosci* 23(3):209–212, 2001.
20. Greisen G: Autoregulation of cerebral blood flow in newborn babies, *Early Hum Dev* 81(5):423–428, 2005.
21. Tyszczuk L, Meek J, Elwell C, et al.: Cerebral blood flow is independent of mean arterial blood pressure in preterm infants undergoing intensive care, *Pediatrics* 102(2 Pt 1):337–341, 1998.
22. Seri I, Abbasi S, Wood DC, et al.: Regional hemodynamic effects of dopamine in the sick preterm neonate, *J Pediatr* 133(6):728–734, 1998.
23. Kluckow M, Evans N: Low superior vena cava flow and intraventricular haemorrhage in preterm infants, *Arch Dis Child Fetal Neonatal Ed* 82:188–194, 2000.
24. Kissack CM, Garr R, Wardle SP, et al.: Cerebral fractional oxygen extraction in very low birth weight infants is high when there is low left ventricular output and hypocarbia but is unaffected by hypotension, *Pediatr Res* 55(3):400–405, 2004.
25. Seri I: Hemodynamics during the first two postnatal days and neurodevelopment in preterm neonates, *J Pediatr* 145:573–575, 2004.
26. Friedman AH, Fahey JT: The transition from fetal to neonatal circulation: normal responses and implications for infants with heart disease, *Semin Perinatol* 17:106–121, 1993.
27. Mahoney LT, Coryell KG, Lauer RM: The newborn transitional circulation: a two-dimensional Doppler echocardiographic study, *J Am Coll Cardiol* 6(3):623–629, 1985.
28. Gentile R, Stevenson G, Dooley T, et al.: Pulsed Doppler echocardiographic determination of time of ductal closure in normal newborn infants, *J Pediatr* 98(3):443–448, 1981.
29. Evans N, Iyer P: Longitudinal changes in the diameter of the ductus arteriosus in ventilated preterm infants: correlation with respiratory outcomes, *Arch Dis Child Fetal Neonatal Ed* 72(3):F156–F161, 1995.
30. Seidner SR, Chen YQ, Oprysko PR, et al.: Combined prostaglandin and nitric oxide inhibition produces anatomic remodeling and closure of the ductus arteriosus in the premature newborn baboon, *Pediatr Res* 50(3):365–373, 2001.
31. Evans N, Iyer P: Assessment of ductus arteriosus shunt in preterm infants supported by mechanical ventilation: effects of interatrial shunting, *J Pediatr* 125:778–785, 1994.
32. Agata Y, Hiraishi S, Oguchi K, et al.: Changes in left ventricular output from fetal to early neonatal life, *J Pediatr* 119:441–445, 1991.
33. Drayton MR, Skidmore R: Ductus arteriosus blood flow during first 48 hours of life, *Arch Dis Child* 62(10):1030–1034, 1987.
34. Kluckow M, Evans N: Low systemic blood flow in the preterm infant, *Semin Neonatol* 6(1):75–84, 2001.
35. Teitel DF: Physiologic development of the cardiovascular system in the fetus. In Polin RA, Fox WW, editors: *Fetal and neonatal physiology*, vol. 2. Philadelphia, 1998, W. B Saunders Company, pp 827–836.
36. Takahashi Y, Harada K, Kishkurno S, et al.: Postnatal left ventricular contractility in very low birth weight infants, *Pediatr Cardiol* 18(2):112–117, 1997.
37. Weindling AM, Kissack CM: Blood pressure and tissue oxygenation in the newborn baby at risk of brain damage, *Biol Neonate* 79(3-4):241–245, 2001.
38. Osborn D, Evans N, Kluckow M: Diagnosis and treatment of low systemic blood flow in preterm infants, *NeoReviews* 5(3):e109–e121, 2004.
39. Gill AB, Weindling AM: Echocardiographic assessment of cardiac function in shocked very low birthweight infants, *Arch Dis Child* 68:17–21, 1993.

40. Kluckow M, Evans N: Relationship between blood pressure and cardiac output in preterm infants requiring mechanical ventilation, *J Pediatr* 129(4):506–512, 1996.
41. Bauer K, Linderkamp O, Versmold HT: Systolic blood pressure and blood volume in preterm infants, *Arch Dis Child* 69(5 Spec No):521–522, 1993.
42. Barr PA, Bailey PE, Sumners J, et al.: Relation between arterial blood pressure and blood volume and effect of infused albumin in sick preterm infants, *Pediatrics* 60(3):282–289, 1977.
43. Lopez SL, Leighton JO, Walther FJ: Supranormal cardiac output in the dopamine- and dobutamine-dependent preterm infant, *Pediatr Cardiol* 18(4):292–296, 1997.
44. Pladys P, Wodey E, Beuchee A, et al.: Left ventricle output and mean arterial blood pressure in preterm infants during the 1st day of life, *Eur J Pediatr* 158(10):817–824, 1999.
45. Ng PC, Lam CW, Fok TF, et al.: Refractory hypotension in preterm infants with adrenocortical insufficiency, *Arch Dis Child Fetal Neonatal Ed* 84(2):F122–F124, 2001.
46. Watterberg KL: Adrenal insufficiency and cardiac dysfunction in the preterm infant, *Pediatr Res* 51(4):422–424, 2002.
47. Hanna CE, Jett PL, Laird MR, et al.: Corticosteroid binding globulin, total serum cortisol, and stress in extremely low-birth-weight infants, *Am J Perinatol* 14(4):201–204, 1997.
48. Scott SM, Watterberg KL: Effect of gestational age, postnatal age, and illness on plasma cortisol concentrations in premature infants, *Pediatr Res* 37(1):112–116, 1995.
49. Sasidharan P: Role of corticosteroids in neonatal blood pressure homeostasis, *Clin Perinatol* 25(3):723–740, 1998.
50. Moise AA, Wearden ME, Kozinetz CA, et al.: Antenatal steroids are associated with less need for blood pressure support in extremely premature infants, *Pediatrics* 95(6):845–850, 1995.
51. Demarini S, Dollberg S, Hoath SB, et al.: Effects of antenatal corticosteroids on blood pressure in very low birth weight infants during the first 24 hours of life, *J Perinatol* 19(6 Pt 1):419–425, 1999.
52. LeFlore JL, Engle WD, Rosenfeld CR: Determinants of blood pressure in very low birth weight neonates: lack of effect of antenatal steroids, *Early Hum Dev* 59(1):37–50, 2000.
53. Leviton A, Kuban KC, Pagano M, et al.: Antenatal corticosteroids appear to reduce the risk of post-natal germinal matrix hemorrhage in intubated low birth weight newborns, *Pediatrics* 91(6):1083–1088, 1993.
54. Bhatt S, Polglase GR, Wallace EM, et al.: Ventilation before umbilical cord clamping improves the physiological transition at birth, *Front Pediatr* 2:113, 2014.
55. Rabe H, Diaz-Rossello JL, Duley L, et al.: Effect of timing of umbilical cord clamping and other strategies to influence placental transfusion at preterm birth on maternal and infant outcomes, *Cochrane Database Syst Rev* 8:CD003248, 2012.
56. Cheifetz IM: Cardiorespiratory interactions: the relationship between mechanical ventilation and hemodynamics, *Respir Care* 59(12):1937–1945, 2014.
57. Trang TT, Tibballs J, Mercier JC, et al.: Optimization of oxygen transport in mechanically ventilated newborns using oximetry and pulsed Doppler-derived cardiac output, *Crit Care Med* 16:1094–1097, 1988.
58. Maayan C, Eyal F, Mandelberg A, et al.: Effect of mechanical ventilation and volume loading on left ventricular performance in premature infants with respiratory distress syndrome, *Crit Care Med* 14(10):858–860, 1986.
59. Skinner JR, Boys RJ, Hunter S, et al.: Pulmonary and systemic arterial pressure in hyaline membrane disease, *Arch Dis Child* 67(4):366–373, 1992.
60. Evans N, Kluckow M: Early determinants of right and left ventricular output in ventilated preterm infants, *Arch Dis Child Fetal Neonatal Ed* 74(2):F88–94, 1996.
61. Chang HY, Cheng KS, Lung HL, et al.: Hemodynamic effects of nasal intermittent positive pressure ventilation in preterm infants, *Medicine (Baltimore)* 95(6):e2780, 2016.
62. Beker F, Rogerson SR, Hooper SB, et al.: The effects of nasal continuous positive airway pressure on cardiac function in premature infants with minimal lung disease: a crossover randomized trial, *J Pediatr* 164(4):726–729, 2014.
63. Skelton R, Evans N, Smythe J: A blinded comparison of clinical and echocardiographic evaluation of the preterm infant for patent ductus arteriosus, *J Paediatr Child Health* 30:406–411, 1994.
64. Evans N, Moorcraft J: Effect of patency of the ductus arteriosus on blood pressure in very preterm infants, *Arch Dis Child* 67:1169–1173, 1992.
65. Fenton AC, Woods KL, Leanage R, et al.: Cardiovascular effects of carbon dioxide in ventilated preterm infants, *Acta Paediatr* 81:498–503, 1992.
66. Roze JC, Tohier C, Maingueneau C, et al.: Response to dobutamine and dopamine in the hypotensive very preterm infant, *Arch Dis Child* 69:59–63, 1993.
67. Seri I, Rudas G, Bors Z, et al.: Effects of low-dose dopamine infusion on cardiovascular and renal functions, cerebral blood flow, and plasma catecholamine levels in sick preterm neonates, *Pediatr Res* 34(6):742–749, 1993.
68. Versmold HT, Kitterman JA, Phibbs RH, et al.: Aortic blood pressure during the first 12 hours of life in infants with birth weight 610 to 4,220 grams, *Pediatrics* 67(5):607–613, 1981.
69. Dempsey EM, Al Hazzani F, Barrington KJ, et al.: Permissive hypotension in the extremely low birthweight infant with signs of good perfusion, *Arch Dis Child Fetal Neonatal Ed* 94(4):F241–F244, 2009.
70. Strozik KS, Pieper CH, Roller J: Capillary refilling time in newborn babies: normal values, *Arch Dis Child Fetal Neonatal Ed* 76(3):F193–F196, 1997.
71. Schriger DL, Baraff L: Defining normal capillary refill: variation with age, sex, and temperature, *Ann Emerg Med* 17(9):932–935, 1988.

72. Tibby SM, Hatherill M, Murdoch IA: Capillary refill and core-peripheral temperature gap as indicators of haemodynamic status in paediatric intensive care patients, *Arch Dis Child* 80(2):163–166, 1999.
73. Osborn DA, Evans N, Kluckow M: Clinical detection of low upper body blood flow in very premature infants using blood pressure, capillary refill time, and central-peripheral temperature difference, *Arch Dis Child Fetal Neonatal Ed* 89(2):F168–F173, 2004.
74. Linshaw MA: Concentration of the urine. In Polin RA, Fox WW, editors: *Fetal and neonatal physiology*, vol. 2. Philadelphia, 1998, W.B. Saunders Company, pp 1634–1653.
75. Miletin J, Pichova K, Dempsey EM, et al.: Bedside detection of low systemic flow in the very low birth weight infant on day 1 of life, *Eur J Pediatr* 168(7):809–813, 2009.
76. Cady Jr LD, Weil MH, Afifi AA, et al.: Quantitation of severity of critical illness with special reference to blood lactate, *Crit Care Med* 1(2):75–80, 1973.
77. Peretz DI, Scott HM, Duff J, et al.: The significance of lacticacidemia in the shock syndrome, *Ann N Y Acad Sci* 119(3):1133–1141, 1965.
78. Rashkin MC, Bosken C, Baughman RP: Oxygen delivery in critically ill patients. Relationship to blood lactate and survival, *Chest* 87(5):580–585, 1985.
79. Vincent JL, Dufaye P, Berre J, et al.: Serial lactate determinations during circulatory shock, *Crit Care Med* 11(6):449–451, 1983.
80. Weil MH, Afifi AA: Experimental and clinical studies on lactate and pyruvate as indicators of the severity of acute circulatory failure (shock), *Circulation* 41(6):989–1001, 1970.
81. Beca JP, Scopes JW: Serial determinations of blood lactate in respiratory distress syndrome, *Arch Dis Child* 47(254):550–557, 1972.
82. Deshpande SA, Platt MP: Association between blood lactate and acid-base status and mortality in ventilated babies, *Arch Dis Child Fetal Neonatal Ed* 76(1):F15–F20, 1997.
83. Graven SN, Criscuolo D, Holcomb TM: Blood lactate in the respiratory distress syndrome: significance in prognosis, *Am J Dis Child* 110(6):614–617, 1965.
84. Butt WW, Whyte HW: Blood pressure monitoring in neonates: comparison of umbilical and peripheral artery measurements, *J Pediatr* 105:630–632, 1984.
85. Colan SD, Fujii A, Borow KM, et al.: Noninvasive determination of systolic, diastolic and end-systolic blood pressure in neonates, infants and young children: comparison with central aortic pressure measurements, *Am J Cardiol* 52(7):867–870, 1983.
86. Emery EF, Greenough A: Non-invasive blood pressure monitoring in preterm infants receiving intensive care, *Eur J Pediatr* 151(2):136–139, 1992.
87. Kimble KJ, Darnall Jr RA, Yelderman M, et al.: An automated oscillometric technique for estimating mean arterial pressure in critically ill newborns, *Anesthesiology* 54(5):423–425, 1981.
88. Lui K, Doyle PE, Buchanan N: Oscillometric and intra-arterial blood pressure measurements in the neonate: a comparison of methods, *Aust Paediatr J* 18(1):32–34, 1982.
89. Park MK, Menard SM: Accuracy of blood pressure measurement by the Dinamap monitor in infants and children, *Pediatrics* 79(6):907–914, 1987.
90. O'Shea J, Dempsey EM, O'Shea J, et al.: A comparison of blood pressure measurements in newborns, *Am J Perinatol* 26(2):113–116, 2009.
91. Dannevig I, Dale HC, Liestol K, et al.: Blood pressure in the neonate: three non-invasive oscillometric pressure monitors compared with invasively measured blood pressure, *Acta Paediatr* 94(2):191–196, 2005.
92. Alverson DC, Eldridge M, Dillon T, et al.: Noninvasive pulsed Doppler determination of cardiac output in neonates and children, *J Pediatr* 101:46–50, 1982.
93. Walther FJ, Siassi B, Ramadan NA, et al.: Pulsed Doppler determinations of cardiac output in neonates: normal standards for clinical use, *Pediatrics* 76:829–833, 1985.
94. Groves AM, Groves AM: Cardiac magnetic resonance in the study of neonatal haemodynamics, *Semin Fetal Neonatal Med* 16(1):36–41, 2011.
95. Stark MJ, Clifton VL, Wright IM, et al.: Microvascular flow, clinical illness severity and cardiovascular function in the preterm infant, *Arch Dis Child Fetal Neonatal Ed* 93(4):F271–F274, 2008.
96. Amir G, Ramamoorthy C, Riemer RK, et al.: Visual light spectroscopy reflects flow-related changes in brain oxygenation during regional low-flow perfusion and deep hypothermic circulatory arrest, *J Thorac Cardiovasc Surg* 132(6):1307–1313, 2006.
97. Takahashi S, Kakiuchi S, Nanba Y, et al.: The perfusion index derived from a pulse oximeter for predicting low superior vena cava flow in very low birth weight infants, *J Perinatol* 30(4):265–269, 2010.
98. Van Laere D, O'Toole JM, Voeten M, et al.: Decreased variability and low values of perfusion index on day one are associated with adverse outcome in extremely preterm infants, *J Pediatr* 178:119–124 e111, 2016.
99. de Waal K, Evans N: Hemodynamics in preterm infants with late-onset sepsis, *J Pediatr* 156(6):918–922, 922e1, 2010.
100. Lou HC, Lassen NA, Friis-Hansen B: Impaired autoregulation of cerebral blood flow in the distressed newborn infant, *J Pediatr* 94(1):118–121, 1979.
101. Victor S, Marson AG, Appleton RE, et al.: Relationship between blood pressure, cerebral electrical activity, cerebral fractional oxygen extraction, and peripheral blood flow in very low birth weight newborn infants, *Pediatr Res* 59:314–319, 2006.
102. Wardle SP, Yoxall CW, Weindling AM: Peripheral oxygenation in hypotensive preterm babies, *Pediatr Res* 45(3):343–349, 1999.

26

103. Perlman JM, McMenamin JB, Volpe JJ: Fluctuating cerebral blood-flow velocity in respiratory-distress syndrome. Relation to the development of intraventricular hemorrhage, *N Engl J Med* 309(4):204–209, 1983.
104. Pryds O, Greisen G, Lou H, et al.: Heterogeneity of cerebral vasoreactivity in preterm infants supported by mechanical ventilation, *J Pediatr* 115(4):638–645, 1989.
105. Wong FY, Leung TS, Austin T, et al.: Impaired autoregulation in preterm infants identified by using spatially resolved spectroscopy, *Pediatrics* 121(3):e604–e611, 2008.
106. Bada HS, Korones SB, Perry EH, et al.: Mean arterial blood pressure changes in premature infants and those at risk for intraventricular hemorrhage, *J Pediatr* 117(4):607–614, 1990.
107. Cunningham S, Symon AG, Elton RA, et al.: Intra-arterial blood pressure reference ranges, death and morbidity in very low birthweight infants during the first seven days of life, *Early Hum Dev* 56(2-3):151–165, 1999.
108. Grether JK, Nelson KB, Emery ES, et al.: Prenatal and perinatal factors and cerebral palsy in very low birth weight infants, *J Pediatr* 128:407–411, 1996.
109. Fanaroff JM, Wilson-Costello DE, Newman NS, et al.: Treated hypotension is associated with neonatal morbidity and hearing loss in extremely low birth weight infants, *Pediatrics* 117:1131–1135, 2006.
110. Heuchan AM, Evans N, Henderson Smart DJ, et al.: Perinatal risk factors for major intraventricular haemorrhage in the Australian and New Zealand neonatal network, 1995-97, *Arch Dis Child Fetal Neonatal Ed* 86(2):F86–F90, 2002.
111. de Vries LS, Regev R, Dubowitz LM, et al.: Perinatal risk factors for the development of extensive cystic leukomalacia, *Am J Dis Child* 142(7):732–735, 1988.
112. Perlman JM, Risser R, Broyles RS: Bilateral cystic periventricular leukomalacia in the premature infant: associated risk factors, *Pediatrics* 97(6 Pt 1):822–827, 1996.
113. Goldstein RF, Thompson Jr RJ, Oehler JM, et al.: Influence of acidosis, hypoxemia, and hypotension on neurodevelopmental outcome in very low birth weight infants, *Pediatrics* 95(2):238–243, 1995.
114. Low JA, Froese AB, Galbraith RS, et al.: The association between preterm newborn hypotension and hypoxemia and outcome during the first year, *Acta Paediatr* 82(5):433–437, 1993.
115. Martens SE, Rijken M, Stoelhorst GM, et al.: Is hypotension a major risk factor for neurological morbidity at term age in very preterm infants? *Early Hum Dev* 75(1-2):79–89, 2003.
116. Pellicer A, Bravo MC, Madero R, et al.: Early systemic hypotension and vasopressor support in low birth weight infants: impact on neurodevelopment, *Pediatrics* 123(5):1369–1376, 2009.
117. Durrmeyer X, Marchand-Martin L, Porcher R, et al.: Hemodynamic EPIPAGE 2 Study Group. Abstention or intervention for isolated hypotension in the first 3 days of life in extremely preterm infants: association with short-term outcomes in the EPIPAGE 2 cohort study, *Arch Dis Child Fetal Neonatal Ed* 102(6):490–496, 2017.
118. Hunt RW, Evans N, Rieger I, et al.: Low superior vena cava flow and neurodevelopment at 3 years in very preterm infants, *J Pediatr* 145(5):588–592, 2004.
119. Plomgaard AM, van Oeveren W, Petersen TH, et al.: The SafeBoosC II randomized trial: treatment guided by near-infrared spectroscopy reduces cerebral hypoxia without changing early biomarkers of brain injury, *Pediatr Res* 79(4):528–535, 2016.
120. Pellicer A, Greisen G, Benders M, et al.: The SafeBoosC phase II randomised clinical trial: a treatment guideline for targeted near-infrared-derived cerebral tissue oxygenation versus standard treatment in extremely preterm infants, *Neonatology* 104(3):171–178, 2013.
121. Noori S, Anderson M, Soleymani S, et al.: Effect of carbon dioxide on cerebral blood flow velocity in preterm infants during postnatal transition, *Acta Paediatr* 103(8):e334–e339, 2014.
122. Rios DR, Kaiser JR: Vasopressin versus dopamine for treatment of hypotension in extremely low birth weight infants: a randomized, blinded pilot study, *J Pediatr* 166(4):850–855, 2015.
123. Subhedar NV: Treatment of hypotension in newborns, *Semin Neonatol* 8(6):413–423, 2003.

CHAPTER 27

Assessment and Management of Septic Shock and Hypovolemia

Koert de Waal and Istvan Seri

- Septic shock in neonates usually presents with high cardiac output and low systemic vascular resistance (i.e., warm shock) and can be accompanied by pulmonary hypertension.
- First-line treatment should target distributive shock with volume and vasopressors.
- Norepinephrine can be considered over epinephrine or dopamine as the vasopressor of first choice due to its superior vasopressor effect and its potential beneficial effects on pulmonary vascular resistance.
- Because of its vasopressor potency, careful but effective titration of norepinephrine is of great clinical importance for optimizing the hemodynamic response and minimizing sudden unwanted swings in blood pressure.
- In cases with signs of vasopressor resistance, hydrocortisone can be started early to enhance the cardiovascular efficacy of catecholamines.
- Early and serial assessments with echocardiography are important to recognize the type of septic shock and follow the changes in hemodynamics in response to treatment.

Infection is a common complication in neonatal intensive care and is associated with significant morbidity and mortality.[1–3] Risk factors include *maternal* factors that can facilitate vertical transmission and the development of early-onset sepsis (<72 hours after birth). Such factors include colonization with group B streptococcus (GBS), prolonged duration of ruptured membranes, and chorioamnionitis. *Neonatal* risk factors with horizontal transmission can cause late-onset sepsis (>72 hours after birth) and include prematurity, vascular catheterization, mechanical ventilation, and other invasive diagnostic and treatment modalities. Infection starts with the presence of susceptibility to and invasion by a pathogen, which can be followed by a systemic inflammatory response with a complex series of molecular and cellular events.[4] Neonates with infection may initially present with minimal signs and symptoms and then progress to sepsis, septic shock, and full-blown multiorgan failure.

To aid in the standardization of observational studies and evaluation of therapeutic interventions in clinical trials, Goldstein et al. presented consensus definitions of the pediatric sepsis continuum.[5] Sepsis is defined as a systemic inflammatory response in the presence of a suspected or proven infection; septic shock is defined as sepsis with cardiovascular organ dysfunction. Details are provided for the clinical definition of a systemic inflammatory response, cardiovascular dysfunction, and organ dysfunction, but it has been difficult to provide neonatal-specific definitions, especially for preterm infants.[6,7] Indeed, the pediatric consensus definitions for sepsis are not accurate in neonates, which is most likely explained by the developmental differences in the systemic inflammatory, cardiovascular, and other organ systems' response to sepsis and the fact that many other common neonatal conditions can mimic sepsis.[8,9]

The Hemodynamic Response to Sepsis

Adults

The hemodynamic response to sepsis is a continuum with different phases; to the clinician, this response will depend on the time of presentation and progress of the disease. In adults, septic shock is primarily a form of distributive shock, characterized by ineffective tissue oxygen delivery and extraction due to inappropriate vasodilatation with preserved or increased cardiac output.[10,11] There is an absolute and/ or relative decrease in central blood volume, with load-driven alterations in left and right ventricular function.[12] However, the heart can also be directly affected by the host immune response or by pathogen toxins, especially in the advanced stages of sepsis. Indeed, a number of mediators and pathways have been shown to be associated with myocardial depression in sepsis, but the precise cause remains unclear. There is currently no evidence supporting global ischemia as an underlying cause of myocardial dysfunction in sepsis in adults.[13] An important hemodynamic aspect of sepsis is the dysfunctional microcirculation.[14,15] Microcapillary obstruction, redistribution of local blood flow, and the inability of the affected cells to extract oxygen from central blood flow even when it has been restored contribute to increased mortality.

Children

The presentation and hemodynamic response to sepsis in children is more variable compared with that in adults. In a prospective observational study, 30 children with suspected fluid-resistant septic shock were assessed within 4 hours after the onset of shock with a noninvasive cardiac output device.[16] Fluid-resistant septic shock secondary to in-hospital acquired infection typically presented with high cardiac output and low systemic vascular resistance (SVR), or warm shock. However, in patients with community-acquired sepsis, a low cardiac output with a high SVR, or cold shock, was predominant. This finding might be explained by the longer interval to diagnosis for community-acquired sepsis and advanced disease progression at the time of admission to the pediatric intensive care unit (PICU). Both types evolved in a heterogeneous manner concerning the findings of cardiac output and SVR, needing frequent revision of the cardiovascular support therapy.[17,18] Importantly, Raj et al. showed that cardiac dysfunction was common in children with septic shock. About one-third of the children had systolic dysfunction as measured by reduced ejection fraction (EF) or fractional shortening (SF) or diastolic dysfunction with an increased Ee′ ratio within 24 hours of admission.[19] The Ee′ ratio represents the ratio of early mitral inflow velocity (E wave) and tissue Doppler–derived mitral annular early diastolic velocity (e′); it is used as an estimate of left ventricular filling pressure. Of note is that—because measures of myocardial function, especially EF and SF are load-dependent—caution should be used in interpreting these data.

Neonates

Early newborn animal studies using rabbits, lambs, or piglets have shown that septic shock consistently presents with reduced cardiac output and increased systemic and pulmonary vascular resistance (PVR).[20–22] Reduced cardiac contractility was found, often independent of a decrease in preload. Doppler echocardiography was only just being introduced in neonatal practice at the time of these studies; hence the experiments were not confirmed in neonates. Yet the clinical presentation of septic neonates fit with the findings of the animal studies. Neonates were described as cold, mottled, and peripherally vasoconstricted, with hypoxia, oliguria, and evidence of organ ischemia—characteristic findings for cold shock.[23–25] When echocardiography became more widely available, clinical studies revealed that cardiac output was often low in shocked hypotensive newborns.[26–29] However, these cohorts described mostly infants with perinatal asphyxia or preterm transition, and the few included neonates with shock with sepsis were not described separately. Interestingly, more recent clinical echocardiography studies in neonates with sepsis have revealed, maybe unexpectedly, that almost all of the studied infants presented with warm shock. De Waal and Evans described a cohort of 20 preterm infants with suspected late-onset infection or necrotizing enterocolitis and at least two clinical signs of cardiovascular compromise. Of the 20 infants, 15 could be classified as having septic shock as they needed greater than 40 mL/kg of volume and/or vasopressor-inotrope support. The infants underwent echocardiography within 2 hours of presentation, which was repeated every 12 hours until clinical recovery or death.[30] All infants presented with high cardiac output and low SVR, with the nonsurvivors showing a rapid decline in cardiac output and an increase in SVR during the first 12 hours of the clinical presentation (Figs. 27.1 and 27.2). This finding was later confirmed in a larger study of 52 preterm infants with

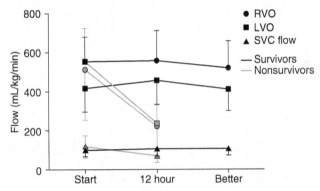

Fig. 27.1 Central blood flows in 20 preterm infants with late-onset sepsis at presentation at 12 hours and when clinically improved (survivors only). The upper limit of right ventricular output (RVO) and left ventricular output (LVO) in well preterm babies (using similar methodology) is estimated to be around 350 to 400 mL/kg/min. *SVC flow,* Superior vena cava flow. (From de Waal K, Evans N: Hemodynamics in preterm infants with late-onset sepsis. *J Pediatr* 156(6):918–922, 2010.)

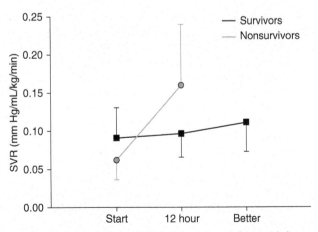

Fig. 27.2 Systemic vascular resistance (SVR) in 20 preterm infants with late-onset sepsis at presentation at 12 hours and when clinically improved. The five nonsurviving infants *(gray lines)* showed a significant increase in SVR after initiation of the treatment within 12 hours after presentation. (From de Waal K, Evans N: Hemodynamics in preterm infants with late-onset sepsis. *J Pediatr* 156(6):918–922, 2010.)

late-onset sepsis or septic shock.[31] Saini et al. also found higher left ventricular output (LVO) in the infants with septic shock but not those with celiac or cerebral blood flow.[31] Using multisite near infrared spectroscopy and echocardiography, van der Laan et al. studied 24 preterm infants with clinically suspected sepsis.[32] They also reported normal to high blood flows and mostly normal renal, cerebral, and intestinal fractional tissue oxygen extraction, indicating that oxygen delivery to the tissues matched cellular demand at the time of study. However, high intestinal fractional tissue oxygen extraction was correlated with low LVO and/or right ventricular output (RVO), suggesting that the intestinal perfusion is most at risk during periods of low cardiac output.[32] Tomerak et al. studied 30 term and preterm newborns with sepsis within 24 hours of presentation and before the initiation of vasopressor-inotropes.[33] EF was marginally increased, and the majority of infants showed diastolic dysfunction as measured by the EA ratio (the ratio between early diastolic and atrium contraction flow velocity) and myocardial performance index (MPI). In a study by Abdel Hady et al., 20 term infants with clinical *and* culture-proven sepsis were measured 1 to 4 days after presentation.[34] Cardiac output was comparable to that in controls, but tissue Doppler revealed reduced systolic annular velocities and increased MPI, suggesting systolic and diastolic dysfunction.

However, there are understandable limitations to these clinical studies. Not all of the included infants had culture-proven infection, and there were only a limited number of infants with early-onset sepsis. Accordingly, at the time of the first hemodynamic assessment, infants could be classified anywhere on the continuum of sepsis, from mild clinical signs to full-blown septic shock. Nevertheless, all currently available clinical data indicate that neonates most often present with warm rather than cold shock, as the early animal studies suggested.

Approach to the Treatment of Neonates With Septic Shock

Treatment of septic shock has seen significant changes over time. Early goal-directed therapy and the implementation of "sepsis bundles" have helped to reduce mortality in adults and children with sepsis.[35–37] Guidelines are also available for neonates with septic shock. The 2012 international guidelines for the management of severe sepsis and septic shock provide recommendations for term newborns but exclude preterm infants.[35] The 2007 clinical practice parameters for hemodynamic support of pediatric and neonatal septic shock by the American College of Critical Care Medicine (ACCCM) do not specifically exclude preterm infants, but most thresholds, diagnostic interventions, and therapeutic end points are derived from the PICU environment.[38]

Acknowledging these limitations, Wynn and Wong added an alternative flow diagram with suggestions for monitoring and treating preterm infants with septic shock (Fig. 27.3).[4] For the treatment of septic shock in newborns, especially with early sepsis, it is important to recognize the variable hemodynamic conditions during the normal transition from fetus to newborn, as detailed in Chapter 1. If septic shock is likely, restoration of blood pressure, blood flow, hypoxia, and acidosis are generally accepted short-term therapeutic end points. The definitive goal when managing a neonate in shock is to restore blood flow and thus oxygen delivery to the tissues so that perfusion and aerobic cellular metabolism matching oxygen demand are restored and preserved. Suggestions for therapeutic end points in neonates include a capillary refill time of less than 2 seconds, normal pulses without differential between peripheral and central pulses, warm extremities, urine output greater than 1 mL/kg/h, low serum lactate, normal central blood flows (cardiac output between 200 and 400 mL/kg/min, superior vena cava [SVC] flow >40 mL/kg/min), a central and mixed venous saturation of more than 70%, and normal mental status.[38] Therapeutic end points in premature neonates have not been established, and some of the suggested hemodynamic measurements have not been validated in preterm infants.

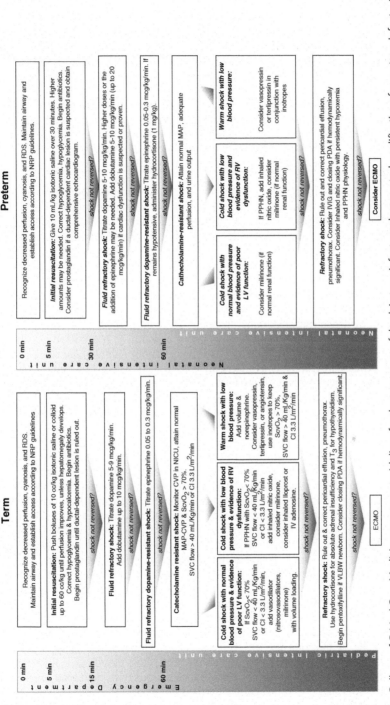

Fig. 27.3 American College of Critical Care Medicine consensus guidelines for the treatment of shock in term infants and suggested modifications for preterm infants. *CI*, Cardiac index; *CVP*, central venous pressure; *ECMO*, extracorporeal membrane oxygenation; *IVIG*, intravenous immunoglobulin; *LV*, left ventricular; *MAP*, mean arterial pressure; *NRP*, Neonatal Resuscitation Program; *PDA*, patent ductus arteriosus; *PPHN*, persistent pulmonary hypertension of the newborn; *RDS*, respiratory distress syndrome; *RV*, right ventricular; *ScvO₂*, central venous oxygen saturation; *SVC*, superior vena cava; *VLBW*, very low birth weight. (From Wynn JL, Wong HR: Pathophysiology and treatment of septic shock in neonates. *Clin Perinatol* 37(2):439–479, 2010.)

As in the current ACCCM guideline, *the following sections provide suggestions for a future update based on accumulated new evidence.* Accordingly, initial resuscitation of septic shock starts with volume boluses of 10 to 20 mL/kg. Repeat boluses might be needed up to 60 mL/kg. The neonatal myocardium is very capable of increasing stroke volume with increasing preload, especially when the ductus arteriosus is open.[27,39,40] Nevertheless, there are some concerns about early volume loading in septic children. Both early and acquired daily fluid overload were independently associated with mortality in children with severe sepsis.[41,42] However, the available data for early volume resuscitation was heavily weighted by one well-conducted trial that enrolled a significant proportion of children with malaria in sub-Saharan Africa, sparking considerable controversy regarding the applicability of the results to different contexts and populations. Routine fluid administration in preterm infants with signs of poor perfusion or hypotension has not been reported to be associated with increased morbidity or mortality, but further trials are needed for the subgroup of neonates and especially preterm neonates with sepsis.

When fluid-refractory shock is present, a vasopressor-inotrope would be the first choice of vasoactive medication if no hemodynamic monitoring is available. Neonatologists are historically most familiar with *dopamine*, and it remains the most commonly used vasoactive medication in transitional hypotension and septic shock.[43–45] Although dopamine is an effective vasopressor in neonates, there is accumulating evidence that dopamine in higher doses (>10 mcg/kg/min) might also increase PVR to the same or even a higher extent as the increase in SVR.[46–49] Although these findings concern preterm neonates with preexisting increased pulmonary blood flow, such as patients with a large PDA with left-to-right shunting, there is no evidence that dopamine decreases PVR in patients with normal or decreased pulmonary blood flow. This is obviously a concern, as it can have possible negative effects on pulmonary blood flow and oxygenation. *Dobutamine* can be added when no echocardiography is available at this point or when low central blood flow is likely. A simple bedside assessment of high versus low cardiac output using Doppler flow velocity would provide the clinician with a targeted choice.[50] Finally, *epinephrine* and *norepinephrine* have also been used as secondary or primary vasoactive drugs in neonates (see the following discussion).

The time to evaluate outcomes of the initial resuscitation with fluids and first-line vasoactive drug administration is set at 60 minutes in early goal-directed guidelines. It is unclear if this time line is feasible and/or appropriate in neonates. Particularly for infants with very low birth weight, infusion rates are low and dead space in a newly inserted central venous line (either umbilical or central venous) can be significant. Manual flushing of vasoactive drugs is not recommended, as this could lead to large fluctuations in blood pressure. Cerebral hyperperfusion following cerebral hypoperfusion is fundamental to the hemodynamic basis of periventricular intraventricular hemorrhage in preterm infants, and rapid changes in blood pressure and flow should be avoided if possible.[51,52] However, careful priming of the infusion line and the use of higher vasoactive drug infusion rates can mitigate some of these concerns.

If shock is resistant to dopamine and/or dobutamine, adding hydrocortisone early in the course of treatment for shock can reduce the duration of vasopressor-inotrope or inotrope use in term and preterm infants (see Chapter 30 for further details).[53,54] Neonates with septic shock often have blood cortisol levels within the normal and not appropriately elevated range, but with increased levels of cortisol precursors suggesting inadequate cortisol synthesis.[55]

Epinephrine is recommended in cold shock and norepinephrine in warm shock if shock remains resistant to first-line therapies, although there is limited evidence to support either therapy in neonates. Heckman et al. showed that epinephrine improved blood pressure in a cohort of 22 shocked very low birth weight infants.[56] Most infants were considered as having an infection, but only 10% had a culture-proven infection. Epinephrine was started 3 days (median) after birth as first- or second-line vasoactive therapy. Cardiac output was not studied, but the authors classified the infants as having cold shock with probable depressed myocardial function and poor organ perfusion. Daga et al. describe nine term and late preterm infants with fluid-refractory septic shock where epinephrine improved the immediate hemodynamic compromise.[57] Tourneux et al. studied 22 term newborns with fluid-refractory and dopamine/dobutamine-resistant early-onset septic shock.[58] Norepinephrine (mean starting dose 0.4 mcg/kg/min) improved blood pressure in all; there was also a suggestion of improved tissue oxygenation as indicated by an increase in urine output and a decrease in blood lactate concentration. Rowcliff et al. presented a cohort of 48 preterm infants with shock.[59] Two-thirds had early- or late-onset septic shock, and most infants received additional vasoactive medications before norepinephrine was started. Normotension was achieved at a median of 1 hour in all but one infant at a median dose of 0.5 mcg/kg/min.

In most studies the infants were treated with a combination of two or three catecholamines. The addition of potent vasoactive drugs like epinephrine or norepinephrine led to an average 10% increase in heart rate. Neonates, and in particular preterm infants, have stiff ventricles with intrinsic poor diastolic function. A further shortening of the ventricular filling time can lead to reduced stroke volume and organ blood flow. It is also possible that catecholamine overload with high SVR contributes to cardiovascular failure and early mortality during sepsis, as seen in a cohort of preterm infants with late-onset sepsis.[30] In a patient with severe shock, an unplanned discontinuation of all four running catecholamines prompted a reduction in heart rate and an acute improvement in oxygenation and blood flow (de Waal, unpublished data). Therefore the targeted increase in SVR in septic neonates with warm shock must be matched with the ability of the myocardium to pump against the increased resistance. This is a delicate balance and can only be achieved with careful and thorough monitoring of blood flow, blood pressure, and tissue oxygenation. The risk of an unwanted increase in SVR beyond the targeted range is especially high when very high doses of vasoactive medications are used, the patient has been started on hydrocortisone and/or starts improving, and cardiovascular adrenergic receptor expression is enhanced. Therefore careful titration of these medications is a fundamental requirement to decrease the chances of side effects and enhance drug effectiveness. The risk of tachycardia might also be reduced by appropriate titration resulting in decreased dose and by replacing one vasopressor-inotrope for another (epinephrine for dopamine or norepinephrine for epinephrine) instead of adding them all together, thus preventing catecholamine overload from occurring.[60,61]

Some neonatal units have changed the choice of first-line vasoactive drug for septic shock from dopamine to epinephrine or norepinephrine depending on the findings on echocardiography. In preterm animal models, the distribution of adrenoceptor subtypes in the myocardium and vasculature is strikingly different from that seen in older animals, and the cardiovascular actions of dopamine and dobutamine might not be adequate at moments of significant hemodynamic compromise.[62,63] Two recent randomized trials in pediatric patients with fluid-refractory septic shock showed that early administration of epinephrine as a first-line drug was associated with increased survival or improved organ function compared with dopamine.[64,65] As detailed earlier, however, neonates show a similar hemodynamic response to sepsis as seen in adults (primarily warm shock) rather than children (primarily cold shock). Indeed, as most neonatal cases with septic shock present while the infant is still in hospital, it would be reasonable to direct the first-line treatment at warm shock. Norepinephrine is superior to dopamine when used to treat septic shock in adults.[66] Furthermore, norepinephrine has additional advantages over dopamine, with an improved SVR:PVR ratio, and can thus be used if sepsis is accompanied by pulmonary hypertension.[47,67,68] However, more data are needed to satisfactorily settle the issue as to whether norepinephrine is superior to epinephrine in neonatal septic shock. Finally, due to norepinephrine's very potent systemic vasoconstrictive effects, careful but effective titration of the medication to the optimum hemodynamic response (improved systemic blood pressure, systemic blood flow, and tissue oxygenation) is of great clinical relevance, since significant and sudden swings in systemic blood pressure and organ blood flow (particularly to the brain) are harmful in neonates, especially in preterm infants.

These changes can simplify the flow diagram for early- and late-onset sepsis in neonates (see Fig. 27.3). A main concern remains the clinician's limited ability to confirm the presence of sepsis early on. Other more common neonatal illnesses, especially those eliciting a nonspecific inflammatory response, can present with hypotension and signs of shock, and it is not clear if aggressive treatment improves long-term outcomes in those situations.[69]

Catecholamine-Resistant Septic Shock (see Chapter 30)

If catecholamine-resistant shock develops, it will be increasingly difficult to manage without information on central blood flow, cardiac shunts, and the presence of pulmonary hypertension. The 2007 guideline suggests central venous pressure monitoring, central or mixed venous saturation measurements, and/or echocardiography to collect the necessary hemodynamic practice parameters. In neonatology and especially for preterm infants, ultrasound remains the most frequently used noninvasive tool to provide the information needed. However, there are other emerging monitoring tools, such as electrical impedance velocimetry, that can be used noninvasively and continuously and do not require the sophistication needed for the use and interpretation of echocardiography (see Chapter 14). In addition, use of the recently developed comprehensive monitoring systems described in Chapter 21 has the potential to provide information on most aspects of neonatal hemodynamics. However, it must be kept in mind that all of the diagnostic tools have their limitations and should only be used with a full understanding of their potentials and pitfalls.

Fluid responsiveness (preload reserve) remains difficult to assess in neonates. Several echocardiographic parameters can reliably be used as a proxy for fluid responsiveness in adults, but they can only be assessed when the patient is on ventilator support and without spontaneous respiratory effort (i.e., during neuromuscular blockade).[70,71] In addition, the normal range of central venous pressure is too variable in neonates and is also dependent on mean airway pressure. Central venous pressure is not a good predictor of fluid responsiveness even in adults and should probably no longer be recommended.[72–74] Central venous oxygen saturation is an invasive measurement but is being replaced by the use of tissue oxygen saturation measurements using near infrared spectroscopy, although much more needs to be understood and more comprehensive clinical information needs to be collected before routine use in patients with septic shock can be recommended.[75,76]

Suggestions for the treatment of catecholamine-resistant shock are mainly unchanged from the 2007 ACCCM guideline. Vasopressin has been well studied in adults with warm shock and is increasingly studied in children and neonates with catecholamine-resistant shock.[77] Neonates with septic shock responded well to vasopressin, but mortality in these cohorts remained high.

Pulmonary hypertension is commonly described in animal models of septic shock. Sepsis-induced acidosis and hypoxia can increase PVR and thus pulmonary artery pressure, with increased right ventricular work. As early animal studies also showed low cardiac output, treatments targeted to provide systemic and pulmonary vasodilatation was tried but with variable results.[78] Inhaled nitric oxide (iNO) is currently the treatment of choice in sepsis-induced pulmonary hypertension during the transitional period, especially when pulmonary blood flow is low. We strongly recommend echocardiography evaluation before starting iNO, as clinical signs of pulmonary hypertension such as a pre- and postductal saturation difference can also become apparent in severe systemic hypotension without high pulmonary pressures. iNO was not effective in adult patients with sepsis and adult respiratory distress syndrome, and it is not known if iNO for sepsis-induced pulmonary hypertension after the transitional period is effective in neonates.[79,80]

In preterm infants with septic shock, the presence of a large patent ductus arteriosus can complicate hemodynamics. Closure with nonsteroidal anti-inflammatory drugs can be attempted if renal function allows and PVR is not elevated, although animal studies could not show benefits from early treatment with prostaglandin synthesis inhibitors in sepsis.[81,82]

Some neonates present with cold shock or change from a high to low cardiac output phenotype during the course of their disease. If these changes are recognized, careful weaning off the vasopressor-inotrope support and replacement with inotropes (dobutamine) and/or lusitropes (milrinone) with appropriate titration of these medications has the potential to reduce the SVR and should be the drugs of choice.

When available, extracorporeal membrane oxygenation (ECMO) should be considered as a final therapeutic option. Although success rates are high, early studies showed a high rate of bleeding complications (especially intraventricular hemorrhage) has earlier been reported in neonates with intractable septic shock.[83] However, ECMO technology has changed over time, and there has been a move from venoarterial to venovenous ECMO, with superior efficacy in infants with sepsis and with lower complication rates. Survival in the studies in neonates and children with sepsis requiring ECMO support varies from 50% to 100%, with neonates showing higher survival as compared with older children.[84–86] Indications to initiate ECMO are not always clear from the publications, but they have included catecholamine-resistant shock and/or respiratory failure with sepsis.

Hypovolemic Shock in Neonates

True hypovolemic shock is rare in neonates and is mostly seen early after birth. Causes include peripartum bleeding from the fetal side of the placenta, fetomaternal hemorrhage, fetofetal hemorrhage, or a postpartum neonatal hemorrhage. With ongoing bleeding, the autonomic sympathetic system is activated with inhibition of the parasympathetic system leading to increased heart rate, cardiac contractility, and arterial and venous tone. Blood volume from the nonvital organs and the venous system will be recruited to help preserve blood flow to the brain, heart, and adrenal glands. The decreased perfusion pressure and increased sympathetic tone associated with epinephrine and norepinephrine release activate the renin-angiotensin-aldosterone system in the juxtaglomerular apparatus of the kidneys. If the bleeding cannot be stopped, severe hypovolemia will finally lead to severe acidosis and myocardial dysfunction, organ failure, and death.

The optimal approach to hemorrhagic hypovolemia in neonates has not been well studied. Most of what is known about physiology and management has been extrapolated from animal and adult data. First-line resuscitation of hemorrhagic shock starts with volume, and the limited available clinical evidence would suggest isotonic saline.[87,88] A second step would be replacing the type of volume lost, in this case blood. Neonates with severe bleeding or anemia may require a massive transfusion with blood products. The definition of a massive transfusion in pediatric patients varies. According to one suggestion, a transfusion of greater than 50% of total blood volume in 3 hours, replacement of greater than 100% of total blood volume in 24 hours, or transfusion to replace an ongoing blood loss of greater than 10% of the total blood volume per minute would qualify as a massive transfusion.[89] Most massive transfusion protocols for adults employ a physiologic 1:1:1 transfusion ratio of red blood cells, plasma, and platelets, but there are limited neonatal data to make recommendations. Importantly, the availability of an institute-specific massive transfusion protocol has the potential to improve outcomes.[90] Neonates in particular are at risk for metabolic derangements and/or coagulopathy after a massive transfusion and should be monitored closely for hypocalcemia, hypomagnesemia, and fluctuations in potassium, glucose, and pH as well as for signs of oozing or bleeding.[91]

There has been a paradigm shift in the approach toward major bleeding in adults. Observational data have shown that aggressive fluid resuscitation increases the risk of mortality, probably by promoting dilution coagulopathy and delayed clot formation due, at least in part, to increased arterial pressure.[92] The currently recommended approach is low-volume fluid resuscitation while maintaining an acceptable level of tissue perfusion with permissive hypotension. Noradrenaline is the first-line vasopressor-inotrope used in adults, as it induces significant venoconstriction as well at the level of the splanchnic circulation in particular. This increases the pressure in capacitance vessels and actively shifts splanchnic blood volume to the systemic circulation.[93] The effect of dopamine on the splanchnic circulation is complex, and the information in the literature is controversial.[94] However, in newborn animal models, dopamine was the most effective vasoactive drug in increasing gut blood flow; it might therefore be considered an alternative to norepinephrine.[46,95] The effect of catecholamines administered during hypovolemia depends to a large extent on the volume of blood in the splanchnic reservoir. When hypovolemia is severe, the physiologic responses to maintain volume and pressure have already emptied the splanchnic reservoir. The use of exogenous catecholamines should thus be limited to a brief period and should not be viewed as a substitute for the immediate replacement of blood volume.

The use of vasopressin may be beneficial in the management of fluid- and transfusion-resistant uncontrolled bleeding. Vasopressin not only restores the depleted intrinsic vasopressin production but also seems to be more effective in maintaining vascular tone compared with catecholamines in a hypovolemic and acidotic environment.[96,97] However, in an infant animal model of hypovolemic shock, the addition of terlipressin did not improve cardiac output or blood pressure 90 minutes after resuscitation.[98] Thus more data are needed before routine vasopressin administration in hypovolemic neonatal shock can be recommended.

Echocardiography can be effectively used to monitor systemic perfusion during hypovolemic shock in neonates. Biventricular low cardiac output, small ventricular internal dimensions in diastole, and increased collapsibility of the large veins (SVC and inferior vena cava) are all indicators of hypovolemia in the early phase of hypovolemic shock. In addition, respiratory variation in aortic blood flow peak velocity remains an important predictor of fluid responsiveness in mechanically ventilated children.[99] However, this parameter has not been validated in neonates. Myocardial dysfunction, independent of the loading condition, is not uncommon with persistent hypovolemia and can be supported with the addition of dobutamine. In addition, monitoring tissue oxygen saturation by the use of near infrared spectroscopy may add important information on organ blood flow distribution and tissue oxygen delivery in neonates with hypovolemic shock.

Finally, the effects of physiologic cord clamping on hemodynamic transition and the volume status of the neonate is discussed in detail in Chapters 4 and 5.

Conclusion

Contrary to what is seen in children, neonatal *septic shock* is mostly diagnosed in its earlier phases as warm, distributive shock. Accordingly, the cardiovascular pathophysiologically targeted first-line management approach includes aggressive fluid resuscitation and the use of a vasopressor-inotrope. Recent data suggest the consideration of careful use of effectively titrated norepinephrine as the potential first choice of a vasopressor-inotrope. In *hypovolemic shock* of the neonate, rapid replacement of the type of the fluid lost, most frequently whole blood, is the key approach, along with appropriate supportive measures and, if available, use of more sophisticated hemodynamic monitoring to follow the patient's response to the treatment.

REFERENCES

1. Stoll BJ, Hansen N, Fanaroff AA, et al.: Late-onset sepsis in very low birth weight neonates: the experience of the NICHD Neonatal Research Network, *Pediatrics* 110(2 Pt 1):285–289, 2002.
2. Stoll BJ, Hansen NI, Higgins RD, et al.: National Institute of Child Health and Human Development. Very low birth weight preterm infants with early onset neonatal sepsis: the predominance of gram-negative infections continues in the National Institute of Child Health and Human Development Neonatal Research Network, 2002-2003, *Pediatr Infect Dis J* 24(7):635–639, 2005.
3. Bizzarro MJ, Raskind C, Baltimore RS, et al.: Seventy-five years of neonatal sepsis at Yale: 1928-2003, *Pediatrics* 116(3):595–602, 2005.
4. Wynn JL, Wong HR: Pathophysiology and treatment of septic shock in neonates, *Clin Perinatol* 37(2):439–479, 2010.
5. Goldstein B, Giroir B, Randolph A: International pediatric sepsis consensus conference: definitions for sepsis and organ dysfunction in pediatrics, *Pediatr Crit Care Med* 6(1):2–8, 2005.

6. Haque KN: Defining common infections in children and neonates, *J Hosp Infect* 65(Suppl 2):110–114, 2007.
7. Wynn JL, Wong HR, Shanley TP, et al.: Time for a neonatal-specific consensus definition for sepsis, *Pediatr Crit Care Med* 15(6):523–528, 2014.
8. Hofer N, Zacharias E, Müller W, et al.: Performance of the definitions of the systemic inflammatory response syndrome and sepsis in neonates, *J Perinat Med* 40(5):587–590, 2012.
9. Wynn J, Cornell TT, Wong HR, et al.: The host response to sepsis and developmental impact, *Pediatrics* 125(5):1031–1041, 2010.
10. Russell JA: Management of sepsis, *N Engl J Med* 355(16):1699–1713, 2006.
11. Casserly B, Read R, Levy MM: Hemodynamic monitoring in sepsis, *Crit Care Clin* 25(4):803–823, 2009.
12. Vieillard-Baron A, Prin S, Chergui K, et al.: Hemodynamic instability in sepsis: bedside assessment by Doppler echocardiography, *Am J Respir Crit Care Med* 168(11):1270–1276, 2003.
13. Merx MW, Weber C: Sepsis and the heart, *Circulation* 116(7):793–802, 2007.
14. Trzeciak S, Rivers EP: Clinical manifestations of disordered microcirculatory perfusion in severe sepsis, *Crit Care* 9(Suppl 4):S20–S26, 2005.
15. Ince C: The microcirculation is the motor of sepsis, *Crit Care* 9(Suppl 4):S13–S19, 2005.
16. Brierley J, Peters MJ: Distinct hemodynamic patterns of septic shock at presentation to pediatric intensive care, *Pediatrics* 122(4):752–759, 2008.
17. Ceneviva G, Paschall JA, Maffei F, et al.: Hemodynamic support in fluid-refractory pediatric septic shock, *Pediatrics* 102(2):e19, 1998.
18. Deep A, Goonasekera CD, Wang Y, et al.: Evolution of haemodynamics and outcome of fluid-refractory septic shock in children, *Intensive Care Med* 39(9):1602–1609, 2013.
19. Raj S, Killinger JS, Gonzalez JA, et al.: Myocardial dysfunction in pediatric septic shock, *J Pediatr* 164(1):72.e2–77.e2, 2014.
20. Meadow WL, Meus PJ: Early and late hemodynamic consequences of group B beta streptococcal sepsis in piglets: effects on systemic, pulmonary, and mesenteric circulations, *Circ Shock* 19(4):347–356, 1986.
21. Peevy KJ, Reed T, Chartrand SA, et al.: The comparison of myocardial dysfunction in three forms of experimental septic shock, *Pediatr Res* 20(12):1240–1242, 1986.
22. Covert RF, Schreiber MD: Three different strains of heat-killed group B beta-hemolytic streptococcus cause different pulmonary and systemic hemodynamic responses in conscious neonatal lambs, *Pediatr Res* 33(4 Pt 1):373–379, 1993.
23. Quirante J, Ceballos R, Cassady G: Group B beta-hemolytic streptococcal infection in the newborn. I. Early onset infection, *Am J Dis Child* 128(5):659–665, 1974.
24. Siegel JD, McCracken Jr GH: Sepsis neonatorum, *N Engl J Med* 304(11):642–647, 1981.
25. Rudinsky B, Bell A, Hipps R, et al.: The effects of intravenous L-arginine supplementation on systemic and pulmonary hemodynamics and oxygen utilization during group B streptococcal sepsis in piglets, *J Crit Care* 9(1):34–46, 1994.
26. Walther FJ, Siassi B, Ramadan NA, et al.: Cardiac output in newborn infants with transient myocardial dysfunction, *J Pediatr* 107(5):781–785, 1985.
27. Simma B, Fritz MG, Trawöger R, et al.: Changes in left ventricular function in shocked newborns, *Intensive Care Med* 23(9):982–986, 1997.
28. Sabatino G, Ramenghi LA, Verrotti A, et al.: Persistently low cardiac output predicts high mortality in newborns with cardiogenic shock, *Panminerva Med* 40(1):28–32, 1998.
29. Gill AB, Weindling AM: Echocardiographic assessment of cardiac function in shocked very low birthweight infants, *Arch Dis Child* 68(1 Spec No):17–21, 1993.
30. de Waal K, Evans N: Hemodynamics in preterm infants with late-onset sepsis, *J Pediatr* 156(6):918–922, 2010.
31. Saini SS, Kumar P, Kumar RM: Hemodynamic changes in preterm neonates with septic shock: a prospective observational study, *Pediatr Crit Care Med* 15(5):443–450, 2014.
32. van der Laan ME, Roofthooft MT, Fries MW, et al.: Multisite tissue oxygenation monitoring indicates organ-specific flow distribution and oxygen delivery related to low cardiac output in preterm infants with clinical sepsis, *Pediatr Crit Care Med* 17(8):764–771, 2016.
33. Tomerak RH, El-Badawy AA, Hussein G, et al.: Echocardiogram done early in neonatal sepsis: what does it add? *J Investig Med* 60(4):680–684, 2012.
34. Abdel-Hady HE, Matter MK, El-Arman MM: Myocardial dysfunction in neonatal sepsis: a tissue Doppler imaging study, *Pediatr Crit Care Med* 13(3):318–323, 2012.
35. Dellinger RP, Levy MM, Rhodes A, et al.: Surviving Sepsis Campaign Guidelines Committee including The Pediatric Subgroup. Surviving sepsis campaign: international guidelines for management of severe sepsis and septic shock, 2012, *Intensive Care Med* 39(2):165–228, 2013.
36. Workman JK, Ames SG, Reeder RW, et al.: Treatment of pediatric septic shock with the surviving sepsis campaign guidelines and PICU patient outcomes, *Pediatr Crit Care Med* 17(10):e451–e458, 2016.
37. Park SK, Shin SR, Hur M, et al.: The effect of early goal-directed therapy for treatment of severe sepsis or septic shock: a systemic review and meta-analysis, *J Crit Care* 38:115–122, 2016.
38. Brierley J, Carcillo JA, Choong K, et al.: Clinical practice parameters for hemodynamic support of pediatric and neonatal septic shock: 2007 update from the american college of critical care medicine, *Crit Care Med* 37(2):666–688, 2009.
39. Clyman RI, Roman C, Heymann MA, et al.: How a patent ductus arteriosus effects the premature lamb's ability to handle additional volume loads, *Pediatr Res* 22(5):531–535, 1987.

27

40. Evans N: Volume expansion during neonatal intensive care: do we know what we are doing? *Semin Neonatol* 8(4):315–323, 2003.
41. Chen J, Li X, Bai Z, et al.: Association of fluid accumulation with clinical outcomes in critically Ill children with severe sepsis, *PLoS One* (7)11, 2016.
42. Ford N, Hargreaves S, Shanks L: Mortality after fluid bolus in children with shock due to sepsis or severe infection: a systematic review and meta-analysis, *PLoS One* 7(8):e43953, 2012.
43. Sehgal A, Osborn D, McNamara PJ: Cardiovascular support in preterm infants: a survey of practices in Australia and New Zealand, *J Paediatr Child Health* 48(4):317–323, 2012.
44. Wong J, Shah PS, Yoon EW, et al.: Inotrope use among extremely preterm infants in Canadian neonatal intensive care units: variation and outcomes, *Am J Perinatol* 32(1):9–14, 2015.
45. Koch L, Bosk A, Sasse M, et al.: Managing neonatal severe sepsis in Germany: a preliminary survey of current practices, *Klin Padiatr* 227(1):23–27, 2015.
46. Cheung PY, Barrington KJ: The effects of dopamine and epinephrine on hemodynamics and oxygen metabolism in hypoxic anesthetized piglets, *Crit Care* 5(3):158–166, 2001.
47. Jaillard S, Houfflin-Debarge V, Riou Y, et al.: Effects of catecholamines on the pulmonary circulation in the ovine fetus, *Am J Physiol Regul Integr Comp Physiol* 281(2):R607–R614, 2001.
48. Liet JM, Boscher C, Gras-Leguen C, et al.: Dopamine effects on pulmonary artery pressure in hypotensive preterm infants with patent ductus arteriosus, *J Pediatr* 140(3):373–375, 2002.
49. Bouissou A, Rakza T, Klosowski S, et al.: Hypotension in preterm infants with significant patent ductus arteriosus: effects of dopamine, *J Pediatr* 153:790–794, 2008.
50. Evans N: Which inotrope for which baby? *Arch Dis Child Fetal Neonatal Ed* 91(3):F213–F220, 2006.
51. Osborn DA, Evans N, Kluckow M: Hemodynamic and antecedent risk factors of early and late periventricular/intraventricular hemorrhage in premature infants, *Pediatrics* 112(1 Pt 1):33–39, 2003.
52. Wong FY, Silas R, Hew S, et al.: Cerebral oxygenation is highly sensitive to blood pressure variability in sick preterm infants, *PLoS One* 7(8):e43165, 2012.
53. Ng PC, Lee CH, Bnur FL, et al.: A double-blind, randomized, controlled study of a "stress dose" of hydrocortisone for rescue treatment of refractory hypotension in preterm infants, *Pediatrics* 117(2):367–375, 2006.
54. Noori S, Friedlich P, Wong P, et al.: Hemodynamic changes after low-dosage hydrocortisone administration in vasopressor-treated preterm and term neonates, *Pediatrics* 118(4):1456–1466, 2006.
55. Khashana A, Ojaniemi M, Leskinen M, et al.: Term neonates with infection and shock display high cortisol precursors despite low levels of normal cortisol, *Acta Paediatr* 105(2):154–158, 2016.
56. Heckmann M, Trotter A, Pohlandt F, et al.: Epinephrine treatment of hypotension in very low birthweight infants, *Acta Paediatr* 91(5):566–570, 2002.
57. Daga SR, Gosavi DV, Verma B: Adrenaline for septic shock in newborn, *Indian Pediatr* 37(7):799–800, 2000.
58. Tourneux P, Rakza T, Abazine A, et al.: Noradrenaline for management of septic shock refractory to fluid loading and dopamine or dobutamine in full-term newborn infants, *Acta Paediatr* 97(2):177–180, 2008.
59. Rowcliff K, de Waal K, Mohamed AL, et al.: Noradrenaline in preterm infants with cardiovascular compromise, *Eur J Pediatr* 175(12):1967–1973, 2016.
60. Germanakis I, Bender C, Hentschel R, et al.: Hypercontractile heart failure caused by catecholamine therapy in premature neonates, *Acta Paediatr* 92(7):836–838, 2003.
61. McNamara PJ: Caution with prolonged or high-dose infusions of catecholamines in premature infants, *Acta Paediatr* 94(7):980–982, 2005.
62. Kim MY, Finch AM, Lumbers ER, et al.: Expression of adrenoceptor subtypes in preterm piglet heart is different to term heart, *PLoS One* 9(3):e92167, 2014.
63. Eiby YA, Shrimpton NY, Wright IM, et al.: Inotropes do not increase cardiac output or cerebral blood flow in preterm piglets, *Pediatr Res* 80(6):870–879, 2016.
64. Ventura AM, Shieh HH, Bousso A, et al.: Double-blind prospective randomized controlled trial of dopamine versus epinephrine as first-line vasoactive drugs in pediatric septic shock, *Crit Care Med* 43(11):2292–2302, 2015.
65. Ramaswamy KN, Singhi S, Jayashree M, et al.: Double-blind randomized clinical trial comparing dopamine and epinephrine in pediatric fluid-refractory hypotensive septic shock, *Pediatr Crit Care Med* 17(11):e502–e512, 2016.
66. De Backer D, Aldecoa C, Njimi H, et al.: Dopamine versus norepinephrine in the treatment of septic shock: a meta-analysis, *Crit Care Med* 40(3):725–730, 2012.
67. Jaillard S, Elbaz F, Bresson-Just S, et al.: Pulmonary vasodilator effects of norepinephrine during the development of chronic pulmonary hypertension in neonatal lambs, *Br J Anaesth* 93(6):818–824, 2004.
68. Schindler MB, Hislop AA, Haworth SG: Postnatal changes in response to norepinephrine in the normal and pulmonary hypertensive lung, *Am J Respir Crit Care Med* 170(6):641–646, 2004.
69. Batton B, Li L, Newman NS, et al.: Eunice Kennedy Shriver National Institute of Child Health & Human Development Neonatal Research Network. Early bloodpressure, antihypotensive therapy and outcomes at 18-22 months' corrected age in extremely preterm infants, *Arch Dis Child Fetal Neonatal Ed* 101(3):F201–F206, 2016.
70. Vignon P, Repessé X, Bégot E, et al.: Comparison of echocardiographic indices used to predict fluid responsiveness in ventilated patients, *Am J Respir Crit Care Med* 195(8):1022–1032, 2017.

71. Gan H, Cannesson M, Chandler JR, et al.: Predicting fluid responsiveness in children: a systematic review, *Anesth Analg* 117(6):1380–1392, 2013.

72. Skinner JR, Milligan DW, Hunter S, et al.: Central venous pressure in the ventilated neonate, *Arch Dis Child* 67(4 Spec No):374–377, 1992.

73. Trevor Inglis GD, Dunster KR, Davies MW: Establishing normal values of central venous pressure in very low birth weight infants, *Physiol Meas* 28(10):1283–1291, 2007.

74. Marik PE, Baram M, Vahid B: Does central venous pressure predict fluid responsiveness? A systematic review of the literature and the tale of seven mares, *Chest* 134(1):172–867, 2008.

75. Weiss M, Dullenkopf A, Kolarova A, et al.: Near-infrared spectroscopic cerebral oxygenation reading in neonates and infants is associated with central venous oxygen saturation, *Paediatr Anaesth* 15(2):102–109, 2005.

76. Ghanayem NS, Wernovsky G, Hoffman GM: Near-infrared spectroscopy as a hemodynamic monitor in critical illness, *Pediatr Crit Care Med* 12(4 Suppl):S27–S32, 2011.

77. Meyer S, McGuire W, Gottschling S, et al.: The role of vasopressin and terlipressin in catecholamine-resistant shock and cardio-circulatory arrest in children: review of the literature, *Wien Med Wochenschr* 161(7–8):192–203, 2011.

78. Walsh-Sukys MC, Tyson JE, Wright LL, et al.: Persistent pulmonary hypertension of the newborn in the era before nitric oxide: practice variation and outcomes, *Pediatrics* 105(1 Pt 1):14–20, 2000.

79. Krafft P, Fridrich P, Fitzgerald RD, et al.: Effectiveness of nitric oxide inhalation in septic ARDS, *Chest* 109(2):486–493, 1996.

80. Trzeciak S, Glaspey LJ, Dellinger RP, et al.: Randomized controlled trial of inhaled nitric oxide for the treatment of microcirculatory dysfunction in patients with sepsis, *Crit Care Med* 42(12):2482–2492, 2014.

81. Peevy KJ, Ronnlund RD, Chartrand SA, et al.: Ibuprofen in experimental group B streptococcal shock, *Circ Shock* 24(1):35–41, 1988.

82. Gibson RL, Truog WE, Henderson Jr WR, et al.: Group B streptococcal sepsis in piglets: effect of combined pentoxifylline and indomethacin pretreatment, *Pediatr Res* 31(3):222–777, 1992.

83. McCune S, Short BL, Miller MK, et al.: Extracorporeal membrane oxygenation therapy in neonates with septic shock, *J Pediatr Surg* 25(5):479–482, 1990.

84. Skinner SC, Iocono JA, Ballard HO, et al.: Improved survival in venovenous vs venoarterial extracorporeal membrane oxygenation for pediatric noncardiac sepsis patients: a study of the Extracorporeal Life Support Organization registry, *J Pediatr Surg* 47(1):63–67, 2012.

85. Ruth A, McCracken CE, Fortenberry JD, et al.: Extracorporeal therapies in pediatric severe sepsis: findings from the pediatric health-care information system, *Crit Care* 19:397, 2015.

86. MacLaren G, Butt W, Best D, et al.: Central extracorporeal membrane oxygenation for refractory pediatric septic shock, *Pediatr Crit Care Med* 12(2):133–136, 2011.

87. Boluyt N, Bollen CW, Bos AP, et al.: Fluid resuscitation in neonatal and pediatric hypovolemic shock: a Dutch Pediatric Society evidence-based clinical practice guideline, *Intensive Care Med* 32(7):995–1003, 2006.

88. Naumann DN, Beaven A, Dretzke J, et al.: Searching for the optimal fluid to restore microcirculatory flow dynamics after haemorrhagic shock: a systematic review of preclinical studies, *Shock* 46(6):609–622, 2016.

89. Diab YA, Wong EC, Luban NL: Massive transfusion in children and neonates, *Br J Haematol* 161(1):15–26, 2013.

90. DeLoughery TG: Logistics of massive transfusions, *Hematology Am Soc Hematol Educ Program* 470–473, 2010.

91. Fasano R, Luban NL: Blood component therapy, *Pediatr Clin North Am* 55(2):421–445, 2008.

92. Rossaint R, Bouillon B, Cerny V, et al.: The European guideline on management of major bleeding and coagulopathy following trauma: fourth edition, *Crit Care* 20:100, 2016.

93. Gelman S, Mushlin PS: Catecholamine-induced changes in the splanchnic circulation affecting systemic hemodynamics, *Anesthesiology* 100(2):434–439, 2004.

94. Noori S, Seri I: Neonatal blood pressure support: the use of inotropes, lusitropes, and other vasopressor agents, *Clin Perinatol* 39(1):221–238, 2012.

95. Nachar RA, Booth EA, Friedlich P, et al.: Dose-dependent hemodynamic and metabolic effects of vasoactive medications in normotensive, anesthetized neonatal piglets, *Pediatr Res* 70(5):473–479, 2011.

96. Morales D, Madigan J, Cullinane S, et al.: Reversal by vasopressin of intractable hypotension in the late phase of hemorrhagic shock, *Circulation* 100(3):226–229, 1999.

97. Anand T, Skinner R: Arginine vasopressin: the future of pressure-support resuscitation in hemorrhagic shock, *J Surg Res* 178(1):321–329, 2012.

98. Urbano J, González R, López J, et al.: Comparison of normal saline, hypertonic saline albumin and terlipressin plus hypertonic saline albumin in an infant animal model of hypovolemic shock, *PLoS One* (3)10:e0121678, 2015.

99. Desgranges FP, Desebbe O, Pereira de Souza Neto E, Raphael D, Chassard D. Respiratory variation in aortic blood flow peak velocity to predict fluid responsiveness in mechanically ventilated children: a systematic review and meta-analysis, *Paediatr Anaesth* 26(1):37–47, 2016.

27

CHAPTER 28

Hemodynamics in the Asphyxiated Neonate and Effects of Therapeutic Hypothermia

Samir Gupta and Yogen Singh

- Hypoxic ischemic (HI) injury occurs in two phases: the acute insult and the subsequent reperfusion injury.
- Impaired cerebral blood flow/oxygen delivery leads to hypoxic-ischemic brain injury, while loss of cerebral autoregulation likely contributes to the insult.
- Two-thirds of infants with moderate to severe HI injury have cardiac dysfunction, potentially contributing to tissue hypoperfusion.
- Significant hemodynamic changes take place during provision of therapeutic hypothermia (TH) and rewarming.
- TH causes bradycardia, decreases cardiac output, and increases systemic and pulmonary vascular resistance, which may lead to or worsen persistent pulmonary hypertension of the newborn.
- Clinician-performed cardiac ultrasound provides more insight into the hemodynamic status of the neonate and aids in delivering pathophysiology-directed treatment.
- There is insufficient evidence to guide the hemodynamic management of babies with HI injury.

Oxygen deprivation before or around the time of birth often results in hypoxia-ischemia (HI) induced brain damage or hypoxic-ischemic encephalopathy (HIE), which remains a common cause of neonatal brain injury across the world, affecting 1 to 3 per 1000 live births in the developed countries. Its incidence is much higher in developing countries, as high as 25 per 1000 having been reported.[1] Despite our improving understanding of the pathophysiology of HIE and the advances in neonatal intensive care in general and in the treatment of moderate to severe birth asphyxia, HIE continues to be associated with significant mortality and long-term neurodisabilities in survivors.[2-6] Ironically, even today, the definition of birth asphyxia remains imprecise.

Various pathophysiological mechanisms that contribute to HI-associated brain injury have been proposed. However, abnormal cerebral blood flow (CBF) and loss/impairment of cerebral autoregulation remain at the center of the HIE process in neonates.[7-9] The disruption in CBF may be acute, chronic, or intermittent, and is most likely to occur as a consequence of interruption in placental blood flow and gas exchange when the fetus is compromised in the perinatal period. Impaired CBF results in hypoxia and anaerobic metabolism in the fetal brain, and overall impairments in tissue oxygen delivery, result in the development of fetal metabolic acidosis.[9] Metabolic acidosis is a fairly consistent finding in neonates reflecting the degree of anaerobic metabolism and severity of hypoxia and/or ischemia during this process.[9,10] The HI-associated neuronal brain injury is closely linked to the initial hypoperfusion and the ensuing reperfusion injury (Fig. 28.1).[11] There are two hemodynamic aspects to the pathological process. The first is the injury to the

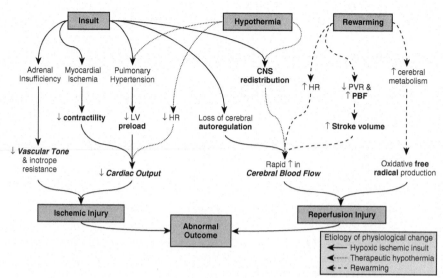

Fig. 28.1   Hemodynamic changes after hypoxic insult, therapeutic hypothermia, and rewarming and the patho-genesis of ischemic and reperfusion injury. *CNS,* Central nervous system; *HR,* heart rate; *LV,* left ventricle; *PBF,* pulmonary blood flow; *PVR,* pulmonary vascular resistance. (Permission from Giesinger RE, Bailey LJ, Deshpande P, McNamara PJ: Hypoxic-ischemic encephalopathy and therapeutic hypothermia: the hemodynamic perspective. J Pediatr 180:22–30, 2017.)

cardiovascular system itself, and the second is the deleterious effect of the impaired cardiovascular function on systemic and organ blood flow (including the CBF) in the postnatal period after the hypoxic/ischemic insult. The injury to the cardiovascular system results from myocardial ischemia and abnormal vasoregulation, as well as from the effects of pulmonary hypertension contributing to further decreases in car-diac output and systemic perfusion. Adrenal insufficiency secondary to immaturity, and the hypoxic/ischemic insult can decrease vascular tone and further exacerbate ischemic injury to the brain. Moreover, the treatment using therapeutic hypothermia (TH) and the ensuing rewarming process can also affect CBF and its autoregulation, as well as the distribution of blood flow in the brain, and potentially exacerbate the reperfusion injury.

The hemodynamic changes secondary to HI can start from fetal life and con-tinue postnatally. The management of cardiovascular pathology in this group of infants is clinician-biased rather than evidence-based. In this chapter we discuss the underlying pathophysiological mechanisms, the principles of hemodynamic assess-ment and management, and how we can utilize current bedside assessment tools to adopt a more objective approach. We will focus on the hemodynamic changes in the asphyxiated infant and the effects of TH on the hemodynamic responses.

Pathophysiology of Hypoxic Ischemic Injury

The fetus exhibits both circulatory and noncirculatory responses to improve tissue oxygen delivery, especially to preserve cerebral perfusion. However, when the dis-ruption of CBF reaches a certain level of severity and/or when the systemic and local adaptive mechanisms become exhausted, neuronal cell death starts. The pattern of neuronal injury depends on the level of the maturity and the severity of the insult. In term infants, severe HI causes selective damage to the sensorimotor cortex, basal ganglia, thalamus, and brain stem. However, in very preterm infants, periventricular white matter is particularly vulnerable to HI, resulting in a different pattern of brain injury characterized by motor, cognitive, sensory, and cortical visual deficits.[1]

HI induced injury occurs in two phases:
1. during the time of the acute insult, and
2. during the recovery period, known as the reperfusion phase.

Acute Injury

The significant reduction in CBF and oxygen delivery in severe cases of HI initiates a cascade of deleterious biochemical events at the cellular level. Hypoxia leads to anaerobic metabolism, an energy-inefficient state, resulting in rapid depletion of high-energy phosphate reserves such as adenosine triphosphate (ATP), and lactic acidosis.[12] This directly affects neuronal cellular function and causes disruption of transcellular ion transfer, leading to intracellular accumulation of sodium, calcium, and water. Inappropriate membrane depolarization results in the release of excessive excitatory neurotransmitters, specifically glutamate, from the axon terminals. Glutamate then activates specific cell surface receptors, resulting in a further influx of sodium and calcium into postsynaptic neurons. Accumulation of calcium in cytoplasm is a consequence of both increased cellular influx and decreased efflux of calcium across the plasma membrane. Moreover, in selected neurons, intracellular calcium also induces the production of nitric oxide (NO), a potent free radical that easily diffuses to adjacent cells causing widespread NO toxicity in susceptible cells. Furthermore, there is also an excessive production of oxygen free radicals from increased fatty acid peroxidation.[12,13]

The combined effect of cellular energy failure, acidosis, glutamate release, intracellular calcium accumulation, excessive production of oxygen free radicals, and NO neurotoxicity disrupts neuronal cell function and, if severe and/or long-lasting, leads to cell death by apoptosis. This process is multifactorial and the severity and duration of this insult determines the extent of cellular injury after HI.[13,14]

Reperfusion Injury (Delayed Brain Damage)

Following resuscitation and circulatory restoration (if properly identified), cerebral perfusion and oxygenation are restored and the recovery phase begins. This phase is characterized by a secondary cerebral energy failure and often occurs 6 to 48 hours after the initial insult. During this phase, blood pH starts to normalize and the cardiorespiratory status often seems stable using "conventional" assessment. However, during this phase there is a decrease in the ratio of phosphocreatine/inorganic phosphate and the intracellular pH also remains acidic, which potentially contributes to further brain injury. Subsequently, acidosis improves, pH normalizes, and the concentration of phosphate metabolites returns to baseline. During the rewarming phase following TH, there is a sudden increase in CBF, potentially worsening the effects of the reperfusion, especially in preterm infants. Studies have shown poor outcome when CBF autoregulation remains impaired, especially during the reperfusion phase of HI.[15,16]

The mechanism of secondary energy failure likely involves mitochondrial dysfunction secondary to extended reactions from the primary insults, and circulatory and endogenous inflammatory mediators contributing to ongoing brain injury. In infants, the severity of the secondary energy failure is correlated with adverse neurodevelopmental outcome.[14,16]

The pathophysiology of HI, phases of brain injury and its management with TH in infants has been well characterized in the literature.[12-17] However, the hemodynamic responses to HI and TH, which play an important role in the process, have not been well studied (Fig. 28.2).

Fetal Cardiovascular Adaptation to Hypoxia-Ischemia

In experimental fetal animal models, initial HI decreases fetal systemic vascular resistance (SVR) by at least 50% to maintain CBF and oxygen delivery to a large extent.[18-20] The decrease in fetal SVR persists until a normal or elevated mean arterial blood pressure is achieved. However, persistent hypoxemia from a severe or ongoing hypoxemic insult can lead to sustained systemic hypotension in the presence of maximal cerebral vasodilation. In such cases, CBF will be reduced.[18-20] In adults, CBF thresholds to cellular injury have been identified,[21,22] but the critical ischemic threshold for a developing brain in neonates remains unclear (see also Chapter 16).

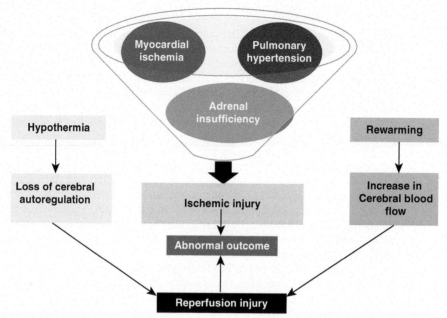

Fig. 28.2   Pathogenesis of hypoxia-ischemia induced injury, and the effects of therapeutic hypothermia and rewarming.

The important cardiovascular manifestations of interruption of placental blood flow have been well described in fetal experimental studies.[23,24] Circulatory failure (shock) develops in two phases: compensated and uncompensated.

1. Compensated phase:
   a. Neuroendocrine compensatory mechanisms ensure redistribution of the initially only somewhat decreased cardiac output to preserve blood flow to the vital organs (brain, myocardium, adrenal gland) while blood flow to the nonvital organs such as kidneys, intestine, and muscles declines
   b. Vasoparalysis with loss of cerebral autoregulation resulting in a pressure-passive cerebral circulation at maximum compensation
2. Uncompensated phase:
   a. When the neuroendocrine compensatory mechanisms become overwhelmed by the ongoing and/or severe HI, systemic hypotension and critically low cerebral perfusion with reduced oxygen delivery, lactic acidosis, and HI tissue damage

The mechanisms involved in the redistribution of blood flow are complex and include peripheral vasoconstriction, neuroendocrine and endocrine factors, and local components.[20,23,25]

Cardiovascular Effects of Hypoxia-Ischemia

Transient myocardial ischemia (and the resultant myocardial dysfunction), which may or may not be clinically symptomatic, occurs in two-thirds of asphyxiated infants. There is no doubt that this is also one of the more common causes of perinatal myocardial infarction.[26,27]

The effects of HI insult on the cardiovascular system are complex, and it is very important to understand the principles of developmental cardiovascular physiology and pathophysiology in these sick infants. Both the primary insult and the ongoing redistribution of blood flow can lead to reduced myocardial perfusion potentially resulting in myocardial ischemia, especially in the sub-endocardial tissue and papillary muscles. The hemodynamic effects of myocardial ischemia may be further impacted by the immaturity of the neonatal myocardium, and decreased myocardial contractility secondary to acidosis and hypoxia.[3,26-28] Hypoxia and acidosis are also potent pulmonary vasoconstrictors and hence increase the pulmonary vascular resistance (PVR), resulting in deleterious effects on the already

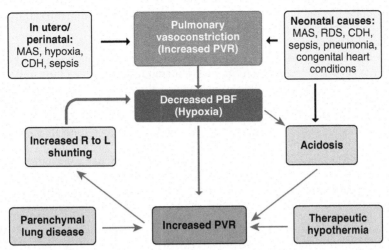

Fig. 28.3 Pathophysiology of persistent pulmonary hypertension of the newborn and effects of hypothermia. *CDH*, Congenital diaphragmatic hernia; *MAS*, meconium aspiration syndrome; *PBF*, pulmonary blood flow; *PVR*, pulmonary vascular resistance; *R to L*, right to left; *RDS*, respiratory distress syndrome.

impaired right ventricular (RV) function. Poor RV function and increased PVR affect left ventricular (LV) filling and function, and thus might impact systemic and cerebral blood flow. In addition, TH also increases PVR and SVR.[28] As a consequence, cardiac function can deteriorate further, although hypothermia also results in reduction of the metabolic needs, and subsequently lower cardiac output and systemic oxygen delivery might suffice. Finally, neonates with HI insult often have associated morbidities such as meconium aspiration syndrome (MAS) and/or sepsis. These conditions themselves may have a negative impact on cardiac function (Fig. 28.3).

The clinical consequences of the cardiovascular effects include low pulmonary blood flow (PBF) because of high PVR and thus increased RV afterload and RV dysfunction, especially when ductal flow is restricted or nonexistent. As mentioned earlier, the resulting decreases in pulmonary venous return lead to low systemic cardiac output and, if not compensated by peripheral vasoconstriction, systemic hypotension. If hypotension is treated with vasopressor-inotropes, systemic blood flow may further decrease if the response to the medication(s) is an overwhelming peripheral vasoconstriction. The impact of the clinical deterioration, the escalation of treatment, and their resultant effect on brain injury remain unknown.

The Cardiovascular System and Central Nervous System injury

The cerebral circulation is particularly sensitive to changes in partial pressure of carbon dioxide and oxygen (Chapter 2). Hypercarbia and/or hypoxia induced by interruption of placental blood flow result in significant increases in CBF. Moreover, the resultant changes in regional blood flow vary widely among the different parts of the brain. For example, the cerebral white matter has a relatively limited vasodilatory response to hypoxia and/or hypercarbia compared with the brainstem and cortical structures.[29]

Autoregulation

In healthy infants, CBF remains constant over a relatively wide range of changes in systemic mean arterial blood pressure (see Chapter 2 for details). In animal models, the fetal autoregulatory curve differs from that of the adult.[9,30] The curve is narrower, particularly at the upper elbow of the curve, and importantly, the normal mean arterial blood pressure in the less mature animal is only marginally above the lower elbow of the autoregulatory curve. In human preterm and term infants, the mean blood pressure value at the lower elbow of the autoregulatory curve, or the blood pressure threshold associated with neuronal dysfunction and then tissue injury are unknown.[31]

Autoregulation is disrupted by hypoxia, hyperoxia, hypocarbia, hypercarbia, and/or acidosis.[32] Severe disruption of autoregulation results in a pressure-passive cerebral circulation. In animal models, the role of the asphyxia-associated impaired CBF autoregulation in the pathogenesis of ischemic cerebral injury has been clearly described. If the same is true for humans, the clinical implications are of importance, as hypotension and decreased cardiac output result in decreases in CBF and thus secondary energy failure and neuronal injury.[33] As expected, this process is more pronounced in the more vulnerable regions of the brain, such as the parasagittal cortex or periventricular white matter.[30] However, in humans, this link between cerebral ischemia and cardiovascular dysfunction is not yet clear, and thus it is not known whether appropriate cardiovascular support and stabilization of CBF improve outcomes in asphyxiated infants.

Cardiovascular Effects of Therapeutic Hypothermia

TH improves outcomes in moderate to severe cases of HIE and is now part of standard care in term and near term infants (>35 weeks of gestation).[34] The cardiovascular effects of TH may be more pronounced in infants with associated conditions such as sepsis and MAS.[35-38] The direct effects of TH on the cardiovascular system include:

1. Moderate bradycardia which may decrease cardiac output[35]
2. An increase in PVR, potentially resulting in the clinical presentation of persistent pulmonary hypertension of the newborn (PPHN) or worsening of PPHN in cases with preexisting PVR elevation
3. Resultant RV dysfunction and decreased RV output, leading to decreases in pulmonary venous return and thus LV filling and LV cardiac output

As a consequence of these effects of TH in an infant already compromised from severe HI, cardiorespiratory support may need to be escalated. This may involve the need for higher airway pressures on the ventilator. Unfortunately, this maneuver, especially in patients with normal lung compliance, may further impair venous return and hence decrease ventricular output. Introduction of vasopressor-inotropes, especially at inappropriately high doses, may impair myocardial perfusion and increase myocardial oxygen demand, potentially resulting in further deterioration of cardiac function (Fig. 28.4).[39]

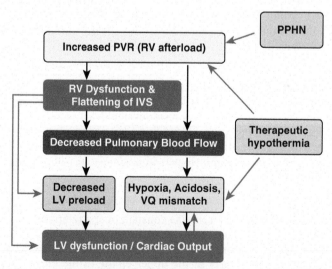

Fig. 28.4   Cardiac function in persistent pulmonary hypertension of the newborn and effect of hypothermia. *IVS,* Interventricular septum; *LV,* left ventricle; *PPHN,* persistent pulmonary hypertension of newborn; *PVR,* pulmonary vascular resistance; *RV,* right ventricle; *VQ mismatch,* ventilation-perfusion mismatch.

Cardiovascular Effects of Rewarming After Hypothermia

As in the case of TH, the cardiovascular effects of rewarming have not been well studied. Accordingly, there is very little published data on the hemodynamic changes during rewarming in neonates. Rewarming decreases PVR and SVR and affects redistribution of cardiac output to the organs. It increases heart rate and cardiac output, although mean blood pressure may decrease or remain unaffected as a consequence of a decrease in diastolic blood pressure. Hence the physiological consequences of rewarming are likely to influence management, such as choice of vasopressor-inotropes/inotropes and fluid management, and might even impact clinical outcomes.[40] In addition, rewarming affects metabolism and clearance of drugs, including cardiovascular medications.[36]

Rewarming certainly has an effect on the cardiovascular status/hemodynamic stability in these sick babies. In addition, studies have shown that infants are more likely to have seizures during the rewarming phase. In a recent study involving 160 asphyxiated infants, 9% developed intra/periventricular hemorrhage during the rewarming phase.[41] Therefore these infants remain particularly vulnerable during the rewarming phase and need to be monitored more closely for any hemodynamic instability. It seems to be a sensible approach to avoid large fluctuations in blood pressure and cardiac output and thus in CBF, especially in the sicker, more vulnerable infant on significant cardiovascular support.

The cardiovascular effects of TH and rewarming, and their subsequent impact on management, clearly needs further assessment in well-designed studies using clinician-performed cardiac ultrasound (CPU) and other advanced cardiorespiratory and neurocritical care monitoring techniques (see Chapter 21).

Clinical Implications

As discussed earlier, HI, TH, and rewarming all affect the cardiovascular system. These physiologic changes present with different clinical signs and symptoms, and have implications on the assessment and management of these infants.

Effect on Heart Rate and Cardiac Output

Hypoxic-ischemic insults often lead to compensatory tachycardia, although severe or terminal insults can lead to bradycardia. Due to the decreased metabolic demand and the direct effects of cooling itself, TH is associated with a decrease in heart rate in all infants, and there is a reduction in cardiac output in up to 62% of infants.[4] The direct effects of cooling on heart rate presenting as sinus bradycardia are mostly due to the decreased repolarization of the sinoatrial node and the diminished influence of the sympathetic autonomic nervous system. It also induces pulmonary and peripheral vasoconstriction, which can affect ventricular filling and afterload, thereby further decreasing cardiac output.[7,36,40] Vasopressor-inotrope and/or inotrope administration to combat hypotension and/or poor myocardial function, respectively, may lead to increases in heart rate and oxygen demand. Inappropriate dosing of these medications may cause excessive tachycardia and decreases in PBF and cardiac output, and adversely affect myocardial contractility.

Rewarming has the opposite effects on the cardiovascular parameters. During the re-warming phase, there is a sometimes sudden increase in the heart rate and cardiac output.[40] These changes, especially if abrupt, may contribute to reperfusion injury in the brain and other organs. These effects can be more pronounced in infants already needing cardiorespiratory support.

Clinical Implications in Asphyxiated Infants With Sepsis and Persistent Pulmonary Hypertension of the Newborn

Hypoxic-ischemic insults can be associated with PPHN, and this may have significant clinical implications in these often critically ill infants. Hypoxia and TH can increase PVR, cause RV dysfunction, cause decrease in cardiac output, and subsequently lead to systemic hypotension and hypoperfusion.[39,42-44] Sepsis, especially when associated with parenchymal lung disease, can have similar effects, but sepsis without parenchymal pathology also presents with tachycardia, increased oxygen demand, and systemic hypotension.[43]

Clinical Assessment of the Asphyxiated Neonate

HI injury often exerts multisystem affects, including impairment of cardiovascular function. It may result in primary pump failure due to direct myocardial ischemic injury, abnormal vasoregulation, or both, and thus present with systemic hypoperfusion and hypotension. Disturbances of transition to extrauterine life and delayed resolution of the high PVR can manifest as maladaptation and pulmonary hypertension. The presence of clinical signs and symptoms of poor perfusion usually reflect the state of uncompensated shock and suggest the presence of HI organ damage of varied severity. It is therefore of importance to diagnose the hemodynamic disturbance early in its compensated phase. Clinician-performed cardiac ultrasound represents one of the essential diagnostic approaches in the care of these neonates. Its use may aid in appropriately targeting the treatment to the needs of the individual patient and could potentially lead to improvements in short- and long-term outcomes in this group of neonates. However, there is little evidence so far to support that this approach indeed results in better outcomes.

Immediate Assessment of Perfusion

The immediate assessment of perfusion in neonates with HI injury can be broadly grouped into assessment during the precooling phase and during TH. In both stages, the principles of assessment remain the same, but the findings should be interpreted according to the phase of the care of the infant.

The assessment of perfusion can be broadly classified into:
- Preload
- Cardiac function
- Afterload
- End organ perfusion
- Capillary perfusion

Furthermore, the assessment targets can be broadly grouped into:
- Clinical assessment
- Noninvasive assessment
- Invasive assessment

Clinical assessment is routinely carried out, but there are inherent limitations as the signs and symptoms mostly become recognizable in the compensated phase of shock (Chapter 1). *Cardiac function and preload* can be assessed by monitoring heart rate and jugular venous pressure, respectively.[45] However, jugular venous pressure is very difficult to gauge in neonates, and hence it is difficult to assess *preload* clinically. In newborn infants, the cardiac output usually changes by variations in *heart rate*. As neonates receiving TH present with sinus bradycardia (see earlier), heart rate monitoring is of limited value to clinically assess changes in cardiac output in these infants. Heart rate variability has also been used for the staging of HIE and outcome prognostication (see Chapter 20). Severe HIE is reported to be associated with lower heart rate variability in the first 24 postnatal hours. In addition, the heart rate is affected by the temperature of the baby and the use of vasopressor-inotropes and inotropes, and hence it is a poor marker for bedside cardiac function.

The *afterload* can be assessed clinically by the blood pressure, but the choice of method may affect the measured values. Invasive blood pressure measurements are encouraged over noninvasive assessments, due to their suggested higher accuracy in critically ill patients (Chapter 3). Blood pressure is affected by gestational and postnatal age, as well as by the severity of the acute insult and hypothermia treatment.[46] Low systolic blood pressure is usually due to cardiac dysfunction. If low systolic blood pressure is recorded, it should be correlated with the requirements for oxygen. Normal oxygenation with low systolic blood pressure primarily reflects LV/RV systolic dysfunction. On the contrary, the finding of low systolic blood pressure and impaired oxygenation should alert the clinician to rule out PPHN with or without LV/RV dysfunction. Low systolic pressure may be seen during TH, but usually it is high enough to maintain adequate tissue perfusion due to the reduced metabolic demand. During TH, the diastolic blood pressure is usually maintained due to peripheral vasoconstriction. If diastolic blood pressure remains persistently low during TH, underlying causes such as sepsis should be ruled out. Mean arterial pressures alone should not be used for decision-making in infants with HIE, as it can delay identification of low systolic blood pressure.[47]

The clinical signs of compensated shock (decreased urine output, prolonged capillary refill time, core-peripheral temperature difference) are of limited value in the neonate immediately following delivery (Chapter 1 and Chapter 26). By the time metabolic acidosis and high lactate are present, shock has entered its uncompensated phase, and organ damage has become more likely. Finally, with active cooling, most of these clinical signs cannot be reliably used to assess perfusion.[46]

The invasive assessments are useful for precise measurements but are either cumbersome or not available routinely on neonatal intensive care units. The exceptions are arterial blood gas measurements and continuous invasive blood pressure recording. The preload can be assessed using central venous pressure measurements. However, its accuracy is questionable at best. End-organ perfusion can be continuously assessed using mixed venous saturations to provide more accurate information on tissue perfusion, but this requires a central line that often is not available in babies on neonatal intensive care units. However, intermittent arterial blood gas analysis provides information on blood gas parameters that can be helpful for routine management of babies with HIE with or without pulmonary hypertension and/or maladaptation. The assessment of metabolic derangement through markers of end organ perfusion such as lactate concentration and the base deficit are helpful, but are late signs that are only present in the uncompensated phase of shock.[4,46]

The interest in *bedside noninvasive assessment of perfusion* to assess various components of the hemodynamic status using various tools and techniques (see Chapters 14, 16 to 18 for details) and even a comprehensive approach (Chapter 21) is now rapidly increasing. Some of these novel approaches, such as near infrared spectroscopy, are of special value for use in neonates with HIE.

Clinician-Performed Cardiac Ultrasound for Hemodynamic Assessment in Neonates With Hypoxic-Ischemic Encephalopathy

Clinician-performed cardiac ultrasound (US) has been increasingly used for the assessment of neonates with HIE, as it provides comprehensive information on the determinants of cardiac function and organ perfusion.[48-54] With an increasing number of neonatologists available to utilize this bedside tool, in addition to providing information on the cardiovascular status and establishing the diagnosis of PPHN, with CPU the clinician can also help assess the response to treatment and more appropriately titrate the vasoactive medications. A number of assessments are available that can be used to assess loading conditions and cardiac function.[51-54] The echocardiographic parameters for hemodynamic evaluation and pulmonary hypertension are summarized in Tables 28.1 and 28.2, respectively. The details of echocardiographic techniques are discussed in Chapters 10 to 13.

Approach to Hemodynamic Management

Most neonates with isolated mild transient myocardial ischemia are asymptomatic and improve spontaneously over time. However, infants with moderate to severe HI often have significant cardiac injury, and hypotension is observed in up to 62% of patients following perinatal asphyxia.[4] Most of the "antihypotensive" medications, when used in inappropriate doses in the given patient, may have adverse cardiac effects such as tachycardia, increased oxygen consumption, decreased systemic blood flow, and alteration of tissue perfusion. Furthermore, studies have demonstrated an association between altered CBF and poor outcome.[55] Hence aggressive

Table 28.1   SUMMARY OF HEMODYNAMIC EVALUATION USING ULTRASOUND

Assessment of preload

- Inferior vena cava variability and collapsibility
- Superior vena cava flow
- Visual assessment of the heart ("eyeballing")

Assessment of cardiac function

- Systolic function
  - Left ventricular systolic function (Fig. 28.5)
    - Fractional shortening measurement (Figs. 28.6 and 28.7)
    - Tissue Doppler imaging (TDI)—anterior/septal walls of mitral valve
  - Right ventricular function
    - TAPSE—Tricuspid annular plane systolic excursion by M-mode
    - Tissue Doppler imaging—tricuspid valve
    - Right ventricular fractional area change
  - Indirect markers of systolic function
    - Left ventricular output (LVO)
    - Right ventricular output (RVO)
- Diastolic function
  - Isovolumetric relaxation time (IVRT measured with TDI)
  - E/A ratio at the mitral and tricuspid valve

Table 28.2   SUMMARY OF ULTRASOUND ASSESSMENT OF PULMONARY HYPERTENSION OF NEWBORN

Assessment of pulmonary hypertension

- Establishing normal structure of heart
- Right ventricular hypertrophy and/or dilatation
- Assessment of right and left ventricular systolic function
- Estimation of pulmonary artery systolic pressure by measuring right ventricular pressure (when cardiac function is normal) = $(4V^2)$ + right atrial pressure; V is the velocity of tricuspid regurgitation (Fig. 28.8)
- Evaluation of shunt across ductus arteriosus and foramen ovale
- Assessment of interventricular septum for flattening/bowing (Fig. 28.9)
- Time to peak velocity/Ejection time of flow in main pulmonary artery (Normal > 0.25)

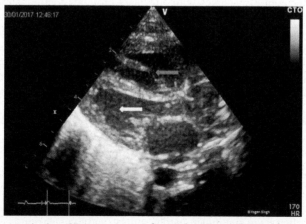

Fig. 28.5   Parasternal long-axis view, 2D image in an infant with HIE and PPHN showing a dilated and hypertrophied right ventricle (marked with *red arrow*), along with a normal looking LV (marked with *yellow arrow*) during therapeutic hypothermia. The patient's poor LV function (illustrated in Fig. 28.6) was, at least in part, due to the decrease in pulmonary blood flow and the resulting poor LV filling. *HIE,* Hypoxic-ischemic encephalopathy; *LV,* left ventricle; *PPHN,* persistent pulmonary hypertension of newborn.

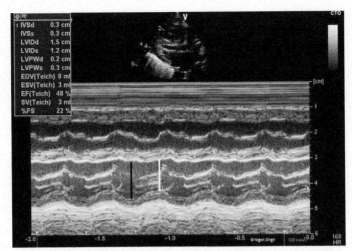

Fig. 28.6 Parasternal long-axis view demonstrating M-mode for an LV study showing poor LV function during therapeutic hypothermia in an infant with hypoxic-ischaemic encephalopathy and persistent pulmonary hypertension of newborn (Echo image taken at the same time as in Fig. 28.5). Left ventricular end diastolic diameter illustrated by the *red line* and left ventricular end systolic diameter by the *yellow line*. *LV,* Left ventricle.

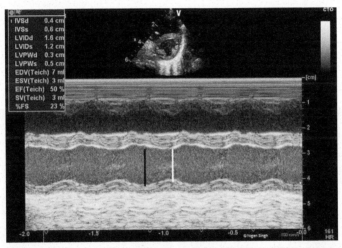

Fig. 28.7 Parasternal short-axis view demonstrating M-mode for an LV study showing poor LV function during rewarming after therapeutic hypothermia in an infant with hypoxic-ischemic encephalopathy and persistent pulmonary hypertension of newborn (same infant as in Figs. 28.5 and 28.6). Left ventricular end-diastolic diameter illustrated by the *red line* and left ventricular end-systolic diameter by the *yellow line*. *LV,* Left ventricle.

volume resuscitation should be avoided after initial resuscitation, except when there is direct evidence of acute hypovolemia. A judicious approach to cardiovascular management should involve a good understanding of the effects of HI, TH, rewarming, and medications on systemic and pulmonary hemodynamics and CBF.

Preload, Pump, and Afterload

Preload, pump, and afterload are affected by the HI insult, TH, the rewarming process, and the medications used to treat hypotension. These infants often have increased PVR and SVR from the underlying pathology, which is further increased by TH.[31-35]

A significant HI insult usually leads to myocardial and endocardial ischemia, which in turn affects myocardial contractility and causes valvular insufficiency, respectively. Neonates with significant cardiac dysfunction can have critically low cardiac output that may be compounded by the TH-induced vasoconstriction and the

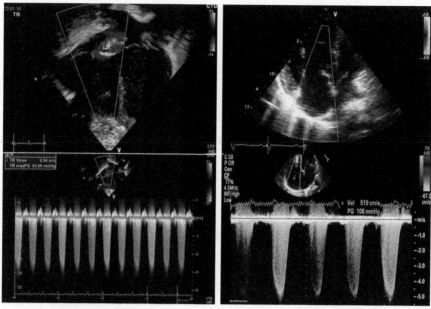

Image a: Mild TR   Image b: Severe TR

Fig. 28.8   Estimation of pulmonary artery pressure by measuring tricuspid regurgitation (TR), which measures the gradient between RV and RA. Image "a" shows mild TR suggestive of mild pulmonary hypertension (estimated pulmonary artery pressure around 40 mm Hg). Image "b" showing severe TR suggestive of severe pulmonary hypertension (estimated pulmonary artery pressure around 110 to 115 mm Hg). Of note is that there are a number of neonates with pulmonary hypertension where TR is not seen. *RA,* Right atrium; *RV,* right ventricle.

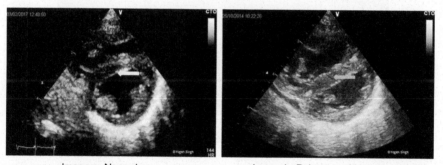

Image a: Normal   Image b: Pulmonary Hypertension

Fig. 28.9   Parasternal short-axis view. Image "a" shows normal LV contour and interventricular septum (IVS); Image "b" shows flattening of the interventricular septum suggestive of systemic/suprasystemic pulmonary artery pressure. The *yellow arrow* in the image "a" shows normal IVS, while the *red arrow* in image "b" reveals flattening of the IVS. *IVS,* Intraventricular septum; *LV,* left ventricle.

associated increased afterload. LV dysfunction results in reduced stroke volume, and thus low cardiac output and dilatation of the LV could also result in mitral regurgitation and left atrial enlargement and, subsequently, persistent venous pulmonary hypertension.[43]

Right ventricle dysfunction causes reduction in RV output. The decrease in PBF results in worsening gas exchange and reduction in LV end-diastolic volume and thus LV output. Persistent RV diastolic dysfunction and tricuspid insufficiency lead to dilatation of the RV, also impairing systemic venous return. Overdistension of the lungs from mechanical ventilation can also reduce systemic venous return. This leads to decreased RV preload, further reducing RV output.[40,41,51] Serial bedside assessment by US provides important information on preload, SVR, PVR, and cardiac function, and allows for targeting the therapy to the underlying pathophysiology (Table 28.3).

Table 28.3 A SUGGESTED APPROACH TO MANAGEMENT OF HEMODYNAMIC CHANGES IN NEONATES WITH HIE RECEIVING TH WITH OR WITHOUT PPHN USING CLINICIAN-PERFORMED CARDIAC ULTRASOUND (FOR PATIENTS WITH PPHN SEE CHAPTER 9 FOR DETAILS)

Echocardiographic Assessment	Therapeutic Goals	Suggested Drug Therapy	Specific Comments
HIE with myocardial dysfunction without evidence for PPHN	1. Myocardial dysfunction with increased SVR—Use drugs to reduce SVR with inotropic effect 2. Myocardial dysfunction with decreased SVR—Use drugs with inotropic *and* vasopressor effect 3. Myocardial dysfunction with refractory hypotension and inappropriate tissue oxygen delivery	a. Milrinone or dobutamine b. Low- to moderate doses of epinephrine Epinephrine or dopamine (± Dobutamine) Add hydrocortisone (Chapter 9)	Use milrinone for at least 2–3 days. Beware of drug clearance if renal impairment and with TH
HIE with PPHN without appreciable myocardial dysfunction	1. Increase systemic blood flow and blood pressure 2. Decrease PVR to increase pulmonary blood flow 3. Refractory hypotension and inappropriate tissue oxygen delivery 4. In the presence of restrictive PDA and inadequate response to above treatment	Low- to moderate-dose epinephrine or dopamine (follow myocardial function closely) • iNO (+ milrinone) ± sildenafil[b] • Consider low-dose norepinephrine[c] or vasopressin[d] if presentation is resistant to iNO + milrinone + sildenafil and optimized ventilation Hydrocortisone (+ vasopressin if no response to HC) Low dose prostaglandin E1	Use milrinone at least until iNO is administered.[a,b] If associated RV or LV dysfunction—aim for specific therapy as below
HIE with PPHN and myocardial dysfunction	1. Increase pulmonary blood flow/decrease PVR 2. Increase systemic blood flow (RV preload) 3. In the presence of restrictive PDA, RV dysfunction and inadequate response to above treatment 4. Refractory hypotension and inappropriate tissue oxygen delivery	• iNO (+ milrinone) ± sildenafil[b] • Consider low-dose norepinephrine[c] (see above) Add dobutamine to iNO, milrinone (±sildenafil) Low dose prostaglandin E1 Hydrocortisone	RV and LV functions are interdependent

[a]Chen B, Lakshminrusimha S, Czech L, et al: Regulation of phosphodiesterase 3 in the pulmonary arteries during the perinatal period in sheep. Pediatr Res 66:682–687, 2009.
[b]Lakshminrusimha S, Konduri GG, Steinhorn RH: Considerations in the management of hypoxemic respiratory failure and persistent pulmonary hypertension in term and late preterm neonates. J Perinatol 36 Suppl 2:S12–S19, 2016.
[c]Tourneux P, Rakza T, Bouissou A, et al: Pulmonary circulatory effects of norepinephrine in newborn infants with persistent pulmonary hypertension. J Pediatr 153:345–349, 2008.
[d]Mohamed A, Nasef N, Shah V, McNamara PJ. Vasopressin as a rescue therapy for refractory pulmonary hypertension in neonates: case series. Pediatr Crit Care Med 15:148–154, 2014.
Maintain optimum hemoglobin levels to improve oxygen delivery.
Optimize therapy for pulmonary vasodilation with appropriate ventilation strategy; surfactant if pulmonary parenchymal disease is present and optimized sedation/analgesia.
Follow hemodynamic changes closely with CPU and comprehensive, continuous hemodynamic monitoring if available (Chapter 21).
CPU, Clinician-performed cardiac ultrasound; *HC,* hydrocortisone; *HIE,* hypoxic-ischemic encephalopathy; *iNO,* inhaled nitric oxide; *LV,* left ventricle; *PDA,* patent ductus arteriosus; *PPHN,* persistent pulmonary hypertension of the newborn; *PVR,* pulmonary vascular resistance; *RV,* right ventricle; *SVR,* systemic vascular resistance; *TH,* therapeutic hypothermia.

As with all medications, cardiovascular medications used in the treatment of neonates with HIE and TH also have side effects, which may be more frequent and/or serious in infants with HIE with or without PPHN. Indeed, in infants in general and in those with HIE and TH in particular, clearance of cardiovascular medications may be reduced. For instance, when milrinone is used, drug accumulation could result in systemic hypotension due to enhanced systemic vasodilatation in these patients.[56,57] Dobutamine is the most commonly used inotrope in neonates, and dopamine along with epinephrine are the most commonly used vasopressor-inotropes.[58] Dobutamine or milrinone might be used as first-line therapy in infants with myocardial dysfunction in patients with HI injury. It improves perfusion by increasing cardiac output.[59,60] However, doses higher than 10 μg/kg/min have the potential to also increase SVR, especially in preterm neonates and in patients without significant adrenergic receptor downregulation.[58] In hypotensive asphyxiated patients without apparent myocardial injury and with vasodilation, dopamine or epinephrine are usually effective in increasing blood pressure and improving systemic and, potentially, pulmonary blood flow.[58] Finally, in severely asphyxiated infants, adrenal insufficiency may occur independently of, or in combination with, other causes of hypotension, potentially resulting in the presentation of volume- and vasopressor-refractory hypotension. In these patients, the addition of hydrocortisone often results in improvement of the cardiovascular status.

In neonates with HIE and coexisting pulmonary hypertension, US evaluation of hemodynamics is considered to be an essential part of routine care of these patients. Although inhaled nitric oxide (iNO) remains the drug of choice to reduce PVR, inotropic, lusitropic, and vasopressor support can be more objectively guided by serial assessment of PVR, SVR, and measures of cardiac function (see Table 28.3). For instance, infants with failing RV function and a restrictive ductus arteriosus on echocardiography may benefit from low-dose prostaglandin E_1 (5 to 10 ng/kg/min) to open the ductus arteriosus and offload the right ventricle.[40,61] Finally, patients with PPHN receiving HT and not responding to advanced conventional therapy may require extra-corporeal membrane oxygenation (ECMO) support. In units where ECMO is not available, nonresponding patients might improve their oxygenation if cooling temperature is increased by 0.5°C first instead of immediately fully abandoning TH. These maneuvers might allow for safer transfer of the critically ill patient to an ECMO center. These practices are variable, as there is no evidence to support the preferred approach, and hence are clinician-biased.

Moreover, cardiorespiratory management strategies are often interdependent on each other, and strategies used for supporting one system could affect the other system. A commonly encountered scenario is overdistension of the lungs, especially with improving parenchymal disease leading to impairment of venous return and thus preload and cardiac output. Parenchymal disease or collapse/atelectasis of the lungs can also increase PVR, resulting in the worsening of hypoxia. On the other hand, underventilation may exacerbate hypoxia and thus impair cardiac function. Therefore cardiorespiratory strategies should be carefully planned and followed, especially with changes in the clinical condition.

Clinical Studies of Hemodynamic Management of Asphyxia and Therapeutic Hypothermia

Randomized control trials (RCTs) of TH in neonates with HIE convincingly demonstrated neurological benefits, especially in neonates with moderate HIE. Accordingly, TH is now part of standard care for moderate or severe HIE in the Western world.[34] There was no statistically significant increase in the incidence of clinically detectable pulmonary hypertension identified in the RCTs. However, these trials were not powered to detect differences in the severity of pulmonary hypertension, and more importantly, in some trials (such as the "Neo.nEURO.network Trial" and the "Infant Cooling Evaluation Trial"), the hemodynamically unstable infants were excluded.[62,63]

In clinical practice, all infants with HIE and PPHN receive therapeutic cooling despite the possibility that, in some patients, pulmonary vasoconstriction may worsen.[64,65] Therefore, in infants with HIE receiving TH, hemodynamic assessment with US and iNO need to be available to diagnose and treat, respectively, the pulmonary hypertension, while still having the benefits of TH.

The use of multiple inotropes and vasopressor-inotropes in the management of these infants is common practice, primarily led by uncertainty rather than need. Such practice may increase the side effects of the pharmacological management, primarily through causing inadvertent rapid changes in systemic and organ blood flow and blood pressure. The current practices are often based on personal experience and preference rather than evidence or, at least, on a management approach guided by thorough monitoring of the hemodynamic status using CPU and comprehensive hemodynamic monitoring (Chapter 21).

Conclusions

The majority of infants with moderate to severe hypoxic insult have cardiac dysfunction and cardiovascular instability. TH is now a standard practice in the treatment of these patients. Both TH and rewarming lead to significant hemodynamic changes that can be further affected by mechanical ventilation, use of inotropes, lusitropes, and vasopressor-inotropes, and other medications used in the treatment of infants with HIE, as well as by comorbidities including pulmonary hypertension and sepsis. Conventional hemodynamic assessment only provides indirect markers of cardiovascular well-being, while CPU and comprehensive hemodynamic monitoring provide more objective information on the hemodynamic status of the patient. In addition, the latter monitoring approaches also better aid in tailoring management to the individual patient's response to treatment. Finally, more research is needed to better understand the hemodynamic changes and the impact of interventions during the acute phases of the HI injury and TH, so that further improvements in short- and long-term neurodevelopmental outcomes can be achieved.

REFERENCES

1. Kurinczuk JJ, White-Koning M, Badawi N: Epidemiology of neonatal encephalopathy and hypoxic-ischaemic encephalopathy, *Early Hum Dev* 86(10):329–338, 2010.
2. Freeman JM, Nelson KB: Intrapartum asphyxia and cerebral palsy, *Pediatrics* 82:240–249, 1988.
3. Martín-Ancel A, García-Alix A, Cabanas F, et al.: Multiple organ involvement in perinatal asphyxia, *J Pediatr* 127:293–786, 1995.
4. Shah P, Riphagen S, Beyene J, Perlman M: Multiorgan dysfunction in infants with postasphyxial hypoxic–ischaemic encephalopathy, *Arch Dis Child Fetal Neonatal Ed* 89:F152–F155, 2004.
5. Lawn JE, Cousens S, Zupan J: 4 million neonatal deaths: when? Where? Why? *Lancet* 365(9462):891–900, 2005.
6. Lawn JE, Kerber K, Enweronu-Laryea C, et al.: 3.6 million neonatal deaths–what is progressing and what is not? *Semin Perinatol* 34(6):371–386, 2010.
7. Shalak L, Perlman JM: Hypoxic-ischemic brain injury in the term infant-current concepts, *Early Hum Dev* 80:125–141, 2004.
8. Low JA, Panagiotopoulos C, Derrick EJ: Newborn complications after intrapartum asphyxia with metabolic acidosis in the preterm fetus, *Am J Obstet Gynecol* 172:805–809, 1995.
9. Goldaber KG, Gilstrap III LC, Leveno KJ, et al.: Pathologic fetal acidemia, *Obstet Gynecol* 78:1103–1107, 1991.
10. King TA, Jackson GL, Josey AS, et al.: The effect of profound umbilical artery acidemia in term neonates admitted to a newborn nursery, *J Pediatr* 132:624–629, 1998.
11. Giesinger RE, Bailey LJ, Deshpande P, McNamara PJ: Hypoxic-ischemic encephalopathy and therapeutic hypothermia: the hemodynamic perspective, *J Pediatr* 180:22–30, 2017.
12. Wyatt JS, Edwards AD, Azzopardi D, Reynolds EO: Magnetic resonance and near infrared spectroscopy for investigation of perinatal hypoxic-ischemic brain injury, *Arch Dis Child* 64:953–963, 1989.
13. Grow J, Barks JD: Pathogenesis of hypoxic-ischemic cerebral injury in the term infant: current concepts, *Clin Perinatol* 29:585–602, 2002.
14. Ferriero DM: Neonatal brain injury, *N Engl J Med* 351:1985–1995, 2004.
15. Lorek A, Takei Y, Cady EB, et al.: Delayed ('secondary') cerebral energy failure after acute hypoxia-ischemia in the newborn piglet: continuous 48-h studies by phosphorus magnetic resonance spectroscopy, *Pediatr Res* 36:699–706, 1994.
16. Roth SC, Baudin J, Cady E, et al.: Relation of deranged neonatal cerebral oxidative metabolism with neurodevelopmental outcome and head circumference at 4 years, *Dev Med Child Neurol* 39:718–725, 1997.
17. Palmer C: Hypoxic-ischemic encephalopathy. Therapeutic approaches against microvascular injury, and role of neutrophils, PAF, and free radicals, *Clin Perinatol* 22:481–517, 1995.
18. Johnson EW, Palahniwk RJ, Tween WA, et al.: Regional cerebral blood flow changes during severe fetal asphyxia produced by slow partial umbilical cord compression, *Am J Obstet Gynecol* 135:45–48, 1979.
19. Jones Jr MD, Sheldon RE, Peeters LL, et al.: Regulation of cerebral blood flow in the ovine fetus, *Am J Physiol* 235:162–166, 1978.
20. Ashwal S, Dale PS, Longo ID: Regional cerebral blood flow: Studies in the fetal lamb during hypoxia, hypercapnia, acidosis and hypotension, *Pediatr Res* 18:13091316, 1984.

21. Powers WJ, Grubb Jr RL, Darriet D, et al.: Cerebral blood flow and cerebral metabolic rate of oxygen requirements for cerebral function and viability in humans, *J Cereb Blood Flow Metab* 5:600–608, 1985.
22. Heiss WD, Rosner G: Functional recovery of cortical neurons as related to the degree and duration of ischemia, *Ann Neurol* 14:294–301, 1983.
23. Cohn EH, Sacks EJ, Heymann MA, et al.: Cardiovascular responses to hypoxemia and acidemia in fetal lambs, *Am J Obstet Gynecol* 120:817–824, 1974.
24. Lassen NA, Christensen MS: Physiology of cerebral blood flow, *Br J Anaesth* 48:719–734, 1976.
25. Morrison S, Gardner DS, Fletcher AJ, et al.: Enhanced nitric oxide activity offsets peripheral vaso-constriction during acute hypoxemia via chemoreflex and adrenomedullary actions in the fetus, *J Physiol* 547:283–291, 2003.
26. Armstrong K, Franklin O, Sweetman D, et al.: Cardiovascular dysfunction in infants with neonatal encephalopathy, *Arch Dis Child* 97:372–375, 2012.
27. Dattilo G, Tulino V, Tulino D, et al.: Perinatal asphyxia and cardiac abnormalities, *Int J Cardiol* 147:e39–e40, 2011.
28. Benumof JL, Wahrenbrock EA: Dependency of hypoxic pulmonary vasoconstriction on temperature, *J Appl Physiol Respir Environ Exerc Physiol* 42:56–58, 1977.
29. Rosenberg AA, Jones Jr MD, Traystman RJ, et al.: Response of cerebral blood flow to changes in PCO_2 in fetal, newborn, and adult sheep, *Am J Physiol* 242:H862, 1982.
30. Tweed A, Cote J, Lou H, et al.: Impairment of cerebral blood flow autoregulation in the newborn lamb by hypoxia, *Pediatr Res* 20:516–519, 1986.
31. McLean CW, Noori S, Cayabyab R, Seri I: In Perlman JM, editor: *Cerebral circulation and hypo-tension in the premature infant-diagnosis and treatment, in questions and controversies in neona-tology-neurology*, 2011, Saunders/Elsevier.
32. Kaiser JR, Gauss CH, Williams DK: The effects of hypercapnia on cerebral autoregulation in venti-lated very low birth weight infants, *Pediatr Res* 58:931935, 2005.
33. Vannucci RC, Towfighi J, Vannucci SJ: Secondary energy failure after cerebral hypoxia-ischemia in the immature rat, *J Cereb Blood Flow Metab* 24:1090–1097, 2004.
34. Azzopardi DV, Strohm B, Edwards AD, et al.: Moderate hypothermia to treat perinatal asphyxial encephalopathy, *N Engl J Med* 361:1349–1358, 2009.
35. Massaro AN, Govindan RB, Al-Shargabi T, et al.: Heart rate variability in encephalopathic newborns during and after therapeutic hypothermia, *J Perinatol* 34:836–864, 2014.
36. Wood T, Thoresen M: Physiological responses to hypothermia, *Semin Fetal Neonatal Med* 20:87–96, 2014.
37. Thomsen JH, Nielsen N, Hassager C, et al.: Bradycardia during targeted temperature management: an early marker of lower mortality and favorable neurologic outcome in comatose out-of-hospital cardiac arrest patients, *Crit Care Med* 44:308–318, 2016.
38. Hochwald O, Jabr M, Osiovich H, et al.: Preferential cephalic redistribution of left ventricular car-diac output during therapeutic hypothermia for perinatal hypoxic-ischemic encephalopathy, *J Pediatr* 164:999–1004, 2014.
39. Nestaas E, Skranes JH, Stoylen A, et al.: The myocardial function during and after whole-body thera-peutic hypothermia for hypoxic-ischemic encephalopathy, a cohort study, *Early Hum Dev* 90:247–252, 2014.
40. Jain A, McNamara P: Persistent pulmonary hypertension of the newborn: physiology, hemodynamic assessment and novel therapies, *Semin Fetal Neonatal Med* 20:262–271, 2015.
41. Zanelli S, Buck M, Fairchild K: Physiologic and pharmacologic considerations for hypothermia ther-apy in neonates, *J Perinatol* 31:377–386, 2011.
42. Al Yazidi G, Boudes E, Tan X, et al.: Intraventricular hemorrhage in asphyxiated newborns treated with hypothermia: a look into incidence, timing and risk factors, *BMC Pediatr* 15:106, 2015.
43. Giesinger RE, McNamara PJ: Hemodynamic instability in the critically ill neonate: an approach to cardiovascular support based on disease pathophysiology, *Semin Perinatol* 40:174–188, 2016.
44. Lapointe A, Barrington KJ: Pulmonary hypertension and the asphyxiated newborn, *J Pediatr* 158 (Suppl 2):e19–e24, 2011.
45. Osborn DA, Evans N, Kluckow M: Clinical detection of low upper body blood flow in very premature infants using blood pressure, capillary refill time, and central-peripheral temperature difference, *Arch Dis Child Fetal Neonatal Ed* 89(2):F168–F173, 2004.
46. Gebauer CM, Knuepfer M, Robel-Tillig E, et al.: Hemodynamics among neonates with hypoxic-ischemic encephalopathy during whole-body hypothermia and passive rewarming, *Pediatrics* 117(3):843–850, 2006.
47. Soleymani S, Borzage M, Seri I: Hemodynamic monitoring in neonates: advances and challenges, *J Perinatol* 30:S38–S45, 2010.
48. Negrine RJ, Chikermane A, Wright JG, Ewer AK: Assessment of myocardial function in neonates using tissue Doppler imaging, *Arch Dis Child Fetal Neonatal Ed* 97(4):F304–F306, 2012.
49. Breatnach CR, Levy PT, James AT, et al.: Novel echocardiography methods in the functional assess-ment of the newborn heart, *Neonatology* 110(4):248–260, 2016.
50. James AT, Corcoran JD, McNamara PJ, et al.: The effect of milrinone on right and left ventricular function when used as a rescue therapy for term infants with pulmonary hypertension, *Cardiol Young* 26(1):90–99, 2016.
51. Breatnach CR, Forman E, Foran A, et al.: Left ventricular rotational mechanics in infants with hypoxic ischemic encephalopathy and preterm infants at 36 weeks' postmenstrual age: a comparison with healthy term controls, *Echocardiography*, December 9, 2016. https://doi.org/10.1111/echo.13421. [Epub ahead of print].

52. Singh Y, Gupta S, Groves AM, et al.: Expert consensus statement 'Neonatologist-performed Echocardiography (NoPE)'-training and accreditation in UK, *Eur J Pediatr* 175:281–287, 2016.
53. Mertens L, Seri I, Marek J, et al.: Targeted neonatal echocardiography in the neonatal intensive care unit: practice guidelines and recommendations for training. Writing group of the American Society of Echocardiography (ASE) in collaboration with the European Association of Echocardiography (EAE) and the Association for European Pediatric Cardiologists (AEPC), *J Am Soc Echocardiogr* 24:1057–1078, 2011.
54. De Boode W, Singh Y, Gupta S, et al.: Recommendations for neonatologist performed echocardiography in Europe: consensus statement endorsed by European Society for Paediatric Research (ESPR) and European Society for Neonatology (ESN), *Pediatr Res* 80(4):465–471, 2016.
55. Wyckoff M, Garcia D, Margraf L, et al.: Randomized trial of volume infusion during resuscitation of asphyxiated neonatal piglets, *Pediatr Res* 61(4):415–420, 2007.
56. McNamara PJ, Shivananda SP, Sahni M, et al.: Pharmacology of milrinone in neonates with persistent pulmonary hypertension of the newborn and suboptimal response to inhaled nitric oxide, *Pediatr Crit Care Med* 14:74–84, 2013.
57. James AT, Corcoran JD, McNamara PJ, et al.: The effect of milrinone on right and left ventricular function when used as a rescue therapy for term infants with pulmonary hypertension, *Cardiol Young* 26(1):90–99, 2016.
58. Noori S, Seri I: Neonatal blood pressure support: the use of inotropes, lusitropes, and other vasopressor agents, *Clin Perinatol* 39:221–238, 2012.
59. Ruffolo Jr RR: The pharmacology of dobutamine, *Am J Med Sci* 294:244–248, 1987.
60. Gupta S, Donn SM: Neonatal hypotension: dopamine or dobutamine? *Semin Fetal Neonatal Med* 19(1):54–59, 2014.
61. Nair J, Lakshminrusimha S: Updates in PPHN: mechanisms and treatment, *Semin Perinatol* 38:78–91, 2014.
62. Simbruner G, Mittal RA, Rohlmann F, Muche R: Systemic hypothermia after neonatal encephalopathy: outcomes of neo.nEURO.network RCT, *Pediatrics* 126:771–778, 2010.
63. Jacobs SE, Morley CJ, Inder TE, et al.: Whole-body hypothermia for term and near-term newborns with hypoxic-ischemic encephalopathy: a randomized controlled trial, *Arch Pediatr Adolesc Med* 165:692–700, 2011.
64. Gunn AJ, Gluckman PD, Gunn TR: Selective head cooling in newborn infants after perinatal asphyxia: a safety study, *Pediatrics* 102:885–892, 1998.
65. Thoresen M, Whitelaw A: Cardiovascular changes during mild therapeutic hypothermia and rewarming in infants with hypoxic-ischemic encephalopathy, *Pediatrics* 106:92–99, 2000.

28

CHAPTER 29

Hemodynamically Based Pharmacologic Management of Circulatory Compromise in the Newborn

Nicholas Evans

- There is little outcome based evidence to guide circulatory support in the newborn.
- In clinical situations of high risk for circulatory compromise, there are a range of hemodynamics.
- A 'one size fits all' approach to neonatal circulatory support is not logical or likely to be successful.
- It is logical to define the individual hemodynamic in a baby and apply therapy logically on the basis of those individual findings.

Shock refers to a circulatory state where the delivery of oxygen to the organs and tissues of the body is inadequate to meet demand. In neonatology, the terms *hypotension* and *shock* have tended to be used synonymously. This is erroneous, and although many shocked babies will be hypotensive, not all hypotensive babies are shocked and not all shocked babies are hypotensive. True shock is uncommon in neonatology, but borderline states of circulatory incompetence are not uncommon.

Circulatory competence depends on adequate systemic blood flow, which is dependent on cardiac output. Cardiac output is the product of stroke volume and heart rate. Stroke volume is determined by preload (positively), myocardial performance (positively), and afterload (negatively, above an individually variable threshold). Thus cardiac output can be increased by increasing stroke volume, heart rate, or both. Blood pressure (BP) is the product of cardiac output and systemic vascular resistance (SVR), so BP can be improved by increasing cardiac output, SVR, or both. Thus neonatal circulatory compromise can result from four basic mechanisms: reduced intravascular volume (low preload), failure of myocardial performance, obstruction in the circulation (high afterload), and loss of vascular tone or distributive disorders of the peripheral circulation. In the first three processes, the main hemodynamic feature is low systemic blood flow, which results in tissue hypoperfusion and hypoxia. In contrast, vasodilatory shock, if myocardial performance keeps up with the increased workload, exhibits a normal or high systemic blood flow. Abnormal distribution of the circulation and microcirculatory alterations play a primary role in the development of tissue hypoxia. Microcirculatory shock is the condition in which the microcirculation fails to support tissue oxygenation in the face of normal systemic hemodynamics.[1] This complexity is magnified many times in the newborn because we are often dealing with a circulation in transition. The fetal channels may not close, leading to blood either bypassing the lungs or recirculating through them, depending on the pressure differentials in the pulmonary and systemic circulation. If the fetal channels do close (as they often do in near-term or term babies) and pulmonary vascular resistance remains high, the circulation may be compromised because the blood cannot get through the lungs to reach the systemic circulation.

These hemodynamics vary between different clinical situations and even among babies in the same clinical situation. As a result, to determine the logical approach to managing shock in an individual baby, there is a need to understand the mechanism of circulatory compromise in that baby and to apply therapy logically on the basis of our understanding of the actions of the pharmacologic agents that are available. This is not an area where a "one size fits all" evidence-based treatment can be applied. In this chapter, I will initially detail what is understood about the pharmacology of the commonly used circulatory support interventions and what evidence of neonatal effect there is about each of them. I will then suggest a logical approach to utilizing these interventions based on hemodynamic scenarios that are commonly found in the newborn in clinical situations of high circulatory risk.

Circulatory Support Interventions

In a recent European-based survey of neonatal circulatory support,[2] the most common first-line interventions were volume expansion (85%), dopamine (62%), dobutamine (18%), both dopamine and dobutamine (18%), epinephrine (2%), and norepinephrine (1%). The same interventions were used with varying frequency as second-line interventions; however, steroids (10%) and milrinone (1%) were also used as second-line interventions. How do these interventions work and what is the evidence that they provide any benefit?

Volume Expansion

Volume expansion is probably one of the most widely used circulatory support interventions despite evidence that true hypovolemia is rare and the fact that we have very little understanding of the effects of volume expansion in a normovolemic infant. Volume expansion will increase preload on the heart. This will be lifesaving in a truly hypovolemic baby; in a normovolemic infant, however, there may well be an immediate increase in cardiac output, the maintenance of this will depend on how long the extra volume stays in the circulation. If volume expansion keeps being pushed, the distribution of extra volume out of the intravascular compartment may well create interstitial edema in the lungs and other organs. Excessive volume expansion in preterm babies may be associated with higher mortality.[3]

Studies have shown that volume expansion in hypotensive preterm babies has little effect on BP.[4] One study in preterm babies with low systemic blood flow showed an immediate increase in systemic blood flow but did not study how long this increase was maintained.[4] Cerebral blood flow, whether studied by xenon extraction[5] or near infrared spectroscopy (NIRS),[6,7] does not seem to be consistently increased by volume in hypotensive preterm infants. Clinical trials of routine early volume expansion in preterm babies with fresh frozen plasma, plasma substitutes, or isotonic saline have shown no improvement in outcomes as compared with no intervention.[8] However, delayed umbilical cord clamping probably provides benefit, in part by facilitating a routine volume expansion with an extra 10 to 20 mL/kg of blood; there is evidence that this intervention does improve outcomes. The benefit of delayed cord clamping in very preterm infants has been confirmed with the results of the large Australian Placental Transfusion Study (APTS). This study showed a reduction in hospital mortality that did not quite reach statistical significance after correction for multiple comparisons.[9] However, when the APTS results are combined with the other randomized clinical trials, a significant reduction in mortality was confirmed, together with less need for blood transfusions.[9a]

The evidence to guide what type of fluid to use in volume expansion is not consistent. Two small trials in preterm babies showed no difference between isotonic saline and 5% albumin in improving BP.[10,11] One slightly larger trial showed that hypotensive preterm babies given 5% albumin were more likely to achieve normal BP and less likely to be given vasopressors than those randomized to saline.[12]

Because relative hypovolemia in the context of a mechanically ventilated baby is difficult to exclude, there is merit in including some volume expansion in a circulatory support protocol. However, volumes in excess of 20 mL/kg should be used with caution. Delayed cord clamping should now be a standard of care in preterm infants.

Dopamine

Dopamine is the naturally occurring catecholamine precursor to noradrenaline. In older children and adults, dopamine has dose-dependent effects. At low doses (2 to 4 μg/kg/min), it stimulates dopaminergic receptors in the coronary, renal, and mesenteric systems, causing vasodilation. At moderate doses (5 to 10 μg/kg/min), it increases myocardial contractility and heart rate by stimulating β_1, β_2, and α receptors. At high doses (10 to 20 μg/kg/min), vascular α-adrenergic stimulation causes an increase in systemic and probably pulmonary vascular resistance. What evidence there is suggests a similar dose-dependent effect in the newborn, particularly the high-dose α-adrenergic effects.

The clinical trial evidence around dopamine is largely related to its effect on BP, and there are consistent data that it is more effective than volume and dobutamine at increasing BP[13,14] and similarly efficacious to epinephrine,[15] steroids,[16] and vasopressin.[17] Much of this effect on BP seems to be due to the vasopressor effect; the evidence around effects on systemic and cerebral blood flow is less consistent.[5] Dopamine at doses between 4 and 10 μg/kg/min increased cardiac output in a cohort of late preterm and term infants, most of whom were asphyxiated.[18,19] In hypotensive preterm babies, Zhang et al. showed no significant effect on cardiac output.[20] Roze et al. showed a reduction in left ventricular (LV) output with a dose of dopamine sufficient to normalize BP,[21] and Osborn et al. showed no change in superior vena cava (SVC) flow with dopamine despite achieving a significant increase in BP.[4] This study showed a rise in LV wall stress (a marker of afterload) on increasing the dose of dopamine from 10 to 20 μg/kg/min, consistent with an α-adrenergic effect at high doses.[22] There is no evidence that this vasoconstriction significantly limits cerebral blood flow. Studies of changes in cerebral blood flow after dopamine, mainly in hypotensive preterm babies and using NIRS surrogate markers of cerebral blood flow, tend to show either increases or no change.

With reference to effects of dopamine on the pulmonary vasculature, the study is limited to preterm babies with patent ductus arteriosus (PDA). Liet et al. showed variable effects on the ratio of systemic-to-pulmonary pressure, but overall there was no change in that ratio.[23] Bouissou et al.[24] showed an increase in pulmonary artery pressure in response to 8 μg/kg/min of dopamine. They also showed an increase in SVC flow, which they suggest may relate to a reduction in PDA shunt.

In summary, dopamine will reliably increase BP, and it probably does this by increasing SVR more than systemic blood flow. The weight of evidence is that dopamine likely increases cerebral blood flow but that higher doses should be used with caution, as high afterload in either the systemic or pulmonary circulation can result in compromise. In addition, dopamine has a broader spectrum of effects on other organs, including the inhibition of thyroid stimulating hormone production in the pituitary gland. This has special clinical relevance for the newborn.

Dobutamine

Dobutamine is a synthetic catecholamine that was modified from isoprenaline to reduce some of the chronotropic effects. Dobutamine has a half-life of about 2 minutes in children and adults and has β_1 and β_2 effects with some α_1 effects; it therefore causes an increase in myocardial contractility and heart rate and some reduction in peripheral vascular resistance. This vasodilatory effect is likely why clinical trials have consistently shown that dobutamine is not as good as dopamine at improving BP in hypotensive preterm babies.[13] Nevertheless, in the few studies that have measured it, dobutamine seems better than dopamine at improving systemic blood flow.[4,21] There was no difference in neurodevelopment at 3 years in the only trial to report this, although the trial was not powered for this outcome.[25] One small randomized trial has compared dobutamine with placebo in babies with low systemic blood flow and showed that systemic blood flow improved in both groups; however, other markers of perfusion were significantly better in babies treated with dobutamine.[26] This study was unable to show any differences or changes in NIRS markers of cerebral blood flow with either dobutamine or placebo. Other observational studies have shown an impact on Doppler markers of organ blood flow, including cerebral blood flow,[27] but the placebo effect in the study by Bravo et al.[26] reminds us that most blood flow parameters will improve spontaneously after about 12 hours of age in very preterm babies. Dobutamine also has dose-related effects, with low doses (<5 µg/kg/min) probably having little effect but with increasing effects from 5 to 20 µg/kg/min. Osborn et al. showed a continuing drop in LV wall stress (afterload) with increases from 10 to 20 µg/kg/min.[22]

In summary, dobutamine has dose-related central inotropic and chronotropic effects with peripheral vasodilation. It is likely to be most effective where there is myocardial dysfunction and/or increased afterload leading to low systemic blood flow. It is unlikely to be effective when hypotension is due to vasodilatation.

Epinephrine (Adrenaline)

Epinephrine has very similar dose-related effects to dopamine with low doses (0.01–0.1 µg/kg/min) primarily stimulating the cardiac and vascular β_1- and β_2-adrenoreceptors, leading to increased inotropy, chronotropy, and conduction velocity as well as peripheral vasodilation. Its inotropic effect is superior to that of dopamine. At doses greater than 0.1 µg/kg/min, epinephrine stimulates the vascular and cardiac α_1 receptors, causing vasoconstriction and increased inotropy, respectively. There has been limited study of the cardiovascular effects of epinephrine in the newborn. The previously cited randomized trial of dopamine and epinephrine in hypotensive preterm babies showed similar effects in improving BP and cerebral oxygenation index, although the epinephrine group had significantly higher lactate and more hyperglycemia than those randomized to dopamine.[15] This is a recognized metabolic effect of epinephrine, which is most likely explained by the drug-induced stimulation of β_2-adrenoreceptors in the liver and skeletal muscle, resulting in decreased insulin release and increases in glycogenolysis, leading to increases in lactate production, respectively. This does have the clinical side effect of rendering the lactate level an unreliable marker of tissue perfusion. This was one of the few neonatal cardiovascular support trials that assessed neurodevelopmental outcome, and it showed no difference between the two groups at 2 to 3 years of age.[28]

In summary, the vasoconstrictive effects of epinephrine make it best suited for the management of vasodilatory shock. As in the case of dopamine, caution should be exercised in using higher doses because of the risk of afterload compromise.

Norepinephrine (Noradrenaline)

Norepinephrine is a naturally occurring sympathomimetic amine that, while having less β_2 receptor stimulatory effects, has mainly strong α agonist effects; it is therefore a potent vasoconstrictor. There is no clinical trial evidence on the use of norepinephrine in the newborn and not much observational data. A retrospective study of norepinephrine use in 48 babies born before 33 weeks' gestation showed that normotension could be achieved in all but one baby at a median dose of 0.5 µg/kg/min. Apart from tachycardia (in 31%), no immediate side effects were observed.[29] One small cohort study showed improved BP in term babies with septic shock refractory to dopamine and dobutamine.[30] An observational study in term babies with pulmonary hypertension suggested that norepinephrine has a beneficial effect on both systemic and pulmonary hemodynamics by causing systemic vasoconstriction and pulmonary vasodilation.[31] There are no long-term safety data on the use of norepinephrine, but it may have a role in refractory vasodilatory shock and in babies with persistent pulmonary hypertension of the newborn (PPHN) and low BP.

Vasopressin

Vasopressin is a naturally occurring hormone that is mainly involved in the regulation of extracellular osmolarity, although it does play a role in regulating the function of the cardiovascular system as well. Indeed, vasopressin also has potent vasoconstrictive effects, and it is this effect that is used in its role in circulatory support. There has been one small randomized trial ($n = 20$) comparing dopamine with vasopressin in hypotensive preterm infants.[17] Outcomes were limited to physiologic parameters and both agents had similar effects in increasing BP whereas vasopressin had less tachycardic effect. Otherwise there are small case series of improvement in BP in preterm babies with inotrope refractory hypotension.[32,33] There is some evidence from animal studies that vasopressin has a vasodilatory effect on the pulmonary vasculature.[34] This would be consistent with the observational report of the use of vasopressin in 10 babies with PPHN refractory to inhaled nitric oxide (iNO).[35] A vasopressin infusion improved BP, reduced oxygenation index, and improved urine output. There are not enough safety data to recommend the routine use of vasopressin, but it may have a role in treating vasodilatory shock refractory to vasopressor-inotropes.

Milrinone

Milrinone is a phosphodiesterase-3 inhibitor that inhibits the degradation of cyclic adenosine monophosphate (cAMP). By increasing the concentration of cAMP, milrinone enhances myocardial contractility, promotes myocardial relaxation, and decreases vascular tone in the systemic and pulmonary circulation. The role of milrinone is best established in preventing and treating low-cardiac-output syndrome (LCOS) after cardiac bypass surgery. A large randomized controlled trial (RCT) has shown that milrinone significantly reduced the incidence of LCOS in a neonatal and pediatric population.[36] The similarities between LCOS and the postnatal drop in systemic blood flow seen in some preterm babies led to a trial of milrinone to prevent low systemic blood flow in preterm babies.[37] This trial showed no difference in the incidence of low systemic blood flow between milrinone and placebo, although milrinone did increase the need for vasopressor-inotropes to support BP and seemed to slow constriction of the ductus arteriosus. There was a pharmacokinetic arm to this study which showed a considerably longer half-life of milrinone in preterm babies than in term babies (10 hours vs. 4 hours).[38] The afterload-reducing properties of milrinone led to an observational study suggesting that milrinone may prevent the afterload compromise which can follow PDA ligation in preterm babies.[39] The pulmonary vasodilatory properties may also explain the observation of improvement in oxygenation and hemodynamics in babies with PPHN refractory to iNO.[40] There is also a small case series of milrinone being used in conjunction with iNO in seven preterm babies with pulmonary hypertension, with improvement in oxygenation index, right ventricle (RV) myocardial function, and pulmonary pressure.[41] Milrinone may have a role in the management of hemodynamics associated with systemic or pulmonary vasoconstriction, but there are not enough safety data to recommend its routine use. It should be used with caution in very preterm babies because of its long half-life and the risk of hypotension.

Hydrocortisone

In a recent review of circulatory support measures in a U.S. pediatric health information system,[42] hydrocortisone was second to dopamine as the most commonly used drug in extremely low birth weight infants (dopamine 83% vs. hydrocortisone 33%). This is surprising as we do not know much about the hemodynamic impact of hydrocortisone apart from the effect on BP, and we know little about the long-term effects when used early to treat BP. Bourchier et al. randomized hypotensive preterm babies to hydrocortisone or dopamine and showed that both had similar effects on BP.[43] Ng et al. randomized preterm babies needing more than 10 μg/kg/min of dopamine to hydrocortisone or placebo and showed faster weaning of inotropes in those treated with hydrocortisone.[44] Efird et al. randomized preterm babies to hydrocortisone or placebo and confirmed that vasopressor use was reduced.[45] To the best of my knowledge only one study has looked at the hemodynamic effects of hydrocortisone. In a cohort of 15 preterm and 5 term babies with hypotension requiring high-dose dopamine, Noori et al. showed that the immediate effect of hydrocortisone on BP was mediated via an increase in SVR without any change in cardiac output or stroke volume. However, later, with weaning of dopamine, there were increases in stroke volume and cardiac output.[46]

None of these studies looked at longer-term outcomes, and the current Cochrane review on corticosteroids to treat hypotension in preterm babies urges caution, concluding: "With long-term benefit or safety data lacking, steroids cannot be recommended routinely for the treatment of hypotension in preterm infants." Although not addressing the circulatory support use of hydrocortisone, there is some reassurance about the short-term safety of hydrocortisone from the large PREMILOC trial ($n = 523$), where the effect of prophylactic low-dose hydrocortisone on chronic lung disease was assessed.[47] A follow-up to this study is in progress, which should provide data on longer-term safety.

There is some evidence of an increased risk of gastrointestinal perforation, particularly when hydrocortisone is used in conjunction with indomethacin. It is prudent to avoid using these two drugs together.

Applying the Evidence in Clinical Practice

The bottom line is that we know a lot about how our interventions affect BP, less about how they affect hemodynamics, and almost nothing about how they affect outcomes. In light of this, it is the author's view that the logical way to approach circulatory support in the newborn is to use an individual or "precision medicine-based" approach. That is, one should try to define the individual hemodynamic as accurately as possible and apply logical treatment based on what we know about the effects of the interventions on physiology.

How to best define individual hemodynamic is controversial. Many neonatologists would still use vital signs, mainly BP, and this will reflect reality for many with limited access to technologies such as Doppler ultrasound and/or NIRS. But to define a hemodynamic one really needs a measure of pressure and flow so that resistance can be estimated and indicate whether it is flow or resistance or both that must be increased to support pressure. How best to define flow is controversial, particularly whether that should be a measure of global systemic flow or a marker of organ (usually brain) blood flow. Both are clearly important; the ideal situation would be to measure systemic and organ blood flow as well BP. Indeed, in the future there may be comprehensive, real-time hemodynamic monitoring as described in Chapter 21. One would also need a measure of preload or volume status, but such a marker remains elusive except in extreme cases of hypovolemia. The author would argue that it is difficult to define an individualized approach to the circulation without any information about what is happening in the organ that drives the circulation and, indeed, the organ one is trying to manipulate with various interventions, the heart. Without this knowledge, one is flying blind.

Cardiac ultrasound assessment of an individual's hemodynamic is complex; the measurements are covered in more detail in Chapters 10 to 13. It is clearly important to document structural normality, fetal channel shunts, volume status, myocardial function, and pulmonary pressure, but the essentials for circulatory support are a measure of BP, a measure of systemic blood flow, and, in some babies, an estimate of pulmonary blood flow. The author uses SVC flow and/or RV output as markers of systemic blood flow and left pulmonary artery velocity as an estimate of pulmonary blood flow. In addition, ideally, information on blood flow distribution to the organs must be available to fully understand the cardiovascular status of the neonate.

Neonatal hemodynamics exist on a continuum, not in discrete categories. Notwithstanding this, there are several patterns of abnormal hemodynamic seen in the newborn. Although these are discussed separately in the following paragraphs, it must be highlighted that there will be overlap between these hemodynamic patterns in individual babies. One should also emphasize the importance of integrating the cardiac ultrasound findings with the clinical history and vital signs to define the likely diagnosis and individual therapeutic needs.

There are essentially five patterns of abnormal hemodynamic found in the newborn. These are summarized in Table 29.1 and are as follows:

1. Hypovolemic hemodynamic (see Chapter 27)

Absolute hypovolemia is rare in the newborn but is seen in the immediate postnatal period in babies who have suffered intrapartum fetal blood loss and, postnatally,

Table 29.1 DIAGNOSIS AND MANAGEMENT OF COMMON NEONATAL HEMODYNAMICS

Hemodynamic	Clinical Situations	Vital Signs	Cardiac US Flow Measures	Other Cardiac US Findings	Management
Hypovolemic hemodynamic	• Perinatal fetal blood loss • Subgaleal hemorrhage • Abdominal emergencies	• Pallor • Tachycardia • Low BP	• Low or low normal SBF depending on degree of volume loss	• *Biventricular poor filling*	• Give 20 mL/kg isotonic saline IV over 5–10 min depending on severity. • If acute blood loss, follow with 20 mL/kg of uncrossmatched O-negative blood (cross match only if time) over 10–30 min depending on severity. • Monitor impact with FBC, coagulation, vital signs, and cardiac US. • Further volume expansion/blood as indicated, consider implementing massive transfusion protocol if ongoing blood loss exceeds 40 mL/kg.[43]
Low systemic flow hemodynamic	• Very preterm infant after less than 12 h • Any baby with a high ventilation/oxygen need • Asphyxia	• Variable, BP low or normal	• *Low SBF*	• Poor myocardial function may be apparent	• Give 10 mL/kg isotonic saline over 30 min. • At the same time, commence dobutamine infusion at 10 μg/kg/min. Monitor response with cardiac US and/or heart rate. • If SBF not improving, increase dobutamine up to 20 μg/kg/min. • If blood pressure remains low, add dopamine 5 μg/kg/min and titrate to minimal acceptable blood pressure. • Review cardiac US at 24 h, particularly in very preterm babies, and wean dobutamine over 4–6 h if flow measures have normalized (which they usually will).

Vasodilatory hemodynamic	• Sepsis
	 • Preterm baby after 24 h, sometimes earlier
	 • Recovery from shock or asphyxia
		• *BP low*
		 • Other vital signs variable
			• Normal or high SBF	• Good myocardial function
				 • Well-filled ventricles
					• If early postnatal in a preterm baby, it may be reasonable to observe, depending on BP and other vital signs. Spontaneous improvement is common.
					 • Otherwise, give 10 mL/kg isotonic saline over 30 min.
					 • Consider more in probable septic shock. At the same time, commence dopamine at 5 μg/kg/min. Monitor impact with BP.
					 • If not improving, increase dopamine in increments of 2 μg/kg/min to a maximum of 15 μg/kg/min in order to achieve a minimally acceptable MBP.
					 • Reduce dopamine in decrements of 1–2 μg/kg/min if MBP goes significantly above the minimally acceptable MBP.
					 • If BP does not improve:
					   • **In septic shock:** Refer to Chapter 27.
					   • **In late preterm hypotension:** if refractory to dopamine, consider hydrocortisone 1 mg/kg q8–12h.

Continued

29

Table 29.1 DIAGNOSIS AND MANAGEMENT OF COMMON NEONATAL HEMODYNAMICS—cont'd

Hemodynamic	Clinical Situations	Vital Signs	Cardiac US Flow Measures	Other Cardiac US Findings	Management
Low pulmonary blood flow (PPHN)	• High FiO_2 with relatively normal lungs (clinically and on CXR)	• Poor oxygenation • BP normal or low • Variable	• Normal or low SBF • *Low mean velocity in LPA*	• Exclude CHD • Dilated poorly contracting RV • Poorly filled LV • *High PAP* • Dominant R-to-L bidirectional shunt through ductus and/or FO	• Commence iNO at 5–10 ppm. Monitor response with oxygenation and cardiac US; both will usually improve. • If low SBF persists, start milrinone (or dobutamine) at 0.2–0.5 μg/kg/min and consider isotonic saline. • If low blood pressure persists, particularly if oxygenation is varying with MBP, consider norepinephrine starting at 0.05 μg/kg/min increasing to 1.0–2.0 μg/kg/min or epinephrine starting at 0.05 μg/kg/min increasing to 1.0–2.0 μg/kg/min depending on BP response.
Normal pulmonary blood flow (PPHN)	• High FiO_2 with abnormal lungs (clinically and on CXR)	• BP normal or low • Other vital signs variable	• Often low SBF on day 1 • *Normal mean velocity in LPA*	• Exclude CHD • Usually normal contractility • *Moderate to high PAP* • Bidirectional shunt through ductus and/or FO	• Optimize respiratory management, surfactant (repeat surfactant even if there is no apparent response), ventilation, etc. • Consider iNO depending on oxygenation and PAP. • Monitor response with oxygenation and cardiac US. The effect of iNO is more variable. • If low SBF, consider starting milrinone (or dobutamine, depending on myocardial function) and consider isotonic saline. • If low blood pressure, particularly if oxygenation is varying with MBP, consider norepinephrine starting at 0.05 μg/kg/min increasing to 1.0–2.0 μg/kg/min or epinephrine starting at 0.05 μg/kg/min increasing to 1.0–2.0 μg/kg/min depending on BP response.

These hemodynamics are not mutually exclusive and babies may have features of more than one hemodynamic. Criteria in italics indicate the key feature of each hemodynamic.
Low systemic blood flow (SBF): RV output <150 mL/kg/min and/or SVC flow <50 mL/kg/min.
Low pulmonary blood flow (PBF): Left pulmonary artery (LPA) mean velocity <20 cm/s.
Minimally acceptable blood pressure: Controversial; I would use MBP above gestational age.

BP, Blood pressure; *CHD,* congenital heart disease; *CXR,* chest x-ray; *FBC,* full blood count; *FiO2,* fraction of inspired oxygen; *FO,* foramen ovale; *iNO,* inhaled nitric oxide; *IV,* intravenous; *LPA,* left pulmonary artery; *LV,* left ventricle; *MBP,* mean blood pressure; *PAP,* pulmonary artery pressure; *PPHN,* persistent pulmonary hypertension of the newborn; *RV,* right ventricle; *SBF,* systemic blood flow; *US,* ultrasound.

with subgaleal bleeds and postsurgical blood loss. Such babies may have a perinatal or clinical history consistent with blood loss and will be pale, invariably tachycardic, and have low BP if they have progressed beyond the compensatory phase. The main cardiac ultrasound finding is dramatically poor biventricular filling, so that the chambers look small and often have an appearance of poor contractility, reflecting low preload. The systemic veins will also be poorly filled and measures of systemic blood flow will be low or low normal depending on the degree of hypovolemia.

Management: Such babies need immediate volume replacement with isotonic saline and blood as soon as available. The latter may have to be un–cross-matched O-negative blood if the urgency of the situation demands it. Babies with ongoing blood loss of more than 40 mL/kg are vulnerable to develop transfusion-related coagulopathy and should be managed according to the principles of a massive transfusion protocol, where platelets and clotting factors are replaced proactively according to a defined schedule (see Chapter 27).[48]

2. Vasodilatory hemodynamic

This pattern of loss of vascular resistance is invariable in hypotensive preterm babies who are more than 24 hours old; it can be seen during the first 24 hours, sometimes in combination with low systemic blood flow (see further on). It is also seen on recovery from shock or severe asphyxia and is the invariable hemodynamic in late late-onset sepsis (see Chapter 27).[49] These babies will either be very preterm or have a clinical history consistent with sepsis or asphyxia. They will be hypotensive and often tachycardic; the impact on other clinical signs and markers of shock such as lactate will depend on severity. The cardiac ultrasound findings will show well-filled ventricles with a good, sometimes hyperdynamic appearance of the myocardial function. Measures of systemic blood flow will be high normal or high, reflecting the loss of resistance. If treatment is delayed, myocardial function will deteriorate as, after a certain period, myocardial oxygen delivery starts failing to meet tissue oxygen demand.

Management: The suggested management of septic shock is covered in detail in Chapter 27; there are overlaps between the management of septic shock and that of postasphyxial vasodilatory shock.

In preterm neonates with vasodilatory hypotension, the first question is whether it needs to be treated. If the hypotension is borderline and there are no changes in the markers of perfusion, such as lactate and/or urine output, then an expectant approach to management may be reasonable. The decision in these cases also depends on the etiology of the vasodilatory shock. For instance, in preterm neonates with suspected sepsis, there should be a lower threshold to initiate cardiovascular support. In babies with BP well below the normal range and/or with other markers of poor tissue perfusion, intervention is indicated. This hemodynamic needs a vasopressor effect. Some volume expansion may help to fill the additional vascular space created by the vasodilation. I would suggest starting some volume expansion (up to 20 mL/kg) as well as dopamine (because there is the most experience with this vasopressor) at 5 µg/kg/min and titrate the infusion rate up in small increments of perhaps 2 µg/kg/min to achieve a minimal acceptable BP. As long as the drug has reached and is being infused into the patient, one does not have to wait for a response longer than approximately 5 minutes to find out if the given dose must be increased again. It is unusual to need more than 10 µg/kg/min but if the BP remains low at higher doses of dopamine (20 µg/kg/min), then consideration can be given to adding another vasopressor because the hypotension may well be resistant to dopamine. Different neonatologists will recommend different vasopressors in this situation, including epinephrine, norepinephrine, and vasopressin as well as hydrocortisone. There is no evidence to guide the choice. My preference would be to add hydrocortisone at 1 mg/kg every 8 hours in that we know a bit more about its hemodynamic effects (e.g., probably vasopressor by potentiating catecholamine receptors), and it covers the risk of relative or absolute adrenocortical insufficiency. Because of hydrocortisone's prolonged half-life in preterm neonates of less than 34 weeks' gestation, dosing every 12 hours has recently been recommended for this patient population as a starting dosage interval with the option of shortening the dosage interval if the increase in BP is not sustained for the 12 hours.[50] After that, I would consider norepinephrine or vasopressin with a preference for the former because there is more reported experience.[29]

3. Low systemic blood flow hemodynamic

This pattern usually reflects absolute or relative myocardial dysfunction. *Relative myocardial* dysfunction means that a myocardium is struggling against increased or, in the case of the preterm myocardium, unfamiliar afterloads. This is the most common pattern of abnormal hemodynamic seen in the very preterm baby in the first 12 hours after delivery (see Chapter 26). It probably reflects maladaptation of the immature myocardium to the higher afterloads of extrauterine life, possibly compounded by the negative circulatory effects of positive-pressure ventilation as well as shunts out of the systemic circulation through the fetal channels and early cord clamping.[51] It is unusual to find this pattern in preterm babies after the first 24 hours, where the abnormal hemodynamic is invariably vasodilatory.[49,51] Low systemic blood flow due to afterload compromise has also been proposed as the pathophysiology of the cardiorespiratory compromise seen after PDA ligation.[52] Low systemic blood flow is found in more mature babies with high ventilator and oxygen requirements, where primary myocardial dysfunction merges with the PPHN hemodynamic discussed below.[53] Low systemic blood flow is also found in clinical situations associated with an injured myocardium, most commonly in the asphyxiated newborn but also in viral myocarditis or congenital cardiomyopathies. The impact of low systemic blood flow on vital signs is variable, particularly in the preterm baby, where BP may be normal. Because of this, recognition of low systemic blood flow often depends on proactive use of cardiac ultrasound in the high-risk clinical situations previously mentioned. The findings on cardiac ultrasound will be low SVC flow (<50 mL/kg/min) and/or low RV output (<150 mL/kg/min) and, particularly in the more mature baby, poor myocardial function, which may well be subjectively apparent as well as assessed by myocardial function measures.

Management: Most of these babies are not hypovolemic but borderline volume status is difficult to exclude and there is some evidence of short-term improvement in systemic blood flow in preterm babies with low systemic blood flow in response to volume.[4] I would therefore suggest some volume expansion in these babies with 10 mL/kg of isotonic saline. The pathophysiology here would indicate the need for augmentation of myocardial function and, particularly if the BP is normal, with an agent that will tend to reduce afterload. At the same time as the volume, I would suggest starting dobutamine at 10 μg/kg/min. One practical difficulty in this situation is how to monitor the effect. Dobutamine may or may not increase BP even though systemic blood flow has improved. Ideally, the cardiac ultrasound should be repeated about an hour after starting the infusion but, experientially, if that option is not available, the dose can be titrated up until a chronotropic effect is seen in the heart rate, as this will make it likely that inotropy has been achieved. Dobutamine has a good dose-response relationship and, unless there is severe tachycardia, doses of up to 20 μg/kg/min are unlikely to do harm. The more mature baby with low systemic blood flow is often quite responsive to dobutamine, but low systemic blood flow in the preterm baby may be refractory to the intervention.[4] If the BP is low, that suggests combined low flow and vasodilation; I would then suggest adding in dopamine at 5 µg/kg/min and titrating up to a minimally acceptable BP. The concept of titrating to a minimally acceptable BP becomes more important during this early postnatal period because of the risk of afterload compromise. There tends to be an assumption that more is better when it comes to BP, so people are quick to start vasopressor-inotropes if the BP is low but slow to reduce them if the BP gets pushed well into the normal range or high.

It is also important to consider the optimal time for weaning inotropes. The natural history of systemic blood flow in preterm and term babies is for flow to improve between 12 and 24 hours of age. There is often a reluctance to wean the vasopressor-inotropes or inotropes and the theoretical risk this creates is that continuing treatment may drive reperfusion in a system that is in spontaneous recovery. I would suggest repeat cardiac ultrasound at 24 hours of age to confirm normal systemic blood flow and then an aggressive wean of the cardiovascular medications over about 4 to 6 hours. If one does not have access to cardiac ultrasound, it is reasonable to wean the inotropes anyway as long as vital signs and other perfusion markers are normal.

The situation in the very preterm baby may be confused by the presence of large left-to-right ductal shunting even at this early time. This moves blood out of the systemic circulation back to the pulmonary circulation, which may be a factor contributing to low systemic blood flow. Management of the PDA is outside the scope of this chapter (see Chapters 22 to 25), but early medical closure of the poorly constricted ductus arteriosus with a large left-to-right shunt could be considered.

4. Persistent pulmonary hypertension hemodynamics (see Chapters 8 and 9). The plural is pointedly used in the title of this subsection because the hemodynamics are as varied as the causes of the high ventilation and oxygen requirements that lead neonatologists to consider PPHN as a diagnosis. It is important to remember that pressure in the pulmonary arterial system is determined by the same factor as in the systemic circulation, which is flow and resistance. Therefore, as in the systemic circulation, pulmonary arterial pressure can be high because flow is high, or resistance is high, or because both are high.

In fact, the hemodynamics here represent a continuum with, at one end, the classic concept of PPHN with high resistance, low pulmonary blood flow, and right-to-left shunts across the fetal channels, while, at the other end, there is normal pulmonary blood flow with varying degrees of increased pulmonary vascular resistance and pressure as well as variable fetal channel shunts. There are some parallels in these hemodynamics with the classic categorization of PPHN into primary (with relatively normal lungs) and secondary (with parenchymal lung disease); primary PPHN is more likely to involve low pulmonary blood flow hemodynamic and secondary PPHN is more likely to involve normal pulmonary blood flow hemodynamic.[53]

4a. PPHN with low pulmonary blood flow

This hemodynamic is commonly seen in term or late preterm babies with idiopathic primary PPHN. Clinically these babies will have increased oxygen requirements that are out of keeping with any parenchymal lung disease; they will often have relatively normal chest x-rays (CXRs) and may have relatively mildly increased work of breathing. This hemodynamic is also found in babies with hypoplastic lungs from conditions such as diaphragmatic hernia, renal anomalies associated with decreased fetal urine production, or premature prolonged rupture of the membranes. It is uncommon in very preterm babies except those born after prolonged oligohydramnios, where this is the invariable hemodynamic. This was traditionally explained as due to pulmonary hypoplasia; however, the responsiveness to iNO suggests a significant reversible component to the pulmonary hypertension in these babies (see case history 4 in Chapter 10).[54,55]

These babies must have congenital heart disease excluded as soon as possible. Assuming that the heart is structurally normal, cardiac ultrasound usually shows evidence of suprasystemic pulmonary pressure with predominantly right-to-left shunting through the ductus (if patent) and bidirectional shunting through the foramen ovale. There will be low-velocity flow in the left pulmonary artery (mean velocity <0.2 m/s), a finding that predicts responsiveness to iNO.[56] Measures of systemic blood flow may be normal, particularly if the flow through the fetal channels is not restricted. If the flow through the fetal channels is restricted, systemic blood flow may be low, with the likely pathophysiology being low pulmonary blood flow restricting systemic blood flow. The LV can only pump what it receives from the RV.

Management (see Chapter 9 for details): The primary problem in this hemodynamic is high pulmonary vascular resistance due to pulmonary vasoconstriction; therefore therapy must be aimed at dilating the pulmonary arterioles. iNO would be the first choice for this and, when this hemodynamic is associated with otherwise normal lungs, there is usually a brisk response to iNO and rapid normalization of the hemodynamic. In babies who are not responsive to iNO, consideration should be given to adding milrinone if the systemic BP is normal or, if the baby has hypotension, norepinephrine. In iNO-unresponsive babies, where the ductus arteriosus is constricting, there is some logic to considering opening the ductus arteriosus with prostaglandin E2. This will serve to decompress the right heart and improve systemic blood flow, albeit with relatively poorly oxygenated blood. In neonates not responding or not having a sustained response to iNO, the addition of sildenafil can be considered as the next step in the management.

4b. PPHN with normal pulmonary blood flow

This hemodynamic is most commonly seen in babies with severe acquired lung disease such as meconium aspiration, pneumonia, or hyaline membrane disease. The main clinical feature is a history and CXR changes consistent with one of these diagnoses. The babies will usually have presented with severe respiratory distress and, when ventilated, will have high oxygen and pressure requirements. These babies must also have congenital heart disease excluded as soon as possible. If the heart is structurally normal, then pulmonary pressures in these babies will be variable and many of these babies will have subsystemic pulmonary artery pressures. Within this group there is a positive relationship between oxygenation index and pulmonary artery pressure, with the most severely affected babies usually having peri- or suprasystemic pulmonary artery pressures.[53] As in the case of pulmonary artery pressures, shunts will be variable but will often have more left-to-right than right-to-left patterns. The ductus arteriosus often constricts early and closes by the second postnatal day. There is a high incidence of low systemic blood flow on the first day with improvement over time, much as seen in very preterm babies.[53]

Management: The primary problem in these babies is pulmonary; the cardiac and pulmonary vascular effects are secondary to the pulmonary disease. With respect to high-pressure ventilation, it is important to remember that inappropriately high positive intrathoracic pressures will have a negative effect on cardiac output and pulmonary artery pressure will have to be higher to drive the blood through the lungs. The primary focus in these babies should be on optimizing respiratory and conventional ventilator management with surfactant, optimizing ventilator settings, or using other modes of ventilation (as indicated). If oxygenation is still poor despite optimized respiratory management, then iNO can be considered depending on the estimated pulmonary artery pressure and the patient's oxygenation status.

The effect of iNO in this hemodynamic is more variable. If systemic blood flow is low, consider dobutamine or milrinone as mentioned above, and if BP is low, particularly if oxygenation varies with the BP changes, consider norepinephrine or epinephrine titrating to the BP response.

Conclusion

In the absence of outcome-based evidence to guide circulatory support in the newborn, it is the author's view that the logical approach is one that uses individual or precision-based therapy. That is, one should try to define the individual's hemodynamic as accurately as possible and apply treatment logically to that hemodynamic based on what we know about the effects of the pharmacologic interventions on cardiovascular physiology. As is the case of all approaches to circulatory support in the newborn, there is no evidence that this will improve outcomes.

REFERENCES

1. Kanoore Edul VS, Ince C, Dubin A: What is microcirculatory shock? *Curr Opin Crit Care* 21(3): 245–252, 2015.
2. Stranak Z, Semberova J, Barrington K, et al.: International survey on diagnosis and management of hypotension in extremely preterm babies, *Eur J Pediatr* 173(6):793–798, 2014.
3. Ewer AK, Tyler W, Francis A, et al.: Excessive volume expansion and neonatal death in preterm infants born at 27-28 weeks gestation, *Paediatr Perinat Epidemiol* 17(2):180–186, 2003.
4. Osborn D, Evans N, Kluckow M: Randomized trial of dobutamine versus dopamine in preterm infants with low systemic blood flow, *J Pediatr* 140(2):183–191, 2002.
5. Lundstrom K, Pryds O, Greisen G: The haemodynamic effects of dopamine and volume expansion in sick preterm infants, *Early Hum Dev* 57(2):157–163, 2000.
6. Kooi EM, van der Laan ME, Verhagen EA, et al.: Volume expansion does not alter cerebral tissue oxygen extraction in preterm infants with clinical signs of poor perfusion, *Neonatology* 103(4):308–314, 2013.
7. Bonestroo HJ, Lemmers PM, Baerts W, et al.: Effect of antihypotensive treatment on cerebral oxygenation of preterm infants without PDA, *Pediatrics* 128(6):e1502–e1510, 2011.
8. Osborn DA, Evans N: Early volume expansion for prevention of morbidity and mortality in very preterm infants, *Cochrane Database Syst Rev* 2:CD002055, 2004.
9. Tarnow-Mordi W, Morris J, Kirby A, et al.: Delayes vs immediate cord clamping in preterm infants, NEJM 377:2445–2455, 2017.
9a. Fogarty M, Osborn DA, Askie L, et al.: Delayed vs early umbilical cord clamping for preterm infants: a systematic review and meta-analysis. AJOG 2017. http://dx.doi.org/10.1016/j.ajog.2017.10.231.
10. Oca MJ, Nelson M, Donn SM: Randomized trial of normal saline versus 5% albumin for the treatment of neonatal hypotension, *J Perinatol* 23(6):473–476, 2003.
11. So KW, Fok TF, Ng PC, et al.: Randomised controlled trial of colloid or crystalloid in hypotensive preterm infants, *Arch Dis Child Fetal Neonatal Ed* 76(1):F43–F46, 1997.
12. Lynch SK, Mullett MD, Graeber JE, et al.: A comparison of albumin-bolus therapy versus normal saline-bolus therapy for hypotension in neonates, *J Perinatol* 28(1):29–33, 2008.
13. Subhedar NV, Shaw NJ: Dopamine versus dobutamine for hypotensive preterm infants, *Cochrane Database Syst Rev* 3:CD001242, 2003.
14. Osborn DA, Evans N: Early volume expansion versus inotrope for prevention of morbidity and mortality in very preterm infants, *Cochrane Database Syst Rev* 2:CD002056, 2001.
15. Pellicer A, Valverde E, Elorza MD, et al.: Cardiovascular support for low birth weight infants and cerebral hemodynamics: a randomized, blinded, clinical trial, *Pediatrics* 115(6):1501–1512, 2005.
16. Ibrahim H, Sinha IP, Subhedar NV: Corticosteroids for treating hypotension in preterm infants, *Cochrane Database Syst Rev* 12:CD003662, 2011.
17. Rios DR, Kaiser JR: Vasopressin versus dopamine for treatment of hypotension in extremely low birth weight infants: a randomized, blinded pilot study, *J Pediatr* 166(4):850–855, 2015.
18. Walther FJ, Siassi B, Ramadan NA, et al.: Cardiac output in newborn infants with transient myocardial dysfunction, *J Pediatr* 107:781–785, 1985.
19. Padbury JF, Agata Y, Baylen BG, et al.: Dopamine pharmacokinetics in critically ill newborn infants, *J Pediatr* 110 (2):293–298, 1987.
20. Zhang J, Penny DJ, Kim NS, et al.: Mechanisms of blood pressure increase induced by dopamine in hypotensive preterm neonates, *Arch Dis Child Fetal Neonatal Ed* 81(2):F99–F104, 1999.
21. Roze JC, Tohier C, Maingueneau C, et al.: Response to dobutamine and dopamine in the hypotensive very preterm infant, *Arch Dis Child* 69:59–63, 1993.
22. Osborn DA, Evans N, Kluckow M: Left ventricular contractility in extremely premature infants in the first day and response to inotropes, *Pediatr Res* 61(3):335–340, 2007.
23. Liet JM, Boscher C, Gras-Leguen C, et al.: Dopamine effects on pulmonary artery pressure in hypotensive preterm infants with patent ductus arteriosus, *J Pediatr* 140(3):373–375, 2002.
24. Bouissou A, Rakza T, Klosowski S, et al.: Hypotension in preterm infants with significant patent ductus arteriosus: effects of dopamine, *J Pediatr* 153(6):790–794, 2008.
25. Osborn DA, Evans N, Kluckow M, et al.: Low superior vena cava flow and effect of inotropes on neurodevelopment to 3 years in preterm infants, *Pediatrics* 120(2):372–380, 2007.

29

26. Bravo MC, Lopez-Ortego P, Sanchez L, et al.: Randomized, placebo-controlled trial of dobutamine for low superior vena cava flow in infants, *J Pediatr* 167(3):572–578.e2, 2015.

27. Robel-Tillig E, Knupfer M, Pulzer F, et al.: Cardiovascular impact of dobutamine in neonates with myocardial dysfunction, *Early Hum Dev* 83(5):307–312, 2007.

28. Pellicer A, Bravo MC, Madero R, et al.: Early systemic hypotension and vasopressor support in low birth weight infants: impact on neurodevelopment, *Pediatrics* 123(5):1369–1376, 2009.

29. Rowcliff K, de Waal K, Mohamed AL, et al.: Noradrenaline in preterm infants with cardiovascular compromise, *Eur J Pediatr*, 175(12):1967–1973, 2016.

30. Tourneux P, Rakza T, Abazine A, et al.: Noradrenaline for management of septic shock refractory to fluid loading and dopamine or dobutamine in full-term newborn infants, *Acta Paediatr* 97(2):177–180, 2008.

31. Tourneux P, Rakza T, Bouissou A, et al.: Pulmonary circulatory effects of norepinephrine in newborn infants with persistent pulmonary hypertension, *J Pediatr* 153(3):345–349, 2008.

32. Bidegain M, Greenberg R, Simmons C, et al.: Vasopressin for refractory hypotension in extremely low birth weight infants, *J Pediatr* 157(3):502–504, 2010.

33. Meyer S, Loffler G, Polcher T, et al.: Vasopressin in catecholamine-resistant septic and cardiogenic shock in very-low-birthweight infants, *Acta Paediatr* 95(10):1309–1312, 2006.

34. Walker BR, Haynes Jr J, Wang HL, et al.: Vasopressin-induced pulmonary vasodilation in rats, *Am J Physiol* 257(2 Pt 2):H415–H422, 1989.

35. Mohamed A, Nasef N, Shah V, et al.: Vasopressin as a rescue therapy for refractory pulmonary hypertension in neonates: case series, *Pediatr Crit Care Med* 15(2):148–154, 2014.

36. Hoffman TM, Wernovsky G, Atz AM, et al.: Efficacy and safety of milrinone in preventing low cardiac output syndrome in infants and children after corrective surgery for congenital heart disease, *Circulation* 107(7):996–1002, 2003.

37. Paradisis M, Evans N, Kluckow M, et al.: Randomized trial of milrinone versus placebo for prevention of low systemic blood flow in very preterm infants, *J Pediatr* 154(2):189–195, 2009.

38. Paradisis M, Jiang X, McLachlan AJ, et al.: Population pharmacokinetics and dosing regimen design of milrinone in preterm infants, *Arch Dis Child Fetal Neonatal Ed* 92(3):F204–F209, 2007.

39. El-Khuffash AF, Jain A, Weisz D, et al.: Assessment and treatment of post patent ductus arteriosus ligation syndrome, *J Pediatr* 165(1):46–52.e41, 2014.

40. McNamara PJ, Shivananda SP, Sahni M, et al.: Pharmacology of milrinone in neonates with persistent pulmonary hypertension of the newborn and suboptimal response to inhaled nitric oxide, *Pediatr Crit Care Med* 14(1):74–84, 2013.

41. James AT, Bee C, Corcoran JD, et al.: Treatment of premature infants with pulmonary hypertension and right ventricular dysfunction with milrinone: a case series, *J Perinatol* 35(4):268–273, 2015.

42. Rios DR, Moffett BS, Kaiser JR: Trends in pharmacotherapy for neonatal hypotension, *J Pediatr* 165(4):697–701.e691, 2014.

43. Bourchier D, Weston PJ: Randomised trial of dopamine compared with hydrocortisone for the treatment of hypotensive very low birthweight infants, *Arch Dis Child Fetal Neonatal Ed* 76(3):F174–F178, 1997.

44. Ng PC, Lee CH, Bnur FL, et al.: A double-blind, randomized, controlled study of a "stress dose" of hydrocortisone for rescue treatment of refractory hypotension in preterm infants, *Pediatrics* 117(2):367–375, 2006.

45. Efird MM, Heerens AT, Gordon PV, et al.: A randomized-controlled trial of prophylactic hydrocortisone supplementation for the prevention of hypotension in extremely low birth weight infants, *J Perinatol* 25(2):119–124, 2005.

46. Noori S, Friedlich P, Wong P, et al.: Hemodynamic changes after low-dosage hydrocortisone administration in vasopressor-treated preterm and term neonates, *Pediatrics* 118(4):1456–1466, 2006.

47. Baud O, Maury L, Lebail F, et al.: Effect of early low-dose hydrocortisone on survival without bronchopulmonary dysplasia in extremely preterm infants (PREMILOC): a double-blind, placebo-controlled, multicentre, randomised trial, *Lancet* 387(10030):1827–1836, 2016.

48. Diab YA, Wong EC, Luban NL: Massive transfusion in children and neonates, *Br J Haematol* 161(1):15–26, 2013.

49. de Waal KA, Evans N: Hemodynamics in preterm infants with late-onset sepsis, *J Pediatr* 156(6):918–922, 2010.

50. Watterberg KL: Hydrocortisone dosing for hypotension in newborn infants: less is more, *J Pediatr* 174, 2016. 23–26 e21.

51. Kluckow M, Evans N: Low superior vena cava flow and intraventricular haemorrhage in preterm infants, *Arch Dis Child Fetal Neonatal Ed* 82:188–194, 2000.

52. El-Khuffash AF, Jain A, Dragulescu A, et al.: Acute changes in myocardial systolic function in preterm infants undergoing patent ductus arteriosus ligation: a tissue Doppler and myocardial deformation study, *J Am Soc Echocardiogr* 25(10):1058–1067, 2012.

53. Evans N, Kluckow M, Currie A: Range of echocardiographic findings in term neonates with high oxygen requirements, *Arch Dis Child Fetal Neonatal Ed* 78(2):F105–F111, 1998.

54. Semberova J, O'Donnell SM, Franta J, et al.: Inhaled nitric oxide in preterm infants with prolonged preterm rupture of the membranes: a case series, *J Perinatol* 35(4):304–306, 2015.

55. Shah DM, Kluckow M: Early functional echocardiogram and inhaled nitric oxide: usefulness in managing neonates born following extreme preterm premature rupture of membranes (PPROM), *J Paediatr Child Health* 47(6):340–345, 2011.

56. Roze JC, Storme L, Zupan V, et al.: Echocardiographic investigation of inhaled nitric oxide in newborn babies with severe hypoxaemia, *Lancet* 344(8918):303–305, 1994.

The Neonate With Relative Adrenal Insufficiency and Vasopressor Resistance

Erika F. Fernandez

- **Relative adrenal insufficiency has become increasingly recognized in sick premature and term neonates, infants, children, and adults.**
- **Relative adrenal insufficiency often presents with cardiovascular insufficiency and increases the risk of morbidity and mortality in all populations.**
- **In general, relative adrenal insufficiency associated with illness and hypotension lasts less than a week in term infants and no longer than 2 weeks in very preterm infants.**
- **Corticosteroids increase blood pressure, but more studies are needed to determine the treatment criteria, dosage, duration, and long-term effects.**
- **Glucocorticoid therapy should be tailored for each patient and account for gestational age, condition, and response of the patient, limiting the exposure as much as possible.**

Hypotension in the neonate is defined as low blood pressure and signs of decreased systemic and organ blood flow and has been shown to be associated with adrenal insufficiency in critically ill patients, including preterm and term neonates. Accordingly, corticosteroids have been increasingly used for the treatment of neonatal hypotension not responding to vasopressor-inotropes.[1-4] Although there is a better understanding of the underlying pathophysiology, clinical presentation, diagnostic criteria, and treatment strategies for adrenal insufficiency-associated neonatal hypotension, data are still lacking on the long-term benefits and risks of steroid use in neonates with adrenal insufficiency-associated cardiovascular compromise.

Adrenal Insufficiency and Relative Adrenal Insufficiency

In 1885 Thomas Addison described manifestations of primary adrenal insufficiency as "general languor and debility, remarkable feebleness of the heart's action, irritability of the stomach…occurring in connection with a diseased condition of the suprarenal capsules…" (http://wehner.org/addison.htm). Currently, more than 150 years after the original description of Addison's disease, these manifestations of adrenal insufficiency extend to the recently described condition of "relative adrenal insufficiency." Relative adrenal insufficiency is defined as a condition when there is inadequate corticosteroid activity compared with the level of illness in a critically ill patient[5-8] and may arise from inadequate cortisol levels resulting from problems anywhere along the hypothalamic-pituitary-adrenal (HPA) axis or from tissue resistance to corticosteroids. Adrenal insufficiency in critically ill patients is also known as "functional adrenal insufficiency," "transient adrenocortical insufficiency of prematurity," or "critical illness-related corticosteroid insufficiency." For the purposes of this chapter, the term "relative adrenal insufficiency" will be used interchangeably with these terms.

Relative adrenal insufficiency is not characterized by structural abnormality of the adrenal glands but by its transience, because the majority of patients who recover will have normal HPA axis function and corticosteroid activity. However, the diagnosis of relative adrenal insufficiency in a critically ill patient should not make one complacent about or underestimate the potentially life-threatening nature of this type of adrenal insufficiency. Higher mortality rates occur in those whose adrenal response to stress is blunted, as evidenced by trauma patients receiving etomidate during surgery.[9] Etomidate, a sedative commonly used for intubation, suppresses cortisol production by inhibiting 11β-hydroxylase activity which leads to adrenal suppression. Since the 1980s, relative adrenal insufficiency has become increasingly recognized in sick premature and term neonates, infants, children, and adults.[10-32]

In this chapter, we will review the incidence and pathophysiology of relative adrenal insufficiency, along with its clinical presentation, the diagnostic considerations, and treatment strategies the neonatologist needs to understand and consider.

Incidence of Relative Adrenal Insufficiency

The overall incidence of relative adrenal insufficiency in *critically ill adult* patients is approximately 20% in general and approximately 60% in patients with severe sepsis and septic shock in particular.[33] Reported proportions of *critically ill pediatric* patients with "inadequate" cortisol response vary widely, from as low as 2% often up to 87%.[27-29,34-36] Overall, in the *critically ill neonate* the incidence is less well understood because there is no consensus on the diagnostic criteria of relative adrenal insufficiency of the ill newborn.[24,27,30,37-48] But, if relative adrenal insufficiency were to be defined by the use of corticosteroid treatment for hypotension, one large multicenter study found that 17% of the 647 term and late preterm newborns with cardiovascular insufficiency received corticosteroids.[1] In another study of 8019 hypotensive infants born between 2011 and 2012 in 43 neonatal intensive care units (NICUs), 18.8% received hydrocortisone.[2] Moreover, in the extremely low birth weight (ELBW) subset of this population, 33.3% received hydrocortisone.[2] However, these data do not reflect on the true incidence of the condition in the newborn population receiving care in the NICU.

Pathophysiology of Relative Adrenal Insufficiency in The Ill Patient

Postulated pathophysiologic mechanisms for relative adrenal insufficiency in ill patients include adrenergic receptor insensitivity due to receptor downregulation (Fig. 30.1), proinflammatory cytokine-mediated suppression of the function of the pituitary and adrenal glands, inadequate HPA axis response to stress, limited adrenal reserve, gestational age-associated immaturity of the adrenal gland, corticosteroid tissue resistance, and limited adrenal perfusion (Fig. 30.2).[16,25,26,49-53]

Prolonged exposure to inflammatory mediators is one of the proposed mechanisms for both vasopressor-resistant hypotension manifesting via receptor downregulation and relative adrenal insufficiency presenting with suppression of the function of the adrenal gland and/or HPA axis. Decreased vascular responsiveness to adrenergic agents is due to downregulation of adrenergic receptors.[54] Downregulation of adrenergic receptors in clinical conditions occurs within hours due to prolonged exposure to intrinsic (stress response) or extrinsic (vasopressor therapy) catecholamines and inflammatory mediators such as nitric oxide (NO), tumor necrosis factor, and other inflammatory cytokines (interleukin [IL]-1, IL-2, IL-6, interferon gamma).[38,55] Thus production of proinflammatory cytokines also contributes to decreased vascular reactivity to catecholamines and thus to the development of vasopressor-resistant hypotension.

Decreased vascular responsiveness to adrenergic stimulation has been described in critically ill patients who meet specific criteria for adrenal insufficiency. Annane et al. have reported worse vascular responsiveness to norepinephrine in adult patients with septic shock presenting with adrenal insufficiency compared with those without the condition.[56] In the scenario in which severe illness has both inflammation and concomitant cortisol insufficiency-associated decreased cardiovascular responsiveness to catecholamines, corticosteroid therapy reestablishes vascular responsiveness and counteracts inflammation.

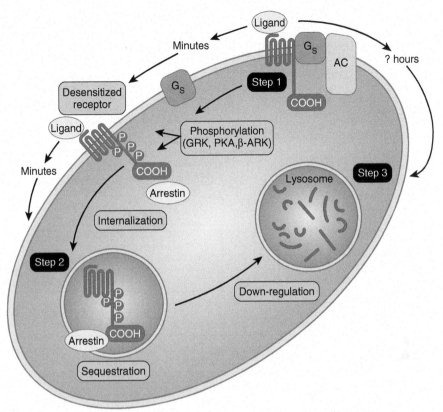

Fig. 30.1   Cellular mechanisms of adrenergic receptor downregulation. Following exposure to agonists, trans-membrane β-adrenergic receptors coupling to the stimulatory guanine nucleotide–binding regulatory proteins (G$_s$) undergo rapid (minutes) and longer-term (hours) regulatory processes induced by the receptor-specific ligands. These processes result in attenuation of the adenylyl cyclase (AC) enzyme and cyclic adenosine monophosphate (cAMP) formation. The initial process includes phosphorylation-regulated functional desensitization due to phosphorylation of the intracellular loops at the carboxyl-terminus of the adrenoreceptor by G-protein coupled receptor kinase (GRK), cAMP-dependent protein kinase A (PKA) and β-adrenergic receptor kinase (β-ARK) **(Step 1)**. Phosphorylation (P) is followed by coupling of the receptor to arrestin and loss of hydrophilic ligand binding. Arrestin promotes internalization of the receptor, which is then targeted for sequestration **(Step 2)** into the cytosolic compartment. The final step, downregulation **(Step 3)** refers to the agonist-induced decrease in the number of the receptors following prolonged exposure to agonists and results in degradation of the receptor presumably via a lysosomal pathway.

Newborns, especially those born prematurely, have unique susceptibilities to relative adrenal insufficiency which is, at least in part, due to the immaturity of their HPA axis and especially the cortical function of the adrenal gland. In addition, the changes in adrenal cortical hormone production, especially cortisol during the transition to extrauterine life and the gestational age-dependent changes in placental 11β-hydroxysteroid dehydrogenase type 2 activity and thus the effect of maternal corticosteroids on fetal corticosteroid production, pose special challenges for the newborn, especially the preterm neonate. Fetal adrenal glands begin to synthetize cortisol de novo only at approximately 22 to 24 weeks' gestation, followed by a steady increase throughout the rest of the pregnancy.[57] Corticotropin-releasing hormone (CRH) production by the placenta also increases throughout gestation, resulting in maternal and fetal serum CRH concentrations at term that are much higher than at any other time in life.[58] Placental CRH stimulates cortisol production in the fetal adrenal gland. At birth, the very high placental CRH production ceases to have an effect on the newborn. The pituitary gland of the newborn which has been exposed to high concentrations of CRH during fetal life may become transiently insensitive to the lower concentrations of CRH produced by the hypothalamus of the neonate. Therefore it may not be able to increase adrenocorticotropic hormone

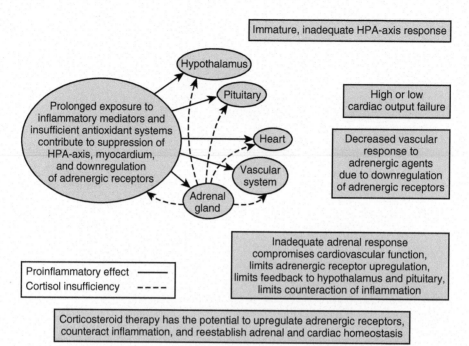

Fig. 30.2 Interaction among the hypothalamic-pituitary-adrenal axis, cardiovascular function, and inflammation. Corticosteroid **therapy** upregulates adrenergic receptor and adenylate cyclase expression and membrane assembly, counteracts inflammation, and reestablishes cardiovascular and adrenal homeostasis. *HPA axis*, Hypothalamic-pituitary-adrenal axis.

(ACTH) production to appropriately stimulate the adrenal gland for several days after delivery. Healthy term newborns tolerate this period of relative HPA insufficiency. However, this situation may predispose the newborn to the development of relative adrenal insufficiency in critical illness. Relative adrenal insufficiency could then contribute to the severity of systemic hypotension and attenuate the response of the cardiovascular system to treatment.

In summary, the physiology and complex regulation of the fetal HPA axis and the sympathoadrenal system and their immaturity at birth, coupled with prolonged exposure to free radicals and the subsequent production of proinflammatory cytokines in critical illness, set the stage for the presentation of adrenal and cardiovascular insufficiency in the acutely ill premature or term infant.

Clinical Presentation of Relative Adrenal Insufficiency and Hypotension

Cardiovascular instability, a key clinical manifestation of relative adrenal insufficiency, may present with hypotension that is either responsive, dependent, or resistant to vasopressor/inotropes and, depending on myocardial function and the loading conditions of the heart, with high or low cardiac output.* Other clinical features of relative adrenal insufficiency may include hyponatremia, hyperkalemia, hypoglycemia, metabolic acidosis, and feeding intolerance (Fig. 30.3). However, the electrolyte and/or metabolic abnormalities are less likely to occur in critically ill patients whose electrolyte and fluid management are tightly controlled.

In addition to cardiovascular instability and the potential electrolyte and metabolic abnormalities, relative adrenal insufficiency is characterized by random and/or stimulated cortisol levels that are inadequate for the degree of illness severity and by rapid clinical and hemodynamic improvement following corticosteroid therapy.[7,30,33,34]

In preterm infants, blood pressure positively correlates with cortisol production rate.[71] Thus patients with low random or basal serum cortisol values are more likely

---

*References 11-19, 21, 23-26, 32, 37, 38, 49, 50, and 59-71.

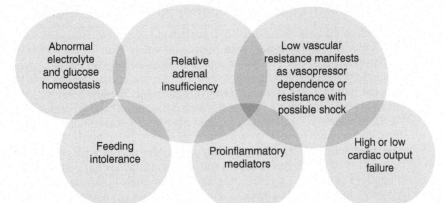

Fig. 30.3 Clinical features and interaction between adrenal insufficiency and cardiovascular function. Severe illness and cardiovascular instability are features of both relative adrenal insufficiency (RAI) and vasopressor-resistant hypotension. RAI may or may not be associated with vasopressor-resistant hypotension and vasopressor-resistant hypotension may or may not be associated with RAI.

to have low blood pressure. In a randomized controlled trial (RCT) of hydrocortisone administration in hypotensive preterm infants, the overall baseline (control) median serum cortisol concentrations were 3.3 and 4.1 µg/dL in the treated and placebo groups, respectively.[34] These values are considered low for the degree of illness severity in preterm infants when compared with the 50th percentile of the serum cortisol values in ill infants (7.2 µg/dL).[4] In 54 surfactant-treated, 1-day-old preterm infants of 24 to 36 weeks' gestation, serum cortisol values were lower in those with left ventricular output less than or equal to 180 mL/min/kg compared with those greater than 180 mL/min/kg.[14,32,72]

The study by Yoder and colleagues in very premature baboons provides the most direct, albeit nonhuman, evidence that relative adrenal insufficiency, cardiovascular insufficiency, and prematurity are related.[73] In earlier studies, this group of investigators documented that the majority of extremely premature baboons, delivered at approximately 67% of baboon gestation (~26 weeks' human gestation), required volume expansion and vasopressor-inotrope therapy to treat the subjects' hypotension, oliguria, and acid-base imbalance. Many of the premature baboons (38%) also required hydrocortisone to successfully treat their hypotension despite receiving vasopressor-inotrope therapy.[74] This group of researchers also demonstrated that decreased urinary free cortisol excretion in the first postnatal day correlated with decreased left ventricular function. Furthermore, hydrocortisone therapy (0.5 to 1.0 mg/kg/day for 1 to 2 days) corrected the hypotension and the left ventricular dysfunction, reduced vasopressor-inotrope requirement and mortality, and increased serum cortisol to levels comparable to those seen in baboons with no evidence of relative adrenal insufficiency or cardiovascular dysfunction.[73]

In term infants, low cortisol values have also been found in association with hypotension. In some studies on late preterm and/or term neonates with refractory hypotension, low median cortisol values were in the range of 4.5 to 11.7 µg/dL.[28,36,75]

Although recent evidence has shown that many infants will respond to corticosteroid treatment regardless of cortisol values, there are reports that show documented low cortisol values in neonates with vasopressor-resistant hypotension *responsive* to corticosteroid treatment.[†] Other studies report a similar presentation of responsiveness to corticosteroids treatment without cortisol data.[14,17,29,62,77] Attenuated cortisol response to adrenal stimulation with ACTH and extremely high random cortisol levels may also represent a clinical presentation in which vasopressor-resistant hypotension is the predominant factor of the cardiovascular collapse.[78]

[†]References 11, 12, 14, 17, 23, 34, 67, and 76.

Relative Adrenal Insufficiency in Preterm Infants

In 1989 Ward and Colasurdo first described ventilated, sick, extremely premature infants who presented with signs consistent with adrenal insufficiency or "Addisonian crisis."[12] These infants had signs of relative adrenal insufficiency, including hypotension, oliguria, hyponatremia, and cortisol values less than 15 μg/dL (414 nmol/L), and responded to hydrocortisone therapy. Since this time, subsequent investigations have further elucidated the clinical and laboratory presentation of relative adrenal insufficiency in ill, hypotensive premature infants.[‡] Investigators have documented two intriguing observations regarding cortisol levels in well and sick premature infants. Many *healthy premature infants* with no signs of relative adrenal insufficiency have random cortisol levels that are not detectable or less than 5 μg/dL (138 nmol/L), a threshold considered to indicate adrenal insufficiency.[§] On the other hand, there is a population of *sick premature infants* with serum cortisol levels similar to or lower than cortisol levels in well preterm or term infants.[¶] The finding that sick premature infants do not have the expected increase in random cortisol levels commensurate with their illness acuity is supportive of the presence of relative adrenal insufficiency in this population.

Further support for relative adrenal insufficiency in the *preterm population* comes from studies that have found that adrenal insufficiency results from immature cortisol synthesis in the adrenal gland. Ng et al. reported normal pituitary response to CRH but blunted adrenal response in sick premature infants with vasopressor-resistant hypotension and low serum cortisol values. These findings led Ng et al. to speculate that, in preterm neonates, the adrenal gland was responsible for the adrenal insufficiency.[23] Findings from other investigators support this notion because sick premature infants have been found to have low random cortisol levels, elevated cortisol precursors, and blunted response to ACTH stimulation.[ǁ] Watterberg et al. reported that compared with term infants, sick premature infants had higher cortisol precursor concentrations (17α-OH pregnenolone, 17α-OH progesterone, and 11-deoxycortisol) and lower serum cortisol concentrations. In another, small, prospective study of infants born at less than 30 weeks' gestation, Huysman et al. demonstrated that critically ill, ventilated infants, compared with less sick, nonventilated infants, had lower cortisol levels, elevated cortisol precursor levels of 17-hydroxyprogesterone, and insufficient cortisol response to ACTH (0.5 μg/kg) stimulation.[66] Korte et al. also reported an abnormal adrenal response to cosyntropin (ACTH) in 51 ventilated, premature infants of less than 32 weeks' gestation who had baseline cortisol levels of less than 5 μg/dL (138 nmol/L). Among the 51 infants, 64% and 37% had inadequate cortisol response (<9 μg/dL) to stimulation with 0.1 and 0.2 μg/kg cosyntropin, respectively.[24]

Evidence of Relative Adrenal Insufficiency in Sick Late Preterm and Term Infants

There is growing evidence that a significant number of ill term and late preterm infants also exhibit evidence of adrenal insufficiency.[28,29,36,82,88-90] In 1972 Gutai et al. were one of the first groups of authors to describe suboptimal cortisol responses to illness in a small number of stressed term newborn infants.[91] Indeed, there was no difference in the median random cortisol value between the 12 ill infants (5.2 μg/dL) and 28 healthy newborns (4.1 μg/dL), but all infants responded to 5 units of ACTH appropriately. A subsequent study by Thomas et al. found that 27% of ill term newborns studied had basal cortisol less than 2 μg/dL, and only 33% of these infants had an appropriate response to ACTH (>18 μg/dL).[82] In the first study to investigate cardiovascular responses to dexamethasone in hypotensive term newborn infants, Tantivit et al. reported that five of the seven infants studied had cortisol values less than 10 μg/dL.[35] All of these infants responded to dexamethasone administration

---

[‡]References 11-14, 17, 18, 21, 23, 29, 31, 64, 66, 67, and 79-81.
[§]References 13, 19, 20, 24, 31, 34, 66, and 79-84.
[¶]References 11-13, 20, 34, 79, 80, 83, 85, and 86.
[ǁ]References 24, 31, 79, 80, 83, 84, 86, and 87.

with prompt hemodynamic stabilization. In 2000 Pittinger et al. described low cortisol values in sick infants with congenital diaphragmatic hernia and found that 79% had random cortisol levels of less than 7 μg/dL.[90] Two of the four critically ill patients had an inappropriately low cortisol response to cosyntropin. On the other hand, Soliman et al. found an overall increase in basal circulating cortisol concentrations by twofold to threefold in neonates with sepsis and respiratory distress.[29] Yet, more than 30% of these infants had cortisol values suggestive of relative adrenal insufficiency (<15 μg/dL). Patients with lower basal cortisol levels and peak cortisol responses to ACTH had higher mortality. Recent reports also suggest that, similar to preterm infants, critically ill late preterm and term infants with hypotension may have problems with adrenal synthesis of cortisol as higher cortisol precursor levels have been documented in those presenting with vasopressor-resistant hypotension.[92] In a larger, prospective, observational study, 35 sick late preterm and term infants on mechanical ventilation had a median random cortisol level of 4.6 μg/ dL, a value very low for the degree of illness.[36] These infants also had relatively low ACTH values but demonstrated appropriate cortisol responses to ACTH stimulation (1 μg/kg), suggesting they had secondary adrenal insufficiency, a mechanism different from the adrenal insufficiency of the sick very low birth weight (VLBW) infant.

Duration of Relative Adrenal Insufficiency

Speculation about the duration of relative adrenal insufficiency in different patient populations is based on the duration of hormone replacement therapy and serum cortisol levels. *In adults*, Hoen et al.[39] and Annane et al.[26] reported that relative adrenal insufficiency and/or vasopressor dependency may be sustained for several days, weeks, or even beyond 1 month in patients with sepsis or hemorrhagic shock from trauma.

In *preterm infants*, Colasurdo et al. found that in nine sick infants of 26 weeks' gestation with clinical symptoms of relative adrenal insufficiency and low cortisol levels (mean, 251 ± 102 nmol/L −9.1 ± 3.7 μg/dL), there was reversal of clinical signs within 2 days.[11] Since then, based on serum cortisol data or response to corticosteroids, studies have reported inconsistent findings for the presumed duration of relative adrenal insufficiency. Ng et al. reported that inadequate cortisol response on postnatal day 7 in sick VLBW infants had resolved by day 14.[85] In contrast, Guttentag et al. reported that no increase in either cortisol or ACTH serum levels occurred through the first 14 days in response to critical illness.[31] If duration of relative adrenal insufficiency was based on the response to hormone replacement therapy, according to an earlier study by Gaissmaier and Pohlandt, a single dose of dexamethasone would be effective in reversing vasopressor-resistant hypotension in sick premature infants.[76] In addition, Ng et al. reported that 79% of preterm infants less than 32 weeks' gestation with refractory hypotension receiving hydrocortisone for 5 days were successfully weaned from vasopressor support by 72 hours of age compared with only 33% who were receiving placebo.[34] Hochwald et al. also showed that a 2-day course of hydrocortisone compared with placebo significantly decreased dopamine exposure by 34 hours versus 67 hours (*P* = .04).[93] Similarly, Efird et al. reported that prophylactic hydrocortisone therapy for 5 days (vs. placebo) in ELBW infants reduced the use of vasopressors during the first two postnatal days.[94] On the other hand, in very premature baboons with relative adrenal insufficiency and vasopressor-resistant hypotension at a gestational age approximately equivalent to human gestation of 26 weeks, there was no decrease in urinary free cortisol levels over the first 2 postnatal weeks (the entire duration of the study).[73]

In *term ill infants*, Economou et al. found that, in 4 of 15 infants who were "low cortisol responders" relative to their illness, this state lasted until the fifth postnatal day.[88] In a more recent study of critically ill newborn infants with refractory hypotension, Baker et al. used cortisol levels and the presence of hemodynamic instability to determine the duration of relative adrenal insufficiency and thereby the duration of hydrocortisone replacement therapy.[75] Sixty-one term infants received 3.5 median days of hydrocortisone therapy, whereas the 37 extremely preterm infants enrolled in the study remained on hydrocortisone for a median of 15 days. In another study, 1-day-old term and late preterm ill infants with random low cortisol values of less than 15 μg/dL received longer courses of treatment with hydrocortisone for hypotension compared with those with higher cortisol values (5 vs. 2.5 median days).[28] Kamath et al. found a high incidence (67%) of cortisol values of less than 15 µg/dL in hypotensive infants with congenital diaphragmatic hernia, all of whom received hydrocortisone for 10.9 ± 7.0 days.[89] Thus it seems that the duration of relative adrenal insufficiency varies with age, disease severity, etiology, and response to treatment. In general, relative adrenal insufficiency seems to last less than a week in term infants and no longer than 2 weeks in very preterm infants irrespective of whether it is defined by cortisol values or by the short-term cardiovascular response to corticosteroid replacement therapy.

Late-onset Relative Adrenal Insufficiency-Associated Hypotension

Most reports of relative adrenal insufficiency are in critically ill newborn infants in the first postnatal days. There is some evidence that adrenal insufficiency can also occur later in life (4 to 7 days of age) in ill newborn infants with respiratory distress or sepsis.[29] A survey in Japan found that approximately 4% of VLBW infants were receiving postnatal corticosteroid therapy after 7 days of age with symptoms suggestive of relative adrenal insufficiency, including hypotension and high cortisol precursors.[95]

Relative Adrenal Insufficiency and Outcomes

In addition to hypotension, transient adrenal insufficiency in the newborn population is associated with other morbidities as well. Term infants born with meconium-stained amniotic fluid who presented with respiratory distress had lower ACTH and cortisol levels than did infants with meconium-stained amniotic fluid without respiratory distress.[96] In another study, cortisol levels of less than 17 µg/dL were associated with more bronchopulmonary dysplasia and increased length of hospital stay.[40] In addition, a number of studies found an association in sick, extremely premature infants between relative adrenal insufficiency, diagnosed by low cortisol values and/or elevated cortisol precursors, and increased pulmonary disease severity and subsequent chronic lung disease.[19,20,24,40,66,84,85,97-102] Relative adrenal insufficiency has also been associated with the presence of patent ductus arteriosus.[19] Of note is that these findings reveal only an association between low serum cortisol values and morbidity, and causation has not been documented.

Diagnosis of Adrenal Insufficiency

The reported incidence of relative adrenal insufficiency is obviously influenced by the *criteria used for "adequate" and "inadequate" cortisol response or cortisol production.* In critically ill adults the proposed criterion for diagnosing relative adrenal insufficiency is a change in total serum cortisol levels of less than 9 µg/dL following 250 µg of cosyntropin administration or a random total cortisol of less than 10 µg/dL (276 nmol/L).[103] Of note is that a cortisol level of less than 10 µg/dL in ill adult patients has high predictive value (0.93) but low sensitivity (0.19) for relative adrenal insufficiency.[104] In their most recent publication on clinical practice parameters for hemodynamic support of pediatric and neonatal septic shock, the American College of Critical Care Medicine propose to maintain "equipoise on the question of adjunctive steroid therapy and thus diagnosis of relative adrenal insufficiency for pediatric and newborn septic shock (outside of classic adrenal insufficiency) pending further trials."[48]

Devising diagnostic criteria for relative adrenal insufficiency *in infants* is particularly challenging because of the relatively little amount of available data.[105] The diagnosis and thus the reported incidence of relative adrenal insufficiency are greatly influenced by the choice of the test. Neonatal investigators most often report isolated, random serum cortisol levels or stimulated serum cortisol levels at specific time points following CRH or ACTH stimulation. Using random cortisol values at the time of stress in VLBW infants, Korte et al. defined normal adrenal function as a random cortisol level of 15 µg/dL (414 nmol/L) and an inadequate serum cortisol as a serum cortisol level less than 5 µg/dL (<138 nmol/L).[24] In critically ill term and late preterm infants, Fernandez et al. showed that those with random cortisol values less than 15 µg/dL had higher blood pressure within 24 hours after hydrocortisone administration.[28] In addition, these infants demonstrated a decreased need for vasopressor-inotropes and had a lower heart rate after hydrocortisone administration compared with those with higher cortisol values. However, debate remains on the use of random cortisol values as a diagnostic tool because total plasma cortisol can have marked hourly variability in both adults and neonates.[106,107] In addition, random cortisol values may not correlate with outcome, response to therapy, or severity of illness.[36,75,106] However, a baseline random cortisol is often the most practical and easiest to obtain in the acute setting of the rapidly deteriorating newborn. In term and late preterm infants, a cutoff random cortisol value of 15 µg/dL is often used.[108] For preterm infants, a recent review has suggested that a serum cortisol value of less than 200 nmol/L (7.25 µg/dL) or the less than 50th percentile for adjusted serum cortisol levels be used to diagnose relative (transient) adrenal insufficiency of prematurity. This value represents the 25th percentile of serum cortisol levels in well VLBW and the 50th percentile in vasopressor-dependent VLBW infants.[108] In his review, PC Ng published a mathematical model which takes into account clinical variables that may change the percentile of the diagnostic serum cortisol.

To further test for relative adrenal insufficiency, some investigators used CRH alone[85,86,98] or CRH followed by ACTH administration.[13] However, investigators more often selected ACTH alone as the stimulating agent with dosages ranging from 0.1 to 62.5 µg/kg.[#] Of note is that adrenal stimulation with supraphysiologic ACTH doses can induce a compromised adrenal gland to produce an "adequate"-appearing serum cortisol response and thus miss the diagnosis of relative adrenal insufficiency.[24] Indeed, ACTH doses at 0.1 to 0.2 µg/kg[24,40,109,110] and perhaps at 0.5 to 1.0 µg/kg[40,66] are more likely to reveal "relative" adrenal insufficiency than higher ACTH doses. Yet, even within the dose range of 0.1 to 1.0 µg/kg, the proportion of sick premature infants with "inadequate" cortisol response (defined as a serum cortisol level of <9 µg/dL) varies greatly. In a study of ventilated VLBW infants of less than 32 weeks' gestation and with random serum cortisol levels of less than 5 µg/dL (138 nmol/L), Korte et al. reported that 64% and 37% of infants had inadequate cortisol response (<9 µg/dL) to ACTH at doses of 0.1 and 0.2 µg/dL, respectively.[24] In a trial of ventilated 3-week-old 25 weeks' gestation *preterm infants*, Watterberg et al. reported 21% and 2% of infants had inadequate cortisol response to 0.1 and 1.0 µg/kg ACTH, respectively.[40] In critically ill *term infants*, after giving 1 µg/kg of ACTH, Fernandez et al. found no infants with a cortisol value of less than 18 µg/dL and all patients increased their serum cortisol by greater than 9 µg/dL.[36] In addition, there was no association between ACTH-stimulated cortisol values and severity of illness, need for vasopressor-inotropes, or days on mechanical ventilation. In nonmechanically ventilated infants with sepsis, Soliman et al. found that, when an ACTH stimulation dose of 250 µg/1.73 m^2 was used, no patients met the criteria of having adrenal insufficiency, whereas 13% of the patients were diagnosed with adrenal insufficiency when 1 µg/1.73 m^2 of ACTH was given.[29] Importantly, patients with lower stimulated cortisol values did have higher mortality. In 2012 Hochwald et al. reported that, if an ACTH stimulation test using a dose of 1 µg/kg is performed in premature infants of less than 29 weeks' gestation with varying degrees of illness in the first 8 postnatal hours, the test could predict those with adrenal insufficiency using hypotension requiring vasopressor-inotrope treatment as a marker.[111] They determined that an ACTH-induced change in cortisol of less than 12% from baseline provided the highest sensitivity (75%) and specificity (93%) for detecting the development of hypotension in this population, On the other hand, random basal cortisol levels did not predict hypotension with an area under the receiver operating characteristic curve (ROC) of 48%.[111]

Free cortisol and not protein-bound cortisol is responsible for the physiologic effects at the cellular level, and it may prove to be a better diagnostic tool for adrenal insufficiency. However, the test to measure free cortisol is not widely available because there are no commercial tests on the market. Yoder et al.[73] measured urinary

---

[#]References 20, 24, 29, 40, 66, 78, 79, 82, 86, 97, 109, and 110.

free cortisol levels in 6-hourly block intervals in their premature baboon model to define the ontogeny of cortisol release over the initial hours and days of postnatal life. They found that urinary free cortisol levels were directly proportional to and highly correlated with plasma cortisol levels.[112] Moreover, urinary free cortisol measurement avoids the potential fluctuations seen in serum cortisol levels and the need for frequent blood sampling.[73] However, one needs to be able to effectively collect timed urine samples, which is not a very practical approach in the NICU. Vezina et al. described unbound cortisol concentrations in critically ill newborns with hypotension requiring vasopressor-inotrope administration.[113] Similar data may serve to better tailor the dosing of hydrocortisone and predict its clinical effects in the future.[113]

The *lack of consensus on diagnostic evaluation and timing of evaluation* is further fueled by the uncertainty about the definition of "adequate" and "inadequate" cortisol response or cortisol production across gestational and postnatal ages for different diagnostic evaluations.[24,40] Indeed, recent studies have continued to complicate the consensus on the utility of adrenal function tests. For instance, Miletin et al. found no correlation between serum cortisol values and superior vena cava (SVC) flow or mean blood pressure.[114] However, this finding might be explained by the lack of our ability to appropriately define the "normal range" for SVC flow and hypotension (see Chapter 3) and by the fact that additional hemodynamic parameters affect the normal range of SVC flow in an individual patient (see Chapters 1 and 11). At present, the validity, reproducibility, and clinical importance of identifying inadequate cortisol response to illness or ACTH at different stimulating doses (0.1, 0.2, 0.5, or 1.0 µg/kg ACTH) in terms of mortality, management, and long-term outcomes requires further study. To further complicate the diagnosis of adrenal insufficiency in the preterm and term neonate, measurements of serum cortisol and the response to ACTH stimulation may be influenced by the various procedures and the testing itself in acutely ill patients.[115] Thus the validity and interpretation of adrenal function tests, especially in the midst of critical illness, is subject to an ongoing debate among adult, pediatric, and neonatal critical care physicians.

Corticosteroid Treatment

Mechanisms of Action of Corticosteroids

The goal of corticosteroid therapy is to maintain homeostasis during stress, minimize organ dysfunction, and ensure appropriate tissue oxygen delivery. The HPA axis and the sympathetic nervous system are the primary mediators of stress response. Under normal conditions, all forms of stress increase hypothalamic CRH followed by pituitary ACTH and thus adrenal cortisol production. The resultant cardiovascular effects of corticosteroids include the maintenance of and/or improvements in myocardial contractility and function, vascular tone, endothelial integrity, and vascular responsiveness to catecholamines and angiotensin II. The sensitivity of the cardiovascular system to endogenous sympathomimetic amines is further increased by the corticosteroid-induced inhibition of the cathechol-O-methyltransferase enzyme limiting sympathomimetic amine metabolism and the decrease in the reuptake of norepinephrine into the sympathetic nerve endings. In addition, corticosteroids attenuate the proinflammatory cytokine response, modulate the immune response, and counteract the inflammatory cascade. Acute exposure to inflammatory cytokines may also increase the affinity of glucocorticoid receptors. In addition, acute exposure to inflammatory cytokines (e.g., IL-1 IL-6, tumor necrosis factor alpha [TNF-α]) can activate the HPA axis, which then attenuates the inflammatory response, and may increase ligand affinity of glucocorticoid and mineralocorticoid receptors. Corticosteroids also reduce vascular permeability in the presence of acute inflammation, decrease the dysregulated production of NO and other vasodilators, and modulate free water distribution within the vascular compartment.[14,49,65,116-118]

Corticosteroids exert their effects through genomic and nongenomic mechanisms.[49,117,118] The genomic actions of corticosteroids reverse vasopressor-refractory hypotension by upregulating cardiovascular α- and β-adrenergic receptors through synthesis and membrane assembly of new receptor proteins, a process that occurs over hours. Other genomic effects include corticosteroid mediation of sympathetic nerve activity and maturational changes in Na^+, K^+-ATPase enzyme activity, myosin fibers, and other components of cardiac muscle.[49,119,120] However, the rapid response of the cardiovascular system to corticosteroids is thought to occur via nongenomic mechanisms through interaction with putative cell membrane-bound steroid receptors and require both glucocorticoid and mineralocorticoid actions.[10]

In summary, via their genomic and nongenomic actions, corticosteroids rapidly sensitize the cardiovascular system to catecholamines. At the cellular and molecular level, corticosteroids exert their cardiovascular effects by increasing catecholamine levels through enhanced catecholamine synthesis and inhibition of catecholamine metabolism and reuptake, by inhibition of prostacyclin and NO synthesis, by increasing intracellular calcium availability leading to enhanced myocardial and vascular smooth muscle cell contraction, and by improving capillary integrity (see Chapter 1).

Corticosteroid Therapy for Cardiovascular Insufficiency

In adults, high-dose, short course, corticosteroid administration confers no benefit and actually possible cause harm in critically ill adult patients with acute lung injury, adult respiratory distress syndrome (ARDS), and septic shock.[7,103] On the other hand, prolonged, low-dose corticosteroid therapy has shown beneficial effects on short-term mortality, ventilation-free days, length of intensive care unit (ICU) stay, multiple organ dysfunction syndrome scores, lung injury scores, and shock reversal without increasing the incidence of significant adverse events.[7,121,122] Accordingly, *corticosteroids are recommended in adults* with catecholamine-refractory shock (norepinephrine at doses of >0.05 to 0.1 μg/kg/min or equivalent dose of vasopressor or vasopressor-inotrope) or having ARDS for greater than 48 hours.[103] In these adult patients a course of stress-dose of hydrocortisone at a dose of 200 to 350 mg/day (approximately 3 mg/kg/day) is recommended for at least 7 days because rapid steroid tapers (2 to 6 days) have been associated with rebound inflammation with increased inflammatory mediator production and the need to reintroduce vasopressor-inotropes and mechanical ventilation.[123,124]

Reversal of shock measured by the timing of withdrawal of vasopressors or vasopressor-inotropes in septic *adult patients* also occurs earlier after receiving hydrocortisone versus placebo (3.3 vs. 5.8 median days).[26] In a group of adults with sepsis and higher illness severity, the median time to vasopressor-inotrope withdrawal with corticosteroids versus placebo also favored the treated group (7 vs. 9 days, respectively).[26]

In preterm infants an updated Cochrane review on *corticosteroids for the treatment of hypotension in preterm infants* concludes that there is insufficient information to give any recommendations based on the four studies with a total of 123 patients enrolled.[125] Another meta-analysis in preterm neonates with hypotension and vasopressor dependence found that hydrocortisone is effective in increasing blood pressure (seven studies, $N = 144$, $r = 0.71$, 95% CI = 0.18 to 0.92) and reducing vasopressor requirement (five studies, $N = 93$, $r = 0.74$, 95% CI = 0.0084 to 0.96).[126] The authors were not able to examine dosing strategy, adverse effects, or any effect on medium- to long-term outcomes because of the limited data available. However, the study's findings were robust; random effects meta-analysis found that the number of new studies needed to cancel out the effects of hydrocortisone on blood pressure increase and the decrease in vasopressor requirement are 78 for blood pressure increase and 47 for reducing vasopressor requirement.

The *time to documented cardiovascular response to hydrocortisone* is often measured in hours in the ill newborn population. Helbock reported an increase in blood pressure as early as 30 minutes and within 2 hours following hydrocortisone therapy (1 mg) in 25- to 26-week gestation infants with vasopressor-resistant hypotension.[67] Based on their case series, Helbock and Ng speculated that the response time for reversal of vasopressor-resistant hypotension may be dose related.[23,67] Gaissmaier and Pohlandt noted improvement in vasopressor-resistant hypotension in 4 to 8 hours following a single injection of dexamethasone.[76] Seri et al.[14] and Noori et al.[62] reported an increase in blood pressure within 2 hours following hydrocortisone or low-dose dexamethasone (0.1 mg/kg) administration, respectively. Mizobuchi found a similar response after a single dose of 2 mg/kg dose of hydrocortisone.[127] Ng et al. showed a difference in the percentage of infants able to be weaned off vasopressor-inotropes by 72 hours between those given hydrocortisone versus placebo (79% vs. 33%, $P = .001$).[128] In 15 newborn infants, Noori et al. studied the hemodynamics following hydrocortisone (2 mg/kg, followed by 1 mg/kg q 12 hours) and showed a significant increase in blood pressure at 6 hours, a parallel increase in systemic vascular resistance, and a decrease in dopamine dosage without initial changes in stroke volume or left ventricular output.[129] The five term infants enrolled in this study showed no response in blood pressure to hydrocortisone but did have lower heart rate and received lower dopamine doses compared to baseline by 48 hours.

In seven *term ill newborn infants* given dexamethasone, 0.2 mg/kg/day, an increase in blood pressure was noted by 4 hours after initial dosing with a concomitant decrease in heart rate and vasopressor dosage.[35] Vasopressors were discontinued in all infants within 72 hours after initiating dexamethasone. In a larger study of ill late pre-term and term neonates, there was a significant change in blood pressure over the first 24 hours after hydrocortisone and an overall decrease in vasopressor dose and heart rate within 12 hours.[28] However, there was no difference in blood pressure response between infants with high or low random cortisol values. In 12 term infants given hydrocortisone for low cardiac output syndrome after cardiac surgery, the blood pressure increased significantly 3 hours after hydrocortisone.[77] Baker et al. also found an increase in blood pressure starting 2 hours after the first dose of hydrocortisone and a decrease in the total vasopressor-inotrope requirement at 6 hours in a study of 117 critically ill term and preterm newborns.[75] In summary, newborn infants appear to respond with improved systemic hemodynamics to corticosteroids within 2 to 6 hours of initiation of treatment and there is no evidence of an exaggerated increase in systemic vascular resistance compromising systemic or organ blood flow.[129]

Pharmacokinetics of Hydrocortisone in the Neonate

The elimination half-life of bound hydrocortisone in neonates is much longer than in adults, reported to be 2 ± 0.3 hours[130] and 61 minutes for free hydrocortisone.[131] In 1962 Reynolds et al. was the first to report pharmacokinetics in five term infants after a bolus of 5 mg/kg of hydrocortisone.[132] The mean peak serum concentration (30 to 80 minutes after dose) was 557 µg/dL, and mean serum half-life was just under 4 hours (range 2.4 to 7.1 hours). In a recent study of unbound hydrocortisone concentrations in 62 preterm infants treated for vasopressor-resistant hypotension, the half-life was 2.9 hours.[113] This is 3 times longer than in the adult population and consistent with other reports on hydrocortisone pharmacokinetics in preterm infants as described in a recent review.[133] As illustrated in this review, high cortisol levels can result from administration of high or "stress" dosing of hydrocortisone because the longer half-life in preterm infants is often not appreciated. In a small pilot study of six infants, hydrocortisone at 0.4 to 0.8 mg/kg/dose resulted in serum cortisol trough levels greater than 20 µg/dL for 8 to 12 hours compared with the median endogenous serum cortisol value in sick ELBW infants of 16 µg/dL at less than 48 hours of age.

Studies of vasopressor-dependent, critically ill newborn infants have used variable hydrocortisone dosing (2 to 3 mg/kg/day), and all have shown an increase in blood pressure, a decrease in volume and vasopressor-inotrope requirement, and a decrease in heart rate without confirmed increases in adverse events.** Of note, doses as low as 1 mg/kg/day of hydrocortisone in preterm infants have been shown to increase blood pressure significantly.[97] In the most recent review, a suggested approach to hydrocortisone dosing in the newborn is outlined and based on studies of clinical responses to dosing and recently published pharmacokinetic data.[133] The suggested approach is to give a test dose of 1 mg/kg for cardiovascular insufficiency after drawing a baseline cortisol value. Although a cortisol level is not always a clear indication of relative adrenal insufficiency, a low

---

**References 14, 21, 28, 34, 75, 126, and 129.

value in the face of critical illness may be suggestive of the need for closer monitoring. If no response in blood pressure or vasopressor requirement is seen within 2 to 4 hours, then give no further doses. If there is a response in blood pressure, then consider giving 0.5 mg/kg q 12 hours for preterm infants or q 6 to 8 hours for late preterm and term infants. In most infants with adrenal insufficiency–associated hypotension, hypotension resolves in less than a few days with only some preterm infants requiring longer treatment. The treatment should be tailored to the infant's clinical condition, and every effort should be made to minimize steroid exposure.

Currently there is increasing supportive evidence for the presence of adrenal insufficiency in ill newborns. However, treatment criteria, dosage, and duration of corticosteroid exposure still need to be better defined. This uncertainty is further fueled by the increases in spontaneous ileal perforations in premature neonates coexposed to either hydrocortisone or dexamethasone and cyclooxygenase inhibitors (i.e., indomethacin), as well as by the documented deleterious effects of early higher-dose dexamethasone on neurodevelopment in preterm neonates.[78,134] However, there are encouraging recent studies on the long-term neurodevelopmental effects of hydrocortisone. Supportive evidence from animal and laboratory studies indicates that unbalanced stimulation of glucocorticoid receptors in the brain induces apoptosis which can be rescued by the addition of a mineralocorticoid.[135] This would explain why dexamethasone, especially when given early and in higher doses (0.5 mg/kg q 12 hours 3 times) during the first 2 postnatal days[136] is associated with significant cerebral pathology (white matter injury, decrease in brain volume, etc.), whereas hydrocortisone seems to be devoid of such effects. Indeed, a meta-analysis of three trials with a total of 411 children found that early low-dose hydrocortisone in preterm infants had no effect on the rate of cerebral palsy and survival without neurosensory or cognitive impairment.[100] In the largest of the three studies, there was a lower incidence of cognitive deficits at 18 to 22 months in former preterm infants who received hydrocortisone early in postnatal life.[137] However, because none of the studies were designed to investigate specifically the population of hypotensive infants and all had long-term neurodevelopment as the primary outcome measure, the studies might have been underpowered and the findings need to be confirmed with appropriately designed RCTs.

Large RCTs designed to evaluate short- and long-term effects of hydrocortisone for the treatment of cardiovascular insufficiency are very challenging to conduct and execute. The Neonatal Research Network has attempted to conduct RCTs on the hemodynamic effects of corticosteroids in sick preterm and term infants with hypotension in the past decade but were unable to enroll patients.[138] Reasons for the low enrollment rates included fewer than anticipated infants with low blood pressure, difficulties in obtaining informed consent within the study window, and lack of physician equipoise. In addition, the enrollment of preterm infants was hampered by high rates of early indomethacin administration. Alternative approaches and creativity in research design may be needed to answer the question of long-term safety and the potential benefits for the thousands of infants currently receiving steroids for hypotension.

Summary

Adequate HPA axis and adrenal function are vital to postnatal adaptation in extremely premature infants and critically ill late preterm and term newborns. Clinical, biochemical, and physiologic evidence indicate that adrenal insufficiency and vasopressor-resistant hypotension are serious conditions in sick preterm and term infants and that these conditions respond to corticosteroid therapy with improvements in cardiovascular status. However, whether this improvement translates to improved mortality and/or short- or long-term morbidity is not known. Yet, recent findings provide important insights into adrenal insufficiency and vasopressor-resistant hypotension and stimulate consideration of mechanisms for adrenal insufficiency and vasopressor-resistant hypotension. Management of the critically ill hypotensive infant remains challenging and requires a better understanding of the pathophysiology of neonatal shock and improvements in our ability to monitor cardiac output, organ blood flow, and tissue perfusion in real time at the bedside (see Chapter 21).

In addition, we still need to improve our understanding of the pathogenesis and epidemiology of adrenal insufficiency and vasopressor-resistant hypotension, especially in terms of the determinants, mechanisms, and characteristics of these conditions, and their relationship with each other and with acute and long-term morbidity/mortality. Ultimately, we need to provide evidence that our interventions also improve clinically meaningful outcomes. Another challenge is to improve the diagnostic methods to assess adrenal function and vasopressor-resistant hypotension and define the criteria for treatment. We need to be able to determine which patient needs therapy, at what dose and for how long, and what evaluations provide the most reliable information early in the course of the disease. Are serum cortisol values the optimal measure of adrenal function? Can one improve diagnostic accuracy and prognosis by combining the findings of different tests? Could serum or urine evaluations of adrenal function further refine the diagnosis? Will simultaneous measurements of inflammatory mediators improve our understanding and guide therapy? By improving our ability to establish accurate and timely diagnosis of adrenal insufficiency, will we be able to target high-risk patients for investigational and clinical interventions and avoid unnecessary exposure of lower-risk infants to corticosteroid therapy?

In addition, the more comprehensive issues to be addressed include identifying the factors that influence the choice of corticosteroid treatment and establishing the dosage, duration, and response to therapy of the individual patient.[139] We also need to find out whether corticosteroid regimens need to be adjusted according to disease severity or the response to treatment to maximize effectiveness and minimize harm. Scientifically and ethically sound research and carefully designed studies will resolve these questions but will also require a different approach than using only large RCTs, such as research establishing a personalized medicine approach starting immediately after or even before delivery (see Chapter 21).

REFERENCES

1. Fernandez E, et al.: Incidence, management, and outcomes of cardiovascular insufficiency in critically ill term and late preterm newborn infants, *Am J Perinatol* 31(11):947–956, 2014.
2. Rios DR, Moffett BS, Kaiser JR: Trends in pharmacotherapy for neonatal hypotension, *J Pediatr* 165(4):697–701.e1, 2014.
3. Sehgal A, Osborn D, McNamara PJ: Cardiovascular support in preterm infants: a survey of practices in Australia and New Zealand, *J Paediatr Child Health* 48(4):317–323, 2012.
4. Ng PC, et al.: A prospective longitudinal study to estimate the "adjusted cortisol percentile" in preterm infants, *Pediatr Res* 69(6):511–516, 2011.
5. Cohen J, Venkatesh B: Relative adrenal insufficiency in the intensive care population; background and critical appraisal of the evidence, *Anaesth Intensive Care* 38(3):425–436, 2010.
6. Cooper MS, Stewart PM: Adrenal insufficiency in critical illness, *J Intensive Care Med* 22(6):348–362, 2007.
7. Marik PE: Critical illness-related corticosteroid insufficiency, *Chest* 135(1):181–193, 2009.
8. Fernandez EF, Watterberg KL: Relative adrenal insufficiency in the preterm and term infant, *J Perinatol* 29(Suppl 2):S44–S49, 2009.
9. de Jong FH, et al.: Etomidate suppresses adrenocortical function by inhibition of 11 beta-hydroxylation, *J Clin Endocrinol Metab* 59(6):1143–1147, 1984.
10. Schneider AJ, Voerman HJ: Abrupt hemodynamic improvement in late septic shock with physiological doses of glucocorticoids, *Intensive Care Med* 17(7):436–437, 1991.
11. Colasurdo MA, H.C.a.G.J, et al.: Hydrocortisone replacement in extremely premature infants with cortisol insufficiency, *Clin Res* 37:180A, 1989.
12. Ward RM, Colasurdo R-D: Addisonian crisis in extremely premature neonates, *Clin Res* 39:11A, 1991.
13. Hanna CE, et al.: Hypothalamic pituitary adrenal function in the extremely low birth weight infant, *J Clin Endocrinol Metab* 76(2):384–387, 1993.
14. Seri I, Tan R, Evans J: Cardiovascular effects of hydrocortisone in preterm infants with pressor-resistant hypotension, *Pediatrics* 107(5):1070–1074, 2001.
15. Briegel J, et al.: Haemodynamic improvement in refractory septic shock with cortisol replacement therapy, *Intensive Care Med* 18(5):318, 1992.
16. Caplan RH, et al.: Occult hypoadrenalism in critically ill patients, *Arch Surg* 129(4):456, 1994.
17. Fauser A, et al.: Rapid increase of blood pressure in extremely low birth weight infants after a single dose of dexamethasone, *Eur J Pediatr* 152(4):354–356, 1993.

18. Reynolds JW, Hanna CE: Glucocorticoid-responsive hypotension in extremely low birth weight newborns, *Pediatrics* 94(1):135–136, 1994.

19. Scott SM, Watterberg KL: Effect of gestational age, postnatal age, and illness on plasma cortisol concentrations in premature infants, *Pediatr Res* 37(1):112–116, 1995.

20. Watterberg KL, Scott SM: Evidence of early adrenal insufficiency in babies who develop bronchopulmonary dysplasia, *Pediatrics* 95(1):120–125, 1995.

21. Bourchier D, Weston PJ: Randomised trial of dopamine compared with hydrocortisone for the treatment of hypotensive very low birthweight infants, *Arch Dis Child Fetal Neonatal Ed* 76(3):F174–F178, 1997.

22. Hanna CE, et al.: Corticosteroid binding globulin, total serum cortisol, and stress in extremely low-birth-weight infants, *Am J Perinatol* 14(4):201–204, 1997.

23. Ng PC, et al.: Refractory hypotension in preterm infants with adrenocortical insufficiency, *Arch Dis Child Fetal Neonatal Ed* 84(2):F122–F124, 2001.

24. Korte C, et al.: Adrenocortical function in the very low birth weight infant: improved testing sensitivity and association with neonatal outcome, *J Pediatr* 128(2):257–263, 1996.

25. Cooper MS, Stewart PM: Corticosteroid insufficiency in acutely ill patients, *N Engl J Med* 348(8):727–734, 2003.

26. Annane D, et al.: Effect of treatment with low doses of hydrocortisone and fludrocortisone on mortality in patients with septic shock, *JAMA* 288(7):862–871, 2002.

27. Menon K, et al.: A prospective multicenter study of adrenal function in critically ill children, *Am J Respir Crit Care Med* 182(2):246–251, 2010.

28. Fernandez E, Schrader R, Watterberg K: Prevalence of low cortisol values in term and near-term infants with vasopressor-resistant hypotension, *J Perinatol* 25(2):114–118, 2005.

29. Soliman AT, et al.: Circulating adrenocorticotropic hormone (ACTH) and cortisol concentrations in normal, appropriate-for-gestational-age newborns versus those with sepsis and respiratory distress: cortisol response to low-dose and standard-dose ACTH tests, *Metabolism* 53(2):209–214, 2004.

30. Ho JT, et al.: Septic shock and sepsis: a comparison of total and free plasma cortisol levels, *J Clin Endocrinol Metab* 91(1):105–114, 2006.

31. Guttentag SH, et al.: The glucocorticoid pathway in ill and well extremely low birthweight infants, *Pediatric Res* 77A, 1991.

32. Scott SM, et al.: Positive effect of cortisol on cardiac output in the preterm infant, *Pediatric Res* 236A, 1995.

33. Annane D: Glucocorticoids in the treatment of severe sepsis and septic shock, *Curr Opin Crit Care* 11(5):449–453, 2005.

34. Langer M, Modi BP, Agus M: Adrenal insufficiency in the critically ill neonate and child, *Curr Opin Pediatr* 18(4):448–453, 2006.

35. Tantivit P, et al.: Low serum cortisol in term newborns with refractory hypotension, *J Perinatol* 19(5):352–357, 1999.

36. Fernandez EF, Montman R, Watterberg KL: ACTH and cortisol response to critical illness in term and late preterm newborns, *J Perinatol* 28(12):797–802, 2008.

37. Rivers EP, et al.: Adrenal insufficiency in high-risk surgical ICU patients, *Chest* 119(3):889–896, 2001.

38. Dimopoulou I, et al.: Hypothalamic-pituitary-adrenal axis dysfunction in critically ill patients with traumatic brain injury: incidence, pathophysiology, and relationship to vasopressor dependence and peripheral interleukin-6 levels, *Crit Care Med* 32(2):404–408, 2004.

39. Hoen S, et al.: Cortisol response to corticotropin stimulation in trauma patients: influence of hemorrhagic shock, *Anesthesiology* 97(4):807–813, 2002.

40. Watterberg KL, et al.: Effect of dose on response to adrenocorticotropin in extremely low birth weight infants, *J Clin Endocrinol Metab* 90(12):6380–6385, 2005.

41. Dickstein G, et al.: Adrenocorticotropin stimulation test: effects of basal cortisol level, time of day, and suggested new sensitive low dose test, *J Clin Endocrinol Metab* 72(4):773–778, 1991.

42. Annane D: Time for a consensus definition of corticosteroid insufficiency in critically ill patients, *Crit Care Med* 31(6):1868–1869, 2003.

43. Arnold J, et al.: Longitudinal study of plasma cortisol and 17-hydroxyprogesterone in very-low-birth-weight infants during the first 16 weeks of life, *Biol Neonate* 72(3):148–155, 1997.

44. Agus M: One step forward: an advance in understanding of adrenal insufficiency in the pediatric critically ill, *Crit Care Med* 33(4):911–912, 2005.

45. Contreras LN, et al.: A new less-invasive and more informative low-dose ACTH test: salivary steroids in response to intramuscular corticotrophin, *Clin Endocrinol (Oxf)* 61(6):675–682, 2004.

46. Hoen S, et al.: Hydrocortisone increases the sensitivity to alpha1-adrenoceptor stimulation in humans following hemorrhagic shock, *Crit Care Med* 33(12):2737–2743, 2005.

47. Marik PE, Zaloga GP: Adrenal insufficiency during septic shock, *Crit Care Med* 31(1):141–145, 2003.

48. Brierley J, et al.: Clinical practice parameters for hemodynamic support of pediatric and neonatal septic shock: 2007 update from the American College of Critical Care Medicine, *Crit Care Med* 37(2):666–688, 2009.

49. Lamberts SW, Bruining HA, de Jong FH: Corticosteroid therapy in severe illness, *N Engl J Med* 337(18):1285–1292, 1997.

50. Annane D, Briegel J, Sprung CL: Corticosteroid insufficiency in acutely ill patients, *N Engl J Med* 348(21):2157–2159, 2003.

30

51. Joosten KF, et al.: Endocrine and metabolic responses in children with meningoccocal sepsis: striking differences between survivors and nonsurvivors, *J Clin Endocrinol Metab* 85(10):3746–3753, 2000.

52. Chrousos GP: The hypothalamic-pituitary-adrenal axis and immune-mediated inflammation, *N Engl J Med* 332(20):1351–1362, 1995.

53. Meduri GU, et al.: Nuclear factor-kappaB- and glucocorticoid receptor alpha-mediated mechanisms in the regulation of systemic and pulmonary inflammation during sepsis and acute respiratory distress syndrome. Evidence for inflammation-induced target tissue resistance to glucocorticoids, *Neuroimmunomodulation* 12(6):321–338, 2005.

54. Briegel J, et al.: Immunomodulation in septic shock: hydrocortisone differentially regulates cytokine responses, *J Am Soc Nephrol* 12(Suppl 17):S70–S74, 2001.

55. Tsuneyoshi I, Kanmura Y, Yoshimura N: Methylprednisolone inhibits endotoxin-induced depression of contractile function in human arteries in vitro, *Br J Anaesth* 76(2):251–257, 1996.

56. Annane D, et al.: Impaired pressor sensitivity to noradrenaline in septic shock patients with and without impaired adrenal function reserve, *Br J Clin Pharmacol* 46(6):589–597, 1998.

57. Liggins GC: The role of cortisol in preparing the fetus for birth, *Reprod Fertil Dev* 6(2):141–150, 1994.

58. McLean M, Smith R: Corticotrophin-releasing hormone and human parturition, *Reproduction* 121(4):493–501, 2001.

59. Seri I, et al.: Cardiovascular response to dopamine in hypotensive preterm neonates with severe hyaline membrane disease, *Eur J Pediatr* 142(1):3–9, 1984.

60. Seri I: Circulatory support of the sick preterm infant, *Semin Neonatol* 6(1):85–95, 2001.

61. Roze JC, et al.: Response to dobutamine and dopamine in the hypotensive very preterm infant, *Arch Dis Child* 69(1 Spec No):59–63, 1993.

62. Noori S, et al.: Cardiovascular effects of low-dose dexamethasone in very low birth weight neonates with refractory hypotension, *Biol Neonate* 89(2):82–87, 2006.

63. Noori S, Seri I: Pathophysiology of newborn hypotension outside the transitional period, *Early Hum Dev* 81(5):399–404, 2005.

64. Ng PC, et al.: Transient adrenocortical insufficiency of prematurity and systemic hypotension in very low birthweight infants, *Arch Dis Child Fetal Neonatal Ed* 89(2):F119–F126, 2004.

65. Keh D, et al.: Immunologic and hemodynamic effects of "low-dose" hydrocortisone in septic shock: a double-blind, randomized, placebo-controlled, crossover study, *Am J Respir Crit Care Med* 167(4):512–520, 2003.

66. Huysman MW, et al.: Adrenal function in sick very preterm infants, *Pediatr Res* 48(5):629–633, 2000.

67. Helbock HJ, Insoft RM, Conte FA: Glucocorticoid-responsive hypotension in extremely low birth weight newborns, *Pediatrics* 92(5):715–717, 1993.

68. Briegel J, et al.: Stress doses of hydrocortisone reverse hyperdynamic septic shock: a prospective, randomized, double-blind, single-center study, *Crit Care Med* 27(4):723–732, 1999.

69. Annane D, et al.: Clinical equipoise remains for issues of adrenocorticotropic hormone administration, cortisol testing, and therapeutic use of hydrocortisone, *Crit Care Med* 31(8):2250–2251, 2003; author reply 2252–2253.

70. Alverson D, et al.: Persistently low cardiac output during the first day of life predicts high mortality in preterm infants with respiratory distress syndrome, *Pediatr Res* 193A, 1995.

71. Arnold JD, et al.: Antenatal glucocorticoids modulate the amplitude of pulsatile cortisol secretion in premature neonates, *Pediatr Res* 44(6):876–881, 1998.

72. Palta M, et al.: Multivariate assessment of traditional risk factors for chronic lung disease in very low birth weight neonates. The Newborn Lung Project, *J Pediatr* 119(2):285–292, 1991.

73. Yoder B, et al.: Impaired urinary cortisol excretion and early cardiopulmonary dysfunction in immature baboons, *Pediatr Res* 51(4):426–432, 2002.

74. Coalson JJ, et al.: Neonatal chronic lung disease in extremely immature baboons, *Am J Respir Crit Care Med* 160(4):1333–1346, 1999.

75. Baker CF, et al.: Hydrocortisone administration for the treatment of refractory hypotension in critically ill newborns, *J Perinatol* 28(6):412–419, 2008.

76. Gaissmaier RE, Pohlandt F: Single-dose dexamethasone treatment of hypotension in preterm infants, *J Pediatr* 134(6):701–705, 1999.

77. Suominen PK, et al.: Hemodynamic effects of rescue protocol hydrocortisone in neonates with low cardiac output syndrome after cardiac surgery, *Pediatr Crit Care Med* 6(6):655–659, 2005.

78. Watterberg KL, et al.: Prophylaxis of early adrenal insufficiency to prevent bronchopulmonary dysplasia: a multicenter trial, *Pediatrics* 114(6):1649–1657, 2004.

79. Hingre RV, et al.: Adrenal steroidogenesis in very low birth weight preterm infants, *J Clin Endocrinol Metab* 78(2):266–270, 1994.

80. Lee MM, et al.: Serum adrenal steroid concentrations in premature infants, *J Clin Endocrinol Metab* 69(6):1133–1136, 1989.

81. Heckmann M, et al.: Reference range for serum cortisol in well preterm infants, *Arch Dis Child Fetal Neonatal Ed* 81(3):F171–F174, 1999.

82. Thomas S, et al.: Response to ACTH in the newborn, *Arch Dis Child* 61(1):57–60, 1986.

83. al Saedi S, et al.: Reference ranges for serum cortisol and 17-hydroxyprogesterone levels in preterm infants, *J Pediatr* 126(6):985–987, 1995.

84. Watterberg KL, Gerdes JS, Cook KL: Impaired glucocorticoid synthesis in premature infants developing chronic lung disease, *Pediatr Res* 50(2):190–195, 2001.

D

85. Ng PC, et al.: Reference ranges and factors affecting the human corticotropin-releasing hormone test in preterm, very low birth weight infants, *J Clin Endocrinol Metab* 87(10):4621–4628, 2002.
86. Bolt RJ, et al.: The corticotrophin-releasing hormone test in preterm infants, *Clin Endocrinol (Oxf)* 56(2):207–213, 2002.
87. Linder N, et al.: Longitudinal measurements of 17alpha-hydroxyprogesterone in premature infants during the first three months of life, *Arch Dis Child Fetal Neonatal Ed* 81(3):F175–F178, 1999.
88. Economou G, et al.: Cortisol secretion in stressed babies during the neonatal period, *Horm Res* 40(5–6):217–221, 1993.
89. Kamath BD, Fashaw L, Kinsella JP: Adrenal insufficiency in newborns with congenital diaphragmatic hernia, *J Pediatr* 156(3):495–497.e1, 2010.
90. Pittinger TP, Sawin RS: Adrenocortical insufficiency in infants with congenital diaphragmatic hernia: a pilot study, *J Pediatr Surg* 35(2):223–225, 2000; discussion 225–226.
91. Gutai J, et al.: Adrenal response to physical stress and the effect of adrenocorticotropic hormone in newborn infants, *J Pediatr* 81(4):719–725, 1972.
92. Khashana A, et al.: Cortisol intermediates and hydrocortisone responsiveness in critical neonatal disease, *J Matern Fetal Neonatal Med* 1–5, 2016.
93. Hochwald O, Pelligra G, Osiovich H: Adding hydrocortisone as 1st line of inotropic treatment for hypotension in very low birth weight infants: authors' reply, *Indian J Pediatr* 81(9):988, 2014.
94. Efird MM, et al.: A randomized-controlled trial of prophylactic hydrocortisone supplementation for the prevention of hypotension in extremely low birth weight infants, *J Perinatol* 25(2):119–124, 2005.
95. Masumoto K, et al.: Comparison of serum cortisol concentrations in preterm infants with or without late-onset circulatory collapse due to adrenal insufficiency of prematurity, *Pediatr Res* 63(6):686–690, 2008.
96. Prasanth K, et al.: Adrenocorticotropic hormone and cortisol levels in term infants born with meconium-stained amniotic fluid, *J Perinat Med* 42(6):699–703, 2014.
97. Watterberg KL, et al.: Prophylaxis against early adrenal insufficiency to prevent chronic lung disease in premature infants, *Pediatrics* 104(6):1258–1263, 1999.
98. Ng PC, et al.: The pituitary-adrenal responses to exogenous human corticotropin-releasing hormone in preterm, very low birth weight infants, *J Clin Endocrinol Metab* 82(3):797–799, 1997.
99. Ng PC, et al.: Early pituitary-adrenal response and respiratory outcomes in preterm infants, *Arch Dis Child Fetal Neonatal Ed* 89(2):F127–F130, 2004.
100. Peltoniemi O, et al.: Pretreatment cortisol values may predict responses to hydrocortisone administration for the prevention of bronchopulmonary dysplasia in high-risk infants, *J Pediatr* 146(5):632–637, 2005.
101. Watterberg KL, et al.: Links between early adrenal function and respiratory outcome in preterm infants: airway inflammation and patent ductus arteriosus, *Pediatrics* 105(2):320–324, 2000.
102. ott SM, Cimino DF: Evidence for developmental hypopituitarism in ill preterm infants, *J Perinatol* 24(7):429–434, 2004.
103. Marik PE, et al.: Recommendations for the diagnosis and management of corticosteroid insufficiency in critically ill adult patients: consensus statements from an international task force by the American College of Critical Care Medicine, *Crit Care Med* 36(6):1937–1949, 2008.
104. Annane D, et al.: Diagnosis of adrenal insufficiency in severe sepsis and septic shock, *Am J Respir Crit Care Med* 174(12):1319–1326, 2006.
105. Aucott SW: The challenge of defining relative adrenal insufficiency, *J Perinatol* 32(6):397–398, 2012.
106. Venkatesh B, et al.: Evaluation of random plasma cortisol and the low dose corticotropin test as indicators of adrenal secretory capacity in critically ill patients: a prospective study, *Anaesth Intensive Care* 33(2):201–209, 2005.
107. Metzger DL, et al.: Characterization of pulsatile secretion and clearance of plasma cortisol in premature and term neonates using deconvolution analysis, *J Clin Endocrinol Metab* 77(2):458–463, 1993.
108. Ng PC: Adrenocortical insufficiency and refractory hypotension in preterm infants, *Arch Dis Child Fetal Neonatal Ed*, 2016.
109. Karlsson R, et al.: Adrenocorticotropin and corticotropin-releasing hormone tests in preterm infants, *J Clin Endocrinol Metab* 85(12):4592–4595, 2000.
110. Karlsson R, et al.: Timing of peak serum cortisol values in preterm infants in low-dose and the standard ACTH tests, *Pediatr Res* 45(3):367–369, 1999.
111. Hochwald O, Holsti L, Osiovich H: The use of an early ACTH test to identify hypoadrenalism-related hypotension in low birth weight infants, *J Perinatol* 32(6):412–417, 2012.
112. Trainer PJ, et al.: Urinary free cortisol in the assessment of hydrocortisone replacement therapy, *Horm Metab Res* 25(2):117–120, 1993.
113. Vezina HE, et al.: Population pharmacokinetics of unbound hydrocortisone in critically ill neonates and infants with vasopressor-resistant hypotension, *Pediatr Crit Care Med* 15(6):546–553, 2014.
114. Miletin J, et al.: Serum cortisol values, superior vena cava flow and illness severity scores in very low birth weight infants, *J Perinatol* 30(8):522–526, 2010.
115. Sweeney DA, et al.: Defining normal adrenal function testing in the intensive care unit setting: a canine study, *Crit Care Med* 38(2):553–561, 2010.
116. Oppert M, et al.: Low-dose hydrocortisone improves shock reversal and reduces cytokine levels in early hyperdynamic septic shock, *Crit Care Med* 33(11):2457–2464, 2005.

30

117. Seri I, Evans JR: Why do steroids increase blood pressure in preterm infants? *J Pediatr* 136(3):
     420–421, 2000.
118. Shenker Y, Skatrud JB: Adrenal insufficiency in critically ill patients, *Am J Respir Crit Care Med*
     163(7):1520–1523, 2001.
119. Segar JL, et al.: Effect of antenatal glucocorticoids on sympathetic nerve activity at birth in preterm
     sheep, *Am J Physiol* 274(1 Pt 2):R160–R167, 1998.
120. Wang ZM, et al.: Glucocorticoids stimulate the maturation of H,K-ATPase in the infant rat stomach,
     Pediatr Res 40(5):658–663, 1996.
121. Annane D, et al.: Corticosteroids in the treatment of severe sepsis and septic shock in adults: a sys-
     tematic review, *JAMA* 301(22):2362–2375, 2009.
122. Tang BM, et al.: Use of corticosteroids in acute lung injury and acute respiratory distress syndrome:
     a systematic review and meta-analysis, *Crit Care Med* 37(5):1594–1603, 2009.
123. Briegel J, et al.: Low-dose hydrocortisone infusion attenuates the systemic inflammatory response
     syndrome. The Phospholipase A2 Study Group, *Clin Investig* 72(10):782–787, 1994.
124. Sprung CL, et al.: Hydrocortisone therapy for patients with septic shock, *N Engl J Med* 358(2):
     111–124, 2008.
125. Subhedar NV, Duffy K, Ibrahim H: Corticosteroids for treating hypotension in preterm infants,
     Cochrane Database Syst Rev (1):CD003662, 2007.
126. Higgins S, Friedlich P, Seri I: Hydrocortisone for hypotension and vasopressor dependence in pre-
     term neonates: a meta-analysis, *J Perinatol* 30(6):373–378, 2010.
127. Mizobuchi M, et al.: Effect of hydrocortisone therapy on severe leaky lung syndrome in ventilated
     preterm infants, *Pediatr Int* 54(5):639–645, 2012.
128. Ng PC, et al.: A double-blind, randomized, controlled study of a "stress dose" of hydrocortisone for
     rescue treatment of refractory hypotension in preterm infants, *Pediatrics* 117(2):367–375, 2006.
129. Noori S, et al.: Hemodynamic changes after low-dosage hydrocortisone administration in vasopres-
     sor-treated preterm and term neonates, *Pediatrics* 118(4):1456–1466, 2006.
130. Czock D, et al.: Pharmacokinetics and pharmacodynamics of systemically administered glucocorti-
     coids, *Clin Pharmacokinet* 44(1):61–98, 2005.
131. Perogamvros I, et al.: Corticosteroid-binding globulin regulates cortisol pharmacokinetics, *Clin
     Endocrinol (Oxf)* 74(1):30–36, 2011.
132. Reynolds JW, Colle E, Ulstrom RA: Adrenocortical steroid metabolism in newborn infants. V.
     Physiologic disposition of exogenous cortisol loads in the early neonatal period, *J Clin Endocrinol
     Metab* 22:245–254, 1962.
133. Watterberg KL: Hydrocortisone dosing for hypotension in newborn infants: less is more,
     J Pediatr 174:23–26.e1, 2016.
134. Paquette L, et al.: Concurrent use of indomethacin and dexamethasone increases the risk of sponta-
     neous intestinal perforation in very low birth weight neonates, *J Perinatol* 26(8):486–492, 2006.
135. Hassan AH, et al.: Exacerbation of apoptosis in the dentate gyrus of the aged rat by dexamethasone
     and the protective role of corticosterone, *Exp Neurol* 140(1):43–52, 1996.
136. Shinwell ES, et al.: Early postnatal dexamethasone treatment and increased incidence of cerebral
     palsy, *Arch Dis Child Fetal Neonatal Ed* 83(3):F177–F181, 2000.
137. Watterberg KL, et al.: Growth and neurodevelopmental outcomes after early low-dose hydrocorti-
     sone treatment in extremely low birth weight infants, *Pediatrics* 120(1):40–48, 2007.
138. Batton BJ, et al.: Feasibility study of early blood pressure management in extremely preterm infants,
     J Pediatr 161(1):65–69.e1, 2012.
139. Aucott SW: Hypotension in the newborn: who needs hydrocortisone? *J Perinatol* 25(2):77–78,
     2005.

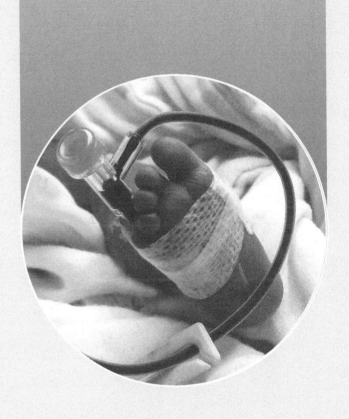

CHAPTER 31

Neonates With Critical Congenital Heart Disease: Delivery Room Management and Stabilization Before Transfer to the Cardiac Intensive Care Unit

Jay D. Pruetz, Jodie K. Votava-Smith, and Linda Tesoriero

- Most prenatally diagnosed congenital heart disease (CHD) does not require emergent neonatal care.
- Critical forms of CHD require emergent stabilization and intervention in the first hours after delivery.
- Critical forms of CHD can benefit most from active perinatal and delivery room management.
- Risk stratification strategies for CHD can help guide neonatal management in cases of complex CHD.
- Fetal echocardiography can be used to determine which critical CHD lesions will need emergent neonatal intervention.
- Current areas of research include evaluation of fetal echocardiographic markers used for assessing CHD severity and fetal interventions to improve postnatal outcomes.

Introduction to Prenatal Evaluation of Congenital Heart Disease and the Definition of Critical Congenital Heart Disease

The incidence of congenital heart disease (CHD) is estimated at about 8 per 1000 live births,[1] while more severe forms of CHD affect about 3 out of 1000 live births.[2] Severe forms of CHD include those which require early medical, surgical, or catheterization based interventions in the first postnatal days to weeks, generally in concert with multidisciplinary subspecialty care including pediatric cardiologists, cardiothoracic surgeons, neonatologists, and pediatric cardiac intensivists. Since the first reports of using ultrasound to prenatally diagnose CHD more than 3 decades ago,[3] there have been remarkable advances in ultrasound technology allowing for high-resolution assessment of fetal cardiac anatomy, function, and rhythm.

Transition at birth from fetal to postnatal circulation involves lung expansion and a drop in pulmonary vascular resistance, loss of the low-resistance placenta from the circulation with a resultant increase in systemic vascular resistance, loss of the fetal intracardiac shunts, and shift to reliance on oxygenation by the lungs rather than the placenta.[4] CHD lesion types with inadequate aortic or pulmonary outflow are termed "ductal dependent," given the need for flow through the ductus arteriosus to provide or augment either pulmonary or systemic blood flow. Postnatally, medical therapy with prostaglandin E1 (PGE1) is needed to maintain ductal patency, with the eventual need for surgical- or catheter-based intervention to provide a more stable source of pulmonary or systemic blood flow (see Chapter 32). The most critical forms of CHD have an additional element of instability with the perinatal transition. These can be grouped into four categories, including (1) lack of adequate pulmonary egress, found in obstructed total anomalous pulmonary venous return (TAPVR) and subtypes of hypoplastic left heart syndrome (HLHS) with intact or restrictive atrial septum; (2) inadequate intracardiac mixing of oxygenated blood to the systemic circulation in some cases of d-transposition of the great arteries (d-TGA) with restrictive atrial shunting; (3) an associated anomaly of the airway which compromises the ability to ventilate such as severe cases of Ebstein anomaly and tetralogy of Fallot (TOF) with absent pulmonary valve (APV); and (4) inadequate cardiac output in cases of severe fetal arrhythmias or diminished cardiac function either in isolation or in combination with CHD. These critical forms of CHD can be predicted with fetal echocardiographic findings, which then allows for careful planning of maternal care to optimize the delivery and provide targeted postnatal care.

Perinatal Management Strategies to Optimize Postnatal Transition

The goals of active prenatal planning and perinatal management for neonates with CHD are a well-coordinated transition from fetal life to postnatal care, minimizing mortality and morbidity, and ensuring a stable preoperative clinical status. Additional benefits include adequate time for parental education, expanded prenatal evaluation, and mobilization of psychosocial support systems. Action plans must take into account the underlying cardiac anatomy, anticipated physiologic changes during the transition from fetal to postnatal life, the speed at which patients may become critically unstable, and the need for emergent neonatal intervention. Risk stratification systems are designed for multiple levels of CHD severity and are used to select the appropriate medical center for delivery, mode of delivery (MOD), level of perinatology and neonatology services available, and capability for immediate access to cardiology and cardiothoracic surgery care. The transportation of infants with critical CHD to a higher-level cardiac care center for delivery and postnatal care has been shown to improve outcomes and is associated with lower overall health care costs.[5-7] Of note is that it is not recommended to deliver patients with CHD prematurely, as prematurity and low birth weight can have a significant negative impact on outcomes.[8-10] Given this data, the current recommendations are to deliver these patients at 39 weeks' gestation. A prenatal diagnosis of CHD may alter the chosen MOD and has been shown to result in elevated rates of elective C-section for many forms of CHD.[11-13] However, there is little evidence to show that altering MOD improves outcomes for CHD patients and studies have shown that vaginal birth is well tolerated in this population.[13-15] Thus, changes in delivery timing and MOD should only be made in order to provide rapid postnatal stabilization and intervention in the most critical of cases.

Active perinatal management of critical CHD is now practiced by many centers across the United States and Europe using similar risk stratifying schemes with recommended care plans.[16-19] These classification systems are based on regional practice patterns and designed to identify patients that require specialized treatment in the delivery room (DR) and cardiac intervention in the first hours after delivery (Table 31.1 and 31.2). The cardiovascular disease severity scales are based on the anatomic severity of CHD, need for postnatal intervention, complexity of intervention, and overall prognosis. The level of care (LOC) is typically assigned first by the cardiologist, according to the CHD severity, and is then reviewed and agreed upon with the entire maternal fetal medicine team. Each LOC is linked with a specific coordinated action plan and detailed perinatal recommendations for delivery and DR management such as need for PGE, transport, and intervention. Risk stratification and management systems using LOC for neonates prenatally diagnosed with CHD have been shown to be highly accurate at predicting the postnatal care and need for emergent intervention at birth.[18,20] These classification strategies have been highly reproducible, with the exception of d-TGA, due to the difficulty determining the risk

Table 31.1 DEFINITION OF LEVEL OF CARE ASSIGNMENT AND COORDINATED ACTION PLAN

LOC	Definition	Example CHD	Prenatal Planning	Delivery	DR Recommendations
1	CHD without physiologic instability in first weeks of life	1. Shunt lesions (e.g., ASD, VSD, AVSD)	Arrange outpatient cardiology evaluation	Spontaneous vaginal delivery	Routine DR management
2	CHD with physiologic stability in DR but requiring postnatal intervention/surgery before discharge	1. Benign arrhythmias 2. Ductal-dependent lesions or lesions with complex physiology likely to require neonatal intervention/surgery (e.g., HLHS, PA/IVS, truncus arteriosus) 3. Nonsustained or controlled tachyarrhythmias	Create plan of care for DR stabilization and neonatal management by local hospital with transport to pediatric cardiac center	Spontaneous vaginal delivery versus induction near term	Neonatologist in DR; initiate PGE at low dose for ductal-dependent lesions
3	CHD with expected instability requiring immediate specialty care in DR before anticipated stabilizing intervention/surgery	1. HLHS/RFO 2. d-TGA/RFO 3. Severe Ebstein anomaly with dilated right ventricle and low RV pressure 4. TOF/APV with RV and/or LV dysfunction and cardiac shift 5. Sustained tachyarrhythmias or CHB with heart failure	Create plan of care to include specialized pediatric cardiology team in DR and interventional/surgical team on standby	Planned induction usually at 39 weeks with "bailout" C/S if necessary for care coordination	Neonatologist and pediatric cardiology specialists in DR; stabilizing medications predetermined by care plan
4	CHD with expected instability requiring immediate specialty care and urgent intervention/surgery in DR to improve chance of survival	1. HLHS/IAS 2. d-TGA/severe RFO or IAS with abnormal DA flow 3. Severe Ebstein anomaly or TOF/APV with hydrops 4. Tachyarrhythmias/bradyarrhythmias with hydrops	Create multidisciplinary plan of care to include delivery at medical center with high-level obstetrical and pediatric cardiac services available and with specialized care team in DR and interventional/surgical team ready	Planned C/S at a medical center with high-level obstetrical and pediatric cardiac and other pediatric subspecialty services available usually at 38–39 weeks or sooner if there is evidence of fetal distress or hydrops; maternal risk determined by obstetrician (delivery of such cases at medical centers with high-level adult and complex pediatric services)	Specialized care team in DR Stabilizing medications/equipment predetermined by care plan

APV, Absent pulmonary valve; *ASD,* atrial septal defect; *AVSD,* atrioventricular septal defect; *CHB,* complete heart block; *CHD,* congenital heart disease; *C/S,* cesarean section; *DR,* delivery room; *DA,* ductus arteriosus; *HLHS,* hypoplastic left heart syndrome; *LOC,* level of care; *LV,* left ventricular; *PA/IVS,* pulmonary atresia with intact ventricular septum; *PGE,* prostaglandin E; *RV,* right ventricular; *RFO,* restrictive foramen ovale; *TOF,* tetralogy of Fallot; *VSD,* ventricular septal defect.
From Donofrio, MT, Skurow-Todd, K, Berger JT, et al: Risk-stratified postnatal care of newborns with congenital heart disease determined by fetal echocardiography: *J Amer Soc Echocardiogr* 2015;28(11):1339–1349.

31

E

Table 31.2 LEVEL OF CARE ASSIGNMENT AND COORDINATING ACTION PLAN

LOC	Definition	Example CHD	Delivery Recommendations	DR Recommendations
P	CHD in which palliative care is planned	CHD with severe/fatal chromosome abnormality or multisystem disease	Arrange for family support/palliative care services Normal delivery at local hospital	
1	CHD without predicted risk of hemodynamic instability in the DR or first days of life	VSD, AVSD. mild TOF	Arrange cardiology consultation or outpatient evaluation Normal delivery at local hospital	Routine DR care Neonatal evaluation
2	CHD with minimal risk of hemodynamic instability in DR but requiring postnatal catheterization/surgery	Ductal-dependent lesions, including HLHS, critical coarctation, severe AS, IAA, PA/IVS, severe TOF	Consider planned induction usually near term Delivery at hospital with neonatologist and accessible cardiology consultation	Neonatologist in DR Routine DR care, initiate PGE if indicated Transport for catheterization/surgery
3	CHD with likely hemodynamic instability in DR requiring immediate specialty care for stabilization	d-TGA with concerning atrial septum primum (note: it is reasonable to consider all d-TGA fetuses without an ASD at risk) Uncontrolled arrhythmias CHB with heart failure	Planned induction at 38–39 weeks; consider C/S if necessary to coordinate services Delivery at hospital that can execute rapid care, including necessary stabilizing/life-saving procedures	Neonatologist and cardiac specialist in DR, including all necessary equipment Plan for intervention as indicated by diagnosis Plan for urgent transport if indicated
4	CHD with expected hemodynamic instability with placental separation requiring immediate catheterization/surgery in DR to improve chance of survival	HLHS/severely RFO or IAS d-TGA/severely RFO or IAS and abnormal DA Obstructed TAPVR Ebstein anomaly with hydrops TOF with APV and severe airway obstruction Uncontrolled arrhythmias with hydrops CHB with low ventricular rate, EFE, and/or hydrops	C/S in cardiac facility with necessary specialists in the DR usually at 38–39 weeks	Specialized cardiac care team in DR Plan for intervention as indicated by diagnosis; may include catheterization, surgery, or ECMO
5	CHD in which cardiac transplantation is planned	HLHS/IAS; CHD including severe Ebstein anomaly; CHD, or cardiomyopathy with severe ventricular dysfunction	List after 35 weeks of gestation C/S when heart is available	Specialized cardiac care team in DR

APV, Absent pulmonary valve; *AS*, aortic stenosis; *ASD*, atrial septal defect; *AVSD*, atrioventricular septal defect; *CHB*, complete heart block; *CHD*, congenital heart disease; *C/S*, cesarean section; *d-TGA*, transposition of the great arteries, *DA*, ductus arteriosus; *DR*, delivery room; *ECMO*, extracorporeal membrane oxygenation; *EFE*, endocardial fibroelastosis; *HLHS*, hypoplastic left heart syndrome; *IAA*, interrupted aortic arch; *IAS*, intact atrial septum; *LOC*, level of care; *PA/IVS*, pulmonary atresia/intact ventricular septum; *PGE*, prostaglandin E; *RFO*, restrictive foramen ovale; *TAPVR*, total anomalous pulmonary venous return; *TOF*, tetralogy of Fallot; and *VSD*, ventricular septal defect.
From Donofrio MT, Moon-Grady AJ, Hornberger LK, et al: Diagnosis and treatment of fetal cardiac disease: a scientific statement from the American Heart Association. *Circulation* 129(21):2183–2242, 2014.

for postnatal atrial level restriction and the result was to upgrade all d-TGA cases to LOC 4 status.[20] Table 31.3 shows a comparison of various published CHD risk stratification systems, while Table 31.4 depicts an example of one of the classification systems, which we have termed "Emergent Neonatal Cardiac Intervention" (ENCI) risk categories (see Table 31.4).[19]

Table 31.3   COMPARISON CHART OF DIFFERENT PUBLISHED CONGENITAL HEART DISEASE RISK CLASSIFICATION SYSTEMS

Characteristics of Various CHD Severity Scales and Coordinating Care Plans	Donofrio et al., 2004	Berkley et al., 2009	Davey et al.,[a] 2014	Pruetz et al., 2014	Slodki et al., 2016	AHA Statement Donofrio et al., 2014
Level description	LOC 1–4	Care plans 1–5	LOC 1–7	ENCI Level 1–4	Severest, severe, urgent, planned	LOC 1–5, palliative care (P)
Palliative care	N	Y	Y	N	N	Y
Delivery site	Y	Y	N	Y	N	Y
Mode of delivery	Y	Y	N	Y	Y	Y
Prostaglandin E1	Y	Y	Y	Y	Y	Y
Neonatology care	Y	Y	Y	Y	Y	Y
Multispecialty care team	Y	Y	Y	Y	Y	Y
Level of instability	Y	N	N	Y	Y	Y
Need for emergent intervention	Y	Y	N	Y	Y	Y
Need for transport/transfer	N	N	N	N	N	Y

[a]This is a Fetal Cardiovascular Disease Scale and does not include coordinating actions plans.
AHA, American Heart Association; *CHD,* congenital heart disease; *ENCI,* emergent neonatal cardiac intervention; *LOC,* level of care.

Table 31.4   EMERGENT NEONATAL CARDIAC INTERVENTION CLASSIFICATION SYSTEM AND MANAGEMENT GUIDELINE[a]

ENCI Level	High Risk	PGE	Mode of Delivery an Issue	NICU Acuity Level	Neonatology Present in Delivery Room	Cardiology, CT Surgery, CTICU, OR/ Cath Lab on Standby	Examples
1	No	No	No	Low	No	No	ASD, VSD, Mild PS
2	No	No	No	Medium	Possibly	No	CAVC, TOF/ PS, Truncus Arteriosus
3	Possibly	Yes	Possibly	High	Yes	Possibly	HLHS, d-TGA/ VSD, PA/IVS
4	Yes	Yes	Yes	High	Yes	Yes	d-TGA/RAS, Obstructed TAPVR

[a]A four-level classification system for prenatally diagnosed congenital heart disease that takes into consideration both the level of postnatal clinical acuity and need for emergent postnatal intervention.
ASD, Atrial septal defect; *CAVC,* complete atrioventricular canal; *Cath,* catheterization; *CT,* cardiothoracic; *CTICU,* cardiothoracic intensive care unit; *d-TGA,* d-transposition of the great arteries; *HLHS,* hypoplastic left heart syndrome; *NICU,* neonatal intensive care unit; *OR,* operating room; *PA/IVS,* pulmonary atresia with intact ventricular septum; *PGE,* prostaglandin E; *PS,* pulmonary stenosis; *RAS,* restrictive atrial septum; *TOF,* tetralogy of Fallot; *VSD,* ventricular septal defect.
From Pruetz JD, Carroll C, Trento LU, et al: Outcomes of critical congenital heart disease requiring emergent neonatal cardiac intervention, *Prenat Diagn* 34(12):1127–1132, 2014.

1. **LEVEL ONE, Low Risk:** The lowest LOC is for CHD that does not cause hemodynamic instability in the newborn and is not expected to require specialized care or intervention in the newborn period. These patients can deliver at a hospital capable of providing care for babies with mild forms of CHD. MOD is not an issue and no special care is needed in the DR. Examples include atrial septal defect (ASD), ventricular septal defect (VSD), and mild valve abnormalities.
2. **LEVEL TWO, Intermediate Risk:** These newborns have potential for hemodynamic instability and need for postnatal evaluation by subspecialists, but low risk

for neonatal intervention. These patients should deliver at a facility with access to subspecialty consultation if needed and neonatology involvement at birth as needed. Thus delivery should occur in a facility in close proximity to a center with pediatric cardiology support and a Level III neonatal intensive care unit (NICU) with a regional transfer agreement with a children's hospital. MOD may be an issue if signs of congestive heart failure or hydrops are present. Examples include complete atrioventricular septal defect, aortic arch obstruction, moderate valve abnormality, truncus arteriosus, and TOF with expected mild to moderate level of pulmonary stenosis.

3. **LEVEL THREE, Moderate Risk:** These patients require neonatal intervention in the first days to weeks after delivery and include all ductal dependent lesions. These deliveries should be highly coordinated and occur at or nearby tertiary care centers with a high level of neonatal and cardiac expertise. If early intervention is likely or there is increased risk for high acuity at birth, delivery by induction or scheduled C-section should be considered to provide a window of anticipated delivery. MOD must also take in to account any evidence of congestive heart failure or hydrops. The cardiac intensive care unit (ICU), cardiology, and cardiothoracic surgery should be made aware of the patient well in advance. The transport team should be notified and on standby, to expedite the transfer. Examples include d-TGA with VSD, HLHS without restrictive atrial septum (RAS), severe aortic or pulmonary valve abnormalities (including single ventricles), unobstructed TAPVR, TOF with APV without lobar emphysema, Ebstein anomaly without hydrops, and complete heart block (CHB) with adequate heart rate (HR) (>60 bpm).

4. **LEVEL FOUR, High Risk:** The highest level is reserved for patients requiring immediate or emergent intervention, within hours after birth, and in whom severe instability is anticipated. The perinatal care should be highly coordinated in order for all resources to be available at the time of birth. These patients should deliver via scheduled C-section to minimize time to treatment with the necessary subspecialists on standby to care for the newborn. Ideally the delivery could occur in a highly specialized labor and delivery unit in a children's hospital for immediate intervention.[18,21] However, few programs have this capability and most still rely on transfer of the newborn from a connected or nearby maternity hospital. If transfer is needed, the transport team should also be on standby at the delivery institution. The baby must be adequately stabilized and monitored for transport, but performance of procedures in the delivery room must be balanced with the need to get the baby to intervention with minimal delay. Cardiac ICU, cardiology, and cardiothoracic surgery should be notified again immediately upon confirmation of birth. The operating room and/or cardiac catheterization laboratory should be on standby. Examples include obstructed TAPVR, HLHS with RAS, d-TGA with RAS, TOF/APV with lobar emphysema, severe Ebstein anomaly with hydrops or uncontrolled arrhythmia and unstable CHB with very low ventricular rate (<50 bpm), decreased myocardial function, or hydrops fetalis.

Delivery Room Management and Stabilization

This section will review specific cardiac lesions detailing the recommended prenatal planning, perinatal recommendations, and DR management.

Ductal-Dependent Lesions (Pulmonary Atresia, Interrupted Aortic Arch, Aortic Coarctation, Hypoplastic Left Heart Syndrome with Atrial Septal Defect)

Cardiac defects expected to be *postnatally ductal dependent for pulmonary blood flow* either can be isolated (pulmonary stenosis/atresia with intact ventricular septum), or can occur as a part of TOF or a complex single ventricle lesion. Prenatal prediction of postnatally ductal-dependent pulmonary blood flow includes evaluation for antegrade pulmonary blood flow, reversed flow in the ductus arteriosus (e.g., prenatally directed from the aorta to the pulmonary arteries), pulmonary valve size with z-score less than −3, and a pulmonary-to-aortic valve annulus ratio less than 0.6.[22-24] Cardiac defects expected to be postnatally *ductal dependent for systemic blood flow* include severe aortic stenosis/atresia, interrupted aortic arch (IAA), hypoplastic aortic arch, and suspected coarctation of the aorta. These lesions can occur in isolation or in combination with single ventricle defects such as HLHS. Prenatal predictors of postnatally ductal-dependent systemic blood flow include systolic flow reversal in the transverse aortic arch, left-to-right atrial shunting across the foramen ovale, and hypoplasia of the distal transverse aortic arch.[22,25-27] All of these lesions will require neonatal intervention, but are unlikely to require specialized DR care or emergent intervention in the first 24 hours of postnatal life. They should have neonatology involvement and require initiation of PGE after birth.

Postnatal care for complex cardiac patients requires preparation of the DR resuscitation team, NICU, and ancillary services (diagnostic imaging) prior to the delivery. The use of established DR room guidelines and checklists ensures a consistent approach to the stabilization of cardiac patients pending transfer to a surgical center. Team leaders should conduct a predelivery meeting with staff to review the CHD diagnosis, plan of care, and assign team member roles for the resuscitation/stabilization. Equipment, intravenous (IV) access devices, emergency medications, cardiac medication infusions (such as PGE), and IV fluids should be prepared. Many steps outlined here will recur in the postnatal management of neonates with different forms of CHD, with variations based on the underlying diagnosis.

Delivery room management begins by following the basic steps of neonatal resuscitation to assess the infant's respiratory effort, circulation, and color. ENCI Level-3 patients are not at high risk for respiratory decompensation due to their underlying cardiac lesion after delivery, so elective intubation based on the cardiac diagnosis alone is not recommended. As with any neonate, the decision to intubate should be based on the assessment of the clinical respiratory and circulatory status with the use of premedication ("rapid sequence intubation") if the intervention is not required on an emergent basis. Pulse oximetry should be initiated immediately after birth to guide judicious oxygen use in the DR with the goal of establishing preductal saturations based on the diagnosis: greater than 94% in patients with coarctation versus 75% to 85% in patients with HLHS and open septum. Ongoing circulatory assessment includes evaluation of HR, color, pulses, and central capillary refill. Once the patient has been assessed and stabilized in the DR, further stabilization should take place in the NICU prior to transfer out of the unit or facility.

Cardiovascular monitoring can be further facilitated by placing umbilical venous (UVC) and arterial catheters (UAC). A UAC is used to directly monitor arterial blood pressure (BP) and obtain arterial laboratory samples. A UVC provides a secure method of monitoring central venous pressure (CVP), infusing IV medications, and delivering nutrition. X-ray or ultrasound verification of the central line position must be performed prior to use or transfer to avoid complications of catheter malposition (extravasation, cardiac tamponade, hepatic injury, etc.). Once IV access is secured, an infusion of PGE concentrated to 20 µg/mL at a dose of 0.025 µg/kg/min should be started in a central line (UVC) or peripheral IV placed in an upper extremity to optimize medication transfer to the ductal tissue. Apnea and hypotension are known side effects of PGE which can manifest early. If the patient becomes apneic, respiratory stabilization is required using elective intubation with premedication and radiographic confirmation of the endotracheal tube position. Circulatory monitoring should continue with close attention to BP, urine output, and lactate levels. Transient hypotension can be managed with isotonic saline boluses of 10 mL/kg that may be repeated. Further BP stabilization may require the use of inotropic-lusitropic or vasopressor-inotropic support, as appropriate, to avoid repetitive volume bolus administration leading to volume overload. Maintenance fluid goals initiated with 10% dextrose at a total fluid goal of 80 mL/kg/day provide a glucose infusion rate of 5.5 mg/kg/min, which should maintain euglycemia in most term neonates. Following stabilization, care can be endorsed to the receiving facility and the neonatal transport team contacted.

Hypoplastic Left Heart Syndrome With Restrictive or Intact Atrial Septum

Restriction of the foramen ovale is a severe and often fatal complication of HLHS occurring in 6% to 20% of HLHS cases.[28-30] Prenatal identification of this high-risk subset of HLHS fetuses is crucial in order to coordinate the delivery, such that intervention to create an adequate atrial communication, via either cardiac catheterization or surgical intervention, can be performed in the first few minutes to hours after delivery.[18,31] Pulsed Doppler interrogation of fetal pulmonary venous flow with measurement of the forward-to-reverse velocity time integral (VTI) is the most sensitive predictor of critically restrictive foramen ovale in HLHS (Fig. 31.1).[32] This measurement evaluates the magnitude of flow reversal during atrial systole and provides an estimate of left atrial hypertension. Risk stratification categorizes pulmonary vein Doppler forward-to-reverse VTI ratio greater than 5 as a low-risk group, between 3 and 5 as moderate risk, and less than 3 high risk, with likely need for urgent intervention after birth.[19,20] Neonates at the highest risk require a well-organized plan and close cooperation between pre- and postnatal

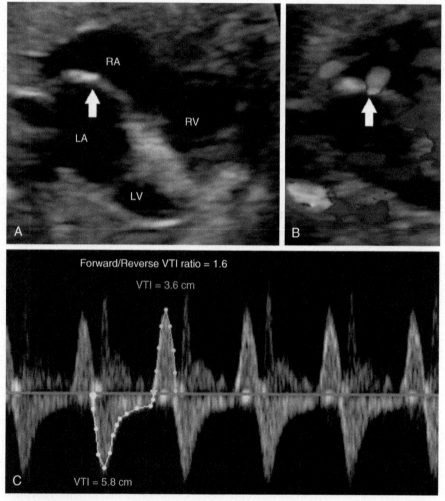

Fig. 31.1 Fetal echocardiogram images demonstrating HLHS with highly restrictive atrial septum. (A) Two-dimensional image showing thick atrial septum *(arrow)* bowing from left atrium *(LA)* to right atrium *(RA)*. (B) Color Doppler image of tiny left to right foramen ovale shunt *(red* flow marked with *arrow)*. (C) Pulmonary vein pulsed Doppler waveform of the same fetus demonstrating measurement of forward flow *(green)* and prominent atrial systolic reversal *(blue)*, with forward/reverse velocity time integral *(VTI)* ratio of 1.6 indicating highly restrictive atrial septum. *LV,* Left ventricle; *RV,* right ventricle.

caregivers. The perinatal plan should involve a highly coordinated delivery via scheduled C-section to minimize time to treatment with the necessary subspecialists on standby to care for the newborn. In some centers, the delivery takes place in a specialized labor and delivery unit within the children's hospital for immediate intervention, but if transfer is needed, the transport team should be ready on standby and an operating room or cardiac catheterization laboratory prepped and ready to receive the patient.

As previously noted, the postnatal care of complex cardiac patients requires preparation of the DR resuscitation team, NICU, and support services such as radiology and the neonatal transport team. Due to the high acuity of ENCI Level-4 patients, these services should be on standby in the NICU prior to the delivery in order to expedite patient handoff after the initial stabilization. A standardized approach to care with optimized communication and predelivery preparation are even more important in the early management of these high-risk patients. Of note, delayed umbilical cord clamping at present is not recommended in these patients, who are anticipated to require immediate resuscitation for respiratory and/or cardiac compromise at birth. Evaluation begins by assessing the infant's HR, respiratory effort, circulation, and color. Early elective endotracheal intubation is recommended in these patients due to the high risk for respiratory decompensation within the first hour after delivery. Pulse oximetry should be initiated immediately after birth to guide judicious oxygen use in the DR, with the goal of establishing preductal saturations in the range of 75% to 85%. In the event of bradycardia or cardiac compromise, a low-lying UVC should be immediately placed for the administration of emergency medications and IV fluids. Once the patient has been assessed and stabilized in the DR, further stabilization including radiographic confirmation of endotracheal tube and/or line placement should take place in the NICU prior to transfer. Recommendations for vascular access, prostaglandin infusion, circulatory monitoring, and fluids are outlined in the section covering ductal-dependent lesions.

Management strategies for these patients include maneuvers to promote right-to-left shunting across the PDA to facilitate systemic blood flow. Steps to keep pulmonary vascular resistance from dropping quickly include avoiding the excess use of oxygen by targeting preductal saturations in the range of 75% to 85%, avoiding systemic hypertension by targeting a mean BP equal to the weeks of gestation with a maximum of 5 to 10 points above this level, and maintaining the hematocrit greater than 40% to temper pulmonary blood flow through viscosity. Close circulatory monitoring of HR, BP, pulses, and capillary refill remains ongoing throughout stabilization. Other markers of systemic perfusion, such as pH, lactate levels, and urine output, should also be followed. Once stabilized, the patient should be transferred to a cardiac center in an expedited manner by a highly trained neonatal transport team.

D-Transposition of the Great Artery With Restrictive Atrial Septum

Neonates with d-TGA have pulmonary and systemic circulations in parallel rather than in series, causing them to rely on intracardiac mixing of oxygenated blood into the systemic circulation, generally at the level of the atrial septum. Neonates with d-TGA and inadequate mixing at the atrial septum can be profoundly hypoxemic, and may require an urgent balloon atrial septostomy (BAS) by an interventional cardiologist to open the atrial septum. Differentiating which fetuses with d-TGA will have postnatal restriction of the atrial septum can be challenging. Several studies have shown that fetal echocardiographic assessment of atrial septal movement and excursion can be useful to predict cases at risk for postnatal atrial septal restriction.[33-35] The predictive factors include hypermobility of the septum primum and bowing into the left atrium by more than 50% (Fig. 31.2), as well as diminished mobility, with an angle of less than 30 degrees between the atrial septum and bowing septum primum.[34-36] Abnormal ductus arteriosus shunting patterns in d-TGA, including constriction, bidirectional flow, and reversal (see Fig. 31.2), can predict profound postnatal pulmonary hypertension and risk for neonatal death.[35,37] However, our predictive capabilities remain suboptimal, such that the recent American Heart Association guidelines state that given the current lack of reliable markers to determine postnatal instability with high specificity and sensitivity, all babies with d-TGA should be delivered in anticipation of needing urgent BAS.[7,12,36] Perinatal planning should include discussions of transfer of care to a higher level center and delivery by C-section or induction to expedite the time to intervention.

As in the case of other ENCI Level-4 patients, the resuscitation team, equipment, and medications should be prepared prior to delivery as stated in the previous sections. Radiology services and a neonatal transport team should be on standby in the NICU in order to expedite the patient's initial stabilization and transfer. Again, delayed umbilical cord clamping is not recommended due to the need for expedited resuscitation that includes early elective intubation. Initial DR management begins with assessment of the infant's respiratory effort, HR, circulation, and color. Pulse oximetry initiated immediately after birth should guide oxygen use with the goal of establishing preductal saturations in the range of 75% to 85%. Early elective intubation is recommended, as these patients are at high risk for respiratory decompensation in the first minutes to hours after delivery and also require airway stabilization

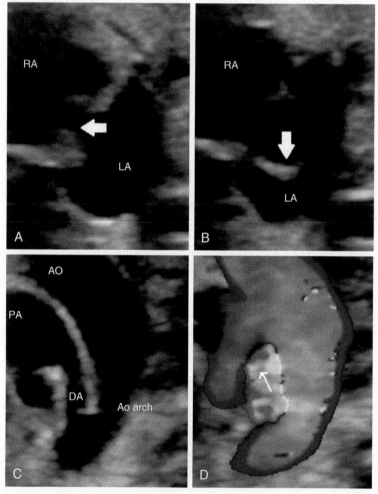

Fig. 31.2   D-Transposition of the great arteries (d-TGA) with restrictive atrial septum. Fetal echocardiogram images of patient with d-TGA with findings concerning for postnatal atrial septal restriction. (A) and (B) show hypermobile atrial septum (marked with *arrows*) which flops between the right atrium (*RA*) in panel A and left atrium (*LA*) in panel B. (C) Two-dimensional image of aortic arch and ductus arteriosus (*DA*) in the same fetus; note that the aorta (*Ao*) is located anteriorly as it comes off the right ventricle and pulmonary artery (*PA*) posteriorly off the left ventricle. (D) Color Doppler shows antegrade aortic arch flow (*blue*) and retrograde DA flow (*red*) marked with *arrow*.

prior to atrial septostomy. Detailed circulatory assessment should be ongoing during resuscitation and stabilization. In the event of bradycardia or cardiac compromise, an emergent low-lying UVC should be placed for the administration of emergency medications such as epinephrine and IV fluid boluses. A low-lying UVC offers emergency central access in seconds, and its vascular pathway can later be repurposed to facilitate access for a BAS if needed. Line placement must be verified by x-ray prior to further use or transfer to avoid complications of malpositioned catheters. Recommendations for PGE infusion, circulatory monitoring, administration of fluids, and following markers of systemic perfusion are outlined in the previous sections.

Strategies to improve pulmonary blood flow and avoid persistent pulmonary hypertension include optimizing oxygenation while avoiding/treating factors that can cause pulmonary vasospasm: metabolic or respiratory acidosis, systemic hypotension, hyperviscosity, and pain or agitation. Ongoing communication between the neonatology team leader, pediatric cardiology, and the transportation team is vital in expediting the transfer of patient care following the initial stabilization phase.

Congenital Heart Disease With Airway Compromise: Tetralogy of Fallot With Absent Pulmonary Valve Syndrome and Severe Ebstein Anomaly

TOF with APV syndrome is characterized by the absence or severe dysplasia of the pulmonary valve leaflets with severe pulmonary valve insufficiency. There is generally some degree of valvar pulmonary stenosis, but the hallmark is free pulmonary insufficiency with resultant aneurysmal dilatation of the branch pulmonary arteries, sometimes to a massive degree. The dilated pulmonary arteries compress the bronchi, resulting in varying degrees of bronchomalacia. The ductus arteriosus is often absent in this syndrome, but it is not known whether this is part of the defect or a consequence of the fetal hemodynamics.[4] There is a high risk for in utero demise, which is thought to be secondary to right ventricular and right atrial dilatation affecting ductus venosus and venous pressures imposing a risk for hydrops. Airway obstruction due to severely dilated branch pulmonary arteries can cause extrinsic compression of the bronchi leading to "hyperinflation" of the lungs and lobar emphysema due to fetal lung fluid trapping. This can be seen on prenatal ultrasound, as it causes a severe axis shift of the heart in the chest and cardiac displacement, and can also be seen by fetal magnetic resonance image (Fig. 31.3).[38,39]

Preparation for the postnatal care and expedited transfer of ENCI Level-4 patients with antenatal diagnosis of TOF with APV involves the steps previously outlined in the section on HLHS with RAS/IAS. Additional steps must also be taken

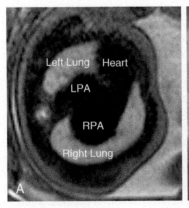 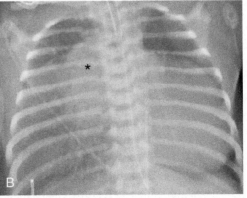

Fig. 31.3   (A) Fetal magnetic resonance image demonstrating axial plane through fetal thorax in a patient with Tetralogy of Fallot with absent pulmonary valve syndrome. The branch pulmonary arteries are massively dilated and the bronchi were not visible. The cardiac apex is deviated leftward. (B) Chest radiography of the same patient taken postnatally, demonstrating visible bulge of dilated RPA (*), lung hyperinflation, and interstitial lung disease in the setting of severe bronchomalacia. *LPA*, Left pulmonary artery; *RPA*, right pulmonary artery,

to prepare for these patients who may be hydropic with limited antegrade pulmonary blood flow and emphysematous lungs, making effective oxygenation and ventilation a challenge following delivery. Large pleural effusions or significant abdominal ascites can impinge upon lung expansion affecting alveolar ventilation and the appropriate establishment of functional residual capacity, which limits gas exchange in general and oxygenation in particular. Preparation in the DR should include a setup for pleurocentesis, paracentesis, pericardiocentesis, and chest tube placement. Again, delayed cord clamping is not recommended for reasons previously stated. Early intubation for hydropic patients is of great importance because the ability to establish effective respirations and systemic oxygenation will likely be further diminished by the presence of generalized edema, pleural effusions, and ascites. Assessment of perfusion and cardiac function should be followed as outlined previously in the section on HLHS with RAS/IAS. The resuscitation team must know the location and size of effusions prior to delivery and be prepared to evacuate the fluid if a limited response to endotracheal positive pressure ventilation is noted. The aspirated fluid should be sent for analysis (glucose, protein, cell count, culture). Pneumothorax is a known potential complication of pleurocentesis and should be considered in neonates with respiratory deterioration after the procedure.

Pulse oximetry should be used to target pre-ductal oxygen saturations between 75% and 85%. In the event of bradycardia or poor perfusion, an emergency low-lying UVC should be placed for the administration of emergency medications such as epinephrine and IV volume boluses. After the initial stabilization, the patient should be moved to the NICU for further stabilization, including appropriate central line placement and optimized respiratory management. There is potential for difficulty with ventilation from both the airway anomalies and inadequate antegrade pulmonary perfusion. PGE is not typically useful, as most cases have an absent ductus arteriosus. Extracorporeal membrane oxygenation (ECMO) may be needed for stabilization in cases of severe hypoxemia. Ventilation strategies for patients with emphysematous lungs should focus on modalities that minimize gas trapping and positioning the patient to decrease bronchial impingement. A trial of conventional ventilation may be employed using a low normal respiratory rate (30 breaths/min), inspiratory time to expiratory time ratio of 1:1.15 to optimize oxygenation, higher positive inspiratory pressure (PIP, 25 to 30 cm H_2O), and adequate peak end-expiratory pressure (7 to 8 cm H_2O) to keep airways stented open during exhalation and prevent collapse or gas trapping. The patient can also be positioned prone to alleviate bronchial compression from the engorged branch pulmonary arteries. If conventional ventilation fails, appropriately used high-frequency oscillatory ventilation (HFOV) or, if available, high-frequency jet ventilation (HFJV) offers a more effective method of ventilation in cases complicated by gas trapping and air leaks, as compared with conventional ventilation. With the use of HFOV or HFJV, ventilation is optimized with the use of lower peak and mean airway pressures compared with conventional ventilation, allowing emphysematous lung tissue to decompress and heal.[40] A study using HFJV has also reported a positive effect on cardiac output, which can be compromised by marked gas trapping, decreasing venous return to the heart.[41] X-ray confirmation of the position of the endotracheal tube and umbilical lines, ongoing hemodynamic monitoring, and communication with the transport team should be carried out as described earlier.

Ebstein anomaly involves displacement of the tricuspid valve deep into the right ventricular cavity leading to severe tricuspid regurgitation, right atrial enlargement, and ventricular dysfunction. These fetuses are at high risk for development of fetal heart failure and hydrops related to elevated CVP,[42] as well as risk for atrial tachyarrhythmia. Severe tricuspid regurgitation can result in massive cardiomegaly, which can pose a risk for the development of pulmonary hypoplasia (Fig. 31.4). Prenatal echo findings can help identify risk factors for poor outcome such as pulmonary regurgitation and cardiac enlargement, but it is not able to accurately predict the highest risk cases in which rapid deterioration in the perinatal period can be anticipated (see Fig. 31.4).[43] Preparing for the postnatal care of patients with severe Ebstein anomaly with hydrops should be carried out as described previously for ENCI Level-4 patients with the additional anticipated challenges to adequate ventilation

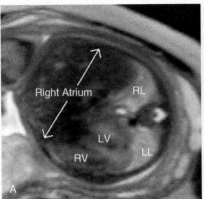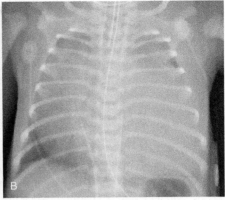

Fig. 31.4   (A) Fetal magnetic resonance image demonstrating axial plane through fetal thorax in patient with severe Ebstein anomaly with massive right atrial dilatation (right atrium width marked with *arrows*) and resultant bilateral lung hypoplasia. (B) Chest radiograph of the same patient taken postnatally, demonstrating severe cardiomegaly with wall-to-wall cardiac silhouette. *RV,* Right ventricle; *LV,* left ventricle; *RL,* right lung; *LL,* left lung.

and oxygenation due to various severity of pulmonary hypoplasia, severe edema, effusions, decreased pulmonary blood flow, and compromised cardiac output due to ventricular dysfunction and tachyarrhythmias. Antiarrhythmic medications and infusions should be prepared prior to delivery if there is a known fetal arrhythmia, and a defibrillator equipped with neonatal pads should be readily available should the need for synchronized cardioversion or defibrillation arise. The published algorithms for the management of arrhythmias delineated by the Pediatric Advanced Life Support program should be followed in these cases.[44]

Cases in which pulmonary hypoplasia is suspected can be given a trial of gentle conventional ventilation that begins in the DR and focuses on using a low-moderate PIP during resuscitation up to 20 to 25 cm H_2O, increasing respiratory rate to 40 to 60 breaths per minute with IT of 0.3 to 0.4 seconds. PIP should be adjusted based on the patient's lung compliance and oxygen titration based on continuous pulse oximetry with pre-ductal saturation goals of 75% to 85%. The team should be prepared to evacuate any significant effusions via pleurocentesis or paracentesis in an attempt to improve oxygenation and ventilation as outlined previously. If the trial with conventional ventilation is unsuccessful due to hypoxemia, hypercapnia, or air leaks, then a transition to HFOV or HFJV is indicated. Cautious titration of the mean airway pressure with close radiographic follow-up should be used to avoid hyperinflation, which can lead to gas trapping, air leaks, decreased venous return to the heart, and decreased pulmonary blood flow. Strategies to improve oxygenation and perfusion in these patients include PGE infusion, decreasing pulmonary vascular resistance (see previous section and consider the use of inhaled nitric oxide), and adding vasopressor-inotropes and/or lusitropes (dopamine and milrinone). Caution should be used in the selection of vasoactive medications in patients with severe Ebstein anomaly because they are at risk for supraventricular tachyarrhythmias (SVT) that can potentially degenerate into life-threatening ventricular arrhythmias.[45] As previously stated, central line placement, ongoing assessments of hemodynamic status, and radiographic confirmation of the position of the central lines and the endotracheal and chest tubes should be completed prior to the hand-off of patient care or facility transfer.

Bradyarrhythmias: Complete Heart Block

Immune-mediated, congenital CHB is prenatally diagnosed in mothers that test positive for SSA/SSB antibodies. These fetuses usually have normal anatomic structure of the heart, but are at risk of developing hydrops, fetal demise, and preterm delivery when the fetal HR drops too low for adequate oxygen delivery to the fetus. After delivery, these infants may need pacing depending on the resting HR and clinical status. However, many of these neonates will not require any immediate intervention

E

or placement of a permanent pacer until later in life. Prenatal findings that denote an increased risk are fetal HR less than 50 bpm, signs of fetal heart failure, and hydrops.[46] Preparing for the delivery of patients with CHB requires preparation prior to delivery as discussed previously. Additional elements to consider include preparation of cardiac medication infusions for vasopressor-inotropic and chronotropic support in cases presenting with bradycardia and hemodynamic instability. Initial DR assessment includes evaluation of the neonate's respiratory effort, HR, circulation, and color. Pulse oximetry should be performed immediately after birth in order to guide oxygen use with the goal for preductal saturations in the 85% to 95% range by 10 minutes after delivery, as delineated in the NRP algorithms.[47] Patients with a documented, long-standing baseline ventricular rate of 55 to 60 bpm or greater than 60 bpm who do not exhibit signs of respiratory or circulatory compromise do not require early elective intubation or chest compressions. However, they do require ongoing hemodynamic monitoring with close attention to systemic perfusion. After initial stabilization in the DR, further NICU evaluation of stable, term neonates includes a 12 Lead electrocardiogram, echocardiogram, and cardiology consultation within 24 hours of birth.

Patients whose antenatal course is complicated by a HR less than 50 bpm, decreased heart function, or hydrops should be approached as ENCI Level-4 patients. Detailed preparations should be carried out in addition to arranging for expedited transfer to a facility with the ability to provide a higher LOC. Early elective intubation followed by the evacuation of any effusions impinging on ventilation or perfusion should be addressed as soon as possible following delivery. Assessments of respiratory and hemodynamic stability should be ongoing during expedited central line placement and confirmation of line and tube positions. Those with imminent need for pacing and/or pacemaker placement for HR less than 55 bpm, significant hemodynamic instability, or wide complex escape rate (QRS duration >120 ms) should be transferred immediately to a higher LOC.[48] For profound bradycardia or hypotension, epinephrine infusion should be initiated at a starting dose of 0.01 µg/kg/min with titration of the dose to the desired effect. An alternative medication to consider would be isoproterenol at a starting dose of 0.02 to 0.05 µg/kg/min. Some unstable patients may require transcutaneous pacing under the guidance of a pediatric cardiologist, which can be accomplished with the use of neonatal defibrillator pads, connected to a manual external defibrillator.

Consideration for Fetal Therapy/Intervention

In the current era of fetal intervention/therapy there exists the potential for lessening the acuity at neonatal presentation of CHD and improving the preoperative clinical condition by altering the disease state prenatally. Although appropriately designed, controlled trials have not been performed yet and might not even be feasible; findings of large case series suggest that balloon valvuloplasty of the aortic valve in cases of critical aortic stenosis might prevent progression to HLHS, resulting in a more stable biventricular circulation at birth.[49,50] These patients may go from being ductal dependent at birth to not requiring a PGE infusion and possibly avoiding neonatal surgery. HLHS with RAS can be stabilized with prenatal/fetal intervention by the creation of an atrial communication using either balloon septostomy or interatrial stent placement in the fetus.[51] This has the potential to improve the physiology, stabilize the newborn, and avoid the need for emergent surgical- or catheter-based septostomy in the first hours after delivery. Medical fetal therapy with digoxin for fetal congenital heart failure (CHF), antiarrhythmia drugs for fetal SVT, and fetal transfusion all have the potential to reverse hydrops and fetal CHF improving fetal status prior to delivery and resulting in improved neonatal outcomes.[36] Emerging therapies such as implantable fetal pacemakers for congenital CHB may help carry a pregnancy to term or near term and reverse fetal hydrops, resulting in a better clinical status at birth prior to permanent pacemaker implantation.[52,53]

Summary/Conclusions

Neonates with critical CHD are at increased risk of mortality and morbidity due to their underlying condition and the compromise that postnatally begins in the delivery room.[18] While advancements in scanning technology and enhanced screening guidelines continue to increase prenatal detection rates and improve outcomes for patients with CHD, identifying which newborns are at greatest risk for needing emergent neonatal cardiac intervention still presents a challenge. Critical CHD requires a highly coordinated perinatal plan and DR management strategy for appropriate stabilization and immediate transfer to the cardiac care team. From the time of initial diagnosis of critical CHD, there should be a comprehensive care plan developed based on the anticipated postnatal acuity level and need for emergent intervention. Active perinatal strategies and DR protocols, as well as close multidisciplinary collaboration, hold the promise of improving the approach to complex CHD. In the future, innovative fetal therapies may alter outcomes of critical CHD, and allow for a less critical transition from fetal to postnatal life. However, until that is fully realized, the best possibility for a good outcome is a well-developed and executed perinatal plan.

REFERENCES

1. Montana E, Khoury MJ, Cragan JD, et al.: Trends and outcomes after prenatal diagnosis of congenital cardiac malformations by fetal echocardiography in a well defined birth population, Atlanta, Georgia, 1990–1994, *J Am Col Cardiol* 28(7):1805–1809, 1996.
2. Hoffman JI, Kaplan S: The incidence of congenital heart disease, *J Am Col Cardiol* 39(12):1890–1900, 2002.
3. Kleinman CS, Hobbins JC, Jaffe CC, et al.: Echocardiographic studies of the human fetus: prenatal diagnosis of congenital heart disease and cardiac dysrhythmias, *Pediatrics* 65(6):1059–1067, 1980.
4. Rudolph AM: *Congenital Diseases of the Heart: Clinical-Physiological Considerations*, ed 3, Chichester, UK; Hoboken, NJ, 2009, Wiley-Blackwell.
5. Anagnostou K, Messenger L, Yates R, et al.: Outcome of infants with prenatally diagnosed congenital heart disease delivered outside specialist paediatric cardiac centres, *Arch Dis Child Fetal Neonatal Ed* 98(3):F218–221, 2013.
6. Jegatheeswaran A, Oliveira C, Batsos C, et al.: Costs of prenatal detection of congenital heart disease, *Am J Cardiol* 108(12):1808–1814, 2011.
7. Morris SA, Ethen MK, Penny DJ, et al.: Prenatal diagnosis, birth location, surgical center, and neonatal mortality in infants with hypoplastic left heart syndrome, *Circulation* 129(3):285–292, 2014.
8. Costello JM, Polito A, Brown DW, et al.: Birth before 39 weeks' gestation is associated with worse outcomes in neonates with heart disease, *Pediatrics* 126(2):277–284, 2010.
9. Cnota JF, Gupta R, Michelfelder EC, et al.: Congenital heart disease infant death rates decrease as gestational age advances from 34 to 40 weeks, *J Pediatr* 159(5):761–765, 2011.
10. Wertaschnigg D, Manlhiot C, Jaeggi M, et al.: Contemporary outcomes and factors associated with mortality after a fetal or neonatal diagnosis of ebstein anomaly and tricuspid valve disease, *Can J Cardiol* 32(12):1500–1506, 2016.
11. Trento LU, Pruetz JD, Chang RK, et al.: Prenatal diagnosis of congenital heart disease: impact of mode of delivery on neonatal outcome, *Prenat Diagn* 32(13):1250–1255, 2012.
12. Peterson AL, Quartermain MD, Ades A, et al.: Impact of mode of delivery on markers of perinatal hemodynamics in infants with hypoplastic left heart syndrome, *J Pediatr* 159(1):64–69, 2011.
13. Peyvandi S, Nguyen TA, Almeida-Jones M, et al.: Timing and mode of delivery in prenatally diagnosed congenital heart disease- an analysis of practices within the University of California Fetal Consortium (UCfC), *Pediat Cardiol* January 11, 2017.
14. Walsh CA, MacTiernan A, Farrell S, et al.: Mode of delivery in pregnancies complicated by major fetal congenital heart disease: a retrospective cohort study, *J Perinatol* 34(12):901–905, 2014.
15. Reis PM, Punch MR, Bove EL, et al.: Obstetric management of 219 infants with hypoplastic left heart syndrome, *Am J Obstet Gynecol* 179(5):1150–1154, 1998.
16. Berkley EM, Goens MB, Karr S, et al.: Utility of fetal echocardiography in postnatal management of infants with prenatally diagnosed congenital heart disease, *Prenat Diagn* 29(7):654–658, 2009.
17. Slodki M, Respondek-Liberska M, Pruetz JD, et al.: Fetal cardiology: changing the definition of critical heart disease in the newborn, *J Perinatol* 36(8):575–580, 2016.
18. Donofrio MT, Levy RJ, Schuette JJ, et al.: Specialized delivery room planning for fetuses with critical congenital heart disease, *Am J Cardiol* 111(5):737–747, 2013.
19. Pruetz JD, Carroll C, Trento LU, et al.: Outcomes of critical congenital heart disease requiring emergent neonatal cardiac intervention, *Prenat Diagn* 34(12):1127–1132, 2014.
20. Soroka M, Respondek-Liberska M, Slodki M: EP07.07: Atrioventricular septal defect: what can we predict for neonates based on prenatal diagnosis - retrospective analysis of 97 cases from a tertiary centre for fetal cardiology, *Ultrasound Obstet Gynecol* 48(Suppl 1):293, September 2016.
21. Rychik J, Tian Z: *Fetal Cardiovascular Imaging a Disease-Based Approach*, Philadelphia, PA, 2012, Elsevier/Saunders. https://www.clinicalkey.com/dura/browse/bookChapter/3-s2.0-C2009034218X.

31

22. Berning RA, Silverman NH, Villegas M, et al.: Reversed shunting across the ductus arteriosus or atrial septum in utero heralds severe congenital heart disease, *J Am Col Cardiol* 27(2):481–486, 1996.
23. Quartermain MD, Glatz AC, Goldberg DJ, et al.: Pulmonary outflow tract obstruction in fetuses with complex congenital heart disease: predicting the need for neonatal intervention, *Ultrasound Obstet Gynecol* 41(1):47–53, 2013.
24. Arya B, Levasseur SM, Woldu K, et al.: Fetal echocardiographic measurements and the need for neonatal surgical intervention in tetralogy of fallot, *Pediatr Cardiol* 35(5):810–816, 2014.
25. Hornberger LK, Sahn DJ, Kleinman CS, et al.: Antenatal diagnosis of coarctation of the aorta: a multicenter experience, *J Am Col Cardiol* 23(2):417–423, 1994.
26. Makikallio K, McElhinney DB, Levine JC, et al.: Fetal aortic valve stenosis and the evolution of hypoplastic left heart syndrome: patient selection for fetal intervention, *Circulation* 113(11):1401–1405, 2006.
27. Matsui H, Mellander M, Roughton M, et al.: Morphological and physiological predictors of fetal aortic coarctation, *Circulation* 118(18):1793–1801, 2008.
28. Atz AM, Feinstein JA, Jonas RA, et al.: Preoperative management of pulmonary venous hypertension in hypoplastic left heart syndrome with restrictive atrial septal defect, *Am J Cardiol* 83(8):1224–1228, 1999.
29. Rychik J, Rome JJ, Collins MH, et al.: The hypoplastic left heart syndrome with intact atrial septum: atrial morphology, pulmonary vascular histopathology and outcome, *J Am Col Cardiol* 34(2):554–560, 1999.
30. Vlahos AP, Lock JE, McElhinney DB, et al.: Hypoplastic left heart syndrome with intact or highly restrictive atrial septum: outcome after neonatal transcatheter atrial septostomy, *Circulation* 109(19):2326–2330, 2004.
31. Cheatham JP: Intervention in the critically ill neonate and infant with hypoplastic left heart syndrome and intact atrial septum, *J Interv Cardiol* 14(3):357–366, 2001.
32. Michelfelder E, Gomez C, Border W, et al.: Predictive value of fetal pulmonary venous flow patterns in identifying the need for atrial septoplasty in the newborn with hypoplastic left ventricle, *Circulation* 112(19):2974–2979, 2005.
33. Punn R, Silverman NH: Fetal predictors of urgent balloon atrial septostomy in neonates with complete transposition, *J Am Soc Echocardiogr* 24(4):425–430, 2011.
34. Maeno YV, Kamenir SA, Sinclair B, et al.: Prenatal features of ductus arteriosus constriction and restrictive foramen ovale in d-transposition of the great arteries, *Circulation* 99(9):1209–1214, 1999.
35. Jouannic JM, Gavard L, Fermont L, et al.: Sensitivity and specificity of prenatal features of physiological shunts to predict neonatal clinical status in transposition of the great arteries, *Circulation* 110(13):1743–1746, 2004.
36. Donofrio MT, Moon-Grady AJ, Hornberger LK, et al.: Diagnosis and treatment of fetal cardiac disease: a scientific statement from the American Heart Association, *Circulation* 129(21):2183–2242, 2014.
37. Talemal L, Donofrio MT: Hemodynamic consequences of a restrictive ductus arteriosus and foramen ovale in fetal transposition of the great arteries, *J Neonatal Med* 9(3):317–320, 2016.
38. Sun HY, Boe J, Rubesova E, et al.: Fetal MRI correlates with postnatal CT angiogram assessment of pulmonary anatomy in tetralogy of fallot with absent pulmonary valve, *Congenit Heart Dis* 9(4):E105–109, 2014.
39. Chelliah A, Berger JT, Blask A, et al.: Clinical utility of fetal magnetic resonance imaging in tetralogy of fallot with absent pulmonary valve, *Circulation 12* 127(6):757–759, 2013.
40. Keszler M, Donn SM, Bucciarelli RL, et al.: Multicenter controlled trial comparing high-frequency jet ventilation and conventional mechanical ventilation in newborn infants with pulmonary interstitial emphysema, *J Pediatr* 119(1 Pt 1):85–93, 1991.
41. Carlon GC, Ray Jr C, Pierri MK, et al.: High-frequency jet ventilation: theoretical considerations and clinical observations, *Chest* 81(3):350–354, 1982.
42. Pruetz JD, Votava-Smith J, Miller DA: Clinical relevance of fetal hemodynamic monitoring: perinatal implications, *Semin Fetal Neonatal Med* 20(4):217–224, 2015.
43. Freud LR, Escobar-Diaz MC, Kalish BT, et al.: Outcomes and predictors of perinatal mortality in fetuses with ebstein anomaly or tricuspid valve dysplasia in the current era: a multicenter study, *Circulation* 132(6):481–489, 2015.
44. de Caen AR, Berg MD, Chameides L, et al.: Part 12: pediatric advanced life support: 2015 American Heart Association guidelines update for cardiopulmonary resuscitation and emergency cardiovascular care, *Circulation* 132(18 Suppl 2):S526–542, 2015.
45. Giamberti A, Chessa M. The tricuspid valve in congenital heart disease.
46. Eliasson H, Sonesson SE, Sharland G, et al.: Isolated atrioventricular block in the fetus: a retrospective, multinational, multicenter study of 175 patients, *Circulation* 124(18):1919–1926, 2011.
47. Weiner GM, Zaichkin J, Kattwinkel J, et al.: *Textbook of Neonatal Resuscitation*. ed 7.
48. Glatz AC, Gaynor JW, Rhodes LA, et al.: Outcome of high-risk neonates with congenital complete heart block paced in the first 24 hours after birth, *J Thorac Cardiovasc Surg* 136(3):767–773, 2008.
49. Freud LR, McElhinney DB, Marshall AC, et al.: Fetal aortic valvuloplasty for evolving hypoplastic left heart syndrome: postnatal outcomes of the first 100 patients, *Circulation* 130(8):638–645, 2014.
50. Moon-Grady AJ, Morris SA, Belfort M, et al.: International fetal cardiac intervention registry: a worldwide collaborative description and preliminary outcomes, *J Am Col Cardiol* 66(4):388–399, 2015.
51. Marshall AC, van der Velde ME, Tworetzky W, et al.: Creation of an atrial septal defect in utero for fetuses with hypoplastic left heart syndrome and intact or highly restrictive atrial septum, *Circulation* 110(3):253–258, 2004.
52. Zhou L, Vest AN, Chmait RH, et al.: A percutaneously implantable fetal pacemaker. Conference proceedings: Annual International Conference of the IEEE Engineering in Medicine and Biology Society. IEEE Engineering in Medicine and Biology Society, *Annual Conference* 2014:4459–4463, 2014.
53. Bar-Cohen Y, Loeb GE, Pruetz JD, et al.: Preclinical testing and optimization of a novel fetal micropacemaker, *Heart Rhythm* 12(7):1683–1690, 2015.

CHAPTER 32

Catheter-Based Therapy in the Neonate With Congenital Heart Disease

Karim Assaad Diab, Bassel Mohammad Nijres, and Ziyad M. Hijazi

- Transcatheter cardiac interventions currently provide a wide range of different therapeutic or palliative alternatives to surgeries in neonates.
- Common catheter-based procedures in neonates include balloon atrial septostomy, balloon valvotomies, perforation of atretic valves, stenting of obstructed vessels, and device closure of abnormal communications.
- Interventional cardiac catheterizations are not risk free; common complications can include bleeding, arrhythmia, cardiac perforation, device embolization, vascular access injuries, and even death.
- With growing experience in the field coupled with numerous advances in the available low-profile instruments and devices, simple and complex interventional cardiac catheterizations have been performed successfully and more safely in recent years.

Over the past five decades, interventional cardiac catheterization has significantly evolved in the management of pediatric patients with congenital heart disease (CHD), particularly in the neonatal period. Since the first successful catheter-based therapeutic procedure in 1966 by Rashkind and Miller who performed a balloon atrial septostomy (BAS or Rashkind procedure) in an infant with transposition of the great arteries without a thoracotomy,[1] several advances in catheter-based technologies and techniques have been achieved that allowed cardiac catheterization to play a major role in treating both adults and children with congenital and acquired cardiovascular diseases. In the neonatal period, a wide variety of transcatheter interventions are commonly performed, either as palliation or therapy, and either as an alternative to surgical intervention or in coordination with surgery in what has been termed "hybrid" procedures, allowing transcatheter interventions on even the smallest patients.

Among these catheterization procedures are creation or enlargement of atrial communications to improve cardiac mixing, balloon valvuloplasty to treat congenital pulmonary or aortic valvular stenosis, balloon angioplasty or stenting of vessels, such as coarctation of the aorta, ductal stenting in ductal dependent lesions, perforation of the atretic valve, and device closure of the ductus arteriosus. This chapter describes various catheter-based therapies that are currently performed in neonates born with CHD.

Indications for Cardiac Catheterization in the Neonate and Potential Complications

During the past three decades, the indications for pediatric cardiac catheterization have undergone significant changes. With the increasing accuracy of noninvasive diagnostic tools, including echocardiography, computed tomography, and magnetic resonance imaging, cardiac catheterization is no longer considered a mainstay diagnostic tool for most cardiac anomalies, except on rare occasions or when accurate hemodynamic measurements are needed. On the other hand, with the advent of new instruments, it has become more common to perform cardiac catheterization for interventional purposes. This is particularly true in the neonate, where interventional cardiac catheterization can offer successful alternative options to cardiac surgery with potentially lower mortality and morbidity. In addition, for certain conditions, it can be used effectively as an alternative or adjunct to surgical procedures ("hybrid" procedures). Thus, currently, the indications for catheterizations are more likely to be for catheter-based therapies rather than diagnostic purposes in patients with CHD.[2-6]

The indications for cardiac catheterization usually fall into one of the following categories:

1. Determine the anatomic diagnosis: This could be the case in patients with limited echocardiographic windows, such as patients with lung pathology, as in chronic lung disease (CLD), resulting in poor visualization of cardiac structures. It could also be needed to further delineate structures usually not well seen with echocardiography, such as vascular abnormalities in the systemic or pulmonary circulation, or presurgical and postsurgical intervention, such as with systemic to pulmonary arterial collaterals.
2. Obtain complete hemodynamic evaluation to guide medical and surgical management, such as assessing pulmonary vascular resistance in a patient with pulmonary hypertension or CHD.
3. Perform interventional procedures, such as closure of atrial or ventricular septal defects, occlusion of vascular structures, such as patent ductus arteriosus (PDA), stenting of PDA or narrowed vessels, perforating or balloon dilating atretic or stenotic valves, respectively, and atrial septostomy to facilitate better systemic and pulmonary blood mixing.[2-7]

Although cardiac catheterization is relatively safe, it can be associated with significant complications, particularly in neonates and small infants. These can be divided into two groups:

1. *Major complications.* These are significant adverse events that typically lead to compromise needing significant intervention, such as cardiopulmonary resuscitation. Examples include complete heart block, structural injury from intervention related to cardiac perforation or device embolization, vessel perforation, central nervous system (CNS) complications, and death.
2. *Minor complications.* These tend to be transient and can include blood loss requiring transfusion, hypotension requiring fluid resuscitation or vasopressor-inotrope administration, deep venous thrombosis, pulse loss requiring heparin or a stronger agent such as a tissue plasminogen activator, transient heart block, dysrhythmias requiring treatment, metabolic acidosis due to decreased oxygen delivery to the tissues, and balloon rupture. Vascular complications can be either major or minor and can be particularly common in neonates due to their small vessel sizes. These possible complications deserve special attention and will be discussed more thoroughly in the next section.

Nowadays, with the increased survival of low birth weight infants, advanced technology, smaller sheath sizes, and better intracatheterization monitoring, low birth weight neonates can undergo catheter interventions more safely, though the complication rate is still higher compared with larger infants.[2,8] Recently, Mobley et al.[8] analyzed the complication rate in neonates in relation to their weight. The overall incidence of complications was higher in neonates weighing less than 2.5

kg compared with those weighing greater than 2.5 kg (34.8% vs. 17.6%, $P = .023$). This higher overall rate was a result of a greater proportion of minor complications 34.8% in small neonates versus 16.9% in larger ones ($P = .021$). However, the percentage of neonates having at least one major complication was the same in both groups (2.2%).

Vascular Access

Femoral arterial and venous access are traditionally the methods of choice for cardiac catheterization in infants using either the right or the left groin. In small newborns, umbilical arterial and venous vessels can also be used usually up to 7 days of age. Other alternative routes for arterial access include carotid, brachial, and axillary arteries. Alternative venous access sites include internal jugular vein, subclavian vein, axillary vein, and transhepatic venous access. Alternative vascular access is occasionally required due to the lack of femoral vascular patency or the need to position the catheter at a particular trajectory not provided through the traditional femoral access. The use of alternative access is safe and effective for performing a wide variety of interventions. In addition, its use may improve the results of selected complex interventional procedures.[6,9,10]

Recently, Choudhry and colleagues[10] reported on the successful percutaneous access through the carotid artery using a 21-gauge Doppler needle (Smart Needle) under ultrasound guidance in infants less than 3 months of age. This route can allow the use of larger sheaths (up to 6-French) with no documented arterial occlusions or neurologic sequelae. Using the carotid approach, the catheter can be maneuvered easily in the left heart structures with potentially less technical difficulty.

In more recent years, interventional congenital cardiologists and congenital cardiovascular surgeons have collaborated to obtain access to even larger, more central vessels or even direct access into the cardiac chambers for catheter-based therapies employing "hybrid" procedures.

Complications of vascular access sites account for the majority of adverse events associated with neonatal cardiac catheterization.[11–13] Injury to the vessel and/or the surrounding area may occur with either venous or arterial access sites, although more significant acute and long-term sequelae are more common with arterial access. In general, vascular injury is more likely in smaller neonates when using large sheaths or catheters, when a patient is on anticoagulation, and after interventional procedures. Complications may include arterial spasm and/or thrombosis causing chronic occlusion, significant tearing or severing of the vessel with extravasation of blood into the surrounding tissue, hematoma, "false" or pseudoaneurysm formation, and creation of an arteriovenous fistula. The frequency of vascular complications has decreased with alterations in access techniques, improvements in availability of size-appropriate equipment for neonates, and meticulous management of the access site following the procedure. With the frequent use of indwelling central venous catheters and/or arterial cannulations and the need for repeated procedures in these small patients (and vessels), the incidence of chronic occlusion of these vessels has increased, necessitating the use of less "standard" access sites and approaches for catheter-based procedures in these patients. These include use of the umbilical vein (in the immediate newborn period), subclavian or jugular veins, or hepatic veins (transhepatic approach) for venous access, or the umbilical artery, the carotid artery (usually via a cut-down technique), the axillary artery for alternative arterial access, or the use of "hybrid" procedures.[9,13–18]

Balloon Atrial Septostomy and Septoplasty

Since Rashkind first performed BAS in 1966 in an infant with transposition of the great arteries, the safety and efficacy of this procedure has been well established and has become a lifesaving procedure for patients with CHD who require improved atrial level mixing of blood or atrial decompression. This is typically needed for patients with D-transposition of the great arteries, particularly with intact ventricular septum (IVS) and some forms of double outlet right ventricle (RV). With the use of prostaglandin infusion, the need for BAS has become less urgent as mixing can at times be adequately improved by keeping the ductus patent. Although initial BAS procedures were performed using fluoroscopic guidance, it was Allan and colleagues who first described performing BAS under echocardiographic guidance in 1982.[19] Since then, improvements in echocardiographic imaging have allowed most neonatal BAS procedures to be performed at the bedside under echocardiographic guidance if the atrial septum anatomy is "straightforward" and the septum is not intact.[20] When atrial communication is not present, most centers perform BAS in the catheterization laboratory using either fluoroscopic guidance with biplane imaging alone or, alternatively, fluoroscopy with transthoracic echocardiography (TTE) or transesophageal echocardiography (TEE) to better visualize the septum when septal perforation is required prior to creation of an atrial communication. When possible, TEE imaging is preferred because the ultrasonographer's hand does not interfere with the fluoroscopic image during the procedure. In small infants in whom a pediatric/infant TEE probe may be too large, successful transesophageal imaging using an intracardiac echo catheter (AcuNav, Acuson/Siemens, Mountain View, California) has been reported.[21] Femoral venous access is preferred to umbilical vein access due to the complexity of the intervention and the more direct course from the femoral vein to the atrial septum. Once access has been obtained in the intubated, sedated neonate, a balloon septostomy catheter is advanced via an introducer sheath to the inferior vena cava and right atrium, across the patent foramen ovale (PFO), and into the left atrium usually under direct visualization using TTE imaging. Once the position of the catheter tip is confirmed to be in the body of the left atrium (and not in a pulmonary vein or across the mitral valve), the balloon at the tip of the catheter is slowly inflated with sterile saline/contrast mixture while simultaneously pulling the balloon back against the left atrial side of the atrial septum. The amount of saline/contrast mixture used to fill the balloon is dependent upon the type of septostomy catheter, the actual size of the left atrium, and the desired size of the resultant septal defect and is usually 2.5 to 3 mL. Next, the balloon inflation lock is secured and the catheter is firmly and rapidly pulled into the right atrium, aiming to produce a tear in the septum primum. Once the balloon has been pulled across the septum, it is quickly deflated so as not to obstruct systemic venous inflow from the inferior vena cava. The procedure may be repeated using serial increases in the inflation volume to fill the balloon until an adequate defect is created or until the maximum volume of the septostomy catheter or the maximum balloon size the left atrium will accommodate has been reached. Once the septostomy procedure has been performed, two-dimensional (2-D) echocardiography and Doppler interrogation are performed to assess the resultant defect size and determine the presence and severity of any residual atrial level restriction to blood flow or mixing. Further echocardiographic assessment of the cardiac function, as well as for evidence of pericardial effusion or damage to any of the cardiac structures, is also recommended following BAS.

Although complications are not common, there have been reports of embolization of balloon fragments or air bubbles in the event of balloon rupture during the procedure (it should be noted here that careful de-airing of the balloon during preparation for BAS should take place to prevent air embolization if balloon rupture should occur). Other complications associated with BAS include heart block or other serious arrhythmias, mitral or tricuspid valve injury, thromboembolic events, such as stroke, and inferior vena cava or pulmonary vein tear or rupture. Death has also occurred. Careful and appropriate echocardiographic imaging prior to and during balloon inflation can decrease the risk of valvular and/or vascular tears or ruptures from occurring. The success rate of BAS in newborns is over 98%, with a procedural mortality of less than 1% and an incidence of major complications reported on the order of 0% to 3%.[22–24] Hemodynamic improvement is usually noted immediately after a successful BAS with increased oxygen saturations and a decrease in the interatrial gradient. Restenosis after BAS is rarely seen.

Some reports have suggested that there is an association between preoperative brain injury in neonates with transposition and performance of BAS.[24–26] Recently, Mukherjee and colleagues reported that there was a significant, positive association between the Rashkind procedure and the diagnosis of stroke when comparing infants with transposition who either did or did not undergo a BAS procedure. However, the lack of temporal data regarding the timing of BAS and the diagnosis of stroke limited the investigators' ability to prove causation.[24] In contrast, others have recently published reports that BAS was not associated with an increased risk of clinical stroke, but that there was an increased incidence of preoperative periventricular leukomalacia (PVL) in neonates with transposition of the great arteries that had longer time to surgical repair and/or lower arterial oxygenation prior to intervention.[27,28] These authors also suggested that BAS was protective against PVL when the procedure resulted in timely improvement in arterial oxygenation.[27] Further studies are needed to better evaluate and define risk factors for preoperative brain injury in this patient population, which may include minimal oxygen saturation after birth and/or length of time from birth to BAS and improvement in systemic oxygenation.[29]

Atrial Septoplasty

Creation or enlargement of an atrial communication in neonates presenting after the immediate newborn period may be difficult due to the presence of a thick or intact atrial septum. Other infants, such as those with hypoplastic left heart syndrome (HLHS), may have malalignment of the atrial septum which is often associated with restriction of pulmonary venous return (Fig. 32.1A). In patients such as these, standard BAS techniques may not be sufficient to create a nonrestrictive atrial communication and other transcatheter techniques may be required. When the septum is intact, perforation of the septum to access the left atrium is required. Historically, this was, and often still is, performed using a Brockenbrough needle to puncture the septum. In recent years, radiofrequency (RF)-assisted septal perforation has been reported using a 0.024-inch diameter wire with a 0.016-inch diameter metal tip (Baylis Medical, Montreal, Canada) attached to a dedicated RF generator (Baylis Radiofrequency Generator, Montreal, Canada). The wire is passed within a coaxial catheter that is, in turn, passed within a guide catheter or long introducer sheath/dilator, which has been placed with its tip adjacent to (and in contact with) the right atrial side of the septum. Perforation with this RF wire can be achieved with the application of 5 to 10 W of energy for 2 to 5 seconds.[30,31] Once mechanical or RF-assisted perforation of the septum and access into the left atrium is achieved, subsequent sequential static balloon dilation ("septoplasty") is performed, starting with small-diameter balloons, followed by serially larger diameter balloons to a maximum balloon diameter

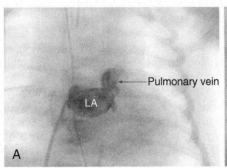
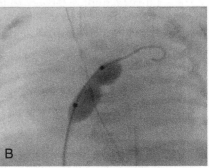

Fig. 32.1   (A) Left atrial (LA) angiogram in a patient with hypoplastic left heart syndrome with restrictive atrial septum. Hand injection demonstrates complete filling of the left atrium with opacification of a dilated left lower pulmonary vein. The left atrium is small without much egress of dye into the right atrium. (B) Balloon septoplasty of the atrial septum in a patient with hypoplastic left heart syndrome with restrictive atrial septum. The balloon catheter is positioned in the mid-septum over a wire positioned with the wire tip in the pulmonary vein. There is a discrete waist in the balloon seen in the region of the thick atrial septum.

of typically 10 to 12 mm in neonates.[31] When there is a PFO, but the septum is thick or malaligned, septal perforation is often performed in a more "favorable" position along the septum with subsequent septoplasty. The use of coronary and peripheral cutting balloons (Boston Scientific, IVT, San Diego, California) or high-pressure angioplasty balloons has also been reported to be a safe and effective option for septoplasty in neonates (see Fig. 32.1B).[32–34] Finally in patients with difficult septal anatomy, an intravascular stent implantation at the atrial septum to maintain septal patency has provided effective palliation until surgical intervention or transplant can be achieved.[35–37]

Pulmonary Balloon Valvuloplasty for Critical Pulmonary Stenosis

Neonates not diagnosed in utero with the suspicion of critical pulmonary valvular stenosis usually present within the first 24 to 48 hours of life with progressive cyanosis as the ductus arteriosus closes. There is typically an outflow murmur from the stenotic valve. Cyanosis is due to persistent right-to-left shunting at the PFO in the presence of a hypertensive and hypertrophied noncompliant RV. By definition, critical pulmonary valve stenosis is ductal dependent as adequate pulmonary blood flow and oxygenation are dependent on systemic-to-pulmonary artery shunting via the ductus. Management of these infants requires the initiation of a PGE-1 infusion to maintain ductal patency and to augment pulmonary blood flow. Currently, percutaneous balloon valvuloplasty is the initial procedure of choice for neonates with critical or severe pulmonary stenosis. These patients typically have a normal-sized tricuspid valve annulus, a tripartite RV, and a normal pulmonary valve annulus. The RV may be hypoplastic or the cavity may be relatively small due to the often severe right ventricular hypertrophy. The main pulmonary artery usually has evidence of poststenotic dilation from the jet of blood across the stenotic valve and there is almost always predominant right-to-left shunting at the atrial level (PFO) due to the stiff, noncompliant RV. In patients with severe pulmonary stenosis that is not ductal dependent with no significant stenosis or suprasystemic RV pressures or cyanosis, balloon valvotomy is usually delayed beyond the neonatal period.

Careful 2-D echocardiographic and Doppler assessment of these patients prior to any interventions is of the utmost importance. Echo evaluation should include assessment of the RV anatomy, tricuspid valve annulus z-score, and measurements of the pulmonary valve annulus in preparation for catheter-based therapy. Balloon valvuloplasty procedures for critical or severe pulmonary stenosis in the neonate are performed in the cardiac catheterization laboratory usually with the patient intubated and sedated or under general anesthesia. A femoral venous approach is typically utilized, although this procedure has also been performed using umbilical venous access in very small neonates. After hemodynamic assessment, a right ventricular angiogram is performed to assess the size of the right ventricular cavity, the outflow tract, and the pulmonary valve annulus. The valve leaflets and annulus are best demonstrated on a straight lateral projection. This projection is also used for determining the annular diameter. An end-hole catheter is positioned with its tip in the RV outflow tract and a floppy-tipped torque wire is used to cross the stenotic orifice of the valve. When the ductus is patent, the wire is often able to be maneuvered across it into the descending aorta for more stable wire (and balloon) position during the procedure. A balloon diameter to valve annulus diameter (balloon-annulus) ratio of 1:1.2 is used for pulmonary valvuloplasty. The balloon is inflated and deflated rapidly after having been positioned over the wire and across the valve. Inflation times are typically less than 10 seconds. During inflation, a waist is seen in the mid-portion of the balloon at the level of the stenotic valve, and this waist disappears with full inflation of the balloon. The balloon is removed over the wire and follow-up hemodynamic data are obtained to reassess the pulmonary valve gradient. With a PDA, the valve gradient may not accurately quantify the valve gradient that may persist. If the right ventricular pressure is still suprasystemic, valvuloplasty may be repeated using a larger diameter balloon as long as a safe and appropriate balloon-annulus ratio is used. At the end of the procedure, a final right ventricular angiogram is performed to assess for any damage to the RV, tricuspid valve apparatus, and/or pulmonary artery and to assess the location of any residual obstruction.

Following successful balloon valvuloplasty, most patients will have sufficient antegrade pulmonary blood flow to tolerate discontinuation of the PGE-1 infusion and subsequent closure of the ductus. However, many will continue to have predominant right-to-left shunting at the atrial level until the right ventricular compliance improves. In some cases, this may take 3 to 4 weeks with multiple attempts of trialing off and restarting PGE-1 infusion for systemic saturations that drop consistently to or below the 75% to 80% range due to decreased ductal-level pulmonary blood flow in conjunction with a restricting or closing ductus. Most successful balloon valvuloplasty procedures result in some amount of pulmonary insufficiency. This is well tolerated in most infants and some have reported a beneficial effect of pulmonary insufficiency promoting right ventricular growth.[38,39] With regression of the right ventricular hypertrophy, improvement of the ventricular compliance, and growth of the RV, the amount of right-to-left shunting at the atrial level decreases over time; adequate saturations are achieved and patients are able to be maintained off PGE-1 infusion. Saturations continue to increase as these right ventricular changes continue or with spontaneous closure of the PFO. A small percentage of infants with critical pulmonary stenosis who have undergone a successful balloon valvuloplasty procedure may still be unable to maintain adequate pulmonary blood flow and systemic saturations off PGE-1 infusion greater than 4 weeks following valve dilation. In the past, these patients have undergone surgical placement of a Blalock-Taussig shunt to augment pulmonary blood flow. Some centers have gone on to perform ductal stenting in the catheterization laboratory to maintain ductal patency and augmented pulmonary blood flow off PGE-1 infusion in these patients. This is more commonly the case in patients with membranous pulmonary valve atresia following perforation of the valve with subsequent balloon valvuloplasty (see later).

Holzer and colleagues recently reported using a multicenter registry on 304 balloon pulmonary valvuloplasty procedures performed in eight institutions over a 34-month period. The median age at intervention was 2 months with 39% of procedures performed in the first month of postnatal life. Procedural success was achieved in 82% of all procedures, being defined as either a reduction in peak systolic valvar gradient to less than 25 mm Hg or greater than 50% reduction of the valve gradient or reduction of right ventricular systolic pressure ratio by 50%. There was a trend toward lower procedural success with moderate to severe thickening of the pulmonary valve (72%). Minor adverse events were documented in 10% of procedures, while moderate, major, or catastrophic adverse events were documented in 2% of procedures. However, there were no deaths.[40]

Pulmonary valvotomy can also be used in patients with other congenital lesions to improve pulmonary blood flow. This can be applied as a palliative procedure, for example, in patients with tetralogy of Fallot or other forms of RV outflow tract obstruction with severe cyanosis and hypoplastic pulmonary arteries that preclude early repair. In these cases, stenting the RV outflow tract is usually necessary. A recent report by McGovern et al. demonstrated successful results with alleviation of RV outflow tract obstruction and resolution of hypercyanotic spells, allowing growth of the pulmonary arteries and successful repair at a later stage without the need for a systemic-to-pulmonary shunt.[41]

Perforation of the Pulmonary Valve in Pulmonary Atresia and Intact Ventricular Septum

Pulmonary atresia (PA) with IVS is a complex disorder that is not only characterized by membranous or muscular atresia of the right ventricular outflow tract (RVOT) but also significant heterogeneity of the right ventricular morphology. The coronary artery anatomy also may be affected in this disorder with in utero development of connections between the RV and the subepicardial coronary arteries (RV to coronary artery sinusoids or fistulas), predisposing these patients to abnormal coronary circulations. Prognosis is related to the severity of the coronary circulation abnormalities as well as to tricuspid valve anatomy and function.[42,43] Prior to transcatheter or surgical intervention, careful assessment of the right heart and coronary anatomy must take place. Newborns with this disorder are obviously dependent on ductal flow and therefore PGE-1 infusion is initiated immediately after birth. TTE is performed for initial assessment. If it is clear that the tricuspid valve and/or RV are severely hypoplastic and that biventricular repair will not be an option, then plans for a palliative surgical shunt are made. In these patients, assessment of the atrial septum to determine adequacy of the atrial communication is made as restriction at the atrial level may lead to poor cardiac output and BAS should be considered. Cardiac catheterization with angiography to assess the coronary artery circulation is usually still performed in these patients, even when there is no plan for right ventricular decompression as patients with severe coronary artery abnormalities may be ultimately managed with cardiac transplantation.[44] In patients where the echocardiographic assessment of right heart adequacy is less clear and/or when relief of the RVOT is considered, cardiac catheterization and angiography are performed to help characterize the size of the right ventricular cavity and outflow tract as well as to define coronary artery anatomy and determine whether coronary circulation is dependent on high right ventricular pressures (right ventricular dependent coronary artery circulation; RVDCC). In patients with RVDCC, relief of the RVOT may result in a catastrophic event due to inadequate perfusion of the myocardium with a sudden drop in the systolic pressure of the RV (i.e., coronary perfusion pressure in patients with RVDCC), resulting in myocardial ischemia, infarct, or death. If RVDCC is not present, then the decision to perform transcatheter relief of the RVOT with or without ductal stenting or surgical relief with placement of a systemic-to-pulmonary shunt is entertained.[45]

It is very important that procedures involving perforation of the membranous valve be performed using a high-quality, biplane x-ray imaging system. Infants should be intubated and sedated and, if necessary, paralyzed so that they do not move during the procedure. Historically, perforation of the atretic pulmonary valve was performed using the stiff end of a guidewire.[46,47] However, the use of a stiff wire tip in the RVOT of a neonate was often associated with significant and severe adverse events, such as perforating the anterior part of the outflow tract, bleeding, the need for emergent surgical procedures, and death.[47] Laser energy was the first energy source to be used for valvar perforations. Unfortunately, the laser beam would perforate any tissue in its path beyond and/or adjacent to the valve as the depth of laser penetration is difficult to control.[48,49] RF energy is less powerful than laser energy, but is easier to control and has more recently been used to perforate atretic valve tissue.[45,50]

The development of a small, flexible coaxial catheter and wire system (Baylis Medical) that could be advanced within small (4-French) catheters positioned with the tip in the RVOT just beneath the atretic pulmonary valve made it possible to deliver RF energy that was confined to the tip of the wire at the membranous valve for perforation. It is very important to clearly define the anatomy of the RVOT as well as the main pulmonary artery by angiography in preparation for this procedure. Operators often use permanent thoracic landmarks and image "roadmaps" in an attempt to avoid inadvertently perforating outside the boundaries of the RVOT. Some advocate placing a retrograde catheter from the aorta across the ductus with its tip in the main pulmonary artery just above the atretic valve for something to aim at. Others have described passing a snare wire (Amplatz Gooseneck; Microvena, Vadnais Heights, Minnesota) within the retrograde catheter and opening it within the main pulmonary artery to act as a "target" as well as to delineate the boundaries of the pulmonary artery lumen (Fig. 32.2A).[51] Only 5 to 10 W of energy applied for 2 seconds is needed to perforate the tissue. Once perforation has been performed, the wire and coaxial catheter are advanced into the main pulmonary artery. The RF wire can then be

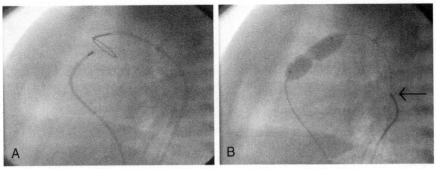

Fig. 32.2 (A) Lateral plane cine fluoroscopy demonstrating a snare wire (Amplatz Gooseneck; Microvena, Vadnais Heights, Minnesota) passed retrograde from the aorta across the ductus to the main pulmonary artery to act as a "target" as well as to delineate the boundaries of the pulmonary artery lumen during radiofrequency (RF) perforation of an atretic pulmonary valve in this patient with pulmonary atresia with intact ventricular septum. (B) Lateral plane cine of balloon pulmonary valvuloplasty in an infant with pulmonary atresia with intact ventricular septum after successful RF perforation. The wire has been snared in the descending aorta (arrow) to gain wire stability for a subsequent balloon valvuloplasty procedure.

exchanged for a floppy-tipped guidewire that can be maneuvered across the ductus into the descending aorta. The snare may also be used to secure the wire tip in the descending aorta and provide maximum wire stability for tracking balloon catheters over it during subsequent valvuloplasty (see Fig. 32.2B). As described in patients with critical pulmonary stenosis, serial dilations with incremental balloon diameters may be necessary for successful valvuloplasty. Postprocedure angiography is performed to assess for any injury of the tricuspid valve apparatus, RV outflow tract, main pulmonary artery, or ductus. Due to the nature of the atretic valve, free pulmonary insufficiency is present following a successful procedure. Also, at this point, consideration of whether pulmonary blood flow will require augmentation by either ductal stenting or surgical shunt placement is made, although many centers may observe patients clinically following valvuloplasty and before implanting a stent or placing a shunt. It is possible that, if the RV is only mildly hypoplastic and if the tricuspid valve function is normal, adequate pulmonary blood flow will have been established by the perforation or valvuloplasty procedure and that the infant may tolerate cessation of the PGE-1 infusion and closure of the ductus without the need for further catheter-based or surgical procedures.

Success of this procedure has been reported by many centers.[52,53] Complications are similar to those associated with pulmonary balloon valvuloplasty for critical pulmonary valve stenosis. Agnoletti and colleagues reported the long-term results in 33 newborns who underwent successful perforation or valvuloplasty procedures for PA or IVS. Of these patients, 50% needed surgery in the neonatal period while an additional three patients had elective surgery beyond the neonatal period for augmentation of pulmonary blood flow.[52]

Schwartz et al.[54] reported on the outcomes and predictors of reintervention in these patients after RF perforation and balloon pulmonary valvuloplasty in 23 patients. All procedures were successful with no major complications and 29% of patients did not require subsequent interventions, 9% required subsequent balloon dilation of the pulmonary valve, and 20% received an additional blood supply for the pulmonary circulation (Blalock-Taussing shunt or PDA stent), while 42% required surgical RVOT augmentation. They found that postvalvuloplasty pulmonary valve gradient was predictive of the subsequent need for RVOT intervention.

More recently, some centers have adopted a hybrid approach for these patients involving perventricular pulmonary valve perforation. Early results showed that this can be a safe and feasible alternative to the surgical approach with the advantages of avoiding cardiopulmonary bypass in the neonatal period, direct access to the RVOT, and lower risk for complications and perforation.[55]

Balloon Aortic Valvuloplasty in Critical Aortic Stenosis

There is often considerable variability in the cardiac anatomy and morphology of infants born with aortic valve stenosis. Defects may range from isolated valvar stenosis with normal annulus size and variable valve morphologies to multiple associated left-sided obstructive lesions or variants of HLHS. When the left ventricle (LV) has been hypertensive in utero, endocardial scarring (fibrosis) also may be present, which has separate acute and long-term implications. In cases of small left heart structures associated with valvar stenosis, it is often difficult to decide on the most appropriate management plan. Decisions must first include whether the left heart structures will be able to sustain a biventricular circulation or whether univentricular palliation will be necessary. If biventricular circulation is considered, then one must decide whether to perform transcatheter balloon dilation of the valve versus surgical valvotomy. Most previous reports have shown comparable results between balloon aortic valvuloplasty (BAV) and surgical valvuloplasty with respect to primary outcomes of survival, efficacy at relieving aortic stenosis, and frequency of important complications, including aortic insufficiency (AI).[56–58] McElhinney et al. also reported that those patients with initially small left heart structures had worse subacute outcomes, and that reinterventions for residual or recurrent aortic stenosis or iatrogenic AI was more common among early survivors of neonatal BAV, particularly in the first year after BAV.[56] Data obtained from the Congenital Heart Surgeons Society database showed a greater likelihood of significant AI with BAV when compared with surgical valvuloplasty, but residual stenosis was more often seen in the surgical group. However, the mortality rate and the risk of reintervention were similar.[57]

When the decision for transcatheter balloon valvuloplasty for severe or critical aortic stenosis in a neonate has been made, most procedures are performed in the cardiac catheterization laboratory under general anesthesia, although there have been reports of percutaneous aortic balloon valvuloplasty being performed at the bedside under echocardiographic guidance using a carotid artery approach.[59,60] Many of these infants present in cardiac failure and/or in a low output state, requiring mechanical ventilation, inotropic support, and PGE-1 infusion to augment systemic blood flow via right-to-left shunting at the ductus. Aortic balloon dilation has been performed using both a prograde or retrograde approach by either venous or arterial access, respectively. Most commonly, a femoral or umbilical artery approach is utilized. Considerations regarding the use of the umbilical artery include the tortuosity of the catheter course to the aortic valve compared with a more direct course from the femoral artery. However, use of the femoral artery increases the risk of significant vascular injury and/or occlusion, especially in very small infants. Reports have suggested that the route from a carotid artery (retrograde) approach is most direct and improves ability (and therefore procedure time) to pass a wire across the stenotic valve orifice for subsequent balloon valvuloplasty. However, there is at least a theoretically increased risk of acute and long-term sequelae from carotid artery injury at the access site, irrespective of whether a percutaneous or surgical cut-down is used.[59–61] Once access has been obtained, the patient is heparinized and hemodynamic data are obtained. LV and ascending aortic angiography is performed for careful assessment of LV size and function, the nature of LV outflow obstruction, aortic valve annulus size, coronary artery anatomy along with quantification of AI if present, and assessment of aortic arch anatomy. Next, wire position across the aortic valve is achieved, most often using a floppy-tipped, "torqueable" wire via an end-hole catheter from a retrograde approach. Once the wire is in place with the tip curled in the LV, the angioplasty catheter is passed over the wire and positioned across the valve (Fig. 32.3). In contrast to the larger balloon-annulus ratios recommended for pulmonary valve dilations, a balloon-annulus ratio of 80% to 90% is recommended for aortic valve dilation to minimize the risk of resultant AI.[62]

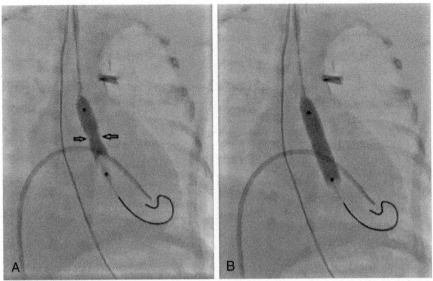

Fig. 32.3   Aortic valvuloplasty in an infant weighing 1.8 kg using a Tyshak II 5 mm × 2 cm balloon. (A) During balloon inflation, notice the waist *(arrows)* at the site of the aortic valve. (B) No residual waist noticed after full balloon inflation.

Recent studies report success rates for BAV of 87% to 97%.[63,64] A recent multicenter study by Torres and colleagues on aortic balloon valvuloplasty showed this procedure to be safe and effective at all ages with success rates of 87% in infants younger than 1 month of age.[65] In assessment for predictors of outcome, there were no significant predictors for patients younger than 1 month of age, although nonelective procedures and PGE-1 infusion at time of procedure tended to be associated with inadequate outcome (defined as a residual gradient of ≥45 mm Hg and ≥3 grade change in AI). For patients older than 1 month of age, a history of complex two-ventricle anatomy and prior transcatheter and/or surgical interventions were associated with inadequate outcome. In this report, high severity adverse events were more frequent in patients younger than 1 month of age (18%) versus those older than 1 month (5%) with no catastrophic events in either group. Most common severe adverse events were significant arrhythmias, pulse loss, and cardiac perforation in a neonate.[65]

Transcatheter Management of Neonatal Coarctation

Coarctation of the aorta accounts for about 5% to 8% of CHD lesions and usually affects the aortic aspect of the insertion of the ductus arteriosus (aortic isthmus).[66] Theoretically, it might be explained by an abnormal migration of the ductal smooth muscle cells into the periductal area early in fetal life.[67] Neonates with critical coarctation may present with circulatory collapse when the ductus closes. Less severe obstructions may present with congestive heart failure, systemic hypertension in the upper extremities, diminished lower extremity pulses, differential cyanosis, or symptoms secondary to other associated defects. For neonates presenting with cardiac shock, stabilization by maximizing cardiac output should be attempted vigorously. This includes starting PGE-1 infusion to maintain the patency of PDA and improve the perfusion of the descending aorta as well as administering intravenous fluids, inotropes, and sedation and correcting the metabolic acidosis along with provision of respiratory support as needed.[68]

Balloon angioplasty has been used for managing coarctation since the early 1980s. There is strong evidence supporting its use beyond the neonatal period as an effective and safe alternative to surgery in both native and recurrent postoperative coarctation. In addition, many reports have concluded that balloon angioplasty

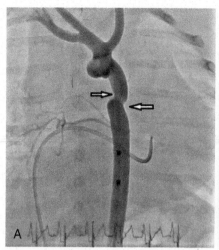
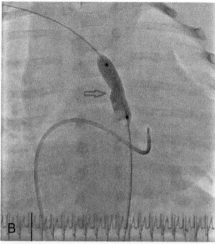

Fig. 32.4   (A) Aortoangiogram using a 4-French marked pigtail showing the recoarcted area in a 5 kg infant who had surgical coarctation repair in the neonatal period. (B) Balloon angioplasty showing the recoarcted area *(arrows)* in a 5-kg infant using a "Tyshak II balloon" (stiff balloon) after securing the supporting wire in the right subclavian. Notice the waist at the middle of the balloon *(arrow)* during inflation.

should be considered the treatment of choice for all patients with postoperative reco-arctation.[69–72] In the current era, the role of balloon angioplasty for native coarctation in neonates remains controversial due to the higher incidence of early restenosis, the need for multiple interventions, potential serious vascular injury and limb ischemia, and the incidence of aneurysm formation when compared with surgical treatment for the same diagnosis and patient population.[73–77] Furthermore, follow-up data comparing both groups up to 3 years postintervention are consistent with improved arch growth in neonates receiving surgical intervention.[73] Thus, most often a primary balloon angioplasty procedure is only recommended under special circumstances and as a palliative treatment for neonatal coarctation of the aorta. It should be considered whenever surgery is contraindicated or carries a high complication rate. This is especially true in very low birth weight neonates with critical coarctation and left ventricular dysfunction with multiorgan failure. In that setting, emergency primary balloon angioplasty can be very effective in acutely relieving heart failure and systemic perfusion and improving acidosis, and hence, decreasing mortality and morbidity and providing a bridge to surgery. Successful and safe balloon angioplasty has been reported in small neonates weighing as low as 790 g.[78] However, the rate of developing recoarctation in primary balloon angioplasty in neonates is much higher (>50% in the vast majority of studies)[73,78–80] compared with surgically treated patients.

The procedure is usually carried out under general anesthesia in a retrograde manner. After recording the gradient across the arch, a biplane aortogram is obtained with contrast injection proximal to the narrowed area (Fig. 32.4A). Measurements are then made at different points of the aorta in order to select the size of balloon to be used for dilatation. The size of the balloon selected should be no more than 1 to 2 mm larger in diameter than the smallest normal aortic diameter proximal to the coarctation and not larger than the size of the aorta at the level of the diaphragm. The dilation balloon catheter is tracked over a stiff wire until the center of the balloon is placed at the middle of the coarcted segment. Balloon inflation is then performed and should be complete and continued until reaching the maximum pressure of the balloon or disappearance of the waist on the balloon (see Fig. 32.4B). Then, the balloon is rapidly deflated. Re-dilation can be carried out if the result of the initial dilation is suboptimal.

In addition to the vascular access complications, aortic wall injury occurs in approximately 10% of cases[70] with aneurysm formation, aortic dissection, or intimal tear. Therefore, adequate heparinization is critical to prevent clot formation.

Although CNS complications are extremely rare, they might have a devastating outcome. These complications can be eliminated by avoiding placing the distal end of the supporting wire (stiff wire) in the carotid or vertebral arteries and appropriate flushing of the catheters to prevent clot formation and air embolism. Moreover, maximum pressure of the balloon should not be exceeded in any circumstance in order to avoid balloon rupture, which may lead to embolization of balloon fragments or air bubbles.[68,70]

Although stenting has been shown to be effective and safe in adults and older children with coarctation, it is not suitable for small infants due to the lack of stents that can be dilated to a potential diameter suitable for the adult aorta to compensate for somatic growth.[81–84] The invention of newer biodegradable stents in the future could expand the application of transcatheter stenting procedures to neonates with native coarctation of the aorta.

Ductal Stenting in Ductal-Dependent Pulmonary Circulation

Stenting the ductus can be necessary in order to either improve pulmonary blood flow or in order to support systemic blood flow. Stenting of the ductus arteriosus to augment or maintain adequate pulmonary blood flow in newborns with cyanotic heart defects was first attempted with the introduction of coronary artery stents in the early 1990s.[85,86] However, these early cases were complicated by the use of delivery systems manufactured for adult procedures that were often too large and quite difficult to maneuver in small infants. Advances in stent and catheter technologies have allowed a wider variety of stent sizes, lower profile balloons, and more flexible delivery systems, making previously very difficult and risky catheter-based therapies an alternative to surgical interventions for neonates with CHD. In many centers throughout the world, ductal stenting is utilized as an alternative first-stage palliation to surgical placement of a systemic-to-pulmonary artery shunt in neonates with cyanotic CHD.[87–89] Reports have shown that ductal stenting may now be performed with relatively low risk, especially when performed in patients with restrictive but dual-sourced pulmonary blood flow.[90] Although in many centers, surgically created systemic-to-pulmonary shunts are still the treatment of choice for neonates with cyanotic CHD, others consider ductal stenting as a way to delay or avoid the need for a surgical shunt and the associated postoperative morbidities and complications that may occur. There are no definite exclusion criteria in regard to ductal morphology, although most feel that a very tortuous ductus (one making a loop of greater than 270-degree curves) or those associated with significant pulmonary artery branch stenosis should be considered poor candidates.[85–90] In addition, stenting the ductus in the setting of ductal dependent systemic circulation is usually entertained as part of the hybrid approach in the treatment of HLHS and its variants. Discussion of this procedure, which involves stenting the ductus and placement of bilateral pulmonary artery bands, is beyond the scope of this chapter.

The acceptance of alternative vascular access sites has further decreased procedure-related morbidity and vascular injuries. When performed in conjunction with perforation and/or valvuloplasty of the pulmonary valve, often ductal stenting may be performed via an antegrade approach using venous access. Femoral arterial access is also often used, but may not allow the appropriate-sized delivery system necessary for this procedure in very small infants. Also, a typical ductus in patients with PA often arises off the underside from the transverse arch and may be difficult to access from a retrograde arterial approach. Alternative access sites may include a carotid artery, accessed via cut-down, or axillary artery using a percutaneous approach. The access sites are typically chosen based on ductal origin and shape, as well as the site that favors the straightest or most direct course toward the ductal origin from the arch.[85,88]

These procedures are typically performed under general anesthesia or deep conscious sedation with assisted ventilation. There is no consensus as to when PGE-1 infusion should be discontinued prior to stent placement. Alwi and colleagues[91] stopped PGE-1 infusion 6 to 12 hours before stent implantation except in those patients who remained PGE-1 dependent with a ductus being the sole source of pulmonary blood flow or when the ductus was significantly stenotic.[85] Angiography is performed to demonstrate aortic arch and head vessel anatomy, and the origin and course of the ductus, as well as to further assess pulmonary artery anatomy. As discussed earlier, the procedure may be performed using an antegrade approach from venous access or from a retrograde arterial approach. Once the most appropriate approach has been selected, the access achieved and the introducer sheath placed, an end-hole catheter with a preformed curve at the tip is used to access the origin of the PDA. A floppy-tipped, torque-controlled wire is used to cross the ductus and the tip is stabilized distal in one of the branch pulmonary arteries. Premounted (either self-expanding or balloon-expandable) coronary stents are usually chosen for ductal stenting. With the wire in place, the coronary stent is passed over the wire and positioned in the ductus. Small hand injections of contrast are usually possible via the side arm of the delivery sheath to assess stent position prior to deployment. Follow-up angiography is performed to confirm satisfactory stent placement after deployment. Additional stents may be required to cover the full extent of the ductus. Any ductal tissue not stented will be at risk of early stenosis and therefore must be stented. Additional stents are telescoped one within another at deployment (Figs. 32.5 and 32.6). Patients are heparinized once vascular access has been obtained. Most continue heparin administration for 24 to 48 hours following the procedure. Long-term antiplatelet therapy with either aspirin (2 to 5 mg/kg/day) or clopidogrel (0.2 mg/kg/day) has been recommended.[90–92]

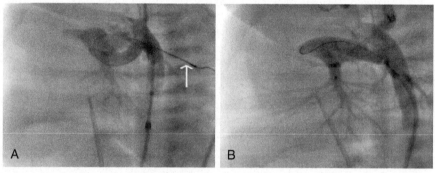

Fig. 32.5 (A) Angiography of a tortuous duct supplying the pulmonary artery. A floppy guidewire is positioned in a left lower lobe artery via the left axillary artery *(arrow)*. Angiography was performed via a second catheter advanced from the right femoral artery to the proximal descending aorta. (B) A premounted stent has been deployed in the ductus arteriosus via a retrograde approach from the femoral artery.

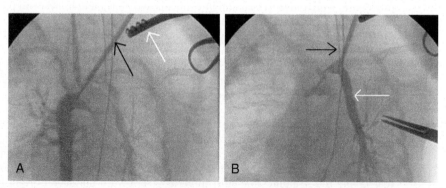

Fig. 32.6 (A) Transcarotid approach via surgical cut-down to the left common carotid in preparation for ductal stenting of a ductus off the left innominate artery in a patient with tetralogy of Fallot with a right aortic arch and left pulmonary artery (LPA) arising from a left-sided patent ductus arteriosus. The *black arrow* points to a sheath in the left carotid and the *white arrow* to surgical retractors used during carotid cut-down. (B) A premounted stent has been successfully deployed in the ductus arteriosus via the left carotid artery with resultant patency of the LPA. The *black arrow* demonstrates a carotid sheath and the *white arrow* the stented ductus.

Early restenosis of ductal stent(s) should be expected with patients presenting with a drop in systemic oxygen saturation on follow-up. Close surveillance and follow-up of these patients are imperative. Repeat cardiac catheterization is recommended when there has been a significant drop in the systemic saturations or prior to surgical intervention. In a recent report by Schranz and colleagues, ductal stenting was achieved in 58 newborns (27 of whom were truly ductal-dependent) between 2003 and 2009 with no procedure-related mortality. Of the 27, 3 required an acute surgical shunt and 4 of the remaining 24 required surgical shunts during midterm follow-up, with 2 others requiring stent redilation. A total of 23 patients went on to have surgical palliation or biventricular repair.[89] Similar results have been reported by others.[91,92]

Similarly, Mallula et al. reported on the successful use of ductal stenting in neonates with PA/IVS and found that the procedure was successful in 92.3% of the cases.[93]

Device Closure of the Patent Ductus Arteriosus in the Neonate

PDA is a relatively common CHD occurring at an incidence of 1 in 2000 live births in children born at term.[94] In addition, it is more common in preterm neonates and can result in significant heart failure and increased morbidity, including an increased risk of intraventricular hemorrhage, necrotizing enterocolitis, and CLD.[95-99]

The first transcatheter closure of a PDA was carried out by Porstmann et al. in 1967.[100] Since then, various PDA devices, sheaths, and low-profile delivery systems have been developed. Nowadays, transcatheter closure of the PDA is considered the standard of care beyond the neonatal period. In addition, it has been recently performed successfully as an alternative to surgical closure even in very small preterm infants.[101,102]

Transcatheter PDA closure can also be done via either the anterograde (venous) or retrograde (arterial) approach, with the former being preferred in very small infants in order to decrease the risk of vascular complications. All patients undergo cardiac catheterization under general anesthesia in a biplane catheterization laboratory. A biplane anteroposterior and lateral descending aortogram is performed to evaluate the size, position, and shape of the ductus. A 4-French introducer sheath can be tracked over a 0.025-inch guidewire across the RV into the pulmonary artery. Then, it can be manipulated to cross the PDA with the tip seating in the descending aorta. After delineating the anatomy and landmarks of the PDA (Fig. 32.7A), the appropriate device is chosen and deployed. After deploying the device and before detaching it from the delivery system, a descending aortogram is performed to confirm the position and stability of the device (see Fig. 32.7B). A repeat aortogram is then performed 10 minutes after the release to assess the degree of residual shunt (Fig. 32.8).

Echocardiographically guided transcatheter PDA closure also was described recently when surgical closure is contraindicated or when transporting unstable infants carries a high risk. This approach can be carried out at the bedside using venous access only, sparing infants the complications potentially associated with arterial access. In addition, it has been shown to be safe and feasible in premature infants weighing less than 1500 g.[101,103]

There are many different devices that can be potentially used to close the PDA in children and infants. These include coils, vascular plugs, and Amplatzer Duct Occluder. The decision on which device to use is dependent on the preference of the operator, the device availability, the PDA type, the ampulla size (aortic end of the PDA), the narrowest pulmonary diameter, the length of the PDA and the descending aorta, the patient size, and the size of the delivery system. The rule of thumb is to use the smallest available delivery system, which is currently 4-French, and to avoid arterial access whenever possible. This is critical, especially in premature neonates as the vascular complications are correlated inversely with their weight.[104] In general, for a small PDA with its narrowest point of less than 2 mm, closure can be achieved by deploying a coil, or an Amplatzer Duct Occluder II device. For a large PDA, other devices may be preferred, such as a vascular plug or an Occlutech duct

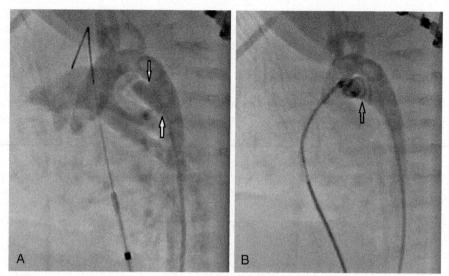

Fig. 32.7   (A) Lateral view showing a patent ductus arteriosus (PDA; *arrows*) in a neonate following contrast injection in the aortic arch using a pigtail catheter. (B) Lateral view after contrast injection in the aortic arch following deployment of a coil in the PDA *(arrow)* before detaching the delivery system. It shows good position of the coil with no residual shunt across the PDA.

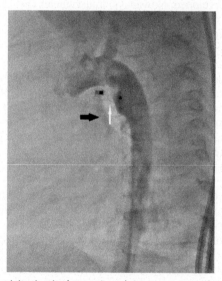

Fig. 32.8   Lateral view of contrast injection in the aortic arch in a neonate with patent ductus arteriosus following deployment of a 6 × 4 mm Amplatzer Duct Occluder II *(white arrow)* with small residual shunt *(black arrow)*.

occluder. These devices usually will be seated within the duct with no retention discs protruding outside the PDA, which could potentially interfere with the flow in the descending aorta or the left pulmonary artery.[105–107]

ADO devices (St. Jude Medical, Plymouth, Minnesota), which are generally safe to use in older children, can be problematic in smaller infants due to the risk of occluding the aorta by the bulky retention discs. Therefore, for this group of very small infants, coil closure may be the preferred and safest approach. Coils can be delivered entirely within the PDA with no protruding parts. Francis and colleagues described successful coil occlusion of the PDA in eight preterm infants with a median birth weight of 1040 g (range 700 g to 1700 g) with no significant complications.[108]

The new ADO II AS with its small articulated retention discs (these discs are only 1 to 1.5 mm larger than the central occlusive part) is a promising device to use in small infants, providing an excellent ductal closure rate via a low-profile delivery system using a 4-French delivery sheath. Although it has not been approved by the U.S. Food and Drug Administration yet, it has been proven to be effective with a low complication rate. Its use in small infants weighing as low as 1700 g was demonstrated in both animal and human studies.[101,102]

Compared to surgical closure, transcatheter PDA closure is associated with lower risk and fewer adverse outcomes directly related to the intervention. However, it is unknown at present if the medical complications following surgical ligation of the PDA, including systemic hypotension and significant worsening of the patient's pulmonary status, also occur after transcatheter PDA closure in preterm infants. Most common complications specifically related to the device include device embolization or malposition and flow obstruction in the descending aorta and/or left pulmonary artery, creating iatrogenic coarctation and/or left pulmonary artery stenosis.[101,104,107] Of note, safety concerns with transcatheter closure are higher in smaller infants; complications, such a coil or device malposition, arrhythmia, and/or hypotension requiring intervention, occur more frequently in infants weighing less than 6 kg compared to larger infants (adverse event rate 27% vs. 8%).[104,109] With growing experience and further advances in robust lower profile sheaths and delivery systems, transcatheter device closure of the PDA will likely be the treatment of choice for PDA closure in both term and premature neonates.

Future Applications

Biodegradable stents will have a bright future for applications in neonates and small infants. Using these stents will obviate the need for subsequent surgical removal or the need for replacement with larger stents and will potentially eliminate or decrease the need for further reinterventions.

These stents consist of an absorbable magnesium alloy with a novel design that allows for radial strength of the stent without measurable recoil after implantation. In animal studies, complete degradation of the stents has been noted by 3 months postimplantation.[110,111] There is a case report on the use of a biodegradable stent in a 3-week-old neonate with recurrent coarctation following surgical repair. Although immediate relief of gradient was achieved, repeat intervention was required at 3 weeks after stent implantation due to significant aortic obstruction at the level of the biodegradable stent.[112]

Some additional potential applications also include stenting hypoplastic or occluded branch pulmonary arteries or stenting aortopulmonary collaterals to increase pulmonary flow in patients with PA with multiple collaterals.[113–115]

As suggested by many investigators, the ideal biodegradable stent should have the following characteristics: it should provide complete relief of obstruction and allow the vessel wall to remodel to the diameter of the stent, and the degradation process should be 100% completed with no residues. It is presumed that as the stent is naturally absorbed, the vessel wall would continue to grow normally without the need for additional reinterventions.[116,117]

One of the important limitations of applying current coronary biodegradable stents in neonates is that the largest expanded diameter of these stents is generally small (up to 4 mm). Treatment of coarctation of the aorta or pulmonary artery stenosis in a newborn would require a stent, which can be expanded to 6 to 8 mm.[117] However, our group is working in our animal laboratory on larger biodegradable stents for use in neonates. These stents are made of a poly-L-lactic acid and most, if not all, are drug coated.

Conclusion

Therapeutic cardiac catheterization procedures represent a major component of the treatment strategy for neonates with CHD. A wide variety of catheter interventions are becoming feasible in the neonatal period as an alternative or adjunct to surgical procedures. In our opinion, long-term follow-up of these patients following such interventions will demonstrate the utility of these procedures in this patient population.

REFERENCES

1. Rashkind WJ, Miller WW: Creation of an atrial septal defect without thoracotomy: a palliative approach to complete transposition of the great arteries, *JAMA* 196:991, 1966.

2. Simpson JM, Moore P, Teitel DF: Cardiac catheterization of low birth weight infants, *Am J Cardiol* 87(12):1372–1377, 2001.

3. Rhodes JF1, Asnes JD, Blaufox AD, et al.: Impact of low body weight on frequency of pediatric cardiac catheterization complications, *Am J Cardiol* 86(11):1275–1278, 2000.

4. Huhta JC, Glasow P, Murphy DJ, et al.: Surgery without catheterization for congenital heart defects: management of 100 patients, *J Am Coll Cardiol* 9:823–829, 1987.

5. Shim D, Lloyd TR, Crowley DC, et al.: Neonatal cardiac catheterization: a 10-year transition from diagnosis to therapy, *Pediatr Cardiol* 20:131–133, 1999.

6. Taqatqa Anas, Saleh Lutfi, Gupta U, et al.: Cardiac catheterization in children: diagnosis and therapy. In Abdulla RI, editor: *Heart Diseases in Children: A Pediatrician's Guide*, New York, 2011, (Chapter 5), Springer.

7. Sheikh N: Pediatric catheterization protocol, *Mymensingh Med J* 24(3):638–648, 2015.

8. Mobley MM, Stroup RE, Kaine SF: Comparative risk of cardiac catheterisations performed on low birth weight neonates, *Cardiol Young* 23(5):722–726, 2013.

9. Davenport JJ, Lam L, Whalen-Glass R, et al.: The successful use of alternative routes of vascular access for performing pediatric interventional cardiac catheterization, *Catheter Cardiovasc Interv* 1;72(3):392–398, 2008.

10. Choudhry S, Balzer D, Murphy J, et al.: Percutaneous carotid artery access in infants <3 months of age, *Catheter Cardiovasc Interv* 87(4):757–761, 2016.

11. Mehta R, Lee KJ, Chaturvedi R, et al.: Complications of pediatric cardiac catheterization: a review in the current era, *Catheter Cardiovasc Interv* 1;72(2):278–285, 2008.

12. Agnoletti G, Bonnet C, Boudjemline Y, et al.: Complications of paediatric interventional catheterisation: an analysis of risk factors, *Cardiol Young* 15(4):402–408, 2005.

13. Cassidy SC, Schmidt KG, van Hare GF, et al.: Complications of pediatric cardiac catheterization: a 3-year study, *J Am Coll Cardiol* 19:1285–1293, 1992.

14. Sapin SO, Linde LM, Emmanouilides GC: Umbilical vessel angiocardiography in the newborn infant, *Pediatrics* 31:946–951, 1963.

15. Giusti S, Borghi A, Redaelli S, et al.: The carotid arterial approach for balloon dilation of critical aortic stenosis in neonates—immediate results and follow-up, *Cardiol Young* 2:155–160, 2008.

16. Schranz D, Michel-Behnke I: Axillary artery access for cardiac interventions in newborns, *Ann Pediatr Cardiol* 1(2):126–130, 2008.

17. Johnson JL, Fellows KE, Murphy JD: Transhepatic central venous access for cardiac catheterization and radiologic intervention, *Cathet Cardiovasc Diagn* 35(2):168–171, 1995.

18. Shim D, Lloyd TR, Beekman RH: Transhepatic therapeutic cardiac catheterization: a new option for the pediatric interventionalist, *Catheter Cardiovasc Interv* 47:41–45, 1999.

19. Allan LD, Leanage R, Wainwright R, et al.: Balloon atrial septostomy under two dimensional echocardiographic control, *Br Heart J* 47:41–43, 1982.

20. Zellers TM, Dixon K, Moake L, et al.: Bedside balloon atrial septostomy is safe, efficacious, and cost-effective compared with septostomy performed in the cardiac catheterization laboratory, *Am J Cardiol* 189(5):613–615, 2002.

21. Hill SL, Mizelle KM, Vellucci SM, et al.: Radiofrequency perforation and cutting balloon septoplasty of intact atrial septum in a newborn with hypoplastic left heart syndrome using transesophageal ICE probe guidance, *Cathet Cardiovasc Interv* 64:214–217, 2005.

22. Mok Q, Darvell F, Mattos S, et al.: Survival after balloon atrial septostomy for complete transposition of great arteries, *Arch Dis Child* 62:549–553, 1987.

23. Mullins CE: Balloon atrial septostomy. In Mullins CE, editor: *Cardiac Catheterization in Congenital Heart Disease: Pediatric and Adult*, Malden, MA, 2006, Blackwell Publishing, pp 378–392.

24. Mukherjee D, Lindsay M, Zhang Y, et al.: Analysis of 8681 neonates with transposition of the great arteries: outcomes with and without Rashkind balloon atrial septostomy, *Cardiol Young* 20(4):373–380, 2010.

25. McQuillen PS, Hamrick SE, Perez MJ, et al.: Balloon atrial septostomy is associated with preoperative stroke in neonates with transposition of the great arteries, *Circulation* 113(2):280–285, 2006.

26. McQuillen PS, Barkovich JA, Hamrick SEG, et al.: Temporal and anatomic risk profile of brain injury with neonatal repair of congenital heart defects, *Stroke* 38:736–741, 2007.

27. Petit CJ, Rome JJ, Wernovsky G, et al.: Preoperative brain injury in transposition of the great arteries is associated with oxygenation and time to surgery, not balloon atrial septostomy, *Circulation* 119(5):709–716, 2009.

28. Applegate SE, Lim DS: Incidence of stroke in patients with d-transposition of the great arteries that undergo balloon atrial septostomy in the University Healthsystem Consortium Clinical Data Base/Resource Manager, *Catheter Cardiovasc Interv* 76:129–131, 2010.

29. Beca J, Gunn J, Coleman L, et al.: Pre-operative brain injury in newborn infants with transposition of the great arteries occurs at rates similar to other complex congenital heart disease and is not related to balloon atrial septostomy, *J Am Coll Cardiol* 53(19):1807–1811, 2009.

30. Justino H, Benson LN, Nykanen D: Transcatheter creation of an atrial septal defect using radiofrequency perforation, *Cathet Cardiovasc Interv* 54:83–87, 2001.

31. Du Marchie Sarvaas GJ, Trivedi KR, et al.: Radiofrequency-assisted atrial septoplasty for an intact atrial septum in complex congenital heart disease, *Catheter Cardiovasc Interv* 56:412–415, 2002.
32. Holzer RJ, Wood A, Chisolm JL, et al.: Atrial septal interventions in patients with hypoplastic left heart syndrome, *Catheter Cardiovasc Interv* 72(5):696–704, 2008.
33. Pedra CA, Neves JR, Pedra SR, et al.: New transcatheter techniques for creation or enlargement of atrial septal defects in infants with complex congenital heart disease, *Catheter Cardiovasc Interv* 70:731–737, 2007.
34. Gossett J, Rocchini A, Lloyd T, et al.: Catheter-based decompression of the left atrium in patients with hypoplastic left heart syndrome and restrictive atrial septum is safe and effective, *Catheter Cardiovasc Interv* 67:619–624, 2006.
35. Rupp S, Michel-Behnke I, Valeske K, et al.: Implantation of stents to ensure an adequate interatrial communication in patients with hypoplastic left heart syndrome, *Cardiol Young* 17(5):535–540, 2007.
36. Leonard Jr GT, Justino H, Carlson KM, et al.: Atrial septal stent implant: atrial septal defect creation in the management of complex congenital heart defects in infants, *Congen Heart Dis* 1(3):129–135, 2006.
37. Danon S, Levi D, Alejos J, et al.: Reliable atrial septostomy by stenting of the atrial septum, *Catheter Cardiovasc Interv* 66:408–413, 2005.
38. Berman W, Fripp RR, Raisher BD, et al.: Significant pulmonary valve incompetence following over-size balloon pulmonary valveplasty in small infants: a long-term follow-up study, *Cathet Cardiovasc Intervent* 48(1):61–65, 1999.
39. Velvis H, Raines KH, Bensky AS, et al.: Growth of the right heart after balloon valvuloplasty for critical pulmonary stenosis in the newborn, *Am J Cardiol* 79:982–984, 1997.
40. Holzer R, Kreutzer J, Hirsch R, et al.: Balloon pulmonary valvuloplasty prospective analysis of pro-cedure related adverse events and immediate outcome—results from a multicenter registry, *Cathet Cardiovasc Intervent* 76:S3–S36, 2010.
41. McGovern E, Morgan CT, Oslizlok P, et al.: Transcatheter stenting of the right ventricular outflow tract augments pulmonary arterial growth in symptomatic infants with right ventricular outflow tract obstruction and hypercyanotic spells, *Cardiol Young* 26(7):1260–1265, 2016.
42. Akagi T, Benson LN, Williams WG, et al.: Ventriculo-coronary arterial connections in pulmonary atresia with intact ventricular septum, and their influences on ventricular performance and clinical course, *Am J Cardiol* 72:586–590, 1993.
43. Hanley FL, Sade RM, Blackstone EH, et al.: Outcomes in neonatal pulmonary atresia with intact ventricular septum: a multiinstitutional study, *J Thorac Cardiovasc Surg* 105:406–423, 1993.
44. Guleserian KJ, Armsby LB, Thiagarajan RR, et al.: Natural history of pulmonary atresia with intact ventricular septum and right-ventricle-dependent coronary circulation managed by the single ventricle approach, *Ann Thorac Surg* 81(6):2250–2257, 2006.
45. Walsh MA, Lee KJ, Chaturvedi R, et al.: Radiofrequency perforation of the right ventricular out-flow tract as a palliative strategy for pulmonary atresia with ventricular septal defect, *Catheter Cardiovasc Interv* 69(7):1015–1020, 2007.
46. Latson L: Nonsurgical treatment of a neonate with pulmonary atresia and intact ventricular sep-tum by transcatheter puncture and balloon dilation of the atretic valve membrane, *Am J Cardiol* 68(2):277–279, 1991.
47. Gournay V, Piechaud JF, Delogu A, et al.: Balloon valvotomy for critical stenosis or atresia of pulmonary valve in newborns, *J Am Coll Cardiol* 26:1725–1731, 1995.
48. Parsons JM, Rees MR, Gibbs JL: Percutaneous laser valvotomy with balloon dilatation of the pulmonary valve as primary treatment for pulmonary atresia, *Br Heart J* 66(1):36–38, 1991.
49. Qureshi SA, Rosenthal E, Tynan M, et al.: Transcatheter laser-assisted balloon pulmonary valve dilation in pulmonic valve atresia, *Am J Cardiol* 67(5):428–431, 1991.
50. Hausdorf G, Schulze-Neick I, Lange PE: Radiofrequency-assisted "reconstruction" of the right ventricular outflow tract in muscular pulmonary atresia with ventricular septal defect, *Br Heart J* 69:343–346, 1993.
51. Asnes JD, Fahey JT: Novel catheter positioning technique for atretic pulmonary valve perforation, *Cathet Cardiovasc Interv* 71:850–852, 2008.
52. Agnoletti G, Piechaud JF, Bonhoeffer P, et al.: Perforation of the atretic pulmonary valve. Long-term follow-up, *J Am Coll Cardiol* 41:1399–1403, 2003.
53. Hirata Y, Chen J, Quaegebeur J, et al.: Pulmonary atresia with intact ventricular septum: limitations of catheter-based intervention, *Ann Thorac Surg* 84:574–580, 2007.
54. Schwartz MC, Glatz AC, Dori Y, et al.: Outcomes and predictors of reintervention in patients with pulmonary atresia and intact ventricular septum treated with radiofrequency perforation and balloon pulmonary valvuloplasty, *Pediatr Cardiol* 35(1):22–29, 2014.
55. Zampi JD, Hirsch-Romano JC, Goldstein BH, et al.: Hybrid approach for pulmonary atresia with intact ventricular septum: early single center results and comparison to the standard surgical approach, *Catheter Cardiovasc Interv* 83(5):753–761, 2014.
56. McElhinney D, Lock J, Keane J, et al.: Left heart growth, function, and reintervention after balloon aortic valvuloplasty for neonatal aortic stenosis, *Circulation* 111:451–458, 2005.
57. McCrindle BW, Blackstone EH, Williams WG, et al.: Are outcomes of surgical versus transcatheter balloon valvotomy equivalent in neonatal critical aortic stenosis? *Circulation* 104(Suppl I):152–158, 2001.

32

58. Mosca RS, Iannettoni MD, Schwartz SM, et al.: Critical aortic stenosis in the neonate: a comparison of balloon valvuloplasty and transventricular dilation, *J Thorac Cardiovasc Surg* 109:147–154, 1995.

59. Weber HS: Catheter management of aortic valve stenosis in neonates and children, *Catheter Cardiovasc Interv* 67(6):947–955, 2006.

60. Weber HS, Mart CR, Myers JL: Transcarotid balloon valvuloplasty for critical aortic valve stenosis at the bedside via continuous transesophageal echocardiographic guidance, *Catheter Cardiovasc Interv* 50(3):326–329, 2000.

61. Fischer DR, Ettedgui JA, Park SC, et al.: Carotid artery approach for balloon dilation of aortic valve stenosis in the neonate: a preliminary report, *J Am Coll Cardiol* 15:1633–1636, 1990.

62. Sholler GF, Keane JF, Perry SB, et al.: Balloon dilation of congenital aortic valve stenosis: results and influence of technical and morphological features on outcome, *Circulation* 78:351–360, 1988.

63. Lofland GK, McCrindle BW, Williams WG, et al.: Critical aortic stenosis in the neonate: a multi-institutional study of management, outcomes, and risk factors; Congenital Heart Surgeons Society, *J Thorac Cardiovasc Surg* 121:10–27, 2001.

64. Han RK, Gurofsky RC, Lee KJ, et al.: Outcome and growth potential of left heart structures after neonatal intervention for aortic valve stenosis, *J Am Coll Cardiol* 50(25):2406–2414, 2007.

65. Torres A, Bergersen L, Marshal AL, et al.: Aortic balloon valvuloplasty in the 21st century: procedural success, efficacy and adverse events: results of a multicenter registry (C3PO), *Circulation* 122:A14392, 2010.

66. Beekman RH: Coarctation of the aorta. In Emmanouilides GC, Riemenschneider TA, Allen HD, et al.: *Moss and Adams' Heart Disease in Infants, Children and Adolescents*, ed 5, Baltimore, 1995, Williams and Wilkins, pp 1111–1133.

67. Ho SY, Anderson RH: Coarctation, tubular hypoplasia, and the ductus arteriosus: histological study of 35 specimens, *Br Heart J* 41:268–274, 1979.

68. Mullins CE: Dilation of coarctation of the aorta native and re/residual coarctation. In Mullins CE, editor: *Cardiac Catheterization in Congenital Heart Disease: Pediatric and Adult*, Malden, MA, 2006, Blackwell Publishing, pp 454–471.

69. Tynan M, Finley JP, Fontes V, et al.: Balloon angioplasty for the treatment of native coarctation: results of valvuloplasty and angioplasty of congenital anomalies registry, *Am J Cardiol* 65:790–792, 1990.

70. Harris KC, Du W, Cowley CG, et al.: Congenital Cardiac Intervention Study Consortium (CCISC). A prospective observational multicenter study of balloon angioplasty for the treatment of native and recurrent coarctation of the aorta, *Catheter Cardiovasc Interv* 83(7):1116–1123, 2014.

71. Fawzy ME, Fathala A, Osman A, et al.: Twenty-two years of follow-up results of balloon angioplasty for discreet native coarctation of the aorta in adolescents and adults, *Am Heart J* 156:910–917, 2008.

72. Hijazi ZM, Fahey JT, Kleinman CS, et al.: Balloon angioplasty for recurrent coarctation of the aorta, *Circulation* 84:1150–1156, 1991.

73. Fiore AC, Fischer LK, Schwartz T, et al.: Comparison of angioplasty and surgery for neonatal aortic coarctation, *Ann Thorac Surg* 80(5):1659–1664, 2005.

74. Dilawar M, El Said H, El-Sisi A, et al.: Safety and efficacy of low-profile balloons in native coarctation and recoarctation balloon angioplasty for infants, *Pediatr Cardiol* 30:404–408, 2009.

75. Früh S, Knirsch W, Dodge-Khatami A, et al.: Comparison of surgical and interventional therapy of native and recurrent aortic coarctation regarding different age groups during childhood, *Eur J Cardiothorac Surg* 39:898–904, 2011.

76. Rodés-Cabau J, Miró J, Dancea A, et al.: Comparison of surgical and transcatheter treatment for native coarctation of the aorta in patients > or = 1 year old. The Quebec Native Coarctation of the Aorta study, *Am Heart J* 154:186–192, 2007.

77. Cowley CG, Orsmond GS, Feola P, et al.: Long-term randomized comparison of balloon angioplasty and surgery for native coarctation of the aorta in childhood, *Circulation* 111(25):3453–3456, 2005.

78. Rothman A, Galindo A, Evans WN, et al.: Effectiveness and safety of balloon dilation of native aortic coarctation in premature neonates weighing < or = 2,500 grams, *Am J Cardiol* 105(8):1176–1180, 2010.

79. Bouzguenda I, Marini D, Ou P, et al.: Percutaneous treatment of neonatal aortic coarctation presenting with severe left ventricular dysfunction as a bridge to surgery, *Cardiol Young* 19:244–251, 2009.

80. Al-Ammouri I, Jaradat S, Radwan J: Severe coarctation of the aorta in a 900 g donor of twin-twin transfusion newborn with successful repeated transcatheter angioplasty: a case report, *Cardiol Young* 25(2):394–397, 2015.

81. Ringel RE, Vincent J, Jenkins KJ, et al.: Acute outcome of stent therapy for coarctation of the aorta: results of the Coarctation of the Aorta Stent trial, *Catheter Cardiovasc Interv* 1;82(4):503–510, 2013.

82. Butera G, Manica JL, Marini D, et al.: From bare to covered: 15-year single center experience and follow-up in trans-catheter stent implantation for aortic coarctation, *Catheter Cardiovasc Interv* 83(6):953–963, 2014.

83. Schaeffler R, Kolax T, Hesse C, et al.: Implantation of stents for treatment of recurrent and native coarctation in children weighing less than 20 kilograms, *Cardiol Young* 17:617–622, 2007.

84. Mohan UR, Danon S, Levi D, et al.: Stent implantation for coarctation of the aorta in children or = 1 year old. The Quebec Native Coarctation of the Aorta study, *Am Heart J* 154:186–192, 2007.
85. Kutty S, Zahn E: Interventional therapy for neonates with critical congenital heart disease, *Cathet Cardiovasc Interv* 72:663–674, 2008.
86. Coe JY, Olley PM: A novel method to maintain ductus arteriosus patency, *J Am Coll Cardiol* 18:837–841, 1991.
87. Santoro G, Gaio G, Palladino MT, et al.: Stenting of the arterial duct in newborns with duct-dependent pulmonary circulation, *Heart* 94(7):925–929, 2008.
88. Mahesh K, Kannan BR, Vaidyanathan B, et al.: Stenting the patent arterial duct to increase pulmonary blood flow, *Indian Heart J* 57(6):704–708, 2005.
89. Schneider M, Zartner P, Sidiropoulos A, et al.: Stent implantation of the arterial duct in newborns with duct-dependent circulation, *Eur Heart J* 19(9):1401–1409, 1998.
90. Schranz D, Michel-Behenke I, Heyer R, et al.: Stent implantation of the arterial duct in newborns with a truly duct-dependent pulmonary circulation: a single-center experience with emphasis on aspects of the interventional technique, *J Intervent Cardiol* 23:581–588, 2010.
91. Alwi M, Choo KK, Latiff HA, et al.: Initial results and medium-term follow-up of stent implantation of patent ductus arteriosus in duct-dependent pulmonary circulation, *J Am Coll Cardiol* 44:438–445, 2004.
92. Gibbs JL, Uzun O, Blackburn ME, et al.: Fate of the stented arterial duct, *Circulation* 99:1621–2625, 1999.
93. Mallula K, Vaughn G, El-Said H, et al.: Comparison of ductal stenting versus surgical shunts for palliation of patients with pulmonary atresia and intact ventricular septum, *Catheter Cardiovasc Interv* 85(7):1196–1202, 2015.
94. Mitchell SC, Korones SB, Berendes HW: Congenital heart disease in 56,109 births: incidence and natural history, *Circulation* 43:323–332, 1971.
95. Gersony WM: Patent ductus arteriosus in the neonate, *Pediatr Clin North Am* 33:545–560, 1986.
96. Jim WT, Chiu NC, Chen MR, et al.: Cerebral hemodynamic change and intraventricular hemorrhage in very low birth weight infants with patent ductus arteriosus, *Ultrasound Med Biol* 31:197–202, 2005.
97. Coombs RC, Morgan ME, Durbin GM, et al.: Gut blood flow velocities in the newborn: effects of patent ductus arteriosus and parenteral indomethacin, *Arch Dis Child* 65:1067–1071, 1990.
98. Bancalari E: Changes in the pathogenesis and prevention of chronic lung disease of prematurity, *Am J Perinatol* 18:1–9, 2001.
99. Brooks JM, Travadi JN, Patole SK, et al.: Is surgical ligation of patent ductus arteriosus necessary? The Western Australian experience of conservative management, *Arch Dis Child Fetal Neonatal Ed* 90:235–239, 2005.
100. Porstmann W, Wierny L, Warnke H: Catheter closure of patent ductus arteriosus: 62 cases treated without thoracotomy, *Radiol Clin North Am* 9:203–218, 1971.
101. Kenny D, Morgan GJ, Bentham JR, et al.: Early clinical experience with a modified amplatzer ductal occluder for transcatheter arterial duct occlusion in infants and small children, *Cathet Cardiovasc Interv* 82:534–540, 2013.
102. Bass JL, Wilson N: Transcatheter occlusion of the patent ductus arteriosus in infants: experimental testing of a new Amplatzer device, *Catheter Cardiovasc Interv* 83(2):250–255, 2014.
103. Bentham J, Meur S, Hudsmith L, et al.: Echocardiographically guided catheter closure of arterial ducts in small preterm infants on the neonatal intensive care unit, *Catheter Cardiovasc Interv* 77(3):409–415, 2011.
104. El-Said HG, Bratincsak A, Foerster SR, et al.: Safety of percutaneous patent ductus arteriosus closure: an unselected multicenter population experience, *J Am Heart Assoc Cardiovasc Cerebrovasc Dis* (6)2:e000424, 2013.
105. Philip R, Rush Waller III B, Agrawal V, et al.: Morphologic characterization of the patent ductus arteriosus in the premature infant and the choice of transcatheter occlusion device, *Catheter Cardiovasc Interv* 87:310–317, 2016.
106. Promphan W, Qureshi SA: What interventional cardiologists are still leaving to the surgeons? *Front Pediatr* 4:59, 2016.
107. Baspinar O, Sahin DA, Sulu A, et al.: Transcatheter closure of patent ductus arteriosus in under 6 kg and premature infants, *J Interv Cardiol* 28(2):180–189, 2015.
108. Francis E, Singhi AK, Lakshmivenkateshaiah S, et al.: Transcatheter occlusion of patent ductus arteriosus in pre-term infants, *JACC Cardiovasc Interv* 3(5):550–555, 2010.
109. Perez KM, Laughon MM: What is new for patent ductus arteriosus management in premature infants in 2015? *Curr Opin Pediatr* 27(2):158–164, 2015.
110. Heublein B, Rohde R, Kaese V, et al.: Biocorrosion of magnesium alloys: a new principle in cardiovascular implant technology, *Heart* 89:651–656, 2003.
111. Di Mario C, Griffiths H, Goktekin O, et al.: Drug-eluting bioabsorbable magnesium stent, *J Interv Cardiol* 17:391–395, 2004.
112. Schranz D, Zartner P, Michel-Behnke I, et al.: Bioabsorbable metal stents for percutaneous treatment of critical recoarctation of the aorta in a newborn, *Catheter Cardiovasc Interv* 67:671–673, 2006.
113. Zartner P, Cesnjevar R, Singer H, et al.: First successful implantation of a biodegradable metal stent into the left pulmonary artery of a preterm baby, *Catheter Cardiovasc Interv* 66(4):590–594, 2005.

32

114. Zartner P, Buettner M, Singer H, et al.: First biodegradable metal stent in a child with congenital heart disease: evaluation of macro and histopathology, *Catheter Cardiovasc Interv* 69(3):443–446, 2007.

115. McMahon CJ, Oslizlok P, Walsh KP: Early restenosis following biodegradable stent implantation in an aortopulmonary collateral of a patient with pulmonary atresia and hypoplastic pulmonary arteries, *Catheter Cardiovasc Interv* 69(5):735–738, 2007.

116. Ma J, Zhao N, Betts L, et al.: Bio-adaption between magnesium alloy stent and the blood vessel: a review, *J Mater Sci Technol* 32(9):815–826, 2016.

117. Alexy RD, Levi DS: Materials and manufacturing technologies available for production of a pediatric bioabsorbable stent, *Biomed Res Int* 2013:137985, 2013.

E

Index

A

Note: Page numbers followed by "f" refer to illustrations; page numbers followed by "t" refer to tables; page numbers followed by "b" refer to boxes.